Principles of
Neurosurgery

SECOND EDITION

Commissioning Editor: Rebecca Schmidt Gaertner
Project Development Manager: Hilary Hewitt
Project Manager: Prepress Projects Ltd, Aoibhe O'Shea
Illustration Manager: Mick Ruddy
Illustrators: Jenni Miller, Robin Dean, Marion Tasker, Lynda Payne
Design Manager: Jayne Jones
Cover design: Stewart Larking
Marketing Managers: Jemma Zighed, Rob Kolton

Principles of
Neurosurgery

SECOND EDITION

Edited by

Setti S Rengachary MD FRCSC
Professor and Vice-Chairman
Department of Neurosurgery
Wayne State University
Detroit, MI
USA

Richard G Ellenbogen MD FACS
Professor and Chairman
Department of Neurological Surgery
University of Washington School of Medicine;
Theodore S Roberts Endowed Chair in Neurological Surgery
Children's Hospital and Regional Medical Center and Harborview Medical Center
Seattle, WA
USA

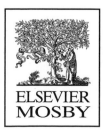

ELSEVIER
MOSBY

Edinburgh   London   New York   Oxford   Philadelphia   St Louis   Sydney   Toronto   2005

ELSEVIER
MOSBY

An affliliate of Elsevier Limited

© Mosby Year-Book Europe Limited 1994
© 2005 Elsevier Limited. All rights reserved.

The right of Setti Rengachary and Richard Ellenbogen to be identified as editors of this work has been asserted by them in accordance with the Copyright, Desings and Patents Act 1988

First edition 1994
Second edition 2005
Reprinted 2005 (twice)

ISBN 0 7234 3222 8

British Library Cataloguing in Publication Data
A catalogue record for this book is available from the British Library

Library of Congress Cataloging in Publication Data
A catalog record for this book is available from the Library of Congress

Notice
Medical knowledge is constantly changing. Standard safety precautions must be followed, but as new research and clinical experience broaden our knowledge, changes in treatment and drug therapy may become necessary r appropriate. Readers are advised to check the most current product information provided by the manufactactureer of each drug to be administered to verify the recommended dose, the method and duration of administration, and contraindications. It is the responsibility of the practitioner, relying on experience and knowledge of the patient, to determine dosages and the best treatment for each individual patient. Neither the Publisher nor the editors assume any liability for any injury and/or damage to persons or property arising from this publication.
The Publisher

Printed in China
Last digit is print number: 9 8 7 6 5 4 3

The publisher's policy is to use **paper manufactured from sustainable forests**

CONTENTS

CONTRIBUTORS

Ramin Abdolvahavi MD
Chief Resident in Neurosurgery
Wayne State University
Detroit, MI, USA

Ossama Al-Mefty MD
Professor and Chairman
Department of Neurosurgery
University of Arkansas for Medical Sciences
Little Rock, AR, USA

Anthony M Avellino MD
Assistant Professor of Neurological Surgery
University of Washington School of Medicine
Children's Hospital and Regional Medical Center
Seattle, WA, USA

Issam A Awad MA MD MSc FACS
Professor of Neurosurgery
Northwestern University Medical School
Chicago, IL;
Attending Neurosurgeon
Evanston Northwestern Healthcare
Evanston, IL, USA

H Hunt Batjer MD
Michael J Marchese Professor and Chair
Department of Neurological Surgery
Northwestern University Medical School
Chicago, IL, USA

Allan J Belzberg BSc MD FRCSC
Associate Professor of Neurosurgery
Johns Hopkins School of Medicine
Baltimore, MD, USA

Bernard R Bendok MD
Assistant Professor of Neurological Surgery
Northwestern University Medical School
Chicago, IL, USA

Christopher M Bono MD
Assistant Professor of Orthopedic Surgery
Boston University School of Medicine;
Attending Spine Surgeon
Boston Medical Center
Boston, MA;
Attending Spine Surgeon
Quincy Medical Center
Quincy, MA, USA

Gavin Wayne Britz MD
Assistant Professor of Neurological Surgery
University of Washington School of Medicine
Harborview Medical Center
Seattle, WA, USA

Jacques Brotchi MD PhD
Professor of Neurosurgery
Universitie libre de Bruxelles
Erasme Hospital
Brussels, Belgium

Jeffrey A Brown MD
Professor of Neurosurgery
Wayne State University
Detroit, MI, USA

Paul D Brown MD
Assistant Professor of Radiation Oncology
Mayo Clinic and Foundation
Rochester, MN , USA

Daniel P Cahill MD PhD
Resident in Neurosurgery
Massachusetts General Hospital
Boston, MA, USA

James P Chandler MD
Assistant Professor of Neurological Surgery
Northwestern University Medical School
Chicago, IL, USA

E Antonio Chiocca MD PhD
Chairman, Department of Neurosurgery
Dardinger Family Professor of Oncologic Neurosurgery
Director of Neurosurgical Services
The Ohio State University Medical Center
James Cancer Hospital and Solove Research Institute
Columbus, OH, USA

Andrew T Dailey MD
Associate Professor of Neurological Surgery
University of Washington School of Medicine
Harborview Medical Center
Seattle, WA, USA

Rajeev Deveshwar MD
Department of Neurosurgery
Wayne State University
Detroit, MI, USA

Dragan F Dimitrov MD
Resident in Neurosurgery
Duke University Medical Center
Durham, NC, USA

James M Ecklund MD FACS LTC(P) MC USA
Professor and Chairman
Neurosurgery Program, National Capital Consortium
Walter Reed Army and National Naval Medical Centers and
Uniformed Services University of the Health Sciences
Washington, DC, USA

Richard G Ellenbogen MD FACS
Professor and Chairman
Department of Neurological Surgery
University of Washington School of Medicine;
Theodore S Roberts Endowed Chair in Neurological Surgery
Children's Hospital and Regional Medical Center and
Harborview Medical Center
Seattle, WA, USA

Daniel R Fassett MD MBA
Resident in Neurosurgery
University of Utah Hospital
Salt Lake City, UT, USA

Richard Fessler MD
Director of Endovascular Neurosurgery
Assistant Clinical Professor of Neurosurgery
Wayne State University
Detroit, MI, USA

Allan H Friedman MD
Guy L Odom Professor and Chairman
Division of Neurosurgery
Duke University Medical Center
Durham, NC, USA

Georg Fries MD
Assistant Professor of Neurosurgery
Johannes Gutenberg University
Mainz, Germany

Fred H Geisler MD PhD
Neurosurgeon
Illinois Neuro-Spine Center at Rush-Copley Medical Center
Aurora, IL, USA

Christopher C Getch MD
Assistant Professor of Neurological Surgery
Northwestern University Medical School
Chicago, IL, USA

James Tait Goodrich MD PhD
Director, Division of Pediatric Neurosurgery
Children's Hospital at Montefiore;
Professor of Clinical Neurosurgery, Pediatrics, Plastics, and
Reconstructive Surgery
Albert Einstein College of Medicine
Bronx, NY, USA

Gerald A Grant MD
Director of Pediatric Neurosurgery
Wilford Hall Medical Center
Lackland Air Force Base
San Antonio, TX, USA

Lance Gravely MD
Chief Resident in Neurological Surgery
Northwestern University Medical School
Chicago, IL, USA

Bernard H Guiot MD
Associate Professor of Neurosurgery
University of South Florida
Tampa, FL, USA

Griffith R Harsh IV MD MBA
Director, Stanford Brain Tumor Center
Professor of Neurosurgery
Stanford University Hospital
Stanford, CA, USA

Robert F Heary MD
Associate Professor of Neurological Surgery
University of Medicine and Dentistry of New Jersey
New Jersey Medical School;
Director, The Spine Center of New Jersey
Neurological Institute of New Jersey
Newark, NJ, USA

Stephen J Hentschel MD
Fellow, Department of Neurological Surgery
The University of Texas MD Anderson Cancer Center
Houston, TX, USA

Jason Heth MD
Skull Base Neurosurgery Fellow
University of Arkansas for Medical Sciences
Little Rock, AR, USA

Roman Hlatky MD
Fellow in Neurosurgical Oncology
Wayne State University
Detroit, MI, USA

Martin C Holland MD
Associate Professor of Neurological Surgery
University College of San Francisco Medical School;
Chair of Neurosurgery
San Francisco General Hospital
San Francisco, CA, USA

Robert F Keating MD
Chief of Pediatric Neurosurgery
Children's National Medical Center
Washington, DC, USA

Suzanne Kempisty RN
Director of Clinical Trials
Department of Neurosurgery
University of Cincinnati
Mayfield Clinic
Cincinnati, OH, USA

Michael Lim MD
Resident in Neurosurgery
Stanford University Hospital
Stanford, CA, USA

Geoffrey SF Ling MD PhD LTC(P) MC USA
Professor and Interim Chair of Neurology
Director, Critical Care Medicine, Anesthesiology, and Surgery
Uniformed Services University of the Health Sciences
Bethesda, MD, USA

John D Loeser MD
Professor of Neurological Surgery and Anesthesiology
University of Washington School of Medicine
Seattle, WA, USA

Robert J McBroom MD
University of Toronto
St Michael's Hospital
Toronto, ON, Canada

Ian E McCutcheon MD
Professor of Neurosurgery
The University of Texas MD Anderson Cancer Center
Houston, TX, USA

Paul N Manson MD
Professor and Chairman
Department of Plastic Surgery
Johns Hopkins School of Medicine
Baltimore, MD, USA

Nevo Margalit MD
Department of Neurosurgery
St. Luke's–Roosevelt Hospital
New York, NY, USA

Neil A Martin MD
Professor and Chairman of Neurological Surgery
University College of Los Angeles Medical Center
Los Angeles, CA, USA

Christian Matula MD
Professor of Neurosurgery
University of Vienna
Vienna, Austria

Minesh P Mehta MD
Professor and Chair of Human Oncology
University of Wisconsin Medical School
Madison, WI, USA

Ehud Mendel MD
Associate Professor of Neurosurgery
The University of Texas MD Anderson Cancer Center
Houston, TX, USA

Ralph Mobbs MD
Fellow, Centre for Minimally Invasive Neurosurgery
Prince of Wales Private Hospital
Sydney, NSW, Australia

Raj Narayan MD
Frank H Mayfield Professor and Chairman
Department of Neurosurgery
University of Cincinnati
Mayfield Clinic
Cincinnati, OH, USA

Kent C New MD PhD
Senior Resident in Neurosurgery
Duke University Medical Center
Durham, NC, USA

W Jerry Oakes MD
Professor of Neurosurgery and Pediatrics
University of Alabama at Birminghan
Children's Hospital of Alabama
Birmingham, AL, USA

Jeffrey G Ojemann MD
Associate Professor of Neurosurgery
University of Washington School of Medicine;
Director, Surgical Epilepsy
Children's Hospital and Regional Medical Center
Seattle, WA, USA

Richard K Osenbach MD
Assistant Professor of Neurosurgery
Duke University Medical Center
Durham, NC, USA

Nelson M Oyesiku MD PhD FACS
Associate Professor of Neurosurgery
Emory University School of Medicine
Atlanta, GA, USA

Dachling Pang MD FACS FRCSC
Professor of Neurosurgery
University of California
Davis, CA;
Chief, Regional Center for Pediatric Neurosurgery
Kaiser Permanente Hospital
Oakland, CA, USA

Andrew T Parsa MD PhD
Assistant Professor of Neurological Surgery
University College of San Francisco Medical School
San Francisco, CA, USA

Rakesh R Patel MD
Assistant Professor of Human Oncology
University of Wisconsin Medical School
Madison, WI, USA

Axel Perneczky MD
Professor of Neurosurgery
Johannes Gutenberg University
Mainz, Germany

Richard G Perrin MD FACS FRCSC
University of Toronto
St Michael's Hospital
Toronto, ON, Canada

Joseph Petronio MD
Pediatric Neurosurgeon
Gillette Children's Specialty Healthcare
St. Paul, MN, USA

Bruce E Pollock MD
Professor, Department of Neurological Surgery and
Division of Radiation Oncology
Mayo Clinic and Foundation
Rochester, MN, USA

Kalmon Post MD
Professor and Chairman
The Mount Sinai Medical Center
New York, NY, USA

Ash Pradhan MD
Resident in Neurosurgery
Duke University Medical Center
Durham, NC, USA

Setti S Rengachary MD FRCSC
Professor and Vice-Chairman
Department of Neurosurgery
Wayne State University
Detroit, MI, USA

Ali Rezai MD
Co-Chairman, Center for Neurological Restoration
Cleveland Clinic Foundation
Cleveland, OH, USA

Robert C Rostomily MD
Associate Professor of Neurological Surgery
University of Washington School of Medicine
University of Washington Medical Center
Seattle, WA, USA

S Clifford Schold Jr MD
Professor and Chair
Department of Interdisciplinary Oncology
Associate Center Director for Clinical Affairs
H Lee Moffit Cancer Center
Tampa, FL, USA

Chandranath Sen MD
Chairman, Department of Neurosurgery
St. Luke's–Roosevelt Hospital
New York, NY, USA

Raj K Shrivastava, MD
Attending Neurosurgeon
Center for Cranial Base Surgery
St. Luke's–Roosevelt Hospital
New York, NY, USA

Andrew E Sloan MD
Associate Professor of Neurosurgery
Department of Interactive Oncology
H Lee Moffitt Cancer Center
Tampa, FL, USA

Robert A Solomon MD
Professor and Chairman of Neurological Surgery
Neurological Institute
Columbia University
New York, NY, USA

Sherman C Stein MD
Clinical Professor of Neurosurgery
University of Pennsylvania School of Medicine
Hospital of the University of Pennsylvania
Philadelphia, PA, USA

Leslie N Sutton MD
Professor of Neurosurgery
University of Pennsylvania School of Medicine;
Chief, Neurosurgery
Children's Hospital of Philadelphia
Philadelphia, PA, USA

Charles Teo, MD
Director, Centre for Minimally Invasive Neurosurgery
Prince of Wales Private Hospital
Sydney, NSW, Australia

Wolfgang A Tomé PhD
Associate Professor in Medical Physics
University of Wisconsin Medical School
Madison, WI, USA

R Shane Tubbs MS PA-C PhD
Assistant Professor of Neurosurgery
University of Alabama at Birmingham
Children's Hospital of Alabama
Birmingham, AL, USA

Dennis A Turner MA MD
Professor of Neurosurgery and Neurobiology
Duke University Medical Center
Durham, NC, USA

Marcelo D Vilela MD
Skull Base Neurosurgery Fellow
University of Washington School of Medicine
University of Washington Medical Center
Seattle, WA, USA

Marion L Walker MD
Professor of Neurosurgery and Pediatrics
University of Utah;
Chairman, Division of Pediatric Neurosurgery
Primary Children's Medical Center
Salt Lake City, UT, USA

Paul P Wang MD
Resident in Neurosurgery
Johns Hopkins School of Medicine
Baltimore, MD, USA

John C Wellons III MD
Assistant Professor of Neurosurgery and Pediatrics
University of Alabama at Birmingham
Children's Hospital of Alabama
Birmingham, AL, USA

G Alexander West MD PhD
Associate Professor of Neurological Surgery
Oregon Health and Science University
Portland, OR, USA

Jack E Wilberger MD
Professor of Neurosurgery
Drexel University College of Medicine;
Chair, Department of Neurosurgery
Allegheny General Hospital
Pittsburg, PA, USA

Christopher E Wolfla MD
Associate Professor of Neurosurgery
The Esther and Ted Greenberg Endowed Chair of Neurosurgery
University of Oklahoma Health Sciences Center
Oklahoma City, OK, USA

Martin Zonenshayn MD
Assistant Professor of Neurological Surgery
Weill Medical College of Cornell University
New York, NY, USA

DEDICATION

This edition is dedicated to the house officers in clinical neurosciences throughout the world who sacrifice themselves to keep our cherished patients safe.

And to Dhanalakshmi, Usha, Dave, and Shama.
SSR

And to the loves of my life: Sandy, Rachel, Paul, and Zach . . . thank you for my happiness.
RGE

PREFACE

Concern for man and his fate must always form the chief interest of all technical endeavors . . . Never forget this in the midst of your diagrams and equations.

Albert Einstein

Principles of Neurosurgery is in its second edition due, in part, to popular demand by our students. It is for those students that this book is intended. There is a host of excellent neurosurgery reference texts currently available; our volume is meant to be comprehensive without being encyclopedic. It is the editors' desire to make the complex subject of neurosurgery slightly more comprehensible to medical students and house officers in the clinical neurosciences. The chapter topics represent both basic core areas and novel subject matter in the rapidly evolving field of neurosurgery. Our intention is to present to these students a modern, broad overview of the subject of neurosurgery in a readable and visually attractive style.

The success of this book rests upon a team of world class contributing scholars, known for their expertise in their field, combined with dedicated and highly skilled artists employing cutting-edge art technology. The second edition enlists many new and international contributions from neurosurgeons, representing a greater breadth of experience than may be found in the first edition. The team that crafted this text set out to create a book with extraordinary visual appeal for the subject matter through clear and concise explanations, beautiful color illustrations, simple tables, and illustrative photographs. The addition of clinical pearls is intended to distill the contents of each chapter and further illuminate the important lessons contained therein. The text, combined with the artists' illustrations, provides the major fabric from which we hope the student new to neurosurgery can grasp the subjects more easily. It is our ultimate goal that this learning process be substantive, long-lived, and enjoyable. This book is designed to be a combination of science and art, with the humble goal of improving our students' knowledge so that they will make better physicians.

We would like to thank the incredible team of innovative editors and superbly talented artists assembled by Elsevier, without whom this text would never have reached fruition. The list is meant to be inclusive but not definitive. We thank Paul Fam, Rebecca Schmidt Gaertner, Hilary Hewitt, Aoibhe O'Shea, Gillian Whytock, Mick Ruddy, Jenni Miller, Robin Dean, Marion Tasker, and Lynda Payne for their skill, patience, and sense of humor.

Setti S Rengachary
Richard G Ellenbogen
2004

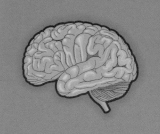

LANDMARKS IN THE HISTORY OF NEUROSURGERY

James Tait Goodrich

If a physician makes a wound and cures a freeman, he shall receive ten pieces of silver, but only five if the patient is the son of a plebeian or two if he is a slave. However it is decreed that if a physician treats a patient with a metal knife for a severe wound and has caused the man to die – his hands shall be cut off. – Code of Hammurabi

Landmarks in the history of neurologic surgery are the focus of this chapter. After reading it, perhaps the neurosurgeon will explore more carefully the subsequent chapters in this volume to avoid having his or her "hands cut off."

To identify major trends in neurosurgery I have organized its history into a series of rather arbitrary periods. In each era the key themes, personalities, and neurosurgical techniques developed and used will be discussed. This review focuses on concepts and ideas in the hope of stimulating further reading in the subject.

PREHISTORIC PERIOD: THE AGE OF TREPHINATION

Prehistoric surgery, compared with its modern successor, lacked several essentials: an understanding of anatomy, recognition of the concept of disease, and comprehension of the origin of illness in an organic system. The failure to grasp these vital principles retarded the practice of medicine and surgery. The art of surgery, and in particular that of neurosurgery, was not even recognized as a discrete specialty until the 20th century.

There remain in many collections around the world examples of the earliest form of neurosurgery – skull trephination. Many arguments and thoughts have been advanced as to the origin and surgical reasons for this early operation – to date no satisfactory answers have been found. Issues of religion, correction of head injuries, release of demons, treatment of headaches, etc. have all been offered. Unfortunately no archaeological materials have surfaced to provide the modern reader with an answer. Nevertheless the skills of these early surgeons were quite remarkable. Many of the trephined skulls show evidence of healing, proving that these early patients survived the surgery. Figure 1.1 shows an example of an early cranioplasty where an inventive surgeon placed a piece of gold as a cranioplasty which was well healed by the time of this patient's death. In the Americas the tumi was the most common instrument used to perform a trephination and many examples of these instruments exist today in museum collections (Figure 1.2).

EGYPTIAN AND BABYLONIAN MEDICINE: EMBRYONIC PERIOD

The Egyptian period covers some 30 successive dynasties, with a claim to have produced the earliest known practising physician – Imhotep (1300 BC). For the modern scholar interested in studying medical and surgical material from this epoch there are only three existing documents available of any relevance. These are the Ebers, Hearst, and Edwin Smith papyri, two of which are considered below.[1,2]

We know that anatomical dissection was performed in this period but an examination of Egyptian papyri also shows that the practice of medicine was based largely on magic and superstition. Therapeutic measures depended on simple principles, most of which allowed nature to provide restoration of health with little intervention. In cases of injury the Egyptians realized that immobilization was important in injuries to extremities and they prescribed splints for that purpose. Their materia medica was impressive, as their substantial pharmacopeias attest.

Written some five hundred years after Hammurabi, and the oldest medical text believed to exist (including about 107 pages of hieratic writing), the Ebers papyrus is of interest for its advocacy of surgical practice.[2] It describes, for example, the removal of tumors, and recommends the surgical drainage of abscesses.

The Edwin Smith papyrus, written after 1700 BC in the time of the New Kingdom, is considered to be the oldest book on surgery *per se* and comprises a papyrus scroll 15 feet in length and 1 foot in width (4.5 m by 0.3 m; Figure 1.3).[1] A total of 48 cases are discussed in this document, including those with injuries to the spine and cranium. Each case is considered with a diagnosis followed by a formulated prognosis. Owing to the scholarly work of James Breasted this papyrus has been translated from the original, which is in the possession of the New York Historical Society, and published in a limited edition.[1]

Other than the isolated cases found in these papyrus fragments, little can be gleaned on the actual practice of neurosurgery. It is evident from these writings that the Egyptian physician recognized head injury and would elevate a skull fracture if necessary. But it was not until the development of the Greek schools that the management and codification of head injury began.

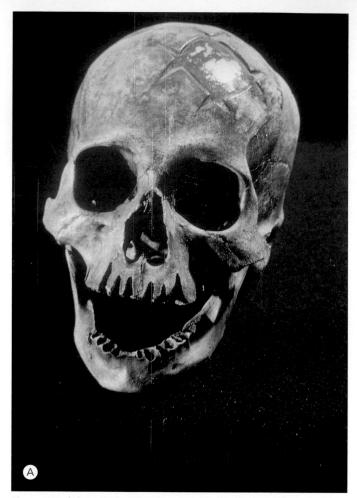

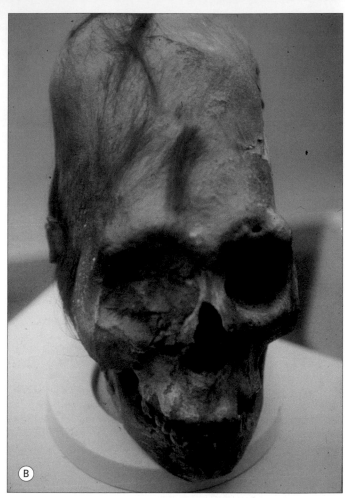

Figure 1.1 **(A)** An early cranioplasty done with a gold inlay which is well healed. From the Museum of Gold, Lima, Peru. **(B)** A well-healed frontal trephination performed on an early Peruvian patient, circa 600 AD. From the Paracas area, Lima, Peru.

GREEK AND EARLY BYZANTINE PERIOD: THE ORIGINS OF NEUROSURGERY

The intellectual development of neurosurgery begins during the golden age of Greece. During the ancient period there were no surgeons who restricted themselves *in stricto sensu* to "neurosurgery." Head injuries, however, appear to have been plentiful, the result of wars and internecine conflicts, as recorded by Herodotus and Thucydides as well as by Homer. War was then, as now, the principal source of material for the study and treatment of head injury.

The earliest medical writings from this period are generally thought to be those attributed to Hippocrates (460–370 BC), that most celebrated of the Asclepiadae (Figure 1.4).[3] Hippocrates was the first to describe a number of neurologic conditions, many of them resulting from battlefield injuries. He understood that the location of the injury to the skull was important. The vulnerability of the brain to injury was categorized from lesser to greater by location, with injury to the bregma representing a greater risk than injury to the temporal region, which in turn was more dangerous than injury to the occipital region.[4]

One of the most interesting observations from this school comes from the *Aphorisms*, which include one of the earliest descriptions of subarachnoid hemorrhage: "When persons in good health are suddenly seized with pains in the head, and straightway are laid down speechless, and breathe with stertor, they die in seven days, unless fever comes on."[5]

Hippocrates described the use of the trephine. He argued for trephination in brain contusions but not in depressed skull fractures (the prognosis was too grave) and cautioned that it should never be performed over a skull suture because of the risk of injury to the underlying dura. In the same spirit he recommended "watering" the trephine bit well to prevent overheating and injury to the dura.

In the section on "Wounds of the Head," Hippocrates warned against incising the brain, as convulsions can occur on the opposite side. He also warned against making a skin incision over the temporal artery, as this could lead to contralateral convulsions (or perhaps severe hemorrhage from the skin). He understood simple concepts of cerebral localization and appreciated the serious prognosis in head injury.

From the region of the Bosporus to the crowded schools of Alexandria came Herophilus of Chalcedon (*fl.* 335–280 BC), the great early anatomist. Unlike his predecessors, Herophilus dissected human bodies in addition to those of animals – more than 100 by his own account. Herophilus engaged in the arduous

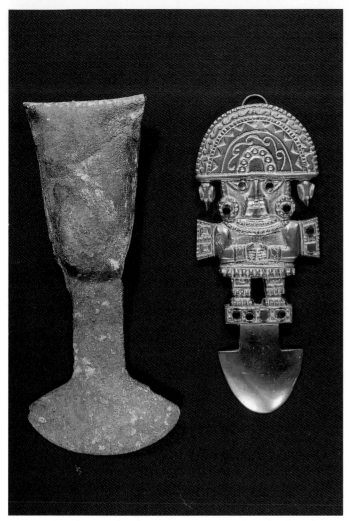

Figure 1.2 Early example of Peruvian tumis, a ceremonial style and a functional – used to perform early trephinations.

task of developing an anatomic nomenclature and forming a language of anatomy. He traced the origin of nerves to the spinal cord and divided them into motor and sensory tracts. He made the important differentiation of nerves from tendons, which were often confused at that time. He was among the first to describe in detail the ventricles and venous sinuses of the brain, in particular the confluens sinuum or *torcular Herophili*. He described for the first time the choroid plexus, so named by him for its resemblance to the vascular membrane of the fetus. Herophilus described in detail the fourth ventricle and noted the peculiar arrangement at its base, which he called the "calamus scriptorius" because it "resembles the groove of a pen for writing." Among his many other contributions was his recognition of the brain as the central organ of the nervous system and the seat of intelligence.[6]

Herophilus is also remembered for introducing one of the longest-standing errors in anatomic physiology: the rete mirabile, (Figure 1.5)[7] a structure present in artiodactyls but not in humans, which acts as an anastomotic network at the base of the brain. This structure was to become important in early physiologic theories of human brain function. The rete mirabile was later described in detail by Galen of Pergamus and canonized by Arabic and medieval

scholars. Not until the 16th century, with the authoritative accounts of Vesalius and Berengario da Carpi, was its absence in humans recognized.

Though Aulus Cornelius Celsus (25 BC–AD 50) was not a surgeon, as a medical encyclopedist he had an important influence on surgery. He reviewed the rival medical schools of his time – dogmatic, methodic, and empiric – fairly and with moderation. As counsel to the emperors Tiberius and Gaius (Caligula), he was held in great esteem. His book, *De re medicina*,[8] is one of the earliest extant medical documents after the Hippocratic writings. It is elegantly written and has therefore had a large influence on medical history. In fact, when printing was introduced in the 15th century, Celsus' works were printed before those of Hippocrates and Galen.

In the field of neurosurgery Celsus made a number of interesting observations. *De re medicina* contains an early description of an epidural hematoma resulting from a bleeding middle meningeal artery.[8] He recommended that the surgeon always operate on the side of greater pain and place the trephine where the pain is best localized. Considering the innervation of the dura and its sensitivity to pressure, this has proved to be a good clinical suggestion. He also provided accurate descriptions of hydrocephalus and facial neuralgia. He knew that a fracture of the cervical spine can cause vomiting and difficulty in breathing, whereas injury of the lower spine can cause weakness or paralysis of the leg, as well as urinary retention or incontinence.

Rufus of Ephesus (*fl.* AD 100) lived during the reign of Trajan (AD 98–117) in the beautiful city of Ephesus. Because so many of Rufus' manuscripts survived, they heavily influenced the medieval compilers. As a result of his great skill as a surgeon, many of his surgical writings were transcribed during the 16th century.[9] Rufus' description of the membranes covering the brain is classic. He distinguished between the cerebrum and cerebellum, and described the corpus callosum. He understood the anatomy of the ventricular system and gave details of the lateral ventricle; he also described the third and fourth ventricles, as well as the aqueduct of Sylvius. Rufus also provided anatomic descriptions of the pineal gland and hypophysis, and his accounts of the fornix and the quadrigeminal plate are accurate and elegant. He also described the optic chiasm and recognized that it is related to vision. The singular accuracy of Rufus' studies must be credited to his use of dissection (mostly monkeys) in an era during which most Greeks abhorred anatomic dissection.

Galen of Pergamus (Claudius Galenus, AD 129–200) needs little introduction to a medical audience. He was an original investigator, compiler, and codifier, as well as a leading advocate of the doctrines of Hippocrates and the Alexandrian school. As physician to the gladiators of Pergamus he had access to many human subjects, particularly with traumatic injuries.

His experience as a physician and his scientific studies enabled Galen to make a variety of contributions to neuroanatomy. He differentiated between the pia mater and the dura mater. He described the corpus callosum, the ventricular system, the pineal and pituitary glands, and the infundibulum. He predated Alexander Monro *Secundus* (1733–1817) in describing the structure later called the foramen of Monro. He also gave an accurate description of the aqueduct of Sylvius. He performed such anatomic experiments as transection of the spinal cord, which led him to describe loss of function below the level of the lesion. In the pig he sectioned the recurrent laryngeal nerve and recognized that hoarseness was a consequence (Figure 1.6). Moreover, Galen made the first recorded attempt at identifying

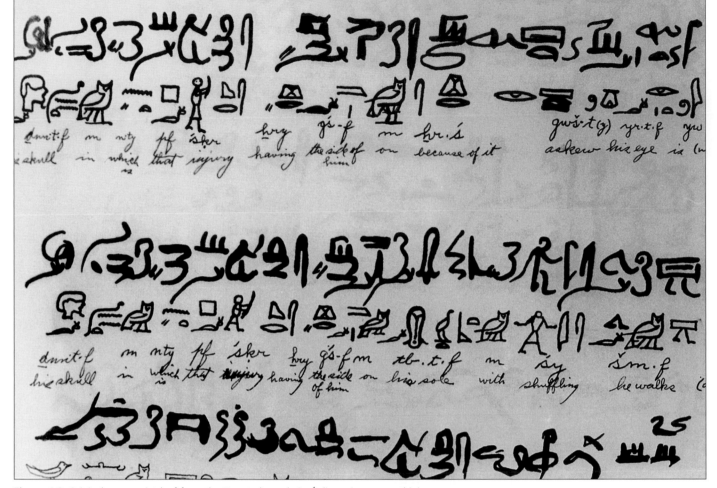

Figure 1.3 Original manuscript leaf from the Breasted translation[1] discussing a neural injury.

and numbering the cranial nerves. He actually demonstrated 11 of the 12 nerves, but he combined several, thus arriving at a total of only seven. He regarded the olfactory nerve as merely a prolongation of the brain and hence did not count it.[10]

Galen held original views concerning the brain's functions. He believed that the brain controlled intelligence, fantasy, memory, and judgment. This was an important departure from the teaching of earlier schools, Aristotle's for example. Galen discarded Hippocrates' notion that the brain is only a gland and attributed to it the powers of voluntary action and sensation.

In neurology, Galen made a number of important observations. He recognized that cervical injury can cause disturbance in arm function. In a study of spinal cord injury, Galen detailed a classic case of what is today known as Brown–Séquard syndrome – i.e. a hemiplegia with contralateral sensory loss in a subject with a hemisection of the cord.[11] Galen's description of the symptoms and signs of hydrocephalus is classic – it enabled him to predict which patients had a poor prognosis. Galen was much more liberal about head injury than Hippocrates, arguing for elevation of depressed skull fractures, fractures with hematomas, and comminuted fractures. Galen recommended removing the bone fragments, particularly those pressing into the brain. Galen was also more optimistic than Hippocrates about brain injuries, commenting "we have seen a severely wounded brain healed." He

provided an extensive description of the safe use of the trephine, pointing out that the dura should not be violated.

Paul of Aegina (AD 625–690), trained in the Alexandrian school, was the last great Byzantine physician. He was a compiler of works in both the Latin and Greek schools, and his writings were consulted well into the 17th century. More importantly, he was a skilled surgeon to whom patients came from far and wide. He venerated the teachings of the ancients as tradition required, but he introduced his own techniques with good results. His classic work, *The Seven Books of Paul of Aegina*, contains an excellent section on head injury and the use of the trephine.[12,13] Paul classified skull fractures in several categories: fissure, incision, expression, depression, arched fracture, and, in infants, dent. In dealing with fractures he used an interesting skin incision: two incisions intersecting one another at right angles, giving the Greek letter X, with one leg of the incision incorporating the scalp wound. The patient's ear was to be stuffed with wool so that the noise of the trephine would not cause distress. The wound was dressed with a broad bandage soaked in oil of roses and wine, with care taken to avoid compressing the brain.[13]

In discussing hydrocephalus Paul of Aegina introduced the concept of the man-handling midwife. He was the first to suggest the possibility that an intraventricular hemorrhage might cause hydrocephalus:

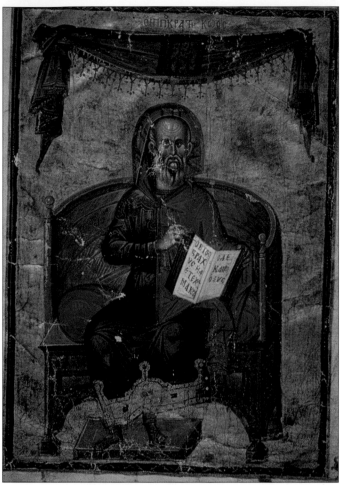

Figure 1.4 An early depiction of Hippocrates. Bibliothèque Nationale, Paris, France.

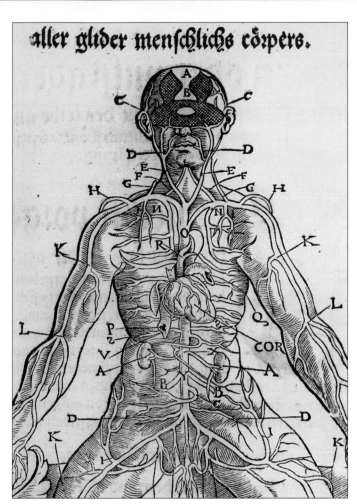

Figure 1.5 Illustrated example of the rete mirabile, from Ryff.[7]

The hydrocephalic affection ... occurs in infants, owing to their heads being improperly squeezed by midwives during parturition, or from some other obscure cause; or from the rupture of a vessel or vessels, and the extravasated blood being converted into an inert fluid ... (Paulus Aeginetes)[13]

Several of the instruments that Paul designed for neurosurgical procedures can be seen in his earlier manuscripts. Elevators, raspatories, bone biters, all came from this period, and trephine bits with conical styles and different biting edges were introduced by Paul. His wound management was also quite sophisticated – he used wine (helpful in antisepsis, although this concept was then unknown) and stressed that dressings should be applied with no compression to the brain. Paul's influence on Arabic medicine, in particular on Albucasis, who is discussed below, was enormous.

ARABIC AND MEDIEVAL MEDICINE: SCHOLARSHIP AND SOMNOLENCE

From approximately AD 750 to AD 1200 the major intellectual centers of medicine were the Arabic and Byzantine cultures. As western Europe revived after AD 1000, the study of surgery and medicine returned there as well.

Arabic scholarship

Arabic schools translated and systematized the surviving Greek and Roman texts. Thanks to their incredible zeal, the best of Greek medicine was made available to Arabic readers by the end of the ninth century. Unfortunately, a rigid scholastic dogmatism became characteristic. Also, the translators too frequently rendered their favorite view instead of that of the author.

Arabic medicine flourished from the 10th century through to the 12th century. Among the most illustrious scholars were Avicenna, Rhazes, Avenzoar, Albucasis, and Averroes. In the writings of these great physicians one sees an extraordinary effort to canonize the writings of their Greek and Roman predecessors. Arab scholars and physicians served as guardians and academics of what now became Hippocratic and Galenic dogma, while the wonderful advances in surgery and anatomy developed by the Alexandrians, among others, were lost or ignored.

Physicians rarely performed surgery in this era. It was expected that the physician would write learnedly and speak *ex cathedra*, but assign the menial task of surgery to an individual of a lower class, that is, to a surgeon.

Arabic medicine did introduce great medical traditions – bedside medicine and teaching. But the lack of dissection and the practice of surgery by individuals of substantially less status than

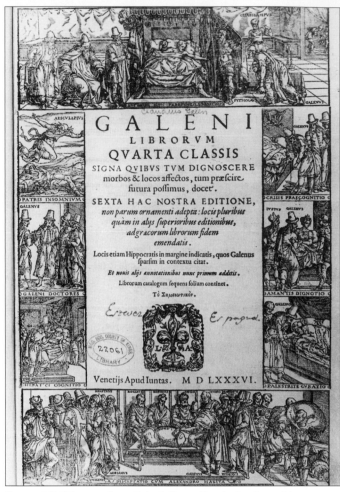

Figure 1.6 Title page from Galen's *Opera Omnia*, Juntine edition, Venice. The border contains a number of allegorical scenes showing the early practice of medicine. The lower panel shows Galen performing his classic study on the recurrent laryngeal nerve.

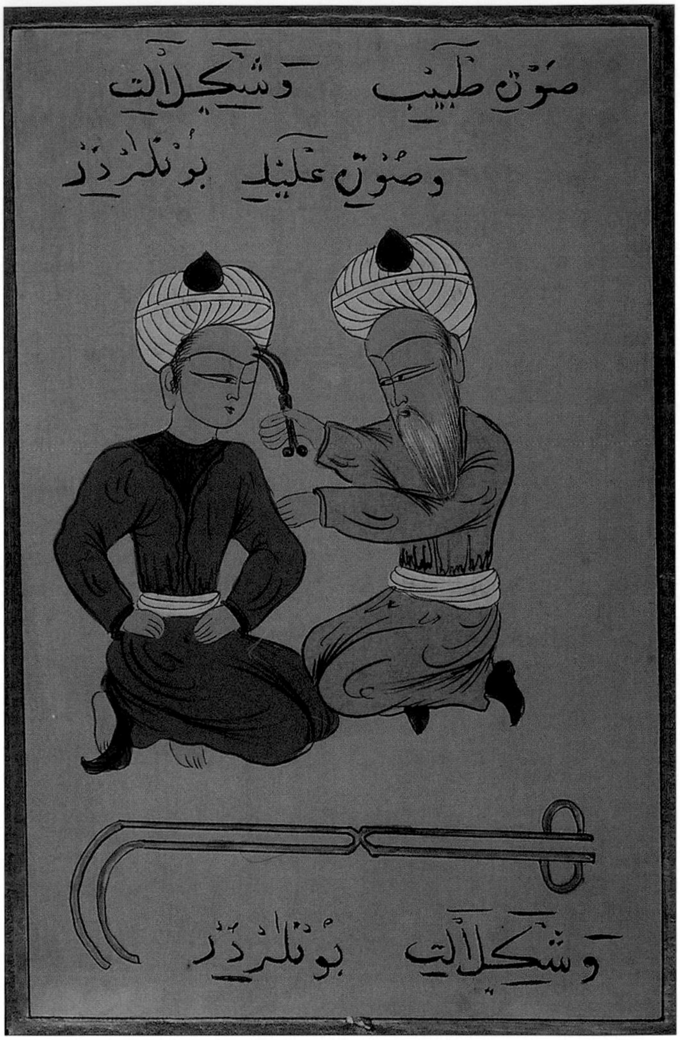

Figure 1.7 Muslim physician applying cautery – from the *Imperial Surgery*.[14]

physicians reduced interest in surgery. The only major contribution to surgery was the reintroduction of the Egyptian technique of using hot cautery to control bleeding. Regrettably, the hot cautery was often used instead of the scalpel to create surgical incisions – a rather destructive way to proceed (Figure 1.7).

The writings of Rhazes (Abu Bakr Muhammad ibn Zakariya' al-Razi, 845–925) indicate that he was a scholarly physician, loyal to Hippocratic teachings and learned in diagnosis. Although primarily a court physician and not a surgeon, his writings on surgical topics remained influential through the 18th century.[14] Rhazes was one of the first to introduce the concept of concussion. Head injury, he wrote, is among the most devastating of all injuries. He advocated surgery only for penetrating injuries of the skull; the outcome was almost always fatal. Rhazes understood that a skull fracture, because it causes compression of the brain, requires elevation to prevent lasting injury.

Avicenna (Abu 'Ali al-Husayn ibn 'Abdallah ibn Sina, 980–1037), the famous physician and philosopher of Baghdad, was known as the "second doctor" (the first being Aristotle). His works were translated into Latin and were a dominant force in the major European universities well into the 18th century. He disseminated the Greek teachings so persuasively that their influence is felt to this day. In his major work, *Canon medicinae*, an encyclopedic effort founded on the writings of Galen and Hippocrates, the observations reported are mostly clinical, bearing primarily on materia medica (Figure 1.8).[15] Within Avicenna's *Canon* are a number of interesting neurologic findings, such as the first accurate clinical explanation of epilepsy, for which treatment consisted of various medicants and herbals. It appears that Avicenna conducted anatomic studies inasmuch as he gives a correct anatomic discussion of the vermis of the cerebellum and the "tailed nucleus," now known as the caudate nucleus. His greatest contribution may be his translation of Galen's collected works.

In the Arab tradition Albucasis (Abu 'l-Qasim ibn 'Abbas al-Zahrawi, 936–1013) was a great compiler as well as a serious scholar, whose writings (some 30 volumes!) were focused mainly on surgery, dietetics, and materia medica. In the introduction to his *Compendium*[16] there is an interesting discussion of why the Arabs had made such little progress in surgery. He attributed it to a lack of anatomic study and inadequate knowledge of the classics. He popularized the frequent use of emetics as prophylaxis against placing ligatures, and then in essence ripping it out! Albucasis recognized the diagnosis of spinal injury, particularly dislocation of the vertebrae: in total subluxation, with the patient showing involuntary activity (passing urine and stool) and flaccid limbs, he appreciated that death was almost certain. Some of the methods he advocated for reduction of lesser spinal injuries, depending on combinations of spars and winches, were rather dangerous. He held that bone fragments in the spinal canal should be removed.

For hydrocephalus (which he, like Paul of Aegina, associated with the midwife grasping the head too roughly) Albucasis recommended drainage, although he noted that the outcome was almost always fatal. He attributed these poor results to "paralysis" of the brain from relaxation. With regard to the site for drainage, Albucasis noted that the surgeon must never cut over an artery, as hemorrhage could lead to death. In the child with hydrocephalus he would "bind" the head with a wrap and then put the child on a "dry diet" with little fluid – a progressive treatment plan for hydrocephalus.[17,18]

An important figure in the history of surgery, and one who bridged the Arabic and medieval schools, was Serefeddin Sabuncuoglu (1385–1468). Sabuncuoglu was a prominent Ottoman surgeon who lived in Amasya, a small city in the northern region of Asia Minor, part of present day Turkey (Figure 1.9). This was a glorious period for the Ottoman Empire and Amasya was a major center of commerce, culture, and art. While working as a physician at Amasya Hospital he wrote a medical book entitled *Cerrahiyyetü'l-Haniyye* [*Imperial Surgery*], which is considered the first colored illustrated textbook of Turkish medical literature, at the age of 83.[19,20] There are only three known copies of this original manuscript, two are in Istanbul and the third at the Bibliothéque Nationale in Paris.[19] The book consists of three chapters dealing with 191 topics, all dealing with surgery. Each topic consists of a single, poetical sentence in which the diagnosis, classification, and surgical technique of a particular disease is described in detail. This book is unique for this period in that virtually all the surgical procedures and illustrations were drawn in color, even though drawings of this type were prohibited in the Islamic religion.

MEDIEVAL EUROPE

Constantinus Africanus (1020–1087) introduced Arabic medicine to the school of Salerno and thus to Europe (Figure 1.10). He had studied in Baghdad, where he came under the influence of the Arabists. Later, he retired to the monastery at Monte Cassino and there translated Arabic manuscripts into Latin, albeit rather inaccurately. Thus began a new wave of translation and transliteration of medical texts, this time into Latin.[21] His work allows one to gauge how much medical and surgical knowledge was lost or distorted by multiple translations, particularly of anatomic works. It is also notable that Constantinus reintroduced anatomic dissection with the annual dissection of a pig. Unfortunately the anatomic observations that did not match those recorded in the Greek classics were ignored! Surgical education and practice continued to slumber (Figure 1.11).

Roger of Salerno (*fl.* 1170) was a surgical leader in the Salernitan tradition, the first writer on surgery in Italy. His work on surgery was to have a tremendous influence on the medieval period (Figure 1.12). His *Practica chirurgiae* offered some interesting surgical techniques.[22] Roger introduced an unusual technique of checking for a tear of the dura or for cerebrospinal

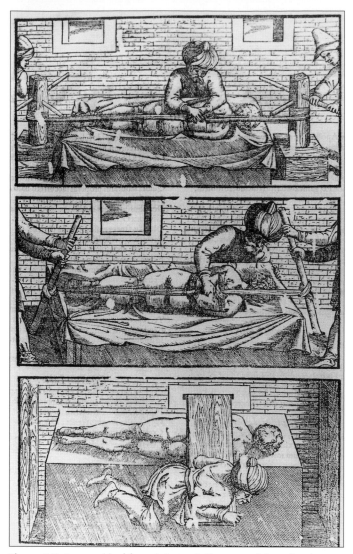

Figure 1.8 Engraved leaf from Avicenna's *Canon medicinae* showing an Arabic physician manipulating a spinal injury. From Avicenna, 1556.[15]

disease, a practice that survived, as "purging," into the 19th century.

The final section of the *Compendium* is a lengthy summary of surgical practice at that time.[16–18] This work was used extensively in the schools of Salerno and Montpellier and hence was an important influence in medieval Europe. Illustrations of surgical instruments to accompany the text describing their use were a unique feature. Many of the instruments were designed by Albucasis, and some were based on those described by Paul of Aegina. His design of a "nonsinking" trephine is classic (he placed a collar on the trephine to prevent plunging), the basis of many later instrument designs.

Albucasis' treatise on surgery is an extraordinary work – a rational, comprehensive, and well-illustrated text designed to teach the surgeon the details of each treatment, including the types of wound dressings to be used. Yet one can only wonder how patients tolerated some of Albucasis' techniques. For chronic headache he applied a hot cautery to the occiput, burning through the skin but not the bone. Another headache treatment he described required hooking the temporal artery, twisting it,

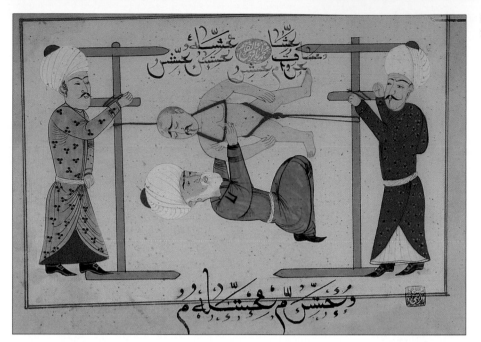

Figure 1.9 Illustration of surgery from Sabuncuoglu *Imperial Surgery*

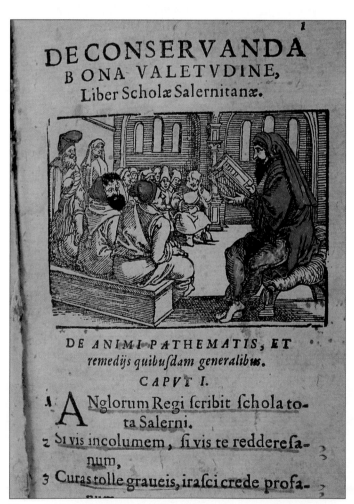

Figure 1.10 Constantinus Africanus giving a lecture to students on a series of Galenic lectures.

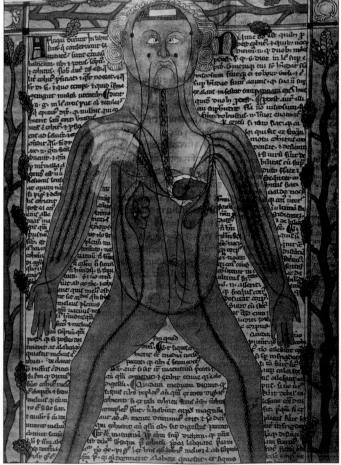

Figure 1.11 One of the "five-figure series," showing a medieval understanding of the circulatory and nervous system with the rete mirabile illustrated.

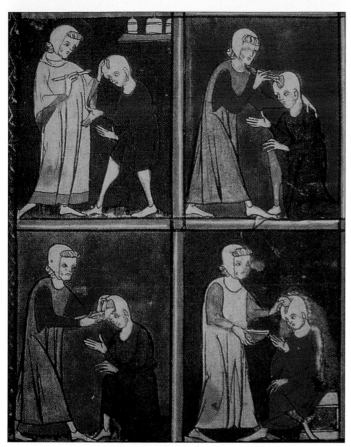

Figure 1.12 Craniotomy being performed by Roger of Salerno (medieval manuscript – Bodleian Library, Oxford, UK).

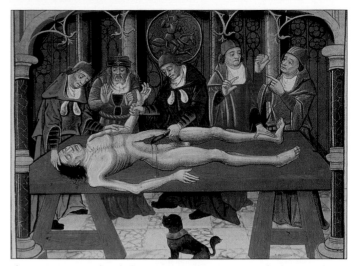

Figure 1.13 A medieval physician attending to a an early dissection. Attributed to Bartholomeeus Anglicus. Late 14th century manuscript from the Bibliothèca Nationale, Paris, France.

fluid (CSF) leakage in a patient with a skull fracture by having the patient hold his or her breath (Valsalva maneuver) and watching for a CSF leak or air bubbles. A pioneer in the techniques of managing nerve injury, he argued for re-anastomosis of severed nerves, and he paid particular attention to alignment. Several chapters of his text are devoted to the treatment of skull fractures.

> When a fracture occurs it is accompanied by various wounds and contusions. If the contusion of the flesh is small but that of the bone great, the flesh should be divided by a cruciate incision down to the bone and everywhere elevated from the bone. Then a piece of light, old cloth is inserted for a day, and if there are fragments of the bone present, they are to be thoroughly removed. If the bone is unbroken on one side, it is left in place, and if necessary elevated with a flat sound (spatumile) and the bone is perforated by chipping with the spatumile so that clotted blood may be soaked up with a wad of wool and feathers. When it has consolidated, we apply lint and then, if it is necessary (but not until after the whole wound has become level with the skin), the patient may be bathed. After he leaves the bath, we apply a thin cooling plaster made of wormwood with rose water and egg.[22]

Roger of Salerno offered little new in the field of anatomy, contenting himself with recapitulating earlier treatises, in particular those of Albucasis and Paul of Aegina. He strongly favored therapeutic plasters and salves; fortunately he was not a strong advocate of the application of grease to dural injuries. Citing the writings of *The Bamberg Surgery*,[23] he advocated trephination in the treatment of epilepsy (Figure 1.13).

An unusually inventive medieval surgeon, Theodoric Borgognoni of Cervia (1205–1298) is remembered as a pioneer in the use of aseptic technique – not the "clean" aseptic technique of today but rather a method based on avoidance of "laudable pus." He attempted to discover the ideal conditions for good wound healing; he concluded that they comprised control of bleeding, removal of contaminated or necrotic material, avoidance of dead space, and careful application of a wound dressing bathed in wine (Figure 1.14).

His surgical work, written in 1267, provides one of the best views of medieval surgery.[24] He argued for meticulous (almost Halstedian!) surgical techniques. The aspiring surgeon was to train under competent surgeons and be well read in the field of head injury. Interestingly, he argued that parts of the brain could be removed through a wound with little effect on the patient. He appreciated the importance of skull fractures, especially depressed ones, recognizing that they should be elevated. Punctures of the dura, he believed, could cause abscess and convulsions. To assist the patient in tolerating surgery, he developed his own "soporific sponge," which contained opium, mandragora, hemlock, and other ingredients. It was applied to the nostrils until the patient fell asleep. This may well have been better, for both patient and surgeon, than no medication (Figures 1.15, 1.16).

The ablest Italian surgeon of the 13th century, professor at the University of Bologna, William of Saliceto (1210–1277) wrote a *Chirurgia*[25] which was highly original, though it does show the influence of Galen and Avicenna. William replaced the Arabic technique of incision by cautery with the surgical knife. He also devised techniques for nerve suture. In neurology, he recognized that the cerebrum governs voluntary motion and the cerebellum involuntary function.

Leonard of Bertapalia (1380?–1460) was a prominent figure in 15th century surgery. He came from a small town near Padua and established an extensive, lucrative practice there and in nearby Venice. He was among the earliest proponents of anatomic research – in fact, he gave a course of surgery in 1429 that

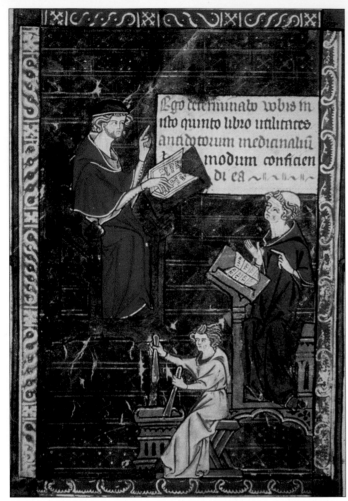

Figure 1.14 Medieval scene of the professor lecturing *ex cathedra* to a student, attributed to Gerard of Cromona, a translator of Avicenna *Canon Medicinae*. Paris, France circa 1320. Bibliothèca Nationale.

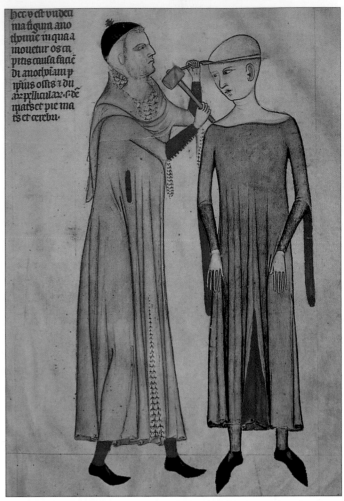

Figure 1.15 Medieval anatomist performing a dissection of the head. From Guido de Papia *Anathmia* circa 1325. Musèe Condé, Chantilly, France.

included the dissection of an executed criminal. Leonard appears to have had a strong interest in injuries of the head – he devoted a third of his book to surgery of the nervous system.[26,27] He considered the brain the most precious organ, regarding it as the source of voluntary and involuntary functions. His insights into skull fractures were remarkable: Always avoid materials that might cause pus, never use a compressive dressing that might drive bone into the brain, and if a piece of bone pierces the brain, remove it.

Lanfranchi of Milan (c.1250–1306), a pupil of William of Saliceto, continued his teacher's practice of using a knife instead of cautery. In his *Cyrurgia parva* he pioneered the use of suture for repairs.[28] He offered classic guidelines for performing trephination in skull fractures and "release of irritation" of dura. He even developed a technique of esophageal intubation for surgery, a technique not commonly practiced until the 20th century.

Guy de Chauliac (1298–1368) was the most influential surgeon of the 14th and 15th centuries and a writer of rare learning and fine historical sense. Guy de Chauliac's *Ars chirurgica* was copied and translated into the 17th century; in fact it was the principal didactic surgical text up to that time.[29,30]

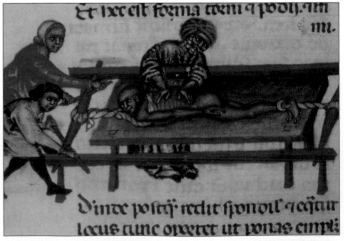

Figure 1.16 Medieval spine distraction for vertebral dislocation injury.

The discussion of head injuries in his *Ars chirurgica* reveals the breadth of his knowledge and intellect. He noted that the head should be shaved prior to surgery to prevent hair from getting into the wound and interfering with primary healing. When dealing with depressed skull fractures he advocated putting wine into the depression to assist healing – an interesting early form of antisepsis. He categorized head wounds into seven types and described the management of each in detail. A scalp wound requires only cleaning and debridement, whereas a compound depressed skull fracture must be treated by trephination and elevation. He advocated repair by primary suture and claimed good results. He used egg albumin to provide adequate hemostasis, always a difficult problem for surgeons.

SIXTEENTH CENTURY: ANATOMIC EXPLORATION

In the 16th century a whole range of new surgical concepts were developed. Physicians and surgeons rediscovered basic investigative techniques. The introduction of anatomic dissection of humans had the most profound influence – great figures like Leonardo da Vinci, Berengario da Carpi, Johannes Dryander, Andreas Vesalius, and others re-explored the human body. Anatomic errors, many ensconced since the Greco-Roman era, were corrected, and great interest in surgery developed. The radically inventive research of the Renaissance laid the foundations of modern neurosurgery.

Leonardo da Vinci (1452–1519) was the quintessential Renaissance man. Multitalented, recognized as an artist, an anatomist, and a scientist, Leonardo went to the dissection table so as better to understand surface anatomy and its bearing on his artistic creations. On the basis of these studies he founded iconographic and physiologic anatomy.[31–33] A well-read man, familiar with the writings of Galen, Avicenna, Mondino, and others, he also appreciated their errors.

In his anatomic studies Leonardo provided the first crude diagrams of the cranial nerves, the optic chiasm, and the brachial and lumbar plexuses. Leonardo made the first wax casting of the ventricular system and in so doing obtained the earliest accurate view. His casting technique involved removing the brain from the calvarium and injecting melted wax through the fourth ventricle. Tubes were placed in the lateral ventricles to allow air to escape. When the wax hardened he removed the brain, leaving a cast behind – simple but elegant (Figure 1.17).

In connection with his artistic studies he developed the concept of "antagonism" in muscle control. His experimental studies included sectioning a digital nerve and noting that the affected finger no longer had sensation, even when placed in a fire. Unfortunately, Leonardo's great opus on anatomy, which was to be published in some 20 volumes, never appeared.[34] From 1519, the year of Leonardo's death, until the middle of the 16th century, his anatomic manuscripts circulated among Italian artists through the guidance of Francesco da Melzi, Leonardo's associate. Later they were lost, and were rediscovered only in the 18th century, by William Hunter.

Ambroise Paré (1510–1590), a poorly educated and humble Huguenot, became one of the greatest figures in surgery; indeed, he is considered the father of modern surgery. As a result of long military experience he was able to incorporate a great deal of practical knowledge into his works. He published in the vernacular rather than Latin, thus allowing wider dissemination of his work. Paré was a popular surgeon with royalty. The fatal injury sustained by Henri II of France was an important case, from which some insight into Paré's understanding of head injury can be obtained. Paré attended the king and was present at the autopsy. The patient developed a subdural hematoma. Paré's clinical observations included headache, blurred vision, vomiting, lethargy, and decreased respiration. Using the clinical observations and the history, Paré postulated that the injury was due to a tear in one of the bridging cortical veins. An autopsy confirmed the findings.

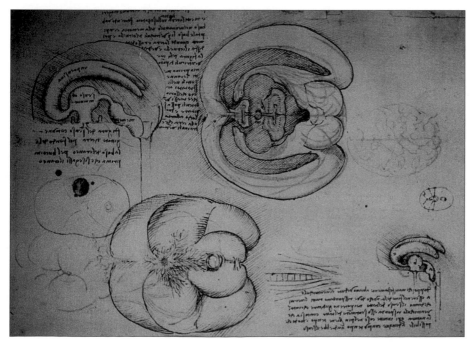

Figure 1.17 From Leonardo's anatomic codices: using a wax casting Leonardo was able to outline the ventricular system. From da Vinci L, 1911–1916.[31]

Among Paré's surgical works,[35,36] the part on the brain best reflects contemporary practice. Book X is devoted to skull fractures. Paré advanced an interesting technique of elevating a depressed skull fracture using the Valsalva maneuver: "… for a breath driven forth of the chest and prohibited passage forth, swells and lifts the substance of the brain and meninges where upon the frothing humidity and sanies sweat forth."[36] This maneuver enabled the expulsion of blood and pus.

His surgical techniques also demonstrate a remarkable advance over previous writers. Paré provided an extensive discussion on the use of trephines, shavers, and scrapers (Figure 1.18). He described the removal of osteomyelitic bone, incising the dura and evacuating blood clots and pus, procedures previously carried out with great trepidation. He advocated debridement, emphasizing that all foreign bodies must be removed. Paré's most useful advance in surgery was the discovery that boiling oil should not be used in gunshot wounds. Rather, he made a dressing of egg yolk, rose oil, and turpentine, which he found greatly improved wound healing and dramatically reduced morbidity and mortality. He also discarded the use of hot cautery to control bleeding, substituting the use of ligatures, which enhanced healing and reduced blood loss, particularly in amputations.

In 1518 a remarkable book by Giacomo Berengario da Carpi (1460–1530) appeared.[37] This book came about because of Berengario's success in treating Lorenzo de'Medici, Duke of Urbino, who had received a serious cranial injury and survived. In a dream shortly after this episode Berengario was visited by the god Hermes Trismegistus (Thrice-Great Mercury), who encouraged him to a write a treatise on head injuries. As a result his marvelous *Tractatus* appeared, the first printed work devoted solely to treating injuries of the head. Not only are original surgical techniques discussed but also illustrations of the cranial instruments for dealing with skull fractures (Figure 1.19). Berengario introduced the use of interchangeable cranial drill bits for trephination. Included in the text are a number of case histories with descriptions of the patients, methods of treatment, and clinical outcomes. This work remains our best 16th century account of brain surgery.

Berengario, like Leonardo da Vinci, was an excellent anatomist who gave one of the earliest and most complete discussions of the ventricular system. He provided early descriptions of the pineal gland, choroid plexus, and lateral ventricles. His anatomic illustrations are believed to be the first published from actual anatomic dissections. In addition his anatomic writings were among the first to challenge dogmatic belief in the writings of Galen and others.

A striking and beautifully illustrated work appeared in 1536 (with an expanded version in 1537) written by a professor of medicine from Marburg, Johannes Dryander (Johann Eichmann, 1500–1560).[38,39] This work contains 16 plates showing successive Galenic dissections of the brain (Figure 1.20). The dura mater, cortex, and posterior fossa are illustrated in detail. Dryander performed public dissections of the skull, dura, and brain, the results of which he published in this little monograph. Despite inaccuracies in the work, reflecting medieval scholasticism, it can be considered the first textbook of neuroanatomy.

Volcher Coiter (1534–1576) was an army surgeon and city physician at Nuremberg who had the good fortune to study under Fallopius, Eustachius, and Aldrovandi. These scholars provided the impetus for Coiter's original anatomic and physiologic investigations. He described the anterior and posterior spinal roots and distinguished gray from white matter in the spinal cord. His interest in the spine led him to conduct anatomic and pathologic

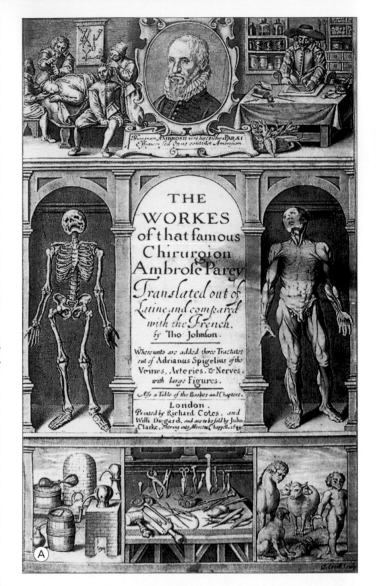

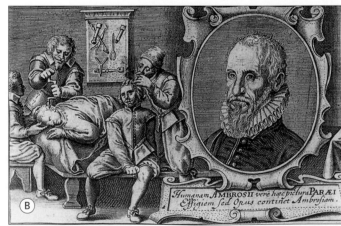

Figure 1.18 (A) Title page from the English translation of Paré, showing some early neurosurgical instruments. From Paré A, 1649. **(B)** Trephination scene from the title of Pare's work enlarged.[36]

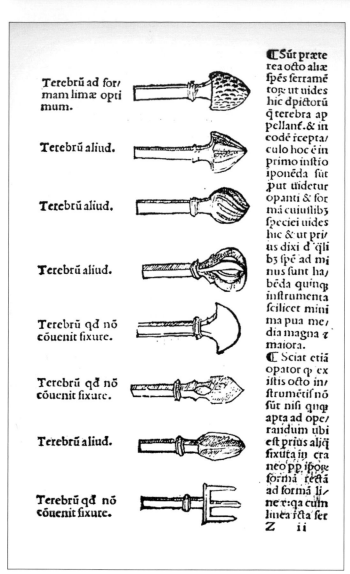

Figure 1.19 Woodcut from Berengario da Carpi's *Tractatus de Fractura Calvae* showing early neurosurgical instruments – the trephines show a sophisticated design to avoid plunging. From Berengario da Carpi, 1518.[37]

studies of the spinal cord, including a study on the decerebrate model. He performed a number of experiments on living subjects. He trephined the skulls of birds, lambs, goats, and dogs, and was the first to associate the pulsation of the brain with the arterial pulse. He even opened the brain and removed parts of it, reporting no ill effects – an early, surprising attempt at cerebral localization.[40]

Using a combination of surgical skill and a Renaissance flair for design, Giovanni Andrea della Croce (1509?–1580)[41] produced some beautifully engraved scenes of neurosurgical operations, performed in family homes, especially in the bedrooms; most being simple trephinations (Figure 1.21). Croce also designed a number of trephination instruments, some of which improved on their predecessors. His trephine drill was rotated by means of an attached bow, in the manner of a carpenter's drill. Various trephine bits with conical designs are proposed and illustrated. The illustrations of surgical instruments include elevators for lifting depressed bone.

Croce's writing is mainly a compilation of important authorities from Hippocrates to Albucasis, but his recommendations for treatment and his instrumentation are surprisingly modern.

A discussion of surgery in the 16th century would not be complete without mention of the great anatomist, Andreas Vesalius (1514–1564). Rejecting the views of his Galenic teachers, Vesalius provided a new and dramatic approach to anatomic dissection. Following on the theme of earlier 16th century anatomists like Berengario da Carpi, Vesalius argued that dissection should be performed by teachers, not by prosectors. His anatomic descriptions are his own observations rather than an interpretation of the Galenic writings.

Vesalius' masterpiece, *De Humani Corporis Fabrica*,[42] has a section on the anatomy of the brain that presents detailed anatomic discussions with excellent illustrations (Figure 1.22). Vesalius noted that "heads of beheaded men are the most suitable [for study] since they can be obtained immediately after execution with the friendly help of judges and prefects."[43]

Vesalius was primarily a surgeon and the section of text on the brain and the dural coverings discusses mechanisms of injury and how the various membranes and bone have been designed to protect the brain. Interestingly, close examination of several of the illustrated initial letters in the text shows little cherubs performing trephinations! Vesalius made an interesting early contribution to hydrocephalus: In Book 1 is a discussion of "Heads of other shape" where he provides the following early description of a child with hydrocephalus:

> … at Genoa a small boy is carried from door to door by a beggar woman, and was put on display by actors in noble Brabant in Belgium, whose head, without any exaggeration, is larger than two normal human heads and swells out on either side.[42]

In the second edition (1555) of his work,[44] Vesalius describes a second case, that of hydrocephalus in a young girl whom he noted to have a head "larger than any man's," at autopsy he noted the removal of nine pounds of water. As a result of these studies Vesalius made the important observation that fluid (i.e. cerebrospinal fluid) collects in the ventricles and not between the dura and skull. Despite these clinical observations Vesalius offered no insight into any effective treatment, either surgical or medical.

A remarkable work on anatomy by Charles Estienne (1504–1564) appeared in Paris in 1546.[45] Although published 3 years after Andreas Vesalius' work, the book had actually been completed in 1539, but legal problems delayed publication. This work contains a wealth of beautiful anatomic plates with the subjects posed against sumptuous, imaginative Renaissance backgrounds (Figure 1.23). The anatomic detail is not as good as that of Vesalius and the book repeats many of the errors of Galen, but the plates on the nervous system are quite graphic. Despite some errors, they detail the anatomy of the skull and brain more accurately than previous works.

SEVENTEENTH CENTURY: ORIGINS OF NEUROLOGY

The 17th century, like the Renaissance, was a period of spectacular growth in science and medicine. Isaac Newton, Francis Bacon, William Harvey, and Robert Boyle made important contributions in physics, experimental design, the discovery of the circulation of blood, and physiologic chemistry. Open public communication of

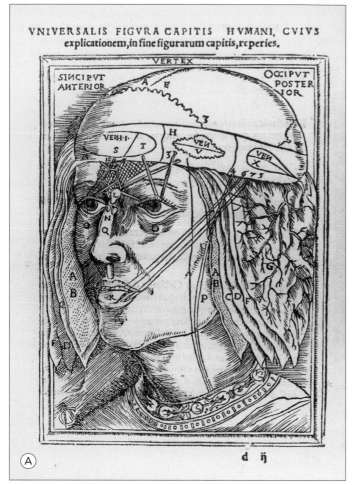

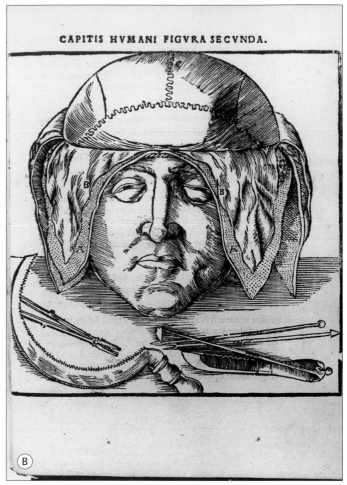

Figure 1.20 **(A)** Illustration from Dryander's *Anatomie* showing a dissection of the head and illustrations of the cell doctrine. **(B)** Illustration from Dryander's *Anatomie* showing a dissection of the skull and brain. From Dryander J, 1537.[38]

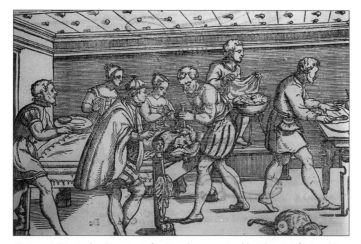

Figure 1.21 A classic scene of a Renaissance trephination performed in a noble's elegantly furnished home – from Croce's classic monograph on surgery.[41]

scientific ideas came with the advent of scientific societies (e.g. the Royal Society of London, the Académie des Sciences in Paris, and the Gesellschaft Naturforschenden Aerzte in Germany), which elevated scientific education and improved the exchange of scientific information.

The figure most remembered for his original investigation of the brain is Thomas Willis (1621–1675), after whom the circle of Willis is named (Figure 1.24). A fashionable London practitioner, educated at Oxford, Willis published his *Cerebri Anatome* in London in 1664 (Figure 1.25).[46] This book was the most accurate anatomic study of the brain up to that time. He was assisted in this work by Richard Lower (1631–1691), who showed that when parts of the "circle" were tied off, the anastomotic network still provided blood to the brain. The engravings were done by the prominent London personality, Sir Christopher Wren (1632–1723).

Willis introduced the concept of "neurology," or the doctrine of neurons, using the term in a purely anatomic sense. The word did not enter general use until Samuel Johnson defined it in his dictionary of 1765, according to which neurology encompassed the entire field of anatomy, function, and physiology. The circle of Willis was also detailed in other anatomic works of this period by Vesling,[47] Casserius,[48] Fallopius,[49] and Humphrey Ridley.[50]

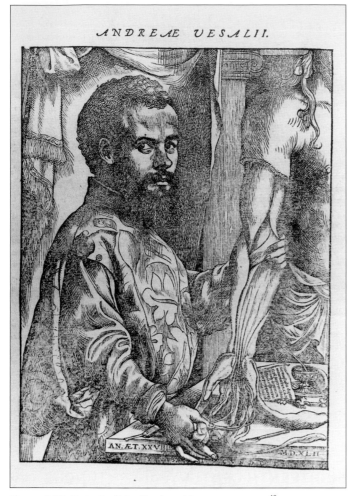

Figure 1.22 Portrait of Vesalius from his *magnum opus*.[42]

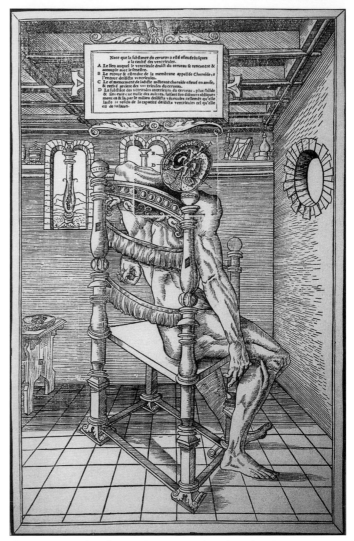

Figure 1.23 A plate from Estienne's *De Dissectione* showing a neurologic dissection of the brain. From Estienne C, 1546.[45]

Humphrey Ridley (1653–1708) produced an important anatomic work on the brain, written in the vernacular and widely circulated (Figure 1.26).[50] Ridley was educated at Merton College, Oxford, and at the University of Leiden, where he received his doctorate in medicine in 1679. At the time his work on the brain appeared, many ancient theories of the brain remained prevalent. Shifting away from the earlier cell theory, however, 17th century anatomists recognized the brain as a distinct anatomic entity. Instead of residing within the ventricles, cerebral function was thought now to be a property of the brain parenchyma.

Ridley recorded a number of original observations in his volume on brain anatomy. He conducted his anatomic studies on freshly executed criminals, most of whom had been hanged, causing vascular engorgement of the brain and hence allowing easier identification of the anatomy. His description of the circle of Willis was even more accurate than Willis's and included a complete account of both the posterior cerebral artery and the superior cerebellar artery. The anastomotic principle of this network was even further elucidated. His understanding of the deep nuclei and, in particular, the anatomy of the posterior fossa, was superior to that of Willis. In addition, Ridley gave a thorough description of the arachnoid membrane. Of interest is Ridley's

erroneous argument in favor of the belief that the rete mirabile exists. The first accurate description of the fornix and its pathways appears in this monograph.

Although Wilhelm Fabricius von Hilden (1560–1634) had received a classical education in his youth, family misfortune did not allow him a formal medical education. Following the apprenticeship system then prevalent, he studied the lesser field of surgery. Fortunately, the teachers he selected were among the finest wound surgeons of the day. With this education, he had a distinguished career in surgery, during which he made a number of advances.

His large work, *Observationum et Curationum*, included over 600 surgical cases and a number of important and original observations on the brain.[51] Congenital malformations, skull fractures, techniques for bullet extraction, and field instruments were described. He performed operations for intracranial hemorrhage (with cure of insanity), vertebral displacement, congenital hydrocephalus, and occipital tumor of the newborn; he also carried out trephinations for abscess and a cure of an old aphasia. He even removed a splinter of metal from the eye using a magnet, a cure that enhanced his reputation.

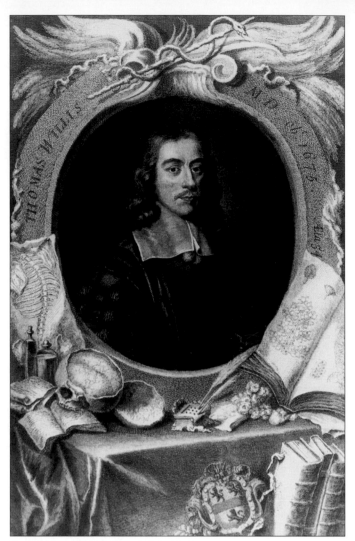

Figure 1.24 Thomas Willis (1621–1675).

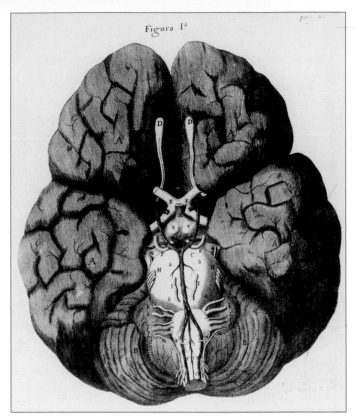

Figure 1.25 A depiction in Willis's *Cerebri Anatome* of what is now called the circle of Willis. From Willis T, 1664.[46]

Johann Schultes (Scultetus) of Ulm (1595–1645) provided in his *Armamentarium Chirurgicum XLIII* the first descriptive details of neurosurgical instruments to appear since those published by Berengario in 1518.[52] This work was translated into many languages, influencing surgery throughout Europe. Its importance lies in the exact detail of surgical instrument design and in the presentation of tools from antiquity to the present. Many of the instruments illustrated are still in use today. In addition, Scultetus gave details of operations for dealing with injuries of the skull and brain (Figure 1.27).

James Yonge (1646–1721) was among the first since Galen to argue emphatically that "wounds of the brain are curable." Appropriately enough, Yonge's remarkable little monograph was entitled *Wounds of the Brain Proved Curable*.[53] Yonge was a Plymouth naval surgeon, remembered mostly for his flap amputation technique. In his monograph Yonge gives a detailed account of a brain operation on a child aged 4 years with extensive compound fractures of the skull from which brain tissue issued forth. The surgery was a success and the child lived. Yonge also included reports on more than 60 cases of brain wounds that he found in the literature, beginning with Galen, which had been cured.

EIGHTEENTH CENTURY: ADVENTUROUS SURGEONS

The 18th century was a period of intense activity in the medical and scientific world. Chemistry as a true science was propelled forward by the work of Priestley, Lavoisier, Volta, Watt, and many others. Clinical bedside medicine, essentially lost since the Byzantine era, was reintroduced by Thomas Sydenham, William Cullen, and Herman Boerhaave. Diagnostic examination of the patient advanced in this period; especially notable is Auenbrugger's introduction of percussion of the chest. Withering introduced the use of digitalis for cardiac problems. Edward Jenner provided the world with cowpox inoculation for smallpox, reducing the terror of this scourge.

Percival Pott (1714–1788) was the greatest English surgeon of the 18th century. His list of contributions, several of which apply to neurosurgery, is enormous. His work *Remarks on That Kind of Palsy of the Lower Limbs Found to Accompany a Curvature of the Spine* describes the condition now known as Pott's disease.[54] His clinical descriptions are excellent, with the gibbous and tuberculous condition of the spine well outlined. Interestingly, he failed to associate the spinal deformity with the paralysis. He also described an osteomyelitic condition of the skull with a collection of pus under the pericranium, now called Pott's puffy tumor. Pott felt strongly that these lesions should be trephined to remove the pus and decompress the brain.

In the ongoing argument over whether to trephine, Pott was a strong proponent of intervention (Figures 1.28, 1.29). In his classic work on head injury,[55] Pott appreciated that symptoms of

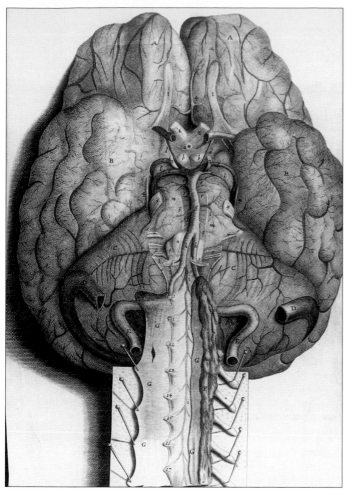

Figure 1.26 "Circle of Willis" as detailed by Ridley[50] – an anatomically more correct rendition than that of Willis.

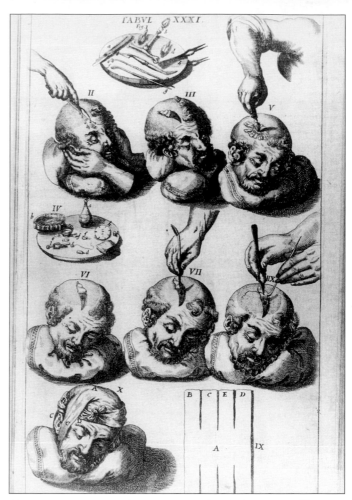

Figure 1.27 Neurosurgical instruments as detailed by Scultetus.[52]

head injury were the result of injury of the brain and not of the skull. He made an attempt to differentiate between "compression" and "concussion" injury of the brain.

> The reasons for trepanning in these cases are, first, the immediate relief of present symptoms arising from pressure of extravasated fluid; or second, the discharge of matter formed between the skull and dura mater, in consequence of inflammation; or third, the prevention of such mischief, as experience has shown may most probably be expected from such kind of violence offered to the last mentioned membrane …
>
> In the … mere fracture without depression of bone, or the appearance of such symptoms as indicate commotion, extravasation, or inflammation, it is used as a preventative, and therefore is a matter of choice, more than immediate necessity.[55]

Pott's astute clinical observations, bedside treatment, and aggressive management of head injuries made him the first modern neurosurgeon. His caveats, presented in the preface to his work on head injury, still hold today.

John Hunter (1728–1793) was one of the most remarkable and talented figures in English medicine. His knowledge and skills

in anatomy, pathology, and surgery and his dedication to his work allowed him to make a number of important contributions. He had minimal formal education, though Percival Pott was an early teacher. In his book *A Treatise on the Blood, Inflammation, and Gun-Shot Wounds*,[56] Hunter drew on his years of military experience (he served as a surgeon with the British forces during the Spanish campaign of 1761–1763). Unfortunately, the section on skull fractures took up only one paragraph and offered nothing original. However, his discussion of vascular disorders was quite advanced, with an appreciation of the concept of collateral circulation. His views on this subject grew out of his observations on a buck whose carotid artery he tied off; the response was, of course, development of collateral circulation.

Benjamin Bell (1749–1806) was among the most prominent and successful surgeons in Edinburgh. He was one of the first to emphasize the importance of reducing pain during surgery. His text, *A System of Surgery*,[57] is written with extraordinary clarity and precision, qualities that made it one of the most popular surgical texts in the 18th and 19th centuries. In the section on head injury there is an interesting and important discussion of the differences between concussion, compression, and inflammation of the brain – each requiring different modes of treatment.[57] Bell stressed the importance of relieving compression of the brain,

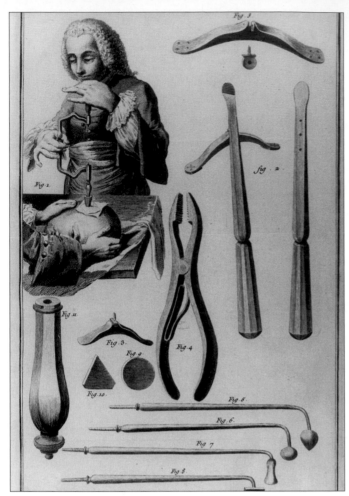

Figure 1.28 An 18th-century trephination in Diderot's *Encyclopédie*.

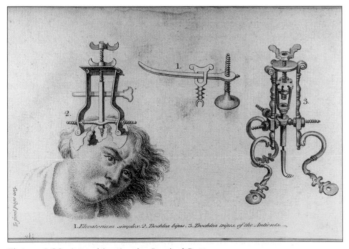

Figure 1.29 A trephination by Percival Pott.

whether it be caused by a depressed skull fracture or pressure caused by pus or blood – a remarkably aggressive approach for this period (Figure 1.30). Bell was among the first to note that hydrocephalus is often associated with spina bifida. His treatment of a myelomeningocele involved placing a ligature around the base

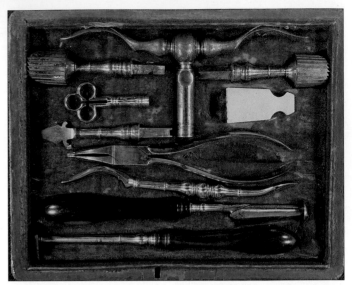

Figure 1.30 A French 18th century travelling trephine set with all the tools necessary for a trephination.

of the myelomeningocele sac. The concept of an epidural hematoma and its symptoms were appreciated by Bell; he argued for a rapid and prompt evacuation. His discussion of the symptoms of brain compression caused by external trauma is classic.

> A great variety of symptoms ... indicating a compressed state of the brain [among which] ... the most frequent, as well as the most remarkable, are the following: Giddiness; dimness of sight; stupefaction; loss of voluntary motion; vomiting; an apoplectic stertor in the breathing; convulsive tremors in different muscles; a dilated state of the pupils, even when the eyes are exposed to a clear light; paralysis of different parts, especially of the side of the body opposite to the injured part of the head; involuntary evacuation of the urine and faeces; an oppressed, and in many case an irregular pulse ... (volume 3, chapter 10, section 3).[57]

Lorenz Heister (1683–1758) produced another of the most popular surgical textbooks of the 18th century. A German surgeon and anatomist (a common combination at the time), he published his *Chirurgie* in 1718. It was subsequently translated into a number of languages and circulated widely.[58] The wide range of surgical knowledge it communicated and its many illustrations made it popular. In the treatment of head injury Heister remained conservative with regard to trephination (Figure 1.31). In wounds involving only concussion and contusion, he felt trephination to be too dangerous. Considering the risk of infection and injury to the brain, this was not too far off the mark.

> XXVII. But when the Cranium is so depressed, whether in Adults or Infants, as to suffer a Fracture, or Division of its Parts, it must instantly be relieved: the Part depressed, which adheres, after cleaning the Wound, must be restored to its Place, what is separated must be removed, and the extravasated Blood be drawn off through the Aperture ... (p. 100).[58]

Heister introduced a number of techniques that proved most useful. To control scalp hemorrhage he used a "crooked needle and

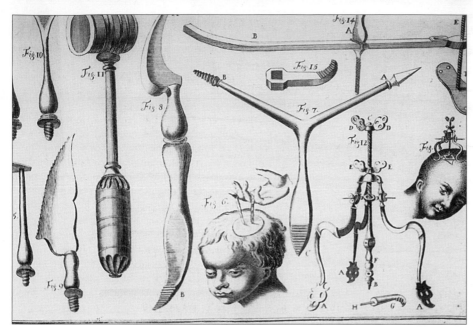

thread" that when placed and drawn tight reduced bleeding. He also pointed out that when the assistant applied pressure to the skin, edge bleeding could be reduced. In spinal injuries Heister argued for exposing the fractured vertebrae and removing fragments that damaged the spinal marrow, even though he recognized that grave outcomes of such attempts were not uncommon.

Francois-Sauveur Morand (1697–1773) published a monograph that describes one of the earliest operations for abscess of the brain. Morand had a patient, a monk, who developed an otitis and subsequently mastoiditis with temporal abscess.[59] He trephined over the carious bone and discovered pus. He placed a catgut wick within the wound, but it continued to drain. He reopened the wound and this time opened the dura (a very adventurous maneuver for this period) with a cross-shaped incision and found a brain abscess. He explored the abscess with his finger, removing as much of the contents as he could, and then instilled balsam and turpentine into the cavity. He placed a silver tube for drainage, and as the wound healed he slowly withdrew the tube. The abscess healed, and the patient survived.

Domenico Cotugno (1736–1822) was a Neapolitan physician who offered a small monograph in which he gave classic descriptions of cerebrospinal fluid (CSF) and sciatica[60] (Figure 1.32). He performed a number of experiments on the bodies of some 20 adults. Using the technique of lumbar puncture, he was able to demonstrate the characteristics of CSF. In *De Ischiade Nervosa Commentarius* he demonstrated the "nervous" origin of sciatica, differentiating it from arthritis, with which it was generally equated at that time. Cotugno discovered the pathways of CSF, showing that it circulates in the pia-arachnoid interstices and flows through the brain and spinal cord via the aqueduct and convexities. He also described the hydrocephalus *ex vacuo* seen in cerebral atrophy.

In 1709, a small, and now very rare, monograph by Daniel Turner (1667–1741) appeared.[61] The book was entitled *A Remarkable Case in Surgery: Wherein an Account is given of an uncommon Fracture and Depression of the Skull, in a Child about Six Years old; accompanied with a large Abscess or Aposteme upon*

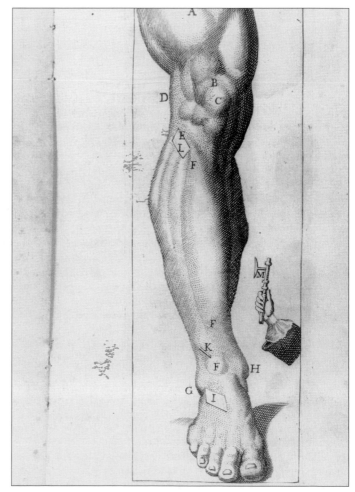

Figure 1.32 From Cotugno's monograph on sciatica.[60]

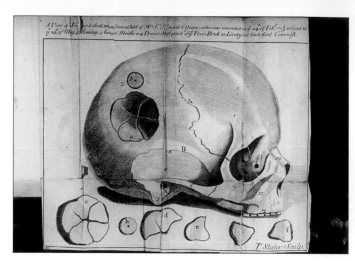

Figure 1.33 A child with a severe skull fracture. From Turner D, 1709.[61]

the Brain ... (Figure 1.33). This rather poignant piece of writing is perhaps our best view of the treatment of brain injuries in the early 18th century.

The case is most disturbing to read, written in the frank and somewhat verbose style of this period. Turner was "... called in much hast, to a Child about the Age of Six Years ... wounded by a Catstick ... He was taken up for dead and continued speechless for some time." Turner examined the head, found a considerable depression, and arrived at the prognosis that the child was in great danger. He sent for the barber to shave the head; while waiting for the barber he opened a vein in the arm to bleed the child, taking about 6 ounces. The patient regained consciousness, vomiting and complaining of a headache. Turner chose to delay surgery. But finding the child the next day still vomiting, restless, and hot, he decided on an exploration. Through a typical X incision he found "the Bones were beat thro' both meninges into the substance of the brain." He elevated the bone and found "... a cavity sufficient to contain near two Ounces of Liquor." Postoperatively the patient was awake with "... a quick pulse, thirst and headache ... but no vomiting. He was very sensible." He visited the child the next day and found him still feverish but without other symptoms. He removed the dressings and realized the extent of the fracture, which had been only partially elevated. He now took a trephine, removed what bone he thought it was safe to remove, and applied a clyster.

A careful report of the operation follows, including a description of a piece of bone that flew across the room upon elevation. Four pieces of bone were removed. The dura now pulsated nicely. The wound was cleaned out with soft sponges soaked in claret. The patient was carried to bed and refreshed with "two or three Spoonfulls of his Cephalic Julep." Despite all this effort and although the patient was doing well, upon removing the dressings "an offensive smell" and fetid matter were noted. A consultant's advice was to redress the wound. Instead, Turner opened the right jugular vein and bled 6 ounces. A vesicatory was also applied to the neck and an emollient clyster given in the evening. The next day Turner was still not satisfied with what was happening, and so he re-explored the wound, venting a great deal of purulent matter.

This patient was to have several additional explorations for removal and drainage of pus. Cannulas were placed for drainage and the wound carefully tended, but despite all this the patient died after 12 weeks.

Louis Sebastian (also listed as Nicolas) Saucerotte (1741–1814) was first surgeon to the King of Poland and later a surgeon in the French Army. As has often been the case in the history of neurosurgery, war provided Saucerotte with training and the opportunity for insight into the management of head injury. He reintroduced the concept of the contre-coup injury. In a review of head injury, he described in detail a series of intracranial injuries and their symptoms, including compression of the brain due to blood clot.[62] Saucerotte described a classic case of incoordination, including opisthotonos and rolling of the eyes, as a result of a cerebellar lesion. He divided the brain into "areas" of injury, pointing out that areas of severe injury are at the base of the brain, while injuries of the forebrain are the best tolerated.

During the 18th century there was a remarkable change in the approach to surgery of the brain. Surgeons became much more aggressive in their management of head injuries and the clinical symptoms associated with brain injury were better recognized.

NINETEENTH AND TWENTIETH CENTURIES: ANESTHESIA, ANTISEPSIS, AND CEREBRAL LOCALIZATION

Three major innovations made possible the great advances in neurosurgery during the 19th century. Anesthesia allowed patients freedom from pain during surgery, antisepsis and aseptic technique enabled the surgeon to operate with a greatly reduced risk of postoperative complications caused by infection, and the concept of cerebral localization helped the surgeon make the diagnosis and plan the operative approach.

In the first half of the century, improvements in surgical technique and neuropathology helped prepare the way for these innovations. John Abernethy (1764–1831) succeeded John Hunter at St Bartholomew's Hospital and followed his tradition of experimentation and observation. Abernethy's surgical technique did not differ from that of his predecessors; what is remarkable in his *Surgical Observations*[63] is the thoughtful, very thorough discussion of all the mechanisms of injury to the brain and spinal cord. He performed one of the earliest known procedures for removal of a painful neuroma. The neuroma was resected and the nerve re-anastomosed; the pain resolved and sensation returned, proving the efficacy of the anastomosis.

Sir Charles Bell (1774–1842), a Scottish surgeon and anatomist, was a prolific writer. He was educated at the University of Edinburgh and spent most of his professional career in London. He is remembered for many contributions to the neurosciences, including the differentiation of the motor and sensory components of the spinal root. He wrote a number of works on surgery, many of which were beautifully illustrated with his own drawings. These hand-colored illustrations were unrivaled at the time in detail, accuracy, and beauty (Figure 1.34). This is one of the earliest works with detailed illustrations to assist the surgeon in mastering neurosurgical techniques.

In describing a trephination Bell gave a view of the technique as practiced in 1821:

Let the bed or couch on which the patient is lying be turned to the light – have the head shaved – put a wax-cloth on the pillow – let the pillow be firm, to support the

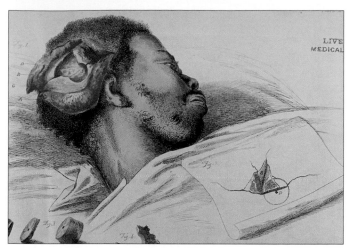

Figure 1.34 Charles Bell's illustrations of repair of a depressed skull fracture, with bone fragments removed shown at the base of the illustration. From Bell C, 1821.[64]

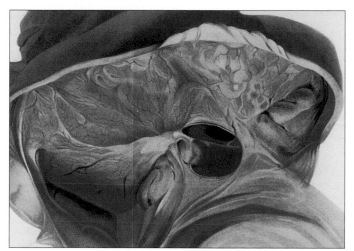

Figure 1.35 A child with hydrocephalus as illustrated by Richard Bright.[65]

patient's head. Put tow or sponge by the side of the head – let there be a stout assistant to hold the patient's head firmly, and let others put their hands on his arms and knees.

The surgeon will expect the instruments to be handed to him in this succession – the scalpel; the rasparatory; the trephine; the brush, the quill, and probe, from time to time; the elevator, the forceps, the lenticular (p. 6).[64]

Also in the first half of the 19th century, a number of industrious individuals provided the basis for study of neuropathologic lesions. Several excellent atlases appeared, beautifully colored and pathologically correct. Among the best known are those of Robert Hooper, Jean Cruveilhier, Robert Carswell, and Richard Bright (Figure 1.35). Cruveilhier's is the most dramatic in appearance.[65]

Jean Cruveilhier (1791–1874) was the first occupant of a new chair of pathology at the University of Paris. He had at his disposal an enormous collection of autopsy material provided by the deadhouse at the Salpêtrière and the Musée Dupuytren, on the basis of which he made a number of original descriptions of pathologies of the nervous system, including spina bifida (Figure 1.36), spinal cord pathology, cerebellopontine angle tumor, disseminated sclerosis, muscular atrophy, and perhaps the best early description of meningioma. This work was published in a series of fascicles issued over 13 years.[66] The detailed descriptions by Cruveilhier and others provided the basis for the later cerebral localization studies. An understanding of tumors and their clinical–pathologic effects on the brain was critical for the later development of neurosurgery and neurologic examination. Harvey Cushing was the first to call attention to Cruveilhier's accuracy in pathology and clinical correlation. He used portions of Cruveilhier's works in his treatise on acoustic neuromas and his classic meningioma work.[66–68]

Anesthesia

Various methods of reducing sensibility to pain were tried by surgeons over the centuries. Mandrake, cannabis, opium and other narcotics, the "soporific sponge" (saturated with opium), and alcohol had all been tried. In 1844, Horace Wells, a dentist in Hartford, Connecticut, introduced the use of nitrous oxide in dental procedures; however, the death of one of his patients stopped him from investigating further. At the urging of W.T.O. Morton, J.C. Warren used ether on 16 October 1846, to induce a state of insensibility in a patient, during which a vascular tumor of the submaxillary region was removed. Similar efforts were undertaken in the United Kingdom by J.Y. Simpson, who preferred chloroform, introduced in 1847, as an anesthetic agent. There were many arguments about which was the best agent. However, the end result was that the surgeon did not need to restrain the patient or operate at breakneck speed, and patients were free of pain during the procedure.

Antisepsis

Even with the best surgical technique, three-minute (!) trephinations, the patient might well die postoperatively of suppuration and infection. Fever, purulent material, brain abscess, and draining wounds, all defeated the best surgeons. No surgeon could open the dura mater without inviting disaster until the risk of infection could be reduced.

Surgery was revolutionized when, using concepts developed by Louis Pasteur, Joseph Lister introduced antisepsis in the operating room (Figure 1.37). For the first time a surgeon, using aseptic technique and a clean operating theater, could operate on the brain with a reasonably small likelihood of infection. The steam sterilizer, the scrub brush, and Halsted's rubber gloves truly heralded a revolution in surgery.

Cerebral localization

To make a diagnosis of a brain lesion or brain injury was not meaningful until the concept of localization was formulated (Figure 1.38). Before the 1860s, the brain was thought to act as a single unit. Then during the 1860s several investigators, including G.T. Fritsch and E. Hitzig[69] as well as Paul Broca (Figure 1.39), introduced the concept that each part of the brain corresponds to a particular function.

Paul Broca (1824–1880) conceived the idea of speech localization in 1861.[70] His studies were based on the work by Ernest Auburtin (1825–1893?), who had as a patient a gentleman who attempted suicide by shooting himself through the frontal

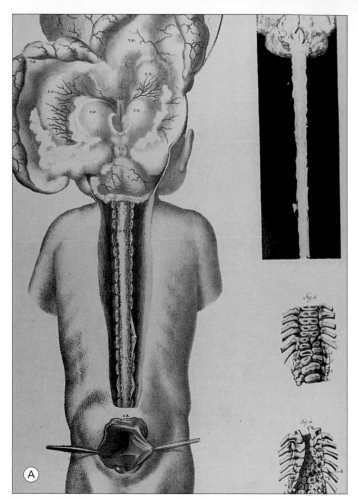 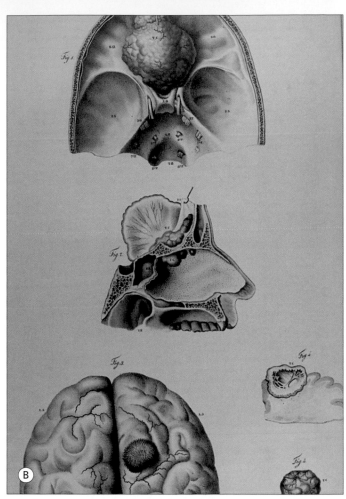

Figure 1.36 (A) Plate showing a child with spina bifida and hydrocephalus: an excellent example of the quality of pathologic illustrations in the first half of the 19th century. From Cruveilhier J, 1829–1842.[66] **(B,C)** Examples of meningiomas. From Cruveilhier J, 1829–1842.[66]   *Continued*

region. He survived, but was left with a defect in the left frontal bone. Through this defect Auburtin was able to apply a spatula to the anterior frontal lobe and with pressure abolish speech, which returned when the spatula was removed. The clinical implications were immediately recognized by Auburtin. Broca further localized speech in an epileptic patient who was aphasic and could only emit the utterance "tan," for which the patient became named. At autopsy, Broca found softening of the third left frontal convolution, and from this he postulated the cerebral localization of speech.[70,71] Later, Karl Wernicke (1848–1904) identified a different area of the brain where speech was associated with conduction defects.[72]

These studies led to an explosion of research on the localization of brain function, such as the use of ablation by David Ferrier (1843–1928).[73] John Hughlings Jackson (1835–1911), the founder of modern neurology, demonstrated important areas of function by means of electrical studies and developed the concept of epilepsy.[74] Robert Bartholow (1831–1904), working in Ohio, published a series of three cases of brain tumors in which he correlated the clinical observations with the anatomic findings.[75]

Bartholow later performed an amazing clinical study correlating these types of pathologic findings. In 1874 he took under his care a lady named Mary Rafferty who had developed a large cranial defect, which had in turn exposed portions of each cerebral hemisphere. Through these defects he electrically stimulated the brain; unfortunately she subsequently died of meningitis. Bartholow records that "two needles insulated were introduced into left side until their points were well engaged in the dura mater. When the circuit was closed, distinct muscular contractions occurred in the right arm and leg."[76] Bartholow stimulated a number of different areas, carefully recording his observations. These clinical observations supported his postulated functional localizations in the brain. The ethics of his studies, though, might be called into question today!

Advances in surgical techniques

The surgical personalities of the 19th century were quite varied and in most cases very talented. Until the end of the 19th century, neurosurgery was not specialized; brain operations were performed by general surgeons, top-hatted, bewhiskered, and always pontifical!

Sir Rickman Godlee (1859–1925) (Figure 1.40) removed one of the most celebrated brain tumors, the first to be successfully diagnosed by cerebral localization, in 1884.[77] The patient, a man by the name of Henderson, had suffered for 3 years from focal

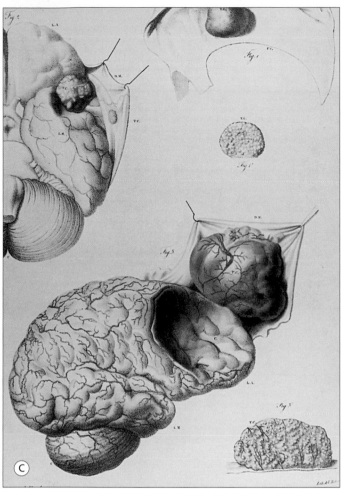

Figure 1.36, cont'd.

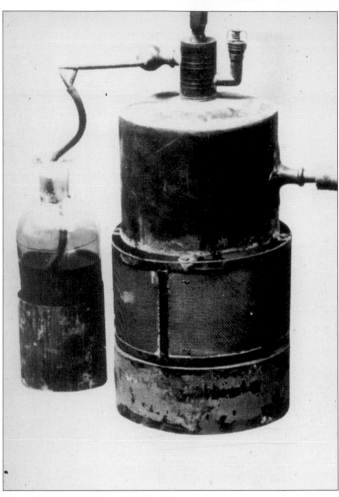

Figure 1.37 Early Lister carbolic acid sprayer.

motor seizures. They started as focal seizures of the face and proceeded to involve the arm and then the leg. In the 3 months prior to surgery the patient also developed weakness and eventually had to give up his work. A neurologist, Alexander Hughes Bennett, basing his conclusions on the findings of a neurologic examination, localized a brain tumor and recommended removal to the surgeon. Godlee made an incision over the Rolandic area and removed the tumor through a small cortical incision. The patient survived the surgery with some mild weakness and did well, only to die a month later from infection. The operation was observed by Bennett, the physician who had made the diagnosis and localization, and by J. Hughlings Jackson and David Ferrier, two local neurologists, all of whom were extremely interested in whether the cerebral localization studies would provide results in the operating theater. The results were good; this operation was a landmark in the progress of neurosurgery.

Sir William Gowers (1845–1915) was one of an extraordinary group of English neurologists. Using some of the recently developed techniques in physiology and pathology, he made great strides in refining the concept of cerebral localization. Gowers was noted for the clarity and organization of his writing; his works remain classics.[78–80] Such studies allowed surgeons to consider operating on the brain and spine for other than desperate conditions.

Sir Victor Alexander Haden Horsley (1857–1916) was another English general surgeon who furthered the development of neurosurgery during this period. Horsley began his experimental studies on the brain in the early 1880s, during the height of the cerebral localization controversies. He worked with Sharpey-Schäfer in using faradic stimulation to analyze and localize motor functions in the cerebral cortex, internal capsule, and spinal cord of primates.[81] In a classic study with Gotch (in 1891), using a string galvanometer, he showed that electrical currents originate in the brain.[82] These experimental studies showed Horsley that localization was possible and that operations on the brain could be conducted safely using techniques adapted from general surgery. In 1887, working with William Gowers, Horsley performed a laminectomy on Gowers' patient, Captain Golby, a 45-year-old army officer. Golby was slowly losing function in his legs from a spinal cord tumor. Gowers localized the tumor by examination and suggested to Horsley where to operate; the tumor, a benign "fibromyxoma" of the fourth thoracic root, was successfully removed.[83]

Horsley made a number of technical contributions to neurosurgery, including the use of beeswax to stop bone bleeding. He performed one of the earliest operations for craniostenosis and relief of increased intracranial pressure. For patients with

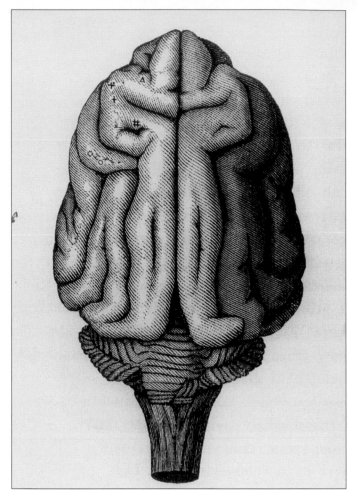

Figure 1.38 Illustration of the exposed cortex of a dog's brain showing sites of cortical stimulation. From Fritsch GT, Hitzig E, 1870.[69]

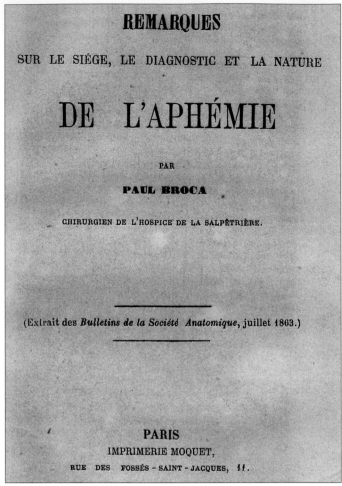

Figure 1.39 Paul Broca (1824–1880): a pioneer in cerebral localization studies presenting here one of his classic studies on aphasia and cerebral localization.

inoperable tumors he developed the decompressive craniectomy. He also developed the technique of sectioning the posterior root of the trigeminal nerve for pain relief, an early effective treatment for trigeminal neuralgia. Using his technical gifts he helped Clarke design the first useful stereotactic unit for brain surgery (Figure 1.41). The Horsley–Clarke stereotactic frame has inspired all subsequent designs.[84]

During World War I, Horsley was sent to Mesopotamia to help develop hygienic procedures in a desert outpost. Ironically, he died within 2 days of arrival after contracting a severe desert fever.

Sir Charles A. Ballance (1856–1936) was a noted English surgeon who received his medical education at University College, London. Ballance was a true pioneer in neurosurgery, performing the first mastoidectomy with ligation of the jugular vein. He was one of the first to graft and repair the facial nerve. In his classic work on brain surgery Ballance sets forth many ideas that were quite modern for an early 20th century monograph.[85] The book was developed from a series of Lettsomian Lectures given in 1906, which contain a series of three lectures on cerebral membranes, tumors, and abscesses. Ballance's treatise recognized and described chronic subdural hematoma with great accuracy and detailed an operative success. Additional successful operations included one for subdural hygroma. Ballance routinely used the

recently introduced lumbar puncture for cases of head injury and suppurative meningitis. An interesting and apparent cure of congenital hydrocephalus was recorded by Ballance using a technique that included ligation of both common carotids. In his treatment of brain abscesses Ballance urged evacuation of the abscess with drainage recommended; in some cases he felt that complete enucleation of an abscess was advisable. Ballance devoted 243 pages of his monograph to a discussion of brain tumors and noted a wide operative experience with 400 such lesions. One of his most important cases, and one only recently recognized in the literature, involved a patient who was well in 1906 from whom he removed "a fibrosarcoma from the right cerebellar fossa" in 1894, i.e. an acoustic neuroma, this would appear to be one of the earliest surgeries for an angle tumor[86] (Figure 1.42). In a rather profound comment on surgical operations for tumors Ballance had a hopeful outlook and stated "... I am convinced that the dawn of a happier day for these terrible cases has come."

William Macewen (1848–1924), a Scottish surgeon and pioneer in the field of neurosurgery, successfully accomplished a brain operation for tumor on 29 July 1879 (Figure 1.43). Using meticulous technique and the recently developed neurologic examination, he localized and removed a periosteal tumor from

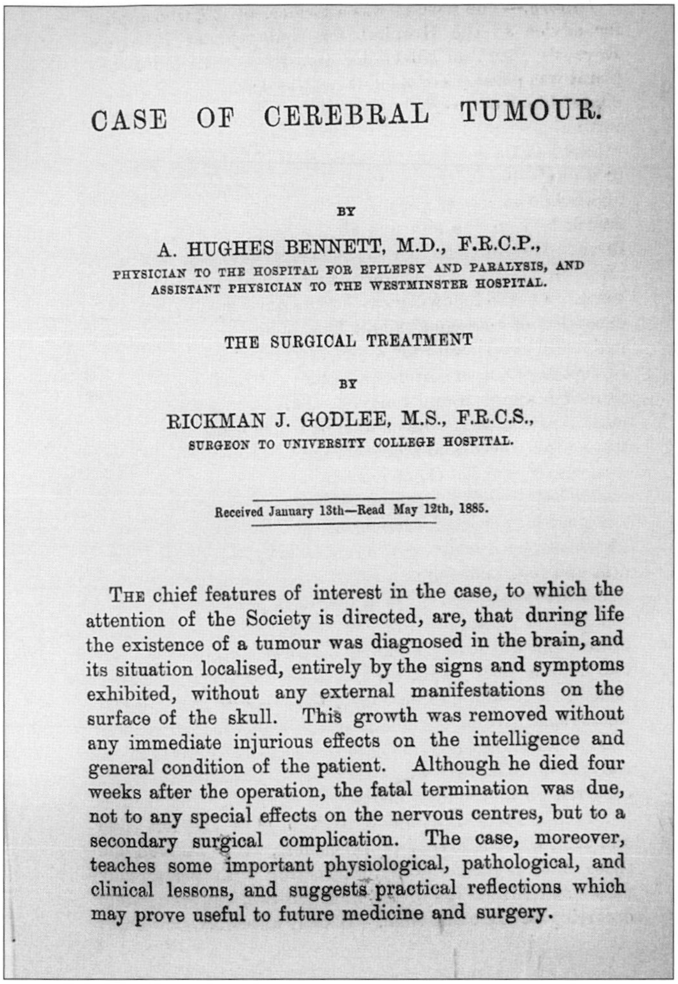

CASE OF CEREBRAL TUMOUR.

BY

A. HUGHES BENNETT, M.D., F.R.C.P.,
PHYSICIAN TO THE HOSPITAL FOR EPILEPSY AND PARALYSIS, AND
ASSISTANT PHYSICIAN TO THE WESTMINSTER HOSPITAL.

THE SURGICAL TREATMENT

BY

RICKMAN J. GODLEE, M.S., F.R.C.S.,
SURGEON TO UNIVERSITY COLLEGE HOSPITAL.

Received January 13th—Read May 12th, 1885.

THE chief features of interest in the case, to which the attention of the Society is directed, are, that during life the existence of a tumour was diagnosed in the brain, and its situation localised, entirely by the signs and symptoms exhibited, without any external manifestations on the surface of the skull. This growth was removed without any immediate injurious effects on the intelligence and general condition of the patient. Although he died four weeks after the operation, the fatal termination was due, not to any special effects on the nervous centres, but to a secondary surgical complication. The case, moreover, teaches some important physiological, pathological, and clinical lessons, and suggests practical reflections which may prove useful to future medicine and surgery.

Figure 1.40 Title page of the classic paper on an operation for brain tumor by Bennett and Godlee.[77]

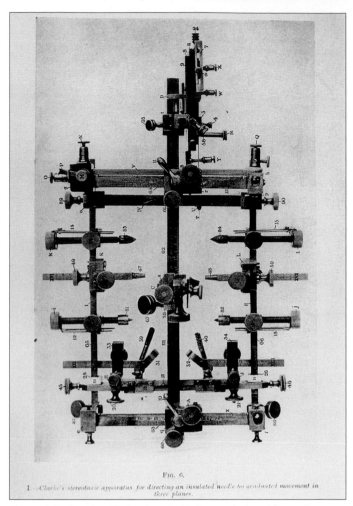

FIG. 6.

I.—Clarke's stereotaxic apparatus for directing an insulated needle by graduated movement in three planes.

Figure 1.41 Horsley–Clarke stereotactic frame, designed for and never used on humans but which nevertheless gave the idea for the modern stereotactic frame.[84]

over the right eye of a 14-year-old. The patient went on to live for 8 more years, only to die of Bright's disease; at autopsy no tumor was detected. By 1888, Macewen had operated on 21 neurosurgical cases with only three deaths and 18 successful recoveries – a remarkable change from earlier studies. He considered his success to be the result of excellent cerebral localization and good aseptic techniques. Macewen's monograph on pyogenic infections of the brain and their surgical treatment, published in 1893,[87] was the earliest to deal with the successful treatment of brain abscess. His morbidity and mortality statistics are as good as those in any series reported today. Without good results, the neurologist of that era was hesitant to recommend surgery; Macewen helped immensely to make the case for performing operations on the brain that had previously been considered too dangerous.

Joseph Pancoast (1805–1882) produced one of the most remarkable 19th century American monographs on surgery in the era just before the introduction of antisepsis and anesthesia[88] (Figure 1.44). Pancoast spent his academic career in Philadelphia, Pennsylvania, where he was physician and visiting surgeon to the Philadelphia Hospital. He later became professor of surgery and anatomy at Jefferson's Medical College in 1838. Pancoast's *Treatise* has 80 quarto plates comprising 486 lithographs with striking surgical details. These plates remain to this day some of the most well-executed and graphical illustrations of different surgical techniques The lithographs are exceedingly graphic, so much so that numbers 69 and 70 were often removed by religious purists because of their depiction of the female genitalia. The section on head injury and trauma clearly demonstrates the techniques of trephination and the elevation of depressed fractures. Pancoast was one of the first to devise an operation for transecting the fifth nerve for trigeminal neuralgia

Fedor Krause (1857–1937) was a general surgeon whose keen interest in neurosurgery made him the father of German neurologic surgery. His three-volume atlas on neurosurgery, *Surgery of the Brain and Spinal Cord* published in 1909–1912, was one of the first to detail the techniques of modern neurosurgery; it has since been through some 60 editions[89] (Figure 1.45). Krause, like William Macewen, was a major proponent of aseptic technique in neurosurgery. His atlas describes a number of interesting techniques. The "digital" extirpation of a meningioma is graphically illustrated. A number of original neurosurgical techniques are reviewed, including resection of scar tissue for treatment of epilepsy. Krause was a pioneer in the extradural approach to the gasserian ganglion for treatment of trigeminal neuralgia. He

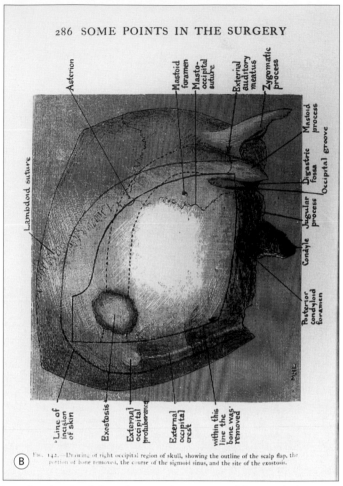

Figure 1.42 **(A)** Title page from Ballance's monograph on brain surgery. **(B)** Illustration showing Ballance's approach to a successful removal of acoustic neuroma.[85]

pioneered the transfrontal craniotomy in addition to transection of the VIII nerve for severe tinnitus. To deal with tumors of the pineal region and posterior third ventricle he pioneered the supracerebellar-infratentorial approach. Krause was the first to suggest that tumors of the cerebellopontine angle (e.g. acoustic neuromas) could be operated on safely. Interestingly, Krause retired to Rome, where he gave up neurosurgery and continued his greatest love, playing the piano. When asked what he would most like to be remembered for, it was not as a neurosurgeon but rather as a classical pianist.

Antony (Antoine) Chipault (1866–1920) has remained an obscure historical figure in neurosurgery yet nevertheless he was one of the pioneers and was once considered the potential father of French neurosurgery. Chipault was named at birth Antonie Maxime Nicolas Chipault on 16 July 1866 in the town of Orleans, France. His father was a surgeon and he began his medical studies in Paris at the age of 18. He initially qualified as a gynecologist but later became interested in neurology. He became initially interested in the anatomy of the spine and published a now rare seminal monograph *Etudes de Chirurgie Médullaires*.[90] In 1891 he began working with Professor Duplay at the l'Hotel Dieu under whom he became interested in craniocerebral pathology. In 1894 he published his classic work on surgery of the spine and spinal cord. Chipault published a series of papers on the brain and spinal

cord including writings on Pott's disease, osteoplastic craniotomy, spinal trauma, posterior root section for pain, surgical treatment of brain tumors and hemorrhage among other subjects. He made a number of technical innovations in neurosurgery, including introducing the removal of the underlying dura in meningiomas, a new laminectomy technique, plus development of small clamps for closing a scalp incision. He treated hydrocephalus by tapping the ventricles through a burr hole, and proposed a scheme of craniectomies for treatment of craniosynostosis (Figure 1.46). He pioneered the use of wires and steel splints in the stabilization of the spine in trauma and deformities. In 1894 his surgical masterpiece appeared *Chirurgie opératoire du systéme nerveux* – an extremely popular work that was translated into English, Spanish, Italian, German, Romanian, and Serbo-Croat.[91] He also introduced one of the first journals devoted to surgery of the spine and brain – *Les Travaux de Neurologie Chirurgicale*. Despite this illustrious career he dropped out of sight in 1905 ceasing all writing and works in neurosurgery. The cause is thought to be the onset of paraplegia, the etiology of which remains unknown. Chipault moved with his family to the Jura mountains near Orchamps. He died in 1920 at the age of 54 in total obscurity, a state in which he still remains.

William W. Keen (1837–1932), professor of surgery at Jefferson Medical College in Philadelphia, was one of the

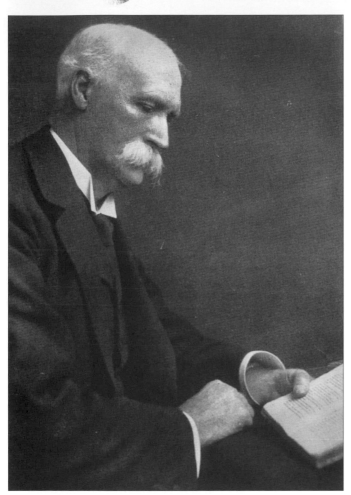

Figure 1.43 William Macewen (1848–1924).

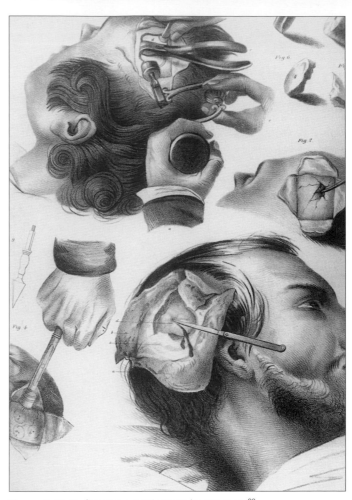

Figure 1.44 Performing a craniectomy by Pancoast.[88]

strongest American advocates for the use of Listerian techniques in surgery, advancing the concepts of surgical bacteriology, asepsis, and antisepsis. A description of Keen's surgical set-up provides a contemporary view of this innovative surgeon's approach to antisepsis:

> All carpets and unnecessary furniture were removed from the patient's room. The walls and ceiling were carefully cleaned the day before operation, and the woodwork, floors, and remaining furniture were scrubbed with carbolic solution. This solution was also sprayed in the room on the morning preceding but not during the operation. On the day before operation, the patient's head was shaved, scrubbed with soap, water, and ether, and covered with a wet corrosive sublimate dressing until the operation, then ether and mercuric chloride washings were repeated. The surgical instruments were boiled in water for 2 hours, and new deep-sea sponges (elephant ears) were treated with carbolic and sublimate solutions before usage. The surgeon's hands were cleaned and disinfected using soap and water, alcohol, and sublimate solution (pp. 1001–1002).[92]

One of the earliest American monographs on neurosurgery, *Linear Craniotomy*, was prepared by Keen.[93] He described the difficult differentiation between microcephalus and craniosynos-

tosis. He then performed, in 1890, one of the first operations for craniostenosis in America. He developed a technique for treatment of spastic torticollis by division of the spinal accessory nerve and the posterior roots of the first, second, and third spinal nerves.[94] He was also responsible for introducing the Gigli saw, first described in Europe in 1897, into American surgery in 1898.[95,96]

The first American monograph devoted to brain surgery was written not by a neurosurgeon but by the New York neurologist Allen Starr (1854–1932) (Figure 1.47).[97,98] Starr was Professor of Nervous Diseases at Columbia and an American leader in neurology. He trained in Europe, working in the laboratories of Erb, Schultze, Meynert, and Nothnagle, experiences that gave him a strong foundation in neurologic diagnosis. Working closely with Charles McBurney (1845–1913), a general surgeon, he came to the realization that brain surgery not only could be done safely but was necessary in the treatment of certain neurologic problems (Figure 1.48).[99] He summarized his views in the preface:

> Brain surgery is at present a subject both novel and interesting. It is within the past five years only that operations for the relief of epilepsy and of imbecility, for the removal of clots from the brain, for the opening of abscesses, for the excision of tumors, and the relief of intra-cranial pressure have been generally attempted … It is the object

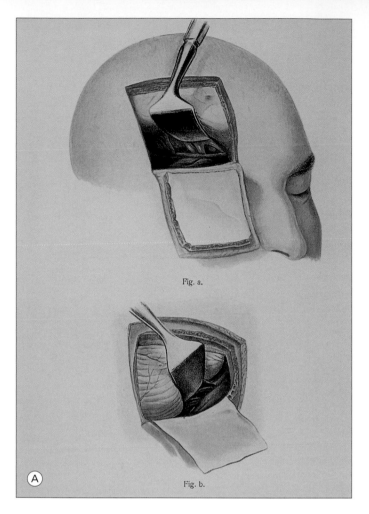

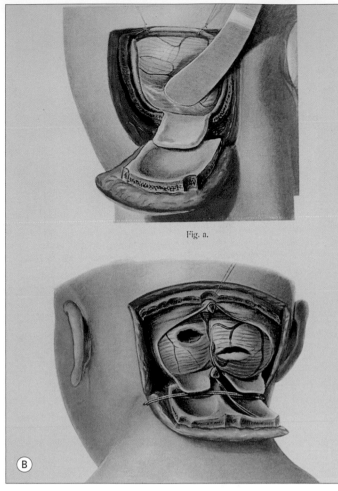

Figure 1.45 **(A)** Krause illustrating a frontal craniotomy. **(B)** Krause illustrating an osteoplastic posterior fossa craniotomy. **(C)** Krause "digitally" removing a brain tumor.[89]

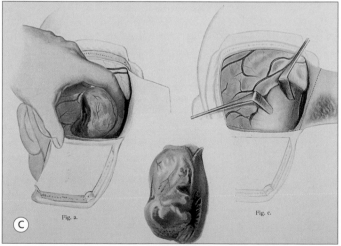

of this book to state clearly those facts regarding the essential features of brain disease which will enable the reader to determine in any case both the nature and situation of the pathological process in progress, to settle the question whether the disease can be removed by surgical interference, and to estimate the safety and probability of success by operation.[97]

Starr was highly regarded by surgeons. In 1923 Harvey Cushing, reviewing one of his own cases, commented about Allen Starr:

I am confident that if Allen Starr, in view of his position in neurology and his interest in surgical matters, had taken to the scalpel rather than the pen we would now be thirty years ahead in these matters, and I am sure his fingers must

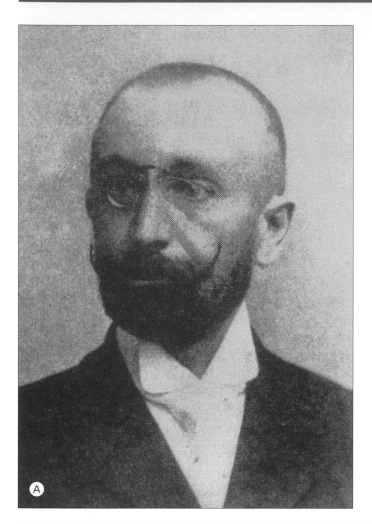

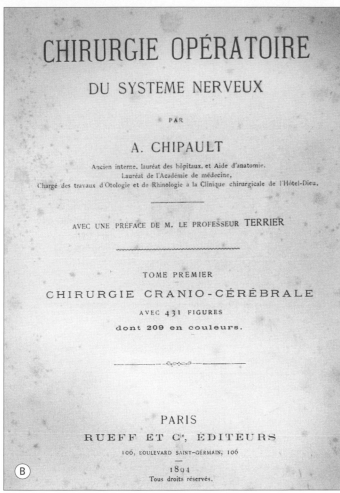

CHIRURGIE OPÉRATOIRE

DU SYSTEME NERVEUX

PAR

A. CHIPAULT

Ancien interne, lauréat des hôpitaux, et Aide d'anatomie.
Lauréat de l'Académie de médecine,
Chargé des travaux d'Otologie et de Rhinologie à la Clinique chirurgicale de l'Hôtel-Dieu.

AVEC UNE PRÉFACE DE M. LE PROFESSEUR TERRIER

TOME PREMIER
CHIRURGIE CRANIO-CÉRÉBRALE
AVEC 431 FIGURES
dont 209 en couleurs.

PARIS
RUEFF ET Cᵉ, ÉDITEURS
106, BOULEVARD SAINT-GERMAIN, 106

1894
Tous droits réservés.

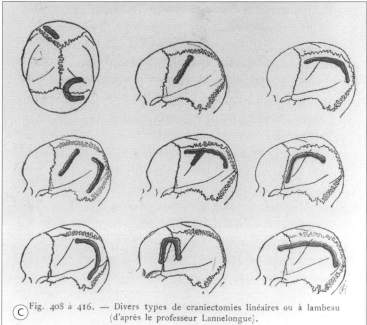

Fig. 408 à 416. — Divers types de craniectomies linéaires ou à lambeau
(d'après le professeur Lannelongue).

Figure 1.46 (A) Chipault. (B) Titlepage from Chipault monograph on surgery of the nervous system.[91] (C) Chipault schema for treating craniosynostosis.[91]

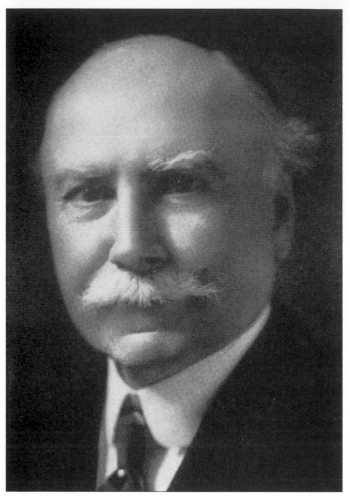

Figure 1.47 Allen Starr (1854–1932).

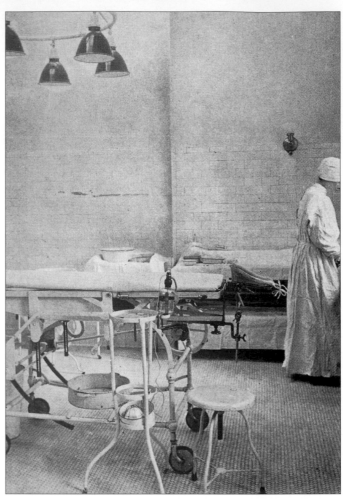

Figure 1.48 Operating room at the New York Neurological Institute, *circa* 1910.

many times have itched when he stood alongside an operating table and saw the operator he was coaching hopelessly fumble with the brain.[100]

Harvey William Cushing (1869–1939) is considered the founder of American neurosurgery (Figure 1.49). Educated at Johns Hopkins under one of the premier general surgeons, William Halsted (1852–1922), Cushing learned meticulous surgical technique from his mentor. As was standard then, Cushing spent time in Europe; he worked in the laboratories of Theodore Kocher in Bern, investigating the physiology of CSF. These studies led to his important monograph in 1926 on the third circulation.[101] It was during this period of experimentation that the cerebral phenomenon of increased intracranial pressure in association with hypertension and bradycardia was defined; it is now called the "Cushing phenomenon." While traveling through Europe he met several important surgical personalities, including Mcewen and Horsley. They provided the impetus for him to consider neurosurgery as a full-time endeavor.

Cushing's contributions to the literature of neurosurgery are too extensive to be listed in this brief chapter. Among his most significant work is a monograph on pituitary surgery published in 1912.[102] This monograph inaugurated a career in pituitary studies.

Cushing syndrome was defined in his final monograph on the pituitary, dated 1932.[103] In a classic monograph, written with Percival Bailey in 1926, Cushing brought a rational approach to the classification of brain tumors.[104] His monograph on meningioma, written with Louise Eisenhardt in 1938, still remains the standard for the profession.[105]

Cushing retired as Moseley Professor of Surgery at Harvard in 1932. By the time he completed his 2000th brain tumor operation,[106] he had unquestionably made some pre-eminent contributions to neurosurgery, based on meticulous, innovative surgical techniques and the effort to understand brain function from both physiologic and pathologic perspectives. An ardent bibliophile, Cushing spent his final years in retirement as Stirling Professor of Neurology at Yale, where he put together his extraordinary monograph on Andreas Vesalius.[107] Cushing's life has been faithfully recorded by his close friend and colleague John F. Fulton.[108]

Walter Dandy (1886–1946), who trained under Cushing at Johns Hopkins, made a number of important contributions to neurosurgery. Based on Luckett's serendipitous finding of air in the ventricles after a skull fracture,[109] Dandy developed the technique of pneumoencephalography (Figure 1.50).[110–112] This technique provided the neurosurgeon with the opportunity to localize the

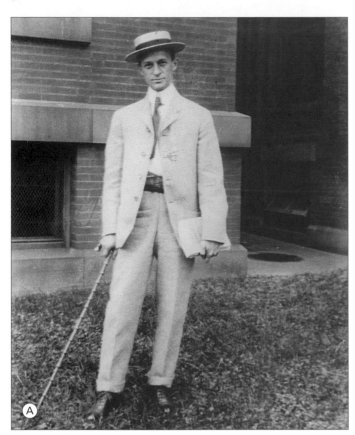

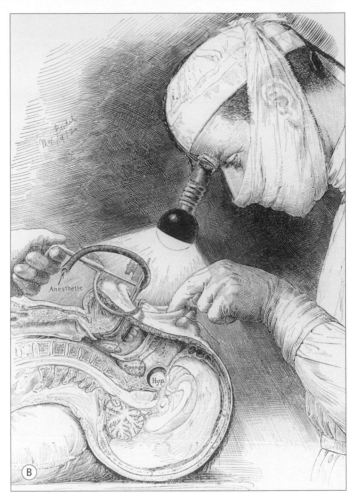

Figure 1.49 **(A)** Cushing as a dapper young man in training. **(B)** Harvey Cushing operating transsphenoidally – from his S. Weir Mitchell lecture.

tumor by analyzing the displacement of air in the ventricles.[112] A Philadelphia neurosurgeon, Charles Frazier, commented in 1935 on the importance of pneumoencephalography and the difference it made in the practice of neurosurgery.

> Only too often, after the most careful evaluation of the available neurologic evidence, no tumor would be revealed by exploration, the extreme intracranial tension would result in cerebral herniation to such an extent that sacrifice of the bone flap became necessary, and subsequently the skin sutures would give way before the persistent pressure, with cerebral fungus and meningitis as inevitable consequences. But injection of air has done away with all these horrors. The neurologist has been forced to recognize its important place in correct intracranial localization and frequently demands its use by the neurosurgeon.[113]

Dandy was an innovative neurosurgeon, far more aggressive in style and technique than Cushing. He was the first to show that acoustic neuromas could be totally removed.[114,115] He devoted a great deal of effort to the treatment of hydrocephalus.[116,117] He introduced the technique of removing the choroid plexus to reduce the production of CSF.[118] He was among the first to attack cerebral aneurysms by obliterating them using snare ligatures or

metal clips.[119] His monograph on the third ventricle and its anatomy remains a standard to this day, with illustrations that are among the best ever produced.[120]

In the field of spinal surgery, two important American figures appeared in the first quarter of the 20th century: Charles Elsberg (1871–1948), Professor of Neurosurgery at the New York Neurological Institute, and Charles Frazier (1870–1936), Professor of Surgery at the University of Pennsylvania. Work in the 19th century by J. L. Corning had shown that lumbar puncture can be performed safely.[121] H. Quincke popularized this procedure, and from there spinal surgery developed.[122,123]

Charles Frazier's book on spinal surgery, published in 1918, was the most comprehensive work on the subject available;[124] he summarized much of the existing literature and established that spinal surgery could be performed safely. His experience in World War I led him to devote his career to neurosurgery.

Charles Elsberg was another pioneer in spinal surgery. His techniques were impeccable and led to excellent results. By 1912 he had reported on a series of 43 laminectomies and by 1916 he had published the first of what were to be three monographs on surgery of the spine.[125,126] He introduced the technique of myelotomy, allowing a intramedullary tumor to deliver itself, so the tumor could be removed later, at a second-stage procedure

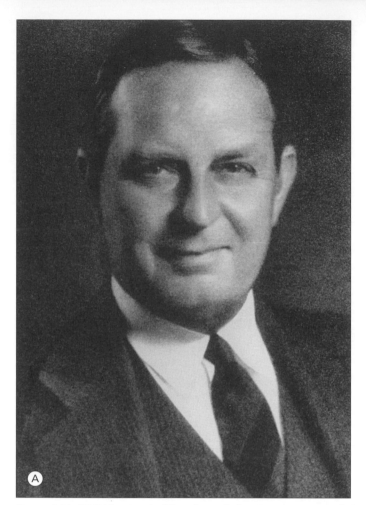

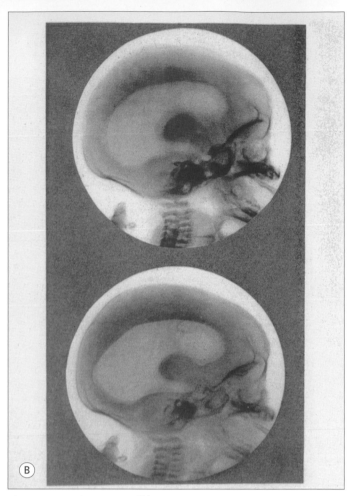

Figure 1.50 (A) Walter Dandy. **(B)** Radiograph showing pneumoencephalography. From Dandy WE, 1918.[114]

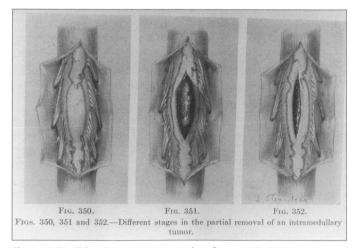

Figs. 350, 351 and 352.—Different stages in the partial removal of an intramedullary tumor.

Figure 1.51 Elsberg's two-stage procedure for removing an intramedullary tumor. A myelotomy is made at the first operation over the tumor. The pressure of the tumor causes its extrusion; then in a later operation the surgeon can remove the extruded tumor safely. (From Elsberg CA. *Tumors of the Spinal Cord*. New York: Hoeber; 1925: 381.)[134]

(Figure 1.51). He worked with a fierce intensity and was always looking for new techniques. Working with Cornelius Dyke, a neuro-radiologist at the New York Neurological Institute, he treated spinal glioblastomas with directed radiation in the operating room after the tumor had been exposed! These procedures were performed with the patients receiving only local anesthesia. During the half-hour therapy, while the radiation was being delivered, the surgeon and assistants stood off in the distance behind a glass shield.[127]

Leo Davidoff (1898–1975) was one of the prodigies of 20th century neurosurgery (Figure 1.52). Starting from humble origins in Lithuania, the son of a cobbler, he emigrated to the United States with his eight siblings. As a teen Davidoff worked in a factory to support his family; the factory's manager admired his skill and dedication and sponsored his education – leading to his graduation from Harvard University in 1916. He completed his medical degree at Harvard in 1922 as an AOA (the national honor society for graduating medical students) member. Davidoff trained under Harvey Cushing and became one of his most popular students, not always an easy achievement with Cushing's personality. When Cushing was once asked who he would allow to

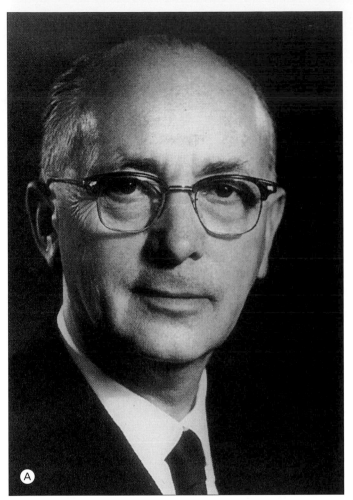

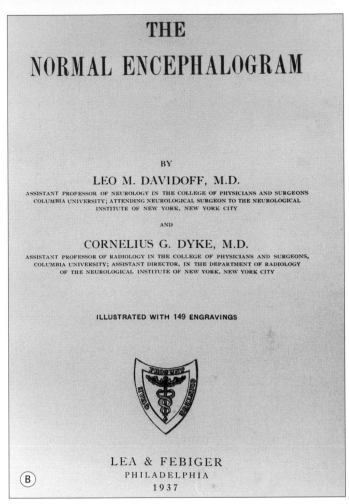

THE
NORMAL ENCEPHALOGRAM

BY

LEO M. DAVIDOFF, M.D.

ASSISTANT PROFESSOR OF NEUROLOGY IN THE COLLEGE OF PHYSICIANS AND SURGEONS
COLUMBIA UNIVERSITY; ATTENDING NEUROLOGICAL SURGEON TO THE NEUROLOGICAL
INSTITUTE OF NEW YORK, NEW YORK CITY

AND

CORNELIUS G. DYKE, M.D.

ASSISTANT PROFESSOR OF RADIOLOGY IN THE COLLEGE OF PHYSICIANS AND SURGEONS,
COLUMBIA UNIVERSITY; ASSISTANT DIRECTOR, IN THE DEPARTMENT OF RADIOLOGY
OF THE NEUROLOGICAL INSTITUTE OF NEW YORK, NEW YORK CITY

ILLUSTRATED WITH 149 ENGRAVINGS

LEA & FEBIGER
PHILADELPHIA
1937

Figure 1.52 (A) Leo Davidoff. **(B)** Title page from Davidoff's monograph on the normal encephalogram.[128] **(C)** Titlepage from Davidoff's monograph on the abnormal pneumoencephalogram.[129]
Continued

operate on him for a brain tumor his reponse was "Well I guess I would have Davey [Davidoff] do it." Davidoff initially joined the staff of the New York Neurological Institute with Charles Elsberg in 1929. Here he began his seminal studies on the normal anatomy seen in pneumoencephalograms utilizing the hundreds of pneumoencephalograms performed at the Neurological Institute. In 1937 he issued a classic monograph with Cornelius Dyke (1900–1943), *The Normal Encephalogram*.[128] This work, and a later publication with Bernard Epstein (1908–1978) *The Abnormal Encephalogram* (1950),[129] became two of the most important neuroradiological texts, remaining influential for over 30 years. Davidoff's meticulous and detailed studies led him to be called the father of neuroradiology. He left the Neurological Institute in 1937 when Bryon Stookey became chief, moving on to Brooklyn to the Jewish Hospital. Davidoff became chief of neurosurgery at Montefiore Hospital in 1945, working with Houston Merritt in neurology and Harry Zimmerman in neuropathology. He later became instrumental in the founding of the Albert Einstein College of Medicine, becoming the first chairman of neurosurgery in 1955. Davidoff was charter member of the Harvey Cushing Society and served as president of the American Association of Neurological Surgeons from 1956 to 1957. Davidoff was

described by his staff as a hard taskmaster, punctual, demanding, and critical. His operating room was meticulous and organized, with no unnecessary sound or speech allowed. Never one to raise his voice, a mere look, even behind a surgical mask could be a chilling experience for the new house officer or scrub nurse. His legacy remains in over 200 scientific publications, his pioneering work in neuroradiology and his total commitment to the highest standards in patient care and resident training.

Besides the pioneering techniques of Dandy, Cushing, and others, a number of diagnostic techniques were introduced whereby the neurosurgeon could localize lesions less haphazardly, thereby shifting the emphasis from the neurologist to the neurosurgeon. One such technique, myelography using opaque substances, was brought forward by Jean Athanase Sicard (1872–1929).[130] Using a radio-opaque iodized oil, the spinal cord and its elements could be outlined on X-ray. Antonio Caetano de Egas Moniz (1874–1955), Professor of Neurology at Lisbon, perfected arterial catheterization techniques and the cerebral angiogram in animal studies. To do this required that a number of iodine compounds be studied, many of which caused convulsions and paralysis in laboratory animals. However, his ideas were sound and by 1927 angiography, used in combination with pneumoencephalography, offered the

THE ABNORMAL PNEUMOENCEPHALOGRAM

BY

LEO M. DAVIDOFF, M.D.

Director of Neurological Surgery, Beth Israel Hospital, New York City; Clinical Professor of Neurosurgery, New York University—Postgraduate Medical School

AND

BERNARD S. EPSTEIN, M.D.

Associate Radiologist, The Jewish Hospital of Brooklyn, Brooklyn, N.Y. and Instructor in Clinical Radiology, Long Island College of Medicine

695 ILLUSTRATIONS ON 289 FIGURES

LEA & FEBIGER
PHILADELPHIA
1950

(C)

Figure 1.52, cont'd.

neurosurgeon the first detailed view of the intracranial contents.[131,132]

In 1929, Alexander Fleming (1881–1955) published a report on the first observation of a substance that appeared to block the growth of a bacterium. This substance, identified as penicillin, heralded a new era of medicine and surgery.[133] With World War II, antibiotics were perfected in the treatment of bacterial infection, reducing even further the risk of infection during craniotomy.

CONCLUSION

The first half of the 20th century brought the formalization of the field of neurosurgery. In the 1920s, Elsberg, Cushing, and Frazier persuaded the American College of Surgeons to designate neurosurgery as a separate specialty. It has taken some 5000 years of constant study and the experience of generations to make neurosurgery what it is today.

In the new millennium the neurosurgery patient can have a painless operation with minimal risk of infection, and surgery will rarely be in the wrong location. Thanks to magnetic resonance imaging and computed tomography, the localization of neurologic problems is hardly an issue. This is a far cry from our Asclepiad fathers, who could only whisper secret incantations and provide herbal medicaments that rarely worked.

REFERENCES

1. Breasted JH. *The Edwin Smith Papyrus. Published in Facsimile and Hieroglyphic Transliteration with Translation and Commentary.* Chicago, IL: University of Chicago Press; 1930
2. Ebers Papyrus. *The Papyrus Ebers. The Greatest Egyptian Medical Document.* Translated by B. Ebbell. Copenhagen: Levin & Munksgard; 1937.
3. Hippocrates [Foesio A, translator/ed.] *Magni Hippocratis Medicorum Omnium Facile Principis, Opera Omnia Quae Extant.* Geneva: Samuel Chouet; 1657–62.
4. Hippocrates [Leonicenus N, Laurentianus L, translators] *Aphorismi, cum Galeni Commentariis; Praedictiones, cum Galeni Commentariis.* Paris: Simon Sylvius; 1527.
5. Clarke E. Apoplexy in the Hippocratic writings. *Bull Hist Med* 1963; 37: 301.
6. Marx KFH. *Herophilus: ein Beitrag zur Geschichte der Medicin.* Verlag der D. R. Marrschen und Runsthandlung: Karlsruhe und Baden; 1838.
7. Ryff W. *Des Aller Furtefflichsten … Erschaffen. Das is des Menchen … Warhafftige Beschreibund oder Anatomi.* Strasbourg: Balthassar Beck; 1541.
8. Celsus. *Medicinae Libri VIII.* Venice: Aedes Aldi et Andreae Asulani Soceri; 1528.
9. *Medicae Artis Principes post Hippocratem et Galenum.* Geneva: Henri Estienne; 1567.
10. Galen. *Omnia Quae Extant Opera in Latinum Sermonem Conversa,* 5th edn. Venice: Juntas; 1576–7.
11. Galen. Experimental section and hemisection of the spinal cord (taken from De locis affectibus). *Ann Med Hist* 1917; 1: 367.
12. Paulus Aeginetes. *Opus de Re Medica Nunc Primum Integrum.* Köln: Joannes Soter; 1534.
13. Paulus Aeginetes [Adams F, translator] *The Seven Books of Paulus Aegineta.* London: Sydenham Society; 1844–7.
14. Rhazes. *Opera Parva.* Lyons: Gilbertus de Villiers, Johannis de Ferris; 1511.
15. Avicenna. *Liber Canonis, de Medicinis Cordialibus, et Cantica.* Basel: Joannes Heruagios; 1556.
16. Albucasis. *Liber Theoricae Necnon Practicae Alsaharavii.* Augsburg: Sigismundus Grimm & Marcus Vuirsung; 1519.
17. Albucasis [Spink MS, Lewis GL [translators/eds] *Albucasis on Surgery and Instruments.* Berkeley, CA: University of California Press; 1973.
18. Al-Rodhan NRF, Fox JL. Al-Zahrawi and Arabian neurosurgery, 936–1013 AD. *Surg Neurol* 1986; 25: 92–5.
19. Sabuncuoglu, S. *Cerrahiyyetü'l-Haniyye Imperial Surgery* [translated from Arabic]. Ottoman Empire circa 15th century. From a later copied manuscript in the author's collection, circa 1725. See also *Cerrahiyyetü'l-Haniyye*. Paris: France Bibliothéque Nationale; 1465, Suppl Turc No 693.
20 Elmaci I. Color illustrations and neurosurgical treatments of Serefeddin Sabuncuoglu in the 15th century. *Neurosurgery* 2000; 47: 947–54.
21. Constantinus Africanus. *Constantini Africani Post Hippocratem et Galenum.* Basel: Henricus Petrus; 1536.
22. Roger of Salerno. Practica chirurgiae. In: *Guy de Chauliac Cyrurgia … et Cyrurgia Bruni, Teodorici, Rolandi, Lanfranci, Rogerii, Bertapalie.* Venice: Bernardinus Venetus de Vitalibus; 1519.
23. Corner G [translator] The Bamberg Surgery. *Bull Inst Hist Med* 1937; 5: 1–32.
24. Theodoric Bishop of Cervia [Campbell E, Colton J, translators] *The*

Surgery of Theodoric, ca. AD 1267. New York, NY: Appleton-Century-Crofts; 1955–66.

25. William of Saliceto. *Chirurgia*. Venice: F di Pietro; 1474.

26. Leonard of Bertapalia. Chirurgia. In: *Guy de Chauliac Cyrurgia … et Cyrurgia Bruni, Teodorici, Rolandi, Lanfranci, Rogerii, Bertapalie*. Venice: Bernardinus Venetus de Vitalibus; 1519.

27. Leonard of Bertapalia [Ladenheim JC, translator] *On Nerve Injuries and Skull Fractures*. Mount Kisco, NY: Futura Publishing; 1989.

28. Lanfranchi of Milan. Chirurgia. In: *Guy de Chauliac Cyrurgia … et Cyrurgia Bruni, Teodorici, Rolandi, Lanfranci, Rogerii, Bertapalie*. Venice: Bernardinus Venetus de Vitalibus; 1519.

29. Guy de Chauliac. Chirurgia magna. In: *Guy de Chauliac Cyrurgia … et Cyrurgia Bruni, Teodorici, Rolandi, Lanfranci, Rogerii, Bertapalie*. Venice: Bernardinus Venetus de Vitalibus; 1519.

30. Guy de Chauliac. *Guy de Chauliac (AD 1363) on Wounds and Fractures*. Translated by W. A. Brennan. Chicago, IL: published by translator; 1923.

31. Leonardo da Vinci. *Quaderni d'Anatomia*. Christiania: Jacob Dybwad; 1911–1916.

32. Hopstock H. Leonardo as an anatomist. In: Singer C (ed.). *Studies in the History of Medicine*. Oxford: Clarendon Press; 1921.

33. Leonardo da Vinci [Keele KD, Pedretti C, eds] *Corpus of the Anatomical Studies in the Collection of Her Majesty the Queen at Windsor Castle*. New York, NY: Harcourt Brace Jovanovich; 1979.

34. Goodrich JT. Sixteenth century Renaissance art and anatomy: Andreas Vesalius and his great book – a new view. *Medical Heritage* 1985; 1: 280–8.

35. Paré A [Guillemeau J, translator] *Opera*. Paris: Jacobus Du Puys; 1582.

36. Paré A [Johnson T, translator] *The Workes of That Famous Chirurgion Ambroise Parey*. London: Richard Coates; 1649.

37. Berengario da Carpi J. *Tractatus de Fractura Calvae Sive Cranei*. Bologna: Hieronymus de Benedictus; 1518.

38. Dryander J. *Anatomiae*. Marburg: Eucharius Ceruicornus; 1537.

39. Hanigan WC, Ragen W, Foster R. Dryander of Marburg and the first textbook of neuroanatomy. *Neurosurgery* 1990; 26: 489–98.

40. Coiter V. *Externarum et Internarum Principalium Humani Corporis Partium Tabulae Atque Anatomicae Exercitationes Observationesque Variae*. Nürnberg: Theodoricus Gerlatzenus; 1573.

41. Croce GA della. *Chirurgiae Libri Septem*. Venice: Jordanus Zilettus; 1573.

42. Vesalius A. *De Humani Corporis Fabrica Libri Septem*. Basel: Joannes Oporinus; 1543.

43. Vesalius A [Singer C, translator/ed.] *Vesalius on the Human Brain*. London: Oxford University Press; 1952.

44. Vesalius A. *De Humani Corporis Fabrica*. Basel: Oporinus, 1555

45. Estienne C. *De Dissectione Partium Corporis Humani Libri Tres*. Paris: Simon Colinaeus; 1546.

46. Willis T. *Cerebri Anatome: Cui Accessit Nervorum Descriptio et Usus*. London: J. Flesher; 1664.

47. Vesling J. *Syntagma Anatomicum*, 2nd edn. Padua: Paulus Frambottus; 1651.

48. Spiegal A van de, Casserius G. *De Humani Corporis Fabrica Libri Decem, Tabulis XCIIX Aeri Incisis Elegantissimis*. Venice: Evangelista Deuchinus; 1627.

49. Fallopius G. *Observationes Anatomicae*. Venice: Marcus Antonius Ulmus; 1561.

50. Ridley H. *The Anatomy of the Brain, Containing Its Mechanisms and Physiology: Together With Some New Discoveries and Corrections of Ancient and Modern Authors Upon That Subject*. London: Samuel Smith; 1695.

51. Fabry W. *Observationum et Curationum Chirurgicarum Centuriae*. Lyons: J. A. Huguetan; 1641.

52. Scultetus J. *Armamentarium Chirurgicum XLIII*. Ulm: Balthasar Kühnen; 1655.

53. Yonge J. *Wounds of the Brain Proved Curable, Not Only by the Opinion and Experience of Many (the Best) Authors, but the Remarkable History of a Child Four Years Old Cured of Two Very Large Depressions, With the Loss of a Great Part of the Skull, a Portion of the Brain Also Issuing Thorough a Penetrating Wound of the Dura and Pia Mater*. London: Henry Faithorn and John Kersey; 1682.

54. Pott P. *Remarks on That Kind of Palsy of the Lower Limbs, Which is Frequently Found to Accompany a Curvature of the Spine*. London: J. Johnson; 1779.

55. Pott P. *Observations on the Nature and Consequences of Wounds and Contusions of the Head, Fractures of the Skull, Concussions of the Brain*. London: C. Hitch and L. Hawes; 1760.

56. Hunter J. *A Treatise on the Blood, Inflammation, and Gun-Shot Wounds*. London: J. Richardson; 1794.

57. Bell B. *A System of Surgery*. Edinburgh: C. Elliot; 1783–1788.

58. Heister L. *A General System of Surgery in Three Parts*. London: W. Innys; 1743.

59. Morand F-S. *Opuscules de Chirurgie*. Paris: Guillaume Desprez; 1768–72.

60. Cotugno D. *De Ischiade Nervosa Commentarius*. Napoli: Fratres Simonii; 1764.

61. Turner D. *A Remarkable Case in Surgery: Wherein an Account is Given of an Uncommon Fracture and Depression of the Skull, in a Child About Six Years Old; Accompanied With a Large Abscess or Aposteme Upon the Brain. With Other Practical Observations and Useful Reflections Thereupon. Also an Exact Draught of the Case, Annex'd. And for the Entertainment of the Senior, but Instruction of the Junior Practitioners, Communicated*. London: R. Parker; 1709.

62. Saucerotte N. *Mélanges de Chirurgie*. Paris: Gay; 1801.

63. Abernethy J. *Surgical Observations*. London: Longman, Rees, Orme, Brown, and Greene; 1809–10.

64. Bell C. *Illustrations of the Great Operations of Surgery*. London: Longman, Rees, Orme, Brown, and Greene; 1821.

65. Bright R. *Report of Medical Cases*. London: Longman, Rees, Orme, Brown, and Greene; 1827.

66. Cruveilhier J. *Anatomie Pathologique du Corps Humain*. Paris: J.-B. Baillière; 1829–42.

67. Flamm ES. The neurology of Jean Cruveilhier. *Med Hist* 1973; 17: 343–53.

68. Bakay L. Historical vignette: Cruveilhier on meningiomas (1829–1842). *Surg Neurol* 1989; 32: 159–64.

69. Fritsch GT, Hitzig E. Über die elektrische Erregbarkeit des Grosshirns. *Arch Anat Physiol Wiss Med* 1870: 300–332.

70. Broca P. Remarques sur le siège de la faculté du language articulé suivie d'une observation d'aphémie (perte de la parole). *Bull Soc Anat Paris* 1861; 36: 330–57.

71. Broca P. Perte de la parole: ramollissement chronique et destruction partielle du lobe antérieur gauche du cerveau. *Bull Soc Anthropol Paris* 1861; 2: 235–8.

72. Wernicke C. *Der aphasische Symptomenkomplex*. Breslau: M. Cohn & Weigert; 1874.

73. Ferrier D. *The Functions of the Brain*. London: Smith, Elder and Co.; 1876.

74. Taylor J (ed.). *Selected Writings of John Hughlings Jackson*. New York, NY: Basic Books; 1958.

75. Bartholow R. Tumours of the brain: clinical history and comments. *Am J Med Sci* 1868; 110(ns): 339–59.

76. Bartholow R. Experimental investigations into the functions of the human brain. *Am J Med Sci* 1874; 67: 305–13.

77. Bennett AH, Godlee RJ. Excision of a tumour from the brain. *Lancet* 1884; 2: 1090–1.

78. Gowers WR. *The Diagnosis of Diseases of the Spinal Cord*. London: J. and A. Churchill; 1880.

79. Gowers WR. *Epilepsy and Other Chronic Convulsive Diseases*. London: J. and A. Churchill; 1881.

80. Gowers WR. *Lectures on the Diagnosis of Diseases of the Brain*. London: J. and A. Churchill; 1886–8.

81. Horsley VAH, Sharpey-Schäfer EA. A record of experiments upon the functions of the cerebral cortex. *Philos Trans R Soc Lond Biol* 1889; 179: 1–45.

82. Gotch F, Horsley VAH. On the mammalian nervous system, its functions, and their localisation determined by an electrical method. *Philos Trans R Soc Lond Biol* 1891; 182: 267–526.

83. Gowers WR, Horsley VAH. A case of tumour of the spinal cord: removal; recovery. *Med Chir Trans* 1888; 71: 377–430.

84. Horsley VAH, Clarke RH. The structure and functions of the cerebellum examined by a new method. *Brain* 1908; 31: 45–124.

85. Ballance CA. *Some Points in the Surgery of the Brain and its Membranes*. London: Macmillan; 1907.

86. Stone JL. Sir Charles Ballance Pioneer British Neurological Surgeon. *Neurosurgery* 1999; 44: 631–2.

87. Macewen W. *Pyogenic Infective Diseases of the Brain and Spinal Cord*. Glasgow: J. Maclehose & Sons; 1893.

88. Pancoast J. *A Treatise on Operative Surgery; Comprising a Description of the Various Processes of the Art, Including all the New Operations; Exhibiting the State of Surgical Science in its Present Advanced Condition*. Philadelphia, PA: Carey and Hart; 1844.

89. Krause F, Haubold H, Thorek M, [translators] *Surgery of the Brain and Spinal Cord Based on Personal Experiences*. New York, NY: Rebman Co.; 1909–12.

90. Chipault A. *Etudes de Chirurgie Médullaire*. Paris: Felix Alcan; 1894

91. Chipault A. *Chirurgie Opératoire du Systéme Nerveux*. Paris: Rueff et Cie; 1894–5.

92. Stone JL. W.W. Keen: America's pioneer neurological surgeon. *Neurosurgery* 1985; 17: 997–1110.

93. Keen WW. *Linear Craniotomy*. Philadelphia, PA: Lea Bros and Co.; 1891.

94. Keen WW. A new operation for spasmodic wry neck, namely, division or exsection of the nerves supplying the posterior rotator muscles of the head. *Ann Surg* 1891; 13: 44–7.

95. Keen WW. On the use of the Gigli wire saw to obtain access to the brain. *Philadelph Med J* 1898; 1: 32–3.

96. Bingham WF. W.W. Keen and the dawn of American neurosurgery. *J Neurosurg* 1986; 64: 705–17.

97. Starr MA. *Brain Surgery*. New York: William Wood & Co.; 1893.

98. Starr MA. Discussion on the present status of the surgery of the brain, 2: a contribution to brain surgery, with special reference to brain tumors. *Trans Med Soc NY* 1896; 119–34.

99. McBurney C, Starr MA. A contribution to cerebral surgery: diagnosis, localization and operation for removal of three tumors of the brain, with some comments upon the surgical treatments of brain tumors. *Am J Med Sci* 1893; 105(ns): 361–87.

100. Cushing H. Neurological surgeons, with the report of one case. *Arch Neurol Psychiatr* 1923; 10: 381–90.

101. Cushing H. *The Third Circulation: Studies in Intracranial Physiology and Surgery*. London: Oxford University Press; 1926.

102. Cushing H. *The Pituitary Body and Its Disorders: Clinical States Produced by Disorders of the Hypophysis Cerebri*. Philadelphia, PA: JB Lippincott Co.; 1912.

103. Cushing H. *Papers Relating to the Pituitary Body, Hypothalamus, and Parasympathetic Nervous System*. Springfield, IL: Charles C. Thomas Publisher; 1932.

104. Bailey P, Cushing H. *A Classification of the Tumors of the Glioma Group on a Histogenetic Basis With a Correlated Study of Prognosis*. Philadelphia, PA: JB Lippincott Co.; 1926.

105. Cushing H, Eisenhardt L. *Meningiomas: Their Classification, Regional Behavior, Life History and Surgical End Results*. Springfield, IL: Charles C. Thomas Publisher; 1938.

106. Cushing H. *Intracranial Tumors: Notes Upon a Series of Two Thousand Verified Cases With Surgical Mortality Percentages Pertaining Thereto*. Springfield, IL: Charles C. Thomas Publisher; 1932.

107. Cushing H. *A Bio-Bibliography of Andreas Vesalius*. New York, NY: Schuman; 1943.

108. Fulton JF. *Harvey Cushing: A Biography*. Springfield, IL: Charles C. Thomas Publisher; 1946.

109. Luckett WH. Air in the ventricles following a fracture of the skull. *Surg Gynaecol Obstet* 1913; 17: 237–40.

110. Dandy WE. Ventriculography following the injection of air into the cerebral ventricles. *Ann Surg* 1918; 68: 5–11.

111. Dandy WE. Röntgenography of the brain after the injection of air into the spinal canal. *Ann Surg* 1919; 70: 397–403.

112. Dandy WE. Localization or elimination of cerebral tumors by ventriculography. *Surg Gynecol Obstet* 1920; 30: 329–42.

113. Frazier CH. Fifty years of neurosurgery. *Arch Neurol Psychiatr* 1935; 34: 907–22.

114. Dandy WE. An operation for the total extirpation of tumors in the cerebellopontine angle: a preliminary report. *Bull Johns Hopkins Hosp* 1922; 33: 344–5.

115. Dandy WE. An operation for the total removal of cerebello-pontine (acoustic) tumors. *Surg Gynecol Obstet* 1925; 41: 129–48.

116. Dandy WE, Blackfan DD. An experimental and clinical study of internal hydrocephalus. *JAMA* 1913; 61: 2216–17.

117. Dandy WE, Blackfan DD. Internal hydrocephalus: an experimental, clinical and pathologic study. *Am J Dis Child* 1914; 8: 406–82.

118. Dandy WE. An operative procedure for hydrocephalus. *Bull Johns Hopkins Hosp* 1922; 33: 189–90.

119. Dandy WE. Intracranial aneurysm of the internal carotid artery cured by operation. *Ann Surg* 1938; 107: 654–9.

120. Dandy WE. *Benign Tumors of the Third Ventricles*. Springfield, IL: Charles C. Thomas Publisher; 1933.

121. Corning JL. Spinal anesthesia and local medication of the cord. *NY Med J* 1885; 42: 483–5.

122. Quincke HI. Die Lumbalpunction des Hydrocephalus. *Berl Klin Wochenschr* 1891; 28: 929–33, 965–8.

123. Quincke HI. Die diagnostische und therapeutische Bedeutung der Lumbalpunction: klinischer Vortrag. *Dtsch Med Wochenschr* 1905; 31: 1825–8, 1869–72.

124. Frazier C. *Surgery of the Spine and Spinal Cord*. New York, NY: Appleton; 1918.

125. Elsberg CA. Surgery of intramedullary affections of the spinal cord: anatomic basis and technic with report of cases. *JAMA* 1912; 59: 1532–6.

126. Elsberg CA. *Diagnosis and Treatment of Surgical Diseases of the Spinal Cord and Its Membranes*. Philadelphia, PA: WB Saunders Co.; 1916.

127. Pool L. *The Neurological Institute of New York, 1909–1974, With Personal Anecdotes*. Lakeville, CT: Pocket Knife Press; 1975: 59.

128. Davidoff L, Dyke C. *The Normal Pneumoencephalogram*. Philadelphia, PA: Lea & Febiger; 1937.

129. Davidoff L, Epstein B. *The Abnormal Pneumocephalogram*. Philadelphia, PA: Lea & Febiger, 1950.

130. Sicard JA, Forestier J. Méthode radiographique d'exploration de la cavité épidurale par le lipiodol. *Rev Neurol* 1921; 37: 1264–6.

131. Moniz CE. L'encéphalographie artérielle: son importance dans la localisation des tumeurs cérébrales. *Rev Neurol* 1927; 2: 72–90.

132. Moniz CE. *Diagnostic des Tumeurs Cérébrales et Épreuve de l'Encéphalographie Artérielle*. Paris: Masson & Cie; 1931.

133. Fleming A. On the antibacterial action of cultures of a Penicillium, with special reference to their use in the isolation of *B. influenzae*. *Br J Exp Pathol* 1929; 10: 226–36.

134. Elsberg CA. *Tumors of the Spinal Cord*. New York: Hoeber; 1925: 381.

ADDITIONAL READING

Bakay L. *An Early History of Craniotomy From Antiquity to the Napoleonic Era*. Springfeld, IL: Charles C. Thomas Publisher; 1985.

Ballance CA. *A Glimpse Into the History of the Surgery of the Brain*. London: Macmillan and Co; 1922.

Bucy PC, [ed.] *Neurosurgical Giants: Feet of Clay and Iron*. New York, NY: Elsevier; 1985.

Clarke E, Dewhurst K. *An Illustrated History of Brain Function*. Oxford: Sandforn; 1972.

Clarke E, O'Malley CD. *The Human Brain and Spinal Cord: A Historical Study Illustrated by Writings from Antiquity to the Twentieth Century*. Berkeley, CA: University of California Press; 1968.

Gurdjian ES. *Head Injury from Antiquity to the Present, With Special Reference to Penetrating Head Wounds*. Springfield, IL: Charles C. Thomas Publisher; 1973

Haymaker W, Schiller F. *The Founders of Neurology*, 2nd edn. Springfield, IL: Charles C. Thomas Publisher; 1970.

Horrax G. *Neurosurgery: An Historical Sketch*. Springfield, IL: Charles C. Thomas Publisher; 1952.

Leonardo RA. *History of Surgery*. New York, NY: Froben Press; 1943.

McHenry LC. *Garrison's History of Neurology, Revised and Enlarged, With a Bibliography of Classical, Original and Standard Works in Neurology*. Springfield, IL: Charles C. Thomas Publisher; 1969.

Meyer A. *Historical Aspects of Cerebral Anatomy*. London: Oxford University Press; 1971.

Poynter FNL, [ed.] *The History and Philosophy of Knowledge of the Brain and Its Functions*. Springfield, IL: Charles C. Thomas Publisher; 1958.

Rose FC, Bynum WF. *Historical Aspects of the Neurosciences: A Festschrift for Macdonald Critchley*. New York, NY: Raven Press; 1982.

Spillane JD. *The Doctrine of the Nerves: Chapters in the History of Neurology*. Oxford: Oxford University Press; 1981.

Sachs E. *The History and Development of Neurological Surgery*. New York, NY: Hoeber; 1952.

Soury J. *Le Système Nerveux Central: Structure et Fonctions, Histoire, Critiques des Théories et des Doctrines*. Paris: Georges Carré; 1899.

Walker AE. *A History of Neurological Surgery*. Baltimore, MD: Williams & Wilkins; 1951.

Wilkins RH, Brody IA. *Neurological Classics*. New York, NY: Johnson Reprint Co.; 1973.

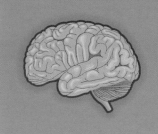

CLINICAL EVALUATION OF THE NERVOUS SYSTEM

2

Gerald A Grant and Richard G Ellenbogen

There are only two sorts of doctors; those who practice with their brains and those who practice with their tongues.

– Sir William Osler

INTRODUCTION

The analytical approach required to bring a patient with a neurological problem from diagnosis to surgery is much akin to the work a detective must perform to solve a mystery. While the evolution of magnetic resonance imaging (MRI) may cause the student to view history-taking skills or that of the neurological examination as superfluous, this is simply not an accurate reflection of the neurosurgeon's intellectual responsibility. Thus, neurosurgeons around the world are still trained to hone their analytical and interpersonal skills, so that they may elicit a history and an examination to provide a context for the radiological examination. The history and neurological examination is still the centerpiece in the evaluation of a patient with a surgically correctable neurological disease. The neurosurgeon's job requires basic investigative work, a thorough knowledge of neuroanatomy, appropriate utilization of the currently available diagnostic tools, and lastly, substantial interpersonal skills. Correctly identifying the neurological problem is one of the most satisfying parts of a neurosurgeon's job, for it is a mandatory skill that must precede a successful surgical outcome for the patient. It is what everything we do is built upon.

NEUROLOGICAL HISTORY

It is a common medical school teaching that acquiring an accurate medical history can help the clinician secure the correct diagnosis in approximately 90% of all patients. Historical information obtained by a skilled clinician, more often than not, will uncover a patient's entire anatomical and etiologic illness. The history is followed by the neurological examination, which should simply confirm dysfunction of the organ system one has already decided is abnormal, prior to reliance on sophisticated neuroimaging. It is paramount that the astute clinician masters the skill of anatomical localization in the nervous system. This complex but beautiful system is composed of ten subsystems (from a practical standpoint): cortex, pyramidal tracts, basal ganglia, brainstem, cranial nerves, cerebellum, spinal cord, nerve roots, peripheral nerves, and muscle. Understanding each subsystem of the nervous system is equivalent to mastering the anatomy of one entire internal organ. Many of the subsystems stretch over long distances both

vertically (i.e. pyramidal tracts, posterior columns) or horizontally (i.e. cortex, cranial nerves, brainstem), which can complicate accurate anatomic localization. To evaluate the functional state of the nervous system, the neurosurgeon requires a basic knowledge of the pertinent anatomy as well as an understanding of the role of ancillary imaging and laboratory tests. Apart from the optic nerve head, which can be evaluated by a funduscopic examination, the rest of the nervous system is hidden from direct observation, and therefore, at the clinical level, disease must be usually inferred from a disorder of normal function.

FOCAL CORTICAL SIGNS

We will begin this tour at the top with the cerebral cortex and then continue down the line. In general, conversation with the patient during the course of the examination will elicit the cortical deficits that are obvious. The ability to talk and respond to questions in a sensible and coherent fashion reveals a great deal about the cerebral cortices. Asking a patient to perform a simple task such as reading a newspaper to the examiner, requires activation of an incredibly complex set of neural circuits. In so doing, the examiner is able to test the visual system, cranial nerves and the motor and sensory systems as well as higher cortical function. This seemingly straightforward, everyday task helps the examiner quickly close down on a wide spectrum of neurological functions that may be affected by the patient's disease. More subtle cortical deficits require meticulous testing, often by neuropsychological examinations, the interpretation of which requires specific training. Neuropsychological examinations are performed more commonly in the pre- and postoperative stages of modern neurosurgical intervention. It is simply not sufficient to know if the patient did "OK" after complex intracranial surgery. It is important to understand what subtle deficits existed preoperatively, and how well the deficits improved postoperatively, or which new deficits will require active rehabilitative intervention to improve after surgery.

In broad strokes, the examiner must understand two major types of pathognomonic cortical signs: focal and bihemispheric. Focal cortical signs direct the examiner to a specific area of cortex in one hemisphere, or bihemispheric, in both hemispheres. Certain portions of the cerebral hemispheres are also termed "silent" areas, because the localizing evidence for lesions here may be absent.[1,2]

Left occipital lobe dysfunction produces a right homonomous hemianopia (loss of the right half of a visual field), although loss of this field can theoretically result from a lesion of the left optic tract or left thalamic lateral geniculate body. A right or left hemianopia can therefore result from any retrochiasmal lesion (behind the chiasm). Color dysnomia (inability to name colors) is the result of an interruption of fibers streaming from the occipital lobe to Wernicke's area, the comprehension center in the left temporal lobe. In 98% of right-handed people, Wernicke's area is located in the left temporal lobe. In most left-handed people, Wernicke's area is located in either the left temporal lobe alone or in both temporal lobes.[3,4] In only a minority of left-handed people is Wernicke's area confined to the right temporal lobe. A lesion in Wernicke's area results in a sensory or receptive aphasia characterized by fluent speech filled with gibberish words. Written words come from the occipital cortex, while spoken words come from both temporal lobes. A mistake in naming results in a paraphasia and is often the result of a lesion in the posterior–superior temporal lobe, but can have quite variable localization. Adjacent to Wernicke's area in the temporal lobe is another area called the "dysnomia center," which shows variable localization from person to person. Another pathognomonic sign of temporal lobe dysfunction is a focal, temporal lobe seizure, described as fits consisting of a sense of fear, smell, pleasure, or déjà vu. Another common manifestation of temporal lobe seizures is the automatism, a brief episode of automatic behavior during which the patient is unaware of his surroundings and is unable to communicate with others. Patients with complex partial seizures may experience sudden unpleasant smells (e.g. burning rubber) of brief duration which constitute olfactory auras. Temporal lobe dysfunction may also cause a superior quadrantopia (loss of a quarter of the visual field), described as a "pie in the sky," as a result of a disruption of the optic radiations, called Meyer's loop, which dip into the temporal lobe. Pathognomonic signs of left parietal dysfunction include right-sided cortical sensory loss, right-sided sensory-motor seizures, or a Gerstmann syndrome, characterized by finger agnosia (inability to recognize one's fingers), acalculia (inability to calculate numbers), right/left confusion, and agraphia without alexia (an ability to read but not write). Another sign of left parietal cortical dysfunction is cortical sensory loss and results in agraphesthesia (inability to identify numbers written on his/her skin). Sensory seizures may spread up or down the sensory strip and have been described as the Jacksonian march. The movement, usually clonic, begins in one portion of the body, for example, the thumb or fingers, and spreads to involve the wrist, arm, face, and leg on the same side along the stereotypical pattern of cortical organization termed the homunculus (Figure 2.1). A Todd's paralysis may then occur following the attack, with the same distribution. Left frontal lobe dysfunction can result in Broca's aphasia, also known as motor or expressive aphasia, and is characterized by halting, slow, and nonfluent speech.[5] Speech lesions in the arcuate fasciculus, a dense bundle of fibers connecting Wernicke's area to Broca's, prevents patients from repeating phrases but does not impair comprehension (Table 2.1). Lesions of the corpus callosum prevent the interhemispheric transfer of information, so a patient cannot follow instructions with his/her left hand but retains the ability to perform these same instructions with the right hand. Another syndrome of the corpus callosum is "alexia without agraphia" (inability to read but retained ability to write) and is caused by a lesion extending from the left occipital lobe and into the splenium. The right frontal lobe, despite its size, is a relatively silent lobe, other than loss of speech intonation (inflection and emotion in speech). The areas of major clinical importance are the motor strip (area 4), the supplementary motor area (area 6), the frontal eye fields (area 8), and the cortical center

Table 2.1 Classification of dysphasias

Lesion	Deficit	Aphasia type
Temporal	Retained repetition and fluency, no comprehension, no naming	Transcortical sensory
Wernicke's	Retained fluency, no comprehension, repetition, or naming	Wernicke's
Parietal	Retained comprehension and fluency, no repetition	Conduction
Broca's	Retained comprehension, no fluency, repetition, or naming	Broca's
Frontal	Retained comprehension and repetition, no fluency or naming	Transcortical motor

for micturition (medial surface of the frontal lobe). Frontal lobes play a major role in personality and acquired social behavior. Frontal lobe dysfunction may result in loss of drive, apathy, loss of personal hygiene, inability to manage one's family affairs or business, and disinhibition. The right parietal lesions cause a characteristic disturbance of space perception and left-side neglect. Signs such as lethargy, stupor, coma, disorientation, confusion, amnesia, dementia, and delirium often result from bihemispheric dysfunction and are not derived from a simple focal cortical lesion.[1] These bihemispheric lesions will be addressed in a later chapter.

PYRAMIDAL TRACT

The pyramidal tract begins in the motor strip of the cortex and courses downward through the brain and into the spinal cord. In the hemispheres, it is called the coronal radiata and then becomes the internal capsule, cerebral peduncle, and pyramidal tract which crosses at the medulla–spinal cord junction, and finally in the spinal cord becomes the corticospinal tract. Functionally, a lesion anywhere along this tract can produce the same long tract signs. Signs of pyramidal tract dysfunction include spasticity, weakness, slowing of rapid alternating movements, hyperreflexia, and a Babinski sign.[6] Muscle tone is examined by manipulating the major joints and determining the degree of resistance. Spasticity is one type of increased tone (resistance of a relaxed limb to flexion and extension). Muscle strength is graded from 0–5 using the grading system shown in Table 2.2.

Acute lesions anywhere along the pyramidal tract may also produce flaccid hemiparesis, at least initially, with spasticity developing later. If the whole area of cortex supplying a limb is damaged, the extrapyramidal pathways may be unable to take over and an acute global flaccid weakness of the limb can occur. Pyramidal tract lesions typically produce weakness of an arm and leg, or face and arm, or all three together. Facial weakness may manifest with a slight flattening of the nasolabial fold, however, the forehead will not be weak (frontalis muscle) since the muscles on each side of the forehead have dual innervation by both cerebral hemispheres (corticopontine fibers). The less affected muscles are the antigravity muscles (wrist flexors, biceps, gluteus maximus, quadriceps, and gastrocnemius). Specific tests of grouped muscle strength can also be quite useful (Table 2.3):

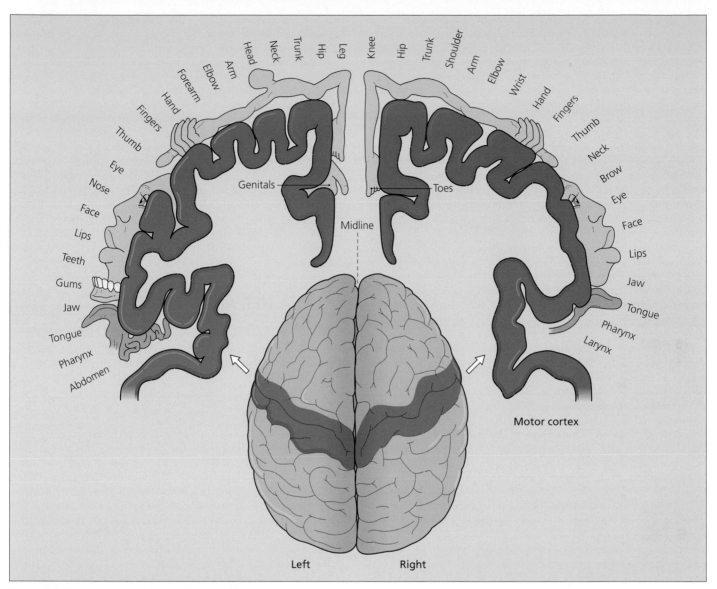

Figure 2.1 Somatosensory and motor homunculi.

Table 2.2 MRC Scale for muscle strength grading

Grade	Strength
0	No muscle contraction
1	Flicker or trace of contraction
2	Active movement with gravity eliminated
3	Active movement against gravity
4	Active movement against gravity and resistance
5	Normal power

Table 2.3 Deep tendon reflexes

Reflex	Segmental level	Peripheral nerve
Biceps	**C5**–6	Musculocutaneous
Triceps	C6,**C7**,C8	Radial
Brachioradialis	C5–C7	Radial
Quadriceps	L2,**L3**,L4	Femoral
Achilles	L4,L5,**S1**,S2	sciatic

Roots in bold type indicate spinal segment with greatest contribution.

pronator drift (arms outstretched with the palms up), standing on each foot, hopping on one foot, walking on toes (gastrocnemius), walking on heels (tibialis anterior), and deep knee bend (proximal hip muscles). Typically, pyramidal lesions often cause rapid alternating movements to become slowed but accuracy is preserved.

This is in contrast to cerebellar lesions (see below), which can result in fast but inaccurate, sloppy movements.

Reflexes can also be quite important in detecting subtle pyramidal tract lesions, especially if asymmetric. Reflexes are graded by a numerical system: 0 an absent reflex, trace is palpable but not visible, 1+ is hypoactive but present, 2+ is normal, 3+ is hyperactive, 4+ implies unsustained clonus, and 5+, sustained clonus. Clonus is a series of rhythmic involuntary muscle contractions induced by sudden stretching of a spastic muscle such as at the ankle. The cutaneous reflex (abdominal twitch obtained when you gently stroke someone's abdomen) and the cremasteric reflex (L1, L2 innervation; retraction of the testicle upward with a brush along the inner thigh) may also be lost in pyramidal tract lesions. The abdominal cutaneous reflexes in the upper quadrant of the abdomen are mediated by segments T8 and T9; the lower by T10 to T12. If for example, the lower abdominal reflexes are absent but the upper are preserved, the lesion may be between T9 and L1. The Hoffman reflex is reflective of hyperreflexia and spasticity on that side and suggests pyramidal tract involvement. The Babinski reflex is the best-known sign of disturbed pyramidal tract function. The Babinski reflex is an important sign of upper motor neuron disease, but should not be confused with a more delayed voluntary knee and toe withdrawal due to oversensitive soles of the feet.[7] The Babinski reflex is sought by stroking the lateral border of the sole of the foot, beginning at the heel and moving toward the toes. The stimulus should be firm but not painful. The abnormal response, referred to as the Babinski sign, consists of immediate dorsiflexion of the big toe and subsequent separation (fanning) of the other toes. When planar responses produce equivocal results, a related reflex may be tested by stroking the lateral aspect of the dorsum of the foot, and is known as the Chaddock sign.

In general, the more spasticity is present, the more likely the pyramidal tract lesion is in the spinal cord, especially if the spasticity is bilateral.[8] Conversely, it is unusual for a pyramidal tract lesion in the spinal cord to produce a hemiparesis or monoparesis. A hemiparesis that involves the face places the lesion somewhere above the facial nucleus, although if the hemiparesis spares the face, the lesion need not be below the facial nucleus. Mild or more chronic hydrocephalus may also cause impressive pyramidal tract dysfunction in the legs more than in the arm fibers. Bladder axons also become stretched by the dilated ventricles associated with hydrocephalus and cause urinary urgency and incontinence. Finally, it should be remembered that the spinal cord terminates normally at the level of the L1–L2 vertebral body and therefore, neurologically L5 is anatomically in the lower thoracic region.

THE EXTRAPYRAMIDAL SYSTEM

Unlike the pyramidal tracts which govern strength and fine dexterity, the basal ganglia govern the speed and spontaneity of movements. Two basic patterns emerge with basal ganglia dysfunction: either too much or not enough movement. The number one characteristic of a basal ganglia tremor is its presence at rest and disappearance with movement, in contrast to a cerebellar tremor which is minimal at rest and exaggerated with movement (intention tremor). The strength and deep tendon reflexes are normal in extrapyramidal diseases and there is no Babinski sign. However, the tone is either hypotonic as occurs in choreiform disorders, or increased (rigid), as in the bradykinetic (slowness of movements) varieties with rachety rigidity appropriately called cogwheeling. Choreiform movements are involuntary random jerky movements of small muscles of the hands, feet, or face and may be proximal enough to cause the whole arm to jerk gently. If instead of the small distal muscles, the larger more proximal

muscles involuntarily flinch, the patient may have ballismus. Ballismus can be unilateral, but chorea is almost always bilateral. Athetoid movements are slower, more continuous, and sustained, and may involve the head, neck, limb girdles, and distal extremities. Dystonic movements resemble a fixation of athetoid movements involving larger portions of the body. Torticollis, or torsion of the neck, is an example of a neck dystonia that is the result of the continuous contraction of the sternocleidomastoid muscle on one side. Postural and gait abnormalities of extrapyramidal disease are most diagnostic in patients with Parkinson's disease (tremor, bradykinesia, and rigidity).[9] A blank expression and infrequent blinking, walking with a leaning forward posture and a festinating gait (running–shuffling feet) are typical findings of a Parkinson's patient. Once in gear, the initially bradykinetic patient may have difficulty stopping. At the same time, the patient's hand is coarsely shaking at three times a second and the patient's speech is also devoid of normal changes in pitch and cadence.

CRANIAL NERVES (I–XII)

There are 12 cranial nerves but only III to XII enter the brainstem (I and II do not). Diagnosing a cranial neuropathy is only the beginning, since the lesion may lie anywhere along the course of the cranial nerve.

Cranial nerve I

Cranial nerve I, the olfactory nerve, begins at the cribriform plate and travels back underneath the frontal lobe to the temporal lobe without relaying in the thalamus. To test olfaction, test each nostril independently and avoid using a caustic substance such as ammonia which tests the trigeminal nerve (V) in addition to the olfactory nerve due to irritation of the nasal mucosa. An olfactory groove tumor may present with unilateral anosmia (loss of smell), although the most likely explanation is local nasal obstruction. Foster–Kennedy syndrome is characterized by ipsilateral anosmia, ipsilateral scotoma with optic atrophy (direct pressure on the optic nerve), and contralateral papilledema (elevated intracranial pressure) and is classically due to an olfactory groove or medial sphenoid wing meningioma. Loss of smell can also complicate up to 30% of head injuries as a result of shearing of the nerves as they pass through the cribriform plate.

Cranial nerve II

The second cranial nerve, the optic nerve, is the most complex. Visual acuity, color vision, Marcus Gunn pupil, visual fields, and direct ophthalmoscopic observation must all be assessed. Visual acuity is affected early in optic neuropathies, since 20–25% of all optic fibers come from the macula and travel in the center of the nerve. If the patient's visual acuity is not 20/20 and cannot be improved by refraction (looking through a pinhole in a piece of cardboard is a good bedside test), then the visual impairment is most likely neurologic. The size, shape, and symmetry of the pupils in moderate lighting conditions should be noted. If the pupils are unequal it is important to decide which pupil is the abnormal one. One frequent mistake is to investigate for the cause of the dilated pupil on one side, because the larger pupil is always the more impressive, even though the patient actually has a constricted pupil on the opposite side because of a Horner syndrome. If there is ptosis of the eyelid on the side of the small pupil, the patient may have Horner syndrome, although if the ptosis is on the side of the large pupil, the patient may have an ipsilateral partial third nerve lesion. Furthermore, the light and accommodation reflexes will be normal in a Horner syndrome and impaired in a partial III nerve lesion. Whenever a patient is found to have a widely dilated pupil that is fixed to light and accommodation without accompanying ptosis, there is a possibility of a pharmacologic pupil (e.g. atropine drops instilled into the eye). A Marcus Gunn pupil (afferent pupillary defect), a form of optic nerve dysfunction, is elicited by the swinging flashlight test: shine a dim light into the right eye, and note how small the right pupil constricts (left pupil also constricts). Swing the light over to the left eye and carefully note the left pupil. If the very first reaction of that pupil is dilation instead of maintaining its previous small size, then there may be left optic nerve dysfunction, i.e. an afferent papillary defect (Figure 2.2). The examiner must ignore "hippus," which is a normal phasic instability of the pupil with waves of alternating constriction and dilatation. An optic nerve lesion can be corroborated with visual fields and direct fundoscopy which will both be discussed below in the dedicated neuro-ophthalmology section.

Cranial nerves III, IV, and VI

The IIIrd cranial nerve, or oculomotor nerve, is one of the three nerves that move the eye, the others being the IVth (trochlear) and the VIth (abducens) cranial nerves. Defective adduction and elevation with outward and downward displacement of the eye suggests a IIIrd nerve palsy. The IIIrd nerve also innervates the levator palpebrae superioris, the muscle that opens the eyelid. Parasympathetic fibers travel within the superior and medial

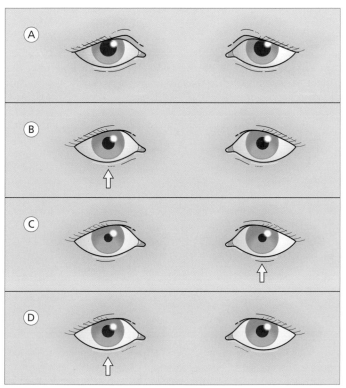

Figure 2.2 Marcus Gunn pupil is a pupil that paradoxically dilates with direct light (↑).

perimeter of the IIIrd nerve to constrict the iris and stimulate the ciliary body to round up the lens. As a general rule, if the pupil is affected, the cause is more likely to be surgical (compressive) and if spared, the cause is more likely to be medical (diabetes, cranial arteritis, arteriosclerosis, syphilis, migraine). A compressive lesion, like an aneurysm, selectively injures these superficially situated parasympathetic fibers, producing a dilated pupil with ptosis and painful ophthalmoplegia. In contrast, diabetes more often causes a pupil-sparing, painless ophthalmoplegia by damaging the interior motor axons through arterial thrombosis.[10] The sympathetics supply Müller's muscle which also slightly elevates the eyelid and when injured causes the upper eyelid to droop and results in ptosis and miosis (eyelid droop and a dilated pupil), i.e. Horner syndrome. If the sympathetic nerves to the eye are interrupted prior to the carotid bifurcation, ipsilateral facial anhidrosis (no sweating) may also result. Some of the sympathetics also ascend the common carotid and follow the external carotid onto the face to stimulate the facial sweat glands.

If the pupils do not react to light, the anatomic differential diagnosis includes the afferent limb (retina, optic nerves, optic tracts) and the efferent limb (pretectum, Edinger–Westphal nucleus, parasympathetic fibers in the oculomotor nerves, and the pupillary constrictor muscle in the iris). A pupil able to accommodate to near vision but not react to light is referred to as an "Argyll Robertson pupil" and has been classically seen in patients with tertiary syphilis. This, of course, is a rare finding because of the decrease in this disease over the past century. Light-near dissociation is also seen in "Adie's pupil," which is usually unilateral and is caused by parasympathetic dysfunction. When parasympathetic innervation is first lost in Adie syndrome, the pupil is relatively large, but with time and reinnervation the pupil constricts. This is a curious but benign disorder of unknown cause, usually affecting one eye and results from injury or illness to the ciliary ganglion, usually inflammatory in nature. Pineal region tumors can also damage the midbrain pretectum and cause light-near dissociation. Pineal region tumors more classically damage the midbrain upgaze center and cause a constellation of dorsal midbrain signs called Parinaud syndrome: (1) impaired upward or downward gaze; (2) bilateral light-near dissociation; (3) pupillary dilatation; and (4) retraction of the eyelids.

In general, nystagmus can be due to labyrinthine or brainstem/cerebellar pathology and may be central or peripheral, and is defined in the direction of the fast movement (Table 2.4). Upbeat or downbeat nystagmus is almost always of central origin, and represents disrupted connections between the cerebellum and brainstem (Chiari malformations, basilar invagination, platybasia, or a midline cerebellar lesion such as medulloblastoma in children). Horizontal nystagmus is more commonly peripheral in origin, especially if the patient can stop the nystagmus by fixating on a target. Two axes of nystagmus, as seen in rotary nystagmus, suggest a disturbance of two semicircular canals. Opsoclonus is another form of nystagmus and is characterized by chaotic, repetitive, saccadic movements in all directions, preventing fixation and has also been termed "dancing eyes."[11] In an adult, opsoclonus is associated with postinfectious encephalopathy as well as with carcinomas of the lung or breast, although in younger children it has been described in association with neuroblastoma. The presence of optokinetic nystagmus can be used to confirm cortical vision; its absence, however, is inconclusive.[12] When the optokinetic tape (a series of vertical black lines on a white background) is pulled from the patient's left to his/her right, the right parieto-occipital lobe tracks the target to the right (smooth pursuit, slow

Table 2.4 Classification of nystagmus

Nystagmus type	Characteristics	Location of pathology	Possible etiologies
Upbeat	Upbeating nystagmus	Cerebellar vermis	Cerebellar or medullary lesion, Wernicke's encephalopathy
Downbeat	Downbeating	Cervicomedullary junction	Chiari I malformation, basilar invagination, syringobulbia, foramen magnum lesion, multiple sclerosis, Wernicke's encephalopathy
Convergence-retraction	Convergence motions and simultaneous retraction of globes into orbits	Rostral midbrain, pretectum, posterior third ventricle	Pineal tumors
Ocular bobbing	Downward jerk with slow drift back into primary position	Pons	Pontine tegmentum hemorrhage or stroke
Ocular flutter	Rapid back and forth saccades, associated with ocular dysmetria	Cerebellum	Neuroblastoma, occult lung or breast carcinoma
Opsoclonus	Continuous, involuntary, random chaotic saccades (dancing eyes), continues during sleep	Cerebellum, dentate nucleus	Neuroblastoma, occult lung or breast carcinoma
Ocular dysmetria	Overshoot or undershoot on rapid refixation, side to side oscillation, fast component towards the side of lesion	Cerebellum	MS
Monocular nystagmus	Vertical	Eye	Acquired blindness
Congenital nystagmus	Horizontal jerk, remains horizontal even in upgaze and downgaze	Eye	Congenital
Spasmus nutans	Torticollis, head nodding, and pendular nystagmus	Unknown	Developmental, 6 months–3 years

phase). The eyes saccade left to track each newly arriving target (fast phase). In right parieto-occipital lesions, smooth pursuit (slow phase) to the right is lost. Occipital strokes because of a posterior cerebral artery infarct do not usually impair optokinetic nystagmus. A tumor, in contrast, may cross vascular boundaries and interrupt smooth pursuit generators.

Looking left involves two cranial nerves: the left VIth (left lateral rectus) and the right IIIrd (right medial rectus) (Figure 2.3). There are three classic signs of a pontine medial longitudinal fasciculus (MLF) lesion, or internuclear ophthalmoplegia: (1) weakness of the contralateral medial rectus muscle causing paralysis of adduction on lateral gaze, since the MLF cannot transmit its message to the IIIrd nerve to pull the eye medially; (2) nystagmus in the abducting eye; and (3) the retained ability to converge, demonstrating that the reason for medial rectus weakness on adduction is not in the IIIrd nerve or muscle itself. In the setting of a IIIrd nerve lesion, the eye will be deviated downwards (secondary depressant action of superior oblique) and outwards (lateral rectus action) and the diplopia would improve when testing lateral gaze in the affected eye.

A IVth or trochlear nerve lesion causes weakness of the superior oblique muscle and results in a compensatory head tilt away from the side of the affected eye to compensate for the diplopia. The diplopia is particularly troublesome on looking downward and especially troublesome when the patient is walking downstairs. In children, this head tilt may be misdiagnosed as

torticollis and is called the Bielschowsky's sign. This move causes compensatory intorsion of the good eye and thus permits the patient to align his eyes so they no longer have double vision from the IVth nerve paresis.

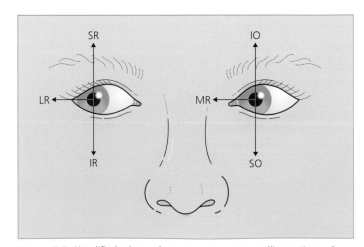

Figure 2.3 Simplified scheme for testing the major pulling actions of extraocular muscles. IO = inferior oblique; IR = inferior rectus; LR = lateral rectus; MR = medial rectus; SO = superior oblique; SR = superior rectus.

A VIth or abducens nerve palsy is the most disabling eye movement abnormality since the diplopia persists in nearly all directions of gaze. At rest, the affected eye is pulled medially by the unopposed action of the medial rectus muscle. Multiple sclerosis is the most common cause of an isolated VIth nerve palsy due to a plaque in the brainstem. The VIth nerve takes a ventral course from the pontine tegmentum over the petrous ridge to the dorsum sellae and into the cavernous sinus lateral to the carotid nerve and medial to cranial nerves III, IV, V1 and V2. A posterior fossa tumor can cause hydrocephalus which can also stretch the VIth nerve over the petrous tip and cause diplopia. As the VIth nerve has a rather long course, it is the most vulnerable cranial nerve to closed head injury. Benign transient VIth nerve palsies can also occur in children following mild infections. More severe cases of mastoiditis (Gradenigo syndrome) can cause ear pain and a combination of VIth, VIIth, VIIIth, and occasionally Vth nerve lesions. These symptoms must be differentiated from Ramsay Hunt syndrome (geniculate herpes zoster), in which there is vesicular eruption in the ear and a VIIth nerve palsy.

Cranial nerve V

The Vth cranial nerve, the trigeminal, controls both sensory and motor function: sensation of the forehead and face (including inside the mouth), and strength of chewing muscles (temporalis, masseter, pterygoids). It is important to recognize that there is a large area over the angle of the jaw supplied by nerve roots C2 and C3 and that patients with nonorganic sensory loss over the face usually claim anesthesia extending to the line of the jaw and the hairline (Figure 2.4). When testing for a corneal reflex, a wisp of cotton wool should not be allowed to cross in front of the pupil or the patient will see it and blink (false positive). In addition, both eyes should shut simultaneously if the corneal reflex is present. A depressed or absent corneal reflex can be an early physical sign of an acoustic neuroma in the cerebellopontine angle. Intracavernous lesions (i.e. aneurysms, meningiomas, carotid–cavernous fistulas,

and pituitary tumors) can all cause facial numbness. However, jaw numbness does not typically occur with cavernous sinus lesions since V_3 does not enter the cavernous sinus like nerves III, IV, VI, V_1 and V_2. Patients suffering from lightning jabs of terrible facial and jaw pain, often precipitated by a trigger point along the gums or lips, may have trigeminal neuralgia.[13] The cardinal feature of trigeminal neuralgia is pain without any objective neurological abnormality (i.e. sensory or motor dysfunction). The cause is thought to be an arterial or venous loop which pulsates against the trigeminal nerve at the pontine root entry zone or sometimes a small plaque of brainstem demyelination as in multiple sclerosis, although attacks of trigeminal pain may occur with any tumor of the cerebellopontine angle or petrous apex. Although herpes zoster can affect any nerve in the body, the thoracic roots are usually affected in younger age groups, although in the elderly, the virus has a predilection for V_1.

Cranial nerve VII

The VIIth nerve, the facial, controls all the facial and forehead muscles. The VIIth nerve does not contribute to normal eye opening but instead contributes to forced eye opening. Paralysis of facial movement including both the cheek and forehead on one side of the face, both volitional and emotional, indicates a lesion in the VIIth nerve (peripheral) somewhere between the pontine facial nerve nucleus and the facial muscles. In general, if the forehead is spared, then the facial paralysis is "central" and is the result of a lesion in the descending corticopontine upper motor neuron. Eye closure and forehead movement will remain relatively intact because the intact hemisphere pathways provide adequate cross-innervation. Recent evidence also suggests that upper facial motor neurons receive little direct cortical input, whereas lower facial neurons do and are therefore more affected.[14] As the facial nerve leaves its nucleus in the brainstem, other nerves piggyback it on their way to the lacrimal gland, stapedius muscle (dampens loud noises in the ear), and the taste buds along the anterior two-thirds of the tongue. Ipsilateral loss of taste and tear production, and the presence of hyperacusis (noises sound too loud) confirm that the patient's facial weakness is the result of lower motor neuron dysfunction. Most often, an acute peripheral facial weakness without associated sensory loss is the result of Bell's palsy, a poorly understood acute inflammatory attack on the facial nerve within the facial canal. This disorder has an excellent prognosis for recovery within weeks or months. Blepharospasm is a recurrent involuntary spasm of forceful eye closure (both eyes) with some spread into other facial muscles. Hemifacial spasm is characterized by recurrent spasms of one side of the face and is most likely the result of an irritation of the facial nerve as it leaves the brainstem by a pulsating arterial loop.[14,15]

Cranial nerve VIII

The VIIIth or acoustic nerve relays hearing to the brainstem from the cochlea as well as balance information from the labyrinth. The early loss of speech discrimination amidst background noise raises the suspicion to a diagnosis of an acoustic neuroma. The closest nerve to the VIIIth nerve is the facial nerve, however, after the acoustic nerve, the most common nerve to be affected is the trigeminal nerve. There is a relative loss of higher tones in nerve deafness whereas lower tones are lost in middle-ear deafness. A tuning fork is also helpful to distinguish between in nerve deafness hearing loss due to middle-ear disease (conductive deafness) and

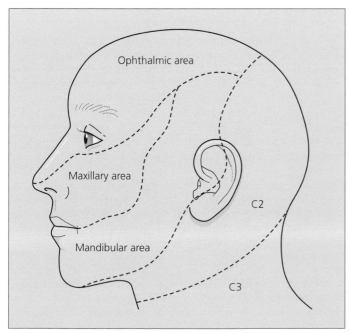

Figure 2.4 Diagrammatic representation of the cutaneous nerve supply of the head.

that due to VIIIth nerve damage (sensorineural deafness). For the Rinne test, a tuning fork is held on the mastoid while the opposite ear is masked. A Rinne "positive" test is when the tuning fork can still be heard in front of the ear but no longer heard on the mastoid and is the normal situation (air conduction > bone conduction). For the Weber test, a tuning fork is placed on the vertex and if heard equally in both ears, then hearing is normal. In conductive deafness, the fork will be heard more loudly in the affected ear, and in sensorineural hearing loss the fork will not be heard in the affected ear. It is also important to recognize that unilateral temporal lobe lesions do not produce hearing loss. After the VIIIth nerve enters the brainstem, spoken words are directed to both sides of the brainstem and ascend to both temporal lobes. Disturbances in the vestibular system may occur in the labyrinth (i.e. Meniere's disease) or in the nerve (acoustic neuroma, petrous temporal bone fracture), or in the temporal lobe of the brain (epilepsy). Meniere's disease is characterized by a triad of recurring attacks of vertigo associated with tinnitus and progressive deafness.

Cranial nerves IX, X, and XI

The IXth or glossopharyngeal nerve controls primarily sensation of the posterior tongue and pharynx. The only muscle supplied by the nerve is the stylopharyngeus muscle which cannot be easily tested clinically, although there is much overlap of the vagal and glossopharyngeal sensory supply to the pharynx. The Xth or vagus nerve is the longest of the cranial nerves. It is primarily motor and when weak can cause ipsilateral vocal cord paralysis. Paralysis of one vocal cord can lead to hoarseness, loss of voice volume, and an inability to cough explosively. Unilateral palatal or pharyngeal palsies may even be asymptomatic. The XIth cranial nerve, the spinal accessory, has two parts, the spinal part which exits the upper cervical spinal cord and tracks up through the foramen magnum into the posterior fossa where it joins the accessory part of nerve XI exiting the medulla. The spinal accessory then does a U-turn back through the jugular foramen to innervate the ipsilateral sternocleidomastoid (SCM) and trapezius muscles. To test the left SCM, ask the patient to put his/her chin on their right shoulder. Try to pull the face back over to the left and feel the left SCM. The left SCM muscle therefore pulls the head to the right and the trapezius muscle helps shrug the shoulders and elevate the arm above the horizontal. Torticollis is caused in part by intermittent contractions of the sternocleidomastoid muscle on the opposite side.

Cranial nerve XII

The XIIth nerve, the hypoglossal, supplies the tongue muscle and damage results in ipsilateral tongue atrophy. On attempted tongue protrusion, the tongue deviates toward the weak side, due to the unopposed genioglossus muscle. Bilateral weakness or paralysis of the tongue is more common than unilateral paralysis and may be caused by amyotrophic lateral sclerosis or in myasthenia gravis, although in the latter, no wasting or fasciculations accompany the weakness. Tongue fasciculations may be present normally when the tongue is resting quietly on the floor of the mouth.

CEREBELLUM

The smooth end efficient performance of volitional movements depends on the coordination of agonist and antagonist muscles,

acting in synergy. A failure of a group of muscles to act harmoniously is a sign of cerebellar dysfunction. Dysdiadochokinesis is characterized by difficulty in performing rapid alternating movements. Dysmetria is the difficulty in reaching a target accurately or past-pointing. The rate, rhythm, amplitude, and smoothness of movement may all be affected in cerebellar disease. A relatively common cerebellar tremor, called titubation, affects elderly people with a rapid, fine, bobbing motion of the head. The side-to-side imbalance of cerebellar ataxia is in contrast to the front-to-back imbalance of Parkinsonian patients. However, unlike the crossed pyramidal and extrapyramidal systems, the right cerebellar hemisphere controls the right arm and right leg and vice versa. Often a cerebellar tremor is present with the arms outstretched (postural tremor), but the tremor almost always worsens with intention (intention tremor). Speech is also affected in cerebellar disorders, causing ataxia of speech called scanning speech. In addition, the inability to perform finger-to-nose movements or to tandem walk is characteristic of cerebellar dysfunction. Postural instability can be best evaluated by the Romberg test which is a nonspecific test of vestibular function and often used to demonstrate loss of joint position sense. A positive test is when the patient falls with his eyes closed when standing with his feet together. In unilateral vestibular or cerebellar disease, the patient sways toward the damaged side.

Saccades are tested by having a patient glance back and forth between two targets about a foot apart. A patient with ocular dysmetria who consistently overshoots the target is likely to be suffering from cerebellar dysfunction. Lesions of one cerebellar hemisphere may cause coarse nystagmus when the patient gazes toward the side of the lesion. The most extreme example of fixation instability is opsoclonus, which is most likely of cerebellar origin. Opsoclonus classically occurs in infants with neuroblastoma and is described as lightning-fast random eye movements often called "dancing eyes."

SPINAL CORD, NERVE ROOTS, AND MUSCLE

The last neural circuits to consider are the spinal cord, nerve roots, and muscles. However, before distinguishing between a root and peripheral nerve lesion it is important to discriminate an upper motor neuron from a lower motor neuron lesion. As discussed above, upper motor neuron signs include spasticity, weakness, slowing of rapid alternating movements, hyperreflexia, and a Babinski sign. Lower motor neuron lesions (root or peripheral nerve) can cause muscular atrophy, fasciculations, hypotonia, or weakness in a particular root or peripheral nerve distribution, and diminished reflexes. To diagnose a myelopathy, the long tract signs need to be combined with root or segmental signs (Figure 2.5). Fasciculations are spontaneous, random contractions of muscle, usually too small to move a joint but visible when the skin over the affected muscle is inspected. However, in order to call a spontaneous muscular twitch a fasciculation, the muscle must be fully at rest. The presence of fasciculations implies a lower motor neuron dysfunction, however, the abnormality may be in the spinal cord (ventral horn) or anywhere along the peripheral nerve up to the point of muscle insertion. Fibrillations are the smallest potentials obtainable from individual muscle fibers and occur in denervated muscle fibers after 3 weeks when the motor neurons supplying a muscle are damaged, either in their cell bodies, the ventral roots, or the peripheral nerve itself.

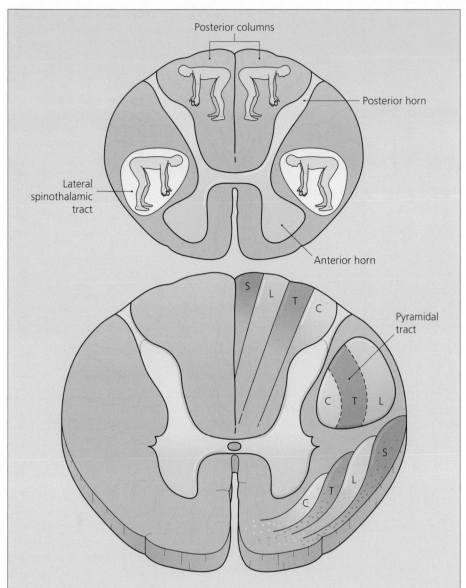

Figure 2.5 The posterior columns and lateral spinothalamic tracts are both somatotopically organized, but the lamination scheme is opposite in the two systems. In the posterior columns, the sacral fibers are mostly medial; in the spinothalamic tracts, the sacral fibers are mostly lateral.

A Brown–Sequard syndrome affects the left or right half of the spinal cord and is characterized by ipsilateral weakness, contralateral pain and temperature loss, and ipsilateral vibration and proprioception loss below the lesion (Figure 2.6). Anterior spinal artery syndrome is characterized by flaccidity followed by spasticity, weakness, slowing of rapid alternating movements, hyperreflexia, and a Babinski sign, as well as bilateral pain and temperature loss below the lesion but no vibratory or proprioceptive loss (dissociated sensory loss).[16] Syringomyelia (slowly expanding cyst of the spinal cord) or a centrally located spinal cord tumor can also cause dissociated sensory loss. A constellation of lower motor neuron signs and upper extremity dissociated sensory loss is virtually pathognomonic of syringomyelia in the cervical spinal cord. A syrinx can be congenital or even post-traumatic and can present in a delayed fashion following a spinal cord injury. Occasionally, the syrinx extends up into the medulla (called syringobulbia) and causes atrophy, fasciculations, and weakness of the tongue and pharynx.[17,18] Vitamin B12 deficiency causes another type of dissociated sensory loss called "combined

systems disease." In this disease, vibration and proprioception are lost but pain and temperature sensation are spared. Lower motor neuron signs may also be present from the peripheral neuropathy due to B12 deficiency. Central cord syndrome is another spinal cord syndrome characterized by post-traumatic quadriparesis (worse in the arms) without sensory loss following a hyper-extension cervical injury. Injury to the ventral horns can cause the lower motor signs in the arms and hands, and injury to the corticospinal tracts results in a spastic quadriparesis.[19]

There are a few pitfalls to consider when examining a patient with a potential myelopathy.[2] First, remember that the pyramidal tracts to the legs terminate neurologically at about L4 (Babinski is extensor hallicus longus: L5) and anatomically at around the T12 vertebral body (Figure 2.7). Therefore, a spastic paraparesis warrants a cervical or thoracic MRI and not a lumbar MRI. A spastic paraparesis does not automatically place the lesion between the thoracic and lumbar regions, since compressive lesions of the upper cervical cord can damage the cord's blood supply and in addition the descending leg fibers in the corticospinal tracts are

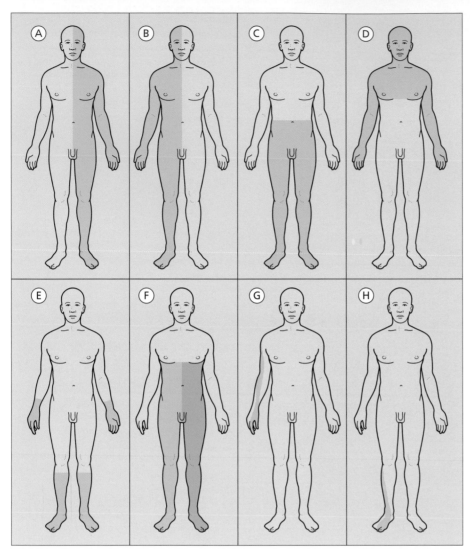

Figure 2.6 Common patterns of organic sensory loss. **(A)** Hemisensory loss as a result of a hemispheric lesion. **(B)** Crossed sensory loss to pain and temperature because of a lateral medullary lesion. **(C)** Midthoracic spinal sensory level. **(D)** Dissociated sensory loss to pain and temperature as a result of syringomyelia. **(E)** Distal, symmetric sensory loss because of peripheral neuropathy. **(F)** Crossed spinothalamic loss on one side with posterior column loss on the opposite side because of Brown–Séquard syndrome. **(G)** Dermatomal sensory loss because of cervical radiculopathy. **(H)** Dermatomal sensory loss due to lumbosacral radiculopathy.

more vulnerable to ischemia than the arm fibers. Second, a hemiparesis sparing the face is not necessarily the result of a cervical myelopathy since a pyramidal tract lesion in the internal capsule can also spare the face. Myelopathies, however, rarely result in a hemiparesis. Third, atrophy of the hands and arms may be the result of a high cervical extramedullary mass at the foramen magnum. An extramedullary mass is one that lies outside the spinal cord, either intradurally or extradurally. It is difficult by history and examination to distinguish an intra- from an extramedullary spinal cord lesion. In general, extramedullary lesions stretch nerve roots and can be more painful than intramedullary lesions and can cause compression of the spinal cord and nerve roots at the affected segment. Also, extramedullary lesions cause more pain in the supine position, which is the opposite of a herniated disk in which lying flat can relieve the pain. Palpation of the spinous processes and straight leg raising will often elicit pain from an extramedullary lesion but not an intramedullary lesion. Intramedullary lesions, in contrast, are more likely to produce atrophy, dissociated sensory loss, and early bowel and bladder problems. Sacral sparing can also be helpful, since the sacral sensory fibers are lateral in the spinothalamic tracts and may not be affected in a patient suffering from an intramedullary lesion.

The cauda equina and conus medullaris syndromes are also important to distinguish from peripheral root symptoms. Lesions at either location interrupt multiple motor and sensory roots to the legs producing bilateral lower extremity atrophy and weakness, depressed reflexes, down-pointing toes, and often a sensory level.

The peripheral nervous system is the final common pathway whatever the movement involved. There are three classes of peripheral nerve lesions, those affecting a single peripheral nerve (mononeuropathy: carpal tunnel), multiple random individual nerves (mononeuropathy multiplex), and all peripheral nerves (polyneuropathy). A diagnosis of mononeuropathy is made by finding mixed motor/sensory loss in the distribution of individual peripheral nerves. A polyneuropathy is diagnosed by the constellation of distal, symmetrical stocking/glove sensory loss or lower motor neuron signs, and absent distal deep tendon reflexes. Electrical studies may also be of value in the diagnosis and prognosis of certain disorders and may help to distinguish between lesions of the motor neuron and the muscle and between spinal and peripheral nerve lesion.

Proximal weakness alone is the most common sign of a myopathy. Patients with proximal weakness waddle, because the hands on their thighs (Gower's sign). Myotonia is a myopathic sign resulting from delayed relaxation after the muscle contracts and occurs in myotonia congenita, myotonic dystrophy, and paramyotonia congenita. As a rule, a myotonic patient shakes your hand and does not let go. In patients with widespread symmetrical weakness, pay attention to any sensory loss so that myopathic weakness is not confused with Guillain–Barré, an acute peripheral neuropathy with some distal vibratory loss and areflexia. Muscles above the shoulders are particularly susceptible to myasthenia gravis and botulism; two illnesses which attack the neuromuscular junction. Patients may present with a pure motor syndrome dominated by ophthalmoplegia, ptosis, weakness of chewing, difficulty sucking through a straw, dysphagia, and tongue weakness, but without pyramidal signs in the arms and legs. Almost any external ophthalmoplegia can be mimicked by myasthenia gravis:[20] internuclear ophthalmoplegia, up- or down-gaze palsy, VIth nerve palsy, and a pupil-sparing IIIrd nerve palsy. Neuromuscular blockade produces "fatigable" weakness which worsens with each contraction.

THE PEDIATRIC PATIENT

The neurological evaluation of the infant or child begins with the birth history, social history, developmental history, family history, and physical examination. The general appearance of the child should be noted, particularly the presence of any dysmorphic features or neurocutaneous abnormalities such as café-au-lait spots, neurofibromas,[21] facial port-wine stain in Sturge–Weber disease, depigmented lesion nevi in tuberous sclerosis, as well as a craniofacial dysmorphism seen with craniosynostosis. It is important to inspect the midline of the neck, back, and pilonidal area for any defects, particularly for small dimples above the level of the gluteal fold in the midline that might indicate the presence of occult spinal dysraphism or a dermal sinus tract. The head should be examined by inspection, palpation, and auscultation. The shape, size, and asymmetry may point to microcephaly, hydrocephalus, craniosynostosis (premature cranial suture fusion), or cerebral atrophy. Maximum head circumference of the head should be recorded on a standard chart according to the patient's age and sex. The charting of the head circumference by the primary-care provider and the neurosurgeon examining that plotted curve are essential parts of the examination and may indicate an intracranial pathology before it becomes symptomatic. The general appearance of the skull, prominence of venous pattern, and palpation of the anterior fontanelle may suggest increased intracranial pressure. The palpation of the anterior fontanelle is another essential part of the neurologic examination. In the sitting position the fontanelle should be concave or sunken; in the supine position it may be more full (Figure 2.8). Intracranial pressure can be estimated within several millimeters of water by palpating the anterior fontanelle. The baby should be laid flat and the head should be gently raised off the examining table. At the point the fontanelle becomes flat, the intracranial pressure equals the extracranial pressure. If one measures the height the head has been raised in millimeters above a horizontal line drawn through the child's heart (the physiologic zero point) then one has a fairly good estimate of the child's intracranial pressure. If the patent anterior fontanelle consistently remains bulging and full when a quiet child is fully erect or sitting than that denotes increased intracranial pressure. An imaging study such as a computed tomography (CT) or MRI of the head is a reasonable

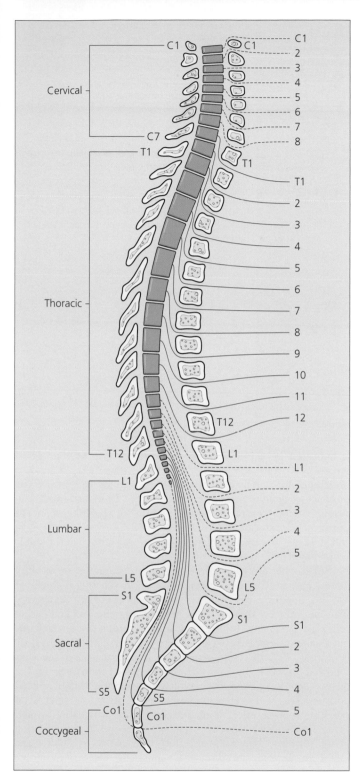

Figure 2.7 Relationship of the spinal cord segments and spinal nerves to the vertebral bodies and spinous processes.

weak gluteus medius muscles allow the pelvis to tilt from side to side. A patient may also have to lean forward and push off with both hands to get up from a chair signifying pelvic girdle weakness. When trying to get up off the floor, children also adapt to pelvic girdle weakness and from the all-fours position, lock both their knees and push their trunk back over their legs by bracing their

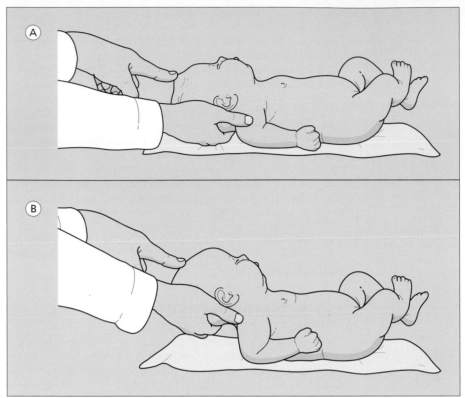

Figure 2.8 Positional changes in appearance of the fontanelle can be used to assess changes in intracranial pressure in children. In **(B)**, as this child's head is raised to 5 cm above the level of the right atrium of the heart (arbitrary physiologic "zero" point), the fontanelle goes from bulging **(A)** to flat. The flat fontanelle means that the intracranial pressure equals the extracranial pressure. Since the height of the head is about 5 cm above the heart, the intracranial pressure is approximately 5 cm of water. This method can be used for estimating the intracranial pressure in a child, with an open fontanelle (younger than 15 months). If the fontanelle is still bulging in the upright position in a quiet baby, this denotes raised intracranial pressure.

option. The anterior fontanelle is often closed by 18–24 months, although the posterior fontanelle closes after 2–3 months. Transillumination of the head with a flashlight in absolute darkness up to the age of approximately 9 months is an old-fashioned but useful way to detect severe hydrocephalus, arachnoid cysts, or subdural effusions at the bedside. However, it has become a lost art and cranial ultrasound has replaced this once important historical diagnostic modality. Percussion of the head, also of historical note, may produce a hollow or "cracked pot" resonance in patients with severe hydrocephalus (Macewen's sign). Cranial nerve examination can be more reliably tested beyond 30 weeks' gestation since prior to that time, the pupillary response to light is not predictably present, and the gag reflex is also not easily elicited. The "blink reflex" is often used to determine the presence of functional vision in small infants but is absent in the newborn. A slight degree of anisocoria is not unusual, particularly in infants and small children. The fundoscopic examination is an essential part of the neurological examination (see below, neuro-ophthalmology). True papilledema with early obliteration of the disc margins and absent pulsations of the central veins is rare in patient's under the age of 2 because of the ability of the expansile skull to dissipate a rise in intracranial pressure. Medulloblastoma, a midline cerebellar tumor which can infiltrate the superior medullary velum, may produce bilateral fourth nerve palsies. A "setting sun sign" (forced downward deviation of the eyes at rest with associated upward gaze palsy; Parinaud syndrome) can also be seen in young children as a result of pressure on the region of the suprapineal recess and quadrigeminal plate due to hydrocephalus.

Muscle tone is examined by passive movement of the joints and extremities, and both sides should be compared. During the first few months of life, normal hypertonia of the flexors of the elbows, hips, and knees occurs. Fine motor development is indicated by the appearance of a pincer grip at the age of 9 months. Careful note should be made of asymmetry or marked preference for one hand or the other in a young child, since the presence of definite hand preference before 24 months may raise suspicions of central nervous system or peripheral nerve impairment. Crawling is normally seen at 9–12 months on average and at 12–15 months the infant begins to walk although the gait is broad-based and unsteady.

Small, choreiform-like movements are common on healthy infants and are transient, emerging at approximately 6 weeks of age and tapering off between 14 and 20 weeks of age. Extremity tone can also be assessed by a number of reflexes. The "grasp reflex" is modulated by the frontal lobes and is present at birth but should disappear between 4 and 6 months. The "Moro reflex" is a primitive startle response and consists of extension of the arms followed by their flexion with simultaneous spreading of the fingers and is elicited by rapidly changing the infant's head position. The Moro reflex is present from birth to 4 months of age. The "rooting reflex" is elicited with gentle stimulation around the mouth which produces turning of the head in the direction of the stimulus. The "Landau reflex" is evaluated by holding the infant in a prone position by supporting his/her abdomen. Normally the head extends and hips flex. If there is weakness of the lower extremities, hip flexion may not occur. Generalized reflexes of the extremities can be elicited beyond 33 weeks' gestation. The Babinski response is a nociceptive reflex elicited by noxious stroking of the lateral aspect of the plantar surface from the heel toward the toes. This response is normal in newborns until the age of 2. However, asymmetry of the Babinski response is abnormal at any age and may reflect an upper motor neuron lesion. Unsustained clonus can also be normal if symmetric, although sustained clonus is suspect at any age.

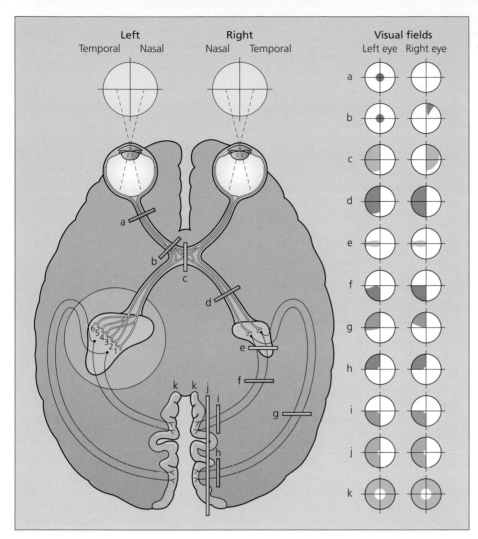

Figure 2.9 Characteristic defects of the visual field produced by lesions at various points along the visual pathways.

NEURO-OPHTHALMOLOGY

No neurological examination is complete without a detailed study of the visual system. Because of the extent of the visual system and its intimate relations with other areas of the brain, much valuable information can be obtained. Color vision is especially important in neuro-ophthalmology in the detection of pregeniculate pathway lesions. The visual field to a red object is interestingly more affected by damage in these areas. Similarly, an optic tract lesion may produce an incongruous hemianopic defect of color vision. The results of confrontation testing are conventionally recorded as seen by the patient, which means reversing the defect as seen by the examiner during confrontation testing. The nature of the field defect should be carefully documented: left central scotoma (optic nerve lesion), bitemporal hemianopia (chiasmatic lesion), right upper quadrantic hemianopia (left temporal), macula-sparing hemianopia (lesions of the optic tract), and right homonomous hemianopia's scotoma lesion (tip of occipital pole) (Figure 2.9). The areas of calcarine cortex subserving the peripheral fields lie anteriorly and those subserving macular vision are concentrated at the extreme tip: the upper fields represented in the lower half below the calcarine sulcus and the lower fields in the upper half of the cortex. Special attention should be paid to whether the defect crosses the horizontal meridian, since retinal

lesions due to vascular occlusion cannot do so. The defect may extend to the blind spot and defects due to vitamin B12 deficiency, toxins, or glaucoma usually extend into it. Lastly, the defect may cross the vertical meridian since organic visual field defects have a sharp vertical edge at the midline. The macula of the retina responsible for central vision is situated to the temporal side of the optic nerve head which then moves centrally into the optic nerve as it joins the chiasm. This papillomacular bundle conveying central vision in the optic nerve is very vulnerable to extrinsic compression by mass lesions. It is equally important to check for an early temporal field cut (contralateral junctional scotoma) in the opposite eye due to damage to the decussating nasal fibers (anterior chiasmatic syndrome of Traquair) (Figure 2.10).

The importance of papilledema is that it is usually associated with raised intracranial pressure, of which it may be the only objective sign. Papilledema (swelling of the optic nerve head) may cause field defects in several ways: enlargement of the blind spot, exudate into the macula, chronic papilledema causing gliosis, papilledema due to hydrocephalus, and a binasal hemianopia, a stretched posterior cerebral artery with cerebral herniation causing a macular-sparing hemianopia. Raised intracranial pressure due to any mass lesion in the brain has to be included in the differential, although conditions interfering with cerebrospinal fluid (CSF) circulation or resorption should also be considered.

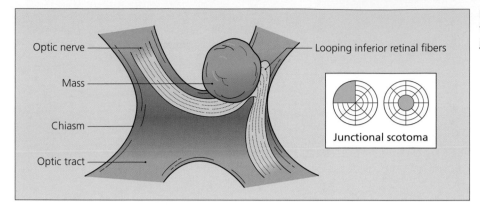

Optic nerve

Mass

Chiasm

Optic tract

Looping inferior retinal fibers

Junctional scotoma

Figure 2.10 A junctional scotoma may result from a mass impinging on the optic nerve at its junction with the chiasm.

Papilledema develops within a day or two after intracranial pressure begins to rise, but will not often be found in the first few hours of such a rise. A similar ophthalmoscopic picture can result from acute retrobulbar neuritis, which is a response of the optic nerve to a variety of toxic and metabolic insults and is commonly seen with an attack of multiple sclerosis (Devic's disease). The classic field defect is a central scotoma and symptomatically, the patient complains that central vision is impaired by a "fluffy ball" or a "steamed-up window" associated with some eye discomfort.

Diplopia may not always be due to extraocular nerve palsies. For example, thyrotoxicosis is characterized by weakness of the superior rectus and lateral rectus muscles as a result of an inflammatory myopathic process. Myasthenia gravis is characterized by diplopia and ptosis of the eyelid which is fatiguable. Diplopia under conditions of fatigue may also be due to lateral strabismus and unmasking of a lifelong squint. The acuity of onset of the diplopia must be determined as well as if there is any variability or remission to help differentiate the above diagnoses. A painful onset may suggest a compressive lesion due to aneurysmal dilatation causing a IIIrd nerve palsy. Associated congestion of the eye may raise the possibility of a granulomatous lesion in the orbit, either pseudotumor or Tolosa–Hunt syndrome (recurrent unilateral orbital pain accompanied by transient extraocular nerve palsies and a high erythrocyte sedimentation rate with a dramatic response to steroids). A caroticocavernous fistula can also cause a painful and red eye which is proptotic and can be associated with rapidly deteriorating visual acuity.

ANCILLARY DIAGNOSTIC TESTS

If a definite diagnosis is not reached either on clinical grounds alone or with the aid of ancillary neurodiagnostic tests, sometimes the best test is said to be a second examination. However, the rapidly increasing sophistication and diagnostic accuracy of neurodiagnostic procedures have challenged the continued need for a detailed and systematic neurological examination.

CT and MRI have revolutionized the diagnostic evaluation of neurologic patients and have eliminated the need for invasive pneumoencephalography and ventriculography. Almost uniformly, an unenhanced (i.e. noncontrast) CT of the brain suffices for patients seen in the emergency room presenting after trauma or with a new neurologic deficit. CT is the best test to rule out the presence of hemorrhage and is more sensitive than MRI for detecting acute blood. CT is also preferable to MRI for the detection of intracranial calcifications. CT angiography (CTA) is

obtained by administering a rapid bolus intravenous contrast that allows the selective imaging of vascular structures, and can be quite useful in the evaluation of subarachnoid hemorrhage to localize aneurysm pathology, carotid stenosis in a patient with transient ischemic attacks, or a traumatic carotid or vertebral dissection. CT is also the study of choice in the evaluation of the skull base and cranial vault (i.e. craniofacial disorders) because of the potential for exquisite bony detail.

MRI is noninvasive and has a number of diverse clinical uses in the evaluation of neurological disorders and without exposure to ionizing radiation. However, as a result of the longer acquisition time and less access to the patient during the study, it is not routinely used for acute trauma or unstable patients. MRI offers superb anatomical detail in the detection of structural causes for neurological dysfunction such as tumors, arteriovenous malformations, demyelinating disease, or stroke. Generally, T1-weighted images provide a better view of structural anatomy, whereas T2-weighted images are exquisitely sensitive to water (hydrocephalus) and cerebral edema and are preferred for the detection of pathology. MRI has been shown superior to CT for the detection and characterization of posterior fossa lesions. MRI has been used to define the anatomy in epilepsy patients with mesial temporal sclerosis or with anomalies of cortical architecture, depict the compression of the trigeminal nerve by a vascular loop, and evaluate CSF flow in patients with Chiari malformation and syringomyelia or normal pressure hydrocephalus. Diffusion-weighted MRI is extremely sensitive to the Brownian motion of water protons and is used in the early evaluation of stroke in evolution. MRA (arteriography or venography) is an excellent way to evaluate the vascular structures and avoids invasive cerebral angiography. MR perfusion techniques have evolved to quantify blood flow to areas of ischemia or hyperemia. MRI can be combined with high-resolution MR spectroscopy to evaluate the spectral peaks obtained that reflect the concentrations of the metabolites and some neurotransmitters in the voxel area under investigation. Spinal MRI is the most efficient way to screen for spinal disease and can be combined with gadolinium contrast in the setting of neoplasia or infection. Functional MRI is useful in the preoperative localization of the motor and somatosensory cortex based on the identification of cortical activation by detecting changes in venous oxygen.

Following fundoscopic and CT or MRI examinations, CSF analysis is indicated in patients suspected of having central nervous system bacterial, fungal, or viral infection as well as subarachnoid hemorrhage. Lumbar CSF pressure recordings are also useful in the diagnosis of pseudotumor cerebri and normal-

Table 2.5 Typical CSF findings in various disorders

Condition	Pressure	Red blood cells/mm³	White blood cells/mm³	Differential	Glucose (mg/dL)	Protein (mg/dL)
Normal	nl	0	0–5	mononuclear	45–80	15–45
Bacterial meningitis	↑	0	500–100 000	Neutrophils	low	↑
Tuberculous meningitis	↑	0	50–500	Mononuclear	low	↑
Viral meningitis	nl to ↑	0	5–500	Mononuclear	nl	15–100
Subarachnoid hemorrhage	nl to ↑	10 000–500 000	↑ in proportion to red blood cells	Mononuclear and neutrophils	nl	↑
Multiple sclerosis	nl	0	0–50	Mononuclear	nl	20–100
Guillain–Barré syndrome	nl	0	0–50	Mononuclear	nl	20–500
Brain tumors	nl to ↑	0	0–100	Mononuclear	nl	Variable (↑ in acoustic schwannoma)

nl = normal; ↑ = elevated.

pressure hydrocephalus, although it is important to recognize that falsely high pressures result when the knees are pressed against the abdomen and when the patient holds his breath. The chief danger of a spinal tap is uncal herniation in patients with raised intracranial pressure because of focal disease. The spinal fluid is normally clear and colorless. Turbidity can result from the presence of leukocytes or bacteria and hemorrhage can result from a "bloody tap" or a subarachnoid hemorrhage. In normal adult CSF, there are 0–4 lymphocytes or mononuclear cells per mm³, and no polymorphonuclear lymphocytes or red blood cells. Polymorphonuclear lymphocytes can be present in the newborn, however they are not normally found in CSF taken from healthy children older than 1 year of age. In general, one white blood cell can be subtracted for every 700 red blood cells in the CSF. The CSF/plasma ratio for glucose is normally 0.60 to 0.80. Low protein content suggests its relative exclusion by the blood–brain or blood–CSF barriers, although high protein levels are found in patients with blood (1000 red blood cells raise the total protein by 1.5 mg/dL) or intraspinal tumors. Among spinal cord tumors, intradural extramedullary tumors such as meningiomas or neurofibromas often have elevated CSF protein greater than 100 mg/dL (Table 2.5).

Angiography now plays a supplementary role in defining the vascularity except in the setting of subarachnoid hemorrhage, a suspected carotid–cavernous fistula, trauma, or in the preoperative planning stages for the treatment of an arteriovenous malformation or for adjuvant preoperative embolization of a tumor. MRA or CT angiography may one day replace the diagnostic capabilities of cerebral angiography if their sensitivity or specificity prove equal to those of angiography, the gold standard.

A positron emission tomography (PET) scan combined with FDG (^{18}F-2-deoxy-D-glucose-6 phosphate) is used clinically in the evaluation of patients with dementia, brain tumors, and epilepsy. FDG is transported into the cell and is not a substrate for further degradation after conversion to glucose-6-phosphate and therefore is an excellent marker of brain metabolism. Patients with dementia often have abnormal PET scans with reduced metabolism in the frontal and parietal regions. FDG-PET techniques have been used to evaluate patients with temporal lobe epilepsy, both ictal and interictal. In general, hypometabolism in the temporal lobe is lateralized to the side of seizure onset interictally, but may be hypermetabolic during the ictal state. Finally, FDG-PET studies have been used in patients with brain tumors to characterize the most malignant component (i.e. hypermetabolic) of a tumor, assess prognosis, and differentiate recurrent tumor from radiation necrosis.

Single photon emission computerized tomography (SPECT) often uses gamma-emitting isotopes, such as technetium (^{99m}Tc), to assess brain perfusion and cerebrovascular reserve. Using HMPAO (hexamethyl-propylene amine oxime) as a marker for cerebral blood flow, cerebrovascular reserve can be determined with or without Diamox, a cerebral vasodilator. HMPAO is lipophilic and crosses the blood–brain barrier and is then rapidly converted to a hydrophilic form and trapped in the brain. SPECT has also proved useful in localizing abnormalities in patients with temporal lobe epilepsy.

Transcranial Doppler ultrasound has been used to record flow velocities from extra- and intracranial arteries. The recorded velocity is not a direct measurement of flow, but proportionality does exist between velocity and flow when the arterial diameter remains constant. Transcranial Doppler ultrasound has been invaluable in its capacity to determine noninvasively the degree of vasospasm after subarachnoid hemorrhage, to evaluate the hemodynamic significance of intracranial stenosis, to monitor changes in autoregulation following closed head injury and microemboli in the circulation, and to assess changes in cerebral blood flow during a carotid endarterectomy or arteriovenous malformation resection.

Electromyography and nerve conduction studies can often aid in the evaluation of neuromuscular disorders or spinal disease, such as herniated discs or spondylosis. A needle electrode is inserted into the muscle and action potentials are generated by muscle activity. Normal resting muscle is electrically silent except for the insertion potential produced by needle insertion. After denervation of the muscle, fibrillation potentials appear. Nerve conduction velocities can be used to differentiate demyelination, axonal degeneration, and also from muscular disorders. Conduction rates of motor nerves can be measured by stimulating the nerve at two points and recording the latency between each stimulus and the muscle contraction. Somatosensory evoked potentials are recorded after stimulation of peripheral nerves and are sensitive to compare side to side.

DIAGNOSIS AND INVESTIGATION OF CEREBRAL TUMORS

History and physical examination remain the gold standard for the initial assessment of any patient suspected of suffering from a primary or secondary cerebral neoplasm. However, the advent of CT and MRI has transformed the investigation.[22] The cardinal symptoms and signs of a cerebral tumor are headache, vomiting, malaise, cognitive decline, and papilledema. These are most commonly seen with posterior fossa tumors or those which have blocked the flow of CSF. However, in general, less than 0.1% of patients referred to the hospital for headaches have a cerebral tumor. Thus, lies the diagnostic dilemma for the primary-care physician. A first (nonfebrile, nonmetabolic-induced) epileptic seizure occurring in a patient warrants an electroencephalogram (EEG) and an imaging study such as an MRI or CT scan. An EEG is of value in the assessment of patients who have presented with an epileptic fit, although it may be misleadingly normal. The EEG does not exclude the presence of epilepsy or organic disease and a single normal EEG is of little value. The basic rhythm observed in an adult is called the alpha rhythm (frequency of 8–13 Hz) and is present when the patient is relaxed with his eyes closed and suppressed when the patient opens his eyes or concentrates.

Angiography retains a small role in the investigation of tumors, particularly in demonstrating and embolizing (occluding) the blood supply of highly vascular tumors such as meningioma, choroid plexus neoplasms, or hemangioblastoma. Adult supratentorial tumors account for 90% of cerebral neoplasms and occur in the lobes in a frequency roughly proportional to the size of the lobe. Unlike in children, 20–30% of cerebral tumors in adults prove to be metastases. Therefore a chest X-ray and careful physical examination are essential.

HEADACHE

Luckily, not all bad headaches are the result of brain tumors and the seriousness of a headache does not correlate with its pathologic severity. All the extracranial structures, including the arteries and muscles, are pain sensitive. Intracranially, the dura and dura-based vessels are pain sensitive, although the brain itself, cortical vessels, and pia-arachnoid, are pain insensitive. Pain can also be referred to the head from other structures sharing its innervation such as the eye, ear, sinuses, and teeth. The temporal pattern of the headache, site and radiation, precipitating, aggravating, and mitigating factors, accompanying symptoms, and family history should all be considered. Classic migraine is fronto-temporal in site, pulsatile, and is often unilateral and accompanied by a prodrome of visual phenomena, nausea, and mood changes. A cluster headache is of very rapid onset, short-lived, and is characterized by pain in and around the eye with associated lacrimation and nasal watering. Nocturnal attacks are more frequent and the attacks are often clustered together for 6–12 weeks. A typical tension headache is characterized by a tight feeling in the sub-occipital muscles which spreads over the top of the head and is exacerbated by stress. A typical pressure headache is one that occurs on waking, is aggravated by bending or coughing, and is not responsive to analgesics. A headache starting after the age of 60 with pain and tenderness over the temporal region may represent temporal arteritis and is associated with a high erythrocyte sedimentation rate, visual impairment, and generalized malaise.

VASCULAR DISEASES

To make the clinical differentiation between a neoplastic or other space-occupying lesion and a stroke one must substantially rely on the temporal history. Following a stroke, it is unusual to find a vessel actually occluded since most occlusions are the result of temporary embolic blockage with rapid subsequent recanalization. Stroke or "brain attack" emphasizes the abrupt onset of symptoms; the single characteristic feature of a vascular accident. It is important to recognize a stuttering onset of symptoms, characterized by repeated identical brief episodes of hemiparesis with full recovery, known as transient ischemic attacks. There are three main types of hemorrhagic strokes: (1) classic hypertensive intracerebral hemorrhage as a result of rupture of one of the peripheral lenticulostriate arteries; (2) hemorrhage associated with a cerebral arteriovenous malformation; and (3) subarachnoid hemorrhage as a result of aneurysms arising from the vessels traversing the subarachnoid space. "Thunderclap" headache, acute nausea, vomiting, and neck stiffness are the hallmarks of both subarachnoid hemorrhage and meningitis. Three considerations should be applied to working up a patient with cerebrovascular disease. (1) Is the extent of the lesion typical of occlusion of an identifiable vessel? (2) Is there any hematological disorder that could have predisposed to or mimicked a cerebrovascular accident? (3) Are there any causative factors or comorbidity such as hypertension, atrial fibrillation, vessel stenosis, or myocardial infarction. If the clinical suspicion is high for a subarachnoid hemorrhage and the CT scan is normal, a lumbar puncture should be performed. Normally the CSF is clear and colorless and therefore if the CSF is pink or bloody, differentiation between a traumatic lumbar puncture and a subarachnoid hemorrhage must be made by performing cell counts on three sequential samples of CSF. Classically, a small amount of CSF is centrifuged and the supernatant is inspected. If the supernatant is xanthochromic, there is a high likelihood that a subarachnoid hemorrhage has occurred. However, an ultra early lumbar puncture (< 2 hours) may precede the window to establish whether or not a subarachnoid hemorrhage has occurred.

HYSTERIA AND MALINGERING

A single disease can often explain all the symptoms and signs, however, a patient may have a variety of diseases, old and new, organic and functional.[2] Although the accuracy of neurodiagnostic tests is superb, it is the additional duty of the neurosurgeon to identify the malingering patient, since hysterical signs present more often in the nervous system than in any other organ system.[2]

Beginning in the cortex, functional signs manifest as seizures, stuttering, amnesia, and coma. The most definitive test for psychogenic seizures is a normal EEG during the ictus or seizure. A postictal EEG should also be abnormal with slowing. If the physician happens to witness a motor seizure, concentrate on the jerking which should have a quick and slow phase (a true jerk) and not simply a tremor. Amnesia when it includes the patient's own name is often hysterical. Hysterical coma can most easily be

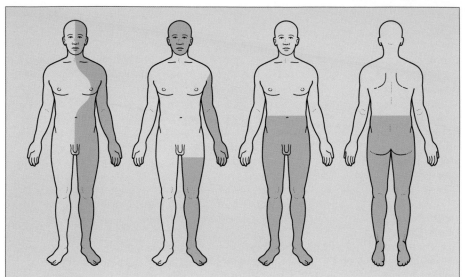

Figure 2.11 Common patterns of nonorganic sensory loss.

diagnosed by performing cold calorics. The presence of nystagmus indicates retained physiologic connections between the brainstem and cortex.

Reactive pupils do not necessarily indicate hysterical blindness, because there may still be a lesion behind the midbrain, damaging the optic radiations or occipital cortex. Normal optokinetic nystagmus in the face of blindness does indicate hysteria or malingering, because optokinetic nystagmus requires intact connections from the retina to the occipital cortex. A constricted visual field should also be cone shaped. Each time the examiner doubles the distance between you and the patient, the intact field should double in diameter and not leave only a central core of retained tunnel vision. Some patients can mimic a VIth nerve palsy by converging their eyes while looking to the side. The tip-off is that convergence also constricts the pupil. Diplopia should often disappear when one covers one eye, however, monocular diplopia does occur in rare cases such as a retinal detachment or lens dislocation.[23]

Eliciting collapsing or ratchety weakness versus true weakness when the muscle gradually gives way can be a challenge. While vigorously testing the strength of an individual muscle, the examiner suddenly lets go. If the muscle fails to spring back to its contracted position, hysterical weakness may be present. When testing grip strength, watch the thumb, since if the flexor pollicus longus does not flex the distal interphalangeal joint, the patient was not really giving maximal effort. The Hoover maneuver is another method of detecting insufficient effort by the patient. After placing one palm under the patient's heel, the examiner asks the patient to lift the other leg against the examiner's other hand. If the examiner does not feel the heel digging into his palm, the patient is not really trying to lift his leg. Hysterically hemiparetic patients also forget that pyramidal lesions selectively weaken the tibialis anterior. Although they drag the leg, there's no circumduction; in fact, they purposely elevate the toe to keep it from scraping the floor. Withdrawal of a limb to pain also belies another common hysterical complaint: marked sensory loss. Hysterical hemihypesthesia may be uncovered by demonstrating nonorganic splitting of vibration at the midline (Figure 2.11). Several nonorganic physical signs have also been described by Waddel, such as pain with gently tapping the lower back or with toe dorsiflexion,[24] and are collectively referred as "Waddel signs."

We hope this review has provided a comprehensive and systematic approach to the evaluation of a patient with a neurological disorder.

REFERENCES

1. Strub R, FW B. *The Mental Status Examination in Neurology.* Philadelphia: F.A. Davis Company; 1985.
2. Patton J. *Neurological Differential Diagnosis.* London: Springer-Verlag; 1998.
3. Ojemann GA. Cortical organization of language. *J Neurosci* 1991; 11: 2281–7.
4. Ojemann GA. Individual variability in cortical localization of language. *J Neurosurg* 1979; 50: 164–9.
5. Damasio AR. Aphasia. *N Engl J Med* 1992; 326: 531–9.
6. Lance JW. The control of muscle tone, reflexes, and movement: Robert Wartenberg Lecture. *Neurology* 1980; 30: 1303–13.
7. Van Gijn J. The Babinski sign and the pyramidal syndrome. *J Neurol Neurosurg Psychiatr* 1978; 41: 865–73.
8. Burke D, Knowles L, Andrews C, Ashby P. Spasticity, decerebrate rigidity and the clasp-knife phenomenon: an experimental study in the cat. *Brain* 1972; 95: 31–48.
9. Rao G, Fisch L, Srinivasan S, *et al.* Does this patient have Parkinson disease? *JAMA* 2003; 289: 347–53.
10. Trobe JD. Isolated pupil-sparing third nerve palsy. *Ophthalmology* 1985; 92: 58–61.
11. Bellur SN. Opsoclonus: its clinical value. *Neurology* 1975; 25: 502–7.
12. Baloh RW, Yee RD, Honrubia V. Optokinetic nystagmus and parietal lobe lesions. *Ann Neurol* 1980; 7: 269–76.
13. Fromm GH, Terrence CF, Maroon JC. Trigeminal neuralgia. Current concepts regarding etiology and pathogenesis. *Arch Neurol* 1984; 41: 1204–7.
14. Loeser JD, Chen J. Hemifacial spasm: treatment by microsurgical facial nerve decompression. *Neurosurgery* 1983; 13: 141–6.
15. Janetta P. Etiology and definitive microsurgical treatment of hemifacial spasm: operative techniques and results in 47 patients. *J Neurosurg* 1977; 47: 321.
16. Schneider RC, Crosby EC, Russo RH, Gosch HH. Chapter 32. Traumatic spinal cord syndromes and their management. *Clin Neurosurg* 1973; 20: 424–92.

CLINICAL PEARLS

Approach to a patient with a neurological disorder

- Step back and observe a patient walk, read, or move in bed before you examine them. If you focus on the deficit you may miss many important details. The examiner must master the skill of listening to the patient. A thorough and artfully elicited history and examination is still essential, and should be used in conjunction with the imaging studies to help direct therapy.

- Signs of pyramidal tract dysfunction include spasticity, weakness, slowing of rapid alternating movements, hyperreflexia, and a Babinski sign. Pyramidal lesions often cause rapid alternating movements to become slowed but accuracy is preserved, in contrast to cerebellar lesions, which can result in fast but inaccurate, sloppy movements.

- A basal ganglia tremor is often present at rest but disappears with movement, in contrast to a cerebellar tremor which is minimal at rest and exaggerated with movement (intention tremor).

- Use caution investigating the cause of the dilated pupil on one side, because the larger pupil is always the more impressive, even though the patient actually has a constricted pupil on the opposite side due to Horner syndrome.

- A compressive lesion, such as an aneurysm, may produce a dilated pupil with ptosis and *painful* ophthalmoplegia, in contrast to a pupil-sparing, *painless* ophthalmoplegia due to diabetes.

- The presence of optokinetic nystagmus can be used to confirm cortical vision and rule out hysterical blindness; its absence, however, is inconclusive.

- A IVth nerve lesion causes weakness of the superior oblique muscle and results in a compensatory head tilt *away* from the side of the affected eye to compensate for the diplopia.

- Note any asymmetry or marked preference for one hand or the other in a young child, since the presence of definite hand preference before 24 months may raise the suspicion of CNS or peripheral nerve impairment.

- Asymmetry of the Babinski response is abnormal at any age and may reflect an upper motor neuron lesion.

17. Bertrand G. Chapter 26. Dynamic factors in the evolution of syringomyelia and syringobulbia. *Clin Neurosurg* 1973; 20: 322–33.
18. Williams B. On the pathogenesis of syringomyelia: a review. *J R Soc Med* 1980; 73: 798–806.
19. Schneider RC. The syndrome of acute central cervical cord injury. With special reference to the mechanism involved in hyperextension injuries of cervical spine. *J Neurosurg* 1954; 11: 546.
20. Engel AG. Myasthenia gravis and myasthenic syndromes. *Ann Neurol* 1984; 16: 519–34.
21. Friedman JM. Neurofibromatosis 1: clinical manifestations and diagnostic criteria. *J Child Neurol* 2002; 17: 548–54; discussion 571–2, 646–51.
22. Jamieson DG, Hargreaves R. The role of neuroimaging in headache. *J Neuroimaging* 2002; 12: 42–51.
23. Keane JR. Neuro-ophthalmic signs and symptoms of hysteria. *Neurology* 1982; 32: 757–62.
24. Waddel G. Nonorganic physical signs in low-back pain. *Spine* 1980; 5: 117.

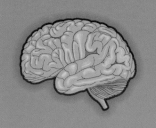

APPLICATIONS OF PRINCIPLES OF CELLULAR AND MOLECULAR BIOLOGY IN NEUROSURGICAL DISORDERS

3

Daniel P Cahill and E Antonio Chiocca

INTRODUCTION

The past two decades have seen striking advances in the fields of molecular and cellular neurobiology. The study of genes and their role in neurosurgical diseases has led to advances in our understanding of the basic biological processes that underlie these diseases. These advances in basic neuroscience will likely accelerate with the recent completion of the human genome draft sequence. The translation of these laboratory discoveries to the clinical arena is the challenge facing neurosurgeons in the next decades. Here we highlight the molecular and cellular principles in various areas of neurosurgery, and discuss the emerging framework of molecular genetic knowledge and its application in clinical neurosurgery.

Neurosurgery, like other areas of modern medicine, has witnessed an increasing focus of research activity on the molecular basis of disease in the last two decades. With the completion of the human genomic DNA sequence and advances in diagnostic and radiological techniques, this trend will continue, yielding important findings for the clinical neurosurgeon. Basic research in molecular and cellular genetics has already seen significant molecular advances in nearly every area of clinical neurosurgery: neurovascular lesions, tumor biology, epilepsy surgery, and spinal surgery. Indeed, the diversity of clinical neurosurgery is reflected in the wide range of molecular biology that has become important to the practicing neurosurgeon.

VASCULAR NEUROSURGERY

The molecular study of neurosurgical vascular lesions has seen notable advances in the last decade. Here we discuss the work on intracranial aneurysms (IA) and cerebral cavernous malformations (CCM). A recurrent theme throughout these fields is the focused study of familial disease for the discovery of the genetic contributors to disease. Once researchers begin to reveal the basic genetic factors that have an impact upon the disease in familial and sporadic instances, the findings can be extended for the general population by appropriate integration into screening modalities or pre-symptomatic treatment.

FAMILIAL INTRACRANIAL ANEURYSMS

For IA, molecular analysis has focused on the study of familial intracranial aneurysm (FIA) in an effort to dissect out the genes which may contribute to the development of an aneurysm.[1,2]

Study of FIA has focused on two broad classes of syndromes (see Table 3.1). The first and most well-defined class contains those patients who are at increased risk from IA as a component of an inherited syndrome such as polycystic kidney disease, a hereditary connective tissue disease syndrome, or a generalized hereditary vasculopathy.[3] The treatment and screening guidance that has arisen from the genetic understanding of these syndromes is familiar to neurovascular surgeons. Nonetheless, it is helpful to consider the key features of these syndromes to better appreciate the basic framework of the future large analyses to come.

The second broad category of familial disease is characterized by familial clustering of intracranial aneurysms and aneurysm rupture in the absence of an obvious systemic syndrome.[4,5] While much less is known about the molecular details affecting the increased risk in these families, it is clear that these clusters of disease hold a great deal of information for the future promise of genetic research in neurosurgery.

INTRACRANIAL ANEURYSMS AND INHERITED DISEASE SYNDROMES

The prototypic FIA syndrome is autosomal dominant polycystic kidney disease [ADPKD, Online Mendelian Inheritance in Man (OMIM); http://www.ncbi.nlm.nih.gov/OMIM entry #173900]. Families segregating ADPKD have an elevated risk for intracranial aneurysm[6–9] and the neurovascular surgeon has become well-versed in the molecular genetics of this disorder in the last decade.

As the underlying genetics of PKD have been uncovered, the molecular complexity of this disease has become apparent.[10] Heritable forms of PKD display genetic heterogeneity across different families, that is to say, mutations in genes located in disparate regions of the genome can produce the same spectrum of clinical disease. The primary inherited locus for PKD, *PKD1*, is localized to chromosome 16.[11] Linkage to this locus accounts for up to 90% of the autosomal dominant form of the disease, with a second locus on chromosome 4,[12] *PKD2*, accounting for most of the remaining cases. The responsible genes have recently been identified,[13–16] with the mutant PKD1 protein product, poly-cystin-1, and the PKD2 protein, polycystin-2, encoding similar large transmembrane proteins that are expressed at the cell surface.

The diverse phenotypic manifestations of PKD arise from a genetic mechanism that highlights an important feature of somatic genetics in disease. An affected individual inherits one defective copy of the gene from one of his or her parents in the standard autosomal dominant mode of transmission – 50% of the parent's

Table 3.1 Features of the two classes of familial intracranial aneurysms. The mutated genes (or genes) underlying the disorder have been identified in most cases of aneurysms that arise as the result of a systemic inherited disease. This molecular definition has allowed better analysis of the clinical syndromes and the development of one gene-one syndrome classifications. Familial clustering in the absence of systemic disease likely represents an amalgam of different disorders, some of which will have as-of-yet unappreciated systemic manifestations. These distinctions will become clearer with the identification of the genes in these clusters

	Syndromic disease associated with intracranial aneurysms	Famlial clusters of intracranial aneurysms
Broad systemic symptoms	Yes – polycystic kidney disease, connective tissue disease, systemic vasculopathy	No
Pattern of inheritance	Autosomal dominant	Heterogeneous
Genetic basis known	Yes	No
Number of genes	One gene – one syndrome	Numerous genes likely
Clinical application of genetic knowledge	Pre-symptomatic testing and screening possible	None yet

children are at risk of inheritance. The remaining normal copy of the gene is mutated in a small percentage of the affected individual's somatic cells (Figure 3.1). The cells sustaining this second mutation give rise to the characteristic phenotypic manifestations of the syndrome.[10,17,18] Thus second-site mutations in renal epithelial cells lead to renal cysts, and it is hypothesized that other phenotypic manifestations are likely the result of similar loss-of-function of the gene at the cellular level.

How do the mutant PKD1 and PKD2 proteins influence the formation of IA? This question is now beginning to be addressed at the molecular level. There is good evidence that the polycystins play a direct structural and functional role in the vascular walls of blood vessels. Studies of mouse models with engineered PKD1 mutations demonstrated marked defects in vascular integrity[19] and histopathologic and RNA analyses of the genes have shown them to be expressed in the cerebral vasculature.[20–22] Consistent with this hypothesized direct effect on the structural integrity of intracranial vessels is the observation of an increased rate of intracerebral arterial dolichoectasia, or aberrant hypergrowth, in patients with PKD.[23,24] It has yet to be shown if second-site mutations in the PKD genes occur in vascular cells and directly contribute to vessel weakening and the development of berry aneurysms.

Interestingly, there seems to be variability in the phenotypic manifestation of the risk for intracranial aneurysm, with some PKD families having a greater incidence of aneurysms than others.[6,25] As molecular studies focus on this variability, the identification of predictive genetic risk factors will allow for the development of proactive screening regimens based on high-resolution computed tomographic angiography or magnetic resonance angiography.[26] In addition, the ability to screen at the molecular level and appropriately diagnose the subset of patients with PKD1 and PKD2 mutations guides the current pre-symptomatic management of these patients and their families. A key component of their appropriate surgical care involves the incorporation of these screening and diagnostic modalities into clinical practice.

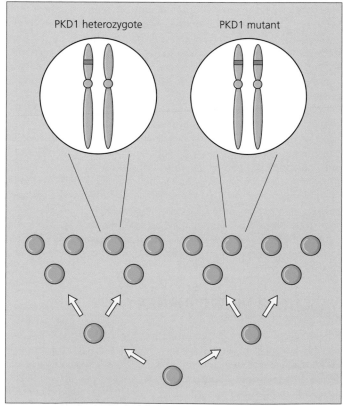

Figure 3.1 PKD1 and polycystic kidney disease somatic genetics. PKD1 is located on the short arm of chromosome 16. In the patient with polycystic kidney disease, one mutant copy (red) is inherited in an autosomal dominant fashion from the affected parent – the vast majority of the cells in the patient are heterozygous for the defect. In some cells, the normal copy of PKD1 on the other parental chromosome is somatically mutated – a mathematical certainty from a statistical point of view – through point mutation, deletion, mitotic recombination, or gene conversion. This clone of cells (red) is homozygously mutant for PKD1. These homozygous cells give rise to the phenotypic features of the syndrome such as renal cysts.

FAMILIAL CLUSTERS OF INTRACRANIAL ANEURYSMS IN THE ABSENCE OF SYSTEMIC DISEASE

As discussed above, a second class of inherited IA syndromes are characterized primarily by familial clustering of IA in the absence of PKD or other obvious connective tissue disorders. Studies have demonstrated a significant increased risk of aneurysm in the family members of patients who present with ruptured aneurysm, consistent with an underlying genetic cause.[4,5]

No gene has yet been identified to account for these clusters of families. However, study of these isolated inherited syndromes may prove to be even more important in the understanding of the genetic risk factors for aneurysms. It is estimated that only 10% of all inherited intracranial aneurysms can be explained by known genes such as *PKD1* or *PKD2*.[1,5] There is likely to be significant genetic heterogeneity between these families, with many different genes contributing in various cases – the search for the responsible genetic loci is in the early stages.[27,28]

CAVERNOUS MALFORMATIONS

With the beginnings of molecular dissection of intracranial aneurysms, one can look to the lessons from the recent research into the basis of CCM (OMIM entry #116860) for an example of how molecular analysis is leading the evolution of clinical management.

There has been striking progress in the molecular analysis of CCM. Cavernous malformations represent a subset of vascular malformation that has no arterial component; they are thus termed angiographically occult malformations. These lesions are characterized by focal capillary and venous growth patterns that hemorrhage internally, giving rise to a classic popcorn-like appearance on radiographic imaging studies. While most patients are asymptomatic, some manifest seizures or headaches as a result of the malformation, leading to neurosurgical excision.

At the outset, detailed familial analyses demonstrated that a subset of cavernous malformations is hereditary.[29,30] In the analysis of the hereditary forms of CCM, it was noted that many of the families with the hereditary syndrome were of Hispanic/Mexican descent. The genetic homogeneity of these families allowed haplotype analysis and linkage disequilibrium to accelerate the mapping of the *CCM1* locus on chromosome 7.[31,32]

Subsequent work led to the identification of mutations in the *Krit1* gene in these patients.[33] Further analysis of non-Hispanic pedigrees suggests that two more genes are likely involved in hereditary forms of the disease.[32] The molecular analysis of the Krit1 protein and its function at the cellular level is at the early stages of biochemical study,[34] revealing the basic molecular instructions to endothelial cells during formation of capillaries and venules.

The lessons drawn from these examples can be broadened beyond familial disease. Many of the patients initially diagnosed with "sporadic" disease likely have a previously unrecognized genetic mutation driving the formation of their CCM.

In the foreseeable future, similar genes will be identified for the risk of FIA. This portends a significant advantage for patients who are at-risk from this devastating disease. Surgical technique is rapidly approaching a time when the initial presenting clinical grade will be one of the factors most predictive of outcome. Discovery of genes contributing to IA is likely to lead to clearer indications for the surgical management of unruptured aneurysms in these high-risk patients and new screening procedures for genetically at-risk individuals. The identification and stratification of pre-symptomatic patients with unruptured aneurysms by genetic screening offers the hope of targeting surgical cure to at-risk individuals. A strongly positive genetic risk predictor will become akin to a "sentinel leak," and pre-symptomatic patients can be offered the benefits of surgery realized prior to the morbidity and mortality of their first aneurysmal rupture.

EPILEPSY

The inherited epilepsy syndromes have seen a true breakthrough in the preceding few years of molecular genetic analyses. The principal lesson has been observed frequently: epilepsy is a disorder of the channels that mediate the intrinsic electrophysiologic properties of neurons. A number of different channel types – sodium, potassium, calcium – are mutant in various forms of congenital epilepsy (see Table 3.2).

Table 3.2 List of channels found in inherited epilepsies. These channels are mutated in the germline of families with clinically-defined inherited epilepsy syndromes. Further analysis is needed before re-classification of these syndromes can commence, based on the underlying molecular genetic causes

Syndrome	Gene	OMIM	Ref.
Benign familial neonatal convulsions	*KCNQ2*	602235	62
	KCNQ3	602232	63
Autosomal dominant nocturnal frontal lobe epilepsy	*CHRNA4*	118504	64
	CHRNB2	118507	65
Generalized epilepsy with febrile seizures plus	*SCN1A*	182389	66
	SCN1B	600235	67
	SCN2A	182390	68
	GABRG2	137164	69
Juvenile myoclonic epilepsy	*CACNB4*	601949	70
	GABRA1	137160	71

Interestingly, the mutations found in these genes are, in most cases, subtle point mutations. It is likely that these mutations have similarly subtle effects on the complex electrophysiologic properties of the neurons in which they are expressed. In the case of *SCN1A*, mutations found in patients with epilepsy appear to prolong sodium-channel opening,[35,36] leading to hyperexcitability and epilepsy predisposition. On the other hand, it is a relative loss-of-function in the potassium channel encoded by the *KCNQ2* gene (mutated in generalized epilepsy syndromes) that appears to lead to hyperexcitability – mutations affect the voltage sensitivity of channel opening.[37,38] Future drugs specifically targeted at modulating the electrophysiology of these neuronal channels will allow for more options in the management of epilepsy.

The next phase in the understanding of epileptogenesis will be the superposition of the structural anatomy of the neuronal connection network on the electrophysiology of these individual channels. The role of the neurosurgeon will initially be guided by standard pre-screening modalities as described above, offering the hope of targeting surgical therapy to those patients who stand to benefit most. As progress continues, however, we can anticipate anatomic mapping of seizure foci with increasing precision to assist in focusing neurosurgical technique to maximize the benefits of an anti-epilepsy procedure.

TUMOR MOLECULAR BIOLOGY

The genetic study of human cancer has witnessed an explosion of discovery in the last two decades, and has now seen the advent of cancer chemotherapeutics targeted at the specific molecular alterations found in human tumors. The study of human brain tumors has similarly benefited from genetic investigation – numerous genes have been identified that are involved in the formation of the range of brain tumors (see Table 3.3).

Similar to the work on epilepsy and intracranial aneurysms, familial study of brain tumors has yielded many insights – for example, the identification of mutations in the *p53* gene in families with classic Li–Fraumeni syndrome (see OMIM entry

#137800). However, there is an additional avenue commonly pursued for the genetic dissection of tumors – the comparison of the tumor cell genome with the normal genome from the affected patient. These types of analyses reveal much about the somatic genetics of tumorigenesis, much like family and hereditary analyses tell us about the inherited genetics of PKD. In one view, a tumor can be seen as a cellular descendent through the somatic genetics of the individual cells in the body.

In brain tumors, as in other cancers, there are two major classes of genes involved in driving tumorigenesis – oncogenes and tumor suppressors. Oncogenes are genes which, when altered in a tumor cell, directly promote the growth of tumors by providing positive signals for tumor growth. An example of this from glioblastomas is the amplified epidermal growth factor receptor (EGFR). Only a single mutation is required to activate an oncogene (Figure 3.2). However, this mutation is usually a very subtle and specific change that leads to a gain-of-function in cellular signaling pathways, and as such, is a rare event in the course of normal cellular division.

Table 3.3 Partial list of oncogenes and tumor suppressor genes mutated in nervous system tumors. This is a partial list of the genes mutated in the pathogenesis of nervous system tumors. A number of other genes have been implicated in the development of brain tumors by alterations in their expression level and methylation status

Tumor type	Gene
Glioblastoma	EGFR
	p53
	PTEN
	p16
Schwannoma	NF1
	NF2
Meningioma	NF2
Malignant rhabdoid tumor	SNF5/INI1
Medulloblastoma	PTCH
	APC

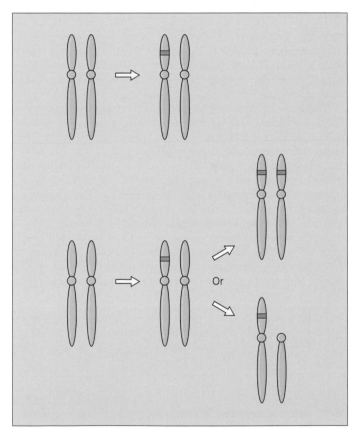

Figure 3.2 Oncogenes and tumor suppressors. Oncogenes drive the growth of tumor cells through an activating, or gain-of-function, mutation in one copy of the gene (pink). This activating mutation is usually targeted to a specific location of the protein. On the other hand, tumor suppressor genes sustain an inactivating mutation or deletion of one copy of the gene (red) and must additionally undergo a loss-of-function mutation or deletion of the remaining normal copy before the brakes on cell growth and division are removed. Since many different types of genetic alterations can inactivate a tumor suppressor gene, the relative contribution of oncogene and tumor suppressor pathways in a tumor appears to be fairly similar.

Tumor suppressors are genes that normally restrain growth or promote the terminal differentiation of cells. In cancers, tumor suppressor gene protein products are mutated, deleted, or inactivated so that the brakes to cell division are removed and the unrestrained growth of the tumor can proceed (Figure 3.2). There are a number of well-established examples of tumor suppressor genes that are targeted in glioblastomas. The *p53* gene is perhaps the most famous example, with *p16* and *PTEN* having an important role in glioblastomas as well.

TUMOR PATHWAYS

It is becoming clear that mutations in these different genes often represent different ways to disrupt a set of core pathways for tumorigenesis.[39] The *PTEN* gene (or *MMAC*) located on chromosome 10 was cloned by classic tumor deletion analyses in 1997[40,41] and it is inactivated in approximately 25–40% of glioblastomas.[42,43] Its inactivation is correlated with higher stage disease[44] and thus poor outcome.

The PTEN protein product encodes a lipid phosphatase and down-regulation of phosphatidylinositol levels. This modulates signaling through phosphatidylinositol-3 kinase and leads to subsequent downstream activation of Akt protein kinase (Figure 3.3). This pathway is thought to be one of the primary effectors of *PTEN*'s tumor suppressive function.[45,46] Given the relatively high rate of mutation of *PTEN* in high-grade glioblastoma, molecularly targeted therapeutics directed against the *PTEN/Akt* pathway hold significant promise in the treatment of these tumors.[47]

Indeed, the *PTEN/Akt* pathway pales only in comparison to another important tumor suppressor pathway in glioblastoma – the *p16/Rb* pathway. Virtually all glioblastomas have inactivated this cell cycle pathway that serves as the molecular brake on DNA synthesis and cell division.[48] It is likely that abrogation of the normal *p16/Rb* pathway is absolutely required for glioblastoma formation and progression and that this represents a uniquely exploitable target for tumor-specific therapy.

THERAPEUTIC TARGETING OF ONCOGENES

The prototypic oncogene involved in glioblastoma is that for EGFR. This gene is frequently amplified in human glioblastomas.[49,50] In addition, it is somatically mutated in cancers and commonly seen in an altered form that has deleted coding exons 2 through 7.[51] Tumors select for these molecular genetic changes through the process of clonal evolution (Figure 3.4). As the unstable tumor genome develops highly variable new cellular subclones during recursive rounds of division, the tumor cell with the greatest survival advantage eventually comes to dominate the population (indicated in red in Figure 3.4).

It is this process of clonal evolution that lies at the core of the development of future molecular therapies against cancer. As we identify the molecular changes that are driving tumor growth, like *EGFR*, these molecules can be specifically targeted pharmacologically. Since the vast majority of the tumor cells in a tumor with *EGFR* amplification are dependent upon continued aberrant *EGFR* signaling for growth, a well-designed anti-*EGFR* therapeutic agent will provide a substantial treatment advance against this tumor.

However, the underlying unstable tumor genome makes it almost inevitable that such targeted agents will ultimately fail because the tumor cell population has a chance to develop new mutations in new pathways to survive and evade the targeted therapy. The war against tumors will be fought at this edge of clonal selection – neurosurgeons and neuro-oncologists will

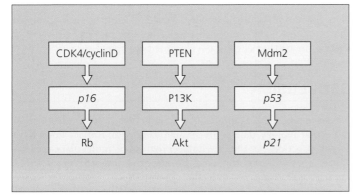

Figure 3.3 Genetic pathways in brain tumors; three primary pathways genetically targeted in brain tumors. The *p16/Rb* pathway is targeted through loss-of-function of *p16* or *Rb*, or oncogenic alteration of the cyclinD–CDK4 complex. The *PTEN/Akt* pathway is usually targeted through deletion of the *PTEN* gene, which leads to increased phosphatidyl inositol 3 kinase (PI3K) activity and Akt activity. The *p53* pathway can be disrupted at many different loci, typically seen is inactivation of *p53* or amplification of the human homolog of *mdm2*.

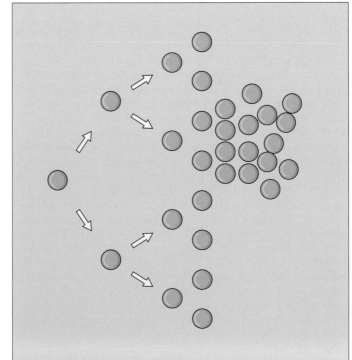

Figure 3.4 Clonal evolution waves. The cells in a tumor have a high rate of genetic instability, giving rise to variant cellular subclones (red) at an appreciable frequency. Once subjected to the selective pressures of the tumor microenvironment, the malignant subclones will undergo selection that results in their outgrowth and eventual predominance within the tumor cell population. Thus the mutational alterations that allowed for survival through the bottleneck of tumor selection become fixed in the final tumor cell population.

employ genetically targeted therapeutics in the first wave, and then attempt to identify the escape routes of tumor subclones to design a second wave of therapy, and so forth.

Biologic agents may also provide a relatively novel avenue for treatment of these tumors. Such agents may comprise immuno-toxins targeted against a tumor-specific antigen, such as tenascin[52] or the transferrin receptor,[53] oncolytic viruses that target onco-genic and/or tumor suppressor pathways,[54] or immunotherapies using dendritic cells or tumor vaccines.[55–57] The first wave of molecularly targeted therapies for brain tumors are directed against oncogenes – the therapeutic agents designed against gene amplifications have progressed more quickly to the clinical arena. Since the *EGFR*, *PTEN*, *p16* and *p53* genes are involved in multiple cancers, it is likely that therapeutic agents useful against these targets will find broad application. Clearly, though the outlook for molecularly targeted agents looks promising, novel therapeutic agents are desperately needed in the treatment of malignant brain tumors.

SPINAL FUSION WITH GROWTH FACTORS

Spinal surgery is encountering major advances in the use of molecular therapeutics with the identification of secreted protein growth factors that direct bone formation. There are a number of new potential therapeutic agents in spinal surgery on the horizon.

In 1988, specific protein growth factors that could induce ecotopic bone formation were identified at the molecular level.[58] In the intervening time, several novel members of this protein family have been identified.[59] These growth factors, termed bone morphogenic proteins (BMPs), are members of the transforming growth factor-β superfamily of signaling molecules. The past decade has seen the identification of numerous bone morphogenic proteins, and the detailed characterization of their effects on bone growth is proceeding rapidly. For example, hereditary mutations in the proteins involved in the BMP signaling pathway have been identified in a number of rare syndromes of chondrodysplasia.[60]

The BMPs are soluble growth factors, and are secreted into the extracellular matrix in the area of future bone growth. BMP signaling proceeds through a typical growth factor receptor complex: the BMP cell surface receptors BMPR-IA, BMPR-IB, and BMPR-II (Figure 3.5). The BMP growth factor ligand binds to the type II receptor, which then forms a complex with a type I receptor, stimulating the serine/threonine kinase activity contained within the intracellular portion of the type I receptor. With this binding of the extracellular ligand, the BMP pathway induces phosphorylation of the downstream effector proteins, known as SMAD proteins. The SMAD proteins, working in concert with other protein effectors, translocate the BMP signal into the nucleus of the target cell. Here transcription factors direct the expression and repression of genes responsible for the developmental and differentiation fates of the cell – driving bone growth and bone formation.[60]

The proposed therapeutic utilization for BMPs is to promote successful bone fusion in surgery to stabilize the weight-bearing elements of the spine, and we are entering an era when one can anticipate the use of these growth factors on a daily basis in surgical procedures. For instance, recent reports have revealed that delivery of the gene for bone morphogenic protein type 9 (*BMP-9*) into human mesenchymal stem cells could be accomplished.[61] These stem cells now started to express *BMP-9*. When injected along the spines of athymic rats, they induced ectopic

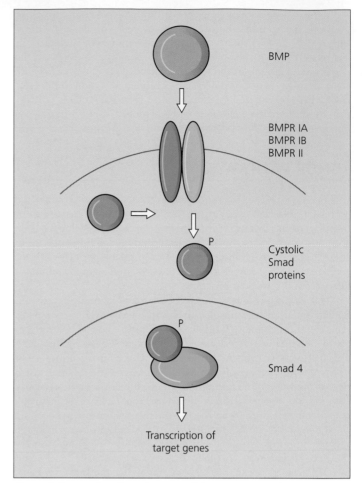

Figure 3.5 BMP signaling. The extracellular BMP growth factor (BMP2 represented here), binds to BMPR type II and recruits the dimerization with a type I receptor. The intracellular kinase activity of the type I receptor activates the b-phosphorylation of cytosolic Smad proteins. These proteins translocate to the nucleus, where they bind to Smad4 and other nuclear co-activating transcription factors and drive the expression of genes required for differentiation.

bone formation, while control cells did not. Clearly, such advances that combine gene- and cell-based therapy provide an exciting avenue for further clinical developments in spinal surgery.

CONCLUSION

Nearly every area of clinical neurosurgery has seen advances in molecular biology that are beginning to have an impact upon day-to-day practice. As the inevitable progress of molecular research carries forward into the next decade, the importance of these findings will continue. It is the appropriate integration of these advances into clinical practice that will be the exciting work of neurosurgery in the coming decades.

ACKNOWLEDGMENTS

We thank members of the Neurosurgical Service at the Massachusetts General Hospital for their helpful comments and discussion.

CLINICAL PEARLS

- Patients and families with polycystic kidney disease or inherited connective tissue diseases have an increased risk of intracranial aneurysm. The identification of the genes causing these syndromes has led to the pre-symptomatic identification of genetically at-risk individuals.

- A strongly positive genetic risk predictor is clinically similar to a "sentinel leak" – the benefits of surgical management can be realized in genetically at-risk patients prior to the morbidity and mortality of the first aneurysmal rupture.

- Epilepsy is a disorder of ion channels. Understanding the anatomy of these channel defects will have an impact on the neurosurgical management of seizure disorders.

- Gene-targeted therapeutic agents are currently under evaluation for the treatment of brain tumors.

- Growth factor and cellular-based therapies provide an exciting avenue for further clinical development in spinal and peripheral nervous system surgery.

REFERENCES

1. Schievink WI. Genetics of intracranial aneurysms. *Neurosurgery* 1997; 40: 651–62; discussion 662–3.
2. Schievink WI. Intracranial aneurysms. *N Engl J Med* 1997; 336: 28–40.
3. Schievink WI. Genetics and aneurysm formation. *Neurosurg Clin N Am* 1998; 9: 485–95.
4. Schievink WID, Schaid J, Rogers HM, Piepgras DG, Michels VV. On the inheritance of intracranial aneurysms. *Stroke* 1994; 25: 2028–37.
5. Ronkainen A, Hernesniemi J, Puranen M, *et al.* Familial intracranial aneurysms. *Lancet* 1997; 349: 380–4.
6. Chapman AB, Rubinstein D, Hughes R, *et al.* Intracranial aneurysms in autosomal dominant polycystic kidney disease. *N Engl J Med* 1992; 327: 916–20.
7. Schievink WI, Torres VE, Piepgras DG, Wiebers DO. Saccular intracranial aneurysms in autosomal dominant polycystic kidney disease. *J Am Soc Nephrol* 1992; 3: 88–95.
8. Rinkel GJ, Djibuti M, Algra A, van Gijn J. Prevalence and risk of rupture of intracranial aneurysms: a systematic review. *Stroke* 1998; 29: 251–6.
9. Belz MM, Hughes RL, Kaehny WD, *et al.* Familial clustering of ruptured intracranial aneurysms in autosomal dominant polycystic kidney disease. *Am J Kidney Dis* 2001; 38: 770–6.
10. Arnaout MA. Molecular genetics and pathogenesis of autosomal dominant polycystic kidney disease. *Annu Rev Med* 2001; 52: 93–123.
11. Reeders ST, Breuning MH, Davies KE, *et al.* A highly polymorphic DNA marker linked to adult polycystic kidney disease on chromosome 16. *Nature* 1985; 317: 542–4.
12. Kimberling WJ, Kumar S, Gabow PA, Kenyon JB, Connolly CJ, Somlo S. Autosomal dominant polycystic kidney disease: localization of the second gene to chromosome 4q13-q23. *Genomics* 1993; 18: 467–72.
13. Consortium EPKD. The polycystic kidney disease 1 gene encodes a 14 kb transcript and lies within a duplicated region on chromosome 16. The European Polycystic Kidney Disease Consortium. *Cell* 1994; 78: 725.
14. Consortium EPKD. The polycystic kidney disease 1 gene encodes a 14 kb transcript and lies within a duplicated region on chromosome 16. The European Polycystic Kidney Disease Consortium. *Cell* 1994; 77: 881–94.
15. Consortium IPKD. Polycystic kidney disease: the complete structure of the PKD1 gene and its protein. The International Polycystic Kidney Disease Consortium. *Cell* 1995; 81: 289–98.
16. Mochizuki T, Wu G, Hayashi T, *et al.* PKD2, a gene for polycystic kidney disease that encodes an integral membrane protein. *Science* 1996; 272: 1339–42.
17. Reeders ST. Multilocus polycystic disease. *Nat Genet* 1992; 1: 235–7.
18. Qian F, Watnick TJ, Onuchic LF, Germino GG. The molecular basis of focal cyst formation in human autosomal dominant polycystic kidney disease type I. *Cell* 1996; 87: 979–87.
19. Kim K, Drummond I, Ibraghimov-Beskrovnaya O, Klinger K, Arnaout MA. Polycystin 1 is required for the structural integrity of blood vessels. *Proc Natl Acad Sci USA* 2000; 97: 1731–6.
20. Griffin MD, Torres VE, Grande JP, Kumar R. Vascular expression of polycystin. *J Am Soc Nephrol* 1997; 8: 616–26.
21. Ong AC, Ward CJ, Butler RJ, *et al.* Coordinate expression of the autosomal dominant polycystic kidney disease proteins, polycystin-2 and polycystin-1, in normal and cystic tissue. *Am J Pathol* 1999; 154: 1721–9.
22. Peters DJ, van de Wal A, Spruit L, *et al.* Cellular localization and tissue distribution of polycystin-1. *J Pathol* 1999; 188: 439–46.
23. Schievink WI, Torres VE, Wiebers DO, Huston J, 3rd. Intracranial arterial dolichoectasia in autosomal dominant polycystic kidney disease. *J Am Soc Nephrol* 1997; 8: 1298–303.
24. Graf S, Schischma A, Eberhardt KE, Istel R, Stiasny B, Schulze BD. Intracranial aneurysms and dolichoectasia in autosomal dominant polycystic kidney disease. *Nephrol Dial Transplant* 2002; 17: 819–23.
25. Watnick T, Phakdeekitcharoen B, Johnson A, *et al.* Mutation detection of PKD1 identifies a novel mutation common to three families with aneurysms and/or very-early-onset disease. *Am J Hum Genet* 1999; 65: 1561–71.
26. Huston J, 3rd, Torres VE, Wiebers DO, Schievink WI. Follow-up of intracranial aneurysms in autosomal dominant polycystic kidney disease by magnetic resonance angiography. *J Am Soc Nephrol* 1996; 7: 2135–41.
27. Onda H, Kasuya H, Yoneyama T, *et al.* Genomewide-linkage and haplotype-association studies map intracranial aneurysm to chromosome 7q11. *Am J Hum Genet* 2001; 69: 804–19.
28. Olson JM, Vongpunsawad S, Kuivaniemi H, *et al.* Search for intracranial aneurysm susceptibility gene(s) using Finnish families. *BMC Med Genet* 2002; 3: 7.
29. Mason I, Aase JM, Orrison WW, Wicks JD, Seigel RS, Bicknell JM. Familial cavernous angiomas of the brain in an Hispanic family. *Neurology* 1988; 38: 324–6.
30. Rigamonti D, Hadley MN, Drayer BP, *et al.* Cerebral cavernous malformations. Incidence and familial occurrence. *N Engl J Med* 1988; 319: 343–7.
31. Dubovsky J, Zabramski JM, Kurth J, *et al.* A gene responsible for cavernous malformations of the brain maps to chromosome 7q. *Hum Mol Genet* 1995; 4: 453–8.
32. Gunel M, Awad IA, Finberg K, *et al.* A founder mutation as a cause of cerebral cavernous malformation in Hispanic Americans. *N Engl J Med* 1996; 334: 946–51.
33. Laberge-le Couteulx S, Jung HH, Labauge P, *et al.* Truncating

mutations in CCM1, encoding KRIT1, cause hereditary cavernous angiomas. *Nat Genet* 1999; 23: 189–93.

34. Zhang J, Clatterbuck RE, Rigamonti D, Chang DD, Dietz HC. Interaction between krit1 and icap1alpha infers perturbation of integrin beta1-mediated angiogenesis in the pathogenesis of cerebral cavernous malformation. *Hum Mol Genet* 2001; 10: 2953–60.

35. Alekov A, Rahman MM, Mitrovic N, Lehmann-Horn F, Lerche H. A sodium channel mutation causing epilepsy in man exhibits subtle defects in fast inactivation and activation in vitro. *J Physiol* 2000; 529: 533–9.

36. Lossin C, Wang DW, Rhodes TH, Vanoye CG, George, AL, Jr. Molecular basis of an inherited epilepsy. *Neuron* 2002; 34: 877–84.

37. Watanabe H, Nagata E, Kosakai A, *et al*. Disruption of the epilepsy KCNQ2 gene results in neural hyperexcitability. *J Neurochem* 2000; 75: 28–33.

38. Dedek K, Kunath B, Kananura C, Reuner U, Jentsch TJ, Steinlein OK. Myokymia and neonatal epilepsy caused by a mutation in the voltage sensor of the KCNQ2 K^+ channel. *Proc Natl Acad Sci USA* 2001; 98: 12272–7.

39. Hahn WC, Weinberg RA. Rules for making human tumor cells. *N Engl J Med* 2002; 347: 1593–603.

40. Li J, Yen C, Liaw D, *et al*. PTEN, a putative protein tyrosine phosphatase gene mutated in human brain, breast, and prostate cancer. *Science* 1997; 275: 1943–7.

41. Steck PA, Pershouse MA, Jasser SA, *et al*. Identification of a candidate tumour suppressor gene, MMAC1, at chromosome 10q23.3 that is mutated in multiple advanced cancers. *Nat Genet* 1997; 15: 356–62.

42. Wang SI, Puc J, Li J, *et al*. Somatic mutations of PTEN in glioblastoma multiforme. *Cancer Res* 1997; 57: 4183–6.

43. Bostrom J, Cobbers JM, Wolter M, *et al*. Mutation of the PTEN (MMAC1) tumor suppressor gene in a subset of glioblastomas but not in meningiomas with loss of chromosome arm 10q. *Cancer Res* 1998; 58: 29–33.

44. Schmidt EE, Ichimura K, Goike HM, Moshref A, Liu L, Collins VP. Mutational profile of the PTEN gene in primary human astrocytic tumors and cultivated xenografts. *J Neuropathol Exp Neurol* 1999; 58: 1170–83.

45. Li J, Simpson L, Takahashi M, *et al*. The PTEN/MMAC1 tumor suppressor induces cell death that is rescued by the AKT/protein kinase B oncogene. *Cancer Res* 1998; 58: 5667–72.

46. Stambolic V, Suzuki A, de la Pompa JL, *et al*. Negative regulation of PKB/Akt-dependent cell survival by the tumor suppressor PTEN. *Cell* 1998; 95: 29–39.

47. Knobbe CB, Merlo A, Reifenberger G. Pten signaling in gliomas. *Neuro-oncology* 2002; 4: 196–211.

48. Ueki K, Ono Y, Henson JW, Efird JT, von Deimling A, Louis DN. CDKN2/p16 or RB alterations occur in the majority of glioblastomas and are inversely correlated. *Cancer Res* 1996; 56: 150–3.

49. Wong AJ, Bigner SH, Bigner DD, Kinzler KW, Hamilton SR, Vogelstein B. Increased expression of the epidermal growth factor receptor gene in malignant gliomas is invariably associated with gene amplification. *Proc Natl Acad Sci USA* 1987; 84: 6899–903.

50. Maher EA, Furnari FB, Bachoo RM, *et al*. Malignant glioma: genetics and biology of a grave matter. *Genes Dev* 2001; 15: 1311–33.

51. Sugawa N, Ekstrand AJ, James CD, Collins VP. Identical splicing of aberrant epidermal growth factor receptor transcripts from amplified rearranged genes in human glioblastomas. *Proc Natl Acad Sci USA* 1990; 87: 8602–6.

52. Cokgor I, Akabani G, Kuan CT, *et al*. Phase I trial results of iodine-131-labeled antitenascin monoclonal antibody 81C6 treatment of patients with newly diagnosed malignant gliomas. *J Clin Oncol* 2000; 18: 3862–72.

53. Hagihara N, Walbridge S, Olson AW, Oldfield EH, Youle RJ. Vascular protection by chloroquine during brain tumor therapy with Tf-CRM107. *Cancer Res* 2000; 60: 230–4.

54. Chiocca EA. Oncolytic viruses. *Nature Reviews Cancer* 2002; 2: 938–50.

55. Ellem KA, O'Rourke MG, Johnson GR, *et al*. A case report: immune responses and clinical course of the first human use of granulocyte/macrophage-colony-stimulating-factor-transduced autologous melanoma cells for immunotherapy. *Cancer Immunol Immunother* 1997; 44: 10–20.

56. Liau LM, Black KL, Prins RM, *et al*. Treatment of intracranial gliomas with bone marrow-derived dendritic cells pulsed with tumor antigens. *J Neurosurg* 1999; 90: 1115–24.

57. Yu JS, Wheeler CJ, Zeltzer PM, *et al*. Vaccination of malignant glioma patients with peptide-pulsed dendritic cells elicits systemic cytotoxicity and intracranial T-cell infiltration. *Cancer Res* 2001; 61: 842–7.

58. Wozney JM, Rosen V, Celeste AJ, *et al*. Novel regulators of bone formation: molecular clones and activities. *Science* 1988; 242: 1528–34.

59. Wozney JM, Rosen V. Bone morphogenetic protein and bone morphogenetic protein gene family in bone formation and repair. *Clin Orthop* 1998; 346: 26–37.

60. Massague J, Blain SW, Lo RS. TGFbeta signaling in growth control, cancer, and heritable disorders. *Cell* 2000; 103: 295–309.

61. Dumont RJ, Dayoub H, Li JZ, *et al*. Ex vivo bone morphogenetic protein-9 gene therapy using human mesenchymal stem cells induces spinal fusion in rodents. *Neurosurgery* 2002; 51: 1239–45.

62. Charlier C, Singh NA, Ryan SG, *et al*. A pore mutation in a novel KQT-like potassium channel gene in an idiopathic epilepsy family. *Nat Genet* 1998; 18: 53–5.

63. Singh NA, Charlier C, Stauffer D, *et al*. A novel potassium channel gene, KCNQ2, is mutated in an inherited epilepsy of newborns. *Nat Genet* 1998; 18: 25–9.

64. Steinlein OK, Mulley JC, Propping P, *et al*. A missense mutation in the neuronal nicotinic acetylcholine receptor alpha 4 subunit is associated with autosomal dominant nocturnal frontal lobe epilepsy. *Nat Genet* 1995; 11: 201–3.

65. De Fusco M, Becchetti A, Patrignani A, *et al*. The nicotinic receptor beta 2 subunit is mutant in nocturnal frontal lobe epilepsy. *Nat Genet* 2000; 26: 275–6.

66. Escayg A, MacDonald BT, Meisler MH, *et al*. Mutations of SCN1A, encoding a neuronal sodium channel, in two families with GEFS+2. *Nat Genet* 2000; 24: 343–5.

67. Wallace RH, Wang DW, Singh R, *et al*. Febrile seizures and generalized epilepsy associated with a mutation in the Na^+-channel beta1 subunit gene SCN1B. *Nat Genet* 1998; 19: 366–70.

68. Sugawara T, Tsurubuchi Y, Agarwala KL, *et al*. A missense mutation of the Na^+ channel alpha II subunit gene Na(v)1.2 in a patient with febrile and afebrile seizures causes channel dysfunction. *Proc Natl Acad Sci USA* 2001; 98: 6384–9.

69. Baulac S, Huberfeld G, Gourfinkel-An I, *et al*. First genetic evidence of GABA(A) receptor dysfunction in epilepsy: a mutation in the gamma2-subunit gene. *Nat Genet* 2001; 28: 46–8.

70. Escayg A, De Waard M, Lee DD, *et al*. Coding and noncoding variation of the human calcium-channel beta-4-subunit gene CACNB4 in patients with idiopathic generalized epilepsy and episodic ataxia. *Am J Hum Genet* 2000; 66: 1531–9.

71. Cossette P, Liu L, Brisebois K, *et al*. Mutation of GABRA1 in an autosomal dominant form of juvenile myoclonic epilepsy. *Nat Genet* 2002; 31: 184–9.

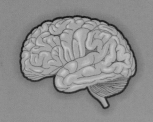

INCREASED INTRACRANIAL PRESSURE, CEREBRAL EDEMA, AND BRAIN HERNIATION

4

Setti S Rengachary

The vertebrate cranium is a rigid structure. The major intracranial contents are the *brain* (including the neuroglial elements and interstitial fluid), *blood* (arterial and venous) and *cerebrospinal fluid* (CSF; Table 4.1). Because the intracranial volume is constant, when an intracranial mass is introduced, compensation must occur through a reciprocal decrease in the volume of venous blood and CSF. This is the Monro–Kellie–Burrows doctrine (Figure 4.1), which has been confirmed by many experimental and clinical observations. Only in children whose sutures have not yet fused can the cranium itself expand to accommodate extra volume. The relative volume of CSF increases with advancing age because of brain atrophy.

To maintain pressure within the physiologic range the venous system collapses easily, squeezing venous blood out through the jugular veins, or through the emissary and scalp veins. CSF, likewise, can be displaced through the foramen magnum into the spinal subarachnoid space. When these compensatory mechanisms have been exhausted, minute changes in volume produce precipitous increases in pressure. This can be demonstrated in an experimental model by inserting a Foley catheter into the epidural space and inflating the balloon gradually. The curve produced by plotting intracranial pressure against volume (Figure 4.2) is initially flat because of the pressure-buffering capacity offered by displacement of CSF and venous blood. Later, there is a precipitous increase in pressure because compensatory mechanisms have been exceeded. Brain parenchyma and arterial blood do not participate, to any significant extent, in the intracranial pressure-buffering mechanism.

Compliance (dV/dP) is the change in volume observed for a given change in pressure. This represents the accommodative potential of the intracranial space. Compliance is high when the cranial cavity will permit the accommodation of a large mass with very little change in pressure. In clinical practice, however, what is measured is *elastance (dP/dV)*, the inverse of compliance; that is the change in pressure observed for a given change in volume. It represents the resistance to outward expansion of an intracranial mass. Elastance can be measured at the bedside by injecting 1 mL of sterile saline through the ventricular catheter in 1 second and observing the change in pressure – an increase of less than 2 mmHg implies low elastance and high compliance. However, the high risk of infection associated with this maneuver precludes its use.

THE BLOOD–BRAIN BARRIER

Not all substances that are carried in the blood reach neural tissue – a barrier blocks the entry of many substances into the brain. This barrier resides in the cerebral capillaries. Its function is to regulate the flow of biologically active substances into the brain and to protect the sensitive neural tissue from toxic materials.

Comparison of the structural differences between somatic capillaries and brain capillaries helps us to understand the anatomic basis of the blood–brain barrier (Figure 4.3). In the somatic capillary, blood components pass freely through the fenestrae between endothelial cells. Also, certain materials are transported directly across the capillary cell wall through bulk transport via pinocytotic vesicles. The endothelial cells of brain capillaries, on the other hand, are connected by tight junctions. These junctions act as a barrier to the passive movement of many substances across the endothelium. There are two mechanisms by which materials may be transported across the endothelial cells. Lipid-soluble substances can usually penetrate all capillary endothelial cell membranes in a passive manner. Amino acids and sugars are transported across the capillary endothelium by specific carrier-mediated mechanisms. A specific transferrin receptor on the brain endothelial cell surface is thought to play a key role in transendothelial transport.

The physiology of the blood–brain barrier is especially important in certain clinical settings. First, when there is a disruption of the blood–brain barrier by any cause, plasma components easily cross the barrier into neural tissue, causing *vasogenic edema*. Second, tight junctions can be transiently opened artificially by the intra-arterial injection of a bolus of an osmotic agent, such as mannitol, which dehydrates the endothelial cells. Recently, bradykinin, or better still its analog RMP-7, has been used for the same purpose. During this brief interval, which lasts for a few hours, certain chemotherapeutic or other agents can be administered that would not otherwise cross the barrier. Third, when mannitol is given intravenously, the concentration in the

Table 4.1 Intracranial contents and their respective volumes

Content	Volume	Percentage of total volume
Brain (70%) and interstitial fluid (10%)	1400 mL	80%
Blood	150 mL	10%
Cerebrospinal fluid	150 mL	10%
Total	1700 mL	100%

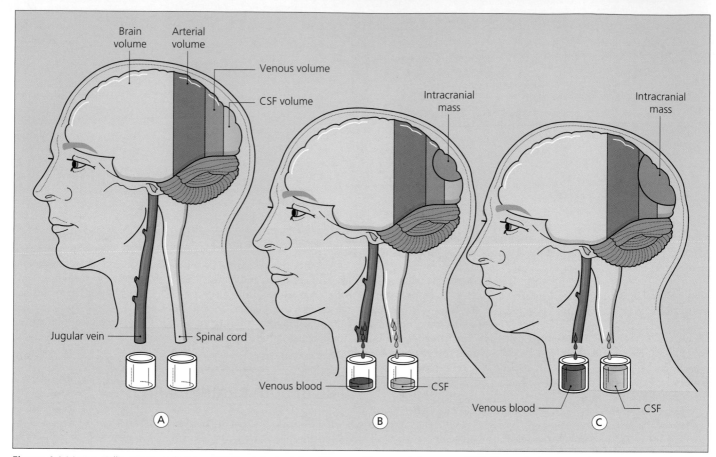

Figure 4.1 Monro–Kellie–Burrows doctrine. **(A)** Physiologic state with normal intracranial pressure (ICP). The major intracranial components are brain (80%), arterial and venous blood (10%), and CSF (10%). The cranium is a rigid container, the intracranial volume is constant, and the normal intracranial contents are shown with ICP within physiologic range (10 to 15 mm Hg). **(B)** Intracranial mass with compensation (normal ICP). This patient has an intracranial mass (space-occupying lesion) of moderate size. Because intracranial volume is constant, the increasing volume caused by the mass is compensated by a decrease in the intracranial content. Venous volume decreases through egress of venous blood from the intracranial cavity into the jugular veins. CSF volume decreases because of egress of CSF through the foramen magnum into the spinal canal. The brain itself is nearly incompressible, and thus no significant change in its volume occurs; neither is there change in arterial volume. Intracranial volume is constant and there is no net rise in ICP (pressure buffering). **(C)** Intracranial mass with decompensation and elevated ICP. The intracranial mass is much larger, beyond the pressure-buffering capacity of venous blood and CSF; there is a net rise in ICP.

cerebral capillary is quite low; however, it is sufficient to create an osmotic gradient between the cerebral tissue and the capillary, allowing withdrawal of interstitial fluid into the capillary lumen. An intact tight junction is necessary for this to occur. If the tight junctions are not intact, mannitol will permeate the neural tissue, preventing the formation of an osmotic gradient.

CEREBRAL EDEMA

Cerebral edema may be defined as a state of increased brain volume as a result of an increase in water content. There are three types of cerebral edema (Table 4.2).

Vasogenic edema is the most common form of brain edema encountered in clinical practice (Figure 4.4). It results from increased permeability of capillaries. The tight junctions between the endothelial cells become incompetent, allowing plasma filtrate to escape into the intercellular space (Figure 4.5). The phenomenon of contrast enhancement in computed tomography

(CT) and magnetic resonance imaging (MRI) scans is, in part, because of the breakdown of the blood–brain barrier and resultant vasogenic edema. Vasogenic edema is most commonly seen with trauma, tumor and abscess. The edema is more marked in white matter than in gray matter.

Cytotoxic edema most commonly results from hypoxia of the neural tissue. The hypoxia affects the ATP-dependent sodium pump mechanism in the cell membrane, promoting an accumulation of intracellular sodium and the subsequent flow of water into the cell to maintain osmotic equilibrium. Thus, the edema is primarily intracellular and affects virtually all cells, including the endothelial cells, astrocytes, and neurons. Because of the swelling of these cells, the interstitial space is considerably narrowed (see Figure 4.5). The two most common causes of cytotoxic edema are tissue hypoxia and water intoxication. The CT scan commonly shows only subtle changes, or indeed no changes at all, indicative of cytotoxic edema in the early phases of ischemic stroke.

Interstitial edema results from transudation of CSF in obstructive hydrocephalus. This is best observed on CT or MRI

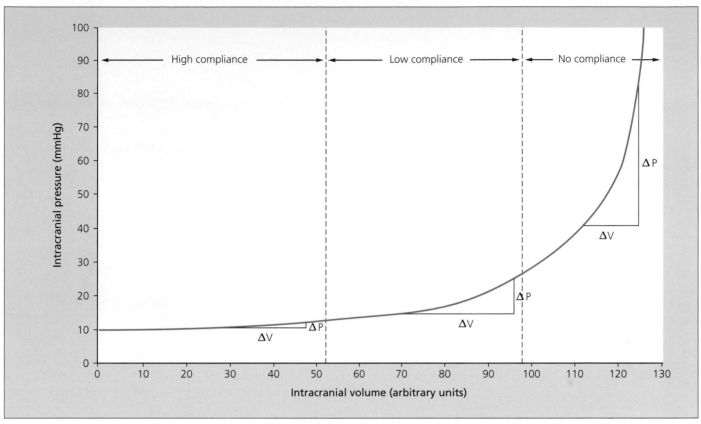

Figure 4.2 Pressure–volume curve. If an intracranial balloon is expanded slowly in a laboratory animal and the ICP and the balloon's volume are plotted, an exponential curve results. In the initial phase there is virtually no increase in ICP because of the compensatory decrease in CSF and venous volumes. The compliance is high (elastance low). With further expansion of the balloon, the ICP begins to rise. Compliance is low (elastance high). In the terminal stages, when the compensatory mechanisms are exhausted, there is a steep rise in pressure (no compliance, highest elastance).

Table 4.2 Types and characteristics of cerebral edema

	Vasogenic edema (extracellular edema)	Cytotoxic edema (intracellular edema)	Interstitial edema
Pathogenesis	Increased capillary permeability	Cellular swelling (neuronal, glial, and endothelial cells)	Increased brain water due to impairment of absorption of CSF
Location of edema	Mainly white matter	Gray and white matter	Transependymal flow of CSF and interstitial edema in the peri-ventricular white matter in hydrocephalus
Composition of edema fluid	Plasma filtrate containing plasma proteins	Increased intracellular water and sodium due to failure of membrane transport	CSF
Extracellular fluid	Increased	Decreased	Increased
Pathologic lesion causing edema	Primary or metastatic tumor, abscess, late stages of infarction, trauma	Early stages of infarction, water intoxication	Obstructive or communicating hydrocephalus
Effect of steroids	Effective	Not effective	Not effective
Effect of mannitol	Effective	Effective	Questionable

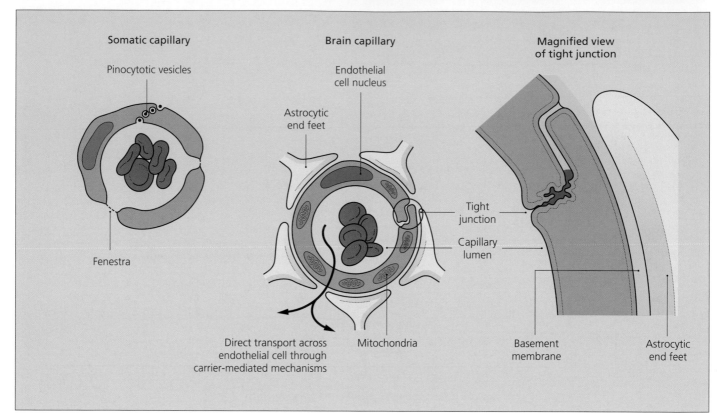

Figure 4.3 Differences between somatic and brain capillaries. In the somatic capillary, fenestrations between endothelial cells allow free flow of plasma components into the tissues. In addition, there is bulky flow of plasma components across endothelial cells via pinocytotic vesicles. In the brain capillary, the endothelial cells are attached to each other by tight junctions. There are no intervening fenestrae. Certain selected plasma components cross the endothelial membrane if they are lipid-soluble; others, such as amino acids and sugars, are transported across the endothelial cells through carrier-mediated mechanism. The large number of mitochondria in the brain endothelial cells generate energy for active transport.

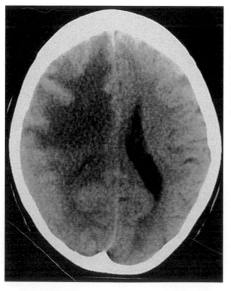

Figure 4.4 CT scan of a patient with vasogenic edema caused by metastatic tumor. Note that the edema involves predominantly the white matter.

scans as periventricular low density areas because of the retrograde transependymal flow of CSF into the interstitial space of the white matter (Figure 4.6). This is most commonly observed in the frontal region. This finding generally indicates active hydrocephalus requiring surgical therapy.

CEREBRAL BLOOD FLOW

Normal cerebral blood flow averages 55 to 60 mL/100 g brain tissue/min. In the gray matter the blood flow is 75 mL/100 g brain tissue/min, whereas in the white matter it is only 45 mL/100 g brain tissue/min. This flow is sufficient to meet the metabolic needs of the brain. The most significant factor that determines cerebral blood flow at any given time is the cerebral perfusion pressure, which is the effective blood pressure gradient across the brain. It is the difference between the incoming mean arterial pressure and the opposing intracranial pressure. The mean arterial pressure is the diastolic pressure plus one-third of the pulse pressure. With increased intracranial pressure there is a tendency for the cerebral perfusion pressure to decrease.

Three major factors regulate cerebral blood flow under physiologic conditions (Figure 4.7): systemic blood pressure, concentration of CO_2 and hydrogen ions in the arterial blood, and oxygen concentration. The ability to maintain blood flow to the brain at a constant level over a wide range of mean arterial pressures (50–160 mmHg) is called autoregulation. When the mean arterial pressure is low, the cerebral arterioles dilate to allow adequate flow at the decreased pressure. Conversely, an increase in systemic blood pressure causes the arterioles to constrict and maintain the flow within physiologic range.

Cerebral blood flow cannot always be regulated. When the mean arterial blood pressure falls below 50 mmHg, such as in

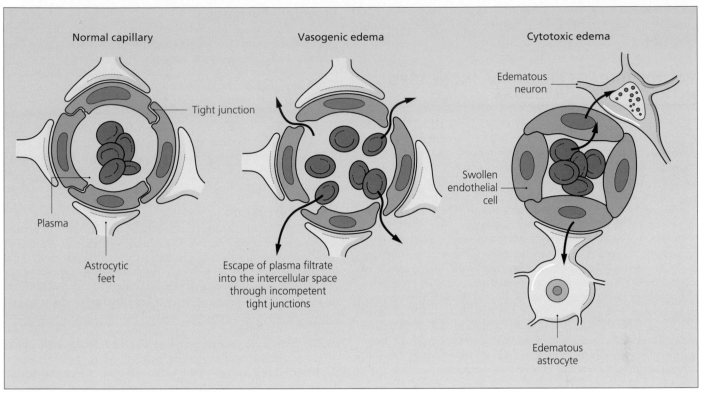

Figure 4.5 Normal appearance of a cerebral capillary contrasted with the changes that occur in vasogenic or cytotoxic edema. Under normal conditions, the intercellular tight junctions are intact. In vasogenic edema, the tight junctions are not competent, allowing leakage of plasma into the interstitial space. In cytotoxic edema, there is a primary failure of ATP-dependent sodium pump mechanism resulting in intracellular accumulation of sodium and secondarily water.

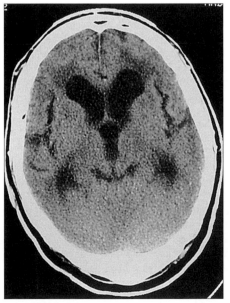

Figure 4.6 CT scan of a patient with active hydrocephalus showing periventricular low density representing transependymal flow of CSF (interstitial edema).

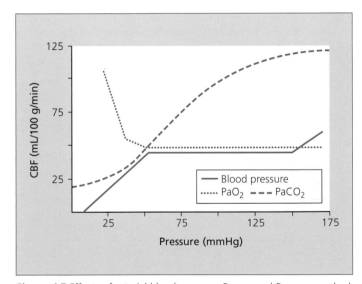

Figure 4.7 Effects of arterial blood pressure, $PaCO_2$, and PaO_2 on cerebral blood flow (CBF).

hypovolemic shock, there is inadequate perfusion of the brain. When the mean arterial pressure exceeds 150 mmHg the autoregulatory system fails. There is a passive increase in blood flow proportionate to the increase in systemic pressure, causing, in extreme cases, exudation of fluid from the vascular system with resultant vasogenic edema. This cascade results in hypertensive

encephalopathy. Carbon dioxide tension is the most potent stimulus for cerebrovascular dilatation. There is a graded increase in cerebral blood flow with an increase from 15 to 80 mmHg PCO_2. Hyperventilation, by decreasing the CO_2 tension in the blood, decreases both cerebral blood flow and cerebral blood volume in the brain. Hypoxia causes cerebrovascular dilatation, which becomes apparent when the oxygen tension in the blood drops down to 50 mmHg, and becomes maximal around 20 mmHg.

PATHOLOGICAL EFFECTS OF INCREASED INTRACRANIAL PRESSURE

Normal intracranial pressure (ICP) ranges from 10 to 15 mmHg (136 to 204 mmH$_2$O). This is primarily contributed by arterial pulsations transmitted to the brain directly and through the choroid plexus. An increase in ICP always occurs when there is a disparity between intracranial volume and the intracranial contents. Common causes of raised ICP are listed in Table 4.3.

An increase in ICP can cause deleterious effects on the brain in two ways. First, brain ischemia may occur when the cerebral perfusion pressure is reduced to critical levels. Second, focal masses can cause distortion and herniation of the brain, resulting in compression of critical brainstem structures. The presence of herniation syndromes with occlusion of the tentorial incisura or the aqueduct further elevates the ICP by blocking CSF pathways. As a general rule, an increase in ICP without a shift of brain structures is better tolerated than an increase secondary to a focal mass. Examples of generalized increased pressure without brain shift include pseudotumor cerebri and chronic hydrocephalus. In these disorders, the patient may or may not have a headache.

TYPES OF BRAIN HERNIATION

The brain is supported by dural folds that prevent undue movements of the brain within the cranial cavity (Figure 4.8). There are two major dural folds – the *falx cerebri* and the *tentorium cerebelli*. The falx cerebri is a sickle-shaped dural fold in the midline that separates the two cerebral hemispheres. The tentorium cerebelli is a tent-shaped dural fold that separates the occipital lobes from the posterior fossa structures. The tentorial incisura, or hiatus, is the dural opening that surrounds the rostral brainstem.

Table 4.3 Common causes of increased intracranial pressure

Pathologic process	Representative examples
Localized masses	Hematomas: epidural, subdural, intracerebral Neoplasms: gliomas, meningiomas, metastases Abscesses Focal edema due to trauma, infarction, tumor
Obstruction to CSF pathways	Obstructive hydrocephalus Communicating hydrocephalus
Obstruction to major venous sinuses	Depressed skull fracture over major venous sinuses, thromboembolic disease from contraceptive pills
Diffuse brain edema or swelling	Encephalitis, meningitis, diffuse head injury, subarachnoid hemorrhage, Reye's syndrome, lead encephalopathy, water intoxication from fluid overload, near-drowning
Idiopathic	Pseudotumor cerebri

Cingulate herniation

A focal mass lesion in the supratentorial compartment exerts progressive pressure locally on the ipsilateral hemisphere. The increase in ICP may not be uniform; it is greatest close to the mass, thus creating a pressure gradient. A supratentorial mass lesion may displace the cingulate gyrus, which is next to the free edge of the falx cerebri, and cause it to herniate under the falx to the opposite side. There is usually displacement of the ventricular system as well (Figure 4.9). The anterior cerebral artery may be compromised by the tight, sharp edge of the falx cerebri. There are no clinical signs and symptoms specific to a cingulate herniation.

Uncal herniation

Uncal herniation is the most dramatic and most common herniation syndrome observed clinically. Uncal herniation is often seen with lesions of the middle cranial fossa, such as acute epidural hematoma, subdural hematoma, temporal lobe contusions, or temporal lobe neoplasms. An expansile mass of the middle fossa causes the uncus, the most inferomedial structure of the temporal lobe, to herniate between the rostral brainstem and the tentorial edge into the posterior fossa (see Figure 4.12). In post-mortem studies, a deep groove may be noticed at the lateral margin of the uncus as a manifestation of the herniation. In some instances, the medial displacement of the brainstem may cause compression of the brainstem against the opposite tentorial edge, producing a notch called Kernohan's notch.

With uncal herniation, the clinical syndrome consists of progressively impaired consciousness, dilated ipsilateral pupil, and contralateral hemiplegia. The impaired consciousness results from compression of the reticular activating system in the rostral brainstem. The dilated pupil is the result of compression of the third nerve, which carries the parasympathetic pupilloconstrictor fibers. Contralateral hemiplegia results from direct compression of the cerebral peduncle, which carries corticospinal fibers to the opposite side. When a Kernohan's notch is present, the hemiplegia will be on the ipsilateral side. In some patients with uncal herniation, the posterior cerebral artery may be compromised, causing secondary infarction of the occipital lobe on one or both sides.

Central transtentorial herniation

In contrast to uncal herniation, which occurs from mass lesions located to the tentorial hiatus, central transtentorial herniation occurs with mass lesions far removed from the tentorial hiatus, such as in frontal, parietal, or occipital areas. Bilateral mass lesions, such as bilateral subdural hematomas, can also cause central herniation. There is a downward displacement of the diencephalon and midbrain centrally through the tentorial incisura (see Figure 4.12). The clinical syndrome in central herniation is not as easily recognizable as that of uncal herniation. The patient with central transtentorial herniation tends to have bilaterally small, reactive pupils, exhibits Cheyne–Stokes respirations, is quite obtunded, and may show loss of vertical gaze.

Tonsillar herniation

Acute tonsillar herniation generally results from acute expansion of posterior fossa lesions. It may result from an ill-advised lumbar puncture in a patient with a mass lesion within the cranial cavity.

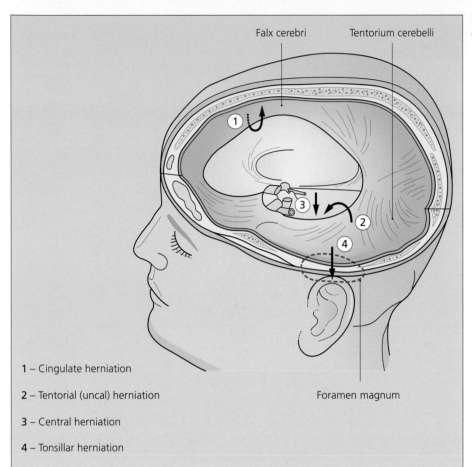

Falx cerebri   Tentorium cerebelli

Foramen magnum

1 – Cingulate herniation

2 – Tentorial (uncal) herniation

3 – Central herniation

4 – Tonsillar herniation

Figure 4.8 Dural folds within the cranial cavity and associated herniation sites.

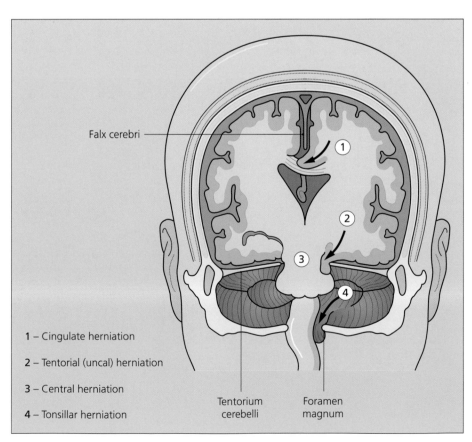

Falx cerebri

1 – Cingulate herniation

2 – Tentorial (uncal) herniation

3 – Central herniation

4 – Tonsillar herniation

Tentorium cerebelli   Foramen magnum

Figure 4.9 Types of brain herniation.

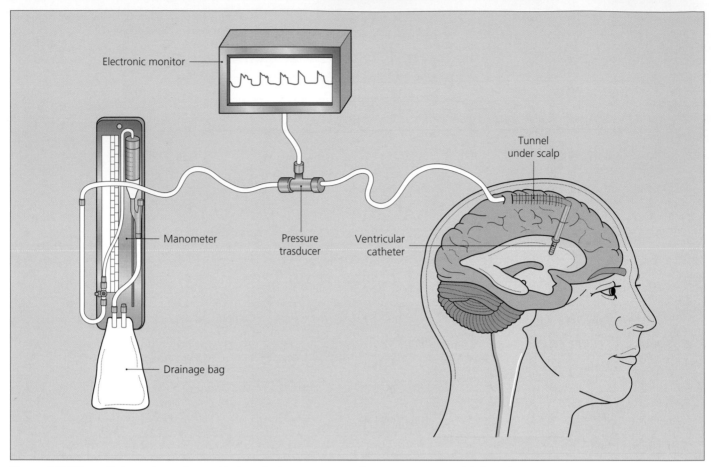

Figure 4.10 ICP monitoring system using ventricular catheter, pressure transducer, manometer, and drainage bag.

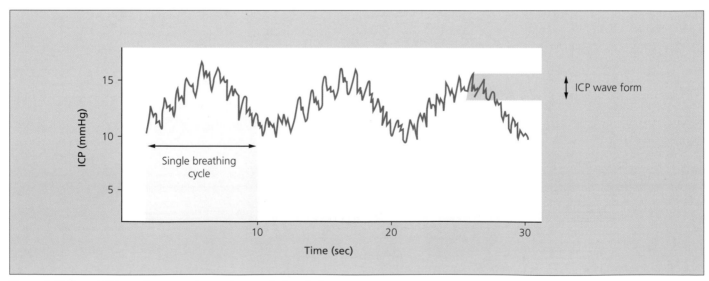

Figure 4.11 Normal ICP waveform superimposed on respiratory rhythm.

The tonsil of the cerebellum herniates through the foramen magnum into the upper spinal canal, compressing the medulla (see Fig. 4.12). The manifestations of acute medullary compression are cardiorespiratory impairment, hypertension, high pulse pressure, Cheyne–Stokes respirations, neurogenic hyperventilation, and impaired consciousness. The patient may have a stiff neck or be in an opisthotonic position. Decorticate or decerebrate posturing may be present as well.

SYMPTOMS AND SIGNS

The most common symptom of increased ICP is headache. It is generalized in nature and is worse at night or when the patient is recumbent, presumably because of the increase in CO_2 tension and increased venous pressure. The pain-sensitive structures within the cranial cavity are the dura and the blood vessels. Focal mass lesions that distort the dura and stretch the vessels tend to cause headache more frequently than diffuse generalized increases in ICP without focal mass effect, such as a pseudotumor cerebri or hydrocephalus. The headache, if present, may be associated with nausea and vomiting. Projectile vomiting is thought to be indicative of an intracranial mass and increased pressure, but clinical experience has shown that all vomiting, regardless of the cause, is projectile and one cannot assign intracranial etiology from the nature of vomiting. The vomiting associated with increased ICP is usually not associated with nausea. Vomiting associated with neurologic signs such as ataxia, papilledema and cranial nerve paralysis is most likely associated with an intracranial lesion. Papilledema is another cardinal sign of increased ICP.

The symptoms of increased ICP vary depending on whether the increased pressure is of a chronic, slowly progressive nature or results from an acute, rapidly evolving lesion, such as a clot that follows trauma. When there is an acute and rapid rise in ICP the patient generally becomes obtunded and there may be signs of brainstem compression from herniation. This is manifested by irregular breathing patterns, decorticate or decerebrate rigidity, hemiplegia, and pupillary inequality.

MONITORING INTRACRANIAL PRESSURE

The most significant factor determining morbidity and mortality in patients with neurosurgical disorders is increased ICP. Continuous ICP monitoring is very useful for assessing intracranial dynamics in patients with suspected increased pressure. There are no clinical indicators that can be used at an early stage of rising ICP to forestall a further rise. The classic clinical indicators described in the literature occur in the end stage and they are not sensitive enough to show subtle changes in pressure. Equally important is the role of ICP monitoring in assessing treatment regimens for increased pressure. The two most common indications for ICP monitoring are closed head injury and subarachnoid hemorrhage. Although significant neurologic impairment can occur in neurosurgical disorders without elevation of pressure (head injury), the vast majority have significant elevation of ICP.

Techniques of monitoring ICP

Intracranial pressure is best measured directly and continuously from the cranial cavity. Although lumbar puncture can indirectly indicate ICP, it is neither safe nor accurate. It is not safe because it might precipitate tonsillar and uncal herniation. It may not be accurate if the subarachnoid pathways in the vicinity of the tentorial incisura are blocked, for then the spinal subarachnoid compartment is isolated from the supratentorial subarachnoid compartment.

There are two commonly used pressure-monitoring systems in contemporary neurosurgical practice. An intraventricular catheter connected to a manometer and a drainage system is the simplest and most economical method and represents the standard against which all other systems are compared. The ventricular catheter ideally should be tunneled under the skin and brought out through a separate stab wound, well away from the ventricular entry site, to minimize the risk of infection, which is the most significant complication of intraventricular pressure monitoring. Using an electronic transducer, the waveform can also be monitored (Figure 4.10). The major advantage of the method is that the ventricular catheter is used not only to measure the pressure, but also as a treatment modality allowing continuous drainage of CSF when the pressure exceeds physiologic limits.

A second method is the use of the fiberoptic transducer-tipped catheter system. The transducer-tipped catheter can be placed within the ventricle or brain parenchyma or in the subdural space, depending on the surgeon's choice and the clinical situation. The pressure monitor gives both digital readout and a waveform. The advantages of this system are that the zero point does not have to be reset with changes in head position because the pressure-sensing transducer is within the cranial cavity, and it is not susceptible to blockage by debris and air bubbles because it is not a fluid-coupled system. The disadvantages of this system, however, are: (1) higher cost; (2) inability to tunnel – the fiberoptic cables tend to break at acute angles, so that extended monitoring using the same port carries a higher risk of infection; (3) baseline drift – with prolonged monitoring the indicated pressures become less reliable; and (4) possible inaccuracy of intraparenchymal pressure readings – there is some concern about whether they truly reflect ICP.

ICP WAVEFORMS

The waveform of normal ICP typically shows three arterial components superimposed on the respiratory rhythm (Figure 4.11). The first arterial wave is the percussion wave, followed by the tidal wave, which ends in the dicrotic notch. This notch is followed by the dicrotic wave. Under physiologic conditions, the percussion wave is the tallest, with the tidal and dicrotic waves having progressively smaller amplitudes (Figure 4.12A). When the ICP rises even to a modest degree (by 20 mmHg) the waveform may change, with the peaks of the tidal or dicrotic waves exceeding that of the percussion wave (Figure 4.12B). Such alterations in the morphology of the pressure tracing indicate decreasing compliance and increasing ICP.

When the ICP waveforms are registered over a period of time, certain trends may become apparent (Figure 4.13). Plateau waves, or type A waves, are characterized by an abrupt elevation in ICP for 5 to 20 min followed by a rapid fall in the pressure to resting levels. The amplitude may reach as high as 50–100 mmHg. Plateau waves may be clinically marked by a decreasing level of consciousness, restlessness, increased tone in the extremities, and tonic–clonic movements. Plateau waves may represent transient surges in ICP secondary to increased cerebral blood volume,

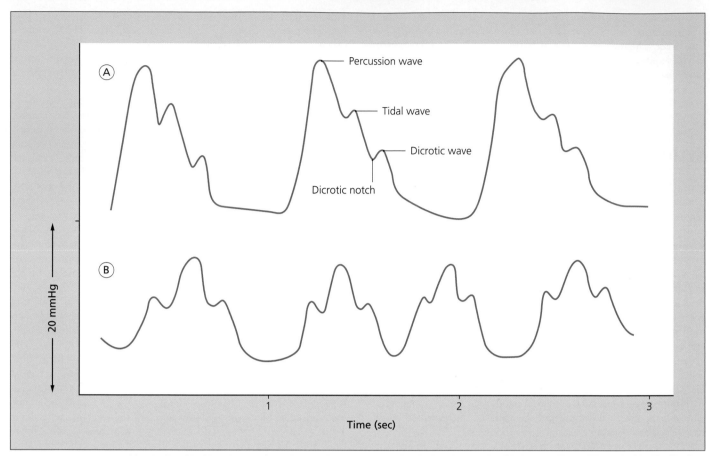

Figure 4.12 (A) ICP waveform under physiologic conditions. Three peaks are generally recognizable. The first, and usually tallest, is the percussion wave, followed by the tidal wave, the dicrotic notch, and the dicrotic wave. Note that the tidal and dicrotic waves have progressively lesser amplitudes than the percussion wave. **(B)** Abnormal intracranial waveform with high ICP. The amplitude of the tidal wave exceeds the amplitude of the percussion wave.

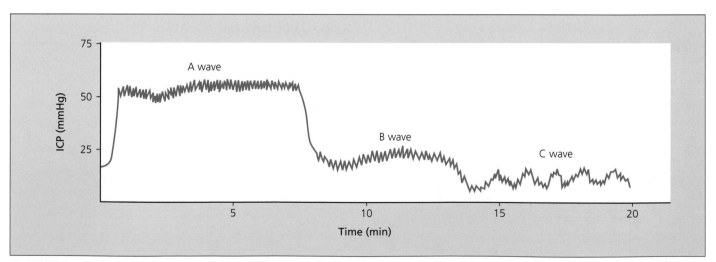

Figure 4.13 Examples of abnormal ICP waveforms with trend recording. Plateau waves, or A waves, are characterized by abrupt elevation in ICP for 5 to 20 min followed by a rapid fall in pressure to the resting level. Plateau waves herald neurologic worsening. B and C waves have questionable clinical significance.

possibly related to CO_2 retention. B waves, which have a frequency of 0.5–2/min, are related to rhythmic variations in breathing. The C waves are rhythmic variations related to the Traub–Meyer–Hering waves of systemic blood pressure and have a smaller amplitude, with a frequency of about 6/min. B and C waves have questionable clinical significance.

MICRODIALYSIS

Brain microdialysis is being used in some centers to investigate brain metabolism in patients with increased ICP and other brain insults. Detailed discussion of this technique is beyond the scope of this chapter.

TREATMENT

The most direct way to normalize raised ICP to the physiologic range is to eliminate its cause. If the increased pressure is the result of a mass effect, such as a blood clot, prompt evacuation of the offending lesion will restore ICP to normal more effectively than any other measure.

Ventricular drainage

Drainage of CSF from the ventricular system is the simplest, most effective, and quickest method of decreasing ICP. The modality is particularly effective in patients with cerebral edema. Experimental work has shown that the vasogenic edema fluid that has extravasated into interstitial space is cleared by diffusion into either the ventricular system or the subarachnoid space. Draining the ventricular fluid and decreasing the intraventricular pressure promotes rapid diffusion of the edema fluid from the site of pathology. This experimental observation provides a logical foundation for the use of ventricular drainage in the management of vasogenic edema. Ventriculostomy is also highly effective in patients who have acute subarachnoid hemorrhage with acute communicating hydrocephalus. In patients with critically increased ICP, a ventricular catheter system can be used not only to monitor pressure continuously, but to drain the ventricular system automatically when the pressure exceeds the upper limits of the physiologic range. In ventilator-dependent patients ventricular drainage may be particularly effective at preventing sharp rises in ICP during suctioning or turning.

Mannitol

Mannitol is the universally used osmotic agent to treat cerebral edema (other osmotic agents such as urea and glycerol are no longer used in contemporary neurosurgical practice). It has many pharmacologic effects, but the most significant one is its osmotic effect. It is not metabolized and it does not cross the blood–brain barrier. It increases serum osmolality and thus helps to draw fluid from the brain parenchyma into the vascular space. The normal serum osmolality is 275–290 mOsm/kg. An increase in serum osmolality of as little as 10 mOsm/kg is enough to have a significant effect on cerebral edema. Mannitol is generally given in small boluses rather than as a continuous drip. The usual dose is 0.25 g/kg at 4 to 6-hour intervals. In addition to the osmotic effect, mannitol decreases CSF production, increases cerebral blood flow and cerebral oxygen consumption, and decreases blood viscosity, thereby improving perfusion. Mannitol is generally effective for 48 to 72 hours. Its use beyond 72 hours in ineffective because mannitol slowly leaks out of the blood vessel, especially in areas of blood–brain barrier breakdown, with resulting loss of osmotic gradient. Serum osmolality and electrolytes should be carefully monitored during mannitol therapy.

Hypertonic saline

Since 2001, hypertonic saline has been increasingly used to control high ICP from brain swelling. Experimental and clinical studies suggest that it may be as effective as mannitol.

Hyperventilation

Hyperventilation causes a fall in ICP by reducing intracranial blood flow and blood volume through vasoconstriction. Hyperventilation is generally initiated for acute management of increased ICP, but sustained hyperventilation as a mode of therapy has not been found to be beneficial because of compensatory mechanisms that come into play. Also, recent studies show that some patients with increased ICP, such as patients with acute head trauma, may have low blood flow to begin with. Hyperventilation in such individuals may worsen the clinical condition. Hyperventilation, if undertaken, should be moderate, bringing the P_{CO_2} down to 28–32 mmHg. Reducing the P_{CO_2} much further will decrease blood flow to critically low levels, compounding the ischemia produced by increased ICP.

Loop diuretics

Furosemide has been used as an adjunct to mannitol because they seem to have a synergistic effect. Furosemide alone, however, cannot be depended on to reduce ICP. Because its primary action is on the kidney, it is not dependent on the intact blood–brain barrier for its effect. It is thought to reduce CSF production as well.

Steroids

Dexamethasone is used for treating chronic increases in ICP, especially those related to vasogenic edema caused by primary or metastatic neoplasms. It is ineffective in the management of vasogenic edema related to head trauma or cerebral infarction. It is thought to stabilize the cell membrane and restore the normal permeability of endothelial cells. This is brought about by inhibition of lysosomal activity, suppression of polyunsaturated fatty acid production that causes edema, and decrease of free radical production. The usual loading dose is 10 mg, given intravenously, followed by 4 mg every 6 hours. When the appropriate therapeutic goal has been achieved, the dose should be slowly tapered over a period of 3–4 days.

Barbiturate coma

Induction of coma with short-acting barbiturates is the last resort in the management of raised ICP when all other measures fail. Its clinical use is controversial. Barbiturates decrease the ICP by several mechanisms. They inhibit the release of fatty-acid peroxidation products by scavenging free radicals from the mitochondrial respiratory chain. They also inhibit cerebral metabolism and reduce cerebral blood flow. The most commonly

CLINICAL PEARLS

- States of impaired consciousness may be expressed using various descriptive terms or, more accurately, using the Glascow Coma Score (GCS).

- The key clinical signs that help in clinical assessment and determination of prognosis are the presense or absence of certain brainstem reflexes such as pupillary response, corneal reflex, oculocephalic and oculovestibular reflexes, and gag reflex.

- CT scan of the head remains the key imaging modality in the rapid assessment of a patient with impaired consciousness.

- All neuroscience practitioners should be familiar with the accepted clinical and ancilllary tests for establishing brain death, based on their institutional criteria.

used drug is thiopental, which is given in a loading dose of 3–10 mg/kg over a 10-min period and a maintenance dose of 1–2 mg/kg/h. The serum level should be maintained at 3–4 mg/L. Patients in barbiturate coma require intensive monitoring of hemodynamic function, ICP, and blood gases. Vasopressors may have to be administered if hypotension results. Barbiturate therapy is usually withdrawn when the ICP normalizes and there is a good intracranial compliance; no clinical indicators are available to dictate termination of therapy.

REFERENCES

1. Wanifuchi H, Schmzu T, Maruyama T. Age-related changes in the proportion of intracranial cerebrospinal fluid space measured using volumetric computerized tomography scanning. *J Neurosurg* 2002; 97: 607–10.

2. Langfitt TW, Weinstein JD, Kassell NF. Cerebral vasomotor paralysis produced by intracranial hypertension. *Neurology* 1965; 15: 622–41.

3. Kroll RA, Neuwelt EA. Outwitting the blood–brain barrier for therapeutic purposes: osmotic opening and other means. *Neurosurgery* 1998; 42: 1083–105.

4. Friden PM. Receptor-mediated transport of therapeutics across the blood–brain barrier. *Neurosurgery* 1994; 35: 294–301.

5. Matsukado K, Inamura T, Nakaro S, Fukui M, Bartus R, Black KL. Enchanced tumor uptake of carboplatin and survival in glioma-bearing rats by intracarotid infusion of bradykinin analog RMP-7. *Neurosurgery* 1996; 39: 125–47.

6. Neuwelt EA, Abbott JN, Drew L, *et al. Neurosurgery* 1999; 44: 604–614.

7. Pollay M, Roberts PA. Blood–brain barrier: a definition of normal and altered function. *Neurosurgery* 1980; 6: 675–85.

8. Ignelzi RJ. Cerebral edema: present perspectives. *Neurosurgery* 1979; 4: 338–42.

9. Fishman RA. Brain edema. *N Engl J Med* 1975; 293: 706–11.

10. Stochetti N, Paparella A, Bridelli F, Bacchi M, Piazzol P, Zuccoli P. A cerebral venous saturation studied with bilateral samples in the internal jugular vein. *Neurosurgery* 1994; 34: 38–47.

11. Van Santbrink H, Maas AIR, Cees JJ, Avezaat CJJ. Continuous monitoring of partial pressure of brain tissue oxygen in patients with severe head injury. *Neurosurgery* 1996; 38: 21.

12. Zauner A, Bullock R, Di X, Young HF. Brain oxygen CO_2, pH, temperature monitoring: evaluation in feline brain. *Neurosurgery* 1995; 37: 1168–75.

13. Vandenbrink WA, van Santbrink H, Steyerberg EW, *et al.* Brain oxygen tension in severe head injury. *Neurosurgery* 2000; 46: 868–82.

14. Raabe A, Stockel R, Hohrerin D, Schoche J. Reliablity of intraventricular pressure measurement with fiber-optic or solid-state transducers: avoidance of methodological error. *Neurosurgery* 1998; 42: 74–83.

15. Raabe A, Tatzauer R, Meyer O, Stockel R, Hohrein D, Schoche J. Reliability of epidural pressure measurement in clinical practice: behavior of three modern sensors during simultaneous ipsilateral intraventicular or intraparenchymal pressure measurement. *Neurosurgery* 1998; 43: 306–15.

16. Gray WP, Palmer JD, Gill J, Gardner M, Iannotti F. A clinical study of parenchymal and subdural miniature strain-gauge transducers of monitoring intracranial pressure. *Neurosurgery* 1996; 39: 927–34.

17. Bavetta S, Norris JS, Wyatt M, Sutcliff JC, Hamlyn PJ. Prospective study of zero drift in fiberoptic pressure monitors used in clinical practice. *J Neurosurg* 1997; 86: 927–30.

18. Piper I, Barnes A, Smith D, Dunn L. The Camino intracranial pressure sensor: is it optimal technology? An internal audit with a review of current intracranial pressure monitoring technologies. *Neurosurgery* 2001; 49: 1158–69.

19. Czosynka M, Czosnyka ZH, Richards HK, Pickard JD. Hydrodynamic properties of extraventricular drainage systems.

20. Kanter MJ, Narayan RK. Intracranial pressure monitoring. *Neurosurg Clin North Am.* 1991; 2: 257–265.

21. Lundberg N. Continuous recording and control of ventricular fluid pressure in neurosurgical practice. *Acta Psychiatr Neurol Scand Suppl.* 1960; 149: 1.

22. Unterberg AW, Sakowitz OW, Sarrafzadeh AS, Benndorf G. Role of bedside microdialysis in the diagnosis of cerebral vasospasm following aneurysmal subarachnoid hemorrhage: *J Neurosurg* 2001; 94: 740–9.

23. Hutchinson PJ, O'Connell MT, Al-Rawj PG, *et al.* Cerebral clinical microdialysis: a methodological study. *J Neurosurg* 2000; 93: 37–43.

24. Reinstrup R, Stahls N, Mellergord P, Uski T, Ungerstedt V, Nordstrom H. Intracerebral microdialysis in clinical practice: Baseline values for chemical markers during wakefulness, anesthesia, and neurosurgery. *Neurosurgery* 2000; 47: 701–13.

25. Zauner A, Doppenberg EMR, Woodward JJ, Choi SC, Young HF, Bullock R. Continuous monitoring of cerebral substrate delivery and clearance: initial experience in 24 patients with severe acute brain injuries. *Neurosurgery* 1997; 41: 1082–97.

26. Zauner A, Daughherty WP, Bullock R, Warner D. Brain oxygenation and energy metabolism. Biological function and pathophysiology. *Neurosurgery* 2002; 51: 289–99.

27. Carter BS, Ogilvy CS, Candia G, Rosas D, Buonanano F. One year outcome after decompressive surgery for massive nondominant hemisphere infarction. *Neurosurgery* 1997; 40: 1168–79.

28. Polin RS, Shaffey ME, Bugaev CA, *et al.* Decompressive bifrontal craniectomy in the treatment of severe refractory posttraumatic cerebral edema. *Neurosurgery* 1997; 41: 84–100.

29. Munch E, Horn P, Schurer L, Piepgras A, Paul T, Schmidek P. Management of severe traumatic brain injury by decompressive craniectomy. *Neurosurgery* 2000; 47: 315–26.

30. Reulen HJ, Grahm R, Spatz M, Klatzo I. Role of pressure gradients and bulk flow in dynamics of vasogenic brain edema. *J Neurosurg* 1977; 46: 24–35.

31. Ohata K, Marmarou A. Clearance of brain edema and macromolecules through the cortical extracellular space. *J Neurosurg* 1992; 77: 387–96.

32. Reulen HJ, Tsuyumu M, Tack A, Fenske AR, Prioleau GR. Clearance of edema fluid into cerebrospinal fluid. *J Neurosurg* 1978; 48: 754–64.

33. Hartwell RC, Sutton LN. Mannitol, intracranial pressure and vasogenic edema. *Neurosurgery* 1993; 32: 444–54.

34. Berger S, Schurer L, Hartl R, Messmer K, Baethman A. Reduction of post-traumatic intracranial hypertension by hypertronic/hyperoncotic saline/dextran and hypertonic mannitol. *Neurosurgery* 1995; 7: 98–109.

35. Qureshi AI, Wilson DA, Traystman RJ. Treatment of elevated intracranial pressure in experimental intracerebral hemorrhage: comparison.

36. Raichle ME, Plum F. Hyperventilation and cerebral blood flow. *Stroke* 1972; 3: 566–75.

37. Bouma GJ, Muizelaar P, Choi SC, Newlon PG, Young HF. Cerebral circulation and metabolism after severe traumatic brain injury: the elusive role of ischemia. *J Neurosurg* 1991; 75: 685–93.

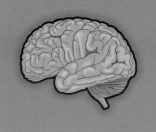

IMPAIRED CONSCIOUSNESS

5

Setti S Rengachary

Coma, or loss of consciousness, may be defined as a loss of awareness of one's self or environment (Table 5.1). The comatose state constitutes an acute neurosurgical emergency and is one of the most frequent reasons for a neurosurgical consultation in the emergency room.[1] Evaluation of the patient, history-taking clinical assessment, basic resuscitation efforts, laboratory investigations and radiologic assessment should occur in rapid sequence or concurrently, if possible; there is no justification for a sequential and leisurely evaluation. The comatose patient poses a challenge to the diagnostic acumen of the physician and the treatment resources available.

A unique feature in the clinical assessment of the comatose patient is the inability to obtain a history from the patient, unless the patient is known to the physician from previous admissions. The history must be obtained from previous medical records, relatives, friends, law-enforcement officials, or anyone else available. The circumstances in which the patient was found by the paramedics may be valuable. Knowing about a history of trauma from a fall, assault, penetrating wound, or automobile accident is helpful. The patient should be searched for empty pill containers. A history of psychiatric illness, suicide attempt, epilepsy, illicit drug use, endocrine or other metabolic disorders, cardiac irregularity, hypertension, vascular disease, or coagulopathy may be helpful in determining the etiology of impaired consciousness.

EMERGENCY MANAGEMENT

First, the airway is inspected. If the patient vomits, the head should be turned to the side to prevent aspiration of matter. Depending on the circumstances, an oral airway, nasal airway, endotracheal tube, or cricothyrotomy may be necessary. Whether to place the patient on a ventilator depends on the blood gases, tidal volume, rate of respirations, oxygen saturation, and level of consciousness. Vital signs, including temperature, pulse, respiratory rate and blood pressure, should be recorded. The head, neck, trunk and extremities are checked for signs of external trauma. Periorbital ecchymosis (raccoon eyes) (Figure 5.1), drainage of clear fluid or blood from the nose, and Battle's sign are all indicative of trauma. The odor of alcohol in inebriation, an ammoniacal odor in uremia, a musty odor in hepatic coma and a spoiled-fruit odor in diabetic coma should be noted, if present. An intravenous line should be started and the appropriate electrolyte solution should be administered. If the patient is hypotensive, other sources of bleeding should be sought (for example, in the

abdominal and pelvic areas). After cervical spine films have been taken to rule out cervical spine trauma, the patient is checked for meningeal signs such as neck stiffness, Kernig's sign, and Brudzinski's sign.

CLINICAL ASSESSMENT

Level of consciousness

Assessing the level of consciousness is of foremost importance.[2] Level of consciousness varies from the patient who is fully alert and is responsive to verbal commands to one who is totally incognizant of the environment and to herself or himself. To assess the level of consciousness, the Glasgow coma scale, which is particularly helpful in patients with head injury, has been devised (see Chapter 18, Table 18.4).[3] The three parameters taken into consideration are eye-opening response, verbal response, and motor response.

Eyelids

Comatose patients have their eyes closed as a result of the tonic contraction of the orbicularis oculi muscles (Figure 5.2). If the eyelids are opened by the examiner they gradually and smoothly close. Hysterical patients cannot mimic this gradual closure, but keep their eyes closed forcibly, resisting opening by the examiner.

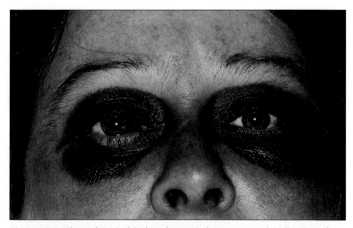

Figure 5.1 Bilateral periorbital ecchymosis (raccoon eyes) indicative of a fracture of the floor of the anterior cranial fossa.

Table 5.1 Terms used to describe altered states of consciousness

Coma
Unawareness of self and environment

Alpha coma
An apparently comatose state in which the patient exhibits EEG rhythms within the alpha-frequency range, paradoxically resembling an awake EEG pattern.[13,14] Alpha coma is generally observed in the following groups of patients: (1) those who survive cardiopulmonary arrest with global ischemic changes in the brain, (2) those with a focal brainstem lesion at or just caudal to the pontomesencephalic junction, and (3) those with metabolic or toxic encephalopathies

Persistent vegetative state
(synonyms: akinetic mutism, coma vigil, neocortical death, apallic syndrome, cerebral death)
A state of wakefulness without the ability to appreciate or respond to external stimuli.

Minimally conscious state (MCS) is a condition with severe impairment of consciousness but does not meet the criteria for coma or persistent vegetative state. In MCS, there is inconsistent but clearly discernible behavioral evidence of consciousness. Patients may evolve to MCS from coma or persistent vegetative state after brain trauma. This condition is often transient but may also exist as a permanent outcome.

Brain death
A comatose state with an irreversible total loss of cerebral and brainstem functions preceding cessation of cardiac activity.

Locked-in state
(synonyms: pseudocoma, ventral pontine syndrome, de-efferented state, cerebromedullospinal disconnection)
A state of unimpaired consciousness with tetraplegia and pseudobulbar paralysis. Patients generally have preserved vertical but absent horizontal eye movements. They respond to verbal stimuli with coded lid movements.

Lethargy
A mild decrease in the level of alertness; patient responds when spoken to but clearly lacks concentration and the attention span is short.

Obtundation
A modest decrease in the level of alertness; patients generally tend to sleep when undisturbed but can be aroused to answer simple questions appropriately.

Stupor
A severe decrease in the level of alertness; patients respond to continuous vigorous stimulation (shaking or shouting) with unintelligible sounds, if any. Verbal responses are absent.

Confusion
Clouded, slow thinking.

Delirium
A hyperactive, agitated, confused state with hallucinations; paranoid ideations and signs of autonomic overactivity.

Syncope (fainting)
Transient loss of consciousness from a reversible, temporary impairment of blood flow to the brain.

Sleep
Cyclic loss of consciousness reversible with stimulation.

Resting position of the eyes

A quick inspection of the eyes at rest may given an idea of the general location of the pathologic lesion (Figure 5.3). Patients with large destructive lesions in the *frontal lobe*, such as an acute intracerebral hematoma, will have conjugate deviation of the eyes away from the side of paralysis, looking toward the lesion. In *deep-seated thalamic lesions* there may be "wrong-way" gaze paresis, i.e. the conjugate deviation may be toward the paralysis and away from the lesion. In *unilateral pontine lesions* the conjugate gaze may imply an internuclear ophthalmoplegia, paresis of individual muscles, or pre-existing tropia or phoria. Spontaneous slow horizontal roving eye movements may indicate a good prognosis in that they usually imply an intact brainstem. They have essentially the same clinical significance as a positive response to the doll's

eye maneuver, which is discussed below. It is to be emphasized that in a deeply comatose patient with a structural lesion in the brain, true nystagmus with fast and slow components is never observed.

Pupils

Examination of pupillary size, equality, and response to light (both direct and consensual) gives valuable information regarding the integrity of the brainstem, especially the midbrain area (Figure 5.4).

Pupillary abnormality is one of the cardinal features differentiating surgical disorders from medical disorders; pupillary abnormalities in a comatose patient generally herald structural

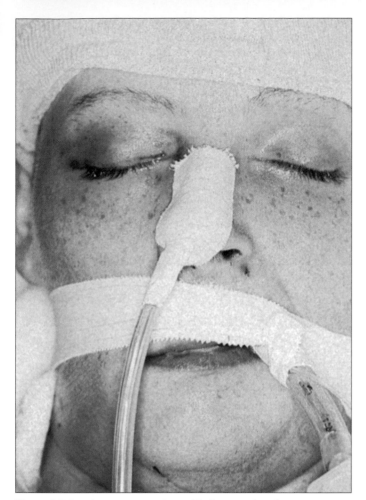

Figure 5.2 Deeply comatose patient with the eyes closed.

changes in the brain, especially the brainstem, whereas in metabolic coma such abnormalities are not observed. In patients who are on a ventilator and who have received paralyzing agents, pupillary examination may be the only objective neurologic test possible. Resting pupillary size is determined under ambient light. In the critical-care setting, the pupils should not be pharmacologically dilated to observe the fundus because this eliminates one of the prime objective means to assess brainstem integrity. One should check for orbital trauma, including injury to the iris that could cause pupillary dilatation; this dilatation has no value for neurologic localization. Previous cataract surgery will impair mobility of the iris and thus the pupillary reaction.

A significant pupillary abnormality that can be encountered in neurosurgical practice is the unilaterally dilated and fixed pupil (see Figure 5.4A, left). This generally indicates uncal herniation with compression of the third cranial nerve at the tentorial edge, resulting in impairment of the parasympathetic pupilloconstrictor fibers within the nerve. Pupillary dilatation can also occur with sudden expansion or rupture of an internal carotid artery aneurysm or because of an intrinsic lesion of the midbrain (for example, acute hematoma). In extreme midbrain compression both pupils become fixed and dilated (Figure 5.5). Fixed and dilated pupils also characterize the terminal stages of brain death, whatever the etiology. *Pontine tegmental lesions* produce small pinpoint pupils with a flicker of reaction to light, which sometimes can be appreciated only with a magnifying lens. *Medullary*

lesions may cause a unilateral Horner syndrome, which is characterized by miosis, ptosis, enophthalmos, and reduced sweating on the face homolateral to the lesion in the brainstem. *Hypothalamic lesions* may also produce Horner syndrome. It is to be emphasized that offerent optic abnormalities, such as an optic nerve transection, do not cause pupillary inequality. In such a situation, the direct response to light may be absent, but the consensual response is intact.

Eye movements

Forced downward deviation of the eyes occurs in lesions of the thalamus or the tectum of the midbrain. This would be associated with nonreactive pupils (Parinaud syndrome). *Skew deviation*, or vertical divergence, follows lesions of the cerebellum or brainstem. *Ocular bobbing*, or conjugate downward movement from the primary position through a very small arc, usually follows lesions in the pontine tegmentum.[4] In such a situation there is usually lateral gaze paralysis.

Disconjugate movements may be seen in cranial nerve paralysis. The two most commonly paralyzed nerves are the sixth nerve, as a result of a generalized increased intracranial pressure, or the third nerve, as a result of uncal herniation.

Oculocephalic reflex (doll's eye movement)

Elicitation of the oculocephalic reflex is a quick bedside test to determine the integrity of the brainstem (Figure 5.6). This brainstem reflex has an afferent limb, a central relay, and an efferent arc. The afferent response is from the vestibular end organs through the vestibular nerve terminating in the vestibular nuclei. The efferent arc is the medial longitudinal fasciculus connecting the nuclei of the third, fourth and sixth cranial nerves on the ipsilateral and opposite sides. In deeply comatose patients with absence of brainstem function, the doll's eye movement is completely abolished (see Figure 5.6D). The whole reflex is inhibited by the cerebral cortex. This reflex cannot be demonstrated in an alert, conscious individual because of the intact inhibitory influences from the cerebral hemispheres. In an unconscious patient, however, the presence or absence of this reflex gives an indication of the integrity of the brainstem. If the brainstem is intact, the eyes lag behind and roll toward the opposite side if the head is briskly turned to one side (see Figure 5.6C). Before eliciting the doll's eye movement, one should be certain that there is no cervical spine injury.

Oculovestibular reflex (ice-water caloric test)

Elicitation of the oculovestibular reflex gives the same information as the doll's eye maneuver. This test is particularly useful in patients who have a head injury and possible an associated spine injury. Before doing the test, one inspects the ear canal to make certain that the tympanic membranes are intact. The head is kept flexed 30° from the horizontal. Approximately 30 mL of ice-cold water is injected into the external auditory canal. In normal, awake individuals stimulation from the cold water induces nystagmus, with the fast component away from the stimulated side. In comatose patients the fast component is lost. Thus, cold caloric stimulation causes slow deviation of the eyes towards the irrigated side (Figure 5.7A) lasting for 2 to 3 minutes before the eye returns to the neutral position. Patients with brainstem damage exhibit no response to cold caloric stimulation; the eyes assume a fixed forward gaze (Figure 5.7B). The caloric test is also helpful for differentiating organic coma from hysterical coma.

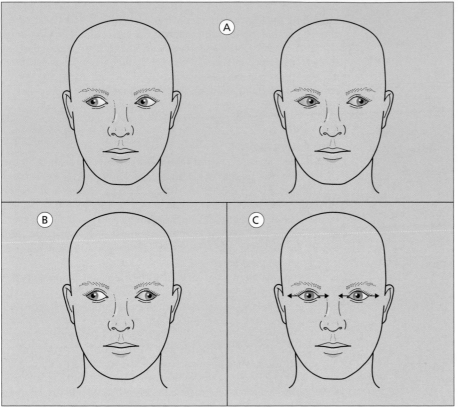

Figure 5.3 Resting position of the eyes. **(A)** *Left*: Patient with a large right frontal destructive lesion. There is tonic conjugate deviation of the eyes toward the lesion away from the paralysis. *Right*: With deep-seated thalamic lesions on the right side, there is "wrong-way" gaze deviation; there is tonic deviation of the eyes away from the lesion and toward the paralysis. With a right pontine lesion there is conjugate deviation of the eyes toward the side of paralysis (not shown). **(B)** A disconjugate gaze may imply an internuclear ophthalmoplegia, paresis of individual muscles, or pre-existing tropia or phoria. **(C)** Spontaneous slow horizontal roving eye movements have a good prognostic value in that they usually imply an intact brainstem.

Hysterical patients will develop nystagmus from caloric testing. Caloric testing may also reveal gaze paralysis, individual muscle paresis, or internuclear ophthalmoplegia. It is to be noted that in metabolic encephalopathy, at least in the early stages, the oculocephalic reflexes are intact.

Respirations

Using bedside observations, clinical neurologists have described several classic patterns of respiration that correlate with various levels of anatomic involvement of the central nervous system. These patterns of respiration have been useful in the clinical evaluation of patients.[5] Most comatose patients with neurosurgical disorders and a Glasgow coma score less than 8 are intubated soon after arrival to ensure adequate oxygenation of the brain. Because these patients are intubated, paralyzed and ventilated, the classic respiratory patterns cannot be observed. However, the standard descriptions of various classic patterns are given for completeness of discussion of the subject.

Cheyne–Stokes respirations are generally seen in patients with diffuse forebrain lesions (Figure 5.8A). Patients with diffuse forebrain lesions are thought to be hypersensitive to normal levels of CO_2. This results in a hyperventilatory phase which blows off CO_2 and results in apnea for a brief period. During the apneic interval CO_2 accumulates to normal levels; thus, cycles of hyperventilation and apnea alternate. Cheyne–Stokes breathing can be seen occasionally for brief periods in a normal individual during sleep. In Cheyne–Stokes respiration the hyperventilation phase is longer than the apnea phase. As a result, the patients are generally alkalotic.

Central neurogenic hyperventilation is a rare phenomenon seen in a head-injured patient with a severe midbrain lesion (Figure 5.8B). In true neurogenic hyperventilation the partial pressure of oxygen (Po_2) is high and that of carbon dioxide (Pco_2) is low. Many episodes of hyperventilation seen in comatose individuals are not true neurogenic hyperventilation but rather are the result of pulmonary edema and aspiration pneumonitis. In such individuals, the Po_2 is below normal in spite of the tachypnea.

Apneustic breathing is characterized by a prolonged pause at full inspiration (Figure 5.8C). This phenomenon is quite rare. It usually reflects a lesion of the mid to caudal pons. Usually it is seen in the patients with brainstem stroke from basilar artery occlusion.

Ataxic breathing occurs in patients with medullary lesions where the respiratory center is located (Figure 5.8D). The breathing is very irregular with deep and shallow breaths occurring randomly. It represents impairment of the orderly cyclic respiratory rhythm. Lesions in the posterior cranial fossa may produce this pattern in the terminal stages.

Cluster pattern is also seen in lower medullary lesions (Figure 5.8E). Clusters of breaths occur in an irregular sequence with varying pauses between clusters. Clustered breathing and gasping respirations occur in end-stage medullary failure.

Motor function

A quick assessment of motor function helps to localize lesions in the nervous system. The patient who can obey orders and perform simple motor tasks on command obviously has intact corticospinal tracts and the related integrative pathways. When asking a patient to squeeze a hand on command, one should make sure that the grasp reflex is not mistaken for volitional contraction. This can be done by asking the patient to release the hand on command. Patients with reflex grasp but without volitional contraction will

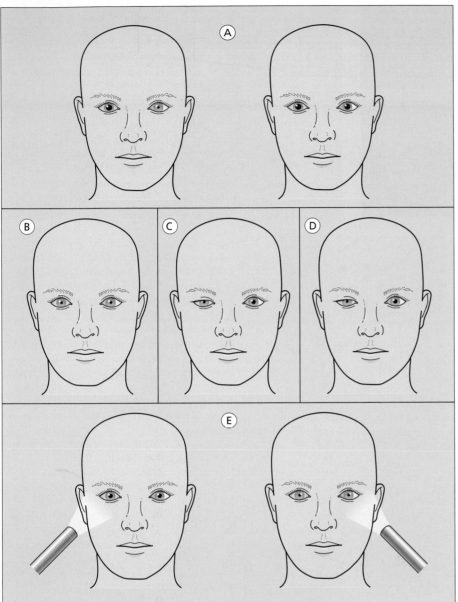

Figure 5.4 (A) Midbrain lesions. *Left*: Third nerve paresis or a unilateral midbrain lesion produces an ipsilaterally dilated pupil. This is generally indicative of uncal herniation. *Right*: Bilaterally fixed and dilated pupils in bilateral midbrain lesions, anoxic encephalopathy, and brain death. **(B)** Pontine lesion: bilaterally small pinpoint pupils. **(C)** Medullary lesions: unilateral Horner syndrome with miosis, ptosis, enophthalmos. **(D)** Hypothalamic lesion producing Horner syndrome. **(E)** Optic nerve injury on the right with no reaction to direct light but with consensual response.

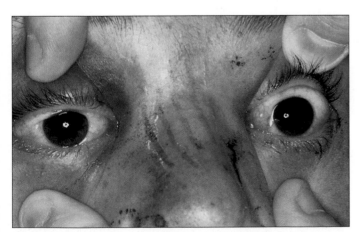

Figure 5.5 Bilaterally fixed and dilated pupils in a deeply comatose patient.

not be able to release the hand on command. A better test is to ask the patients to hold up two fingers. If a patient does not respond to vocal stimuli, a painful stimulus, such as pressure on the supraorbital notch, sternum, or nailbed, should be applied. Usually, the patient moves the extremities defensively to ward off the painful stimulus (Figure 5.9A).

At a lesser level of response, the patient may slightly withdraw the limb from the painful source without any complicated purposeful defensive movements. *Decorticate posturing* (Figure 5.9B), either spontaneously or in response to stimuli, is characterized by flexion of the arms and wrists and extension of the lower extremities. The lesion is generally thought to be in the cerebral white matter, internal capsule and the thalamus. In *decerebrate rigidity* (Figure 5.9C) the patient has the upper and lower extremities in complete extension. In extreme cases the patient may assume an opisthotonic position. In decerebrate posturing, the lesion is slightly more caudal in the upper brainstem. *Flacci-*

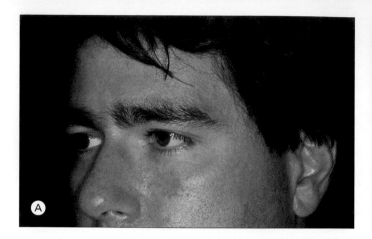

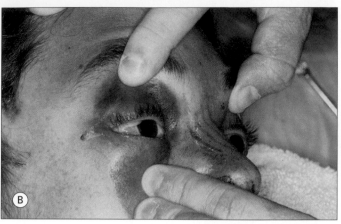

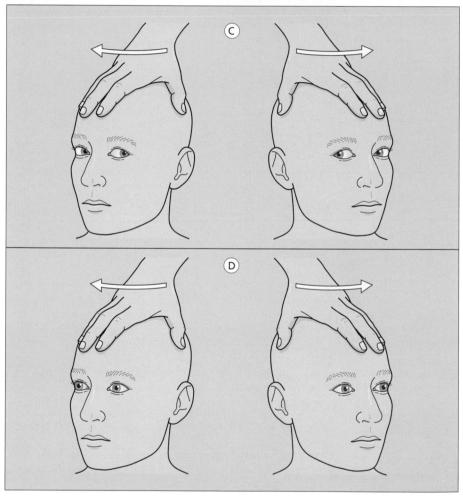

Figure 5.6 Oculocephalic reflex (doll's eye movements). **(A)** In a fully conscious individual, doll's eye movements are absent. The eyes point in the direction in which the head points. **(B)** In an unconscious patient with intact brainstem function, doll's eye movements can be elicited. As one briskly turns the head to one side, the eyes lag behind and roll toward the opposite side **(C)**. In a deeply comatose patient with absent brainstem function the doll's eye movements are absent **(D)**. The eyes have a fixed forward stare and move with the head.

dity of the extremities with no response to any noxious stimuli is seen in moribund patients with medullary failure (Figure 5.9D).

Other brainstem functions

Other commonly tested brainstem reflexes include corneal, gag and cough reflexes. The corneal reflex is tested by lightly touching the edge of the cornea with a wisp of cotton. There is usually prompt eye closure. Intact corneal reflex implies that the facial nerve and the pathway from the first division of the trigeminal

nerve to the facial nerve nucleus are intact. The gag reflex is tested by touching the pharynx with a cotton swab. The cough reflex is tested by suctioning the patient or manipulating the endotracheal tube.

Diagnostic tests

Admission laboratory studies include complete blood count, electrolytes, liver function test, renal function tests, serum alcohol level, and toxic drug screen of both blood and urine. If poisoning

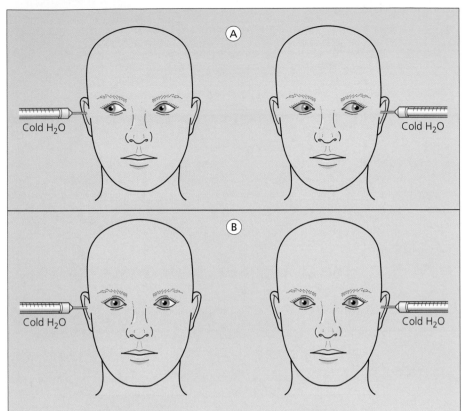

Figure 5.7 Oculovestibular reflex (ice-water caloric test). **(A)** Cold caloric stimulation in a comatose patient causes slow tonic deviation of the eyes toward the stimulated side, if the brainstem is intact. **(B)** With a damaged brainstem, the eyes are immobile despite cold caloric stimulation.

is suspected, gastric lavage is instituted and gastric contents are sent for analysis. A fingerstick blood test for glucose is taken, and if the glucose level is low 50% glucose is administered. The rationale for using 50% glucose blindly in comatose individuals is now being questioned because there is some evidence that high glucose concentrations may increase the infarct size in patients with impending stroke.[6,7]

After initial clinical assessment and drawing of blood samples, a computed tomography (CT) scan is performed without contrast administration. The CT scan has considerable value in patients in coma. A negative CT scan in a coma patient implies a metabolic process such as uremic, diabetic, or anoxic encephalopathy. A structural lesion (for example, intracerebral hematoma, brain tumor, abscess) will be clearly visible on the scan. If the CT scan is normal and the patient has meningeal signs and fever, a lumbar puncture should be performed to rule out meningitis or subarachnoid hemorrhage.

PATHOGENESIS OF COMA

The conscious state depends on the integrity of the reticular activating system in the rostral pons, midbrain and thalamus (Figure 5.10). This system receives collateral input from all the incoming sensory pathways (specific sensory systems). Projection from the rostral end of the reticular activating system from the thalamic nuclei radiate diffusely to the entire cerebral cortex. The thalamocortical connection is bidirectional in that regulatory input to the reticular activating system is directed from the cortex and the input to the cortex is derived from the reticular nuclei. Impairment of consciousness can occur in two types of lesions: focal destruction in the reticular core of the rostral brainstem or a

diffuse lesion in both cerebral hemispheres. Therefore, the causes of impaired consciousness can be broadly classified into four major categories. *Diffuse cortical lesions* can result from hypoxia, hypoglycemia, hyperosmolar coma, acid–base imbalance, uremia, hepatic coma, etc. In this situation the neurons of the cerebral cortex are diffusely affected. *Supratentorial mass lesions*, either extrinsic or intrinsic, in the cerebral hemispheres may cause compression and uncal herniation, which results in compression of the rostral brainstem and thus impairment of the reticular activating system. This is a common mechanism of coma in a neurosurgical setting. *Direct lesions* in the rostral brainstem itself, for example, acute hemorrhage or trauma, may result in coma. *Infratentorial lesions* with secondary compression on the brainstem caused by large cerebellar tumors, large cerebellar hemorrhage, or infarction may impair consciousness.

RELATED STATES

Persistent vegetative state

This state is also called akinetic mutism, coma vigil, neocortical death, apallic syndrome, or cerebral death.[8,9] The term *vegetative* is used because only vegetative or autonomic functions are preserved. In this state patients appear wakeful, but there is no cognitive function. Although they may open their eyes, they do not track and explore the surroundings. Purposeful movements of the eyes in response to commands are absent. These patients do not vocalize or verbalize, their faces are expressionless, and they generally assume a fetal position with the limbs flexed. They do not have any purposeful motion of the extremities in response to noxious stimuli. They continue to have normal spontaneous respirations and normal cardiac and gastrointestinal activity. They

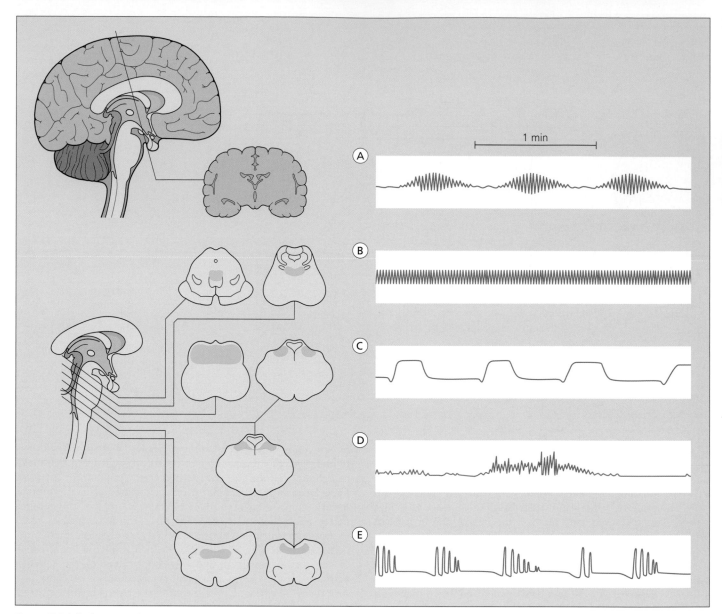

Figure 5.8 (A) Cheyne–Stokes respiration. Periods of hyperventilation alternate with apneic intervals. **(B)** Central neurogenic hyperventilation. **(C)** Apneustic breathing. **(D)** Ataxic breathing. **(E)** Cluster pattern.

are totally dependent for all activities of daily living, including eating, drinking, and attention to personal hygiene. Sleep–wake cycles may remain intact. A positron emission tomographic (PET) scan will show low cerebral metabolic rate for glucose. A patient may enter a persistent vegetative state in one of two ways. A patient may start with a chronic nervous disorder that has a continuous downhill course, such as Alzheimer's disease. Or the patient may suffer an acute insult to the brain that causes coma and may partially recover from the coma only to go into a persistent vegetative state. Most patients in a persistent vegetative state were first comatose.

Locked-in syndrome

The so-called locked-in syndrome, also called pseudocoma, ventral pontine syndrome, deferent state, or cerebromedullospinal disconnection,[10,11] occurs as a result of a lesion in the pons affecting both corticospinal and corticobulbar tracts bilaterally. The distal part of the reticular formation in the pons and tegmentum may be involved but does not appear to be critical in maintaining consciousness. Thus the patient is tetraplegic and has pseudobulbar paralysis and is unable to communicate except by coded blinking motions. Horizontal eye motions are affected as well. The patient is fully conscious because the reticular activating system in the rostral brainstem is intact. This is a very unusual neurologic syndrome and one should be cognizant of it to avoid mistaking this for coma.

Blood flow studies of the cerebral hemispheres in patients with locked-in syndrome and in patients with chronic vegetative state have shown that blood flow is close to normal in the former and considerably decreased in the latter.[12] Figure 5.11 illustrates the location of the lesion in locked-in syndrome.

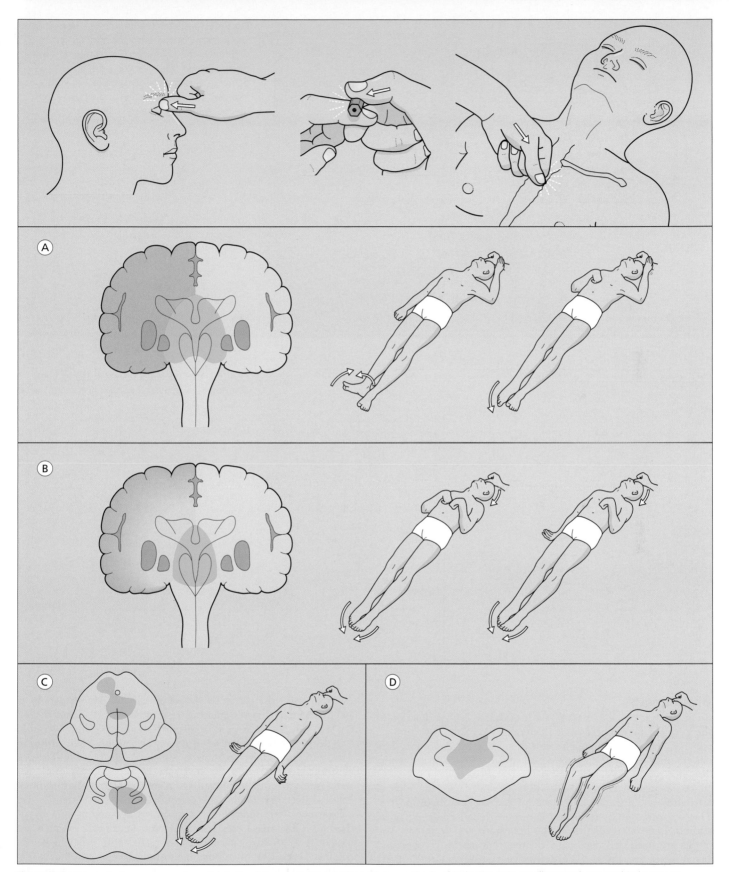

Figure 5.9 Various motor responses to painful stimuli in a comatose patient. Three methods of inducing pain are illustrated: supraorbital pressure, pressure on the finger nailbed with a pencil, and sternal rub. **(A)** With a hemispheric lesion the patient is hemiplegic on the opposite side. The patient has purposeful defensive movements on the nonparalyzed side. **(B)** With a bilateral lesion in the deep white matter and thalamus there is decorticate posturing characterized by flexion of the arms and wrists and extension of the legs. **(C)** With upper brainstem lesions there is decerebrate rigidity – the patient has both upper and lower extremities in extreme extension. **(D)** Medullary lesions produce generalized flaccidity.

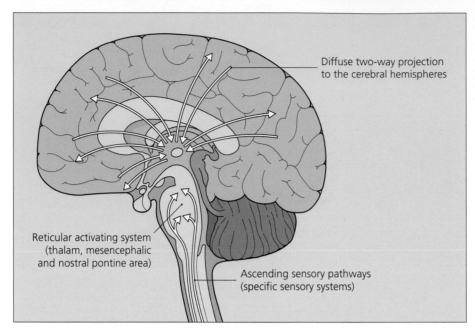

Figure 5.10 Anatomic substrate of consciousness. The anatomy of the reticular activating system is depicted in this illustration. This system receives collateral input from all incoming sensory pathways (specific sensory systems). There is a two-way projection (afferent and efferent) from the reticular core to the cerebral cortex.

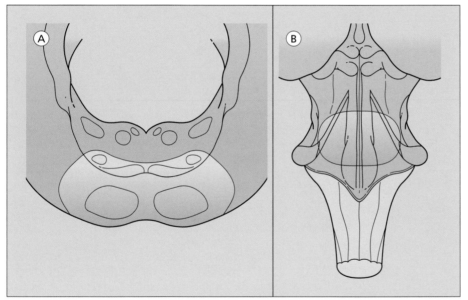

Figure 5.11 Axial (**A**) and coronal (**B**) sections, showing the extent of the lesion in a patient with locked-in syndrome.

Brain death

Brain death is defined as total and irreversible loss of function of the cerebral hemispheres and the brainstem. Some institutions, however, have made minor modifications to this definition. The patient may continue to have some spinal reflex activity, which does not preclude declaring the patient brain dead.

As a general rule, a brain-dead patient lacks the clinical attributes of a functioning brainstem and cerebral hemispheres. This is manifested by coma and unresponsiveness to deep painful stimuli. Reflexes mediated by the brainstem are all absent. The pupils are fixed and maximally dilated. The corneal, cough and gag reflexes are absent. The doll's eye testing and cold caloric stimulation do not induce any response. There are no spontaneous respirations. Apnea can be further tested by disconnecting the patient from the respirator to allow the P_{CO_2} to rise to 60 mmHg.

At this stage the patient who does not initiate breathing is assumed to have no spontaneous respiratory effort. Generally, all the extremities are flaccid, with no response to painful stimuli. The deep tendon reflexes are generally absent, but their presence does not preclude declaration of brain death. Similarly, a withdrawal response in the feet may be present. An EEG will show isoelectric tracing in spite of high-gain setting. Before brain death is declared, it must be ascertained that the patient is not intoxicated with sedative or hypnotic drugs and is not hypothermic. Objective criteria seldom used in clinical practice are radionuclide brain scan and arteriogram, both of which can confirm a total lack of cerebral blood flow.[2]

It is customary when declaring brain death to examine the patient on two occasions, 6 hours apart, to make certain the state is irreversible. After a patient meets the criteria for brain death,

CLINICAL PEARLS

- Impaired consciousness constitutes a neurosurgical emergency. The treating physician should arrive at a rapid diagnosis derived from clinical history, quick neurological assessments, laboratory data and imaging studies.

- The degree of impairment of consciousness in expressed in contemporary practice as the *Glagow Coma Score*.

- Elicitation of brainstem reflexes is a key determinant in assessing depth of impaired consciousness.

- The anatomical substrate of consciousness is the central reticular core of the brainstem and its diffuse projections to the cerebral hemispheres.

within minutes to a few days cardiac activity invariably ceases. Because there is no exception to this rule, it has become customary to declare patients legally dead if they meet the brain-death criteria. Brain-dead patients who continue to have good cardiac function and perfusion are potential organ donors. When the criteria are met and the patient is declared brain-dead, the family should be approached for potential organ donation.

REFERENCES

1. Posner JB. The comatose patient. *JAMA*. 1975; 232: 1313.
2. Fisher CM. The neurological examination of the comatose patient. *Acta Neurol Scand* 1969; 36(suppl.): 273–90.
3. Teasdale G, Jennet B. Assessment of coma and impaired consciousness – a practical scale. *Lancet* 1974; 2: 81.
4. Fisher CM. Ocular bobbing. *Arch Neurol* 1964; 11: 543–6.
5. North JB, Jennet S. Abnormal breathing patterns associated with acute brain damage. *Arch Neurol* 1974; 32: 338.
6. Couten-Meyers G, Myers RE, Schoolfield L. Hyperglycemia enlarges infarct size in cerebrovascular occlusion in cats. *Stroke* 1988; 19: 623–30.
7. Vazquez-Curz J, Vilalta JL, Ferer I, Perez-Gallofre A, Folch J. Progressing cerebral infarction in relation to plasma glucose in gerbils. *Stroke* 1990; 21: 1621–4.
8. Feldman MH. Physiological observations in a chronic case of "locked-in" syndrome. *Neurology* 1971; 21: 459–78.
9. Nordgren RE, Markesbery WR, Fukuda K, Reeves AG. Seven cases of cerebromedullospinal disconnection: the "locked-in" syndrome. *Neurology* 1971; 21: 1140–8.
10. Munsat TL, Stuart WH, Cranford RE. Guidelines on the vegetative state: commentary on the American Academy of Neurology statement. *Neurology* 1989; 39: 123–4.
11. American Academy of Neurology. Position of the American Academy of Neurology on certain aspects of the care and management of the persistent vegetative state patient. *Neurology* 1989; 39: 125–6.
12. Levy DE, Sidtis JJ, Rottenberg DA, *et al*. Differences in cerebral blood flow and glucose utilization in vegetative versus locked-in patients. *Ann Neurol* 1987; 22: 673–82.
13. Iragui VJ, McCuthen CB. Physiologic and prognostic significance of "alpha coma". *J Neurol Neurosurg Psychiatr* 1983; 46: 632.
14. Westmoreland BF, Klass DW, Shargbough FW, Reagan TJ. Alpha-coma: electroencephalographic, clinical, pathologic and etiologic correlations. *Arch Neurol* 1975; 32: 713–18.

ADDITIONAL READING

Albright TD, Jessell TM, Kandell ER, Posner MI. Progess in the neural sciences in the century after Cajal (and the mysteries that remain). *Am NY Acad Sci* 2001; 929: 11–40.

Arbib MA. Coerdution of human consciousness and language. *Am NY Acad Sci* 2001; 929: 195–220.

Bateman DE. Neurological assessment of coma. *J Neurol Neurosurg Psychiatr* 2001; 71(suppl 1): i13–17.

Blackmore S. *Consciousness*. Oxford: Oxford University Press; 2003.

Bone I, Fuller GN. Neurology in practice: sleep and coma. *J Neurol Neurosurg Psychiatr* 2001; 71(suppl 1): i1–2.

Brunia CH. Thalamo cortical relations in attention and consciousness. *Int J Psychophysiol* 2001; 43: 1–4.

Carter R. *Exploring Consciousness*. Berkeley, CA: University of California Press; 2002.

Cartlidge N. States related to or confused with coma. *J Neurol Neurosurg Psychiatr* 2001; 71(suppl. 1):18–19.

Cijona PC, Bosinelli M. Consciousness during dreams. *Conscious Cogn* 2001; 10: 26–41.

Crick F. *Astonishing Hypothesis: The Scientific Search for the Soul*. Carmichael, CA: Touchstone Books; 1995.

Crick F, Koch C. A framework for conscious awareness. *Nat Neurosci* 2003; 6: 119–26.

Deouell LY. Pre-requisites for conscious awareness: dues from electrophysiological and behavioral studies of unilateral neglect patients. *Conscious Cogn* 2002; 11: 546–67.

Edelman GM. *Remembered Present: A Biological Theory of Consciousness*. New York: Basic Books; 1990.

Edelman GM. Consciousness: the remembered present. *Am NY Acad Sci* 2001: 929: 111–22.

Giacino JT, Ashwal S, Childs N, Cranford R, Jennet B, Kate DL. The minimally conscious state: definition and diagnostic criteria. *Neurology* 2002; 58: 349–33.

Hobson JA, Pace-Schott EF. The cognitive neuroscience of sleep, neuronal systems, consciousness and learning. *Nat Rev Neurosci* 2002; 3: 679–93.

John ER. The neurophysics of consciousness. *Brain Res Rev* 2002; 39: 1–28.

Johnson PL, Eckard DA, Chason DP, Bracheisen MA, Batnitsky S. Imaging of acquired cerebral herniations. *Neuroimaging Clin North Am* 2002; 12: 217–28.

Karakatsanis KG, Tsanakas JN. A critique on the concept of brain death. *Issues Law Med* 2002; 18: 127–41.

Kerridge IH, Saul P, Lowe M, McPhee J, Williams D. Death, dying and donation: organ transplantation and the diagnosis of death. *J Med Ethics* 2002; 28: 29–94.

Le Berge D. Attention. Consciousness, and electrical wave activity within the cortical column. *Int J Psychophysiol* 2001; 43: 5–24.

Leon-Carrion J, Van Eckhart P, Dominquez-Morales Melel R. The Locked-in syndrome: a syndrome looking for a therapy. *Brain Injury* 2002; 16: 555–69.

Lloyd D. Functional MRI and the study of human consciousness. *J Cogn Neurosci* 2002; 14: 818–31.

Lombardi F, Tarricco M, Detanti A, Telaro E, Liberati X. Sensory stimulation of brain injured individuals in coma or vegetative state. *Clin Rehabil* 2002; 16: 464–72.

Malik K, Hess DC. Evaluating the comatose patient. Rapid neurologic assessment is key to appropriate management. *Postgrad-Med* 2002; 111: 38–40, 43–6, 49–50.

McAlonan K, Brown VJ. The thalamic reticular nucleus more than a sensory nucleus? *Neuroscientist* 2002; 8: 302–5.

Niedermeyer E. The concept of consciousness. *Ital J Neurol Sci* 1999; 20: 7–15.

O'Connell S. Animal consciousness. *Biologist (London)* 2002; 47: 207–10.

Plum F, Posner J. *The Diagnosis of Stupor and Coma*. Oxford: Oxford University Press; 1982.

Rees G, Krisman G, Koch C. Neural correlates of consciousness in humans. *Nat Rev Neurosci* 2002; 3: 261–70.

Robinson LR, Mickelesen PJ, Tirchvell DL, Lew HL. Predictive value of somatosensory evoked potentials for awakening from coma. *Crit Care Med* 2003; 31: 960–7.

Schiff ND, Plum F. The role of arousal and "gating" systems in the neurology of impaired consciousness. *J Clin Neurophysiol* 2000; 17: 438–92.

Searle JR. *The Mystery of Consciousness*. New York: New York Times Review Books; 1997.

Tassi P, Muzet A. Defining the states of consciousness. *Neurosci Biobehav Rev* 2001; 25: 175–91.

The Brain Trauma-Foundation. The American Association of Neurological Surgeons. The Joint Section on Neurotrauma and Critical Care. Glasgow Coma Scale; Score. *J Neurotrauma* 2000; 17: 563–71.

Wijdidcs EF. The diagnosis of brain death. *N Engl J Med* 2001; 344(16): 1215–21.

Young GB. The EEG in coma. *J Clin Neurophysiol* 2000; 17: 473–85.

Zeman A. Consciousness. *Brain* 2001; 124: 1263–89.

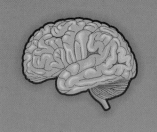

PERIOPERATIVE CARE OF THE NEUROSURGICAL PATIENT

6

Dragan F Dimitrov and Dennis A Turner

This chapter discusses the major principles of preoperative, intraoperative, and postoperative care of neurosurgical patients. Accurate and routine preoperative assessment of the patient's condition improves both preoperative and intraoperative management, minimizes problems in the immediate postoperative course, and substantially decreases the overall surgical risks.

PREOPERATIVE CARE

The general goal of preoperative care is to minimize the surgical risks and to optimize the patient's recuperation and outcome, taking into account patient characteristics and the particular planned procedure.[1-6] Medical problems and risk factors, such as hypertension and diabetes, should be treated prior to surgical intervention, if possible. Perioperative risks, as devised for carotid endarterectomy,[7,8] include neurological, medical, and angiographic or radiological criteria. This system of risk evaluation can be widely applied to neurosurgical procedures.

Preparation includes: (1) preventing problems related to the specific operative approach; (2) evaluating and treating systemic medical risks; and (3) obtaining an informed consent from the patient and family.[6] The extent and timing of this preparation is dictated by the urgency required to alleviate the nervous system abnormalities.

Specific nervous system preparation

The primary goal of preparation is to stabilize abnormalities of the nervous system as much as possible. Even in emergencies, the wait for the operating suite may be 15 to 30 minutes, during which time secondary damage may occur. Table 6.1 lists some of the ways in which the nervous system can be temporarily protected. For example, performing cerebrospinal fluid (CSF) drainage preoperatively may help to stabilize the patient, protecting against damage caused by increased intracranial pressure or secondary brain shift. Conditions that increase risk need to be recognized so that treatment plans can prevent surprising perioperative complications. Many neurological disorders, such as Parkinson's disease and multiple sclerosis, require optimal medical treatment before and during surgery to minimize temporary worsening of the neurological state.

Evaluation and treatment of systemic abnormalities

Table 6.2 lists common systemic risk factors that require evaluation and treatment to ensure optimal safety during anesthesia and the surgical procedure. Some of these abnormalities may even preclude either anesthesia or the procedure until corrected (e.g. severe arrhythmia or coagulation disorders). Other abnormalities may increase the intraoperative risks (e.g. metabolic

Table 6.1 Neurological preoperative risks and management

Nervous system risk factors	Management scheme to decrease risk
Increased ICP	CSF drainage via ventricular or lumbar catheter Steroids: dexamethasone, prednisone, or hydrocortisone Controlled anesthesia induction: hyperventilation Narcotics
Coma	Early intubation, assessment, and systemic stabilization ICP management: CSF drainage, mannitol as needed Treatment of urinary retention: bladder catheter
Seizures	Control of seizures: parenteral medication, with loading of phenytoin (20 mg/kg) or phenobarbital (15 mg/kg) Treatment of status with additional agents as required
Contaminated or open wound	Antibiotics to cover skin contaminants and prompt debridement and secondary closure

Table 6.2 Systemic preoperative risks and management

Systemic risk factors	Management scheme
Cardiovascular	Control of hypertension, hypotension, arrhythmias, vascular compromise
Respiratory	Pulmonary function tests and chest X-ray to assess complicating lesions and need for bronchodilation
Endocrine	Diabetes management, pituitary assessment, steroid coverage for stress management
Hematologic	Coagulation disorders and platelets; anemia evaluation
Gastrointestinal	Risk of aspiration; general nutrition for healing
Genitourinary	Management of urinary infections and drainage
Renal	Need for dialysis in patient with renal compromise
Fluids and electrolytes	Metabolic balance, control of electrolytes
Infection	Identification of source, treatment with antibiotics

imbalance or inadequate nutritional status) but can be managed intraoperatively if necessary. For example, hyperglycemia should be treated with sufficient insulin to lower the blood sugar to less than 250 mg/dL, using an insulin drip and frequent blood sugar measurements. Hypertension should be treated until blood pressure is in the range of 160/90 mmHg or less, to decrease the risk of postoperative intracranial hemorrhage in patients undergoing craniotomy.[9] Platelets may need to be supplemented, if there are abnormalities in platelet number ($< 75\,000/mm^3$) or function that cannot be rapidly corrected. Pulmonary function tests, cardiology consultation as needed for cardiovascular risk assessment, and endocrine evaluation may be required in addition to the standard electrocardiogram (ECG) and serum tests for electrolytes, renal function, blood count, and coagulation factors. The urgency of the procedure must be weighed against the risk of either delay (with the attendant risk of neurological worsening) or inadequate treatment of the systemic complicating factor. From this discussion it should become clear that excellent care of patients with neurological disorders begins with attention to the entire patient.

Pre-existing cardiac disease often requires special preoperative attention. The main role of the neurosurgeon is to identify patients at high risk and initiate the appropriate preoperative and perioperative measures. Factors that are associated with a higher risk of cardiac complications after surgery include: (1) known ischemic heart disease; (2) congestive heart failure; (3) diabetes mellitus; (4) renal insufficiency; (5) poor functional status; and (6) those undergoing high-risk procedures that require long operating room time or involve increased blood loss.[10] Cardiology consultation may be helpful to assess the risk of a major cardiac event with the proposed neurosurgical procedure. This evaluation may clarify that preoperative cardiac revascularization is indicated, or that perioperative medications, such as beta blockers, should be used. There is a growing body of evidence that perioperative beta blockers may be of benefit to a wide patient population in helping to prevent perioperative cardiac events.[11] Cardiology consultation may also clearly identify surgical risks. Some patients may choose to live with a radiculopathy if surgery entails a high risk of myocardial infarction, for example.

Informed consent

Informed consent is a surprisingly new entity in the field of health care, dating back only to 1960, when the Kansas Supreme Court essentially stated that it is the duty of a physician to disclose to patients what other reasonable physicians would do in the same circumstances.[12] In response to patients' desire to be better informed, the courts have significantly expanded this duty over the years. It is important to understand that informed consent is not a document but rather a dialog between physician and patient. The informed consent form simply assures that the dialog has occurred. It is legally assumed that the patient will remember little of this preoperative discussion, therefore the surgeon's documentation that the dialog occurred is critical as the primary record of the informed consent. The more detailed the discussion, the better informed the patient and family will be for what to expect, assuming that bad outcomes or unexpected worsening will inevitably occur. Obviously, informed consent is crucial in high-risk patients and when the benefits of the procedure may only marginally outweigh the risks. Generally any procedure that entails significant risk of morbidity or mortality necessitates documentation of informed consent, although no absolute guidelines exist.

Legally, informed consent consists of four components: duty, breach, causation, and damage.[12] It is the duty of the physician not only to inform the patient but also then to obtain the patient's consent for a given procedure. What information is disclosed while informing the patient remains vague. At best, it is safe to say that physicians are expected to disclose information that any reasonable practitioner would be expected to disclose, or that any reasonable patient would wish to know. The general components of an informed consent discussion are outlined in Table 6.3. Legally, it is clear that the responsibility of obtaining and documenting the consent lies with the person performing the procedure. For procedures often performed solely by a neurosurgical resident, such as placement of a ventriculostomy or lumbar drain, it is the duty of the resident to obtain consent.[12] If the operative plan outlined through the informed consent process is different from what is actually performed, such as a posterior cervical discectomy rather than an anterior approach, legally, a breach of the informed

Table 6.3 Preoperative preparation and informed consent

1. Nature of the condition	Clinical history, examination, diagnostic tests (MRI, CT scan)
2. Proposed treatment and associated possible complications	Possible benefit when balanced against known and/or unexpected risks
3. Alternative forms of treatment	Benefits and risks compared with natural history and proposed treatment, including nonoperative management
4. Complications (a) Temporary (b) Permanent	Pain, infection, steps to correct Neurologic deficits
5. Death	
6. Expected benefit of proposed treatment is not guaranteed	

Table 6.4 Perioperative medication management

Type of medication	Rationale and duration of treatment
Perioperative antibiotics	First dose prior to anesthesia; continue throughout surgery until skin closed, unless infection demonstrated or wound contaminated
Perioperative steroids	Useful for spinal cord injury, brain tumor edema, and increased ICP; dexamethasone 10–20 mg loading, 4–6 mg every 6 hours
Hypertonic solutions	Mannitol 1 g/kg for increased ICP and to help retraction; 3% saline for persistent hyponatremia
Antihypertensives	To prevent immediate postoperative bleeding and for management of subarachnoid hemorrhage
Anticonvulsants	Full preoperative load when risk of seizures exceeds 5% to 10% or after seizure occurs

consent has occurred. If a situation develops where a result occurs that, had the patient had further information and known this might happen, he or she may not have elected to proceed with the operation, it may be argued that the physician caused (causation) the injury. Furthermore, if financial loss can be proven as a result of such a situation, the physician may be held responsible (damages).

It is worth mentioning that there are rare situations where informed consent is waived. The most common situation is when an emergency surgery or life-saving procedure is necessary, and neither family nor guardian is available at the critical time required. Although such situations are complex, it is generally best to do everything possible to save a life in the acute setting, rather than wait for a consenting party.

Preoperative medications

During the preoperative evaluation, the surgeon should determine if additional medications are required to facilitate the intraoperative course and enhance the patient's recovery (Table 6.4). For example, perioperative steroid management may be helpful to decrease cerebral edema or spinal cord injury. The suggested dose of dexamethasone is 10–20 mg intravenously for a loading dose and 4–6 mg every 6 hours before, during, and after the procedure. If the risk of seizures from a primary cortical abnormality is thought to be greater than 5–10%, management with anticonvulsants should be considered. Gram-positive organisms, mainly

Staphylococus aureus, are the causative pathogens in the majority of postoperative infections in clean cases, as a result of contamination of the wound with skin flora. Preoperative antibiotics with Gram-positive bacterial coverage can help reduce the risk of postoperative infections in clean neurosurgery cases.[13–17] The principle is to maintain antibiotic tissue levels during the operation. However, gentleness with tissues, good operating technique in closing tissue layers, and attention to blood supply are fundamental; the surgeon cannot rely on antibiotics to treat infections caused by inadequacies in surgical technique. The current trend is to administer antibiotics directly before and during procedures only, while avoiding the selection for antibiotic-resistant organisms caused by lengthy regimens.[13,17] In contaminated or infected wounds, a full course of antibiotics during and after the procedure may prevent more severe infections and aid healing.

INTRAOPERATIVE CONSIDERATIONS

Medications and anesthetics

Routine preoperative preparation should include an empty stomach (to avoid aspiration) and often sedation, prior to intubation.[6] The risk of increased intracranial pressure (ICP) can be minimized at the time of induction, for example, by spraying lidocaine on the patient's vocal cords or hyperventilating the patient to a P_{CO_2} near 25–27 mmHg (Table 6.5). Muscle paralysis may be contraindicated for certain procedures, particularly those

Table 6.5 Intraoperative medications

Type of medication	Rationale and medication-related problems
Intravenous narcotics	Postoperative sedation may be pronounced clouding neurologic examination, making it difficult to determine true neurologic deficits
Inhalation agents	Increased ICP as a result of venous vasodilatation
Hyperventilation	Maintain low Pco_2 and vasoconstriction
Nitrous oxide	Only as a supplement to other anesthetics
Muscle paralysis agents	For induction and intubation but not when stimulating excitable structures (nerves and brain) for locating muscle or EMG response
Local anesthetics	On vocal cords during induction to decrease ICP and in skin incisions to decrease overall need for general anesthetic
Hypertensives (pressors)	Persistent hypotension intraoperatively

Table 6.6 Intraoperative monitoring

Risk or structure	Type of monitoring performed
Cardiovascular system	Pulse, ECG, pulmonary artery catheter for cardiac output
Blood pressure	Indwelling arterial cannula or external automatic self-inflating cuff
Respiration	End-tidal expired CO_2
Air embolism	End-tidal expired CO_2, precordial Doppler
Specific structure monitoring	Facial nerve stimulation and EMG recording; spinal cord evoked potentials during decompression or fixation; peripheral nerve monitoring during repair; EMG recording during selective rhizotomy

where either a muscle twitch or electromyogram (EMG) response is required to document the status or location of peripheral nerves. Examples of the latter include procedures for nerve root decompression, where a muscle twitch may indicate potential root damage, and surgery for acoustic neuroma, where the facial nerve may be located using an EMG recording prior to direct visualization with the microscope. Medications that protect neural structures from damage, such as steroid protocols, and prophylactic antibiotics should also be continued intraoperatively.

The recommended anesthesia for most neurosurgical procedures is balanced, which includes a mixture of intravenous narcotics, inhalation agents, and nitrous oxide as needed for adequate analgesia. Agents that raise ICP (including most inhalation agents, such as halothane and isofluorane) should be avoided in circumstances where this would be harmful. Of course, the particular circumstances and neurological status of the patient should be considered (e.g. a comatose patient needs only light anesthesia during surgery).

Intraoperative monitoring

Physiological variables should be assessed during induction and intubation, including ECG, arterial pressure, and, if critical, ICP using a ventriculostomy to allow venting of CSF (Table 6.6). End-tidal CO_2 measurements also allow assessment of ventilation adequacy. Other types of physiological monitoring include: (1) evoked potentials to evaluate axonal conduction along pertinent pathways; (2) EMG recording of end-organs associated with the operative field (such as EMG recording of the facial muscles during surgery for acoustic neuroma); (3) monitoring of bladder and anal sphincter function during procedures involving sacral nerve roots or the conus; and (4) evaluation of swallowing during sectioning of the upper cervical nerves and accessory nerves for torticollis. Physiological monitoring may substantially decrease the risk of damage to critical neurological structures in close proximity to the exposure.

Procedures performed on patients in the sitting position, particularly those involving the posterior fossa, require constant vigilance because of the increased risk related to veins unable to collapse under negative pressure. The veins in this category include those embedded in bone (e.g. the mastoid emissary vein), large muscles, and particularly the dural venous sinuses. These veins may remain open regardless of the intraluminal venous pressure. The patient must be monitored constantly. Specific methods to detect air embolism have been developed, including Doppler monitoring of the heart for abnormal mixing of air within its chambers, and end-tidal CO_2 measurement. Air embolism is treated by withdrawing the air through a right atrial catheter, in addition to identifying and stopping the source in the surgical field.

Surgical positioning of the patient

Intraoperative management includes determining the proper surgical position, the types of perioperative monitoring required, and how to minimize complications such as infection, bleeding, and peripheral nerve palsies caused by pressure. For instance, the ulnar nerves should always be carefully padded and the axilla should be well protected during surgery in the lateral position. Figure 6.1 illustrates standard positions. Other positions include extensile exposure for peripheral nerve problems in the upper and lower extremities, the lateral thoracotomy position for exposure of T2–L3 in complex spine procedures, and the lateral retroperitoneal position for lumbar spine procedures. Positioning and the associated monitoring requirements should be discussed with the anesthesiologist either before or at the time of surgery. For example, air embolism is one of the more severe complications associated with the sitting position.[2-4] However, there is even a risk of air embolism in the supine and prone positions, depending on the location of the operative site and the right atrium and central venous pressures.

Continuous surgical management

Identified preoperative risk factors and their treatment paradigms should be continued, such as blood clotting factors needed for coagulopathy. Intraoperative antibiotics, steroids, and anticonvulsants should be maintained. Induced hypo- or hypertension for complex vessel exposure and direct replacement of blood loss to ensure stability may be required. Adequate monitoring can indicate neurological changes during surgery that require the surgeon to make changes in surgical technique. Monitoring techniques that help confirm the level of surgery and the field of exposure, and that delineate the pathologic abnormalities include regular X-ray film, fluoroscopy, intraoperative ultrasound, and angiography. Instances occur in which the operation may be significantly altered or terminated, such as severe bleeding, hypotension, impending cardiac or respiratory instability, or severe air embolism. It is sometimes necessary to implement contingency plans and alternative routes of treatment, such as unplanned intensive care unit (ICU) observation.

POSTOPERATIVE CARE

Postoperative care of the patient should include knowledge of potential complications.[3,4] A thorough understanding of how the central nervous system reacts to stress and anesthesia can help predict an individual patient's response to a situation. For instance, patients with significant pre-existing central nervous system disease often recover slowly from the anesthesia and exhibit a prolonged deficit for the first 6–12 postoperative hours.[18]

Acute postoperative recovery and early problems

The patient's recovery following complex procedures involves either a specialized neurosurgical ICU or a general surgical ICU.[19] Management of cardiac or respiratory instability, CSF drainage (such as with ventriculostomy), ICP management, and care of patients with altered mental status can be facilitated by a knowledgeable ICU staff. In the early postoperative period (particularly the first 48 hours), close observation may help detect early problems, such as postoperative bleeding or hematomas, or local central nervous system problems that may or may not be directly related to the surgical procedure, including dural sinus thrombosis, acute seizures, inappropriate serum dilution, and early assessment for infection (Table 6.7).

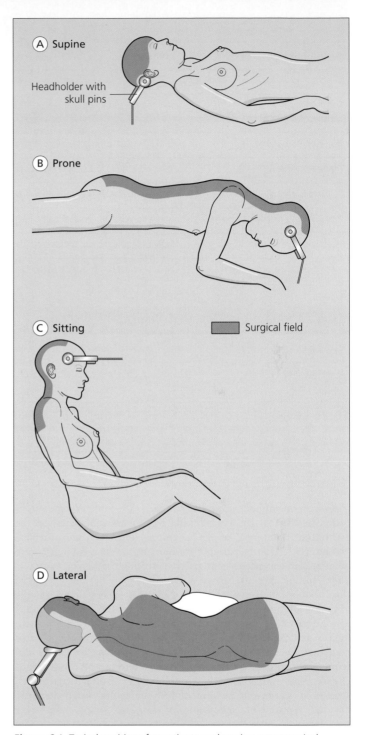

Figure 6.1 Typical positions for patients undergoing neurosurgical procedures, and the regions of access for each particular position (shaded areas). Note that for all craniotomy procedures (apart from those performed supine with a head roll), a headholder with skull pins is used to clamp the patient to the operating room bed securely and prevent damage to the eyes and face. Each position has a number of variations and precautions, discussed more fully in the text. **(A)** Supine position – frontal craniotomies, carotid endarterectomy procedures, anterior cervical discectomy procedures, and transsphenoidal adenomectomy. **(B)** Prone position – posterior occipital and suboccipital craniotomy and craniectomy procedures and cervical, thoracic, and lumbar laminectomy procedures. **(C)** Sitting or lounge position – posterior fossa and cervical spine procedures. **(D)** Lateral or park bench position – posterior fossa and retromastoid craniectomy procedures, lateral thoracotomy and anterolateral lumbar spine approaches, lateral cervical, thoracic and lumbar spine procedures, and lumboperitoneal shunt placement

Table 6.7 Early postoperative problems

Event or disease	Management
Subarachnoid/intraventricular blood	CSF drainage from subarachnoid space
Vasospasm following subarachnoid hemorrhage	Maintain blood volume and pressure
CSF leak from operative site	CSF drainage, proper positioning
Respiratory insufficiency	Treat atelectasis, intubation if severe
Seizures	Remove source of cortical irritation and hemorrhage, if possible
Postoperative clot formation	May require direct evacuation of clot
Infection	Early or late: antibiotics, drainage, debridement
Inappropriate serum dilution	Fluid restriction, hypertonic saline

Table 6.8 Phases and risks of wound healing

1. Risks for poor healing	Prior radiation, diabetes, small vessel disease, previous infection
2. Suture type for closure	Absorbable versus permanent (incision location, use of suture site, likelihood of heavy work dictates type of suture and density of suturing)
3. First 4 days	Inflammatory healing only with no tissue crossbridges
4. Intermediate period	Proliferative changes, cell and collagen turnover, cell migration, and capillary formation
5. Reorganization phase	Continued remodeling and strengthening of wound for up to 2 years

Thromboembolism, which can be a life-threatening complication because of the risk of fatal pulmonary embolism, has an estimated incidence of 24% among elective neurosurgical procedures.[20] Glioma patients are thought to represent a subgroup of neurosurgical patients at particularly high risk. For example, brain tumor patients have a significant reduction in partial thromboplastin times and bleeding times, beginning at the initiation of surgery and lasting into the postoperative period.[21] Much attention has recently been focused on appropriate measures for reducing the risk of thromboembolism after neurosurgical procedures. Graduated compression stockings and sequential compression devices are considered to be the standard of care. Neurosurgeons have been reluctant to add anticoagulants, such as subcutaneous heparin or low molecular weight heparin, despite reports of subcutaneous heparin being safe after craniotomy.[22] However, a combination of subcutaneous low molecular weight heparin combined with compression stockings is more effective than compression stockings alone in preventing thromboembolism, and does not appear to lead to increased rates of bleeding.[23]

Wound healing and activity

Table 6.8 briefly describes the phases of wound healing. The type of sutures used depends on the expected rate of healing and anticipated problems. For example, prior radiation to an incision site may considerably inhibit healing, necessitating several layers of permanent sutures to ensure wound closure. The presence of associated medical diseases, particularly diabetes, will slow the healing process, as will vascular diseases such as arteriosclerosis. However, good operative technique and clear apposition of important layers (such as the fascia and subcutaneous tissues) without overlap or infolding will decrease the chances of wound dehiscence or infection. The surgeon must decide when to mobilize the patient following surgery and what level of activity should be achieved. Ambulation is beneficial and prevents deep venous thrombosis, aspiration, and atelectasis. The advantages of early ambulation, however, have to be balanced against contravening factors, such as the need to prevent CSF leak through a dural incision in some cases, and the maintenance of cervical traction for an unstable spine and postoperative comfort.

The objective of early postoperative care and observation is the management of immediate complications. Later in the postoperative course, the goal is to bring the patient gradually up to the level of functioning that the postoperative neurological status allows. Subsequent rehabilitation or long-term nursing care is necessary for patients who will not return to their preoperative level of independent functioning or who require additional recovery time.

Late postoperative problems

Late postoperative complications include slow but progressive neurological conditions. These conditions include hydrocephalus, deep venous thrombosis and pulmonary embolism, delayed hemorrhage within operative sites, and infection, such as discitis

Table 6.9 Late postoperative complications

Class of complication	Examples of complications
Late infections	Discitis, CSF shunt infections, cranioplasty infections
Late hemorrhage	Hemosiderosis after hemispherectomy
CSF leak	Meningitis following surgery or trauma
Late hydrocephalus	Subarachnoid hemorrhage, posterior fossa surgery
Deep venous thrombosis	Pulmonary embolism and risk of death
Pituitary insufficiency	Thyroid, gonadal, and steroid hormone insufficiency
Late seizures	Late development of epileptic focus because of scar or irritation

(Table 6.9). Constant vigilance is required to recognize and assess problems before they become serious. The surgeon must be aware of the potential problems following the procedure and the time frame in which they occur to improve proper diagnosis and treatment. Thus hydrocephalus several months following a subarachnoid hemorrhage, unexpected thyroid deficiency following a transsphenoidal adenomectomy for a nonsecreting adenoma, or lumbar discitis presenting several weeks after a discectomy procedure should not be unexpected. These complications may seem so remote from the surgery that they are not considered, delaying diagnosis until there is secondary damage or instability (e.g. late hormone insufficiency).

CLINICAL PEARLS

- A systematic and routine approach to preoperative evaluation will decrease intraoperative and postoperative morbidity, and enhance patient recovery.

- Informing the patient clearly as to the goals and objectives of the procedure, the likely outcome, the potential for unexpected events to occur and the likely recovery time will significantly improve the patient's response to the procedure.

- Immediate preoperative preparation and careful operative planning and positioning will facilitate an optimal and smooth intraoperative course.

- Thorough preparation for possible complications during and after surgery may lead to avoidance of risk, and improve outcome even if complications do occur.

- Wound healing problems and possible late postoperative complications may be anticipated occasionally and should be sought and treated before irreversible damage occurs.

CONCLUSION

Many postoperative difficulties can be anticipated and their impact eliminated or ameliorated, with adequate preoperative and intraoperative planning. The goal is to decrease the risks associated with the procedure and to facilitate recovery, maximizing the patient's independent functional capabilities.

REFERENCES

1. Keller TS. Preoperative evaluation of a neurosurgical patient. In: Wilkins RH, Rengachary SS (eds). *Neurosurgery*. New York, NY: McGraw-Hill; 1985: 366–8.
2. Wise BL. *Preoperative and Postoperative Care in Neurological Surgery*. Springfield, IL: Charles C Thomas Publisher; 1978.
3. Horwitz NH, Rizzoli HV. *Postoperative Complications of Intracranial Neurological Surgery*. Baltimore, MD: Williams & Wilkins; 1982.
4. Horwitz NH, Rizzoli HV. *Postoperative Complications of Extracranial Neurological Surgery*. Baltimore, MD: Williams & Wilkins; 1987.
5. Stern WE. Preoperative evaluation; complications, their prevention and treatment. In: Youmans JR (ed.). *Neurological Surgery*. Philadelphia, PA: WB Saunders Co; 1985: 1051–116.
6. Wilkins RH, Odom GL. General operative technique. In: Youmans JR (ed.). *Neurological Surgery*. Philadelphia, PA: WB Saunders Co; 1985: 1136–59.
7. Sundt TM Jr, Sandok BA, Whisnant JP. Carotid endarterectomy: complications and preoperative assessment of risk. *Mayo Clin Proc* 1975; 50: 301–6.
8. Turner DA, Tracy J, Haines SJ. Risk of late stroke and survival following carotid endarterectomy procedures for symptomatic patients. *J Neurosurg* 1990; 73: 193–200.
9. Basali A, Mascha EJ, Kalfas I, Schubert A. Relation between perioperative hypertension and intracranial hemorrhage after craniotomy. *Anesthesiology* 2000; 93: 48–54
10. Fleisher LA, Eagle KA. Lowering cardiac risk in noncardiac surgery. *N Engl J Med* 2001; 345: 1677–82.
11. Auerbach AD, Goldman L. Beta-blockers and reduction of cardiac events in noncardiac surgery. *JAMA* 2002; 287: 1445–7.
12. Scarrow AM, Scarrow MR. Informed consent for the neurosurgeon. *Surg Neurol* 2002; 57: 63–9.
13. Haines SJ. Prophylactic antibiotics. In: Wilkins RH, Rengachary SS (eds). *Neurosurgery*. New York, NY: McGraw-Hill; 1985: 448–52.
14. Bullock R, van Dellen JR, Ketelbey W, Reinach SG. A double-blind placebo-controlled trial of perioperative prophylactic antibiotics for elective neurosurgery. *J Neurosurg* 1988; 69: 687–91.
15. Dempsey R, Rapp RP, Young B, Johnston S, Tibbs P. Prophylactic parenteral antibiotics in clean neurosurgical procedures: a review. *J Neurosurg* 1988; 69: 52–7.
16. Horowitz NH, Curtin JA. Prophylactic antibiotics and wound infections following laminectomy for lumbar disc herniation. *J Neurosurg* 1975; 43: 727–31.
17. Mollman HD, Haines SJ. Risk factors for postoperative neurosurgical wound infections. *J Neurosurg* 1986; 64: 902–6.
18. Albin MS. Neuroanesthesia. In: Wilkins RH, Rengachary SS (eds). *Neurosurgery*. New York, NY: McGraw-Hill; 1985: 384–95.
19. Wirth FP, Ratcheson RA. *Neurosurgical Critical Care*. Baltimore, MD: Williams & Wilkins; 1987.
20. Agnelli G, Piovella F, Buoncristiani P, *et al.* Enoxaparin plus compression stockings compared with compression stockings alone in the prevention of venous thromboembolism after elective neurosurgery. *N Engl J Med* 1998; 339: 80–5.

21. Iberti TJ, Miller M, Abalos A, *et al*. Abnormal coagulation profile in brain tumor patients during surgery. *Neurosurgery* 1994; 34: 389–94.

22. Macdonald RL, Amidei C, Lin G, *et al*. Safety of perioperative subcutaneous heparin for prophylaxis of venous thromboembolism in patients undergoing craniotomy. *Neurosurgery* 1999; 45: 245–51.

23. Agnelli G, Piovella F, Buoncristiani P, *et al*. Enoxaparin plus compression stockings compared with compression stockings alone in the prevention of venous thromboembolism after elective Neurosurgery. *N Engl J Med* 1998; 339: 80–5.

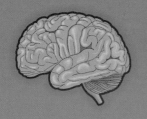

SPINAL DYSRAPHISM

7

Leslie N Sutton

The term *spinal dysraphism* refers to a group of congenital anomalies of the spine in which the midline structures fail to fuse. If the lesion is confined to the bony posterior arches at one or more levels, it is termed *spina bifida*. Simple spina bifida of the lower lumbar spine is a common radiologic finding, especially in children, and by itself carries no significance; in contrast, bony spina bifida may accompany any of several complex anomalies involving the spinal cord, nerve roots, dura, and even the pelvic visceral structures. In these cases, spinal dysraphism constitutes a major source of disability among children and adults.

There are two distinct syndromes of spinal dysraphism: (1) *spina bifida cystica*, which includes the familiar myelomeningocele, is characterized by herniation of elements through the skin as well as the bony defect and is obvious at birth; and (2) *spina bifida occulta*, in which the underlying neural defect is masked by intact overlying skin. The external signs are often subtle; symptoms may not develop until late childhood, or even adulthood, as the result of spinal cord tethering. Included in the latter group are diastematomyelia, lipomyelomeningocele, tethered filum terminale, anterior sacral meningocele, myelocystocele and the caudal regression syndromes. Early recognition of these entities is important, because neurologic function may be preserved only by early (prophylactic) and appropriate surgical intervention.

MYELOMENINGOCELE

Myelomeningocele is the most common significant birth defect involving the spine. Since the early 1980s the prevalence of spina bifida in industrialized countries has been decreasing because of the steadily increasing proportion of affected fetuses that are detected prenatally and electively terminated. The incidence of the condition ranges from less than one case per 1000 live births in the United States to almost nine cases per 1000 in areas of Ireland. The etiology is unknown, but evidence exists for both environmental and genetic influences. A role for genetic risk factors is supported by numerous studies documenting familial aggregation of this condition. In addition, several lines of evidence point to the potential importance of maternal nutritional status as a determinant of the risk for having a child with spina bifida. Indirect evidence for this association is provided by studies indicating that the season of conception, socioeconomic status and degree of urbanization may be related to the risk of spina bifida. In August 1991, the Centers for Disease Control and Prevention (CDC) advised that women with a history of an affected pregnancy should take 4 mg of folic acid daily, starting at the time

they planned to become pregnant, after publication of the Medical Research Council in Britain Vitamin Study Group report.[1] This recommendation was based on a randomized, double-blind, multicenter study performed in Europe which clearly showed the protective effect of periconception folate in reducing the recurrence of spina bifida when ingested by the mothers who had previous births of children with spina bifida. A second randomized, double-blind study was performed in Hungary which demonstrated conclusively the beneficial effects of periconception folic acid intake by mothers on decreasing the incidence of first occurrence of spina bifida.[2] It was anticipated that these recommendations would have a substantial impact on the risk of neural tube defects in the offspring of such women. While this will hopefully be the case it should be noted that the vast majority of affected pregnancies (approximately 95%) occur in women with no history of a prior affected fetus or child (for review, see ref. 3).

Embryologically, the abnormality manifests between 3 and 4 weeks of gestation. At this point in development, the neural plate folds into the neural tube, a process termed *neurulation*. Neurulation begins in the dorsal midline, and progresses cephalad and caudad simultaneously. The last portion of the tube to close is the posterior end (neuropore) at 28 days. Myelomeningocele presumably occurs when the posterior neuropore fails to close, or if it reopens as the result of distension of the spinal cord's central canal with cerebrospinal fluid (CSF). The spinal abnormality is only part of a more widespread complex of central nervous system abnormalities, which also include hydrocephalus, gyral anomalies, and the Chiari II malformation of the hindbrain.

Recent developments in the prenatal diagnosis of fetal anomalies have made antenatal recognition of myelomeningocele commonplace. Families at risk are routinely offered amniocentesis for amniotic alpha-fetoprotein and acetylcholinesterase, which are important in separating open lesions from skin-covered masses, such as myelocystocele. Amniocentesis combined with ultrasound screening has a combined accuracy of more than 90%. Prenatal magnetic resonance imaging, using ultrafast T2-weighted sequences, may also be used to characterize the Chiari II malformation and other associated anomalies.[4] Recent studies indicate that such prenatal imaging studies can help to determine prognosis. Specifically, lesion level determined by prenatal imaging studies appears to predict neurological deficit and ambulatory potential, but not the degree of fetal ventriculomegaly or the extent of hindbrain deformity.[5] Families can be professionally counseled regarding the expected prognosis and decisions about abortion or the new option of fetal closure.

The majority of fetuses with spina bifida that are not electively terminated receive no specific treatment until after birth. In the United States, these babies are generally delivered by cesarean section.[6] The benefit of this approach relative to vaginal delivery has not, however, been clearly demonstrated. Data suggest that if broad-spectrum antibiotics are administered, closure of the myelomeningocele can be safely delayed for up to a week to allow time for discussion with the parents. In most instances, however, the closure is performed within 48–72 hours of birth. The parents should be told the infant's prognosis based on the functional spinal level, and it should be emphasized that closure of the defect is a life-saving measure but will not alter the pre-existing neurological deficits. Pending plans for definitive care, the infant is nursed in the prone position with a sterile, saline-soaked gauze dressing loosely applied over the sac or neural placode.

The initial step in managing the newborn with myelomeningocele is a careful physical examination by a pediatrician and neurosurgeon. A thorough evaluation should reveal associated anomalies, including cardiac and renal defects that might contraindicate surgical closure of the spine defect. A large head or bulging fontanelle suggests active hydrocephalus and indicates the need for a head ultrasound or computed tomography (CT) scan. Stridor, apnea, or bradycardia in the absence of overt intracranial hypertension suggests a symptomatic Chiari II malformation, which carries a poor prognosis. The myelomeningocele is inspected; the red, granular neural placode is surrounded by a pearly "zona epitheliosa" that must be entirely excised to prevent the appearance of a dermoid inclusion cyst. Most myelomeningoceles are slightly oval with the long axis oriented vertically. If the lesion is oriented more horizontally, a horizontal skin closure may be preferable. Neurological examination is difficult in a newborn infant, and it is hard to separate voluntary leg motion from reflex movement. It must be assumed that any leg movement in response to a painful stimulus to that limb is reflexive. Contractures and foot deformity denote paralysis at that segmental level. Virtually all affected neonates have abnormal bladder function, but this is difficult to assess in the newborn. A patulous anus lacking in sensation confirms sacral denervation.

Generally, the back is closed first, and a CSF shunting procedure is deferred unless necessary. In cases with overt hydrocephalus, the back closure and the shunt can be performed at the same time to protect the back closure from CSF leakage. The goal of back closure is to seal the spinal cord with multiple tissue layers to inhibit the entrance of bacteria from the skin and to prevent CSF leakage while preserving neurologic function and preventing tethering of the spinal cord. Accomplishing this goal requires a thorough understanding of the three-dimensional anatomy of the tissue layers involved (Figure 7.1).

Surgical technique

General anesthesia is used, and the patient is placed in the prone position, with rolls under the chest and hips to allow the abdomen to hang freely (Figure 7.2). If the sac remains intact, fluid is aspirated and sent for culture. The surgeon gently attempts to approximate the base of the sac or defect vertically, then horizontally, to determine which direction of closure will produce

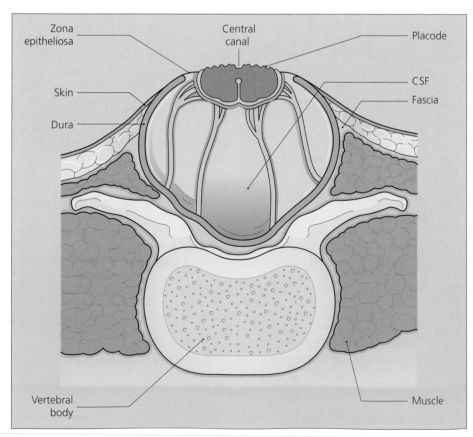

Figure 7.1 Cross-sectional anatomy of a myelomeningocele. The neural placode is visible on the back, usually at the center of the sac. It is separated from the full-thickness skin by a fringe of pearly tissue, the "zone epitheliosa." The neural tissue herniates through a defect in the skin, fascia, muscle, and bone. The dorsal dura and zona epitheliosa converge to attach laterally to the placode, forming the roof of the sac.

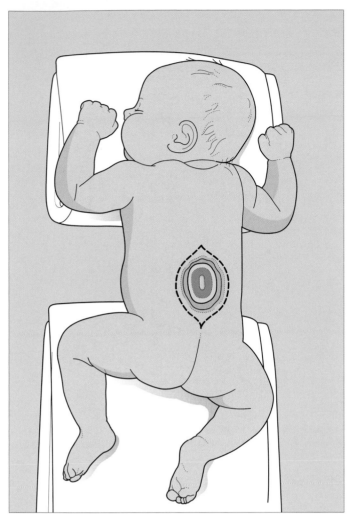

Figure 7.2 Positioning the patient for myelomeningocele closure. The infant is placed in the prone position, with rolls beneath the chest and iliac crests to minimize epidural bleeding. The skin incision is outlined circumferentially on the outside of the zona epitheliosa. A vertical orientation of the elliptical incision is appropriate for most closures.

the smallest skin defect. An elliptical incision is made, oriented along that axis, just outside the junction of the normal, full-thickness skin and the thin, pearly zona epitheliosa. Full-thickness skin forming the base of the sac is viable and should not be excised. The incision is carried through the subcutaneous tissue until the glistening layer of everted dura or fascia is encountered. The base of the sac is mobilized medially until it is seen to enter the fascial defect (Figure 7.3A). The sac is entered by radially incising the cuff of skin surrounding the neural placode. This skin is sharply excised circumferentially around the placode with scissors and discarded (Figure 7.3B). It is important to excise all of the zona epitheliosa to prevent later formation of an epidermoid cyst. At this point, the neural placode is lying freely above the everted dura (Figure 7.4).

In some instances it is appropriate to "reconstruct" the neural placode so that it fits better within the dural canal and a pial surface is in contact with the dural closure to prevent tethering. Interrupted 6-0 sutures approximate the pia-arachnoid-neural junction of one side of the placode with the other, folding the placode into a tube. The central canal is closed along its entire length.

Attention is then directed to the dura, which is everted and loosely attached to the underlying fascia. The dura is undermined bluntly and reflected medially on each side until enough has been mobilized to enable a closure (Figure 7.4). The dura is closed in a watertight fashion using a running suture of 4-0 neurilon. If possible, the fascia is closed as a separate layer by incising it laterally in a semicircle on both sides, elevating it from the underlying muscle, and reflecting it medially. Like the dura, the fascia is closed with a continuous stitch of 4-0 suture material (Figure 7.5). The fascia is poor at the caudal end of a lumbar myelomeningocele as well as with most sacral lesions, thus closure at this level may be incomplete.

The skin is mobilized by blunt dissection with dissecting scissors or a finger. It may be necessary to free up the skin ventrally all the way to the abdomen (Figure 7.5). In most instances, midsagittal (vertical) plane closure is easiest, but occasionally horizontal closure results in less tension. A two-layer closure using vertical interrupted mattress skin sutures is preferred.

Very large lesions require special techniques. Various types of "Z-plasties" and relaxation incisions have been described and may be necessary in very large or difficult lesions. Large circular defects can be closed using a simple rotation flap (Figure 7.6).

Care of the child with a myelomeningocele is life-long; it only begins with the surgical closure. Any deterioration in neurologic function signals a progressive process such as shunt malfunction, hydromyelia, tethered cord, or symptomatic Chiari II malformation. Significant advancements have been made in the treatment of these children over the past two decades, particularly in the widespread use of multidisciplinary teams of specialists to manage their urologic, orthopedic, and other needs. Among those who undergo early back closure, 92% will survive infancy and 86% will be alive 5 years later. Death is the result of problems associated with the Chiari II malformation, restrictive lung disease secondary to chest deformity, shunt malfunction, or urinary sepsis. Approximately 75% of children with myelomeningocele are ambulatory, although most require braces and crutches. Approximately 75% of surviving infants will have normal intelligence (defined as IQ > 80), although only 59–60% of those requiring shunts for hydrocephalus will have normal intelligence.[7]

In a few centers, the fetus with spina bifida may be a candidate for *in utero* treatment, because this condition is routinely detected before 20 weeks of gestation. There is evidence that neurological deterioration occurs during gestation. Normal lower extremity movement can be seen on sonograms of affected fetuses before 17–20 weeks of gestation, while most late-gestation fetuses and newborns have some degree of deformity and paralysis. Such deterioration could be the result of exposure of neural tissue to amniotic fluid and meconium or direct trauma as the exposed neural placode impacts against the uterine wall In theory, such deterioration could be reduced or eliminated by *in utero* closure of the lesion. Animal studies (in which a model for spina bifida is created by laminectomy and exposure of the fetal spinal cord to the amniotic fluid) have demonstrated improved leg function if the lesion is closed before birth. There is also evidence that the Chiari II malformation, which occurs in the vast majority of individuals with spina bifida, is acquired and could potentially be prevented by *in utero* closure.

The first cases of *in utero* spina bifida repair were performed in 1994 using an endoscopic technique. This technique proved

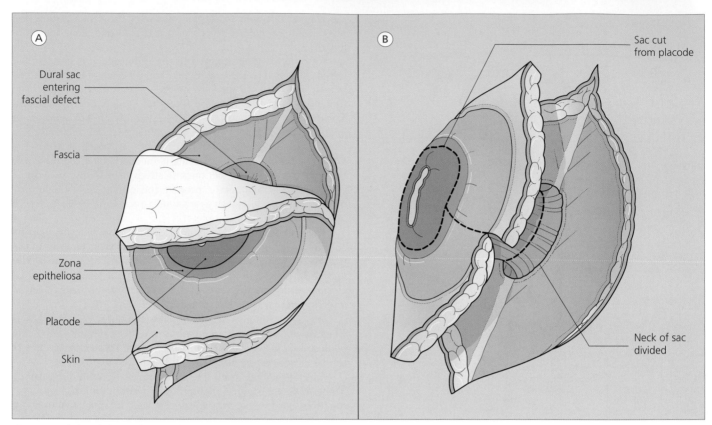

Figure 7.3 (A) Mobilizing the sac. The skin is undermined medially until the dural sac is seen to enter the fascial defect. **(B)** Excising the fringe of skin surrounding the placode. A radial cut is used to enter the sac, and it is continued around the placode to excise the skin. A separate circumferential cut amputates the base of the sac.

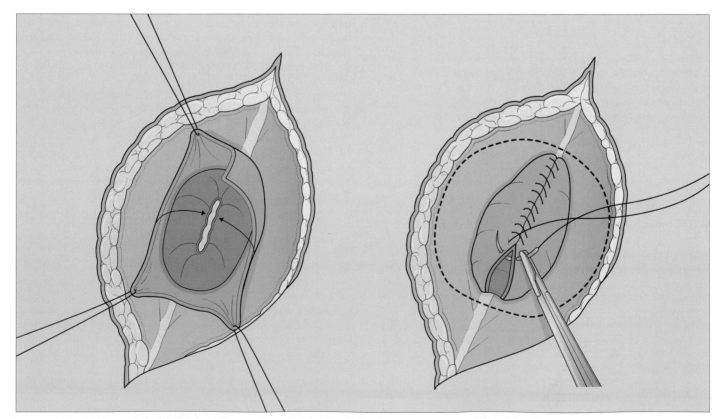

Figure 7.4 Mobilizing and closing the dura. The dura is undermined and closed using a continuous 4-0 nonabsorbable suture.

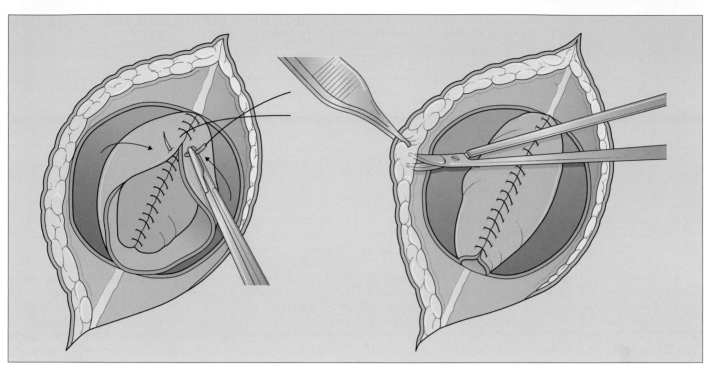

Figure 7.5 The fascial closure. The fascia is closed with a continuous stitch. The caudal end of the repair may be incomplete. Skin is mobilized by blunt dissection with scissors or a finger.

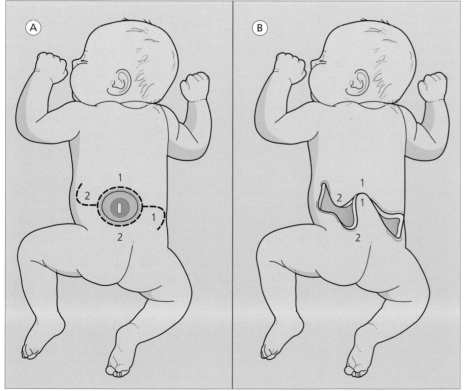

Figure 7.6 Simple rotation flap. **(A)** An S-shaped horizontal incision is made, encompassing the circular defect. **(B)** The points are approximated to the hollows, relieving tension both vertically and horizontally. The resulting skin closure has a W-shape.

unsatisfactory and was quickly abandoned. In 1997, *in utero* repair of spina bifida was performed by hysterotomy at Vanderbilt University and at The Children's Hospital of Philadelphia.[8,9] Fetuses treated *in utero* are delivered by cesarean section because the forces of labor are likely to produce a uterine dehiscence. The early experience at both institutions suggested that relative to babies treated postnatally, those treated *in utero* had a decreased incidence of hindbrain herniation, and possibly a decreased need for shunting. The combined experience at the Children's Hospital of Philadelphia and Vanderbilt, so far, indicates that the incidence of hydrocephalus requiring shunting in patients treated *in utero* is less than in historical controls stratified by spinal level who received standard postnatal care. It is hypothesized that fetal closure of the spinal lesion reduces the need for shunting, by eliminating the leakage of spinal fluid which puts back-pressure on the hindbrain. This allows reduction of the hindbrain hernia and relieves the obstruction of the outflow from the fourth ventricle (for review, see ref. 10).

It is now estimated that over 250 *in utero* spina bifida closures have been performed. The procedure appears to be generally well tolerated by the expectant mothers. Eight children have died from complications associated with uncontrollable labor and premature birth. An analysis of leg function in children treated prenatally revealed no significant difference from a set of historical controls who were treated with conventional postnatal repair.[11] However, many of the children evaluated in this series had lower limb paralysis at the time of the surgery, which may have diluted any possible benefit. Problems with delayed development of dermoid inclusion cysts and tethered cord may adversely affect outcome in the long term.[12] The preliminary experience suggests that children treated *in utero* have the same urodynamic abnormalities that are seen in conventionally treated children with spina bifida. The incidence of the Chiari II malformation, and the need for shunting may be decreased,[13] but there are currently no long-term data.

To date, outcomes for spina bifida babies treated *in utero* have been assessed relative to outcomes in conventionally treated, historical controls.[14] Such comparisons are, however, prone to substantial biases because fetuses that undergo *in utero* closures represent a highly selected subset of cases. In addition, the medical management of spina bifida is continuously improving, making comparisons with historical controls particularly problematic. It is clear that definitive answers about the benefits of fetal closure will only be obtained by a properly designed and conducted randomized trial.

A consortium of three institutions (Children's Hospital of Philadelphia, Vanderbilt, and University of California San Francisco) have undertaken an unblinded, randomized, controlled trial of *in utero* treatment of spina bifida. Pregnant women who receive a prenatal diagnosis of spina bifida between 16 and 25 weeks gestation will be referred to a central screening center. Eligible subjects who consent to participate in the trial, will be assigned to one of the three centers, and randomized to either *in utero* repair at 19–25 weeks gestation or cesarean delivery after demonstration of lung maturity. The primary study endpoints are the need for a shunt procedure at 1 year, and fetal/infant mortality. Secondary endpoints are neurologic function, cognitive outcome, and maternal morbidity. The study will enroll 200 subjects, and is estimated to close in 2006. It is hoped that the trial will be completed before other institutions begin performing *in utero* repair of spina bifida, which at this time remains of unproven benefit.

OCCULT SPINA BIFIDA AND THE TETHERED CORD SYNDROME

Developmental anomalies involving the caudal portion of the neural tube are increasingly important in clinical practice, largely as a result of advances in diagnostic techniques and the consequent change in the philosophy of treatment. Greater awareness of these conditions by pediatricians, orthopedists, and urologists, and the development of magnetic resonance imaging (MRI) have led to earlier recognition of these relatively rare problems.

The term *occult spinal dysraphism* actually encompasses several separate, possibly coexisting, entities. Most of these entities are localized to the lower spine segments and hidden by full-thickness skin. Embryologically, they arise from abnormal retrogressive differentiation of the caudal cell mass, a process by which the previously formed tail structures undergo a precise, ordered necrosis, leaving only the filum terminale, the coccygeal ligament, and the terminal ventricle of the conus as remnants by 11 weeks of gestation. Failure of regression presumably gives rise to the hypertrophied filum terminale; abnormal and incomplete regression result in lipomyelomeningocele. The embryology of diastematomyelia remains poorly understood,[15] but it may involve persistence of the fetal neurenteric canal between the yolk sac and the amniotic cavity, allowing herniation of endodermal elements through a split notochord, and causing migrating mesenchymal elements to form the bony "spike."

Symptoms may have several causes. Abnormal formation of the spinal cord and roots during embryogenesis can result in permanent neurologic deficits, as seen in myelomeningocele. Local masses growing within the spinal canal (lipomas or neurenteric cysts) can cause compression. Tethered cord syndrome, the result of traction on the spinal cord, occurs with any of the entities associated with occult spinal dysraphism. It can also occur in the adult in whom the conus has already completed its ascent.

To recognize occult dysraphic states one must appreciate the significance of the various syndromes that occur in association with the various entities. The *cutaneous syndrome* refers to any midline skin anomaly overlying the lower spine. This anomaly often signals a dysraphic state, and its recognition is especially important in the infant, in whom urologic or orthopedic complaints are not yet manifest. Dimples may be significant if they are at the level of the upper sacral or lumbar spine, but the common coccygeal pit overlying the lowest point of the coccyx in the gluteal fold has no particular significance.[16] The cutaneous abnormality may include the striking "faun's tail" of hair (Figure 7.7), dermal sinus tract, hemangioma (Figure 7.8), or skin-covered fatty mass (Figure 7.9). The *orthopedic syndrome* is apparent at birth or develops progressively in childhood. Common components include high arched feet, clawtoes, unequal leg length, and scoliosis. The *urologic syndrome* should be considered in any infant or small child who has an abnormal voiding pattern, new onset of incontinence after toilet-training, or with urinary tract infection in a child of any age. The *neurologic syndrome* presents as leg muscle atrophy or weakness, numbness of the feet, or radicular lower extremity pain and can occur at any age. In summary, patients may present with any of the above syndromes, but, in general, infants primarily present with skin manifestations, older children present with urologic, neurologic, or orthopedic syndromes, and adults often complain of pain (Table 7.1).[17]

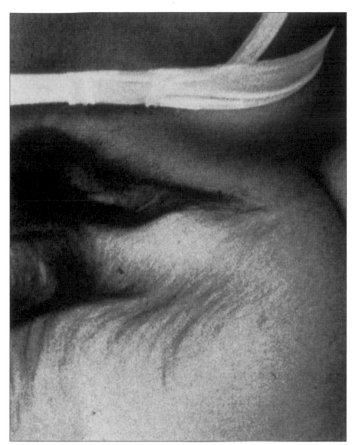

Figure 7.7 Faun's tail. This patch of hair in the midlline overlying the lower spine is highly suggestive of a dysraphic state. It is not associated with any particular entity, and it may occur in lipomyelomeningocele, diastematomyelia, or hypertrophied filum terminale. (Reprinted with permission from Rothman RH, Simeone FA. *The Spine*, 3rd edn. Philadelphia: WB Saunders; 1992.)

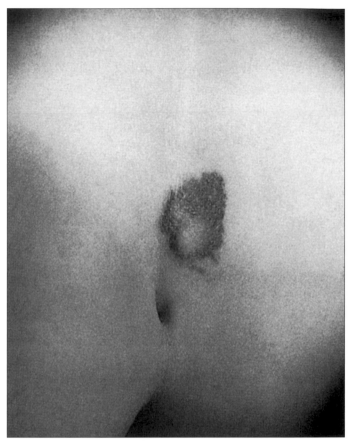

Figure 7.8 Hemangioma and dermal sinus. Dermal sinus tracts overlying the distal sacrum or coccyx are common in normal infants and do not generally represent dysraphic states. Any midline hemangioma or sinus tract over the lumbar spine warrants an investigation. (Reprinted with permission from Rothman RH, Simeone FA. *The Spine*, 3rd edn. Philadelphia: WB Saunders; 1992.)

The current method of choice for a suspected occult spinal dysraphic lesion is MRI scanning, which is usually definitive. In newborn infants the image quality can be suboptimal because of their small size, and if the clinical suspicion is high, a repeat scan at 6 months is indicated. The scan is examined for the level of the conus, which should not be below the L2–L3 interspace, and for the presence of fatty masses, a split cord, and/or a thickened filum. A large distended urinary bladder suggests sacral root dysfunction. In some cases of hypertrophied filum terminale the MRI scan may be equivocal, and if the clinical suspicion is high, surgical exploration may be warranted.[18] Fat in the filum is a frequent incidental MRI finding, and if the conus is at a normal level and there are no clinical indications of a tethered cord, surgery is usually not indicated.

LIPOMYELOMENINGOCELE

Lipomyelomeningocele is one of the more common forms of occult spinal dysraphism seen in pediatric neurosurgical practice. The term is actually a misnomer, because it suggests herniation of

Table 7.1 Presenting symptoms and signs of occult spinal dysraphism

Symptoms/signs	Incidence
Foot deformity	39%
Scoliosis	14%
Gait abnormality	16%
Leg weakness	48%
Sensory abnormality	32%
Urinary incontinence	36%
Recurrent urinary tract infections	20%
Fecal incontinence	32%
Cutaneous abnormality	48%

Adapted from ref. 26.

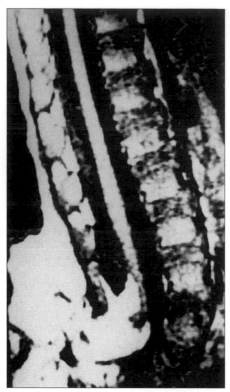

Figure 7.12 MRI of a dorsally inserting lipoma. The mass inserts dorsally within the conus. It extends through a spina bifida defect to be continuous with the subcutaneous mass. (Reprinted with permission from Rothman RH, Simeone FA. *The Spine*, 3rd edn. Philadelphia: WB Saunders; 1992.)

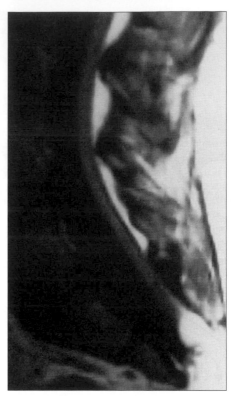

Figure 7.13 MRI of caudal lipoma. The lipoma is entirely within the caudal spinal canal, and the cord is tethered to the caudal portion of the thecal sac. (Reprinted with permission from Rothman RH, Simeone FA. *The Spine*, 3rd edn. Philadelphia: WB Saunders; 1992.)

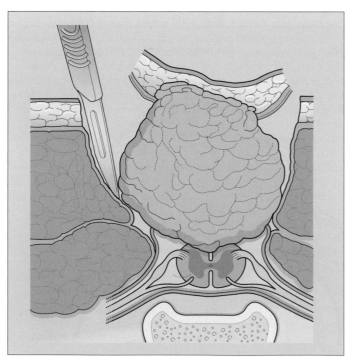

Figure 7.14 Initial exposure of a spinal lipoma. The skin has been elliptically incised around the subcutaneous mass and the incision has been carried to the lumbodorsal fascia. Dissection has proceeded medially, until the stalk of the lipoma is seen entering the spinal canal through the spina bifida and the dural defect.

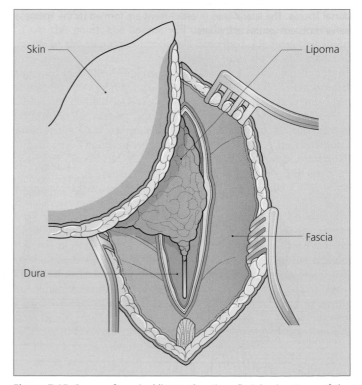

Figure 7.15 Surgery for spinal lipoma (continued). A laminectomy of the lowest intact neural arch has been performed and the dura has been opened at this level. The dural incision is extended caudally until the lipoma is encountered.

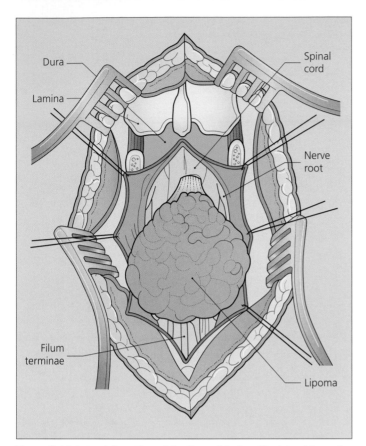

Figure 7.16 Lateral dissection of the lines of fusion. The lateral lines of fusion are sharply incised on either side of the lipoma. A tunnel can usually be formed between the lateral lines of fusion and the nerve roots beneath.

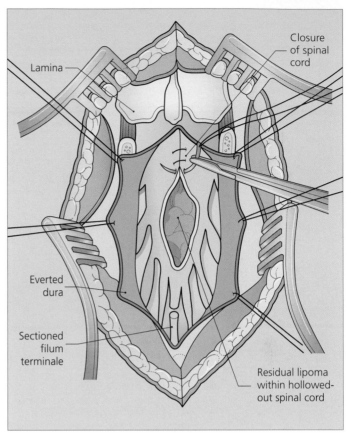

Figure 7.17 Reconstruction of the spinal cord. The lipoma has been largely removed with a CO_2 laser, creating a cavity within the conus. This may be closed with interrupted sutures to prevent re-tethering.

the risks. The major late problem is re-tethering, which is suggested by clinical deterioration, and requires re-exploration.[22]

DIASTEMATOMYELIA AND THE SPLIT CORD MALFORMATIONS

The term *diastematomyelia*, which derives from the Greek word *diastema*, meaning cleft, refers to a congenital splitting of the spinal cord. The term is used to describe the split, not the bony spike that often accompanies the abnormality. Clinically, it presents as tethered cord syndrome.[23] It occurs predominantly in females and most often in the lower thoracic or upper lumbar spine. Most patients have a midline cutaneous abnormality, but it does not necessarily correspond to the level of the cleft. The most common finding is a hairy patch, but a variety of other cutaneous abnormalities are seen. The spinal deformity (kyphoscoliosis), which eventually develops in virtually all patients, is thought to be primarily the result of the bony structure abnormalities, rather than of neurologic involvement.

Pang has suggested a useful classification scheme.[15,23] It is proposed that the term diastematomyelia be replaced by the more general term "split cord malformation" (SCM), which may occur as one of two types: The Type I SCM consists of two hemicords separated by a bony or cartilaginous median septum, with each housed in its own dural sheath. The Type II SCM consists of two

hemicords enveloped in the same dural sheath, and separated by a fibrous septum. Both are associated with tethering.

Neurologic symptoms are the result of spinal cord tethering and may not occur until adulthood, if at all. Symptoms can include back pain, gait disturbance, muscular atrophy, spasticity, or urologic complaints. These abnormalities are not specific, and other conditions, such as spinal cord tumor, Friedrich's ataxia, and syringomyelia, must be considered in the differential diagnosis. Neurologic deterioration can occur following corrective surgery for scoliosis, if spinal cord tethering is not recognized beforehand.

The classic appearance of the SCM on plain spine roentgenograph is a fusiform interpedicular widening of the spinal canal on the anteroposterior view with a midline oval bony mass projecting posteriorly from the vertebral body. The spur is usually not visible on lateral views. CT myelography will clarify the diagnosis, but MRI is currently the primary diagnostic test. The coronal study shows the split nicely, but severe kyphoscoliosis can make the study difficult to interpret. Newer imaging sequences, in which the scan is obtained along the curve of the spine, will probably solve this problem. It is important to evaluate the entire spine so that secondary lesions such as lipomas or hypertrophied fila are not missed.

Clear indications for surgery include progressive neurologic deficit and scoliosis. When performing surgery to untether the cord for scoliosis, it is usually advisable to operate on the SCM first as a separate procedure; removal of the bony spike most often

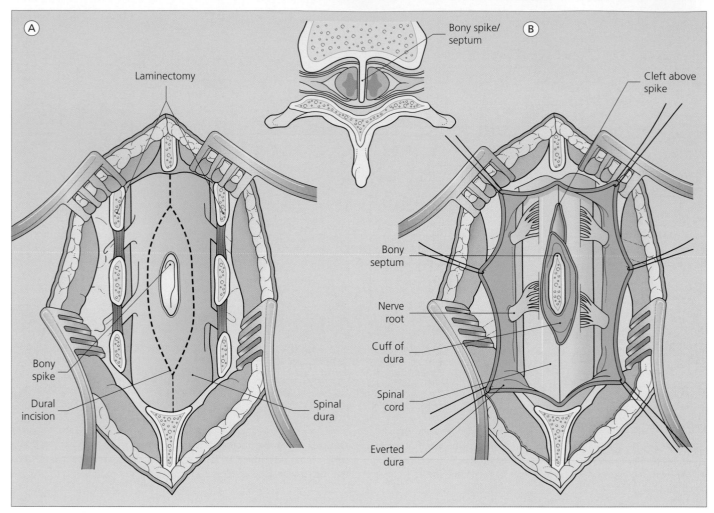

Figure 7.18 **(A)** Diastematomyelia. Full laminectomy has been performed above and below the bony septum and the bone has been removed laterally to expose the dural cleft. The proposed dural incision is shown. **(B)** Diastematomyelia, dura open. The cuff of dura is used to protect the spinal cord as the bony septum is drilled to the level of the vertebral body below. Note that the caudal end of the split cord tightly hugs the inferior surface of the bony spike, suggesting tethering.

results in the temporary loss of evoked potential signals, which can reduce the safety of the orthopedic procedure. The management of the asymptomatic patient remains controversial. Some authors favor prophylactic surgery within the first 2 years in asymptomatic children. Others favor a more conservative approach because of the potential risks of surgery and the significant number of patients who remain asymptomatic (or with stable deficits) throughout growth.

Surgical technique

The patient is positioned as for a standard laminectomy. The paraspinal muscles on either side of the midline are freed and retracted laterally as in any standard laminectomy, but vigorous blunt dissection with a periosteal elevator and sponges is avoided, because spina bifida can coexist with the bony septum. The laminectomy is initiated at least one full segment above and below the septum, and it is carried out around the bony spike itself, exposing the dural cleft (Figure 7.18A). The cleft will usually extend cephalad to the spur but hug it tightly caudally, which indicates tethering. A septal elevator frees the septum from the surrounding dura. The superficial portion of the septum is removed by a rongeur or a high-speed drill that has a diamond burr

within the investing dural sheath, which protects the spinal cord. Once the cleft is decompressed, the dura is opened around the cleft, and all intradural adhesions at the cleft are divided (Figure 7.18B). The dural cuff and the deeper portions of the septum are removed to the level of the anterior spinal canal. It is not necessary or appropriate to close the anterior dura. The posterior dura is closed in a watertight fashion, using a graft if necessary. If an associated hypertrophied filum is suspected, it is divided, using a separate laminectomy if needed.

The procedure should be considered largely prophylactic, although some patients may show neurologic improvement. Complications include worsening of neurologic status and CSF leak. Late deterioration after surgery can be the result of failure to remove the spike completely, failure to address associated lesions or, rarely, of regrowth of the septum.

ANTERIOR SACRAL MENINGOCELE

Anterior sacral meningocele is a relatively rare condition in which there is herniation of the dural sac through a defect in the anterior surface of the spine, usually in the sacrum. The sac is composed of

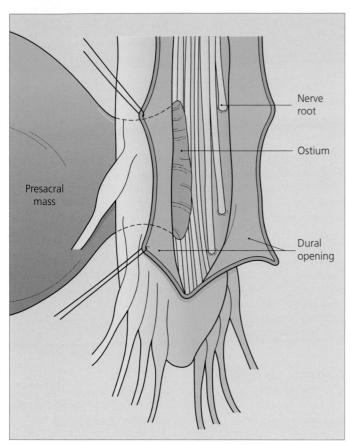

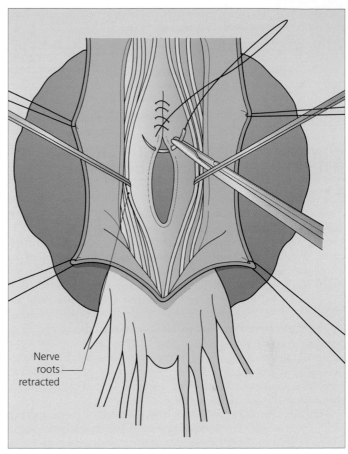

Figure 7.19 Approach to anterior sacral meningocele by sacral laminectomy. The posterior dura is opened longitudinally, exposing the sacral nerve roots and the ostium to the pelvic mass.

Figure 7.20 Anterior sacral meningocele. The nerve roots are retracted, and the ostium is oversewn using a continuous suture. No attempt is made to resect the pelvic mass.

an outer dural membrane and an inner arachnoid membrane. It contains CSF and, occasionally, neural elements. If the sac is large, it may present as a pelvic mass. Most anterior meningoceles are congenital, as evidenced by their appearance in children. Unlike the typical posterior myelomeningocele, there is no association with hydrocephalus or Chiari malformation. The embryology of these lesions is incompletely understood; most likely, the primary problem is a defect in dural development, resulting in a defect through which the arachnoid herniates, resulting in pulsations that erode the bone.

The lesion is more commonly detected in women, but this most likely reflects the gynecologic presentation of a pelvic mass. Symptoms are usually produced by pressure of the presacral mass on adjacent pelvic structures, causing constipation, urinary urgency, dyspareunia, or low back pain. Headache on defecation is occasionally described by children. The cardinal sign is a smooth, cystic mass detected on rectal or pelvic examination.

MRI scanning is the imaging study of choice. When communication between the pelvic cyst and the spinal subarachnoid space is not evident, a metrizamide CT-myelographic study may be indicated.

Surgical treatment of symptomatic lesions is advised because there is no possibility of spontaneous regression, and untreated female patients have a significant risk of pelvic obstruction at the time of labor. Asymptomatic lesions may be followed without operation, if there is no possibility of pregnancy and the lesion does not enlarge on repeated rectal examinations.

Aspiration of the cyst through the rectum or vagina may result in meningitis and should not be performed. If the meningocele is discovered at laparotomy for other reasons, the operation should be terminated and further workup carried out. Surgical treatment via laparotomy has been described, but the sacral laminectomy approach is preferable because it allows visualization of the intraspinal contents of the cyst, resection of adhesions, and sectioning of the filum terminale. The goal of surgery is to untether the spinal cord, decompress the pelvic mass, and obliterate the CSF fistula.

Surgical technique

The surgical technique has been reviewed.[24] Antibiotic coverage and a bowel preparation are begun 48 hours prior to surgery in case bowel perforation occurs. Under general anesthesia the patient is positioned for laminectomy. A lumbosacral laminectomy is performed from L5 to S4, and the posterior dura is opened longitudinally (Figure 7.19). Nerve roots within the dural canal are carefully retracted, and the filum terminale is divided to expose the dural ostium leading to the pelvic sac. If no roots enter the sac and the neck is narrow, the anterior dura is simply oversewn (Figure 7.20). If the sac arises as a caudal extension of the dural sac, and the sacral roots have exited above, the dural sleeve may simply be ligated. If the anterior defect is wide and cannot be mobilized into the field sufficiently for primary closure, digital collapse of the sac through the rectum can be helpful or a fascial graft can be sewn to the edges of the defect. If roots exit through the defect, the dura or graft will have to be plicated around the roots as they exit. The posterior dura is closed. Postoperatively, stool softeners are given to prevent straining. In difficult cases, a second pelvic procedure is required.

The results of surgery described in the literature have generally been good. Complications have included meningitis, CSF leak, and neurologic problems when roots have entered the meningocele sac.

CONGENITAL DERMAL SINUS AND HYPERTROPHIED FILUM TERMINALE

The term *congenital dermal sinus* refers to a group of congenital malformations in which a tubular tract lined with squamous epithelium extends from the skin overlying the spine inward to varying depths. The sinus terminates in the subcutaneous tissue, bone, dura, subarachnoid space, filum terminale, or within an intradural dermoid cyst or neuroglial mass within the spinal cord itself. They occur at all levels within the spine but are most commonly seen in the lower lumbosacral area, where they are frequently confused with simple pilonidal sinuses. Pilonidal sinuses are acquired lesions in adults, believed to be secondary to trauma or chronic inflammation, that have no connection with the subarachnoid space or neural elements. In contrast, a congenital dermal sinus is a significant lesion because it enables skin flora to enter the spinal fluid pathways, resulting in repeated bouts of meningitis. It also causes spinal cord tethering, which leads to progressive neurologic problems. The hallmark of the lesion is a midline cutaneous dimple overlying the lumbosacral spine. There can be other associated cutaneous abnormalities (see Figure 7.10), such as hemangiomas or hairy patches.

A somewhat related condition is the so-called "meningocele manqué," which is believed to represent an incomplete form of open dysraphism in which bands of meninges, fibrous tissue, and some neural tissue tether the cord to a small area of atretic skin on the back.

The radiographic hallmark is a tract extending from the low-lying conus to the cutaneous abnormality. It is now recognized that the spinal cord may be tethered even with the conus at a normal level.[18] This may only be suspected if there are clear clinical symptoms.

Prophylactic surgery is performed as early as possible, even in newborns, to excise the entire tract. When there is clinical evidence of spinal cord compression, MRI scanning is indicated to determine the extent of abscesses or dermoid cysts. In asymptomatic cases, the lesions can simply be explored and the tract followed to its termination. The surgeon undertaking such an operation must be prepared to carry out an extensive intradural dissection, because the tract can extend for a considerable distance. In typical cases, the sinus tract begins at the skin dimple and proceeds cephalad through the soft tissues overlying the spine to traverse the dorsal dura. Once intradural, the tract often becomes continuous with the filum terminale, which is thickened and may contain dermoid elements (Figure 7.21).

Surgical technique

The operation begins with an elliptical skin incision that surrounds the sinus opening and encompasses any abnormal skin surrounding it. The tract is sharply dissected and followed through the defect in the fascia. If the tract appears to continue through the dura, a laminectomy is performed above the level of the tract. If the tract attaches to the dura, the dura is opened above the attachment in

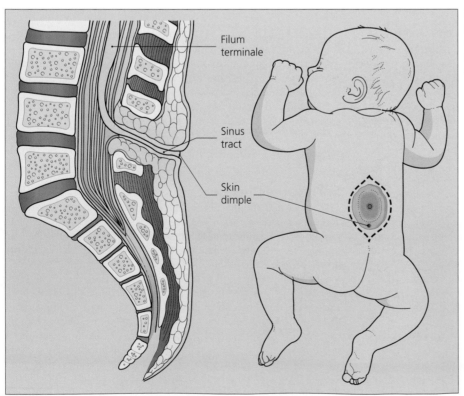

Figure 7.21 Cross-sectional anatomy of typical congenital dermal sinus tract. The tract may extend to any depth but it often continues in a cephalad direction, enters the dura, and becomes continuous with the filum terminale.

Filum terminale

Sinus tract

Skin dimple

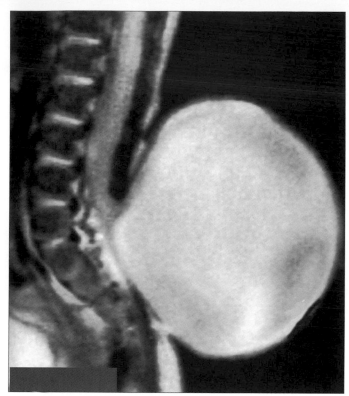

Figure 7.22 Lateral MRI of a terminal myelocystocele. A large, skin-covered lumbosacral mass is seen clinically. The radiographic finding is a cystic mass which is a massively dilated terminal central canal of the spinal cord.

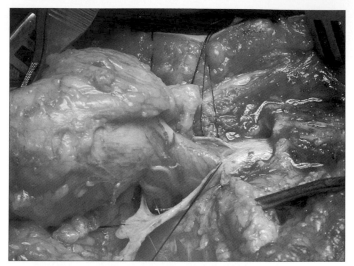

Figure 7.23 Operative photograph of a terminal myelocystocele. The terminal end of the spinal cord protrudes through the dural defect. The surgery consists of amputating this tissue while preserving the anterior roots which remain within the spinal canal.

the midline and incised inferiorly around the point of entry. Any intradural tract must be followed to its termination, even if this involves an extensive laminectomy, because remaining tissue has the capacity to grow into a dermoid inclusion cyst. Intradural dermoids are completely removed, if possible without violating the capsule. If the cyst has ruptured or has been infected, a dense arachnoiditis with scarred nerve roots will prevent complete excision. In this case, judicious intracapsular removal of purulent material and dermoid material is performed, and no attempt is made to remove the scarred capsular wall from the nerve roots. A watertight dural closure is accomplished, except when closure would compress residual infected dermoid cyst material, in which case the dura is left open and the muscle and fascia are closed.

The syndrome of the hypertrophied filum terminale may occur without a cutaneous dimple or sinus tract. If a patient presents with the typical picture of the tethered cord syndrome, an MRI scan is indicated. The scan will demonstrate the low-lying conus, but it may not demonstrate the thickened filum. In these cases, a metrizamide CT-myelogram can demonstrate the pathology, although surgical exploration may be more expeditious.

SACRAL AGENESIS, MYELOCYSTOCELE, AND CLOACAL EXTROPHY

A number of complex anomalies involving the caudal spine have been described, some of which may come to the attention of the neurosurgeon.[25,26] These may involve multiple organ systems, and include imperforate anus, the VATER syndrome (*v*ertebral anomalies, *a*nal imperforation, *t*racheo-*e*sophageal fistula, and *r*enal-*r*adial abnormalities), the OEIS complex (*o*mphalocele, cloacal *e*xtrophy, *i*mperforate anus, and *s*pinal deformities), and sacral agenesis. Any of these conditions may be associated with the tethered cord syndrome.

Some consider these caudal regression syndromes to be a continuum, while others feel that they are distinct entities. The severity of the anomaly determines the likely spinal pathology and the management. Simple imperforate anus is associated with hypertrophy of the filum terminale, and there may be no cutaneous stigmata of this condition. Screening with MRI is often recommended. Sacral agenesis is suspected by flattening of the buttocks, shortening of the intergluteal cleft, and prominence of the iliac crest. The newborn with an omphalocele, ambiguous genitalia, and cloacal extrophy may have an associated skin-covered lumbosacral mass, which may represent a myelocystocele or a lipomyelomeningocele. Myelocystocele may occur in association with these complex syndromes, or in isolation. It is generally considered to be an extreme form of the common *ventriculus terminalis*, which is a normal anatomic variant seen often on MRI scans performed for unrelated indications. The central canal of the terminal spinal cord is massively dilated to form a huge cystic structure, which presents as a skin-covered lumbosacral mass. Fetal ultrasound may confuse a myelocystocele with a cystic myelomeningocele. The spinal cord is invariably tethered. Sacral agenesis is associated with maternal diabetes. Pang has divided these cases into five types, based on the appearance of the sacrum.[26] As a practical matter, one can divide these anomalies into those with a high conus, and those with a low conus. High symmetric sacral agenesis is correlated with a truncated, club-shaped conus ending around T11 or T12. Tethering is not present, although dural canal stenosis has been reported as the cause of delayed deterioration. The lower asymmetric forms of sacral dysgenesis are more likely to have a low-lying tethered cord. Mechanisms of tethering included myelocystocele, lipomyelo-meningocele, or simple hypertrophy of the filum.

Initial management of infants with multisystem anomalies is usually non-neurosurgical, and consists of colostomy, closure of

CLINICAL PEARLS

- Spinal dysraphism refers to anomalies of the spine in which the midline structures do not fuse. Myelomeningocele is the most common significant birth defect involving the spine.

- The prevalence of spina bifida in industrialized countries has been decreasing because of the steadily increasing proportion of affected fetuses that are detected prenatally and electively terminated. In addition, there is strong scientific evidence that the use of preconception folate appears to decrease the risk of developing a neural tube defect such as myelomeningocele.

- Embryologically, the abnormality manifests between 3 and 4 weeks of gestation, during the period called neurulation. The abnormality represents the failure of the posterior neuropore to close properly. Patients with myelomeningocele usually have hydrocephalus and a Chiari II malformation. Surgical closure of the dorsal defect is performed shortly after birth.

- A new surgical procedure of *in utero* closure of the myelomeningocele is being pioneered at several medical centers. The goal is to decrease the incidence of hydrocephalus and hindbrain abnormalities found in this population. Although the preliminary results are promising a randomized trial will be required to assess the efficacy of this unproven treatment option.

- Developmental anomalies involving the caudal portion of the neural tube are increasingly important in clinical practice. This is the result of advances in radiologic diagnostic techniques and a consequent change in the philosophy of treatment, which includes prophylactic cord untethering to prevent neurologic deficits. Greater awareness of the conditions of lipomyelomeningocele, tethered cord, diastematomyelia, and sinus tracts, by pediatricians, orthopedists, and urologists, in concert with the widespread application of MRI have led to earlier recognition of these congenital surgically correctable problems.

an omphalocele, urinary diversion, and reconstruction for tracheo-esophageal fistula. An MRI of the spine is obtained electively, when the infant is stable (Figure 7.22). When the conus is at a normal level, neurosurgical intervention is usually not required. Those cases in which the conus is low lying should undergo tethered cord release at about 3 months of age, or when the systemic condition permits. It is useful to perform the tethered cord release prior to reversing the colostomy, because the wound is protected from fecal contamination. Even infants with high motor levels should undergo prophylactic untethering, because improvement is possible.

Surgery is similar to that for other tethered cord syndromes. Surgery for myelocystocele consists of defining normal anatomy above the sac, and amputating the sac and all of the tissue below the level of the last intact nerve roots with untethering (Figure 7.23). The dural reconstruction may require a graft.

Patients who do not have tethering, or who have undergone successful untethering procedures, should remain with stable deficits. If new signs or symptoms appear, a repeat MRI should be performed to define re-tethering, syrinx formation, or dural constriction. Patients may require long-term management by neurosurgeons, pediatric general surgeons, urologists, and orthopedists.

REFERENCES

1. MRC Vitamin Study Research Group. Prevention of neural tube defects: results of the Medical Research Council Vitamin Study. *Lancet* 1991; 338: 131–7.

2. Czeizel AE, Dudas I. Prevention of the first occurrence of neural-tube defects by periconceptional vitamin supplementation. *N Engl J Med* 1992; 327(26): 1832–5

3. Botto L, Moore C, Khoury M, Erickson J. Neural tube defects. *N Engl J Med* 1999; 341: 1509–19.

4. Simon E, Goldstein R, Coakley F, *et al*. Fast MR imaging of fetal CNS anomalies *in utero*. *Am J Neuroradiol* 2000; 21: 1688–98.

5. Cochrane D, Wilson R, Steinbok P, *et al*. Prenatal spinal evaluation and functional outcome of patients born with myelomeningocele: information for improved prenatal counselling and outcome prediction. *Fetal Diagn Ther* 1996; 11: 159–68.

6. Luthy D, Wardinsky T, Shurtleff D. Cesarean section before the onset of labor and subsequent motor function in infants with myelomeningocele diagnosed antenatally. *N Engl J Med* 1991; 324: 662–6.

7. Sutton L, Charney E, Bruce D, Schut L. Myelomeningocele – the question of selection. *Clin Neurosurg* 1986; 33: 371–82.

8. Adzick N, Sutton L, Crombleholme T, Flake A. Successful fetal surgery for spina bifida. *Lancet* 1998; 352: 1675–6.

9. Tulipan N, Bruner J. Myelomeningocele repair *in utero*. *Pediatr Neurosurg* 1998; 28: 177–80.

10. Sutton L, Sun P, Adzick N. Fetal neurosurgery. *Neurosurgery* 2001; 48: 124–42.

11. Tulipan N, Bruner J, Hernanz-Schulman M, *et al*. The effect of intrauterine myelomeningocele repair on central nervous system structure and neurologic function. *Pediatr Neurosurg* 1999; 31: 183–8.

12. Mazzola C, Albright AL, Sutton L, Tuite G, Hamilton R, Pollack I. Dermoid inclusion cysts and early spinal cord tethering after fetal surgery for myelomeningocele. *N Engl J Med* 2002; 347: 256–9.

13. Sutton L, Adzick N, Bilaniuk L, Johnson M, Crombleholme T, Flake A. Improvement in hindbrain herniation demonstrated by serial fetal magnetic resonance imaging following fetal surgery for myelomeningocele. *JAMA* 1999; 282: 1826–31.

14. Rintoul N, Sutton L, Hubbard A, *et al*. A new look at myelomeningoceles: functional level, vertebral level, shunting, and the implications for fetal intervention. *Pediatrics* 2002; 109: 409–13.

15. Pang D, Dias M, Ahab-Barmada M. Split cord malformation: Part I: A

unified theory of embryogenesis for double spinal cord malformations. *Neurosurgery* 1992; 31.

16. Medina L, Crone K, Kuntz K. Newborns with suspected occult spinal dysraphism: a cost-effectiveness analysis of diagnostic strategies. *Pediatrics* 2001; 108: E101.

17. James H, Walsh W. Spinal dysraphism. *Current Problems in Pediatrics – Spinal Dysraphism*. Chicago, IL: Yearbook Medical Publisher; 1981; XI: 8.

18. Warder D, Oaks W. Tethered cord syndrome: the low-lying and normally positioned conus. *Neurosurgery* 1994; 34: 597–600.

19. Chapman P. Congenital intraspinal lipomas: anatomic considerations. *Childs Brain* 1982; 9: 37–47.

20. Pierre-Kahn A, Lacombe J, Pichon J. Intraspinal lipomas with spina bifida: prognosis and treatment in 73 cases. *J Neurosurg* 1986; 65: 756–61.

21. Kanev P, Bierbrauer K. Reflections on the natural history of lipomyelomeningocele. *Pediatr Neurosurg* 1995; 22: 137–40.

22. Colak A, Pollack I, Albright A. Recurrent tethering: a common long-term problem after lipomyelomeningocele repair. *Pediatr Neurosurg* 1998; 29: 184–90.

23. Pang D. Split cord malformation: II Clinical syndrome. *Neurosurgery* 1992; 31: 481–500.

24. Mapstone T, White R, Takacka Y. Anterior sacral meningocele. Surg Neurol 1981; 16: 44–7.

25. Estin D, Cohen A. Caudal agenesis and associated caudal spinal cord malformations. *Neurosurg Clin North Am* 1995; 6: 377–91.

26. Pang D. Sacral agenesis and caudal spinal cord malformations. *Neurosurgery* 1993; 32: 755–79.

HYDROCEPHALUS IN CHILDREN

Paul P Wang and Anthony M Avellino

8

INTRACRANIAL CONTENTS

For children older than 2–3 years, the cranial fontanelles and sutures are closed, and the skull can be considered a rigid container with a fixed volume. Its contents include the brain bulk (80%), blood volume (10%), and cerebrospinal fluid (CSF) (10%). According to the Monro–Kellie doctrine, intracranial volume is equal to the sum of the volume of brain, blood, CSF, and other mass lesions.[1] Therefore, an increase in volume of any one of these components, such as CSF, can raise intracranial pressure (ICP) and reduce cerebral perfusion pressure and cerebral blood flow.

The major compensatory mechanism within the intracranial vault appears to be the CSF volume, 90% of which is in the subarachnoid spaces and 10% of which is within the ventricular system. This mechanism can be quantified as the volume–pressure intracranial compliance ($\Delta V/\Delta P$ = compliance) or pressure volume index (PVI). The PVI is the volume of fluid injected or withdrawn that would result in a tenfold change in ICP and can be calculated as: $PVI = \Delta V/\log (P_f/P_0)$, where ΔV is volume change, P_f is final ICP, and P_0 is initial ICP. The PVI varies with age; for example, the PVI is 8 mL in an infant but 25 mL in a 14-year-old.[2] Thus a 10-mL addition in volume to the intracranial contents of a 14-year-old may produce a modest and tolerable increase in ICP, but the same addition can be lethal in an infant (Figure 8.1). However, with infants and very young children who have open fontanelles and sutures, the Monro–Kellie doctrine does not apply because the cranial vault can expand with increased volume.[3]

CEREBROSPINAL FLUID

CSF is a clear, colorless fluid that fills the ventricles of the brain and the subarachnoid space that surrounds the central nervous system (CNS). CSF is produced mainly in the choroid plexus within the lateral, third, and fourth ventricles and, to a lesser extent, in the spinal cord. (Figure 8.2). The choroid plexus consists of numerous villi, each composed of single-layer cuboidal epithelial cells surrounding a core of highly vascularized connective tissue. Ultrafiltrate from the capillaries is processed by the epithelial cells and diffuses into the ventricles at a rate of 0.30–0.35 mL/min, or approximately 500 mL/day, in adults and children.[4] CSF production is partially regulated by the enzymes sodium–potassium ATPase and carbonic anhydrase. Certain pathological entities that affect the choroid plexus can influence the production rate of CSF. For example, choroid plexus papillomas can increase CSF production, while ventriculitis can lead to sclerosis of the choroid plexus, which in turn will reduce production. The total CSF volume is approximately 40–50 mL in neonates and 65–140 mL in children.

CSF flows through the pathways displayed in Figure 8.2. It is absorbed by arachnoid villi, which are diverticula of arachnoid that invaginate within the sagittal sinus and nearby major cortical veins. Clusters of arachnoid villi, called arachnoid granulations, are grossly visible. A layer of endothelial cells lines the villi. Water and electrolytes freely traverse the endothelial layer into the systemic circulation, and proteins are actively transported out by pinocytosis.

The mechanism by which CSF exits the central nervous system via arachnoid villi is unclear. The ICP must be greater than 6.8 mmH$_2$O, or no CSF absorption will take place.[2] CSF absorption is normally in equilibrium with CSF production, with the resulting ICP varying with age (Table 8.1).

PATHOPHYSIOLOGY OF HYDROCEPHALUS

Hydrocephalus is the abnormal accumulation of CSF within the ventricles and subarachnoid spaces. It is often associated with dilatation of the ventricular system and increased ICP. The incidence of pediatric hydrocephalus as an isolated congenital disorder is approximately 1/1000 live births. Pediatric hydrocephalus

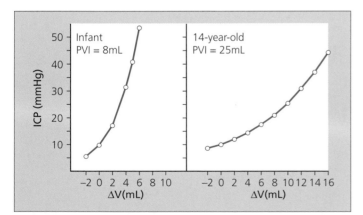

Figure 8.1 Pressure–volume curves of a normal infant (left) and adolescent (right) showing that an infant has less ability to buffer equal increments of volume. (From Shapiro *et al.* 1994,[2] with permission from WB Saunders.)

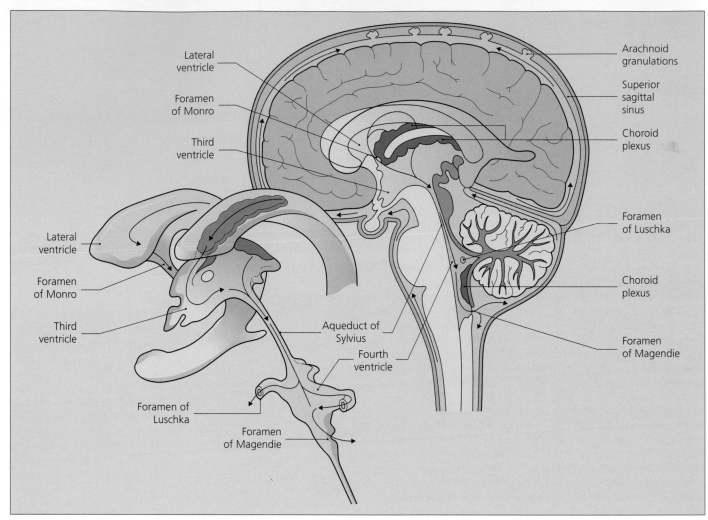

Figure 8.2 Normal CSF pathways.

is often associated with numerous other conditions, such as spina bifida.

Hydrocephalus is almost always a result of an interruption of CSF flow and is rarely because of increased CSF production. Common obstruction sites and etiologies are displayed in Figure 8.3. As ICP rises, CSF absorption increases somewhat, but CSF production remains constant.[5] If progressive ventricular dilatation separates ependymal cells lining the ventricles, interstitial cerebral edema will develop. The CSF will eventually enter the white matter of the brain via bulk flow through the ependymal cells lining the ventricles.

CLASSIFICATIONS

Historically, hydrocephalus has been classified as *obstructive* or *nonobstructive*, a somewhat misleading classification because all forms of hydrocephalus, except hydrocephalus *ex vacuo* (resulting from brain atrophy), involve some form of CSF obstruction. A more commonly used classification differentiates hydrocephalus between *communicating* or *noncommunicating*. Traditionally, this classification was based on whether dye injected into the lateral ventricles could be detected in CSF extracted from a subsequent lumbar puncture. Currently, the term "noncommunicating hydrocephalus" refers to lesions that obstruct the ventricular system, either at the aqueduct of sylvius or basal foramina (i.e. basal foramina of Luschka and Magendie). The term "communicating hydrocephalus" refers to lesions that obstruct at the level of the subarachnoid space and arachnoid villi.

Table 8.1 Normal intracranial pressure by age

Age	ICP range (mmHg)
Neonate	< 2
Infant	1.5–6
Young child	3–7
Adolescent (> 15 years)	< 15
Adult	< 15

(Modified from Greenberg, 2001.[70])

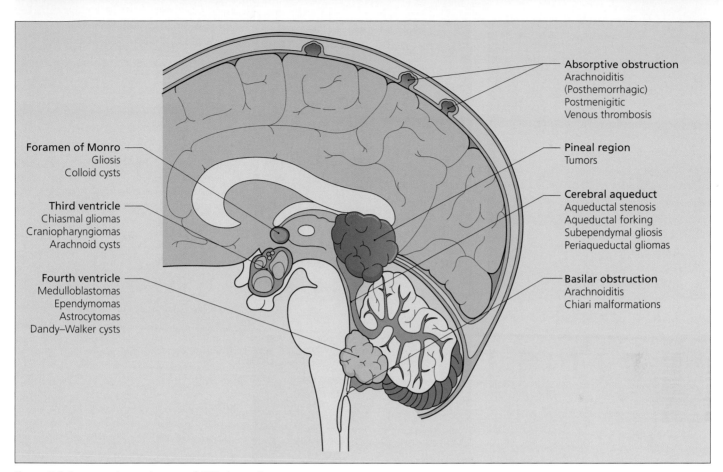

Figure 8.3 Common sites and causes of CSF obstruction.

There are several other less commonly used classifications. Hydrocephalus can be divided into *physiologic*, i.e. secondary to CSF overproduction mainly from choroid plexus tumors, or *nonphysiologic*. However, because such choroid plexus tumors are rare (less than 1% of all brain tumors), this classification has only minor clinical application.. Another classification infrequently employed in the literature describes hydrocephalus as *internal* or *external*, depending on whether the site of obstruction is proximal or distal to the basal foramina. Hydrocephalus can also be classified by etiology and site of obstruction (Figure 8.3).

PATHOLOGY – SITE OF OBSTRUCTION

Lateral ventricles
Choroid plexus tumors are rare in the general population, with an incidence ranging from 0.4 to 0.6% of all CNS tumors.[6] However, within the pediatric population, the incidence is higher, ranging from 1.5 to 3.9% of all pediatric CNS tumors,[7,8] and even higher in children less than 2 years old. Most choroid plexus tumors are choroid plexus papillomas, which usually present within the first 3 years of life. CSF production rates three to four times the normal rate have been documented in children with choroid plexus papillomas.[9] Removal of the papilloma resolves the hydrocephalus in approximately two-thirds of cases. The remaining third probably suffer from obstruction of the aqueduct and/or basal meninges and require a shunt presumably secondary to

preoperative microhemorrhages or postoperative scarring of the arachnoid villae.

A second disorder in the lateral ventricle that can cause hydrocephalus in children is the extremely rare choroid plexus (villous) hypertrophy. Scans demonstrate substantial enlargement of the choroid plexus in the trigones of the lateral ventricles. It is usually associated with ventriculomegaly and is difficult to treat with shunts. Endoscopic coagulation of the choroid plexus or surgical removal of the hypertrophied plexi has been used to successfully treat the hydrocephalus.[10]

Foramina of Monro
Occlusion of one foramen of Monro can occur secondary to a congenital membrane, atresia, or gliosis after intraventricular hemorrhage (IVH) or ventriculitis. The resulting unilateral ventriculomegaly is often occult until after age 6, and may enlarge the ipsilateral hemicalvarium (Figure 8.4).

An iatrogenic functional stenosis of the foramen of Monro can develop in children with spina bifida whose hydrocephalus has been treated with a shunt. The contralateral nonshunted ventricle occasionally expands secondary to deformity of the foramen of Monro.[11] If symptomatic, the patient can be treated with a shunt system having two ventricular catheters, each draining a separate lateral ventricle or an endoscopic fenestration of the septum pellucidum with one ventricular catheter draining subsequently both ventricles.

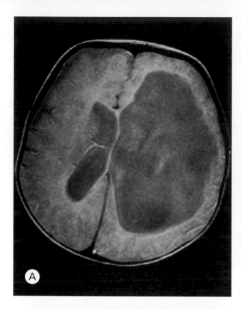
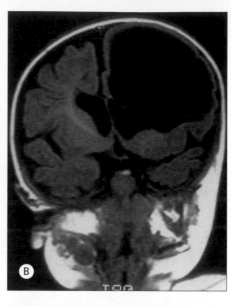

Figure 8.4 (A, B) Unilateral hydrocephalus secondary to posthemorrhagic gliosis of the foramen of Monro.

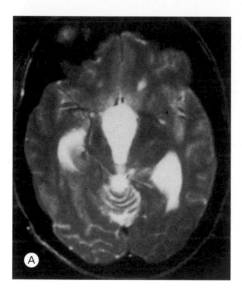
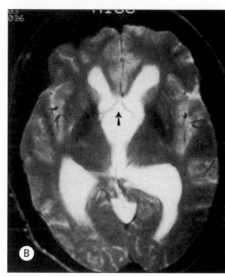

Figure 8.5 (A, B) Arachnoid cyst within the third ventricle. The cyst wall is evident (arrow) at the foramina of Monro.

Third ventricle

Cysts and neoplasms within the third ventricle commonly cause hydrocephalus. Colloid cysts are uncommon neoplasms that present superiorly and anteriorly within the third ventricle, and usually obstruct both foramina of Monro. Considered to be congenital lesions, they can become symptomatic at any age, with the youngest reported case at age 2 months.[12] However, they rarely present within the pediatric population, and are commonly symptomatic between the ages of 20 and 50 years. They can cause either intermittent, acute, life-threatening hydrocephalus or chronic hydrocephalus. They are customarily treated with stereotactic aspiration of the cyst, resection via craniotomy, or endoscopic resection (see Chapter 10).[13–15]

Ependymal and arachnoid cysts within the third ventricle usually present with hydrocephalus in late childhood (Figure 8.5). Patients may present with bobble-head doll syndrome, a rhythmic head nodding at a frequency of two to three times per second.[16] While endoscopic fenestration is a treatment option, they are often treated with a ventricular catheter fenestrated to drain both ventricles and the cyst.[17,18] Dermoid cysts rarely occur in the third ventricle, and are often treated with cyst removal.

The most common pediatric neoplasms that obstruct the third ventricle are craniopharyngiomas and chiasmal-hypothalamic astrocytomas. Hydrocephalus secondary to craniopharyngiomas usually resolves after surgical resection of the tumor; hydrocephalus secondary to third ventricular gliomas usually does not resolve after surgical resection, and shunt placement is often necessary.

Sylvian aqueduct

The normal aqueduct of a neonate is 12–13 mm in length and only 0.2–0.5 mm in diameter.[19] Thus, it is prone to obstruction from a variety of lesions, including congenital aqueductal malformations (i.e. stenosis, forking, septum, or subependymal gliosis) (Figure 8.6), pineal region neoplasms, arteriovenous malformations, and periaqueductal neoplasms.

True aqueductal stenosis, i.e. true luminal narrowing, occurs in

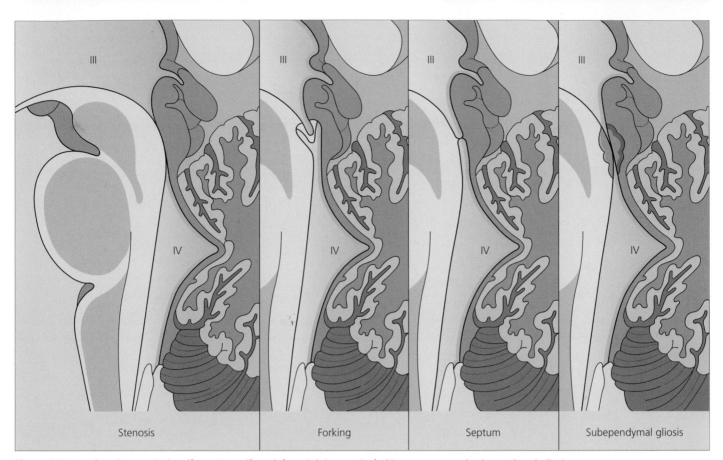

Figure 8.6 Aqueductal congenital malformations: (from left to right) stenosis, forking, septum, and subependymal gliosis.

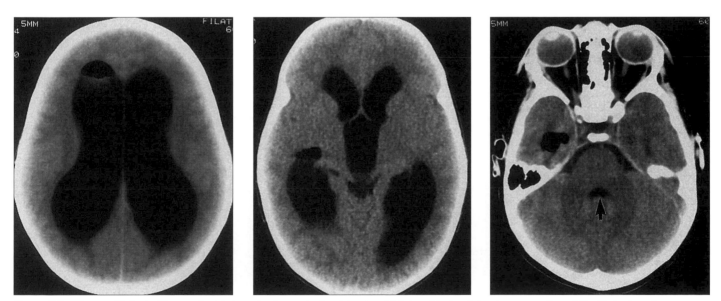

Figure 8.7 CT scan of infant with aqueductal stenosis, demonstrating lateral and third ventricular distension, separation of the thalami, and compression of the cerebral hemispheres . The fourth ventricle (arrow) is normal.

only 4–8% of infants with obstruction of the aqueduct.[20] More common lesions include aqueductal forking, subependymal gliosis secondary to *in utero* infections (e.g. toxoplasmosis), intraventricular hemorrhage, or mumps encephalitis. Hydrocephalus secondary to aqueductal occlusion is generally severe and causes distension of the third ventricle and separation of the thalami, thinning of the septum pellucidum and corpus callosum, and compression of the cerebral hemispheres (Figure 8.7). Less than 2% of cases of congenital aqueductal stenosis are the result of the recessively-inherited X-linked Bickers–Adams–Edwards syndrome, which is associated with flexion–adduction of the thumbs ("cortical thumbs") in 25% of cases.[21]

Any pineal mass can obstruct the aqueduct and produce hydrocephalus. Many pineal region tumors, especially germinomas, are highly radiosensitive; successful tumor irradiation, as well as surgical resection, may adequately treat the obstructive hydrocephalus. Perioperatively, it may be necessary to place an external ventricular drain (EVD).

Low-grade astrocytomas are the most common periaqueductal pediatric neoplasms that cause hydrocephalus. Historically, children with neurofibromatosis have often been diagnosed with "late-onset aqueductal stenosis." However, with the advent of magnetic resonance imaging (MRI), many of these children present with periaqueductal hyperintense T2 signals, indicating low-grade astrocytomas (Figure 8.8).[22]

Fourth ventricle

In infants, the fourth ventricle is the location for obstruction secondary to Dandy–Walker cysts or obliteration of the basal foramina. In older children, neoplasms are a common cause. Such occlusions result in the dilatation of the lateral, third and fourth ventricles above the obstruction. Dandy–Walker cysts are developmental abnormalities characterized by a large cyst in the fourth ventricle lined with pia-arachnoid and ependyma, hypoplasia of the cerebellar vermis, and atrophy of the cerebellar hemispheres (Figure 8.9). Over 85% of children with Dandy–Walker cysts have hydrocephalus.[23]

Pediatric tumors associated with the fourth ventricle commonly present with hydrocephalus. Hydrocephalus is associated with 85% of medulloblastomas, 65% of posterior fossa astrocytomas, 75% of ependymomas, and 25% of brainstem gliomas. Arachnoiditis secondary to either meningitis or subarachnoid hemorrhage can occlude the basal foramina and cause obstructive hydrocephalus. Infants with Chiari II malformations and myelomeningoceles have hydrocephalus secondary to blockage of CSF flow from basilar obstruction.

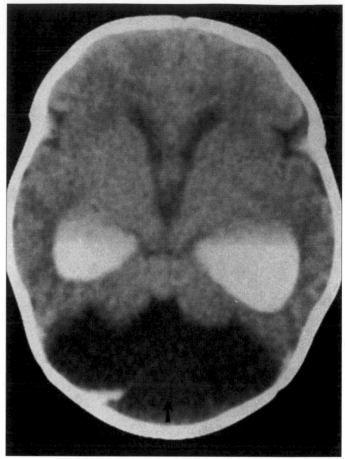

Figure 8.9 Axial CT scan of an infant with a Dandy–Walker cyst (arrow). Iohexal (white) injected into the lateral ventricles did not enter the cyst.

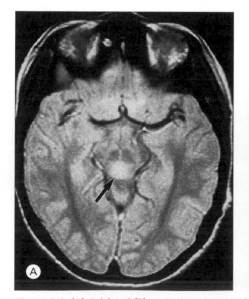
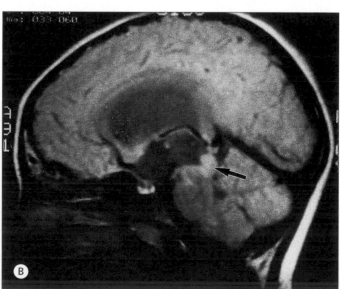

Figure 8.8 **(A)** Axial and **(B)** sagittal MR images demonstrating hydrocephalus secondary to a periaqueductal astrocytoma (arrow). The lesion was not visible on CT scans.

Arachnoid granulations

Sclerosis or scarring of the arachnoid granulations can occur after meningitis, subarachnoid hemorrhage, or trauma. The subarachnoid spaces over the convexities enlarge, thus forming a condition often referred to as "external hydrocephalus" (Figure 8.10). The radiographic imaging from this disorder is often confused with subdural effusions, which are typically bifrontal, or cerebral atrophy, which is rare in children with macrocephaly. Symptomatic external hydrocephalus is treated with a subdural/subarachnoid to peritoneal shunt.

ETIOLOGY, SIGNS, AND SYMPTOMS

Premature infants

Hydrocephalus in premature infants is predominantly caused by IVH. The hemorrhage occurs in the germinal matrix, and can extend into the ventricles and parenchyma depending on its severity. There is a general correlation between the amount of IVH and the likelihood of posthemorrhagic hydrocephalus (PHH).[24] The severity of the hemorrhage or grading system is based on the radiologic appearance of the neonate's brain and ventricles when imaged by ultrasound or computed tomography (CT) scan (see Table 8.2). Grade I and II IVH are often asymptomatic and resolve spontaneously; the higher-grade cases will usually develop PHH within 4 weeks after IVH. The mechanism for PHH is threefold. The blood products within the CSF cause: (1) subependymal gliosis that occludes the narrow cerebral aqueduct, (2) basal arachnoiditis that occludes the basal foramina of Luschka and Magendie, and (3) fibrosis or scarring that occludes the arachnoid granulations.

Because the poorly myelinated premature brain is so easily compressed, premature infants can develop considerable ventriculomegaly before their head circumference increases. Infants with PHH may have no symptoms, or may exhibit increasing spells of apnea and bradycardia (Table 8.3). Poor feeding and vomiting are uncommon signs of hydrocephalus in premature infants. If ventriculomegaly progresses and ICP increases, the anterior fontanelle becomes convex, tense, and nonpulsatile, and the scalp veins distend. As ventriculomegaly persists, the head develops a globoid shape, and the head circumference increases at a rapid, pathologic rate. Head circumference increases 0.5 cm/week in sick premature infants, 1 cm/week in healthy premature infants, and up to 2 cm/week in premature infants with PHH. Lateral rectus palsies and the "setting-sun" sign seen in older infants and children is not a common presentation of PHH because the neonate skull is so distensible and will initially expand to compensate for expanding ventricles.

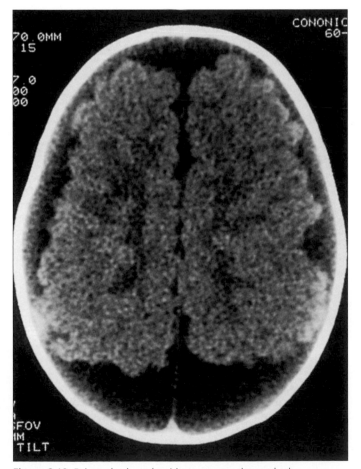

Figure 8.10 Enlarged subarachnoid spaces over the cerebral hemispheres, secondary to impaired CSF absorption.

Table 8.2 Grading system for intraventricular hemorrhage (IVH) in neonates[25]

Grade	Extent of hemorrhage
I	Subependymal germinal matrix hemorrhage
II	IVH without ventricular dilatation
III	IVH with enlargement/dilatation of the ventricle(s)
IV	IVH with parenchymal hemorrhage

Table 8.3 Signs and symptoms of hydrocephalus in children

Premature infants	Infants	Toddlers and older
Apnea	Irritability	Headache
Bradycardia	Vomiting	Vomiting
Tense fontanelle	Drowsiness	Lethargy
Distended scalp veins	Macrocephaly	Diplopia
Globoid head shape	Distended scalp veins	Papilledema
Rapid head growth	Frontal bossing Macewen's sign Poor head control Lateral rectus palsy "Setting-sun" sign	Lateral rectus palsy Hyperreflexia/clonus

Full-term infants

The common causes of hydrocephalus in full-term infants include aqueductal stenosis, Chiari II malformation, Dandy–Walker syndrome, cerebral malformations (e.g. encephaloceles, holoprosencephaly, and hydranencephaly), arachnoid cysts, neoplasms, and vein of Galen malformations. Symptoms include irritability, vomiting, and drowsiness (Table 8.3). Signs include macrocephaly, a convex and full anterior fontanelle, distended scalp veins, cranial suture splaying, frontal bossing, cracked pot sound on percussing over dilated ventricles (positive Macewen's sign), poor head control, lateral rectus palsies, and the "setting-sun" sign, in which the eyes are inferiorly deviated. Paralysis of upgaze and Parinaud's sign herald dilatation of the suprapineal recess.

Normal head circumference for full-term infants is 33–36 cm at birth. Head circumference increases by 2 cm/month during the first 3 months, by 1 cm/month from 4 to 6 months, and by 0.5 cm/month from 7 to 12 months. Head circumference increases that are progressive and rapid, crossing percentile curves on the head growth chart are a stronger diagnostic indicator of hydrocephalus than increases that are consistently above, but parallel to the 95% percentile curve. Papilledema is rare in infants. Chorioretinitis in an infant with hydrocephalus indicates an *in utero* infection, such as toxoplasmosis, cytomegalovirus, or lues.

Older children

Hydrocephalus after infancy is usually secondary to trauma or neoplasms. The predominant symptom is usually a dull and steady headache, which typically occurs upon awakening (Table 8.3). It may be associated with lethargy, and often improves after vomiting. The headaches slowly increase in frequency and severity over days or weeks. Other common complaints include blurred or double vision.

Children presenting with headaches, vomiting, and drowsiness are unfortunately often misdiagnosed as having early meningitis; thus, a CT or MRI scan should be performed to rule out hydrocephalus, hematoma or tumor before a lumbar puncture is attempted. Older children often present with decreased school performance and behavioral disturbances, as well as endocrinopathies (e.g. precocious puberty, short stature, hypothyroidism).

Common signs include papilledema and lateral rectus palsies (unilateral or bilateral). Hyperreflexia and clonus are also seen. Rarely, children with hydrocephalus may experience transient or permanent blindness if the posterior cerebral arteries are compressed against the tentorium. Treatment is urgent if the child becomes lethargic. If the hydrocephalus is severe, Cushing's triad of bradycardia, systemic hypertension, and irregular breathing patterns, as well as autonomic dysfunction, may occur. This triad is rare and often denotes a very severe case of increased ICP requiring emergency treatment.

DIAGNOSTIC STUDIES

Historically, several studies were commonly used before the advent of CT scans in 1976. Skull radiographs demonstrate several diagnostic signs, including cranial suture separation in infants, as well as a beaten copper appearance and enlarged sella in older children. Periventricular punctate calcifications in infants with hydrocephalus indicate *in utero* cytomegalovirus infection, while disseminated calcifications indicate toxoplasmosis. Skull radiographs have since been supplanted by more modern imaging studies.

Other historical procedures include transillumination, ventriculography, and angiography. Angiography is currently used in the investigation of pediatric hydrocephalus, but only in cases with a vascular etiology, such as a vein of Galen malformation or stenosis of the jugular foramina in achondroplastic infants.

Cranial ultrasonography is particularly useful in the evaluation of premature infants with IVH, as well as the detection and monitoring of ventricular size. By measuring through the anterior fontanelle of an infant, ultrasonography can demonstrate lateral and third ventricular morphology, intraventricular clots, and periventricular leukomalacia. However, it cannot image the fourth ventricle or subarachnoid space well.

From 1976 to 1986, CT scanning was the definitive method of diagnosing pediatric hydrocephalus. CT images can accurately demonstrate ventricular size and shape, as well as the presence of blood and calcium deposits. Signs of increased ICP, such as compressed cerebral sulci, obliterated subarachnoid spaces over the convexity, and transependymal resorption of CSF into the white matter (Figure 8.11) can all be detected on CT. With intravenous contrast injections, CT scans can also reveal abnormalities such as tumors and abscesses. CT scans are limited because they can only be performed predominantly in the axial plane, require irradiation, and have considerably less resolution than MRI.

Since 1986, CT has been augmented by the introduction of commercially available MRI, which can project the brain in axial, coronal, and sagittal projections. In addition, MRI can detect transependymal resorption and low-grade gliomas more clearly than CT, as well as determine CSF flow across the aqueduct. However, MRI does not supplant CT entirely because it does not demonstrate calcium as well.

In patients with Dandy–Walker cysts or arachnoid cysts, it is often important to determine whether the cyst communicates with the ventricular system. With an intraventricular injection of water soluble contrast agent into the lateral ventricles, a CT scan obtained 1–4 hours later can evaluate the communication between the ventricles (Figure 8.9, Figure 8.12).

TREATMENT

The treatment of hydrocephalus can be divided into nonsurgical approaches and surgical approaches, which in turn can be divided into nonshunting or shunting procedures. The goals of any successful management of hydrocephalus are: (1) optimal neurological outcome and (2) preservation of cosmesis. The radiographic finding of normal-sized ventricles should not be considered the goal of any therapeutic modality.

Nonsurgical options

There is no nonsurgical medical treatment that definitively treats hydrocephalus effectively. Even if CSF production were to be reduced by 33%, ICP would only modestly decrease by 1.5 cmH$_2$O. Historically, acetazolamide and furosemide have been used to treat hydrocephalus. Although both agents can decrease CSF production for a few days, they do not significantly reduce ventriculomegaly. Acetazolamide, a carbonic anhydrase inhibitor, is needed in large doses (25 mg/kg/day divided into three daily doses), and potential side-effects include lethargy, poor feeding, tachypnea, diarrhea, nephrocalcinosis, and electrolyte imbalances (e.g. hyperchloremic metabolic acidosis, which may require treatment with a systemic alkalizer).[25] While acetazolamide has been used historically to treat premature infants with PHH, recent studies have shown it to be ineffective in avoidance of shunt placement and to be associated with increased neurological morbidity.[26,27] Other nonsurgical therapies tried, which have all been ineffective, include glycerol, isosorbide, radioactive gold, and serial head wraps.

Serial lumbar or ventricular punctures to evacuate CSF are nonsurgical procedures to treat premature infants with PHH. The goal is to temporize the progressive ventriculomegaly with daily aspirations of fluid until the CSF protein levels drop to < 1000 mg/dL and the infant has increased in body size to tolerate operative intervention. If the infant demonstrates continued inadequate CSF absorption, then a shunting procedure is indicated. These temporizing maneuvers are not without controversy, and recent studies have questioned their efficacy.[28] However, the practice is still commonly used in some centers to relieve rising ICPs in the premature infant too small or sick to tolerate placement of a CSF diversion device such as a shunt or reservoir.

Surgical – nonshunting options

Whenever possible, the obstructing lesion that causes the hydrocephalus should be surgically removed. For example, the resection of tumors in the vicinity of the third and fourth ventricle often definitively treats the secondary hydrocephalus. Unfortunately, in most cases of congenital hydrocephalus, the obstructive lesion is not amenable to surgical resection.

For CSF obstruction at or distal to the aqueduct, a potential surgical treatment is the endoscopic third ventriculostomy. By surgically creating an opening at the floor of the third ventricle, CSF can be diverted without placing a shunt. Kamikawa and associates reported a 75% success rate for endoscopic third ventriculostomies among 44 pediatric patients with hydrocephalus secondary to aqueductal stenosis; they also reported statistically

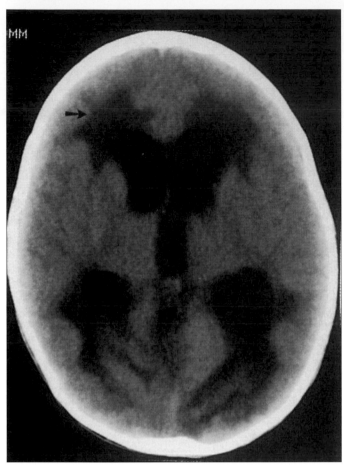

Figure 8.11 Axial CT scan demonstrating transependymal resorption of CSF (arrow) into frontal white matter

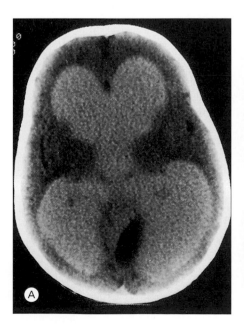
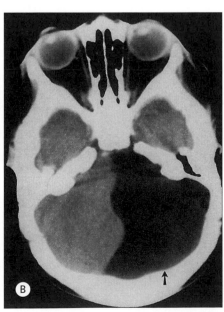

Figure 8.12 Axial CT scans of an infant with hydrocephalus **(A)** secondary to a posterior fossa arachnoid cyst **(B)**. Iohexal injected into the ventricles did not communicate into the cyst (arrow).

significant lower complication rates with the endoscopic procedure when compared with a control group of 44 children treated with conventional shunting procedures.[29] While earlier studies demonstrated that ventriculostomies are of intermediate value in patients with congenital aqueductal stenosis and myelomeningoceles,[30] recent studies suggest that these patients also enjoy high success rates with this procedure.[31,32] Other etiologies with a high success rate with ventriculostomies include tectal plate tumors, posterior fossa tumors, and acquired aqueductal stenosis. Communicating hydrocephalus is not an indication for a third ventriculostomy.

Surgical – CSF shunts

Components

CSF shunts are usually silastic tubes that divert CSF from the ventricles to other body cavities (i.e. peritoneal, atrium or pleural space), where normal physiologic processes can absorb the fluid. Shunts typically have three components: a proximal (ventricular) catheter, a one-way valve that permits flow out of the ventricular system, and a distal catheter that diverts the fluid to its eventual destination. Most shunts have built-in reservoirs that can be percutaneously aspirated for CSF.[33]

Most shunt valves are pressure-differential valves, i.e. they are designed to open at designated pressures and remain open as long as the pressure differential across the valve is greater than the opening pressure. However, some shunts are flow-controlled, where the valve mechanism attempts to keep flow constant in the face of changing pressure differentials and patient position. Valves come in a variety of different pressure and flow settings depending on the manufacturer. A comparison of pressure-differential valves and flow-control valves among infants showed no statistically significant difference in overall shunt lifespan or time to first shunt complication.[34] A recent advance in shunt valve technology has been the introduction of programmable valves. These permit the neurosurgeon to adjust the opening pressure settings of the implanted shunt without the need to subject the patient to an additional surgical procedure to change valves. A comparison study between the programmable valve and the conventional valve found similar efficacy and safety characteristics.[35]

The paths in which a ventricular catheter can be inserted include the frontal, parietal, or occipital approaches[36] (Figure 8.13). There is great controversy on whether a frontal or parietal/occipital approach to placing a ventricular catheter has a lower obstruction rate. There is no clear-cut answer and surgeon's preference plays a significant role in the choice. Ventricular catheters are usually placed in the right nondominant cerebral hemisphere.

Surgical techniques

The local landmarks that guide the placement of the ventricular catheter are demonstrated in Figure 8.13. The length of a frontal ventricular catheter is approximately 4 cm in a full-term infant and 6 cm in an adult. (The exact measurement can be determined via preoperative imaging studies, such as CT and/or MRI.) Patients often outgrow their ventricular catheters, especially between the ages of 6 and 10 years if their shunts were initially placed frontally as infants; this necessitates an additional operation

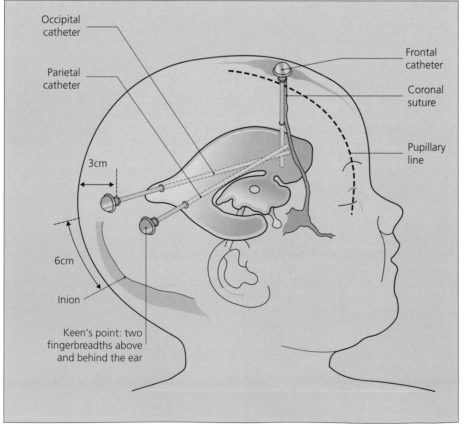

Figure 8.13 Three routes for insertion of ventricular shunt catheters: frontal, parietal, and occipital.

to revise the shunt when the catheter pulls out of the ventricular system. The addition of endoscopic technology was predicted to improve the accuracy of catheter placement in difficult cases;[37] however, randomized studies have not yet demonstrated a distinct advantage of endoscopically placed catheters. Endoscopy does appear to be enormously helpful in fenestrating the septations of loculated ventricles, thus avoiding the necessity of multiple ventricular catheters.

The distal catheters are passed through subcutaneous removable tubes or trocars to their destination sites. The most common site is the peritoneal cavity, which is accessed via a small incision and open dissection or a percutaneous trocar (Figure 8.14). Common sites of insertion include the epigastric midline immediately below the xiphoid process and the lateral edge of the lateral rectus abdominal muscle. For full-term infants and older infants, > 40 cm of the peritoneal catheter can be safely placed within the peritoneal cavity to avoid future distal revisions secondary to the child outgrowing the shunt.

If the peritoneal cavity is an inappropriate site (e.g. recent infection or abdominal adhesions), the next preferred location is the atrium. The most common technique for atrial catheter placement is via a modified Seldinger technique, in which a guidewire and peel-away catheter are inserted into the right atrium under fluoroscopic guidance similar to the placement of a central venous line. The distal shunt tubing is then inserted through the peel-away sheath.[38]

For children > 4–5 years of age, the pleural cavity is also a viable site for distal catheter placement. However, in children < 4 years of age, the absorptive capability of the pleura may be inadequate, and placing a pleural catheter may lead to increasing pleural effusions and respiratory compromise. The gallbladder is another option, but is associated with higher complication rates. However, such ventricle to gallbladder shunts have been successfully used to treat difficult-to-manage cases of pediatric hydrocephalus.[39,40] The subgaleal space is also an option for premature infants with PHH (see below). There are case reports of shunts being successfully placed in the sagittal sinus and other vascular conduits in the body for patients with no other reasonable site of insertion

Treatment of hydrocephalus diagnosed *in utero*

In utero hydrocephalus can often produce head circumferences of > 40 cm, causing complications in childbirth, such as cephalopelvic disproportion and inhibition of labor. If detected by ultrasound, marked fetal hydrocephalus discovered prenatally can be further evaluated with *in utero* MRI scans (Figure 8.15). If the MRI scans demonstrate a severe brain malformation (e.g. holoprosencephaly, hydranencephaly), a cephalocentesis can be performed after prenatal counseling, which results in fetal death in a majority of cases, but allows the safe delivery of the fetus without subjecting the mother to additional risks, such as an extensive uterotomy.

Historically, fetal hydrocephalus has been treated *in utero* with ventriculoamniotic shunts, but the results have been poor, and overall prognosis, which is poor to start with, is not improved by

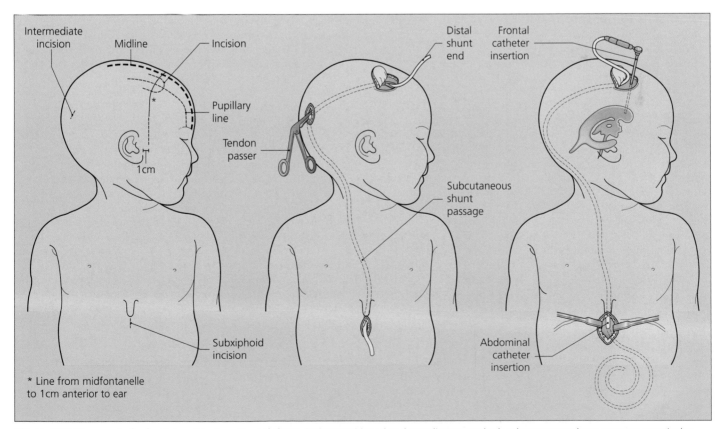

Figure 8.14 Placement of a frontal ventriculoperitoneal shunt. Patient positioned and coordinates marked; subcutaneous shunt passage; ventricular catheter insertion; peritoneal catheter insertion.

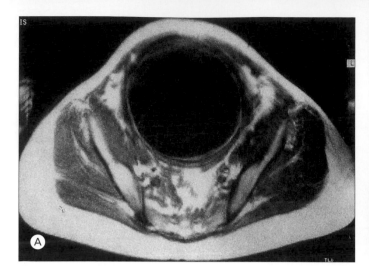

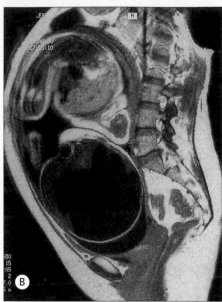

Figure 8.15 Fetal MRI scans demonstrating (A) holoprosencephaly and (B) severe hydrocephalus.

in utero intervention. Currently, cases of fetal hydrocephalus with normal brain morphology are followed with serial ultrasound examinations and delivered via cesarean section when fetal lung maturity becomes adequate. The hydrocephalus is then treated with a shunting procedure, if symptomatic.

Treatment of posthemorrhagic hydrocephalus

Premature infants weighing 0.5–1.5 kg often develop IVH that obstructs the CSF pathways. A treatment algorithm for this type of hydrocephalus used by the authors is presented in Figure 8.16. First, serial lumbar punctures and/or ventricular taps are performed to normalize ICP; approximately 7–15 mL of CSF must be removed daily to adequately temporize PHH. The infant's ICP can be assessed by palpation of the anterior fontanelle and detection of cranial suture splaying; ventriculomegaly can be followed by serial cranial ultrasounds. If the infant's weight is > 1 kg, a ventriculosubgaleal shunt or a ventricular catheter and subcutaneous reservoir can be placed. Ventriculosubgaleal shunts can safely temporize PHH while avoiding external drainage or frequent CSF aspirations (Figure 8.17).[41] A ventricular catheter connected to a subcutaneous reservoir can be accessed for daily CSF aspirations with a risk of infection of less than 5%.[42] A ventriculoperitoneal shunt should be considered when the CSF is cleared of posthemorrhagic debris, CSF protein is < 1000 mg/dL, the infant weighs > 1.5 kg, and the infant has progressive PHH.

Treatment of hydrocephalus associated with myelomeningoceles

Approximately 85% of infants with myelomeningoceles develop symptomatic hydrocephalus, and approximately 50% have obvious hydrocephalus at birth. Treatment is usually with a ventriculoperitoneal shunt, although recent evidence suggests that endoscopic third ventriculostomies may have a useful role.[31] Historically, shunt placement is deferred until after the myelomeningocele is repaired; however, contemporary evidence suggests that the risks of shunt complications are not significantly

increased if the shunt is placed during the same setting as the myelomeningocele closure.[43,44] In many centers the shunt is placed in neonates with ventriculomegaly at the time of the myelomeningocele closure with the hope that a shunt will prevent a CSF leak from the spine site.

In utero surgical repair of myelomeningoceles remains a controversial topic. While it is clear that fetal surgery for myelomeningocele repair increases the risk of premature delivery, there has been some preliminary evidence that it may reduce the likelihood of shunt dependence and Chiari II malformations.[45] This remains an area of active research interest and debate. There is currently, a multi-centered National Institutes of Health Study examining the efficacy and safety of *in utero* repair of myelomeningoceles (see Chapter 7).

Treatment of Dandy–Walker cysts

To treat hydrocephalus secondary to a Dandy–Walker cyst, a contrast study can be performed to determine if the lateral ventricles communicate with the cyst. With no communication, at least two shunts are necessary, one to decompress the cyst and one to drain the ventricular system. With communication, a single shunt in either the lateral ventricle or the cyst could adequately treat the hydrocephalus, although some centers recommend simply shunting both the cyst and ventricle as the initial treatment.[46] A decompressed Dandy–Walker cyst can yield dramatic radiographic results, i.e. cerebellar hemispheres that seem to be severely atrophic are often in reality only severely compressed (Figure 8.18).

Treatment of trapped fourth ventricles

The predominant cause of trapped fourth ventricle is IVH but occasionally meningitis can precipitate it if the cerebral aqueduct and basal foramina have been occluded by gliosis and arachnoid fibrosis, respectively. This entity is often discovered after hydrocephalus is treated with a lateral ventricular shunt, in which the lateral and third ventricles decompress, but the fourth ventricle

Figure 8.16 Algorithm for management of posthemorrhagic hydrocephalus.

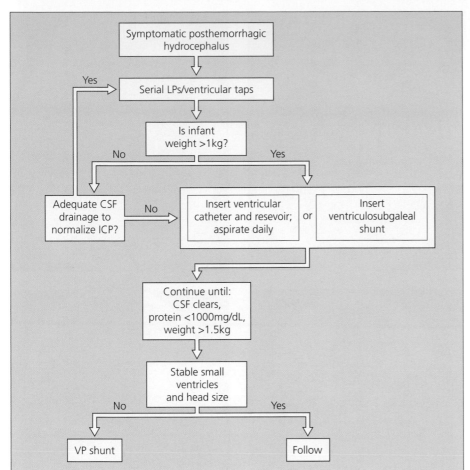

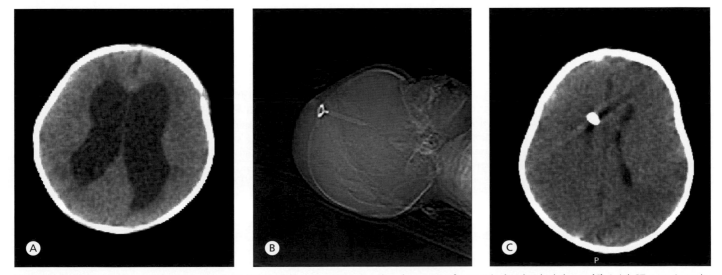

Figure 8.17 (A) Axial CT scan of infant with PHH. **(B)** Skull film demonstrating the placement of a ventriculosubgaleal shunt. **(C)** Axial CT scan 4 weeks after placement of the ventriculosubgaleal shunt.

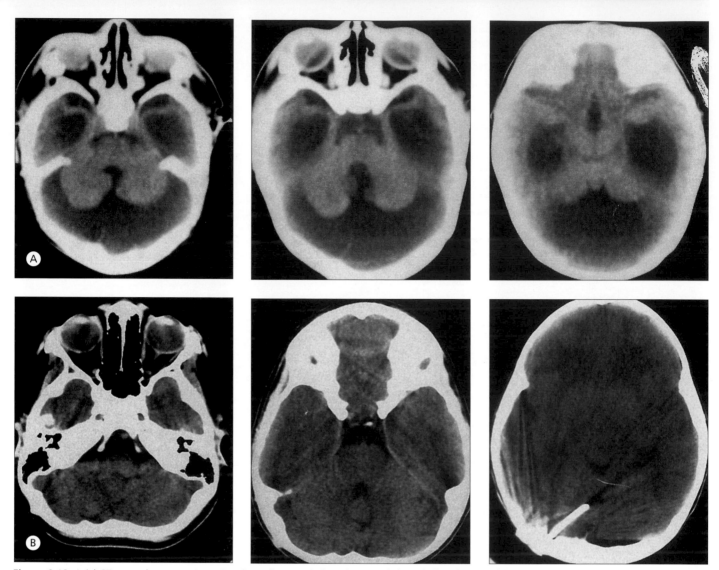

Figure 8.18 Axial CT scans demonstrating a Dandy–Walker cyst before shunting **(A)**, and after shunting **(B)**.

enlarges.[47] Treatment can consist of placement of a fourth ventricular shunt via a paramedian approach (to avoid the midline occipital sinus); however, such shunts are often difficult to place with potentially complicated courses.[48] Alternatively, endoscopic procedures, such as aqueductoplasty or fenestration of the fourth ventricle wall, have been shown to treat trapped fourth ventricles effectively while reducing the revision rate when compared with fourth ventricular shunts.[49]

Treatment of hydrocephalus caused by arachnoid cysts

Most arachnoid cysts are asymptomatic, and do not require treatment. If a cyst is responsible for hydrocephalus, decompressing the cyst with a cystoperitoneal shunt will usually resolve the hydrocephalus as well. Shunts draining arachnoid cysts often require low pressure settings or programmable valves to decompress them adequately.

Treatment of hydrocephalus secondary to posterior fossa tumors

Hydrocephalus secondary to posterior fossa tumors can often be treated without a shunt. An EVD system is surgically inserted in many centers before the posterior fossa tumor resection is performed. It is then left in place postoperatively, and the patient is weaned off the EVD by progressively elevating the height of the drainage bag. When the child demonstrates the ability to tolerate clamping of the ventricular drainage tubing for 24 hours without developing symptoms of ICP or ventriculomegaly on CT scan the EVD can be safely withdrawn. Approximately 25–50% of children cannot tolerate the removal of the EVD. In those patients a ventriculoperitoneal shunt is required.[50]

Treatment of other conditions

Children with severe brain malformations, such as hydranencephaly or holoprosencephaly present ethical dilemmas because of their poor prognosis. On one hand, the introduction of a shunt does not alter their overall course. On the other hand, if left untreated, their heads will expand enormously, leading to significant nursing and care-providing issues. Shunts are often introduced to prevent increasing head circumference, and they generally function well because the proximal catheters lie in large CSF spaces and rarely become obstructed by choroid plexus.

Achondroplastic children may present with ventriculomegaly. Symptomatic patients are traditionally shunted, while the treatment of asymptomatic patients with documented ventriculomegaly or macrocephaly is controversial. Achondroplastic children with hydrocephalus have also been successfully treated with jugular foramen decompression.[51]

While lumboperitoneal shunts can theoretically be used to treat children with communicating hydrocephalus, in practice they are seldom used, except for patients with pseudotumor cerebri and those with difficult to treat hydrocephalus such as the "slit ventricle syndrome." These are children who have an over-drainage problem in which they develop debilitating symptoms from increased ICP after placement of a shunt. A CT scan will often show small, slit-like ventricles and a "tight appearing brain" that does not respond normally to intracranial pressure changes. A lumboperitoneal shunt is often used as an alternative form of CSF drainage to decrease the intracranial pressure and symptoms. However, lumboperitoneal shunts do have some disadvantages in that they are difficult to assess for function, they can induce downward herniation of the hindbrain causing an iatrogenic Chiari malformation, and they are prone to malfunction.

Shunt complications

Shunt complications and failures remain a significant problem in treating hydrocephalus. The goal in treatment of hydrocephalus with a shunt is to decrease intracranial pressure and associated cerebral damage and simultaneously prevent complications associated with the shunting procedure. Shunt complications fall into three major categories: (1) mechanical failure of the device, (2) functional failure because of too much or too little flow of CSF, and (3) infection of the CSF or the shunt device.

In a recent study investigating the performance of two popular shunt valves, the Delta valve (PS Medical-Medtronic) and the Sigma valve (NMT Cordis), the failure rate was noted to be approximately 38% after the first year, 48% after 2 years, 54% after 3 years, and 59% 4 years after shunt placement.[52] A list of shunt complications is outlined in Table 8.4. The two most common complications are infection and obstruction.

Infection

Despite the numerous measures used to decrease the risk of infection, in general, approximately 1–15% of all shunting procedures are complicated by infection. This rate seems to remain constant despite a host of precautions employed, which include the use of systemic and intrashunt antibiotics, iodine-impregnated transparent surgical drapes, covering incisions with Betadine-soaked sponges, glove changes, and using only instruments to handle shunt hardware. Premature infants have an increased risk; the hazard ratio for an infant with gestational age < 40 weeks at the time of surgery is 4.72.[53] There are only a few centers around the world in which shunt infection rates have remained below 1%. Those centers employ precautions that are difficult to duplicate in most hospitals. Approximately three-quarters of all shunt infections become evident within 1 month of placement. Nearly 90% of all shunt infections are recognized within 12 months of the last shunt manipulation, as it is believed that most bacteria are introduced at the time of surgery.

The offending organism is most often a member of the skin flora. *Staphylococcus epidermidis* causes approximately 60% of shunt infections, *Staphylococcus aureus* is responsible for 30%, and coliform bacteria, propionibacteria, streptococci, or *Haemophilus influenzae* cause the remainder. In general, Gram-positive organisms correlate with a better prognosis than Gram-negative organisms.

Common symptoms include irritability and anorexia. Common signs include low-grade fever and elevated C-reactive protein. *Staphylococcus aureus* infections often present with erythema along the shunt track. Infected ventriculoatrial shunts may present with subacute bacterial endocarditis and shunt nephritis, an immune-complex disorder that resembles acute glomerulonephritis.

The literature regarding the usefulness of prophylactic antibiotics is conflicting. Several prospective, randomized, trials demonstrated statistically significant improvement in shunt infection rates when children were treated with systemic oxacillin, systemic trimethoprim-sulfamethoxazole, or intraventricular vancomycin.[54–56] However, similar studies using systemic methicillin or cephalothin demonstrated no significant advantage.[57,58] Regardless of this, prophylactic antibiotics, such as cefazolin, vancomycin or oxacillin, are routinely used in clinical practice.

Treatment usually involves the removal of the infected shunt and placement of an EVD. In the case of some bacterial infections, it is possible to eradicate the infection without removing the shunt.[59] However, *in situ* treatment of shunt infections is fraught with hazards and does not uniformly lead to success. The most

Table 8.4 Shunt complications

Common complications	Uncommon complications			
	Cranial	Subcutaneous	Peritoneal	Atrial
Infection	Subdural hygroma	Shunt migration	Peritonitis	Endocarditis
Obstruction	Subdural hematoma	Shunt disconnection	Pseudocysts	Nephritis
Inadequate flow or overdrainage	Hemiparesis Hematoma	Shunt fracture	Perforation Hernias	

effective and widely used treatment of a shunt infection is to remove the infected hardware and either place no hardware (if tolerated) or place an EVD. The patient is then treated with the appropriate intravenous antibiotics, based on culture and sensitivity results. When the infection is cleared, i.e. (1) 5–7 consecutive daily CSF cultures that are negative, (2) CSF white blood cell count < 50, and (3) CSF protein < 500 mg/dL, a new shunt system is implanted, and the EVD is removed.

Obstruction

Shunt obstruction is another common complication. The clinical presentation can vary greatly. Shunt devices are to be viewed as mechanical devices that can become obstructed or malfunction anywhere in their course, and anytime during their lifetime. The most common scenarios occur weeks, months, or years after insertion, when choroid plexus or debris has occluded the proximal ventricular catheter tip. Another common shunt malfunction scenario is the child who has obstructed his distal catheter or has outgrown his peritoneal catheter and presents with an obstruction after the distal tip has slipped out of the peritoneal cavity. In addition, shunt valves can malfunction, and shunt tubing can break, disconnect or dislodge from its previous location.

Common symptoms of shunt obstruction depend on the age of the child (Table 8.3). A child with a shunt malfunction often presents with signs and symptoms of increased ICP. Infants with a shunt malfunction usually present with irritability, poor feeding, increased head circumference, and/or inappropriate sleepiness. Children with a shunt malfunction usually present with headache, irritability, lethargy, nausea, and/or vomiting. However, it is important to inquire if the signs and symptoms that the child is presenting with are the same as those during a shunt malfunction in the past.[3] The child can present with waxing and waning symptoms, or can alternatively present with a progressively worsening picture that does not improve until the shunt is revised. A child complaining of pain with a clinical picture consistent with shunt obstruction should not be given narcotics because of possible respiratory depression or arrest.

When a shunt malfunction is suspected, neuroimaging studies should be obtained after a careful history and physical examination. A head CT, as well as anteroposterior and lateral skull, chest, and abdominal radiographs, are obtained to evaluate for increased ventricular size and shunt hardware continuity. Even though a majority of children with a shunt malfunction present with increased ventricular size on neuroimaging studies, there are those whose ventricular size does not change because of decreased brain compliance (i.e. "stiff ventricles"). In these children, a shunt tap through the reservoir or valve (see below) is indicated to test the adequacy of CSF flow and the intracranial pressure. Children who are diagnosed with a shunt malfunction are taken promptly to the operating room for shunt revision.[3]

The shunt itself can be examined for evidence of obstruction. The presence of a fluid collection in the subcutaneous tissue in proximity to the shunt track is suggestive. The shunt valve can be "pumped," i.e. compressed several times against the skull, which may provide useful information. A collapse of the valve without quick refilling of CSF may indicate a shunt obstruction. Finally, the shunt reservoir can be accessed by a 23–25-gauge butterfly needle. The presence of spontaneous flow with good respiratory variations up the tubing or in a manometer connected to the butterfly, indicates patency of the ventricular catheter. ICP can then be measured, and normal ICP varies by age (Table 8.1). If there is no CSF flow up the manometer and the ventricles are large, a presumed shunt obstruction is confirmed. In some institutions, a nuclear medicine patency study may be performed to evaluate a presumed shunt malfunction, by occluding the valve and injecting through the butterfly needle a radioactive isotope, such as indium (^{111}In) into the reservoir. The isotope can then be traced from the ventricular system, through the shunt device, and into the distal collection site.

Shunt obstructions/malfunctions are treated by replacing the occluded or nonfunctioning components, or by replacing the entire system. In cases where the clinical picture of obstruction occurs in the presence of small ventricles, the term "slit-ventricle" syndrome has been utilized.[60] This disorder afflicts a small but not insignificant number of children with shunt malfunctions, and can be difficult to diagnose and treat. Often the patient's symptoms worsen when standing and improve when laying flat, which is consistent with an "overdrainage" component to this syndrome. The syndrome is treated in a systematic fashion. First, the diagnosis of migraine or underlying treatable cause is ruled out. If the symptoms and CT scan are consistent with overdrainage, or an intermittent shunt malfunction, a shunt exploration is planned. A shunt revision may include placement of a new catheter or a higher pressure shunt valve. If the child has a programmable valve, the setting of the valve is first increased, thereby avoiding a surgical intervention. As a last resort, and in very rare instances, a decompressive craniectomy can be performed to improve the intracranial compliance of the brain and ventricles.

Uncommon complications

Table 8.4 lists several uncommon shunt complications. Subdural hygromas and hematomas may develop after the insertion of a shunt into a child with very large ventricles and thin cerebral cortical mantles. Treatment of symptomatic subdural hygromas and hematomas consists of changing the shunt valve to a higher pressure setting and/or by introducing a catheter into the effusion and connecting it to the distal shunt system.

Ventricular catheter migration out of the ventricular system occurs if the shunt has not been properly fixed at the burr hole site where it exits the skull. Catheters with reservoirs attached to them theoretically have a lower risk of migration.

Abdominal pseudocysts can develop around the distal end of a peritoneal catheter. They often develop in young children secondary to indolent bacterial infections. In addition to presenting with a clinical picture of shunt infection, the patient may also complain of abdominal pain and distension. They can be diagnosed radiographically via abdominal ultrasound or a CT scan. The cysts may be percutaneously aspirated, and the fluid can be cultured. Given the indolent nature of the likely infections, treatment is no different from any other shunt infection. Ascites, similarly, may be indicative of an indolent infection, or it may be secondary to CSF overproduction and/or inadequate peritoneal absorption. Hernias can also develop within 3 months of shunt insertion, and are treated like any other hernia. Perforation of intraperitoneal organs is a rare but well-recognized complication.

Follow-up

The authors examine children with shunted hydrocephalus every 3 months for the first year following shunt placement, every 6 months in the second year, and then yearly with a follow-up head CT after that. A postoperative CT scan after surgery is obtained to document the baseline size of the patient's shunted ventricles. Infants shunted for massively dilated ventricles may require more than a year before the ventricles stabilize in size. Future CT scans are obtained yearly and as needed to evaluate shunt complications. Children with ventriculoatrial shunts require yearly chest X-rays to monitor the location of the atrial catheter tip.

OUTCOME

The prognosis of pediatric hydrocephalus is dependent more on the underlying brain morphology, as well as other factors, such as IVH, ventriculitis, and perinatal ischemia, than on the severity of the hydrocephalus and ventriculomegaly. The 5-year survival rate of children with congenital hydrocephalus is approximately 90%.[61] Normal intellect has been reported to range from 40 to 65%,[62] but obviously varies widely with each specific etiology.

Before the advent of the CT scan, several studies attempted to investigate the prognosis of shunted versus nonshunted hydrocephalic children. In 1963, Foltz and Shurtleff performed a 5-year study of 113 hydrocephalic children of whom 65 were shunted early, and 48 were not operated on.[63] Based on life-table data projected from birth to 10 years, the shunted children had significantly better survival (61.8% vs. 33.8%) and a higher percentage with an IQ of at least 75 (33.8% vs. 5.5%). Intellectual capacity was found to correlate inversely with duration of increased intracranial pressure. In 1973, Young and colleagues performed an outcome analysis on a series of 147 shunted hydrocephalic children.[64] They discovered a correlation between the width of the child's cerebral mantle and IQ. The IQ distribution approached a normal pattern when a mantle width of 2.8 cm is achieved. They also discovered that prompt and adequate treatment of pure hydrocephalus (without myelodysplasia or severe brain malformation) before 6 months of age nearly always resulted in normal or relatively unimpaired intelligence.

Since the introduction of modern imaging techniques, such as CT and MRI, there have been several studies investigating the outcomes of hydrocephalus secondary to specific etiologies. Op Heij and colleagues followed a case series of 50 children with congenital nonobstructive hydrocephalus and found that IQ was normal (> 80) in 50% of cases and < 55 in 28%.[65] There was no correlation with head circumference or degree of ventriculomegaly. They concluded that degree of intellectual impairment had less to do with the severity of the hydrocephalus and more to do with the severity of underlying anomalies in the CNS and defects in the cyto-architecture of the neocortex.

Infants with PHH have a significantly higher mortality rate when compared with low-birth-weight infants without PHH (16–35% vs. 6.5–13%).[66] When the grade of PHH was taken into account, however, grade I and II PHH was associated with a mortality rate of 9% vs. 49% for grades III and IV. The correlation between PHH grade and severity of neurological disabilities is less clear. Skullerad and Westre found no correlation between neurological development and PHH grade.[67] Between 40 and 60% of all infants with PHH were developmentally normal at 1–2 years of age, and 20–30% already showed major disabilities. Krishnamoorthy and associates, however, stratified the PHH grades and revealed that higher grade PHH was associated with an increased risk of major disability.[68]

Historically, the mortality for infants with Dandy–Walker malformation approached 20–30%. However, in 1990, Bindal and colleagues demonstrated a mortality of only 14% in their series.[69] In cases where the infant was shunted both above and below the tentorium, they reported an increased incidence of shunt failure because of the cyst shunt component. They also reported an average of 6.5 shunt revisions per patient over an average 7 years of follow-up. Lower IQ and neurological developmental delay are seen in children with Dandy–Walker malformations, but they are thought to be most commonly related to associated anomalies in the CNS.

This chapter contains material from the first edition, and we are grateful to the author of that chapter for his contribution.

CLINICAL PEARLS

In these authors' experience:

- Signs and symptoms of progressive hydrocephalus depend on age (Table 8.3).

- Symptomatic posthemorrhagic hydrocephalus should be treated with serial CSF evacuation followed by a ventricular shunt in progressive cases. Subcutaneous reservoirs and ventricular catheters or ventriculosubgaleal shunts may play key roles in temporizing the infant until shunt placement is feasible.

- Symptomatic ventricular shunt malfunction should be evaluated, recognized and treated promptly to avoid undue morbidity.

- Shunt infections currently occur in 1–15% of children who have shunts placed or revised. The majority of infections are detected within the first 1–6 months after a shunt procedure. A high index of suspicion and proximity to a recent shunt manipulation makes this diagnosis more likely.

- The prognosis of pediatric hydrocephalus is dependent primarily on the underlying brain morphology. A child with relatively normal brain organization has a better outcome than a child with abnormal morphology.

REFERENCES

1. Mokri B. The Monro–Kellie hypothesis: applications of CSF volume depletion. *Neurology* 2001; 56: 1746–8.

2. Shapiro K, Morris WJ, Teo C. Intracranial hypertension: mechanisms and management. In: Cheek WR, Marlin AF, McLone DG, *et al.* (eds). *Pediatric Neurosurgery of the Developing Nervous System*, 3rd edn. Philadelphia: WB Saunders; 1994: 307–19.

3. Avellino AM, Carson BS. Increased intracranial pressure. In: Maria BL (ed.) *Current Management in Child Neurology*, 2nd edn. Hamilton: BC Decker; 2002: 481–6.

4. Cutler RWP, Page L, Galicich J, *et al.* Formation and absorption of cerebrospinal fluid in man. *Brain* 1968; 91: 707–20.

5. Lorenzo AV, Page LK, Watters GV. Relationship between cerebrospinal fluid formation, absorption, and pressure in human hydrocephalus. *Brain* 1970; 93: 679–92.

6. Matsuda M, Uzura S, Nakasu S, et al. Primary carcinoma of the choroid plexus in the lateral ventricle. *Surg Neurol* 1991; 36: 294–9.

7. Ellenbogan RG, Winston KR, Kupsky WJ. Tumors of the choroid plexus in children. *Neurosurgery* 1989; 25: 327–35.

8. Ho DM, Wong TT, Liu HC. Choroid plexus tumors in childhood. Histopathologic study and clinico-pathological correlation. *Child's Nervous System* 1991; 7: 437–41.

9. Eisenberg HM, McComb JG, Lorenzo AV. Choroid plexus papilloma. Proof of cerebrospinal fluid overproduction. *J Neurosurg* 1974; 40: 381–5.

10. Philips MF, Shanno G, Duhaime AC. Treatment of villous hypertrophy of the choroid plexus by endoscopic contact coagulation. *Pediatr Neurosurg* 1998; 28: 252–6.

11. Habballah MY, Hoffman HJ. The isolated lateral ventricle. *Surg Neurol* 1987; 27: 220–2.

12. Gemperlein J. Paraphyseal cysts of the third ventricle. Report of two cases in infants. *J Neuropathol Exp Neurol* 1960; 19: 133–4.

13. Camacho A, Abernathey CD, Kelly PJ, et al. Colloid cysts: experience with the management of 84 cases since the introduction of computed tomography. *Neurosurgery* 1989; 24: 693–700.

14. Kondziolka D, Lunsford LD. Stereotactic management of colloid cysts: factors predicting success. *J Neurosurg* 1991; 75: 45–51.

15. Decq P, Le Guerinel C, Brugieres P, et al. Endoscopic management of colloid cysts. *Neurosurgery* 1998; 42: 1288–94.

16. Wiese JA, Gentry LR, Menezes AH. Bobble-head doll syndrome: review of the pathophysiology and CSF dynamics. *Pediatr Neurol* 1985; 1: 361–6.

17. Pierre-Kahn A, Capelle L, Brauner R, et al. Presentation and management of suprasellar arachnoid cysts. J Neurosurg 1990; 73: 355–9.

18. Fritsch MJ, Mehdorn M. Endoscopic intraventricular surgery for treatment of hydrocephalus and loculated CSF space in children less than one year of age. *Pediatr Neurosurg* 2002; 36: 183–8.

19. Emery JL. Intracranial effects of longstanding decompression of the brain in children with hydrocephalus and myelomeningocele. *Dev Med Child Neurol* 1965; 7: 302–9.

20. Milhorat TH, Hammock MK, Chandra RS. The subarachnoid space in congenital obstructive hydrocephalus, II: microscopic findings. *J Neurosurg* 1971; 35: 7–15.

21. Faivre J, Lemarec B, Betagne J, et al. X-linked hydrocephalus, with aqueductal stenosis, mental retardation, and adduction-flexion deformity of the thumbs. *Childs Brain* 1976; 2: 226–33.

22. Spadaro A, Ambrosio D, Mracic A, et al. Nontumoral aqueductal stenosis in children affected by von Recklinghausen's disease. *Surg Neurol* 1989; 26: 487–95.

23. Asa A, Hoffman HJ, Hendrick EB, et al. Dandy–Walker syndrome: experience at the Hospital for Sick Children. *Pediatr Neurosci* 1989; 15: 66–73.

24. Papile LA, Burstein J, Burstein R, et al. Incidence and evolution of subependymal and intraventricular hemorrhage: a study of infants with birth weights less than 1,500 gm. *J Pediatr* 1978; 92: 529–34.

25. Libenson MH, Kaye EM, Rosman NP, et al. Acetazolamide and furosemide for posthemorrhagic hydrocephalus of the newborn. *Pediatr Neurol* 1999; 20: 185–91.

26. Whitelaw A, Kennedy CR, Brion LP. Diuretic therapy for newborn infants with posthemorrhagic ventricular dilatation. *Cochrane Database Syst Rev* 2001; 2: CD002270.

27. Kennedy CR, Ayers S, Campbell MJ, et al. Randomized, controlled trial of acetazolamide and furosemide in posthemorrhagic ventricular dilation in infancy: follow-up at 1 year. *Pediatrics* 2001; 108: 597–607.

28. Whitelaw A. Repeated lumbar or ventricular punctures in newborns with intraventricular hemorrhage. *Cochrane Database Syst Rev* 2001; 1: CD000216.

29. Kamikawa S, Inui A, Kobayashi N, et al. Endoscopic treatment of hydrocephalus in children: a controlled study using newly developed Yamadori-type ventriculoscopes. *Minim Invasive Neurosurg* 2001; 44: 25–30.

30. Jones RFC, Stening WA, Byrydon M. Endoscopic third ventriculostomy. *Neurosurgery* 1990; 75: 865–73.

31. Brockmeyer D, Abtin K, Carey L, et al. Endoscopic third ventriculostomy: an outcome analysis. *Pediatr Neurosurg* 1998; 28: 236–40.

32. Gangemi M, Donati P, Maiuri F, et al. Endoscopic third ventriculostomy for hydrocephalus. *Minim Invasive Neurosurg* 1999; 42: 128–32.

33. Czosnyka Z, Czosnyka M, Richards HK, et al. Laboratory testing of hydrocephalus shunts – conclusion of the UK Shunt evaluation programme. *Acta Neurochir (Wien)* 2002; 144: 525–38.

34. Jain H, Sgouros S, Walsh AR, et al. The treatment of infantile hydrocephalus: "differential-pressure" or "flow-control" valves. A pilot study. *Childs Nerv Syst* 2000; 16: 242–6.

35. Pollack IF, Albright AL, Adelson PD. A randomized, controlled study of a programmable shunt valve versus a conventional valve for patients with hydrocephalus. Hakim-Medos Investigator Group. *Neurosurgery* 1999; 45: 1399–408.

36. Albright AL, Haines SJ, Taylor FH. Function of parietal and frontal shunts in childhood hydrocephalus. *J Neurosurg* 1988; 69: 883–6.

37. Theodosopoulos PV, Abosch A, McDermott MW. Intraoperative fiber-optic endoscopy for ventricular catheter insertion. *Can J Neurol Sci* 2001; 28: 56–60.

38. Britz GW, Avellino AM, Schaller R, et al. Percutaneous placement of ventriculoatrial shunts in the pediatric population. *Pediatr Neurosurg* 1998; 29: 161–3.

39. West KW, Turner MK, Vane DW, et al. Ventricular gallbladder shunts: an alternative procedure in hydrocephalus. *J Pediatr Surg* 1987; 22: 609–12.

40. Ketoff JA, Klein RL, Maukkassa KF. Ventricular cholecystic shunts in children. *J Pediatr Surg* 1997; 32: 181–3.

41. Fulmer BB, Grabb PA, Oakes WJ, et al. Neonatal ventriculosubgaleal shunts. *Neurosurgery* 2000; 47: 80–3.

42. McComb JG, Ramos AD, Platzker ACG, et al. Management of hydrocephalus secondary to intraventricular hemorrhage in the preterm infant with a subcutaneous ventricular catheter reservoir. *Neurosurgery* 1983; 13: 295–300.

43. Miller PD, Pollack IF, Pang D, et al. Comparison of simultaneous versus delayed ventriculoperitoneal shunt insertion in children undergoing myelomeningocele repair. *J Child Neurol* 1996; 11: 370–2.

44. Parent AD, McMillan T. Contemporaneous shunting with repair of myelomeningocele. *Pediatr Neurosurg* 1995; 22: 132–5.

45. Bruner JP, Tulipan N, Paschall RL, et al. Fetal surgery for myelomeningocele and the incidence of shunt-dependent hydrocephalus. *JAMA* 1999; 282: 1819–25.

46. Osenbach RK, Menezes AH. Diagnosis and management of the Dandy–Walker malformation: 30 years of experience. *Pediatr Neurosurg* 1992; 18: 179–89.

47. O'Hare AE, Brown JK, Minns RA. Specific enlargement of the fourth ventricle after ventriculoperitoneal shunt for post-hemorrhagic hydrocephalus. *Arch Dis Child* 1987; 62: 1025–9.

48. Lee M, Leahu D, Weiner HL, et al. Complications of fourth-ventricular shunts. *Pediatr Neurosurg* 1995; 22: 309–13.

49. Teo C, Burson T, Misra S. Endoscopic treatment of the trapped fourth ventricle. *Neurosurgery* 1999; 44: 1257–61.

50. Dias MS, Albright AL. Management of hydrocephalus complicating childhood posterior fossa tumors. *Pediatr Neurosci* 1989; 15: 283–9.

51. Lundar T, Bakke SJ, Nornes H. Hydrocephalus in an achondroplastic child treated by venous decompression at the jugular foramen. Case report. *J Neurosurg* 1990; 73: 138–40.

52. Kestle J, Drake J, Milner R, *et al*. Long-term follow-up data from the Shunt Design Trial. *Pediatr Neurosurg* 2000; 33: 230–6.

53. Kulkarni AV, Drake JM, Lamberti-Pasculli M. Cerebrospinal fluid shunt infection: a prospective study of risk factors. *J Neurosurg* 2001; 94: 195–201.

54. Bayston R, Bannister C, Boston V, *et al*. A prospective randomised controlled trial of antimicrobial prophylaxis in hydrocephalus shunt surgery. *Z Kinderchir* 1990; 45 Suppl. 1: 5–7.

55. Djindjian M, Fevrier MJ, Otterbein G, *et al*. Oxacillin prophylaxis in cerebrospinal fluid shunt procedures: results of a randomized open study in 60 hydrocephalic patients. *Surg Neurol* 1986; 25: 178–80.

56. Blomstedt GC. Results of trimethoprim-sulfa-methoxazole prophylaxis in ventriculostomy and shunting procedures. *J Neurosurg* 1985; 62: 694–7.

57. Rieder MJ, Frewen TC, Del Maestro RF, *et al*. The effect of cephalothin prophylaxis on postoperative ventriculoperitoneal shunt infections. *CMAJ* 1987; 136: 935–8.

58. Schmidt K, Gjerris F, Osgaard O, *et al*. Antibiotic prophylaxis in cerebrospinal fluid shunting: a prospective randomized trial in 152 hydrocephalic patients. *Neurosurgery* 1985; 17: 1–5.

59. Lerman SJ. Haemophilus influenzae infection of cerebrospinal fluid shunts. *J Neurosurg* 1981; 54: 261–3.

60. Epstein F, Lapras C, Wisoff JH. "Slit-ventricle syndrome": etiology and treatment. *Pediatr Neurosci* 1988; 14: 5–10.

61. Amacher AL, Wellington J. Infantile hydrocephalus: long-term results of surgical therapy. *Childs Brain* 1984; 11: 217–29.

62. Dennis M, Fitz CR, Netly CT, *et al*. The intelligence of hydrocephalic children. *Arch Neurol* 1981; 38: 607–15.

63. Foltz EL, Shurtleff DB. Five-year comparative study of hydrocephalus in children with and without operation (113 cases). *J Neurosurg* 1963; 20: 1064–79.

64. Young HF, Nulsen FE, Weiss MH, *et al*. The relationship of intelligence and cerebral mantle in treated infantile hydrocephalus. *Pediatrics* 1973; 52: 38–44.

65. Op Heij CP, Renier WO, Gabreels FJ. Intellectual sequelae of primary non-obstructive hydrocephalus in infancy: analysis of 50 cases. *Clin Neurol Neurosurg* 1985; 87: 247–53.

66. Hanigan WC. Intracranial hemorrhage in the premature infant. In: Wilkens RH, Rengachary SS (eds). *Neurosurgery*. New York: McGraw-Hill; 1996: 3729–32.

67. Skullerad K, Westre B. Frequency and prognostic significance of germinal matrix hemorrhage, periventricular leukomalacia, and pontosubicular necrosis in preterm neonates. *Acta Neuropathol* 1986; 70: 257–61.

68. Krishnamoorthy KS, Kuban KC, Leviton A. Periventricular-intraventricular hemorrhage, sonographic localization, phenobarbital, and motor abnormalities in low birth weight infants. *Pediatrics* 1990; 85: 1027–33.

69. Bindal AK, Storrs BB, McLone DG. Management of the Dandy–Walker syndrome. *Pediatr Neurosurg* 1990–1991; 16: 163–9.

70. Greenberg MS. *Handbook of Neurosurgery*, 5th edn. Lakeland: Thieme; 2001.

9

HYDROCEPHALUS IN ADULTS

Sherman C Stein

INTRODUCTION

Our colleagues who specialize in pediatrics constantly remind us that "children are not simply small adults." Perhaps nowhere is the converse more true than in this chapter; adult hydrocephalics are not simply large children. Their pathophysiology, clinical findings, neuroimaging changes, and responses to shunting all differ, often dramatically, from those in children.

NOMENCLATURE AND EPIDEMIOLOGY

The traditional classification systems used to categorize hydrocephalus in infants and children are of little practical importance in adults. As good as any is that proposed by Gowers over a century ago for adult hydrocephalus,[1] namely acute and chronic, primary (idiopathic) or secondary to a known pathology. Among almost 1000 cases of adult hydrocephalus assembled by Katzman in 1977, 34% were idiopathic.[2] Causes among cases where etiology was determined included subarachnoid hemorrhage (51%), head injury (16%), brain tumor (9%), intracranial surgery (7%), aqueduct stenosis (5%), and meningitis (5%).

A survey in Sweden in the late 1990s revealed almost 900 operations annually for hydrocephalus in adults, 3.4 procedures/ 100 000 population/year.[3] The sex ratio was equal; 90% of the operations were shunts and 7.5% were ventriculostomies. The commonest types of hydrocephalus encountered were normal pressure hydrocephalus (47%), high-pressure communicating hydrocephalus (27%) and aqueduct stenosis (11%)

CLINICAL FEATURES (Table 9.1)

Acute high-pressure hydrocephalus
Almost all cases of acute hydrocephalus in adults occur during the course, or close on the heels, of the causative illness. The hallmark of acute hydrocephalus is elevated intracranial pressure (ICP), manifested by the clinical triad of headache, nausea and vomiting, and papilledema. Headaches tend to be poorly localized or bifrontal and worse when recumbent (maximal ICP when flat). They are relieved by analgesics and upright posture. As the ICP rises, headaches become more likely to awaken the patient from sleep, more severe and recalcitrant to treatment. Nausea and vomiting, like headache, tend to accompany increased ICP. Abdominal pain is rare. Papilledema is much more common as a finding in the hydrocephalus of adults than in that of children. Abducens palsy (uni- or bilateral) and some degree of truncal ataxia may, incorrectly, suggest a posterior fossa lesion (false localizing signs). Episodic visual obscurations ("graying") accompanies dangerous pressure waves and suggests the need for emergent ventricular drainage.

Chronic or normal pressure hydrocephalus (NPH)
Chronic hydrocephalus of adulthood presents more insidiously, often weeks or even years after the inciting cause, sometimes without apparent cause at all. Although the clinical findings are much the same in idiopathic or secondary cases, they are quite different from the acute category. The affected patient exhibits a combination of motor dysfunction, urinary incontinence, and dementia.

The early motor signs are most prominent in the lower extremities and are related to difficulty initiating walking, the so-called "magnet gait" phenomenon (Table 9.2). Steps are slow, shuffling and broad-based. Balance may be lost on turning. Advanced cases show frontal release signs, such as suck and grasp reflexes. Parkinsonian and other dyskinesias have been described. In the early stages of hydrocephalus, the patient is well aware of the urge to void, but urinary incontinence results from an uninhibited bladder and a gait-induced inability to reach the bathroom in time. Ultimately, a lack of awareness of the need to empty bladder or bowels occurs.

Table 9.1 Classification schemes for hydrocephalus occurring in adults

Acute	High pressure	Primary (idiopathic)	Communicating (blockage of the subarachnoid pathways)
Chronic	Normal or low pressure	Secondary to a known pathology (subarachnoid hemorrhage, brain tumor)	Obstruction of intraventricular pathways

Table 9.2 Clinical triad of NPH (normal pressure hydrocephalus)

- Gait disturbance (magnetic, apraxic)
- Urinary incontinence (uninhibited neurogenic bladder)
- Dementia

In contrast to the dementia of Alzheimer's disease, the mental deficit of hydrocephalus is subcortical in origin. The patient appears apathetic and responds slowly to most tasks. If the examiner persists, the inattentive-appearing patient will focus on the task at hand and perform better than expected. This is especially true with abstract thought, language and calculation functions, which are severely impaired in Alzheimer's disease. Although there is great variation in the relative degree of involvement and progression of symptomatology, the motor and mental deficits ultimately converge in a state of abulia (loss or impairment of the ability to make decisions or act independently).

The clinical signs of secondary hydrocephalus are often obscured by those of the underlying illness. The risk of acute hydrocephalus following subarachnoid hemorrhage is approximately 25–30% in recent case series; that of chronic hydrocephalus requiring shunting is 15–20%. The incidence of acute hydrocephalus is greater with a more severe hemorrhage, vasospasm, intraventricular bleed, or pre-hemorrhage hypertension.

The identification of post-traumatic hydrocephalus is especially problematic. The frequent coexistence of hydrocephalus and atrophy after severe head injury can be confusing. Acute post-traumatic hydrocephalus is uncommon, and the focal and cognitive effects of traumatic brain injury may obscure those of chronic post-traumatic hydrocephalus. In one series of almost 100 cases of post-traumatic hydrocephalus, fewer than 15% were acute. Although some ventriculomegaly is seen in the aftermath of 30–75% of severe head injuries, the diagnosis of hydrocephalus is made in only 2–6% of recent patient series.

Hydrocephalus frequently complicates basal meningitis, especially tuberculous and fungal. Fortuitously located brain tumors and parasitic infestations can cause hydrocephalus, the acuteness varying with the degree and location of cerebrospinal fluid (CSF) obstruction.

Some adults with stenosis of the aqueduct of Sylvius of nontumoral origin present with chronic symptoms. First described by Pennybacker, patients with "adult aqueductal stenosis" syndrome are uncommon.[4] Wilkinson and colleagues first called attention to the resemblance of one of their patient's findings to those of NPH.[5] Although many of the patients exhibit intermittent signs of intracranial hypertension or suddenly decompensate, others, especially among the elderly, may have a much more indolent course. In this latter group are the more typical findings of NPH, although hearing loss and unusual gaze palsies have been reported. There is often indirect evidence that the disease is chronic. Some patients have large heads or evidence of chronic skull changes; others have a long history of clumsiness or poor intellectual performance. Except for the occasional case of neurofibromatosis or inflammatory ependymitis, the etiology of adult aqueduct stenosis is rarely evident. Oi and colleagues recently reviewed pathophysiology and treatment of this condition, which they term long-standing overt ventriculomegaly in adults (LOVA).[6]

PATHOPHYSIOLOGY

All secondary adult hydrocephalus begins with increased resistance to CSF flow. Whether the subarachnoid pathways are clogged with blood or purulent material, compressed by tumor, or scarred closed by inflammation, resistance to CSF outflow rises. Attempts to describe this relationship mathematically have been refined over the years.[7]

Oi and associates have emphasized the gradual changes in the hydrodynamic properties of the ventricular system over time, ICP being inversely related to ventricular size.[8] In part, these changes reflect alteration of the properties of the surrounding brain parenchyma. In experimental hydrocephalus, cerebral compliance has been demonstrated to change with ventricular dilatation. There is other evidence that the edema, plastic deformation and shearing forces injure the periventricular white matter and vasculature. This secondary parenchymal damage, which may be permanent in some cases, increases compliance in the walls and predisposes to further ventriculomegaly.

Parenchymal changes in patients with NPH are often primary and consist of hypertensive and atherosclerotic white matter damage. This has the same effect on ventricular compliance as does secondary white matter damage and is not necessarily inconsistent with a good shunt response. The possibility was recently put forward of a vicious cycle of increasing ventriculomegaly and periventricular compliance in NPH, in which both primary and secondary parenchymal damage play a role.[9] Figure 9.1 illustrates the proposed interaction of hydrodynamic and parenchymal factors.

Early explanations of the symptom complex of hydrocephalus in adults were based on stretching of leg and bladder motor fibers in their passage around the distended ventricles. As attractive as this hypothesis may be, motor evoked potentials are normal in these patients, and gait analysis shows no evidence of pyramidal dysfunction in NPH. Other white matter areas may be injured by the mechanisms discussed above. In fact, damage to the deep white matter may be more closely tied to gait disorders than is ventriculomegaly. Another theory, first advanced by Symon in 1975,[10] is that ICP is not truly normal, but is intermittently elevated. Studies employing continuous ICP monitoring have found increases, especially during sleep, in some, but by no means all, suspected NPH patients.

Another possible cause of symptoms in adult hydrocephalus is ischemia, either globally or in the periventricular white matter. It is not clear how much of this is caused by the vascular disease that frequently accompanies NPH or whether it is reversible. Finally, neurochemical imbalance has been postulated, based on observations of excessive or decreased concentrations of various substances in NPH. This raises the intriguing possibility that symptoms are, at least in part, the result of CSF stagnation and toxin accumulation. Hence much of the shunt effect might be due to drainage of these toxins, as has been reported to be the case in Alzheimer's disease by Silverberg and colleagues.[11]

DIAGNOSIS

There are few diagnostic difficulties when acute hydrocephalus complicates the course of a brain tumor or subarachnoid hemorrhage. Neuroimaging studies, indicated because of elevated ICP, show ventricular enlargement, usually with periventricular edema (Figure 9.2).

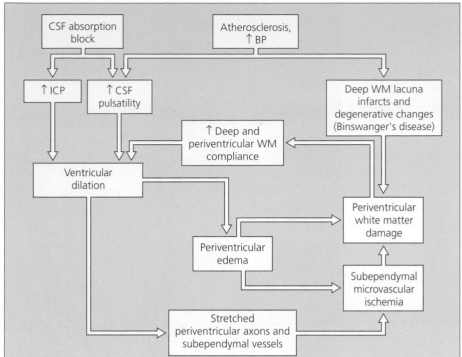

Figure 9.1 Hydrodynamic and parenchymal factors in NPH. Note that both primary white matter damage and CSF absorption block may increase periventricular compliance. After sufficient damage has occurred, the vicious cycle of increasing ventricular growth and further periventricular damage (heavy arrows) continues in the absence of elevated pressure. Adapted with permission from Stein.[9]

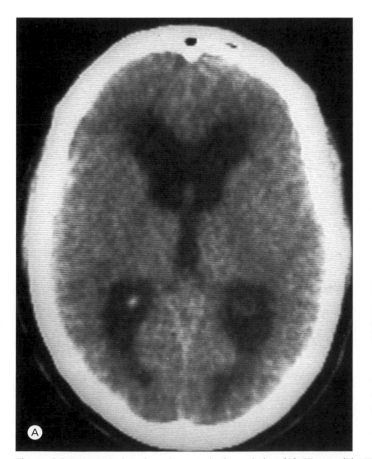

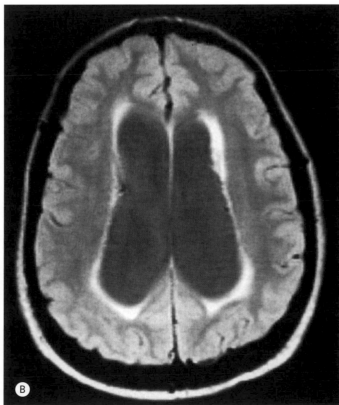

Figure 9.2 Periventricular edema in acute hydrocephalus: **(A)** CT scan, **(B)** MRI scan.

Table 9.3 Potential diagnostic criteria and predictive factors for surgical outcome in normal pressure hydrocephalus

- Nuances in clinical presentation
- Neuropsychological testing
- CT and MRI scans
- Radionuclide cisternogram
- Lumbar dynamic infusion studies
- Response to large volume drainage of CSF through lumbar puncture or continuous lumbar drainage over days
- Continuous ICP monitoring
- CSF flow study across the aqueduct in the MRI
- Cerebral blood flow study
- Evoked potential study
- Biochemical markers
- ? genetic testing

It is much more difficult to distinguish chronic hydrocephalus from other causes of dementia (Table 9.3). This is true of secondary hydrocephalus, in which cerebral atrophy resulting from traumatic or infectious disease may accompany the hydrocephalic process. The distinction is even more difficult in idiopathic NPH. Complicating diseases include especially Alzheimer's disease and deep white matter vascular disease (arteriosclerotic subcortical encephalopathy, vascular dementia with lacunes, Binswanger's disease, leukoariosis). The task is made far more difficult by the relative prevalence of these entities and the frequent coexistence of one or both of with NPH. "In fact," as Vanneste opined, "subcortical arteriosclerotic encephalopathy is much more common than NPH and is the most probable cause of the so-called "classical" triad."[12]

The early diagnostic studies were based on the expected pathophysiology of NPH and lacked any independent confirmation of the disease. They included isotope cisternography, lumbar infusion and pneumoencephalography. None of these techniques proved effective in predicting shunt results. The limitations of pathophysiology were made even more apparent as patients with suspected NPH became the subjects of pathological examination. The relative infrequency of meningeal fibrosis at autopsy and the frequency of parenchymal disease made it clear that there is no pathological "gold standard" for NPH.

In recent years diagnostic efforts have turned to the more practical matter of predicting shunt success, rather than establishing an absolute diagnosis. Clinical features have been promoted as predictive. Many authorities have linked shunt response to the severity of gait disturbance. Others have emphasized that brief symptom duration and a lack of dementia at the onset of symptoms predict shunt success. A specific neuropsychological profile has been promoted.

The introduction of computed tomography (CT) scanning and magnetic resonance imaging (MRI) made it possible to inspect cerebral and ventricular anatomy directly and noninvasively. However, attempts to predict shunt results from the size or shape of the cerebral ventricles and from the convexity subarachnoid spaces have not been widely accepted, nor has the distribution of CSF between the two. Periventricular white matter lesions have been advanced as predictive factors. However, there is no consensus as to whether the white matter signal abnormalities are associated with greater or less likelihood of shunt success. In one recent study, Tullberg and associates were unable reliably to

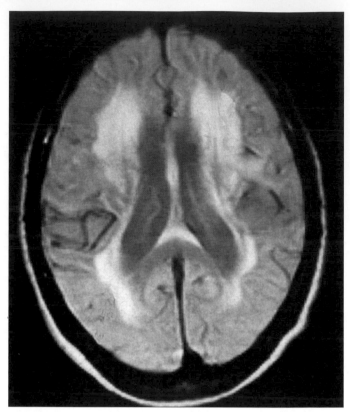

Figure 9.3 Extensive deep and paraventricular white matter lesions (arteriosclerotic subcortical encephalopathy, vascular dementia with lacunes, Binswanger's disease).

distinguish between the white matter changes in NPH and those of Binswanger's disease (Figure 9.3) by MRI scan.[13]

Over the years, continuous ICP monitoring has been employed to seek pressure elevations, especially during sleep. Episodes of high ICP are uncommon but probably predictive. However, it is difficult to justify invasive monitoring, the complications of which are similar to those of shunt insertion. The presence and relative frequency of B-waves have also been investigated. Authorities still disagree about the value of these measurements. There is also equivocal evidence to support the predictive value of the ICP response to CSF infusion as a measure of outflow resistance. The Dutch NPH study has been most often quoted to support the value of CSF outflow resistance as a predictive criterion.[14] Indeed, the response rate to shunting was 92% in the 36 patients whose resistance was above the suggested cutoff of 18 mmHg/mL/min. However, shunting was surprisingly successful in the group of 59 whose resistance was below this level; 66% of them improved. Had high outflow resistance been adopted as a requirement for shunting, these patients would have been denied treatment. CSF pulse–pressure analysis has not proven useful.

Studies of CSF flow are thought by some to predict shunt outcome, although isotope cisternography and clearance studies have been largely discredited. More recent attempts have employed MRI techniques to assay CSF flow through the cerebral aqueduct as a predictor of shunt function (Figure 9.4), higher velocities correlating with greater likelihood of shunt success.[15] Not all investigators are optimistic that this technique will prove useful.

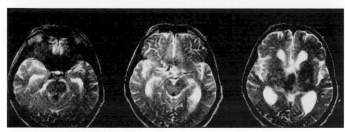

Figure 9.4 MRI images, illustrating CSF flow void involving cerebral aqeduct (center image). The caudal (left image) and proximal (right image), into the fourth and third ventricles, respectively, is thought to be characteristic of NPH. From Krauss JK et al.[20] with permission.

Cerebral bloodflow has been thought to have distinctive regional or global abnormalities in NPH. However, using these changes to predict successful shunt outcome has had mixed success. The same is true when patterns of cerebral metabolism or cerebral bloodflow responses to lowering ICP and/or removing CSF were used. Reports are in conflict as to what autoregulation changes characterize NPH; whether there is a predictive response to Diamox administration is also unclear.

A number of potential biochemical markers of NPH have been reported in CSF. Whether these markers predict shunt response is not known. There is a single report of genetic predisposition to NPH; a higher frequency of the ε-4 allele of the *APOE* gene was found in NPH than in the general population. Evoked potential studies are thought to be predictive in some hands.

Most authorities agree that a temporary clinical improvement following lumbar puncture or CSF drainage suggests a high likelihood that a shunt will result in lasting relief. However, a negative trial is an unreliable predictor. Prolonged lumbar drainage does not appear to offer a better alternative.[16]

One reason for the lack of successful prediction is the pre-selection of candidates for shunting practiced by every investigator. Patients with certain findings are deemed to be unlikely to respond to shunt insertion and are never tested. This creates a self-fulfilling prophecy, precluding knowledge of how the non-shunted patients might have fared. Furthermore, since criteria for shunting vary among studies, accurate comparisons are difficult. A recent meta-analysis suggested that clinical improvement following CSF drainage reliably predicted shunt response, and that enlargement of the subcortical low-cerebral bloodflow area showed promise as a predictor; other reported prediction criteria lacked merit.[17] A multicenter retrospective review in Japan concluded that the heterogeneous nature of the disease made prediction difficult.[18]

We are not yet in a position to state categorical criteria for the diagnosis of idiopathic NPH, nor can we even reliably predict the response to shunting. The following clinical and laboratory findings are accepted by many authorities as being most helpful in predicting shunt success: hydrocephalus of known etiology, gait disturbance appearing earlier and is more prominent than dementia, intermittently elevated ICP, clinical improvement after CSF drainage. Less certain are enlargement of the subcortical low cerebral blood flow area, increased aqueductal flow on MRI and elevated CSF resistance. It must be emphasized that dramatic and durable improvements have accompanied shunting in several

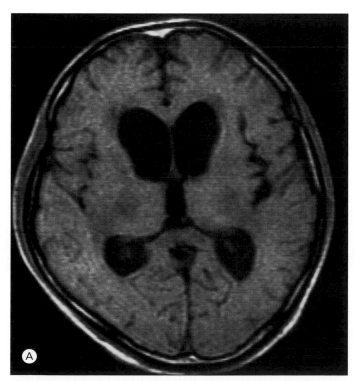

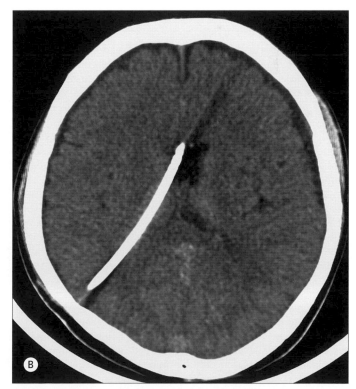

Figure 9.5 A 25-year-old following severe head injury showing gradual ventricular enlargement over several months. **(A)** MRI scan, 6 months post-injury: Glasgow Outcome Scale score = severely disabled. **(B)** CT scan, 8 months post-injury and 1 month following shunting: Glasgow Outcome Scale score = moderately disabled (patient eventually had good outcome).

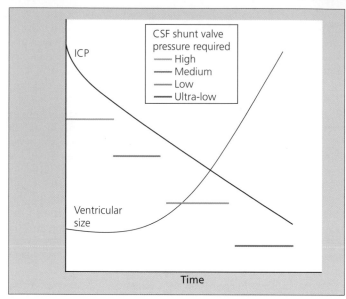

Figure 9.6 Temporal hydrodynamic changes in chronic hydrocephalus. As the cerebral ventricles grow over time, the ICP falls, as does the valve pressure appropriate. From Stein[9] with permission.

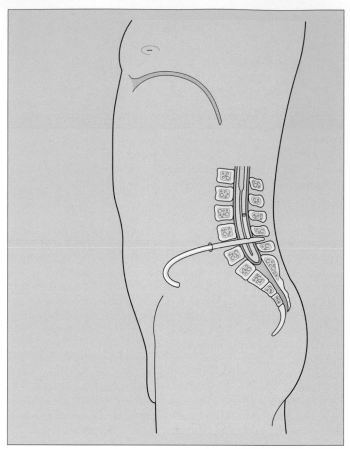

Figure 9.7 Ventriculoperitoneal shunt, used in some cases of communicating hydrocephalus.

patients who lacked any of these positive findings. Conversely, the most promising patient may not remain so. In time, subcortical white matter damage and associated diseases must progress to the point that the deficits are no longer reversible. This adds even more unpredictability to treatment decisions.

MANAGEMENT

As in the pediatric population, treatment of adult hydrocephalus is generally by way of ventriculoperitoneal shunt. Techniques are the same as those in children, the main differences being the longer subcutaneous passage of tubing and the thicker skulls and abdominal walls in adults. Some complications of shunting, such as seizures, shunt malfunction and infection, have similar incidence and presentations in both adults and children. Others, particularly overdrainage problems, are quite different in adults, perhaps because of the closed cranial sutures. Acute subdural hematoma secondary to draining veins being torn by rapid ventricular decompression is unusual, but can be fatal. Much more common are subdural hygromas or chronic hematomas. These collections, which are often asymptomatic, are seen in as many as 17% of shunted adults. If the collections are symptomatic or growing rapidly, treatment options include temporary shunt ligation, valve replacement with a higher pressure or anti-siphon device, hygroma drainage, or shunting. A low-pressure syndrome usually consists of orthostatic headache, neck pain and nausea. It is best treated by increasing drainage pressure or inserting an anti-siphon device.

Most series of post-traumatic hydrocephalus report improvement rates in the range of 50–75%, although Marmarou and associates point out that only a proportion of these are dramatic (Figure 9.5).[19] As many as 30% of these shunts will need to be revised at some point. Programmable valves have been suggested as a way of reducing shunt malfunctions in post-traumatic hydrocephalus.

Shunt results in post-hemorrhagic hydrocephalus vary with the acuteness of onset and clinical status of the patient. Shunting is usually quite successful in treating the hydrocephalus associated with tuberculous meningitis, unless the patient is moribund or has acquired immune deficiency syndrome. As is the case in cryptococcal meningitis, shunt insertion does not spread the infection, nor does it act as a nidus, as long as effective anti-infective medication is administered. The hydrocephalus that accompanies cysticercosis is more difficult to treat; arachnoiditis causes shunt obstruction in approximately 50% of cases. Oral prednisone may prevent shunt malfunction in these patients.

Perioperative steroids and ventricular drainage may reduce the need for shunting after removal of posterior fossa brain tumors. Adult-onset aqueductal stenosis is one condition for which third ventriculostomy has been advocated instead of shunting. Although it has been employed with some success, one report suggests that improvement is only temporary in some cases. Ventricular elastance may be useful in predicting third ventriculostomy effectiveness.

Shunting in idiopathic normal pressure hydrocephalus

As is evident above, diagnosis and selection for shunting is far from straightforward in NPH. Little surprise that the choice of shunt valve pressure is equally problematic. Authorities differ with respect to optimal valve pressure, whether anti-siphon and gravity

CLINICAL PEARLS

- Hydrocephalus occurring in adults is different from that occurring in children in its pathophysiology and clinical manifestations.

- The syndrome of chronic, normal pressure hydrocephalus is unique to adults.

- The classic clinical triad of normal pressure hydrocephalus in adults is gait disturbance, urinary incontinence, and cognitive impairment.

- The diagnostic criteria for normal pressure hydrocephalus remain controversial; equally debatable are the selection criteria for the shunting procedure.

- The complication rate for shunting in normal pressure hydrocephalus is not insignificant; the operative procedure should be undertaken only if prognostic criteria reasonably suggests a favorable outcome, although the predictive ability for success remains controversial and is continuously evolving.

drainage devices improve or worsen outcome. The duration of NPH may explain the variable effects of shunt valve pressures on ventricular decompression (Figure 9.6). Programmable valves and lumbar–peritoneal shunts have been advocated (Figure 9.7). Rates of substantial clinical response are rarely above 30%.[9,17]

Shunting is not without potential problems in this elderly, frail population. Hebb and Cusimano reported a 6% significant complication rate in their literature review.[17] However, they reviewed only the best organized studies; the risks in most case series are closer to 35%.[9]

This chapter contains material from the first edition, and I am grateful to the authors of that chapter for their contribution.

REFERENCES

1. Gowers WR. *A Manual of Diseases of the Nervous System*. Philadelphia: P Blakiston, Son and Co; 1888.
2. Katzman R. Low pressure hydrocephalus. In: Wells CE (ed.). *Dementia*. Philadelphia: F A Davis; 1977.
3. Hoglund M, Tisell M, Wikkelso C. [Incidence of surgery for hydrocephalus in adults surveyed: same number afflicted by hydrocephalus as by multiple sclerosis]. *Lakartidningen* 2001; 98: 1681–5 (in Swedish).
4. Pennybacker J. Stenosis of the aqueduct of Sylvius. *Proc R Soc Med* 1940; 33: 507–12.
5. Wilkinson HA, LeMay M, Drew JH. Adult aqueductal stenosis. Arch Neurol 1966; 15: 643–8.
6. Oi S, Shimoda M, Shibata M, *et al*. Pathophysiology of long-standing overt ventriculomegaly in adults. *J Neurosurg* 2000; 92: 933–40.
7. Hakim CA, Hakim R, Hakim S. Normal-pressure hydrocephalus. *Neurosurg Clin N Am* 2001; 12: 761–73.
8. Oi S. Hydrocephalus chronology in adults: confused state of the terminology. *Crit Rev Neurosurg* 1998; 8: 346–56.
9. Stein SC. Normal-pressure hydrocephalus: an update. *Neurosurg Q* 2001; 11: 26–35.
10. Symon L, Dorsch NW. Use of long-term intracranial pressure measurement to assess hydrocephalic patients prior to shunt surgery. *J Neurosurg* 1975; 42: 258–73.
11. Silverberg GD, Levinthal E, Sullivan EV, *et al*. Assessment of low-flow CSF drainage as a treatment for AD: results of a randomized pilot study. *Neurology* 2002; 59: 1139–45.
12. Vanneste JA. Three decades of normal pressure hydrocephalus: are we wiser now? *J Neurol Neurosurg Psychiatr* 1994; 57: 1021–5.
13. Tullberg M, Hultin L, Ekholm S, *et al*. White matter changes in normal pressure hydrocephalus and Binswanger disease: specificity, predictive value and correlations to axonal degeneration and demyelination. *Acta Neurol Scand* 2002; 105: 417–26.
14. Boon AJ, Tans JT, Delwel EJ, *et al*. Dutch normal-pressure hydrocephalus study: prediction of outcome after shunting by resistance to outflow of cerebrospinal fluid. *J Neurosurg* 1997; 87: 687–93.
15. Luetmer PH, Huston J, Friedman JA, *et al*. Measurement of cerebrospinal fluid flow at the cerebral aqueduct by use of phase-contrast magnetic resonance imaging: technique validation and utility in diagnosing idiopathic normal pressure hydrocephalus. *Neurosurgery* 2002; 50: 534–43.
16. Walchenbach R, Geiger E, Thomeer RT, Vanneste JA. The value of temporary external lumbar CSF drainage in predicting the outcome of shunting on normal pressure hydrocephalus. *J Neurol Neurosurg Psychiatr* 2002; 72: 503–6.
17. Hebb AO, Cusimano MD. Idiopathic normal pressure hydrocephalus: a systematic review of diagnosis and outcome. *Neurosurgery* 2001; 49: 1166–86.
18. Mori K. Management of idiopathic normal-pressure hydrocephalus: a multiinstitutional study conducted in Japan. *J Neurosurg* 2001; 95: 970–3.
19. Marmarou A, Foda MA, Bandoh K, *et al*. Posttraumatic ventriculomegaly: hydrocephalus or atrophy? A new approach for diagnosis using CSF dynamics. *J Neurosurg* 1996; 85: 1026–35.
20. Krauss JK, Regel JP, Vach W, *et al*. Flow void of cerebrospinal fluid in idiopathic normal pressure hydrocephalus of the elderly: can it predict outcome after shunting? *Neurosurgery* 1997; 40: 67–74.

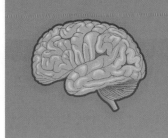

NEUROENDOSCOPY

10

Charles Teo and Ralph Mobbs

INTRODUCTION

Neuroendoscopy is defined as the discipline of applying an endoscope to the treatment of conditions of the central nervous system. There have been four major stages in the development of neuroendoscopy.

The pioneering stage of neuroendoscopy started almost a century ago when the urologist L'Espinasse performed the first endoscopic procedure on the brain (in 1910).[1] He attempted endoscopic coagulation of the choroid plexus to treat a hydrocephalic patient. The next epoch of neuroendoscopy came in the 1920s and 1930s when Dandy and Mixter attempted endoscopic fenestration of the third ventricle for the treatment of hydrocephalus.[2]

The third significant leap in neuroendoscopy came in the early 1970s. Technological advances in optics and electronics allowed the development of both flexible fiber and high-resolution rigid endoscopes that were used successfully for operating within the ventricles.

The current stage of neuroendoscopy has been the explosion of endoscopic third ventriculostomy for the treatment of hydrocephalus and endoscope-assisted minimally invasive surgical procedures which began in the 1980s and 1990s, and continue to this day.

Initially, endoscopic procedures were confined to the ventricles of the brain, which contain the ideal medium: a crystal-clear fluid. However, the endoscope is now used in treating a wide spectrum of neurosurgical pathology, and the indications for neuroendoscopy are rapidly expanding. Neuroendoscopy follows a general trend in neurosurgery of treating disease with minimally invasive techniques to reduce approach-related trauma and to improve visualization of the pathology. In an attempt to minimize operative trauma, the surgeon endeavors to limit the size of the exposure and to avoid unnecessary brain retraction, which can cause damage by increasing local cerebral tissue pressure and decreasing regional cerebral blood flow.[3] This surgery-related trauma may compromise the neurologic outcome after micro-neurosurgical procedures, a factor that is potentially minimized with the use of neuroendoscopy techniques.

The endoscope enhances the surgeon's view by increasing illumination and magnification.[4,5] Endoscopic tumor removal or cerebrospinal fluid (CSF) diversion through endoscopic fenestration may allow patients to undergo a less morbid procedure or to avoid shunt placement. In addition to benefiting the patient, the endoscope is an excellent teaching tool. The anatomical definition and unique angles of view available with the endoscope help

trainee residents to have a better understanding of operations by illuminating anatomico–pathological structures. A comparison of the various magnification modalities is presented following a survey of neurosurgeons (Table 10.1).

We will discuss the applications of endoscopy to intracranial surgery under the following headings:

- equipment;
- endoscopic third ventriculostomy;
- simplification of complex hydrocephalus and intracranial cysts;
- endoscopic applications to neuro-oncology;
- endoscope-assisted microsurgery;
- endoscopic transsphenoidal surgery;
- microvascular decompression;
- miscellaneous applications;
- complications of neuroendoscopy.

EQUIPMENT

It is paramount that the surgeon has a dedicated neuroendoscopy set-up to achieve optimal surgical outcomes. In addition, it is essential to have recording equipment that captures images on video or digital format for later study. The endoscopy tower should include: video camera, camera control units, light source, video recorder, video monitor and a computerized system for storage of video segments or single-picture capture. Endoscope positioning and fixation arms capable of being fastened to the operating table or headrest help the surgeon to avoid arm fatigue, which can disturb eye–hand coordination. Endoscopic instruments include a pair of grabbing forceps and scissors, a coagulation device (either monopolar or bipolar), an irrigation system, and a straight and 30°-angled scope (Figures 10.1, 10.2). In addition, a knowledgeable assistant is essential so that the surgeon can work two-handed (Figure 10.1).

Frameless computerized neuronavigation has been increasingly used in intracranial endoscopic neurosurgery and has proven to be accurate, reliable, and useful in selected intracranial neuroendoscopic procedures to improve the accuracy of the endoscopic approach.[6]

ENDOSCOPIC THIRD VENTRICULOSTOMY

The first attempted endoscopic third ventriculostomy (ETV) was undertaken in 1923.[7] During the investigative period in the

Table 10.1 Comparison of loupe, microscope, and endoscope for neurosurgical procedures

	Loupe	Microscope	Endoscope
Cost	Minimal	Moderate	Moderate
Magnification	Fixed	Variable	Variable
Illumination	With headlight	Superior	Superior
Time to setup	NA	Minimal	Minimal
Scrub staff familiarity	NA	Acceptable	Acceptable
Incision/exposure	Variable	Variable/minimal	Minimal
Surgeon fatigue	Neck, Eye	Eye	Arm
Look around corners?	No	No	Yes (30°, 70°, 110°)
Teaching tool	Poor	Excellent	Excellent
Depth of view	3D	3D	2D (3D possible)

NA, not applicable; 2D, two-dimensional; 3D, three-dimensional.

subsequent decade, the endoscopic technique was restricted by inferior illumination, magnification, and surgical morbidity. The endoscopes were not specifically designed for use within the brain. Technological advances in the 1970s and 1980s produced the much needed improvements in endoscopic instrumentation. Thus, the ETV technique was "rediscovered" in the 1970s and 1980s.[8] There are numerous studies now confirming the high success rate and low complication rate of ETV. It is now considered a safe and effective treatment for obstructive hydrocephalus in selected patients.[9,10] In addition, ETV has numerous potential benefits over the standard shunt procedure, which possesses its own set of inherent risks and complications, including (but not limited to) infection, slit ventricle syndrome, and mechanical malfunction.

Indications for performing ETV are based on computed tomography or magnetic resonance imaging (MRI) findings that demonstrate a noncommunicating-type hydrocephalus with obstruction at the level of, or distal to, the posterior third ventricle. Patients with hydrocephalus from aqueductal stenosis are, in general, excellent candidates for ETV. Although controversial,[11] patients less than 6 months of age have not enjoyed uniformly good results with ETV, and most authors do not advocate the procedure in this group.

ETV has a role in the treatment of hydrocephalus secondary to posterior fossa tumors and is being used for that application in many centers. Neuroendoscopy is being used successfully in pineal tumors simultaneously to treat the associated hydrocephalus by ETV and to biopsy by endoscopy the tumor for diagnosis.[12]

A brief description of ETV is as follows.

Step 1: Patient positioning. The patient is positioned supine with the head slightly flexed. Note the approach angle made by the endoscope (Figure 10.3).

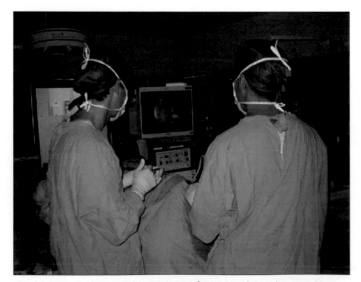

Figure 10.1 An assistant is paramount for successful endoscopy. Note the positioning of the monitor for surgeon comfort.

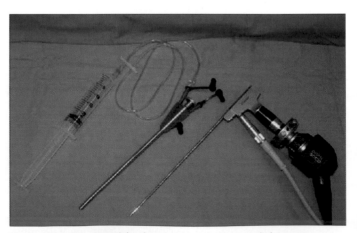

Figure 10.2 The essentials of endoscopy; endoscope, light source, camera, and irrigator for intraventricular surgery.

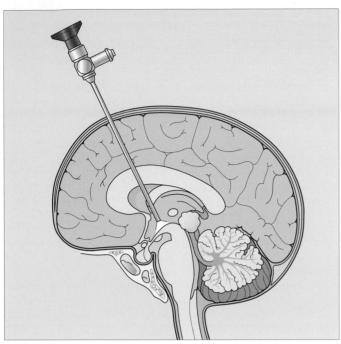

Figure 10.3 The approach angle made by the endoscope for endoscopic third ventriculostomy.

Step 2: Burr hole. A coronal burr hole is performed with the optimal entry position at 3 cm lateral to the midline and 1 cm anterior to the coronal suture[13] (Figure 10.4).

Step 3: Entry into the lateral ventricle. The endoscope is advanced into the lateral ventricle with or without stereotactic assistance, depending on surgeon preference.

Step 4: Entry into the third ventricle. Under direct vision, the endoscope is passed through the foramen of Monro into

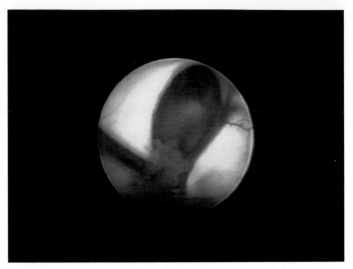

Figure 10.5 The anatomy of the foramen of Monro is helpful to guide the operator from the lateral ventricle into the third ventricle.

the third ventricle. Note that the foramen of Monro can be identified by the thalamostriate vein and choroid plexus (Figure 10.5). The third ventricle is inspected prior to perforation of the floor.

Step 5: Ventriculostomy. The ventriculostomy is placed just posterior to the infundibular recess of the pituitary stalk, anterior to the mamillary bodies. Perforation is either blunt, using the endoscope, or with an instrument followed by balloon catheter dilatation (Figures 10.6–10.8).

Step 6: Inspection and hemostasis. Entry into the prepontine cistern is performed with caution so as to avoid injury to the basilar apex and perforating vessels. Hemostasis with irrigation is achieved until a clear operative field is visualized (Figure 10.9).

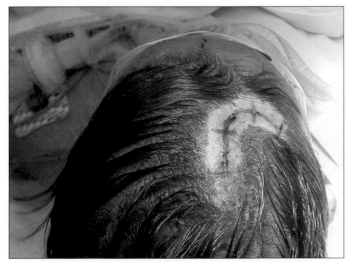

Figure 10.4 An incision is made so that the burr hole is 3 cm lateral to the midline on the right-hand side. A curved incision is prepared so that a shunt/reservoir can be inserted if endoscopic third ventriculostomy is unsuccessful.

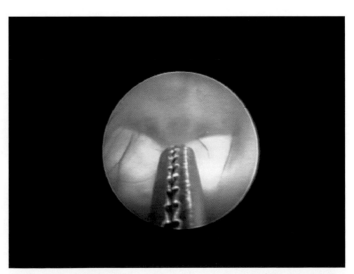

Figure 10.6 A blunt instrument is used to perforate the floor anterior to the mamillary bodies.

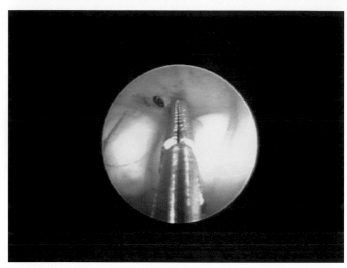

Figure 10.7 The initial fenestration made by the blunt forceps.

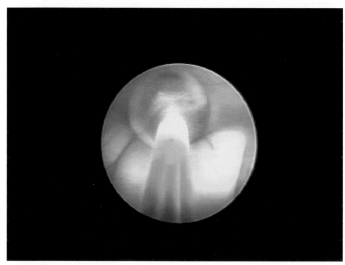

Figure 10.8 The initial fenestration is enlarged with a balloon.

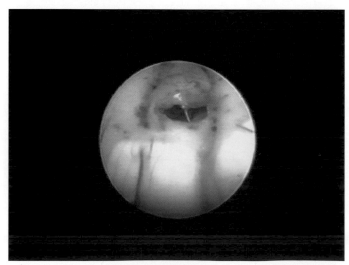

Figure 10.9 The fenestration is complete.

There are several precautions when performing ETV. The anatomy may be altered by tumors, such as a brainstem glioma. This may distort the floor of the third ventricle and displace the basilar artery forward so that the safe zone to penetrate the floor is limited.

Hydrocephalus resulting from tumor obstruction may be relatively acute in onset, with the floor of the third ventricle appearing opaque and non-attenuated. Penetration will be difficult and invariably requires a sharper technique without visualization of the underlying neurovascular structures, which increases the risk.

Also, patients who have been previously shunted are technically more difficult to perform ETV upon, as they have less marked ventricular dilatation, a thicker ventricular floor (Figure 10.10), and often abnormal anatomy. In some patients, an ETV procedure may have to be abandoned if the floor of the third ventricle is too thick, blood is obstructing the endoscopic view, or the basilar artery is sitting directly under or too close to the proposed site of fenestration.

Nevertheless, ETV has an overall success rate of approximately 75% after 3 years but depends on patient selection and the experience of the surgeon. The results of ETV compare favorably with those obtained after shunting, especially in patients with posterior fossa tumors.[14] In addition, ETV would appear to represent an economic advantage over shunting.[15] Table 10.2 outlines some of the studies that have investigated the results of ETV. However, no large multicenter randomized studies have been performed to compare the two modalities in a meaningful manner.

Failure of ETV can occur early or late. Early failure is the result of factors including bleeding around the fenestration site, unnoticed additional arachnoid membranes occluding the flow of CSF, and an inadequate size of the fenestration. Late failure is the

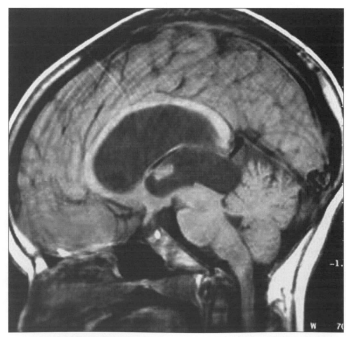

Figure 10.10 A thick third ventricular floor can make endoscopic third ventriculostomy difficult or impossible. Close inspection of the midsagittal magnetic resonance image is important prior to endoscopic third ventriculostomy.

Table 10.2 Results of endoscopic third ventriculostomy for treatment of hydrocephalus

Ref.	n	No. of patients with aqueductal stenosis	Etiology other than aqueductal stenosis	Success rate (%)	Follow-up (months)
Dalrymple and Kelly[40]	85	24	61	87	1–66
Jones et al.[41]	103	NA	NA	61	NA
Choi et al.[42]	81	39	42	91	NA
Hopf et al.[9]	98	40	58	76	26
Cinalli et al.[11]	213	126	87	72	45.5
Gangemi et al.[43]	125	77	48	86	NA
Fukuhara et al.[44]	89	34	55	67	3–62.8

n, number of patients; NA, not available or stated in paper.

result of subsequent closure of the fenestration by gliotic tissue or arachnoid membrane. This problem is potentially serious. There are now several reports in the literature of death following late failure of ETV[16] and this remains a management problem because the failure can occur in a short period of time and may be unpredictable. Tumor progression and inadequate CSF absorption at the level of the arachnoid villi may result in early or late failure. It is not understood why a cohort of patients with open fenestrations exhibits deterioration after months of well-being.[17]

Clinical review is the best assessor of outcome. The significance of postoperative ventricular size remains a controversial point because some patients have persistent ventriculomegaly despite lower intracranial pressure and marked clinical improvement.

Procedure-related complications reported in the literature include bradycardia, hypothalamic dysfunction and hemorrhage from damage to arteries, ependymal veins, or the choroid plexus. The complications fall into two main categories; short-term complications, which are largely intraoperative and technique-related, and long-term complications which occur at a much lower rate.[18] Blunt perforation is less likely to damage vascular structures below the floor, however traction on the lateral walls of the third ventricle, which is associated with blunt manipulation, is thought to account for the transient hypothalamic complications.[19] Those who advocate sharp perforation report less bleeding from the operative site but risk vascular perforation of deeper vessels such as the basilar artery or its perforators. In addition, there have been reports of frontal lobe infarction, subdural hematoma, pseudo-aneurysm formation, epilepsy, pneumoencephalus, syndrome of inappropriate antidiuretic hormone secretion (SIADH), third-nerve palsy and fatal subarachnoid hemorrhage. However, in experienced hands these complications are quite rare.

SIMPLIFICATIONS OF COMPLEX HYDROCEPHALUS AND INTRACRANIAL CYSTS

Patients with shunt infections or intraventricular hemorrhage of prematurity can suffer from compartmentalization of the ventricles often requiring multiple shunt placements. Multiple shunts are not ideal, and are associated with high failure rates and subsequent infections. Endoscopy offers a simple means of communicating isolated CSF spaces and ventricles by membrane fenestration. This can be done through the same burr hole as that for the placement of a ventricular catheter. Fenestration of the septum pellucidum to connect the two lateral ventricles in patients with loculated ventricles will preclude the need for two shunts in the majority of patients.

Many types of cysts can exist within the ventricular system. Arachnoid cysts, although typically extra-axial, can present within the ventricles, as well as choroid plexus cysts, neoplastic cysts and infected cysts (e.g. hydatid and cystercerotic cysts). In many patients, arachnoid cysts can be either endoscopically resected or fenestrated to achieve a successful outcome.

The rapid advances in endoscopic technology have made this the surgical approach of choice for the treatment of most intracranial cysts at our institution. In the preliminary series reported by Walker et al.,[20] nine of 14 children (64%) with arachnoid cysts were successfully treated by endoscopic fenestration through a burr hole, thereby avoiding the need for craniotomy. Even cysts confined to the pituitary fossa are ideally suited to endoscopic transsphenoidal surgery. Ventriculo-cysto-cisternostomy offers long-term decompression of suprasellar arachnoid cysts without the need for shunting (Figure 10.11). The senior author has had success in fenestrating arachnoid cysts, cysts of the cavum velum interpositum, neuroepithelial cysts of the ventricle, colloid cysts and large pineal region cysts. In cases where the ventricles are small, frameless stereotactic guidance has been useful in planning the burr hole placement and trajectory to these cysts. The goal of surgery for arachnoid cysts is symptomatic improvement. This is particularly pertinent with endoscopic fenestration, as the appearance of the cyst on postoperative imaging may be only slightly diminished, despite marked clinical improvement.

ENDOSCOPIC APPLICATIONS TO NEURO-ONCOLOGY

Neuro-oncology provides an ideal venue for the application of endoscopy. The advantages of improved visualization of intraventricular pathology, refined management of tumor-related hydrocephalus, safer biopsies, and minimally invasive removal of intraventricular tumors are invaluable supplements to traditional tumor management. Endoscopy is the next step for surpassing the

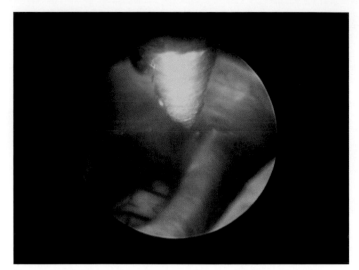

Figure 10.11 Fenestration of a suprasellar cyst: third ventriculostomy is initially performed to gain access to the cyst. Note the basilar artery and cyst wall.

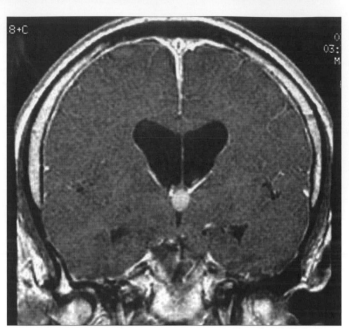

Figure 10.12 Endoscopic techniques are ideal for colloid cyst removal. Coronal magnetic resonance image demonstrating enhancement of a colloid cyst.

limitations of traditional microsurgery and allows the neurosurgeon to view tumor remnants such as those hidden behind eloquent brain tissue, a cranial nerve, or the tentorial edge. Once a tumor is removed, the surgeon can use the endoscope to assess the degree of resection. Often, the same surgery can be carried out through a smaller craniotomy by using the endoscope, in keeping with the concept of minimally invasive, yet maximally effective, surgery.[21] By allowing a more complete removal, endoscopy may improve the survival rates for patients with benign tumors.[22,23] Adjunctive procedures, such as third ventriculostomy and septostomy, can be performed through the same access to manage related problems such as secondary hydrocephalus. Endoscopic tumor removal or CSF diversion may allow patients to avoid shunt placement.

There are very few articles in the neurosurgical literature on the application of endoscopy for the removal of intraventricular tumors. Most of the endoscopic experience has been obtained in the removal of colloid cysts.[24–26] Examples of lesions that may be approached with the endoscope include colloid cysts (Figures 10.12, 10.13), subependymal giant cell astrocytomas, gliomas, subependymomas, and choroid plexus cysts.[27] Most of these lesions are relatively avascular and as a result are amenable to endoscopic treatment. Patients with colloid cysts are appropriate candidates for endoscopic excision at some institutions. The results with these tumors are often good in experienced hands; however, the long-term results in terms of recurrence are not yet available. The burr hole is made so that the scope enters the ventricle as far from the tumor as possible and so that the scope is directly viewing the tumor, not peering from around a corner. The distal approach allows the surgeon to orient himself by identifying normal anatomical structures before encountering the abnormal anatomy. As most of the distal part of the scope is within the ventricle, it also allows the surgeon to move the scope in multiple directions more freely without damaging the surrounding normal brain.

Not all intraventricular tumors should be approached endoscopically. The ideal tumor for endoscopic consideration has the following characteristics:

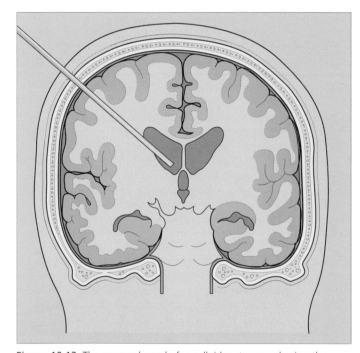

Figure 10.13 The approach angle for colloid cyst removal using the endoscope. A burr hole is made 7 cm from the midline and 8 cm from the nasion. Note: stereotactic guidance is invaluable to plan the best trajectory.

- moderate to low vascularity;
- soft consistency;
- less than 2 cm in diameter;[28]
- associated secondary hydrocephalus;
- histologically low grade.

The principles of endoscopic tumor surgery of the ventricle include:

- A trajectory that avoids eloquent structures but allows a good view of the tumor.
- The outside of the tumor is coagulated with either monopolar electrocautery or a laser.
- Copious irrigation is used both to clear blood and debris and to prevent too much heat from building up inside the ventricle. Cysts are opened and drained, with the contents removed via suction or piecemeal.
- Remaining wall is coagulated and removed piecemeal.
- Hemostasis is obtained with copious irrigation.

With completion of the procedure, the scope is withdrawn while inspecting the tract for intraparenchymal bleeding. Endoscope-assisted microsurgical techniques are particularly applicable to tumors such as sellar tumors, clival chordomas, pineal lesions and intraparenchymal tumors adjacent to the brainstem or cranial base.[29,30]

Considerable benefit is obtained by adding endoscopy to a traditional craniotomy. The tumor pathology frequently extends at acute angles to the cranial base or to the cortical surfaces along which the traditional surgical approach is made. While these avenues are inaccessible to the microscope, which requires a direct line of sight, they are ideal for endoscopy. The degree of retraction required can frequently be lessened substantially by endoscopic examination. When working around the brainstem and cranial nerves, the corridor available to the microscope is often very narrow, as extensive retraction is frequently not an option. The endoscope allows the surgeon to obtain the maximum possible access via the spaces naturally present in the extra-axial compartment.

ENDOSCOPE-ASSISTED MICROSURGERY

This is the most rapidly growing area in endoscopic neurosurgery. Microsurgery evolved to maximize visualization and minimize retraction. Endoscopy allows the neurosurgeon to move another step further towards achieving these goals. Endoscope-assisted microsurgery permits previously inaccessible or poorly accessible tumors located in the skull base, within narrow cavities, deep to key vascular or neural structures, or around corners in the intracranial space, to be clearly visualized and resected. The acutely angled rigid and flexible scopes allow the surgeon to look "around corners" which can be extremely useful in the extirpation of tumors and the clipping of aneurysms. Several approaches to the extra-axial structures of the skull base have been defined to improve visualization without jeopardizing standard microsurgical techniques. The most commonly adopted method is to place the endoscope down the same operative field. This creates no further morbidity but tends to clutter the already limited operative field. To avoid cluttering of instruments down an already limited craniotomy the scope may be inserted through a contralateral burr hole. Access to the subarachnoid space can be achieved through a small supra-orbital incision and then standard microsurgical dissection is performed to identify the pathology. Once the pathology is in view, the scope is fixed in place and attention is focused on the ipsilateral side. This technique, for example, offers excellent visualization of the tips of an aneurysm clip or the contralateral extent of a tumor.

Endoscopy is increasingly used to inspect tumors, tumor resection beds, aneurysms, and other pathology. Various authors have discussed the advantages of endoscopy for these purposes.[18,24,29,31] A summary of the advantages of the endoscope as an adjunct to microsurgery includes:

- Better definition of the normal and pathological anatomy. The endoscope can be used to clarify the anatomy such as key neural or vascular structures. This may be particularly important when working around or within the brainstem, between small perforating vessels, or between the cranial nerves.
- Identification of tumor portions located behind, or adherent to, vital structures. Some portions of tumor which are apparently invasive into the brain have brain–tumor interfaces that can be identified when visualized at more direct angles than is possible with the operating microscope alone.
- Minimization of retraction. The endoscope allows very narrow corridors to be used, reducing the need to displace sensitive structures.
- Assessing adequacy of tumor removal (Figures 10.14–10.16) or aneurysm clip placement.
- As a teaching tool. The endoscope offers a superior and often novel view of the anatomy, which can be beneficial to residents' understanding of the surgical approach. Furthermore, the operating surgeon and the student share the same view, which is not always true even with an operating microscope.

The most dangerous aspect of using the endoscope is the risk of impacting upon structures while introducing the endoscope. It is important to guide the endoscope by viewing it along the length of its barrel, rather than watching the image on the screen. After placing the endoscope into the working area, it is essential to continue to mind the shaft: if the scope is not fixed, then small, barely noticeable movements at the tip can be the result of larger excursions at the back of the scope, which can have potentially

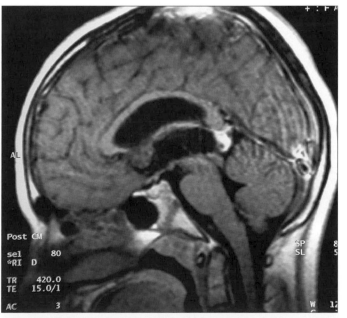

Figure 10.14 Note the enhancing pineal region tumor on the midsagittal magnetic resonance image. Resection was initially planned using the microscope alone.

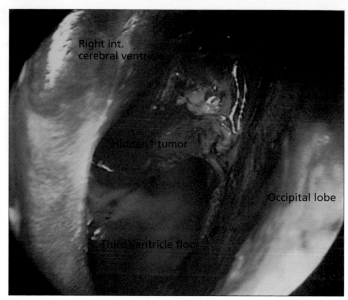

Figure 10.15 Following "complete" resection, a 30° endoscope was introduced which demonstrated residual tumor remnants.

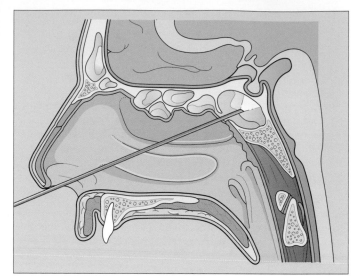

Figure 10.17 Approach made by the endoscope into the sphenoid sinus via the transnasal route.

disastrous consequences. The use of a fixed endoscope holder can aid the surgeon to work with both hands. This will allow the surgeon to use more complex instruments, and will also prevent the endoscope from drifting against vital structures located superficially along the operative corridor.

ENDOSCOPIC TRANSSPHENOIDAL SURGERY

Since the turn of the century, the transsphenoidal route to the pituitary fossa has been advocated as a less invasive means of removing tumors than the transcranial route. However, sinonasal complications are not infrequent, visualization is limited and an

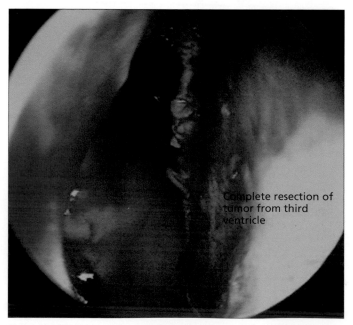

Figure 10.16 Using endoscope-assisted techniques, the "hidden" tumor was resected.

incision through the nose or gum is required. Our otolaryngology colleagues have been mastering the art of sinonasal endoscopy for many years and are comfortable operating in the sphenoid sinus.[32]

It seemed only natural to progress one step further by taking the endoscope through the sphenoid sinus and into the pituitary fossa. The use of the endoscope allows close inspection and differentiation between tumor tissue and glandular remains. This results in microdissection of the tumor with maximum preservation of pituitary function. The angled view of the endoscope aids total gross removal of tumor tissue from the less accessible supra- and parasellar extensions.

There are several benefits of endoscopy over the gold standard which is the microsurgical approach. First, access to the sphenoid sinus is obtained by expanding the osteum after passing the scope directly through the nose. This obviates the need for a sublabial incision and a subperichondrial tunnel. Second, the scope provides better illumination of the surgical field and greater magnification. Third, by changing the angle of the scope from 0° to 30° or 70° one can expand the operative field and even look "around corners" (Figure 10.17). Finally, cluttering of instruments down a limited tunnel, such as the nasal speculum used with the standard microsurgical technique, can be avoided by placing the scope down one nostril and the instruments down the other. When the sphenoid sinus is reached, instruments and technique are similar to the microsurgical approach. Pituitary tumors with or without suprasellar extension can be removed in this fashion. Indeed, visualization is so good (Figure 10.18) that tumors of the parasellar region may also be approached using this technique. The cavernous sinuses, the tuberculum sella and the upper third of the clivus are all within reach of the endoscope (Figure 10.19).

MICROVASCULAR DECOMPRESSION

Endoscope-assisted microvascular decompression (MVD) is a potentially major advancement as improved visualization of the fifth cranial nerve should theoretically increase the number of successful MVDs, and ultimately improve the procedure's success

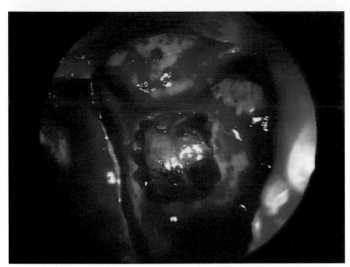

Figure 10.18 The endoscope offers a superior view of the sellar and regions adjacent. Bone removal here is complete, ready for dural opening and resection of tumor.

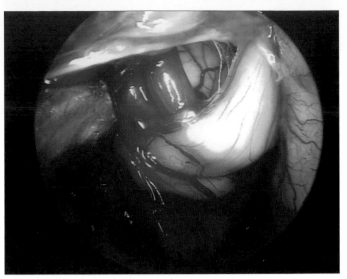

Figure 10.20 A superior view of nerve–vessel conflicts can be achieved with the endoscope. Here the trigeminal nerve is distorted at a right angle by an anterior inferior cerebellar artery (AICA) loop.

rate in both the short and long term. Endoscope-assisted MVD for hemifacial spasm has also been described by some authors.

Endoscope-assisted microsurgery has been shown to improve the surgeon's visualization of structures in the extra-axial space[33] and endoscopic anatomy of the cerebellopontine angle has been published in detail.[34] Our unit has performed over 70 endoscope-assisted MVD procedures since 1994, finding a nerve–vessel conflict in all cases (Figures 10.20–10.22).

As this technique is likely to increase in prominence, we shall describe the operative technique in brief.

- Positioning: lateral decubitus or supine position with the head tilted away as far as their individual neck mobility permitted.
- Craniotomy: a small retrosigmoid craniectomy just inferior to the transverse–sigmoid junction.
- Dura opened and reflected against the sinus.

- Using standard microneurosurgical techniques the trigeminal nerve is identified by gently retracting the cerebellum, releasing CSF from the basal cisterns and lysing the arachnoidal bands.
- Microscopic then endoscopic inspection with a 30° rigid scope.
- If the compressing vessel is seen only with the endoscope, MVD is performed under endoscopic control. If the vessel could be seen clearly with the microscope then the endoscope is used to assess the competency of decompression at the completion of the procedure.
- MVD is achieved by using a small Dacron® patch placed securely between the root entry zone of the nerve and the offending vessel.
- Closure by standard techniques.

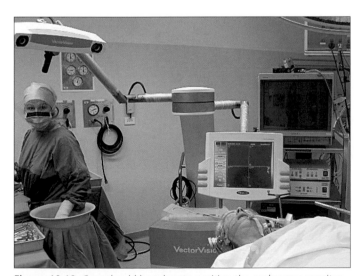

Figure 10.19 Care should be taken to position the endoscope monitor and frameless stereotaxis equipment to aid surgeon comfort and reduce neck fatigue.

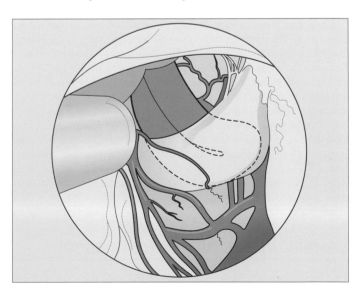

Figure 10.21 The endoscope was used to appreciate the anatomy of the loop in more detail. After endoscopic inspection, the surgeon now has a "mental picture" in far more detail than would be possible with a microscope.

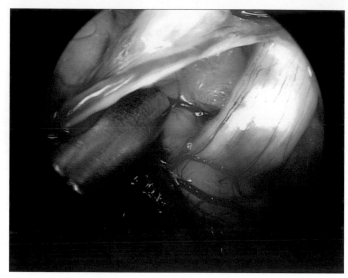

Figure 10.22 Appreciation of the anatomy now enables the surgeon to perform accurate placement of a patch. Note that the tension on the trigeminal nerve is now released.

The current gold standard is exploration with an operating microscope. However, the microscopic view is limited to the line of sight between the craniectomy and the lateral surface of the nerve, whereas compression may occur anywhere around the circumference of the nerve or anywhere along its length. All areas of potential nerve–vessel conflict are easily accessible with the endoscope. Jarrahy and colleagues reported on endoscope-assisted MVD[35] and found that 28% of compressive vessels were seen only with endoscopy. In addition, the treatment of 24% of patients with microscope-guided decompression was found to be inadequate and required revision under endoscopic guidance.

MISCELLANEOUS APPLICATIONS

Hypertensive intracerebral hematomas are usually deep within the basal ganglia, causing neurological deficits that can be limited by evacuation. As they are usually deep, standard surgery involves a cortical incision and retraction. Endoscopy allows aspiration of a hematoma,[36] coagulation of bleeders within the cavity and biopsy of the wall all under direct vision. This may be a reasonable adjuvant or alternative therapy for this patient population.

Some neurosurgeons are offering endoscopic removal of these blood collections through a burr hole (Figure 10.23). They claim adequate hematoma removal, satisfactory control of the bleeding source, lower morbidity, less blood loss, and shorter operating times.[31] There are no randomized data to support these claims to date. Further study on this subject is required. There are, in addition, scattered reports of endoscope-assisted procedures including vestibular neurectomy[37] and posterior fossa decompression.[38]

COMPLICATIONS OF NEUROENDOSCOPY

The endoscope is a powerful tool but, like all tools, it requires experience for safe and effective use. Practice is required to develop the visuomotor skills necessary to guide the tip safely in and out of narrow spaces. If an operation is to be performed primarily using endoscopic techniques, the surgeon must exercise

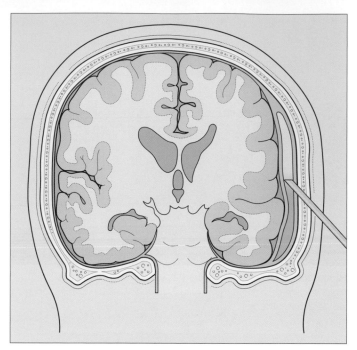

Figure 10.23 Endoscopy can aid in visualizing subdural remnants or loculations via the burr hole exposure.

considerable judgment to determine when the procedure may no longer be possible through an endoscopic approach, and must plan for an open microsurgical approach (Figure 10.24).

A familiarization with the endoscopic perspective and a review of the pertinent microsurgical anatomy is essential before using the endoscope on patients. Used properly, complications directly related to the endoscope can be minimized. It is hypothesized that the incidence of intraoperative complications decreases with experience, while that of the longer-term seqeulae do not, highlighting the steep learning curve with this approach.[39] Lastly, a number of technical issues related to the use of the endoscope have been raised in this chapter. One of the most frequently cited concerns is the fact that the view the endoscope provides is only

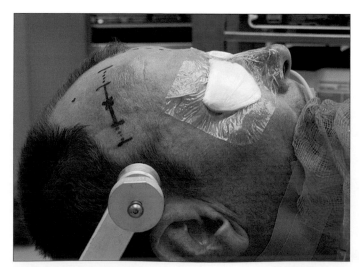

Figure 10.24 An incision is marked for an endoscopic colloid cyst removal. In the event of failure of the endoscopic technique, the dotted line marks the extended incision to perform an open craniotomy.

two-dimensional. Certainly one traverses a steep learning curve in the process of attaining the visuomotor skills necessary to work comfortably using a two-dimensional video image. While disorienting for the novice endoscopist, this theoretical limitation seldom presents much difficulty for most surgeons once they become familiar with it.

CONCLUSIONS

The clear advantages of neuroendoscopy are:

- increased light intensity while approaching an object;
- clear depiction of details in close-up;
- extended viewing angle.

One of the goals of the use of the endoscope is to reduce brain retraction and minimize cortical and nerve manipulation. These characteristics are translated into potential advantages during surgical procedures for deep-seated lesions in narrow spaces. The potential rewards of neuroendoscopy include improved postoperative results, shorter hospitalization times, and fewer postoperative complications. They are striking arguments for the use of this operative technique for specific well-defined indications.

CLINICAL PEARLS

- Neuroendoscopy is a rapidly evolving field which adheres to the principles of minimally invasive surgery: maximum results through minimal exposures with safety by applying superior magnification and illumination. Neuroendoscopy is safe and effective in experienced hands but has a steep visuomotor learning curve. The risks and complications of this technique include vascular or neural injury and may be minimized by developing improved visuomotor skills and applying appropriate case selection. In addition, the surgeon must be prepared to convert a neuroendoscopic procedure into a standard microsurgical procedure if the procedure is not technically feasible with the endoscope.

- The indications for this exciting surgical technique of neuroendoscopy are swiftly expanding from intraventricular pathology to extra-axial pathology. Currently, widely accepted indications of neuroendoscopy include: (1) endoscopic third ventriculostomy for the treatment of hydrocephalus from aqueductal stenosis or posterior fossa tumors; (2) fenestration of loculated ventricles; (3) resection of intraventricular lesions such as cysts, colloid tumors, and small avascular tumors; (4) biopsy of pineal region tumors; (5) resection of pituitary and sellar tumors; (6) treatment of arachnoid cysts and selected extra-axial pathology; and (7) as an adjuvant in endoscope-assisted microsurgery for tumor resection, aneurysm clipping, microvascular decompression and skull-base surgery. This is a powerful tool with increasing applications but known limitations.

REFERENCES

1. L'Espinasse VL. *Neurological Surgery*, 2nd edn. Philadelphia: Lea and Ferbiger; 1943: 442.
2. Dandy WE. An operative procedure for hydrocephalus. *Bull Johns Hopkins Hosp* 1922; 33: 189–90.
3. Yokoh A, Sugita K, Kobayashi S. Intermittent versus continuous brain retraction: an experimental study. *J Neurosurg* 1983; 58: 918–23.
4. Perneczky A, Fries G. Endoscope-assisted brain surgery: Part I Evolution, basic concept, and current technique. *Neurosurgery* 1998; 42: 219–25.
5. Teo C. Endoscopic-assisted tumor and neurovascular procedures. *Clin Neurosurg* 2000; 46: 515–25.
6. Alberti O, Riegel T, Hellwig D, Bertalanffy H. Frameless navigation and endoscopy. *J Neurosurg* 2001; 95: 541–3.
7. Scarff JE. Endoscopic treatment of hydrocephalus: description of a ventriculoscope and preliminary report of cases. *Arch Neurol Psychiatr* 1936; 35: 853–60.
8. Guiot G. Ventriculo-cisternostomy for stenosis of the aqueduct of Sylvis. *Acta Neurochir (Wien)* 1973; 28: 275–89.
9. Hopf N, Grunert P, Fries G, Resch K, Perneczky A. Endoscopic third ventriculostomy: Outcome analysis of 100 consecutive procedures. *Neurosurgery* 1999; 44: 795–804.
10. Buxton N, Ho KJ, Macarthur D, Vloeberghs M, Punt J, Robertson I. Neuroendoscopic third ventriculostomy for hydrocephalus in adults: report of a single unit's experience with 63 cases. *Surg Neurol* 2001; 55: 74–8.
11. Cinalli G, Saint-Rose C, Chumas P, Zerah M, Brunelle F, Lot G, Pierre-Kahn A, Renier D. Failure of third ventriculostomy in the treatment of aqueductal stenosis in children. *J Neurosurg* 1999; 90: 448–54.
12. Teo C, Young R. Endoscopic management of hydrocephalus secondary to posterior third ventricular tumors. *Neurosurg Focus* 1999; 7(4): article 2.
13. Kanner A, Hopf NJ, Grunert P. The "optimal" burr hole position for endoscopic third ventriculostomy: results from 31 stereotactically guided procedures. *Minim Invas Neurosurg* 2000; 43: 187–9.
14. Saint-Rose C, Cinalli G, Roux FE, *et al.* Management of hydrocephalus in paediatric patients with posterior fossa tumours; the role of endoscopic third ventriculostomy. *J Neurosurg* 2001; 95: 791–7.
15. Barlow P, Ching HS. An economic argument in favour of endoscopic third ventriculostomy as a treatment for obstructive hydrocephalus. *Minim Invas Neurosurg* 1997; 40: 37–9.
16. Hader WJ, Drake J, Cochrane D, Sparrow O, Johnson ES, Kestle J. Death after late failure of third ventriculostomy in children. Report of three cases. *J Neurosurg* 2002; 97: 211–15.
17. Tisell M, Almstrom O, Stephenson H, Tullberg M, Wikkelson C. How effective is endoscopsic third ventriculostomy in treating adult hydrocephalus caused by primary aqueductal stenosis? *Neurosurgery* 2000; 46: 104–9.
18. Brockmeyer D, Abtin K, Carey L, Walker ML. Endoscopic third ventriculostomy: an outcome analysis. *Paediatr Neurosurg* 1998; 28: 236–40.
19. Teo C, Jones R. Management of hydrocephalus by endoscopic third ventriculosotomy in patients with myelomeningocele. *Paediatr Neurosurg* 1996; 25: 57–63.
20. Walker ML, Perronio J, Carey CM. Ventriculoscopy. In: Cheek WR (ed.). *Pediatric Neurosurgery*, 3rd edn. Philadelphia: WB Saunders; 1993: 572–81.
21. Perneczky A, Muller-Forell W, van Lindert E, Fries G. *Keyhole Concept in Neurosurgery*. Stuttgart: Thieme; 1999: 120–48.

22. Wallner KR, Gonzales M, Sheline GE. Treatment of oligodendrogliomas with or without post-operative irradiation. *J Neurosurg* 1988; 68: 684–8.

23. Garcia DM, Fulling KH. Juvenile pilocytic astrocytomas of the cerebrum in adults. A distinctive neoplasm with favorable prognosis. *J Neurosurg* 1985; 63: 382–6.

24. Lewis AI, Crone KR, Taha J, *et al*. Surgical resection of third ventricle colloid cyst. Preliminary results comparing transcallosal microsurgery with endoscopy. *J Neurosurg* 1994; 81: 174–8.

25. Teo C. Endoscopic removal of colloid cysts: issues of safety and reliability. *Neurosurg Focus* 1999; 6(4): article 9.

26. Rodziewicz GS, Smith MV, Hodge CJ. Endoscopic colloid cyst surgery. *Neurosurgery* 2000; 46: 655–62.

27. Oka K, Kin Y, Go Y, *et al*. Neuroendoscopic approach to tectal tumors: a consecutive series. *J Neurosurg* 1999; 91: 964–70.

28. Gaab MR, Schroeder HWS. Neurendoscopic approach to intraventricular lesions. *J Neurosurg* 1998; 88: 496–505.

29. Abdullah J, Caemart J. Endoscopic management of craniopharyngioma: a review of 3 cases. *Minim Invas Neurosurg* 1993; 38: 79–84.

30. Cohen AR, Perneczky A, Rodziewciz GS, *et al*. Endoscope-assisted craniotomy: approach to the rostral brainstem. *Neurosurgery* 1995; 36: 1128–30.

31. Gamea A, Fathi M, el-Guindy A. The use of the rigid endoscope in trans-sphenoidal pituitary surgery. *J Laryngol Otol* 1994; 108: 19–22.

32. Perneczky A, Tschabischer M, Resch KDM. *Endoscopic Anatomy for Neurosurgery*. Stuttgart: Thieme; 1998: 91–8.

33. Matula C, Tschabitscher M, Day JD, *et al*. Endoscopically assisted microneurosurgery. *Acta Neurochir (Wien)* 1995; 134: 190–5.

34. Jarrahy R, Berci G, Shahinian HK Endoscope-assisted microvascular decompression of the trigeminal nerve. *Otolaryngol Head Neck Surg* 2000; 123: 218–23.

35. Kim MH, Kim EY, Song JH, Shin KM. Surgical options of hypertensive intracerebral hematoma: stereotactic endoscopic removal versus stereotactic catheter drainage. *J Korean Med Sci* 1998; 13: 533–40.

36. Karakhan VB, Khodnevich AA. Endoscopic surgery of traumatic intracranial haemorrhages. *Acta Neurochir Suppl (Wien)* 1994; 61: 84–91.

37. Wackym PA, King WA, Barker FG, Poe DS. Endoscope-assisted vestibular neurectomy. *Laryngoscope* 1998; 108: 1787–93.

38. Mobbs RJ, Teo C. Endoscopic assisted posterior fossa decompression. *J Clin Neurosci* 2001; 8: 343–4.

39. Teo C, Rahman S, Boop FA, Cherny B. Complications of endoscopic neurosurgery. *Childs Nerv Syst* 1996; 12: 248–53.

40. Dalrymple SJ, Kelly PJ. Computer assisted stereotactic third ventriculostomy in the management of noncommunicating hydrocephalus. *Stereotactic Funct Neurosurg* 1992; 54: 105–10.

41. Jones RF, Kwok BC, Stening WA, Vonau M. The current status of endoscopic third ventriculostomy in the management of non-communicating hydrocephalus. *Minim Invas Neurosurg* 1994; 37: 28–36.

42. Choi JU, Kim DS, Lim SH. Endoscopic surgery for obstructive hydrocephalus. *Yonsei Med J* 1999; 40: 600–7.

43. Gangemi M, Donti P, Maiuri F, Longatti P, Godano U, Mascari C. Endoscopic third ventriculostomy for hydrocephalus. *Minim Invas Neurosurg* 1999; 42: 128–32.

44. Fukuhara T, Vorster SJ, Luciano MG. Risk factors for failure of endoscopic third ventriculostomy for obstructive hydrocephalus. *Neurosurgery* 2000; 46: 1100–11.

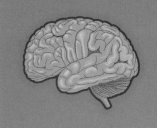

CRANIOSYNOSTOSIS

11

Robert F Keating

INTRODUCTION

Craniosynostosis is the premature closure of a cranial suture which causes abnormal calvarial growth. Virchow, in 1851,[1] was the first to describe premature closure of a cranial suture causing restriction of skull growth perpendicular to the affected suture, and leading to an abnormal cranial contour (Virchow's rule). He subsequently characterized the various craniosynostoses as they related to a specific suture. The surgical release of the affected suture permits normalization of the growth of the skull in the setting of accelerated cerebral growth. This has been a primary objective in contemporary craniofacial surgical reconstruction. Aside from cosmesis, consideration of brain development as well as possible increased intracranial pressure has also become a vital component of the decision-making process. While the likelihood of elevated intracranial pressure remains low for patients with single-suture craniosynostosis, children with multiple suture involvement are at significantly higher risk. This should also be considered in the older patient undergoing surgery for single-suture pathology in association with possible signs and symptoms of intracranial hypertension. Nevertheless, over time progressively earlier recognition of craniosynostosis and its subsequent

treatment have led to improved surgical results with correspondingly decreased perioperative morbidity. With the utilization of biochemical modifiers of bone growth such as bone morphogenic protein and the greater understanding of distraction technology in the craniofacial skeleton, new horizons will inevitably unfold.

HISTORY

Craniosynostosis has long been recognized as an abnormal process originating at the calvarial suture. Early recognition of the importance of the skull sutures and their relationship to head shape was made by many investigators, including Hippocrates, Galen, and Celsus. Sommerring in 1791 first noted that calvarial growth occurred at the suture line and premature suture closure led to restriction of growth perpendicular to the affected suture.[2] Virchow[1] was the first to categorize systematically head shape and associated abnormal suture and he confirmed that calvarial growth would follow a direction perpendicular to the affected suture (Figure 11.1). These observations would stand as principal tenets directing craniosynostosis surgery over the subsequent century. Over time, the relationship between calvarial growth and the skull

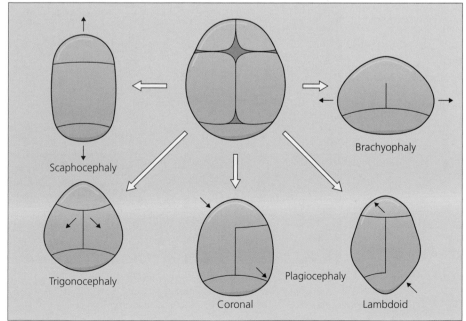

Scaphocephaly

Brachyophaly

Trigonocephaly

Coronal

Plagiocephaly

Lambdoid

Figure 11.1 Restriction of growth at particular sutures will lead to growth perpendicular to the involved suture. In the case of sagittal synostosis, the head will become elongated (scaphocephaly), whereas coronal involvement in turn produces a flattened supraorbital region with compensatory overgrowth over the contralateral frontal region (frontal plagiocephaly). Closure of the metopic suture may produce varying degrees of trigonocephaly with growth now directed in a biparietal direction. Lambdoid craniosynostosis in turn will produce occipital plagiocephaly similar to coronal disease.

base became better appreciated. Moss in 1959 pointed out the importance of the skull base in the promotion and development of the calvarial vault.[3] His contributions included the observation that the cranial base developed prior to the calvarial vault. In addition, he noted that characteristic abnormalities in the cranial base were associated with classical sutural abnormalities. As a result, Moss believed that the skull base was the primary site that predicated calvarial vault growth. Nevertheless, subsequent experimental work in animal models[4–6] demonstrated that restriction of growth at specific sutures resulted in characteristic skull deformities that mimicked shapes seen in simple (non-syndromic) craniosynostosis. As a result, the pathogenesis of craniosynostosis is currently thought to be a combination of skull base and calvarial growth disturbances.

EPIDEMIOLOGY

The incidence of simple or nonsyndromic craniosynostosis varies from 0.25 to 0.60 per 1000 births,[7–11] although higher clinical estimates have been proposed by Tessier[12] (1/1000) as well as Anderson and Geiger[13] (1.6 per 1000). Most often, single-suture synostosis will occur as an isolated phenomenon (except for occasional familial patterns) with an equal frequency in all ethnic populations; however, gender predilection will vary between the different types of suture pathology.

The most common suture involved is the sagittal suture, which accounts for 56–60% of all individuals with craniosynostosis. Males outnumber females 2:1.[4,5,7,14] Closure of the coronal suture (bilateral/unilateral) is demonstrated in approximately 18–29% of series with craniosynostosis[3,7,8] and seen twice as frequently with unilateral versus bilateral involvement. Metopic synostosis occurs in only 4–10% of patients with synostosis whereas "true" lambdoid suture stenosis is a relatively rare event in children, occurring less than 2% of the time[7,8] (see Table 11.1). True lambdoid synostosis is to be distinguished from positional molding or posterior plagiocephaly without synostosis in which there is a flat occiput on the affected side but no premature suture closure. This epiphenomenon appears to be related to the supine sleeping position in young children. The flattening of the back of the head is most often managed successfully in a conservative fashion (discussed in detail later in this chapter).

The majority of isolated craniosynostoses are sporadic, although genetic patterns have been found in 8% of patients with coronal synostosis and in 2% of sagittal synostosis.[5] Autosomal dominant and recessive patterns of inheritance have both been seen with simple craniosynostosis. Although the sporadic nature of simple craniosynostosis makes an accurate prediction of subsequent risk difficult to ascertain, it appears that the risk doubles for future siblings if there are no other family members involved. When one parent and child are affected, the subsequent risk rises to 50%; conversely if both parents are unaffected and two siblings are affected, the risk for additional sibling involvement approaches 25%.[15]

More complex syndromic craniosynostoses, such as Crouzon, Apert, and Pfeiffer syndromes (Figure 11.2), are commonly associated with multiple suture closure (coronal, sagittal, etc.) in addition to other systemic manifestations (Table 11.2). The syndromic variants are much less common than single-suture synostosis and usually represent less than 5% of all patients with craniosynostosis. They are often inherited by an autosomal-dominant mode of transmission.[16]

GENETIC AND ETIOLOGICAL FACTORS

The etiology of craniosynostosis remains elusive because of its heterogeneous nature. Nevertheless, numerous factors are now known to promote or have been implicated in the development of premature closure of the calvarial sutures. Multiple teratogens, genetic mutations, and metabolic as well as hematological disorders have all been associated with craniosynostosis (Table 11.3). More recently, maternal smoking has been associated with isolated craniosynostosis in a study from Sweden.[17]

A better understanding of craniosynostosis has paralleled the advances in molecular genetics which has begun to identify candidate genes and their mutations.[18,19] Genes coding for fibroblast growth factor (FGF) receptors 1 and 2 have been

Table 11.1 Classification of synostosis	
Sagittal	Dolichocephaly, scaphocephaly
Coronal (unilateral)	Anterior plagiocephaly
Coronal (bilateral)	Brachycephaly
Metopic	Trigonocephaly
Lambdoid	Posterior plagiocephaly
Multiple sutures	Cloverleaf, Kleeblatschadel, acrocephaly, oxycephaly

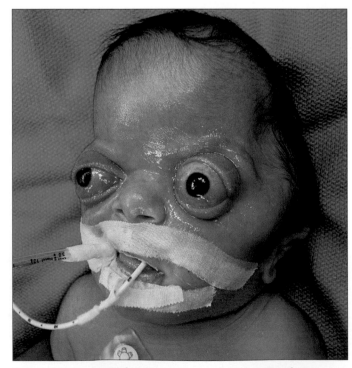

Figure 11.2 Newborn infant born with cloverleaf skull, manifesting characteristic towering and bitemporal expansion with restriction at the supraorbital bar and sphenoid wing in conjunction with severe midfacial hypoplasia and proptosis.

Table 11.2 Craniofacial dysostoses syndromes

Syndrome	Involved suture	Morphological presentation
Crouzon	Coronal, sagittal	Midfacial hypoplasia, shallow orbits, proptosis, hypertelorism
Apert	Coronal, sagittal, lambdoid, etc.	Midfacial hypoplasia, shallow orbits, proptosis, hypertelorism, *symmetrical syndactyly of hands and feet*, choanal atresia, ventriculomegaly, genitourinary/cardiovascular anomalies
Pfeiffer	Coronal, sagittal	Midfacial hypoplasia, proptosis, hypertelorism, *broad great toe/thumb*

Table 11.3 Recognized causes of craniosynostosis

Hematological disorders	Thalassemias
	Sickle cell anemia
	Polycythemia vera
Teratogens	Valproic acid
	Retinoic acid
	Aminopterin
	Diphenylhydantoin
Genetic conditions	
Metabolic disorders	Rickets
	Hyperthyroidism
Mucopolysaccharidoses	Hurler syndrome
	Morquio syndrome
	Mucolipidosis III
β-glucuronidase deficiency	
Malformations	Holoprosencephaly
	Encephalocele
	Microcephaly
	Hydrocephalus (shunted)

demonstrated to be directly involved with Crouzon, Aperts, Pfeiffer and Jackson–Weiss syndromes.[20–24] FGF2 receptors have been observed promoting skeletogenic differentiation of neural crest cells[25] and are thus thought to play an early role in the development of the craniofacial skeleton. FGF2 appears to be an integral component of calvarial osteoblast proliferation and subsequent sutural fusion. Histological analysis of preosteoblastic calvarial cells isolated from infants and fetuses with Apert syndrome[26] demonstrated increased alkaline phosphatase activity when compared with controls, and was consistent with an accelerated maturation rate of bone development. In subsequent studies,[27] fetal rat osteoblasts were cultured with FGF2 and manifested higher proliferation rates while maintaining osteoblast morphology. The same study also demonstrated premature fusion of frontal sutures in FGF2-treated calvarial organ cultures.[23] Other investigators have successfully inhibited previously programmed frontal suture fusion in a murine model via adenoviral vectors transfecting FGF receptor-1 constructs,[28]

demonstrating the eventual potential for *in vivo* modulation of cranial suture activity with growth factors. Alterations in growth factors have also been observed in nonsyndromic craniosynostosis. Gripp and colleagues[29] observed that a subset of patients with unilateral coronal synostosis were positive for a mutation of the FGF receptor 3 gene and subsequently recommend testing of all patients with unilateral coronal synostosis to assess the risk of recurrence. In addition to the numerous FGF receptors, transforming growth factor-β (TGF-β) receptors appear to also be implicated in the development of intrauterine head constraint-related craniosynostosis. Numerous studies have documented up-regulation of TGF-β receptors as well as FGF2 in animal models undergoing intrauterine constraint leading to coronal suture synostosis.[30,31] Such data would support the association between mechanical forces and eventual humoral translation to regulate the balance of growth factors and their input into the growth and development of the craniofacial skeleton. Similar findings have also been seen in patients with persistent lambdoid plagiocephaly. Lambdoid sutures removed from surgical patients who failed conservative therapy for their positional plagiocephaly, subsequently demonstrated elevated levels of TGF-β2 and TGF-β3 at the affected site, whereas the unaffected suture had normal levels.[32] Despite the preponderance of research directed towards the definition of FGF and TGF in the pathogenesis of craniosynostosis, numerous other growth factors have also been implicated in this arena. Epidermal growth factor (EGF), platelet-derived growth factor (PDGF), MSX2 and TWIST transcription factors have also been identified as key molecules in this complicated process.[33–36]

ANATOMICAL AND PATHOLOGICAL CONSIDERATIONS

The growth of the calvarium is dependent upon freedom of movement at involved sutures. Restriction of growth at an affected suture will often give rise to stereotypical shapes manifesting both calvarial undergrowth as well as compensatory overgrowth. It is not precisely known why sutures become immobile in the craniosynostoses. The etiology for craniosynostosis is likely to remain elusive due to its heterogeneous pathogenesis. The calvarium and skull base arise from neural crest cells which surround the rapidly enlarging brain. Dural condensations are first observed at 5–6 weeks' gestation, with subsequent development of islands of cartilage over the dura. These later are transformed into osteoblastic ossification centers which coalesce at defined regions and, as brain growth slows, calvarial bones come together to form sutures.

Studies have shown that sutures are sites of bony adaptation rather than being primary growth centers.[15] Bone growth at a suture can be induced by expansion of the suture, demonstrated experimentally by raising the intracranial pressure. At first, the fibrous sutural ligament is separated and a layer of osteoid is deposited along the suture margin which then mineralizes and is transformed into bone. Successive replication of this process normally results in enlargement of the calvarial bones. On the other hand, compression of a suture (which can be performed experimentally by external mechanical compression) causes bone resorption along the suture margin rather than suture closure.[37,38]

There is some indirect evidence that, in humans, mechanical compression can at least contribute to suture closure.[39,40] There is an increased incidence of craniosynostosis with intrauterine breach positioning and with twins. It is thus believed that external compression from intrauterine crowding may cause fibrosis or ischemia at an involved suture and that this will contribute to premature closure. Postnatal positioning may also have an effect on the site of and progression of suture synostosis. Currently, this is felt to be the pathogenesis of positional molding or nonsynostotic posterior plagiocephaly. Therapeutic approaches include changing a child's position during sleep to help mold the head and improve suture mobility in the first few months of life as well as "helmet therapy," in which a rigid external mold is applied to the skull of a neonate to redirect calvarial growth. These therapies may be beneficial though debated, since they are used on mild cases and the improvement may represent spontaneous resolution as part of the natural history of the process as the children start sitting and walking and spend less time sleeping.

Sutures form by 16 weeks' gestation at the junction of numerous osteogenic fronts and are directly affected by underlying forces of brain growth and dural reflections. These reflections uniformly conform to underlying cortical patterns and will be absent with cerebral hypoplasia which subsequently leads to the absence of suture development at this location. This may in turn lead to the development of secondary craniosynostosis due to the lack of growth vectors at this calvarial location and should not be confused with primary craniosynostosis which is related primarily to premature closure of the affected suture. Such observations have led to proposed hypotheses that underlying tension forces at dural reflections (making up the overlying sutures) act to direct calvarial growth.[41-43] Nevertheless, innumerable experimental observations have also demonstrated the significance of local factors in the development of normal and abnormal suture growth. Sutures and their respective osteogenic fronts removed from their prior biomechanical environment may still form normal sutures.[44] Apoptosis has also been observed[45] at the osteogenic fronts as they approach each other at the sutural interface and thus may help to explain the mechanism of eventual sutural fusion. The significance of other local factors in sutural pathogenesis has been demonstrated by a number of transplantation studies which have removed the suture from its underlying dura and vice versa. Both dural and suture interactions have manifested unusual growth patterns. Transplanted fetal calvarial cells without any corresponding underlying dura will fail to develop a patent suture.[46,47] Patients (neonate) undergoing total calvarial reconstruction will also demonstrate the formation of appropriate sutures with new calvarial growth consistent with an underlying local feedback mechanism at the dural–calvarial interface.[48,49] Growth factors, such as FGF, have also been demonstrated to be involved in the modulation of growth at the suture. Osteoblasts subsequently lay down bone at the edge of the suture in response to underlying extrinsic forces exerted by the developing brain.

There are also components of craniosynostosis which represent arrested embryological development rather than abnormal compensatory growth as well as types that are not directly or mechanically linked to suture closure. These include systemic fibrocartilagenous abnormalities such as syndactyly, renal, skeletal, and cardiac anomalies.

The calvarium grows most rapidly during the first 12 months, with the brain doubling in volume in the first 6 months and again by the second birthday. While calvarial expansion is most pronounced during the first 2 years, growth continues in a linear fashion till the age of 6–7 years, at which time the cranium is 90% of the adult size. Computed tomographically (CT)-determined

intracranial volume has demonstrated that intracranial volume is 95% of the final volume in males at 46 months whereas females reach a similar level at 42 months.[50] Advocates for early surgical correction of craniosynostosis recommend utilization of this differential growth rate to maximize surgical improvement at the involved suture as well as offering the greatest likelihood of improvement at secondary areas of compensatory overgrowth.

DIAGNOSTIC EVALUATION AND IMAGING

Significant craniosynostosis is readily apparent at birth or shortly thereafter, whereas more moderate presentations may become obvious during infancy. Physical findings include premature closure of the anterior fontanelle, peri-sutural ridging (calcification), as well as characteristic calvarial shapes and asymmetries. Normally, the anterior fontanelle can remain open until 12–18 months of age. The history combined with the examination is often confirmatory in an experienced primary-care physician/nurse, or craniofacial surgeon's initial evaluation. Not uncommonly, asymmetric calvarial deformities are often first noted by friends or other family members. While craniosynostosis remains predominantly diagnosed by the physical examination, radiological investigation may be necessary not only for corroboration but to also rule out any associated intracranial abnormalities.

The role of radiological work-up varies amongst clinicians. Many patients arrive with skull X-rays which frequently fail to demonstrate any sutural fusion or conversely, have been interpreted as being abnormal when no obvious deformity exists. Currently, it is not uncommon for prenatal ultrasounds[51-53] to document craniosynostosis *in utero* and fetal magnetic resonance imaging (MRI) (Figure 11.3) at some centers has offered significant prenatal definition in addition to the ultrasound evaluation.

Nevertheless, CT studies remain the most sensitive barometer of bony fusion, although it is important to obtain bone windows as well as appropriate thin slices through the involved suture. The recent advent of three-dimensional CT (3D CT)[54-56] has simplified the diagnosis as well as helped with surgical planning, providing an excellent view of the suture as well as overall head

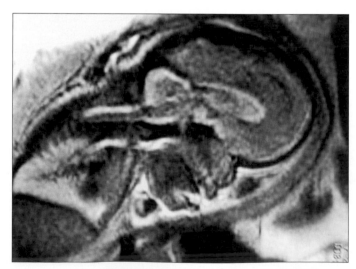

Figure 11.3 Fetal MRI depicting a cloverleaf skull in a 30-week fetus who was born with Pfeiffer syndrome and required a near-total calvarectomy within the first week of life.

shape. Three-dimensional CT is not mandatory, and in some centers is reserved for patients with multiple or complicated suture pathology or when the diagnosis is in question. However, 3D studies may be helpful when demonstration of the skull base is crucial, especially with syndromic patients. It is also important to evaluate the underlying brain to visualize cerebral structures and document the presence of abnormal brain or more importantly to rule out increased intracranial pressure. Unrecognized intracranial abnormalities may exist in a small number of patients and may include hydrocephalus (more common in patients with Crouzon syndrome), partial agenesis of the corpus callosum, holoprosencephaly (seen in patients with trigonocephaly), or focal cortical dysplasias. Boop and colleagues[58] noted that up to 5% of their patients with sagittal synostoses had unappreciated underlying intracranial pathology. Thus, in many centers CT or 3D CT scans are routinely employed. It is very common to see expanded subarachnoid spaces in all types of craniosynostoses,[59] although these spaces usually spontaneously resolve and are not felt to represent an increase in intracranial pressure.

The CT scan may also demonstrate whether there is any radiological evidence for increased intracranial pressure. While increased intracranial pressure remains a clinical diagnosis, and remains uncommon in the setting of isolated suture synostosis, Renier and colleagues[60] have documented that a subset of children (up to 13% depending upon the suture(s) involved) will have elevated intracranial pressure, demonstrated by intracranial monitoring at the time of surgery. While few children will manifest clinical symptoms of increased intracranial pressure (e.g. headache, vomiting, visual changes, developmental delay, feeding problems, etc.), it is not uncommon to visualize erosion of the inner calvarial table on CT scan. The clinical significance of this finding remains unclear. If there is any evidence for elevated pressure, surgical consideration should be expedited. This is especially vital in patients with syndromic synostosis (e.g. Crouzon, Apert, Pfeiffer) who are at a greater risk for hydrocephalus and Chiari malformations, which are associated with increases in intracranial pressure.

THERAPEUTIC CONSIDERATIONS

Surgical indications

The majority of children with simple craniosynostosis are not likely to manifest neurological compromise nor are they expected to have any adverse long-term outcome secondary to restriction of calvarial growth. Thus, for most children with simple craniosynostosis, surgical intervention is made primarily because of cosmetic and psychosocial considerations,[61,62] whereas patients with complex synostoses (syndromic variants) frequently present with a combination of neurological and cosmetic concerns. For children born with an obvious deformity, the likelihood of spontaneous resolution remains low. Presentation at this early stage indicates significant sutural fusion which is unlikely to improve with time and these children are best served by early surgical release[63–71] of the affected suture(s) to produce the best long-term results as well as minimizing secondary midfacial deformations. While there has been debate in the past regarding the appropriate time for correction of simple craniosynostosis, the majority of craniofacial surgeons operate between 3 and 12 months of age. A review by Marchac and colleagues[66] reviewed their craniofacial experience with 983 patients operated on over 20 years and report that children with brachycephalies underwent

frontocranial remodeling between 2 and 4 months of age, whereas children with other craniosynostoses received surgery between 6 and 12 months of age. Additional work by Persing and colleagues[71] demonstrated significantly greater calvarial growth after release of a previously immobilized coronal suture in a rabbit model with earlier surgical intervention. They also found fewer secondary craniofacial abnormalities with the earlier surgical releases. The argument against early surgery includes the fact that re-operation is more common in patients who undergo early surgery than those patients whose operations are delayed until they are 9–12 months of age.

The role of orthotic molding remains controversial at present. Proponents of this approach[37,74,75] argue that in the setting of mild to moderate craniosynostosis, helmet therapy offers a safer and effective alternative. This is perhaps best exemplified in patients with positional molding. Now understood to be secondary to a supine sleeping position,[76,77] which was initially recommended in 1994 by the American Academy of Pediatrics[78] to decrease the incidence of sudden infant death syndrome, positional plagiocephaly without synostosis is predominantly a nonsurgical condition. While the majority of affected infants improve spontaneously with correction of a frequently associated torticollis as well as advancing age and progression of developmental milestones, there nevertheless, remain a small subset of patients(< 7%)[79,80] who may require surgical correction for excellent long-term results.

Timing of surgery

The timing of reconstructive surgery remains controversial and is dependent upon the severity and location of synostosis; though most surgeons prefer to operate between 3 and 9 months of age, with a window up to 15–18 months of age. When children present with mild to moderate degrees of craniosynostosis, the decision to operate is less clear. The age of the child, as well as the severity of calvarial asymmetry, will dictate the rationale for corrective surgery. If the calvarial deformation is mild and the child is approaching 1 year of age, it is unlikely that they will need surgery. The most rapid portion of cerebral and consequently skull growth occurs during the first 6–12 months. Thus the child with a mild degree of deformity at the age of 12 months is unlikely to become significantly more pronounced over time. However, the amount of asymmetry is also likely to remain unchanged as the child grows older. The decision to operate should be made if the family is uncomfortable with the degree of calvarial deformation at that point in time, also remembering the psychosocial issues that will be encountered in the school setting. Nevertheless, it may be prudent to observe the child over a period of time to follow the growth and shape of the calvarium before any surgical decisions are made.

CLINICAL PRESENTATION/THERAPEUTIC CONSIDERATIONS

Metopic synostosis (trigonocephaly)

Clinical features

Premature closure of the metopic suture may lead to the formation of a triangular shaped head, otherwise known as trigonocephaly. While the metopic suture is normally closed by 9 months,[86] examples of physiological closure as early as 3 months have been noted in otherwise normal children.[87] Although the

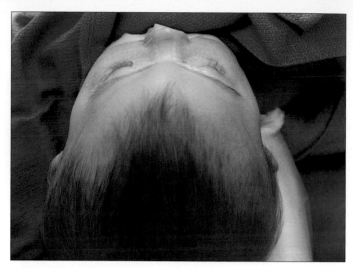

Figure 11.4 A 6-month-old infant with trigonocephaly, manifesting significant ridging over the midline (metopic suture), as well as supraorbital recession and hypotelorism.

presence of metopic synostosis is necessary for the development of trigonocephaly, not all children with premature closure of the metopic suture will develop trigonocephaly. In severe examples of trigonocephaly (Figure 11.4), the child's head will have a prominent "keel" forehead with recession of the lateral orbital rims, hypotelorism, and constriction of the anterior frontal fossa. The degree of severity is considerably variable and will direct the need for, as well as the type of, surgical intervention. Not uncommonly, patients may present with mild ridging of the metopic suture which remains stable and unaccompanied by other manifestations of trigonocephaly. These children are best served by conservative measures.[88]

Mild variants of metopic synostosis may represent familial inheritance[89,90] and have been recently associated with abnormalities of chromosomes 3, 9, and 11[70,91,92] in addition to positional plagiocephaly[93] and Chiari malformations. Tubbs and co-workers[94] found a 30% incidence of Chiari I malformation in the evaluation of patients with simple metopic ridges and postulated that these children were at greater risk secondary to the diminished anterior cranial volume. At the other end of the spectrum lie severe examples of trigonocephaly which not infrequently have associated underlying frontal brain dysmorphology as well as other congenital anomalies.[95] Children born with metopic synostosis comprise approximately 10% of all patients with craniosynostosis and show a male predominance of 3:1.[12–14] The rate of familial inheritance has been demonstrated to be 2–5% and it has been noted, similar for sagittal synostosis, that the rate of concordance in twinning is 7.8%.[96] A number of teratogens have been identified contributing to trigonocephaly, in particular valproic acid. While the majority of patients exhibit nonsyndromal examples of metopic synostosis, a significant number (10–22%) may manifest syndromal features[95,97] and remain at risk for additional congenital concerns as well as difficulty with cognitive function. Furthermore, these individuals not uncommonly demonstrate additional sutural involvement or may fail initial corrective surgical procedures. Although single-suture synostosis has a low incidence of associated mental retardation,[98] trigonocephaly has been observed to have the highest rate.[99] Sidoti and colleagues[100] followed 36 consecutive children with metopic synostosis and evaluated them for cognitive or behavioral disturbances. They found that 63% of their patients demonstrated normal intellect and behavior whereas 25% had mild learning difficulties and 12% had severe problems. They also noted that two children had chromosomal abnormalities. This is most likely related to the increased prevalence of concomitant cerebral abnormalities and is not related to restricted intracranial volume nor intracranial pressure abnormalities. Posnick and associates[90] demonstrated that intracranial volume measurements in patients with single-suture involvement of the metopic as well as sagittal sutures failed to manifest diminished volumes when compared with normal, age- and sex-related children.

Radiological evaluation

Radiographic imaging by plain skull radiographs may demonstrate a hyperostotic, midline metopic suture in addition to hypotelerotic orbits in severe examples of trigonocephaly. Nevertheless, definitive diagnosis is best made by CT which will offer better bone definition while also evaluating the cerebral parenchyma (Figure 11.5). Frontal dysmorphology is most commonly seen in this type of craniosynostosis and may consist of corpus callosum dysgenesis, holoprosencephaly as well as other frontal dysembryogeneses. Patients suspected of harboring a Chiari malformation are best served by an MRI, although CT scans with low cuts through the posterior fossa may also demonstrate a crowded foramen magnum as a result of tonsilar herniation.

Surgical therapeutics

The timing and extent of surgery will be directed by the severity of the frontal changes. The goals of surgery are the normalization of the forehead with reconstitution of a normal supraorbital rim if necessary.[101–106] Individuals presenting solely with a prominent midline keel may be best served by simple contouring of the frontal bone or by removal of the frontal bone flap followed by reconfiguration. These children otherwise demonstrate normal orbital and supraorbital anatomy. Consequently, patients with significant trigonocephaly and hypotelorism will need orbital reconstruction and may also require lateral expansion of the orbits at the same time. Delashaw and colleagues[107] proposed that metopic synostosis and trigonocephaly represent an embryological continuum and directed their surgical approach to deal with the various calvarial deficiencies. More recent modifications have been advocated[108–110] which provide for more radical treatment of the involved sphenoid bone as well as deal with simultaneous correction of the hypotelorism.

The essentials of a bifrontal advancement involve a standard bicoronal incision which will provide adequate exposure of the fronto-orbital region as well as minimizing any postoperative scar. Perioperative antibiotics (Oxacillin 50 mg/kg loading dose, 25 mg/kg intravenous every 6 h for 48 h) as well as steroids (Decadron 0.25 mg/kg intravenous every 6 h for 48 h) are given. Prior to the start of surgery, bilateral tarsorraphies are undertaken. In addition, the incision is infiltrated with 0.5% lidocaine and 1/400 000 parts epinephrine to minimize intraoperative bleeding. The frontal and temporalis regions are dissected in the subgaleal plane leaving the periosteum intact on the surface of the bone which also helps to minimize bleeding. The dissection is taken down to the level of the periorbital tissues, taking care to avoid any injury to the underlying globes. Following exposure of the frontal and orbital regions, the frontal bone is removed, providing access to the intracranial compartment (Figure 11.6A). The supraorbital rim is then removed in one piece to facilitate reconstruc-

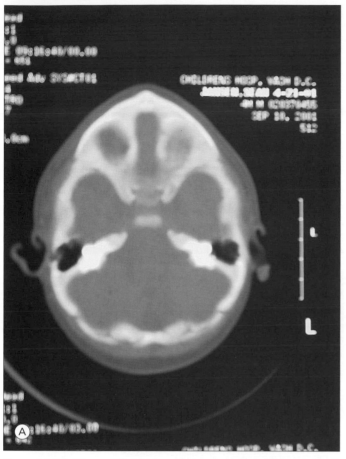 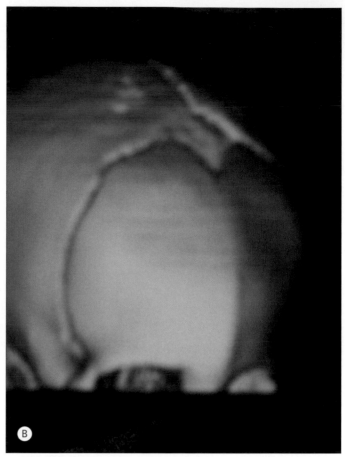

Figure 11.5 A CT scan **(A)** depicting the increased bone thickness over the midline at the region of the metopic suture as well as narrow intraorbital distance consistent with hypotelorism. The 3-D view **(B)** clearly demonstrates the fusion of the metopic suture as well as trigonocephaly.

tion of the previously triangular-shaped supraorbital bar. Care is taken to remove sufficient bone in the region of the sphenoid bone to allow for growth at the midface and orbits. If the orbits require correction of hypotelorism, it will be necessary to displace the lateral walls of the orbit as well as to split the midline and interpose a calvarial bone graft (Figure 11.6B–D). Reconfiguration of the supraorbital bar often requires a midline osteotomy to facilitate a flattened forehead with additional partial-thickness bone cuts at the lateral (pterional) angle to promote normalization of the lateral supraorbital angle. The supraorbital reconfiguration is maintained by the utilization of intervening bone grafts as well as absorbable hardware (Figure 11.6D). Following completion of the supraorbital bar which now functions as a foundation, the frontal bone is reconstructed using the remaining portions of bone. It is often possible to reverse the original frontal bone flap (posterior portion now in an anterior position) to obtain an adequate width and contour with the new frontal bone flap. It is important to provide an adequate enhancement at the pterional region to avoid long-term supratemporal hollowing or recession. Reconstruction may be facilitated by titanium or absorbable hardware. Nevertheless, the patients do remarkably well despite the extensive nature of reconstruction, and surgical morbidity is minimal.

Outcome and complications

The long-term outcome is generally excellent for > 90% of patients[95,111–116] unless there are manifestations of syndromic overlay. Children who initially do well but subsequently develop new metopic ridging, progressive frontal towering or continued laterosuperior fronto-orbital restriction[117] may require additional surgery for normative calvarial configuration. It has also been the author's experience to witness the subsequent development of additional sutural stenosis (sites other than the metopic suture) despite the lack of suture fusion or sclerosis at the time of the initial CT scan.

Surgical morbidity remains low for patients undergoing bifrontal advancements with wound infections, cerebrospinal fluid leaks, post-traumatic encephaloceles (Figure 11.7), orbital or neural injuries being relatively uncommon events. Post-transfusion reactions, as well as hemodynamic instability, constitute a greater danger to the patient and should never be underestimated.

The clinical spectrum of metopic synostosis remains wide. Nevertheless, children with severe deformities usually warrant surgical correction. The type and timing of correction must be tailored to the individual patient and the long-term results are excellent with minimal complications.

Sagittal synostosis (scaphocephaly, dolichocephaly)

Clinical features

Sagittal synostosis is the most common type of single-suture craniosynostosis. With a frequency of 1 per 1000 live births, sagittal synostosis represents 56–58% of reported craniosynostosis

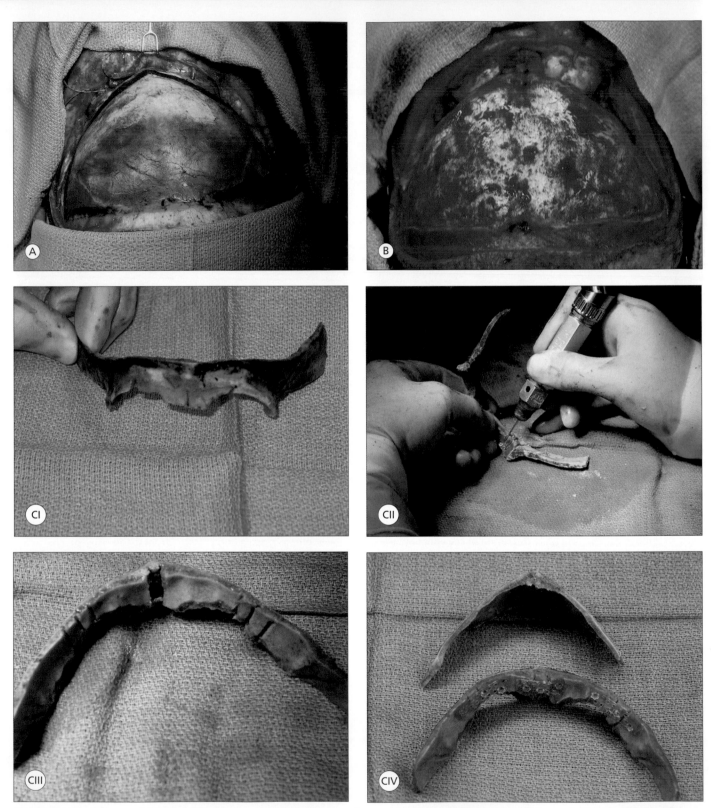

Figure 11.6 (A) Exposure of the frontal bone with synostosis of the metopic suture leading to trigonocephaly. **(B)** Removal of the frontal bone flap demonstrating significant hypotelorism and restricted frontal development. **(C) (I)** Removal of the supraorbital bandeau and subsequent partial osteotomies in the midline **(II and III)** and at the lateral wings to facilitate reconfiguration. A small piece of bone is placed in the midline **(IV)** to maintain a flat frontal contour whereas the lateral partial osteotomies allow for redirection of the lateral wings. **(IV)** Absorbable hardware on the internal surface will maintain the final configuration. After securing the frontal bandeau with absorbable hardware in the midline and lateral **(V)**, the remaining defects are filled with calvarial grafts **(VI)** ensuring a satisfactory frontal contour (avoiding increased towering). Note the degree of supraorbital advancement at the fronto- lateral dural margins **(V)**. **(D)** Frontal reconstruction is facilitated by the utilization of absorbable hardware and reconfigured frontal bone.

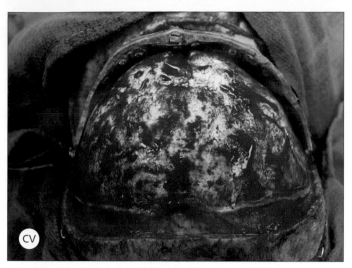

Figure 11.6, *cont'd.*

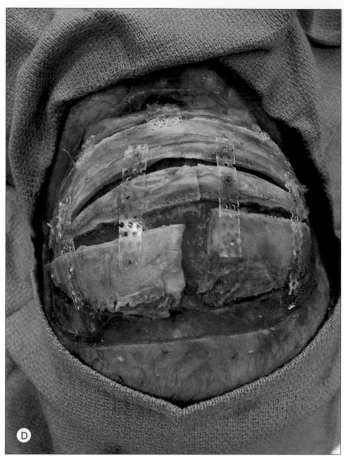

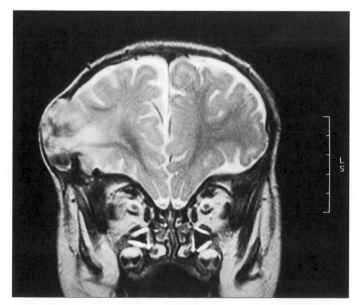

Figure 11.7 The presence of a leptomeningeal cyst after a prior subtotal calvarial reconstruction. This 26-month-old male had numerous episodes of post-surgical head banging with the subsequent development of right frontal swelling and eventual seizure. Dural repair and split-calvarial grafting corrected the problem (no hydrocephalus observed).

cases demonstrating single-suture pathology and manifests a significant male predominance by more than 2:1. Although the majority of cases occur sporadically, occasional familial patterns have been reported. Secondary sagittal closure may also be seen in children with significant ventriculomegaly following shunting procedures for hydrocephalus (~ 1%)[118,119] as well as infants who have undergone serious chronic neonatal illness and associated periods of immobility. Maternal smoking during gestation has also been demonstrated to be associated with an increase in sagittal synostosis when compared with controls.[16]

Children with sagittal synostosis will present with a narrow, elongated skull (*dolichocephaly* – long-headedness, *scaphocephaly* – keel-shaped). Some children also demonstrate characteristics of a "towering" skull (turricephaly). Depending upon the region of greatest premature fusion of the sagittal suture, the child will manifest frontal or occipital bossing, or a combination of both (Figure 11.8). Peri-sutural ridging is often associated at areas of fusion in addition to premature or occasionally delayed closure of the anterior fontanelle. In severe examples of scaphocephaly, these changes will be apparent at birth or may progress at a later age (up to 12–18 months). In older children, secondary changes in the skull base and mid-face constitute a greater surgical challenge.

The majority of children, even those with severe scaphocephaly, fail to manifest neurological abnormalities if only a single suture is involved. However, patients with multiple areas of premature sutural closure often demonstrate an increase in intracranial pressure promoting a more urgent surgical correction.

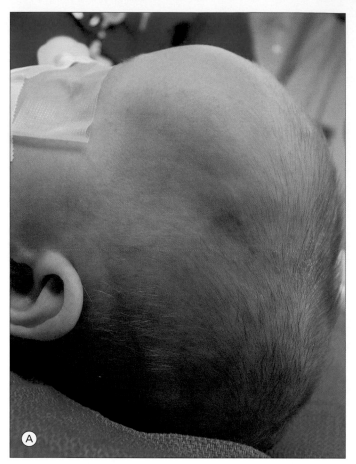 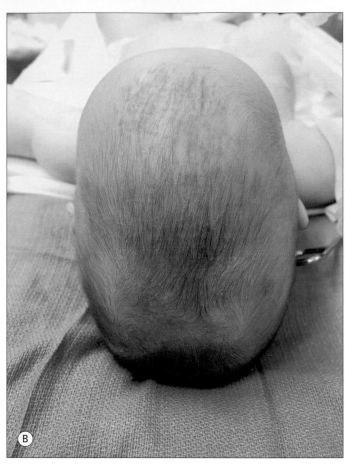

Figure 11.8 Calvarial elongation of a 4-month-old male with scaphocephaly. This child had both frontal **(A)** and occipital **(B)** bossing and underwent a Pi craniectomy with good results.

It has also been shown that a subset of affected individuals may harbor increased intracranial pressure.[120] Nevertheless, most cases of sagittal synostosis constitute a cosmetic and psychosocial problem, although the suggestion of increased intracranial pressure manifested by vomiting, lethargy, headaches, head circumference growth restriction, or developmental delay may warrant a radiological and ophthalmologic work-up. A CT scan with bone windows may demonstrate erosion of the inner table of the calvarium and crowding of the arachnoid cisterns which, when combined with clinical evidence of developmental delay, irritability and restricted skull volumes, remains the most sensitive barometer of this potentially dangerous condition.

Radiological evaluation

Although radiological work-up often starts in the office of the pediatrician with plain skull X-rays, the physical examination is often sufficient. The sagittal ridge can be palpated. There may be early closure of the anterior and/or posterior fontanelle. The yield on plain films may be poor, although good-quality films will demonstrate fusion or ridging of the sagittal suture. Occasionally, concurrent premature fusion of the coronal and/or lambdoid suture may be seen. Typically the calvarium is elongated and manifestations of increased intracranial pressure (e.g. digital markings) may occasionally be seen. In most cases the physical examination and clinical appearance remain the most sensitive and accurate indicators of sagittal synostosis.

All patients identified as requiring surgical correction benefit from a preoperative CT scan in our center. A subset of patients may also demonstrate a classical physical deformation consistent with pathophysiology at the sagittal suture with an otherwise normal radiographic work-up. It has been postulated that these children have "sticky sutures" secondary to microspicules of bone in the involved suture,[38] inhibiting normal growth and development of the calvarium. Nevertheless, these children exhibit similar morphological characteristics to those with clearcut fusion and may also benefit from calvarial reconfiguration in severe examples.

Three-dimensional CT may offer a more accurate depiction of the state of sutural fusion. Unanticipated intracranial pathology is seen in upwards of 5% of patients with sagittal synostosis,[57] including hydrocephalus, agenesis of the corpus callosum, and focal cortical dysplasia. In addition, expanded subarachnoid spaces, often bifrontal, are commonly seen in patients with sagittal synostosis[40,58] (Figure 11.9). Typically, this will resolve spontaneously and does not reflect increased general intracranial pressure.

Surgical therapeutics

The treatment for sagittal synostosis has changed considerably over the past 50 years, with surgical approaches evolving from minimal removal of involved suture and bone to extensive total calvarectomies as well as endoscopic procedures[121,122] and distraction techniques.[123–126] Despite relative long-term experience and

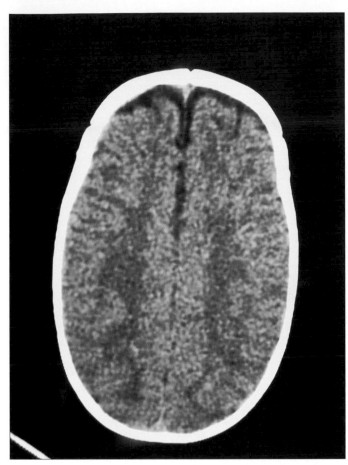

Figure 11.9 A CT scan of a 6-month-old male with sagittal synostosis. In addition to the elongated skull, note the expanded bifrontal subarachnoid spaces.

numerous publications, the "correct" surgical approach remains unclear even today. New techniques continue to be introduced each year[127] and long-term results remain variable. Indications and timing for surgery, as well as extent of bony resection and need for extensive reconstruction, all remain contested.

Currently, controversy continues to surround the optimal timing and choice of surgical procedure for sagittal synostosis. Many craniofacial surgeons recommend early surgery for severely affected children (deformity obvious at birth), to provide a better long-term result, in addition to avoiding the need for eventual extensive calvarial remodeling. However, there is less agreement as to the most appropriate treatment course for children presenting later than 3–6 months of age. Whereas indications for operative intervention are predominantly cosmetic; aesthetic results, recurrence rate, and complications are paramount issues for the surgeon and family.

Consequently, surgical treatment paradigms remain surrounded by controversy. Numerous proponents recommend a minimalist surgical role in contrast to those who favor a more aggressive approach. There is general agreement that earlier surgical intervention leads to better results and may avoid the need for extensive calvarial reconfiguration.[68,129–131] However, there is as yet no consensus on the best type of surgical approach to be used, even at a particular age. A number of simple approaches, proposed as early as 1892,[132–136] advocate the simple removal of the pathologic sagittal suture. Currently, there is a general understanding

that simple synostectomy may be sufficient in patients under the age of 2–3 months. However, patients are not always referred within this time-frame, and criticism has been directed to the overall cosmetic result and persistence of calvarial defects, as well as the increased incidence of restenosis of the sagittal suture.[137–140] Nevertheless, simple synostectomies are best performed by the age of 2–3 months to offer the best results and to minimize overall morbidity. Transfusion may be avoided in certain patients if meticulous hemostasis is maintained, although it is common practice to start transfusing at the initiation of the operation if a significant blood loss (> 10%) is expected in the infant. Numerous modifications to a single-strip craniectomy have also been proposed,[58,141–146] to offer greater biparietal expansion as well as more effective treatment of co-existent frontal or occipital prominences. Overall success of this operation is dependent upon initiation of surgical intervention prior to significant calvarial base and mid-face changes that inevitably occur at a later age. The extremely rapid cerebral growth in infants will help remodel the new calvarial reconfiguration.

The Pi procedure developed by Jane and colleagues[129] is a widely utilized approach for older infants (3–12 months of age) with scaphocephaly. Although multiple modifications with this approach have been proposed, including 12 different variations suggested by Jane depending upon the patient's clinical presentation,[142] the essential operative procedure involves removal of bone along both sides of the sagittal suture as well as bone over the coronal suture (or lambdoid for the reverse Pi) (Figure 11.10). The bone involving the suture as well as overlying the sagittal sinus is left intact to minimize bleeding. While the long-term results are generally excellent, Boop and colleagues reported three children from their series of 85 children operated upon over an 8-year period who had a poor result.[58] Older infants (> 9–12 months of age) as well as those children with significant frontal or occipital prominence will often require more aggressive craniectomies and reconstruction. A number of different approaches have been advocated, ranging from variations of the Pi procedure with wider or additional craniectomies over the lambdoid and/or coronal suture, to total calvarial reconfiguration. The indications for more aggressive surgical intervention with its concomitant increase in morbidity and even mortality remain controversial. Many believe that significant pathology at the skull base, as proposed by Moss[143,144] directs a larger procedure to be undertaken to provide optimal surgical correction, as well as avoiding potential recurrence. Thus, the rationale for total calvarectomy and reconstruction in the setting of severe or late presentation scaphocephaly,[145–150] has been proposed to offer superior cosmetic results with a minimal increase in morbidity. For children beyond the period of maximal cerebral growth (> 12–18 months of age), correction of the cephalic index will require substantial realignment of the calvarium and skull base. This may be accomplished by removal of the frontal and occipital bones as well as both parietal bones with subsequent reconfiguration providing a shortened anteroposterior shape in addition to widening of the biparietal diameter (Figure 11.11). The use of rigid fixation is indispensable in these cases and may provide for greater three-dimensional conformational stability as well as decreased intraoperative time, bleeding, and postoperative infection. Although questions have been raised regarding the use of hardware in the developing infant, there is less controversy in the older patients undergoing total calvarial reconstruction. In addition, the introduction and increasing use of absorbable plates and screws, has mitigated concerns regarding migration and inhibition of calvarial growth.

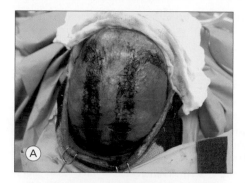

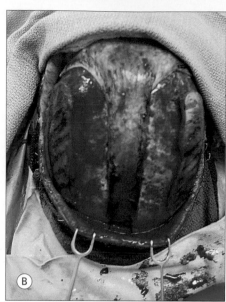

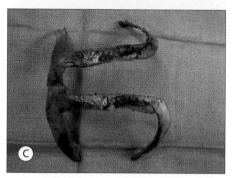

Figure 11.10 A 4-month-old child undergoing a modified Pi procedure. The craniectomies are made along both sides of the sagittal suture and posterior to the coronal/anterior to the lambdoid suture (A). The remaining bone in the midline is then brought forward with two sutures (B) which effectively shortens the antero-posterior length while widening the biparietal diameter, thus improving the cephalic index. The removed bone (C) has the appearance of the Greek symbol Pi and thus its name.

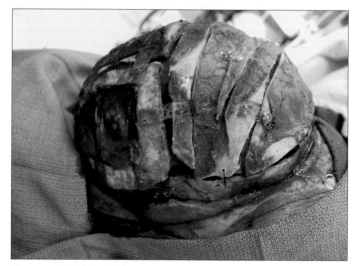

Figure 11.11 Older children with scaphocephaly are best served by a subtotal calvarial reconfiguration. Surgical objectives include widening the biparietal diameter as well as correcting any frontal/ occipital bossing or vertex depression. The use of absorbable plating systems has simplified the reconstruction considerably and they self-absorb over 12–18 months.

The patient presenting in a delayed fashion (after the age of 18–24 months) merits special consideration. Despite the lack of initial concern over the head shape, the significant calvarial deformity may become readily apparent as the child encounters greater social interaction through preschool, daycare, or even later in kindergarten. In addition to the myriad number of psychosocial issues,[151–153] a subset of individuals may also harbor elevated intracranial pressure.[154–158] Older children with significant scaphocephaly, often accompanied by both frontal and occipital bossing in association with mid-vertex depression, should be evaluated closely for any evidence of intracranial hypertension. The presence of headaches (especially exercise-induced), developmental delay, personality shifts, balance difficulties, or visual changes warrant an in-depth search for any other signs of increased intracranial pressure. Routine fundoscopic examination for papilledema is an accurate predictor of raised pressure in the older child but may not be 100% sensitive for the younger child (< 8 years old).[159] Radiological evaluation via CT may manifest early changes seen in association with elevated intracranial pressure; erosion of the inner calvarial table, diminished subarachnoid cisterns, as well as loss of cortical sulcal patterns may be observed in settings of increased pressure. The absence of any of the above signs or symptoms does not preclude the possibility of intracranial hypertension. It has been the author's experience to observe significant intracranial pressure elevations in patients with a paucity of clinical findings who have been monitored for subtle clinical changes or who present with moderate ventriculomegaly amenable to drainage/ monitoring at the time of reconstruction.

The author currently monitors older children undergoing repair of their scaphocephaly if there is any evidence (even subtle) for elevated intracranial pressure in addition to the presence of moderate ventriculomegaly. At the time of monitoring via a ventriculostomy, cerebrospinal fluid drainage is actively employed during calvarial reconfiguration to protect the brain from transient elevations in pressure. At the surgical conclusion, if intracranial pressures are normal (or have returned to a normal baseline), the ventriculostomy is removed prior to closure. In the event of uncertainty regarding persistently elevated intracranial pressure or when the diagnosis of hydrocephalus remains unclear, the ventricular drain may be left in place for postoperative monitoring.

Surgical considerations for delayed repair of scaphocephaly must consider the inherent risks and difficulties in the older child as well as technological challenges in correcting the significant calvarial deformities present at this point. Persistent calvarial defects postoperatively are common and secondary facial deformities remain uncorrected in this group of individuals. Nevertheless, numerous authors propose a variety of approaches for this entity,[160–162] which involve removal of the entire or near-total calvarium in one or two stages while taking into account the possibility of elevated intracranial pressure. Long-term results are considered good to excellent with similar morbidity as seen in the younger patients.

Outcome and complications

Despite countless literature accolades for all types of surgical treatment of scaphocephaly (from simple synostectomy to total calvarectomy), new approaches continue to be proposed on a regular basis for this "resolved" dilemma. Nevertheless, the lack of prospective as well as objective long-term data makes any comparison of results between different techniques relatively difficult.[163] There are, however, an increasing number of studies that address the outcome following surgery for sagittal synostosis. An objective improvement in biparietal intracranial volume was noted by Posnick and colleagues 13–47 months after sagittal osteotomy reconfiguration with graft fixation in eight patients.[164] Marsh and associates also demonstrated that pre- and post-operative cephalic indices were improved in the patients treated with more complex craniectomies.[159] McCarthy and colleagues[88] followed eight children for an average of 25 months after performing five vertex-strip craniectomies and three fronto-orbital advancements, of whom two had originally been treated by strip craniectomy. They considered seven of the eight patients to have had excellent results at the time of follow-up. Kaiser[159] reviewed the results of three different techniques in treating sagittal synostosis: simple, total vertex or more extended craniectomies followed for a mean of 4.7 years. Those children who underwent vertex or extended craniectomies were felt to show the best cosmetic results, although residual calvarial defects were seen in 11% of the children who had undergone more extensive surgery. To date, the longest follow-up after sagittal synostosis surgery is documented by Albright and colleagues.[165] They re-evaluated 25 children operated upon 5–10 years earlier using combinations of midline strip craniectomy, occipital craniectomy and bilateral parietal wedge craniectomies. Examination of these children by an independent investigator showed 23 of 25 children to have an "acceptable" appearance. The results in two children were deemed unacceptable; both were operated on late (3.3 years) and had an involved craniofacial syndrome. A more recent study from Spain[166] followed 210 patients over a 19-year period and noted that the best results were seen in the population < 3 months of age. These children received simple synostectomies leading to excellent outcomes with minimal morbidity.

A retrospective review by Boop and colleagues[58] of 85 children who underwent the Pi procedure revealed that 53% had an excellent correction (surgeon and family were both satisfied) and 43% were considered a good outcome (family alone was satisfied). While the length of follow-up was not clarified, the authors nevertheless felt that the optimum time for this procedure ranged between 3 and 6 months of age, and that the Pi procedure offered a better immediate and long-term correction of scaphocephaly. The three failures in this series were attributed to infants operated upon prior to 2 months of age, and were felt to be related to a more aggressive form of the disease associated with a higher risk of restenosis and poor long-term outcome. A retrospective review of outcome in Pi-plasty patients in Sweden[167] also demonstrated an increase in cephalic index from a preoperative mean of 65% to 72% in the postoperative setting.

Boop and others also reviewed outcome data between simple synostectomy and complex cranial reconstruction in 1996.[58] While direct comparison of the two approaches by the same surgeons was not performed, they nonetheless concluded that the morbidity for the complex procedures was minimally increased when compared with that of simple synostectomy. In addition, cosmesis was felt to be clearly superior in the complex craniectomy population and should "therefore, be considered the treatment of choice for most patients."

In another retrospective review of outcome between children receiving simple strip craniectomy compared with more extensive cranial vault remodeling at the same institution over a 10-year period,[168] no difference was seen in complication rate but a significant improvement in cosmetic outcomes was noted. Patients receiving the more complex surgery were rated excellent 79% versus 41% for the strip craniectomy group. In addition, the synostectomy group manifested calvarial defects in 59% of patients and required additional surgery for poor cosmetic results in two individuals.

Assessment of cranial index (cranial width/cranial length $\times$ 100) was undertaken, comparing patients operated upon before the age of 4 months and later, as well as comparing patients receiving strip craniectomy versus subtotal calvarectomy.[169] A majority of extended strip craniectomy patients did not achieve normal cranial width:length proportions in the first year whereas the percentage of improvement in the subtotal calvarectomy was significantly higher in reaching age-adjusted normal cephalic indices.

The morbidity for the treatment of sagittal synostosis varies according to the type of procedure performed and the age of the patient. Simple synostectomy performed during the first 3 months of life provides minimal surgical risk. However, there is still a risk from anesthesia in an infant, as well as the possibility of inadvertent injury to the sagittal sinus and massive blood loss. While some pediatric neurosurgeons routinely hold blood transfusion for this type of procedure until indicated by blood loss, others feel that transfusion should take place at the start of the case.[67]

Children who undergo more complex craniectomies are often thought to have an increased risk of surgical morbidity, although there are several reports in the literature to the contrary. Children treated by the Pi procedure in the series of 85 patients experienced only three simple dural lacerations, all of which were recognized and repaired without difficulty.[58]

Kanev and Lo[170] noted in their retrospective analysis of 45 patients treated by an extended Pi procedure over 4 years, that complications "compared favorably with other repair techniques." Their average reduction in anteroposterior length was 1.44 cm and their mean blood loss was 96 mL (11 mL/kg). Dural injuries were seen in three patients and one postoperative seizure was observed. McComb's series of 24 patients who underwent biparietal widening and occipital reduction also showed no major operative morbidity.

The majority of patients undergoing extensive craniectomies and calvarial reconfiguration can be expected to require longer surgical procedures as well as needing intraoperative transfusion. The routine practice of offering donor-designated blood (immediate family) to parents of children who undergo this surgery theoretically decreases the potential risk of viral transmission, though it is also effective in reducing parental anxiety. Hentschel and colleagues[171] noted a drop in transfusion rate from 42% to 11% in age/surgery-adjusted patients over time. They attributed this to the acceptance of a lower postoperative hemoglobin level

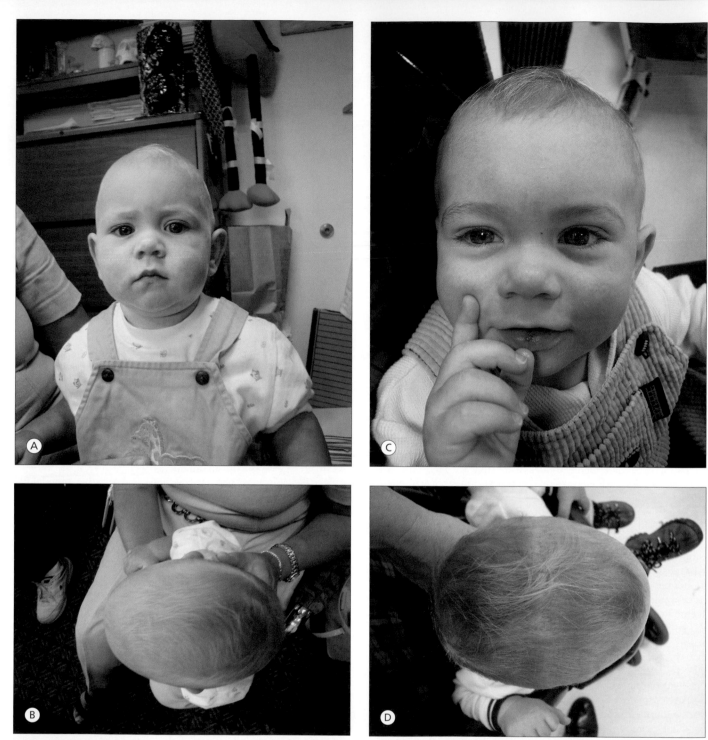

Figure 11.12 Pre **(A,B)** and postoperative **(C,D)** (1 month) photographs of a 13-month-old male with moderate scaphocephaly who underwent an anterior 2/3 calvarectomy to improve his cephalic index and decrease his frontal bossing. Note the peaked nature of his vertex, occasionally seen in patients with a combination of metopic and sagittal involvement, in the preoperative photo.

as well as better surgical technique employing microfibrillar collagen, hypotension, and a coagulating scalpel at skin incision. The use of aprotinen has recently been demonstrated to also significantly decrease the need for transfusion in extensive craniofacial procedures.[172] The majority of larger surgical procedures require less than 1 unit of blood, which has the same risk of viral transmission as a blood loss of 75 cm^3 in an infant requiring a

transfusion after a simple synostectomy. When the differences between simple and complex surgery for sagittal synostosis were reviewed, comparing the need of blood transfusion as well as length of hospitalization and expense,[58] the more complex procedures showed little overall morbidity with improved outcome. The authors felt they easily justified the added length of stay in decreasing the likelihood of recurrence and need for subsequent surgery. In a similar experience, Maugans and colleagues[168] demonstrated an average blood loss of 243 cm³ versus 54 cm³ in more complex sagittal synostosis surgery when compared with strip craniectomy. They also document a 100% transfusion rate compared with 38% for the simple surgical patients.

Endoscope-assisted strip craniectomies in conjunction with cranial orthotic molding helmets being pioneered by Jimenez and colleagues[72] were performed at less than 16 weeks of age in 63% of one series of patients, and offered satisfactory short-term results.

While selection of the correct operative procedure for sagittal synostosis remains controversial, it is becoming increasingly clear that these children may benefit from early surgical intervention (Figure 11.12). Infants in whom synostosis is recognized before the age of 2–3 months, will likely show excellent improvement after simple synostectomy with a lower risk of blood transfusion and minimal perioperative morbidity. Nevertheless, a small number of these patients will eventually require secondary procedures for recurrent sagittal synostosis or unsatisfactory cosmetic outcomes.

A growing number of craniofacial surgeons believe that more extensive craniectomies or total calvarial reconfiguration may offer the best chance of a satisfactory cosmetic outcome with a minimally increased but acceptable risk of morbidity. The envelope will continue to be tested by alternative approaches including endoscopic techniques[173] as well as distraction devices,[130-134] molding helmets,[174] and perhaps even transcutaneous implanted magnets.[175] Nevertheless, the future is likely to bring universal acceptance of resorbable rigid fixation and improved surgical techniques. The type of procedure will likely remain a matter of individual preference and no doubt will continue to undergo scrutiny in the search for the "ultimate" reconstruction.

Coronal synostosis (plagiocephaly/brachycephaly)

Closure of a single coronal suture will manifest as anterior plagiocephaly (in contrast to posterior plagiocephaly seen with lambdoid synostosis) whereas bilateral coronal involvement will lead to brachycephaly. Unilateral plagiocephaly occurs in 1:10 000 live births and constitutes approximately 20–25% of all craniosynostosis. Similar to the lambdoid presentation, coronal positional plagiocephaly is very common and believed to occur in 25–50% of live births secondary to *in utero* molding.[176] More often on the left side of the forehead, positional plagiocephaly is often associated with other congenital conditions secondary to inhibited fetal growth: talipes equinovarus, genovarus, congenital hip dysplasia, micrognathia, and torticollis. Radiological evaluation fails to demonstrate any sutural fusion and the deformity is usually self-limiting, resolving spontaneously.

The patient with true coronal synostosis will manifest a flattened ipsilateral forehead with compensatory overgrowth in the region of the contralateral orbit. The involved side often appears elevated when compared with the other orbit and characteristically is recessed at the orbit as well as forehead, in conjunction with a palpable coronal peri-sutural ridge (Figure 11.13). The presence of a "harlequin" appearance is caused by the superior elevation of the sphenoid wing on skull X-rays and is considered pathognomic for coronal synostosis. The presence of strabismus is common (50–60%) and results from a shortened anterior skull base posteriorly displacing the orbital roof and trochlea which in turn contributes to an imbalance at the superior oblique muscle and decreases its function.[177,178] While correction of the plagiocephaly occasionally improves the strabismus, surgery is frequently needed for ultimate correction. Subsequently, children affected with bilateral closure of their coronal sutures (often syndromic) present with a widened biparietal diameter in addition to frontal towering, known as brachycephaly.

Surgical therapeutics

Surgical indications are predominantly cosmetic although ocular considerations regarding orbital normalization, strabismus and stereoscopic vision may also be important.[179,180] The goal of surgical correction is advancement of the affected orbit with frequent recession of the contralateral orbit, undertaken by a bifronto-orbital advancement.[181-183] Whereas unilateral coronal synostosis presents with bilateral dysmorphic changes, the optimum approach is now believed to be a bilateral correction.[184,185]

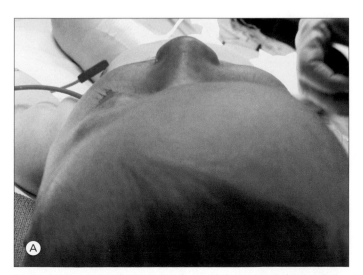
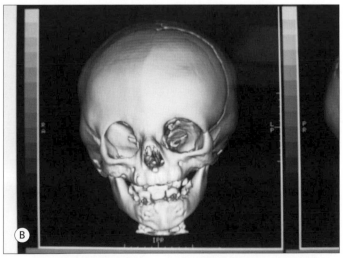

Figure 11.13 A 6-month-old male infant with left coronal plagiocephaly, manifesting significant retrusion over the left orbital and supraorbital region **(A)**. Note the compensatory overgrowth on the contralateral side at the forehead as well as face. **(B)** The three-dimensional CT depicts the elevation of the left orbit as part of the "harlequin" eye.

The timing of surgery however remains controversial with an increasing number of craniofacial surgeons favoring earlier surgery.[62,63,65,68,111,186–189] Surgical intervention is commonly made by 3 months up to 8–10 months with good long-term results in conjunction with minimal morbidity. In addition, to standard bifronto-orbital advancement techniques, endoscopic approaches[71] have been used successfully, as well as the recent introduction of distraction techniques.[190,191]

The surgical approach for both unilateral and bilateral coronal synostosis involves the bilateral release of both coronal sutures while providing a bilateral frontal correction. A standard bicoronal skin incision (after placing bilateral tarsorraphies) is followed by removal of the frontal bone leaving a 1–2 cm wide supraorbital bandeau. Extending the osteotomy posterior to the coronal suture will often provide adequate width on this portion of the bone flap for a satisfactory new frontal reconstruction (when this piece is inverted (Figure 11.14). Care must be taken when performing the osteotomy across the sphenoid wing on the involved side. As seen on plain skull X-rays depicting the characteristic "harlequin" eye, the sphenoid wing is often enlarged as well as elevated. This may in turn lead to technical difficulty when attempting to remove the frontal bone flap while making an osteotomy across the sphenoid wing leading to dural laceration if caution is not exercised. After removal of the frontal bone flap, the orbital bandeau is freed from the orbital roof and lateral orbits with osteotomies taken across the lateral orbit at the fronto-zygomatic suture, through the orbital roof and at the nasion just above the nasofrontal suture. Great care is undertaken to protect the underlying brain as well as orbital contents with judicious placement of retractors. The bandeau is then reconfigured via partial osteotomies at the midline while utilizing absorbable hardware on the interior surface to maintain the newly normalized contour. It is frequently necessary to overcorrect (5–10%) when pushing out the affected side while also providing a sharp turn at the lateral border to provide a satisfactory reconstruction (Figure 11.15). The newly configured supraorbital bar is replaced, often with a mild recession at the unaffected side to compensate for correction of the preoperative compensatory overgrowth. The lateral aspects of the bandeau as well as midline are fixed to the calvarial foundation with rigid fixation (absorbable/titanium hardware) for improved healing and postoperative maintenance of the surgical construct. The frontal bone flap is attached to the supraorbital bar taking care to match the previously overbuilt (5–10%) orbital bandeau on the affected side. It is not uncommon to find varying degrees of recession in the pterional area over time[192,193] and numerous factors have been implicated as contributing to this area of hypodevelopment, including atrophy of the temporalis muscle as well as continued restriction of growth at the affected junction of the coronal and squamosal sutures. For this reason, the sphenoid wing is removed down to the level of the clinoid process to open the suture to the level of the skull base (Figure 11.16) and in the author's experience this has led to a decreased incidence of postoperative hollowing of the supratemporal region. Remaining portions of bone are fixed with absorbable plates or suture, and closure is performed in a routine fashion employing subgaleal drains.

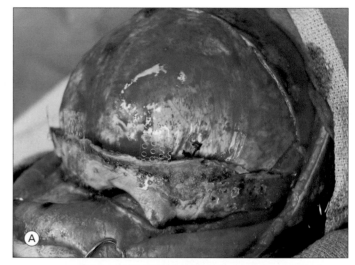

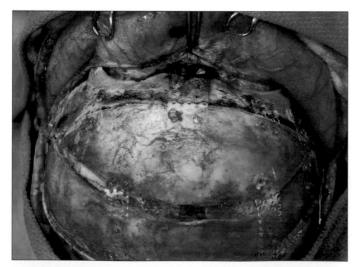

Figure 11.14 After removal and reconfiguration of the frontal bandeau, the frontal bone is returned providing normalization of the forehead. It is often possible to invert the original frontal bone to provide an adequate width and contour for the newly constructed supraorbital region. Absorbable hardware helps to maintain a slight over-correction on the previously affected side.

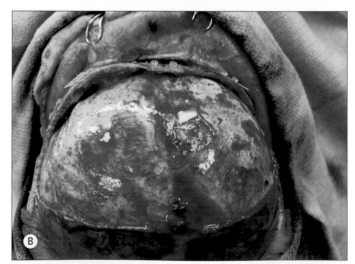

Figure 11.15 (A,B) Reconstruction of the newly configured frontal bandeau utilizing absorbable plates and screws. Note the advancement on the patient's affected left side and mild recession on the contralateral side.

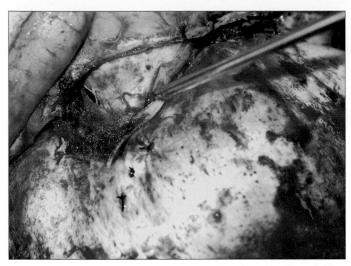

Figure 11.16 The sphenoid wing is over-developed on the affected side in coronal synostosis and is removed to facilitate subsequent growth at this location. Inadequate removal may lead to future restriction at the pterional region.

Outcome and complications

The majority of children undergoing a bifronto-orbital advancement for coronal (unilateral/bilateral) synostosis initially manifest significant improvement at the level of the fronto-orbital involvement. Perioperative morbidity, ranging as high as 6.8%[67] may include wound infection, dural laceration, superficial brain injury, cerebrospinal fluid leak, encephalocele formation, subgaleal hematoma, transfusion reaction, and ocular injury including corneal abrasion. More serious complications, including ischemic brain injury, epidural and subdural hemorrhage, severe transfusion reactions and even death, are considerably less common and have been reported approximating 1%.[194] While most patients with unilateral coronal synostosis demonstrate excellent postoperative results,[194-196] individuals treated for bilateral coronal disease[187,197-199] often require secondary surgery because of the frequent syndromic association. In addition to the common occurrence of supratemporal recession seen in both unilateral and bilateral conditions, patients with bilateral synostosis not infrequently manifest frontal bossing and towering, known as turricephaly. Despite unsatisfactory cosmesis, the presence of turricephaly may indicate underlying increased intracranial pressure as a result of restricted circumferential growth at the skull base or in turn related to the development of hydrocephalus. The presence of towering in conjunction with supraorbital scalloping (recession) should alert the clinician to the possibility of raised intracranial pressure and requires an in-depth evaluation including a head CT with bone windows, opthalmological review and a detailed examination and history inspecting head-circumference growth curves and developmental milestone progression. It is not uncommon for patients with intracranial hypertension to manifest a paucity of clinical signs and symptoms and its recognition thus resides with the clinical acumen of the craniofacial surgeon. Other long-term postoperative concerns involve persistent calvarial deformities including defects in coverage that fail to fill in over time. Defects > 2 cm in patients older than 18–24 months will often persist and may need eventual correction. In older patients (> 18 months) attention is directed to avoiding such calvarial gaps at the surgical conclusion. Persistent

hardware may also be problematic, particularly in patients in whom absorbable hardware was utilized. It is not uncommon for the polylactic/polyglycolic constructs to remain in place for 12–18 months before eventual resorption. In rare individuals, sterile abscesses may develop and subsequently require exploration for debridement. Fortunately, this is a self-limiting process. Nevertheless, the majority of patients do remarkably well and have excellent long-term outcomes.

Lambdoid synostosis (posterior plagiocephaly)

The majority of posterior plagiocephaly seen today represents positional molding or posterior plagiocephaly without synostosis, promoted by a supine sleeping position recommended in the early 1990s after reports appeared in the literature demonstrating a reduced incidence of sudden infant death syndrome with infants placed in this position for their sleeping habits. Early reports of unnecessary surgery culminated in the publication of numerous front-page articles in the lay press and in other media venues. True lambdoid synostosis is a relatively rare event and represents 2–4% of all craniosynostosis. Infants placed in a supine sleeping position appeared to have an increased predilection for persistent flattening over one side of the occiput particularly in the setting of pre-existing torticollis.

Nevertheless, the differentiation between "true" lambdoid synostosis and positional plagiocephaly remains critical when choosing the appropriate course of treatment. A number of investigators[72,200-202] have reviewed their experience with patients presenting with occipital flattening and have noted incidences of "true" lambdoid synostosis ranging from 0.9 to 4%. Despite a few morphological similarities between nonsynostotic and synostotic posterior plagiocephaly, significant morphological differences do exist helping to separate the two entities on clinical grounds.[79,203] Children with lambdoid synostosis characteristically have a trapezoid-shaped head in association with a posteriorly displaced ear, contralateral occipital bossing, and frequently manifest ridging of the lambdoid suture. This is in contrast to the parallelogram-shaped head, anterior displacement of the tragus and ipsilateral frontal bossing usually seen with positional molding or posterio plagiocephaly without synostosis (Figure 11.17). Positional molding or posterior plagiocephaly has been noted to be more common on the right, in males, and is frequently associated with torticollis. Assessment of infants in day-care centers in the Netherlands, evaluated 7609 children below the age of 6 months for positional molding.[204] This extensive screening found an incidence of positional molding in 8.2% of the general population and also noted that firstborns, premature infants and children born in a breech position appeared to be at higher risk. The same study documented that over a 2-year follow-up, 45% of the children continued to manifest occipital asymmetry and 21% had persistent frontal changes in the setting of conservative management. Nevertheless, infants receiving aggressive positional modifications of their sleep habits as well as treatment of any underlying torticollis, in addition to those treated by cranial orthotic correction (Figure 11.18) generally demonstrated satisfactory cosmetic improvement in approximately 95% of affected individuals. Whereas both treatment modalities appear to offer excellent long-term correction of positional molding, it remains unclear today which therapeutic approach offers the greatest efficacy. While a number of studies[205-209] offer data that support their own treatment choice, the results nonetheless remain conflicting. A majority of clinicians presently offer advice and

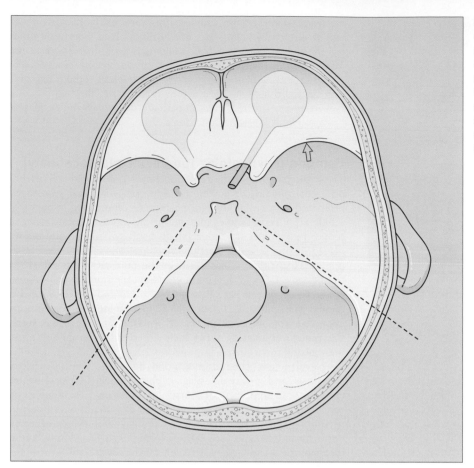

Figure 11.17 Changes at the skull base associated with posititional molding or posteriorl plagiocephaly are consistent with a parallelogram deformity. The petrous ridge as well as tragus are displaced in an anterior direction in addition to compensatory growth of the forehead and occasionally the face. Conversely, true lambdoid synostosis results in a more trapezoid skull and often pulls the tragus in an inferior and posterior direction.

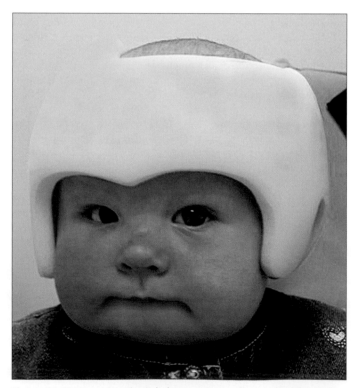

Figure 11.18 Dynamic orthotic helmet used to redirect calvarial growth in children with positional molding or posterior plagiocephaly.

recommend techniques to change the sleeping position and address torticollis issues as an initial course, reserving the orthotic helmets for patients who fail to demonstrate significant improvement.

Surgical therapeutics

Infants with true lambdoid synostosis may benefit from a variety of surgical approaches. Surgical objectives include the release of the affected suture as well as normalization of the posterior calvarial vault. A number of different approaches have been proposed[78–84,210–215] ranging from simple synostectomy, unilateral reconfiguration of the affected occipital region to bilateral occipital reconstruction including the use of an occipital bandeau. The majority of lambdoid surgical candidates have significant parietal and frontal compensatory changes in addition to their occipital deformation and are thus often best served by a more extended calvarectomy and reconstruction, removing both parietal and occipital bone in a bilateral fashion. Patients are positioned in a prone fashion ensuring adequate protection of the orbits. A standard bi-coronal skin incision is undertaken, employing care during the opening to minimize blood loss. Both parietal bone flaps are subsequently removed with osteotomies taken behind the coronal and anterior to the lambdoid sutures. A midline strip of bone is then left to protect the underlying sagittal sinus. After removal of the parietal bone flaps, dissection is carried out at the level of the lambdoid suture under direct visualization, taking great caution at the level of the transverse, sagittal and sigmoid sinuses. Osteotomies are brought to within 1 cm on either side of the midline, with the final cut made after the underlying dura and sinus have been clearly dissected free under direct vision. Inadvertent entry into the sinus, particularly at the region of the asterion, can lead to significant blood loss over a short period and constitutes the greatest risk encountered for this approach. Nevertheless, with appropriate care and attention, this complication may be avoided in the majority of individuals. The removed calvarial plates are then reconfigured to provide adequate normalization of the occipital contour (Figure 11.19) and postoperative fixation may be accomplished with absorbable or titanium microplates and screws; subgaleal drains are routinely employed.

Outcome and complications

Normalization of the posterior cranial vault is satisfactory in > 93% of infants[78,81] and carries minimal morbidity with rare mortality. If surgical correction is undertaken before 15–18 months of age, it is likely that the associated ipsilateral frontal compensatory bossing will normalize over time. Older patients, as well as those with significant frontal deformity, will require more time for correction of distant sites of calvarial deformity and may see changes taking place over 4–5 years. Complications consist of wound infections, transfusion-related problems, hemorrhage, dural injury, and rare intracerebral injury.

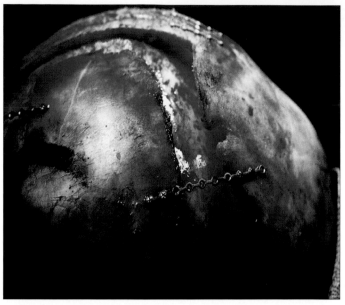

Figure 11.19 Previous removal of parietal and occipital bones will allow reconstruction of the parieto-occipital contour in a normalized fashion. The region of the prior lambdoid suture is left open via the use of rigid fixation.

CLINICAL PEARLS

- Growth of the skull will be arrested in the direction perpendicular to the affected suture (Virchow's rule) and subsequent compensatory growth will occur at the unaffected sutures leading to characteristic calvarial deformations. In addition, the skull base and calvarial development are inter-related and changes at one location may affect the growth parameters at the other location.

- Elevation of intracranial pressure is uncommon in the setting of single-suture craniosynostosis, whereas children with multiple suture involvement (syndromic) are at increased risk for intracranial hypertension and must be followed closely.

- Children with syndromic craniosynostosis suspected of having elevated intracranial pressure may present with irritability, feeding difficulties, failure to thrive, headache, developmental delays, visual changes, calvarial towering, supraorbital recession, or lack of circumferential skull growth. The absence of any of the above does not preclude the possibility of intracranial hypertension and the clinician must remain vigilant for any signs or symptoms of elevated pressure.

- An increasing number of growth factors (FGF, TGF, EGF, PDGF), as well as transcription factors MSX2 and TWIST, have been implicated in the pathogenesis of craniosynostosis and this list will undoubtedly grow in the future as a greater understanding of genetic influences unfolds.

- Positional molding or posterior plagiocephaly without synostosis, promoted by a supine sleeping position, will generally resolve with changes in sleeping position, resolution of associated torticollis or with orthotic devices and is only rarely a surgical condition. True lambdoid synostosis is a rare condition and is characterized by a trapezoid shaped skull versus the parallelogram-shaped skull seen in positional molding.

- The optimal timing of craniosynostosis surgery remains controversial even today, although significant data appear to support better long-term results with earlier surgery (3–9 months). Since the normal brain and skull grow most rapidly in the first 2 years of life, early surgery takes advantage of this rapid period of growth and facilitates skull expansion and cranial volume during a period when this would normally occur.

- Numerous surgical approaches (synostectomy, endoscopic, total calvarial reconfiguration) have been utilized in the treatment of scaphocephaly, each with its own advantages and weaknesses. Overall, the results are excellent with most approaches that increase the biparietal diameter with minimal morbidity, but currently there is no distinct method that offers significant advantage over any other surgical approach.

CONCLUSION

Significant advances over the past decade have contributed to the improvement in diagnosis and treatment of craniosynostosis while concurrently reducing the risks involved in its surgical treatment. An understanding of the genetic underpinnings has allowed investigators an in-depth view of the potential mechanisms involved in the abnormal development of a cranial suture and may eventually lead to new approaches in future treatment.

New surgical treatment methods continue to refine the operative arena, with enhanced cosmetic outcomes and decreasing rates of recurrence. Distraction techniques will undoubtedly play a greater role in the surgical correction of craniosynostosis, as will new bone substitutes. In time, answers will be forthcoming with respect to the appropriate type of surgery for each type of craniosynostosis in addition to the optimum timing for correction. The value of orthotic devices in the setting of positional plagiocephaly will be eventually clarified by objective prospective data. Nevertheless, the future will help to clarify some of the current issues facing the craniofacial surgeon and no doubt will also bring new challenges to the forefront.

This chapter contains material from the first edition, and I am grateful to the authors of that chapter for their contribution.

REFERENCES

1. Virchow R. Uber den Cretinismus, namentlich in Franken, und uber pathologische Schadelformen. *Verh Phys med Gesellsc*
2. Sommerring ST. *Vom Baue des menschlichen Korpers*, 2nd edn. Leipzig: Voss, 1839; 1851; 2: 230–70.
3. Moss ML. The pathogenesis of premature cranial synostosis in man. *Acta Anat (Basel)* 1959; 37: 351–70.
4. Persson KM, Roy WA, Persing JA, *et al*. Craniofacial growth following experimental craniosynostosis and craniectomy in rabbits. *J Neurosurg* 1979; 50: 187–97.
5. Babler WJ, Persing JA. Alterations in cranial suture growth associated with premature closure of the sagittal suture in rabbits. *Anat Rec* 1985; 211: 14A.
6. Persing JA,Babler WJ, Jane JA, *et al*. Experimental unilateral coronal synostosis in rabbits. *Plast Reconstr Surg* 1986; 77: 369–76.
7. Shuper A, Grunebaum M, Reisner SH. The incidence of craniosynostosis in the newborn infant. *Am J Dis Child* 1985; 139: 85–6.
8. Chung CS,Myriatholpoulos NC. Factors affecting risks of congenital malformations: epidemiological analysis. *Birth Defects* 1975; 11: 1–22.
9. Lajeunie E, Le Merrer, Bonaiti-Pellie C, *et al*. Genetic study of nonsyndromic coronal synostosis. *Am J Med Genet* 1995; 55: 500–4.
10. Lajeunie E, Le Merrer, Bonaiti-Pellie C, *et al*. Genetic study of scaphocephaly. *Am J Med Genet* 1996; 62: 282–5.
11. Hunter AGW, Rudd NL. Craniosynostosis I. Sagittal synostosis: its genetics, and associated clinical findings in 214 patients who lacked involvement of the coronal suture. *Teratology* 1976; 14: 185–93.
12. Tessier P. Relationship of craniosynostosis to craniofacial dysostosis, and to faciostenosis – a study with therapeutic implications. *Plastic Reconst Surg* 1971; 48: 224–37.
13. Anderson FM, Geiger LE. Craniosynostosis: a survey of 204 cases. *J Neurosurg* 1965; 22: 229–40.
14. Shillito J Jr, Matson DD. Craniosynostosis: a review of 519 surgical patients. *Pediatrics* 1968; 41: 829–53.
15. Cohen MM Jr. Sutural biology and the correlates of craniosynostosis. *Am J Med Genet* 1993; 47: 581–616.
16. Atkinson FRB. Hereditary craniofacial dysotosis, or Crouzon's disease. *Med Press Circular* 1937; 195: 118–24.
17. Kallen K. Maternal smoking and craniosynostosis. *Teratology* 1999; 60: 146–50.
18. Wilkie AOM, Morriss-Kay GM, Jones EY *et al*. Functions of fibroblast growth factors and their receptors. *Curr Biol* 1995; 5: 500–7.
19. Muenke M, Schell U. Fibroblast growth-factor receptor mutations in human skeletal disorders. *Trends Genet* 1995; 11: 308–13.
20. Jabs EW, Li X, Scott AF. Jackson–Weiss and Crouzon syndromes are allelic with mutations in fibroblast growth factor receptor-2. *Nat Genet* 1994; 8: 275–9.
21. Muenke M, Schell U, Hehr A, *et al*. A common mutation in the fibroblast growth receptor 1 gene in Pfeiffer syndrome. *Nat Genet* 1994; 8: 269–74.
22. Wilkie AOM, Slanet SF, Oldridge M. Apert syndrome results from localized mutations of FGFR2 and is allelic with Crouzon syndrome. *Nat Genet* 1995; 9: 165–72.
23. Ibrahimi OA, Eliseenkova AV, Plotnikov AN, *et al*. Structural basis for fibroblast growth factor 2 receptor activation in Apert syndrome. *Proc Natl Acad Sci USA* 2001; 98: 7182–7.
24. Plomp AS, Hamel BC, Cobben JM, *et al*. Pfeiffer syndrome type 2: further delineation and review of the literature. *Am J Med Genet* 1998; 75: 245–51.
25. Sarkar S, Petiot A, Copp A *et al*. FGF2 promotes skeletogenic differentiation of cranial neural crest cells. *Development* 2001; 128: 2143–52.
26. Lomri A, Lemonnier J, Hott M, *et al*. Increased calvaria cell differentiation and bone matrix formation induced by fibroblast growth receptor 2 mutations in Apert syndrome. *J Clin Invest* 1998; 101: 1310–17.
27. Moursi AM, Winnard PL, Winnard AV *et al*. Fibroblast growth factor 2 induces increased calvarial osteoblast proliferation and cranial suture fusion. *Cleft Palate Craniofac J* 2002; 39: 487–96.
28. Greenwald JA, Mehrara BJ, Spector JA *et al*. In vivo modulation of FGF biological activity alters cranial suture fate. *Am J Pathol* 2001; 158: 441–52.
29. Gripp KW, McDonald-McGinn DM, Gaudenz K, *et al*. Identification of a genetic cause for isolated unilateral coronal synostosis: a unique mutation in the fibroblast growth factor receptor 3. *J Pediatr* 1998; 132: 714–16.
30. Huneko O, Karmacharya J, Ong G, *et al*. Toward an understanding of nonsyndromic craniosynostosis: altered patterns of TGF-beta receptor and FGF receptor expression induced by intrauterine head constraint. *Ann Plast Surg* 2001; 46: 546–54.
31. Kirschner RE, Gannon FH, Xu J, *et al*. Craniosynostosis and altered patterns of fetal TGF-beta expression induced by intrauterine constraint. *Plast Reconst Surg* 2002; 109: 2338–54.
32. Lin KY, Nolen AA, Gampper TJ, *et al*. Elevated levels of transforming growth factors beta 2 and beta 3 in lambdoid sutures from children with persistent plagiocephaly. *Cleft Palate Craniofac J* 1997; 34: 331–7.
33. Pensler JM, Ivescu AS, Radosevich JA. Scaphocephaly: premature closure of the sagittal suture: a localized disorder of cellular metabolism? *Ann Plast Surg* 1998; 40: 48–52.
34. Nah H. Suture biology: lessons from molecular genetics of craniosynostosis syndromes. *Clin Orthodont Res* 2000; 3: 37–45.
35. Jabs EW, Muller U, Li X, *et al*. A mutation in the homeodomain of the human MSX2 gene in a family affected with autosomal dominant craniosynostosis. *Cell* 1993; 75: 443–50.

36. Liu YH, Kundu R, Wu L, *et al*. Premature suture closure and ectopic cranial bone in mice expressing MSX2 transgenes in the developing skull. *Proc Natl Acad Sci USA* 1995; 92: 6137–41.

37. Clarren SK, Smith DW, Hansen JW. Helmut treatment for plagiocephaly and congenital muscular torticollis. *J Pediatr* 1979; 94: 43–6.

38. Clarren SK. Plagiocephaly and torticollis: etiology, natural history, and helmut therapy. *J Pediatr* 1981; 98: 92–5.

39. Ripley AE, Pomatto J, Beals SP, *et al*. Treatment of positional plagiocephaly with dynamic orthotic cranioplasty. *J Craniofacial Surg* 1994; 5: 150–9.

40. Burke MJ, Winston KR, Williams S. Normal sutural fusion and the etiology of single suture craniosynostosis: the microspicule hypothesis. *Pediatr Neurosurg* 1995; 22: 241.

41. Moss ML. Experimental alteration of sutural area morphology. *Acta Anat (Basel)* 1957; 127: 569–90.

42. Smith DW, Tondury G. Origin of the calvaria and its sutures. *Am J Dis Child* 1978; 132: 662–6.

43. Moss ML. Functional anatomy of cranial synostosis. *Childs Brain* 1975; 1: 22–33.

44. Markens IS. Transplantation of the future coronal suture to the dura mater of 3 to 4 month old rats. *Acta Anat (Basel)* 1975; 93: 29–44.

45. Furtwangler JA, Hall SH, Koskinen-Moffet LK. Structural morphogenesis in the mouse calvaria: the role of apoptosis. *Acta Anat (Basel)* 1985; 124: 74–80.

46. Opperman LA, Sweenney TM, Redmon J, *et al*. Tissue interactions with underlying dural mater inhibit osseous obliteration of developing cranial sutures. *Dev Dyn* 1993; 198: 312–22.

47. Opperman LA, Passarelli RW, Morgan EP, *et al*. Cranial sutures require tissue interactions with dura mater to resist osseous obliteration *in vitro*. *J Bone Miner Res* 1995; 10: 1978–87.

48. Drake D, Persing JA, Berman DE, *et al*. Calvarial deformity regeneration following subtotal calvarectomy for craniosynostosis: a case report and theoretical implications. *J Craniofac Surg* 1993; 4: 85–9.

49. Mabutt LW, Kokich VG. Calvarial and suture development following craniectomy in neonatal rabbits. *J Anat* 1979; 129: 413–22.

50. Abbott AH, Netherway DJ, Niemann DB, *et al*. CT-determined intracranial volume for a normal population. *J Craniofac Surg* 2000; 11: 211–23.

51. Van der Ham LI, Cohen-Overbeek TE, Paz y Geuze HD, *et al*. The ultrasound detection of an isolated craniosynostosis. *Prenat Diagn* 1995; 15: 1189–92.

52. Stelniki EJ, Mooney MP, Losken HW, *et al*. Ultrasound prenatal diagnosis of coronal suture synostosis. *J Craniofac Surg* 1997; 8: 252–61.

53. Miller C, Losken HW, Towbin R, *et al*. Ultrasound diagnosis of craniosynostosis. *Cleft Palate Craniofac J* 2002; 39: 73–80.

54. Levi D, Rampa F, Barbieri C, *et al*. True 3D reconstruction for planning of surgery on malformed skulls. *Childs Nerv Sys* 2002; 18: 705–6.

55. Girod S, Teschner M, Schrell U, *et al*. Computer-aided 3-D simulation and prediction of craniofacial surgery: a new approach. *J Craniomaxillofac Surg* 2001; 29: 156–8.

56. Perlyn CA, Marsh JL, Vannier MW, *et al*. The craniofacial anomalies archive at St. Louis Children's Hospital: 20 years of craniofacial imaging experience. *Plast Reconstr Surg* 2001; 108: 1862–70.

57. Cerovac S, Neil-Dwyer JG, Rich P, *et al*. Are routine preoperative CT scans necessary in the management of single suture craniosynostosis? *Br J Neurosurg* 2002; 16: 348–54.

58. Boop FA, Chadduck WM, Shewmake K, Teo C. Outcome analysis of 85 patients undergoing the pi procedure for correction of sagittal synostosis. *J Neurosurg* 1996; 85: 50–5.

59. Chadduck WM, Chadduck JB, Boop FA. The subaracnoid spaces in craniosynostosis. *Neurosurgery* 1992; 30: 867–71.

60. Renier D, Sainte-Rose C, Marchac D, *et al*. Intracranial pressure in craniosynostosis. *J Neurosurg* 1982; 57: 370–7.

61. Pertschuk MJ, Whitaker LA. Psychosocial adjustments and craniofacial malformations in childhood. *Plast Reconstr Surg* 1985; 75: 177–82.

62. Barrit J, Brooksbank M, Simpson D. Scaphocephaly: aesthetic and psychosocial considerations. *Dev Med Child Neurol* 1981; 23: 183–91.

63. Whitaker LA, Bartlett SP, Schut L, *et al*. Craniosynostosis: an analysis of the timing, treatment, and complications in 164 consecutive patients. *Plast Reconstr Surg* 1987; 80: 195–212.

64. Laurent JP, Balasubramanian C, Stal S, *et al*. Early surgical management of coronal synostosis. *Clin Plast Surg* 1990; 17: 183–7.

65. Dhellemmes P, Pellerin P, Vinchon M, *et al*. Surgery for craniosynostosis: timing and technique [French]. *Ann Fr Anesth Reanim* 2002; 21: 103–10.

66. Marchac D, Renier D, Broumand S. Timing of treatment for craniosynostosis and facio-craniosynostosis: a 20-year experience. *Br J Plast Surg* 1994; 47: 211–2.

67. Sloan GM, Wells KC, Raffel C. Surgical treatment of craniosynostosis: outcome analysis of 250 consecutive patients. *Pediatrics* 1997; 100: E2.

68. Shillito J. A plea for early operation for craniosynostosis. *Surg Neurol* 1992; 37: 182–8.

69. McCarthy JG, Cutting CB. The timing of surgical intervention in craniofacial anomalies. *Clin Plast Surg* 1990; 17: 161.

70. Obregon MG, Mingarelli R, Digilio MC, Zelante L, Giannotti A, Sabatino G, Dallapiccola B. Deletion 11q23—>qter (Jacobsen syndrome). Report of three new patients. *Ann Genet* 1992; 35: 208–12.

71. Persing J, Babler W, Winn HR, *et al*. Age as a critical factor in the success of surgical correction of craniosynostosis. *J Neurosurg* 1981; 54: 610–16.

72. Jimenez DF, Barone CM, Cartwright CC, *et al*. Early management of craniosynostosis using endoscopic-assisted strip craniectomies and cranial orthotic molding therapy. *Pediatrics* 2002; 110: 97–104.

73. David LR, Genecov DG, Camastra AA, *et al*. Positron emission tomography studies confirm the need for early surgical intervention in patients with single-suture craniosynostosis. *J Craniofac Surg*. 1999; 10: 38–42.

74. Clarren SK, Plagiocephaly and torticollis: etiology, natural history, and helmut treatment. *J Pediatr* 1981; 98: 92–5.

75. Ripley AE, Pomatto J, Beals SP, Joganic EF, Manwaring KH, Moss SD. Treatment of ositional Plagiocephaly with dynamic orthotic cranioplasty. *J Craniofac Surg* 1994; 5: 150–9.

76. Kane AA, Mitchell LE, Craven KP, *et al*. Observations on a recent increase in plagiocephaly without synostosis. *Pediatrics* 1996; 97: 877–85.

77. Najarian SP. Infant cranial molding deformation and sleep position: implications for primary care. *J Pediatr Health Care* 1999; 13: 173–7.

78. Willinger M, Hoffman HJ, Hartford RB. Infant sleep position and risk for sudden infant death syndrome: report of Meeting held January 13 and 14, 1994, National Institutes of Health, Bethesda, MD. *Pediatrics* 1994; 93: 814–20.

79. Keating RF. Surgical management of posterior plagiocephaly and postional deformation. *Techniques in Neurosurg* 1997; 3: 198–206.

80. David DJ, Menard RM. Occipital plagiocephaly. *Br J Plast Surg* 2000; 53: 367–77.

81. Jimenez DF, Barone CM, Argamaso RV, *et al*. Asterion region synostosis. *Cleft Palate Craniofac J* 1994; 31: 136–41.

82. Goodrich JT, Argamaso R. Labroid stenosis (posterior plagiocephaly) and craniofacial asymmetry: long term outcomes. *Childs Nerv Sys* 1996; 12: 720–6.

83. Jimenez DF, Barone CM. The sunrise technique: the correction of occipital plagiocephaly using bandeau occipital plate and radial osteotomies. *Pediatr Neurosurg* 1995; 22: 162–6.

84. McComb JG. Treatment of functional lambdoid synostosis. *Neurosurg Clin N Am* 1991; 2: 665–72.

85. Dias MS, Klein DM, Blackstrom JW. Occipital plagiocephaly: deformation or lambdoid synostosis? I. Morphometric analysis and results of unilateral lambdoid craniectomy. *Pediatr Neurosurg* 1996; 24: 61–8.

86. Manzanares MC, Goret-Nicaise M, Dhem A. Metopic sutural closure in the human skull. *J Anat* 1988; 161: 203–15.

87. Vu HL, Panchal J, Parker EE *et al*. The timing of physiological closure of the metopic suture: a review of 159 patients using reconstructed 3D CT scans of the craniofacial region. *J Craniofac Surg* 2001; 12: 527–32.

88. McCarthy JG, Glasberg SB, Cutting CB, *et al*. Twenty year experience with early surgery for craniosynostosis: I. Isolated craniofacial synostosis—results and unsolved problems. *Plast Reconstr Surg* 1995; 96: 272–84.

89. Frydman M, Kauschansky A, Elian P. Trigonocephaly: a new familial syndrome. *Am J Med Genet* 1984; 18: 55–9.

90. Posnick JC, Armstrong D, Bite U. Metopic and sagittal synostosis: intracranial volume measurements prior to and after cranio-orbital reshaping in childhood. *Plast Reconstr Surg* 1995; 96: 299–315.

91. Preus M, Vekemans M, Kaplan P. Diagnosis of chromosome 3 duplication q23–qter, deletion p25-pter in a patient with the C (trigonocephaly) syndrome. *Am J Med Genet* 1986; 23: 935–43.

92. Teebi AS, Gibson L, McGrath J, Mey MS, Breg WR, Yang-Feng TL. Molecular and cytogenetic characterization of 9p-abnormalities. *Am J Med Genet* 1993; 46: 288–92.

93. Murarka A, Moore MH. Coincident metopic synostosis and deformational plagiocephaly. *J Craniofac Surg* 1999; 10: 473–4.

94. Tubbs RS, Elton S, Blount JP, *et al*.. Preliminary observations on the association between simple metopic ridging in children without trigonocephaly and the Chiari I malformation. *Pediatr Neurosurg* 2001; 35: 136–9.

95. Schneider EN, Bogdanow A, Goodrich JT, *et al*. Fronto-ocular syndrome: newly recognized trigonocephaly syndrome. *Am J Med Genet* 2000; 93: 89–93.

96. Lajeunie E, Le Merrer M, Marchac D, *et al*. Syndromal and nonsyndromal primary trigonocephaly: analysis of a series of 237 patients. *Am J Med Genet* 1998; 75: 211–15.

97. Collmann H, Sorensen N, Krauss J. Consensus: trigonocephaly. *Childs Nerv Sys* 1996; 12: 664–8.

98. Kapp-Simon KA. Mental development and learning disorders in children with single suture craniosynostosis. *Cleft Palate Craniofac J* 1998; 35: 197–203.

99. Shillito J, Matson DD. Craniosynostosis: A review of 519 surgical patients. *Pediatrics* 1968; 41: 829–53.

100. Sidoti EJ Jr, Marsh JL, Marty-Grames L, *et al*. Long-term studies of metopic synostosis: frequency of cognitive impairment and behavioral disturbances. *Plast Reconst Surg* 1996; 97: 276–81.

101. Anderson FM. Treatment of coronal and metopic synostosis: 107 cases. *Neurosurgery* 1981; 8: 143–9.

102. Marsh JL, Schwartz HG. The surgical correction of coronal and metopic craniosynostosis. *J Neurosurg* 1983; 59: 245–51.

103. Salkind G, Sutton LN, Bruce DA, *et al*. Management of trigonocephaly. *Surg Neurol* 1986; 25: 159–62.

104. Oi S, Matsumoto S. Trigonocephaly (metopic synostosis). Clinical, surgical, and anatomical concepts. *Childs Nerv Sys* 1987; 3: 259–65.

105. Shaffrey ME, Persing JA, Delashaw JB, *et al*. Surgical treatment of metopic synostosis. *Neurosurg Clin N Am* 1991; 2: 621–7.

106. Fearon JA, Kolar JC, Munro IA. Trigonocephaly-associated hypotelorism: is treatment necessary? *Plast Reconstr Surg* 1996; 97: 510–11.

107. Delashaw JB, Persing JA, Park TS, Jane JA. Surgical approaches for the correction of metopic synostosis. *Neurosurgery* 1986; 19: 228–34.

108. Goodrich JT, Hall CD. Metopic synsotosis and trigonocephaly: a spectrum of dysmorphology. In Goodrich JT, Hall CD (eds). *Craniofacial Anomalies: Growth and Development from a Surgical Perspective*. New York: Thieme; 1995: 15–22.

109. Sadove AM, Kalsbeck JE, Eppley BL, Javed T. Modifications in the surgical correction of trigonocephaly. *Plast Reconstr Surg* 1990; 85: 853–8.

110. McCarthy JG, Bradley JP, Longaker MT. Step expansion of the frontal bar: correction of trigonocephaly. *J Craniofac Surg* 1996; 7: 333–5.

111. DiRocco C, Verladi F, Ferrario A. Metopic synostosis: in favor of a "simplified" surgical treatment. *Childs Nerv Sys* 1996; 12: 654–63.

112. Cohen SR, Maher H, Wagner JD *et al*. Metopic synotosis: evaluation of aesthetic results. *Plast Reconstr Surg* 1994; 94: 759–67.

113. Wall SA, Goldin JH, Hockley AD *et al*. Fronto-orbital reoperation in craniosynostosis. *Br J Plast Surg* 1994; 47: 180–4.

114. Posnick JC, Lin KY, Chen P *et al*. Metopic synostosis: quantitative assessment of presenting deformity and surgical results based on CT scans. *Plast Reconstr Surg* 1994; 93: 16–24.

115. Dhellemmes P, Pellerin P, Lejeune JP. Surgical treatment of trigonocephaly. Experience with 30 cases. *Childs Nerv Syst* 1986; 2: 228–32.

116. Albin RE, Hendee RW Jr, O'Donnell RS *et al*. Trigonocephaly: refinements in reconstruction. Experiences with 33 patients. *Plast Reconst Surg* 1985; 76: 202–11.

117. Persing JA, Mayer P, Spinelli H. Prevention of temporal hallowing following fronto-orbital advancement for craniosynostosis. *J Craniofac Surg* 1994; 50: 187–97.

118. Anderson H. Craniosynostosis as a complication after operation for hydrocephalus. *Acta Paediatr Scand* 1966; 55: 192.

119. Pudenz RH, Foltz EL, Hydrocephalus: overdrainage by ventricular shunts: A review and recommendations. *Surg Neurol* 1991; 35: 200.

120. Renier D, Sainte-Rose C, Marchac D, *et al*. Intracranial pressure in craniosynostosis. *J Neurosurg* 1982; 57: 370–7.

121. Jimenez DF, Barone CM. Endoscopic craniectomy for early surgical correction of sagittal craniosynostosis. *J Neurosurg* 1998; 88: 77–81.

122. Cohen SR, Holmes RE, Meltzer HS, Nakaji P. Immediate cranial vault reconstruction with bioresorbable plates following endoscopically assisted sagittal synostectomy. *J Craniofac Surg* 2002; 13: 578–84.

123. Imai K, Kommune H, Toda C, *et al*. Cranial remodeling to treat craniosynostosis by gradual distraction using a new device. *J Neurosurg* 2002; 96: 654–9.

124. Matsumoto K, Nakanishi H, Seike T, *et al*. Application of the distraction technique to scaphocephaly. *J Craniofac Surg* 2000; 11: 172–6.

125. Greensmith AL, Furneaux C, Rees M, *et al.* Cranial compression by reverse distraction: a new technique for correction of sagittal synostosis. *Plast Reconstr Surg* 2001; 108: 979–85.

126. Sugawara Y, Hirabayashi S, Sakurai A, *et al.* Gradual cranial vault expansion for the treatment of craniofacial synostosis: a preliminary report. *Ann Plast Surg* 1998; 40: 554–65.

127. Smith JL, Boaz JC, Eppley BL, *et al.* Late correction of sagittal craniosynostosis: The "Crab Procedure". *American Society of Pediatric Neurosurgeons Annual Meeting*, February 6, 2003.

128. Paul RP, Sugar O. Zenker solution in the surgical treatment of cranial synostosis. *J Neurosurg* 1972; 6: 604–7.

129. Jane JA, Edgerton MT, Futrell JW, *et al.* Immediate correction of sagittal synostosis. *J Neurosurg* 1978; 49: 705–10.

130. McCarthy JG, Epstein F, Sadove M, *et al.* Early surgery for craniofacial synostosi: an 8 year experience. *Plast Reconstr Surg* 1984; 73: 521.

131. McLaurin RL, Matson DD. Importance of early surgical treatment of craniosynostosis: review of 36 cases treated during the first six months of life. *Pediatrics* 1952; 10: 637–50.

132. Lane LC. Pioneer craniectomy for the relief of mental imbecility due to premature sutural closure and microcephalus. *JAMA* 1892; 18: 49.

133. Venes JL, Sayers MP. Sagittal synostectomy: technical note. *J Neurosurg* 1976; 44: 390–2.

134. Albright AL. Operative normalization of skull shape in sagittal synostosis. *Neurosurgery* 1985; 17: 329–31.

135. Olds MV, Storrs B, Walker ML. Surgical treatment of sagittal synostosis. *Neurosurgery* 1986; 18: 345–7.

136. Boop FA, Shewmake K, Chadduck WM. Synostectomy versus complex cranioplasty for the treatment of sagittal synostosis. *Childs Nerv Sys* 1996; 12: 371–5.

137. Marsh JL, Jenny A, Galic M, Picker S, Vannier MW. Surgical management of sagittal synostosis: a quantatative evaluation of two techniques. *Neurosurg Clinics North Am* 1991; 2: 629–40.

138. Greene CS Jr, Winston KR. Treatment of scaphalocephaly with sagittal craniectomy and biparietal morcellation. *Neurosurgery* 1988; 23: 196–202.

139. McComb JG. Occipital reduction—biparietal widening technique for correction of sagittal synostosis. *Pediatr Neurosurg* 1994; 20: 99–106.

140. Vollmer DG, Jane JA, Park TS, *et al.* Variants of sagittal synostosis: strategies for surgical correction. *J Neurosurg* 1984; 61: 557–62.

141. Christophis P, Junger TH, Howaldt HP. Surgical correction of scaphocephaly: experiences with a new procedure and follow-up investigations. *J Maxillofac Surg* 2001; 29: 33–8.

142. Jane JA, Francel PC. The evolution of treatment for sagittal synostosis: a personal record. In Goodrich JT, Hall CD (eds). *Craniofacial Anomalies: Growth and Development from a Surgical Perspective.* New York: Thieme; 1995: 15–22.

143. Moss ML, Salentijn L. The primary role of functional matrices in facial growth. *Am J Orthodont* 1969; 55: 566.

144. Moss ML. Functional anatomy of cranial synostosis. *Child Brain* 1975; 1: 22.

145. Burstein FD, Hudgins RJ, Cohen SR, Boydston WR. Surgical correction of severe scaphocephalic deformites. *J Craniofac Surg* 1994; 5: 228–35.

146. Marchac D, Renier D. *Craniofacial Surgery Craniosynostosis.* Boston: Little, Brown, 1982.

147. Epstein N, Epstein F, Newman G. Total vertex craniectomy for the treatment of scaphalocephaly. *Child Brain* 1982; 9: 309.

148. Hudgins RJ, Burstein FD, Boydston WR. Total calvarial reconstruction for sagittal synostosis in older infants and children. *J Neurosurg* 1993; 78: 119.

149. Pensler JM, Ciletti SJ, Tomita T. Late correction of sagittal synostosis in children. *Plast Reconstr Surg* 1996; 97: 1362–70.

150. Shuster BA, Norbash AM, Schendel SA. Correction of scaphalocephaly secondary to ventricular shunting procedures. *Plast Reconstr Surg* 1995; 96: 1012–19.

151. Barritt J, Brooksbank M, Simpson D. Scaphocephaly: aesthetic and psychosocial considerations. *Dev Med Child Neurol* 1981; 23: 183–91.

152. Magge SN, Westerveld M, Pruzinsky T, *et al.* Long-term neuropsychological effects of saggital craniosynostosis on child development. *J Craniofac Surg* 2002; 13: 99–104.

153. Kapp-Simon KA. Mental development and learning disorders in children with single suture craniosynostosis. *Cleft Palate Craniofac J* 1998; 35: 197–203.

154. Martinez-Lage JF, Alamo L, Poza M. Raised intracranial pressure in minimal forms of craniosynostosis. *Childs Nerv Syst* 1999; 15: 11–16.

155. Cohen SR, Persing JA. Intracranial pressure in single-suture craniosynostosis. *Cleft Palate Craniofac J* 1998; 35: 194–6.

156. Stavrou P, Sgouros S, Willshaw HE, *et al.* Visual failure caused by raised intracranial pressure in craniosynostosis. *Childs Nerv Syst* 1997; 13: 64–7.

157. Tuite GF, Chong WK, Evanson J, *et al.* The effectiveness of papilledema as an indicator of raised intracranial pressure in children with craniosynostosis. *Neurosurgery* 1996; 38: 272–8.

158. Thompson DN, Malcolm GP, Jones BM, *et al.* Intracranial pressure in single-suture craniosynostosis. *Pediatr Neurosurg* 1995; 22: 235–40.

159. Kaiser G, Sagittal synostis: Its clinical significance and the results of three different methods of craniectomy. *Childs Nerv Sys* 1988; 4: 223–30.

160. Weinzweig J, Baker SB, Whitaker LA *et al.* Delayed cranial vault reconstruction for sagittal synostosis in older children: an algorithm for tailoring the reconstructive approach to the craniofacial deformity. *Plast Reconstr Surg* 2002; 110: 397–408.

161. Sutton LN, Bartlett SP, Duhaime AC, *et al.* Total cranial vault reconstruction for the older child with scaphocephaly. *Pediatr Neurosurg* 1993; 19: 63–72.

162. Hudgins RJ, Burstein FD, Boydston WR. Total calvarial reconstruction for sagittal synostosis in older infants and children. *J Neurosurg* 1993; 78: 199–204.

163. Keating RF, Cogen PH. Sagittal synostosis: current approaches to evaluation and treatment. In: Benzel EC, Rengachary SS (eds). *Calvarial and Dural Reconstruction AANS Neurosurgical Topics Series, AANS Publications.* Washington, DC: AANS; 1998: 141–8.

164. Posnick JC, Armstrong D, Bite U. Metopic and sagittal synostosis: intracranial volume measurements prior to and after cranio-orbital reshaping in childhood. *Plast Reconstr Surg* 1995; 96: 299–309.

165. Albright AL, Towbin RB, Shultz BL. Long-term outcome after sagittal synostosis operations. *Pediatr Neurosurg* 1996; 25: 78–82.

166. Alvarez-Garijo JA, Cavadas PC, Vila MM, *et al.* Sagittal synostosis: results of surgical treatment in 210 patients. *Childs Nerv Syst* 2001; 17: 64–8.

167. Guimaraes-Ferreira J, Gewalli F, David L, *et al.* Clinical outcome of the modified pi-plasty procedure for sagittal synostosis. *J Craniofac Surg* 2001; 12: 218–26.

168. Maugans TA, McComb JG, Levy ML. Surgical management of sagittal synostosis: a comparative analysis of strip craniectomy and calvarial vault remodeling. *Pediatr Neurosurg* 1997; 27: 137–48.

169. Panchal J, Marsh JL, Park TS, *et al.* Sagittal craniosynostosis outcome assessment for two methods and timings of intervention. *Plast Reconstr Surg* 1999; 103: 1574–84.

170. Kanev PM, Lo AK. Surgical correction of sagittal craniosynostosis: complications of the Pi procedure. *J Craniofac Surg* 1995; 6: 98–102.

171. Hentschel S, Steinbok P, Cochrane DD, *et al*. Reduction of transfusion rates in the surgical correction of sagittal synostosis. *J Neurosurg* 2002; 97: 503–9.

172. Muraszko KM, D'Errico CC, Buchman SR, *et al*. Efficacy of aprotinin in children undergoing craniofacial surgery. *American Society of Pediatric Neurosurgeons Annual Meeting*, Kona, Hi, February 6, 2003.

173. Barone CM, Jimenez DF. Endoscopic craniectomy for early correction of craniosynostosis. *Plast Reconstr Surg* 1999; 104: 1965–75.

174. Seymour-Dempsey K, Baumgartner JE, Teichgraeber JF, *et al*. Molding helmet therapy in the management of sagittal synostosis. *J Craniofac Surg* 2002; 13: 631–5.

175. Pittman T, Rinehart GC, Hagan R, *et al*. Cranial vault moulding by the transcutaneous activation of implanted magnets. *Pediatr Neurosurg* 1997; 27: 78–83.

176. Graham JM Jr, Badura RJ, Smith DW. Coronal craniostenosis: fetal head constraint as one possible cause. *Pediatrics* 1980; 65: 995–9.

177. Baglioni B, Campos E, Chiesi C, *et al*. Plagiocephaly causing superior oblique deficiency and ocular torticollis. *Arch Opthalmol* 1982; 100: 1093–2001.

178. Gosain AK, Steele MA, McCarthy JG, *et al*. A prospective study of the relationship between strabismus and head posture in patients with frontal plagiocephaly. *Plast Reconstr Surg* 1996; 97: 881–91.

179. Lauer SA, Keating RF. *The Craniosynostoses: A Practical Guide for Ophthalmologists, Advances in Clinical Opthalmology*. Chicago: Mosby; 1996: Vol. 3: 263–290.

180. Lo LJ, Marsh JL, Kane AA, *et al*. Orbital dysmorphology in unilateral coronal synostosis. *Cleft Plalate Craniofac J* 1996; 33: 190–7.

181. Persing JA, Jane JA, Delashaw JB. Treatment of bilateral coronal synostosis in infancy: a holistic approach. *J Neurosurg* 1990; 72: 171–5.

182. Lauritzen C, Friede H, Elander A, *et al*. Dynamic cranioplasty for brachycephaly. *Plast Reconstr Surg* 1996; 98: 7–14.

183. Posnick JC. Unilateral coronal synostosis (anterior plagiocephaly): current clinical perspectives. *Ann Plast Surg* 1996; 36: 430–47.

184. Bartlett SP, Whitaker LA, Marchac D. The operative treatment of isolated craniofacial dysotosis (plagiocephaly): a comparison of the unilateral and bilateral techniques. *Plast Reconstr Surg* 1990; 85: 677–83.

185. Sgouros S, Goldin JH, Hockley AD, *et al*. Surgery for unilateral coronal synostosis (plagiocephaly): unilateral or bilateral correction? *J Craniofac Surg* 1996; 7: 284–9.

186. Hoffman HJ, Hendrick EB. Early neurosurgical repair in craniofacial dysmorphism. *J Neurosurg* 1979; 51: 796–803.

187. Di Rocco C, Verladi F, Sette MP. Early surgical management of coronal and metopic craniosynostosis. *Z Kinderchir* 1981; 34:184.

188. Marsh JI, Schwartz HG. The surgical correction of metopic and coronal craniosynostosis. *J Neurosurg* 1983; 59: 245–233.

189. Marchado HR, Hoffman HJ. Long term results after lateral canthal advancement for unilateral coronal synostosis. *J Neurosurg* 1992; 76: 401–7.

190. Hirabayshi S, Sugawara Y, Sakurai A, *et al*. Frontoorbital advancement by gradual distraction. Technical note. *J Neurosurg* 1998; 89: 1058–61.

191. Kobayshi S, Honda T, Saitoh A, *et al*. Unilateral coronal synostosis treated by internal distraction. *J Craniofac Surg* 1999; 10: 467–72.

192. Losken HW, Pollack IF, Singhai VK. Vascularized fronto-orbital advancement. *J Craniofac Surg* 1996; 7: 107–10.

193. Persing JA, Jane JA, Park TS, *et al*. Floating C-shaped orbital rim advancement in craniosynostosis: preliminary report. *J Neurosurg* 1990; 72: 22–6.

194. Pollack IF, Losken HW, Fasick P. Diagnosis and management of posterior plagiocephaly. *Pediatrics* 1997; 99: 180–5.

195. Hoffman HJ. Procedure of lateral canthal advancement for the treatment of coronal synostosis. *Childs Nerv Sys* 1996; 12: 678–82.

196. Breugem CC, van Zeeman BJ. Retrospective study of nonsyndromic craniosynostosis treated over a 10-year period. *J Craniofac Surg* 1999; 10: 140–3.

197. Wagner JD, Cohen SR, Maher H, *et al*. Critical analysis of results of craniofacial surgery for nonsyndromic bicoronal synostosis. *J Craniofac Surg* 1995; 6: 32–9.

198. Donauer E, Bernardy M, Neuenfeldt D. T-bone plasique for treatment of brachy-turricephaly. *Acta Neurochir (Wien)* 1993; 120–31.

199. Persing JA, Jane JA. Treatment of syndromic and nonsyndromic bilateral coronal synostosis in infancy and childhood. *Neurosurg Clin N Am* 1991; 2: 655–63.

200. Mulliken JB, Van der Woude DL, Hansen M, *et al*. Analysis of posterior plagiocephaly: deformational versus synostotic. *Plast Reconstr Surg* 1999; 103: 371–80.

201. Huang MH, Gruss JS, Clarren SK, *et al*. The differential diagnosis of posterior plagiocephaly: true lambdoid synostosis versus positional molding. *Plast Reconst Surg* 1996; 98: 765–76.

202. Ellenbogen RG, Gruss JS, Cunningham ML. Update on craniofacial surgery: the differential diagnosis of lambdoid synostosis/posterior plagiocephaly. *Clin Neurosurg* 2000; 47: 303–18.

203. Boere-Boonekamp MM, van der Linden-Kuiper LT. Positional preference: prevalence in infants and follow-up after two years. *Pediatrics* 2001; 107: 339–43.

204. Carson BS, Munoz D, Gross G, *et al*. As assistive device for the treatment of positional plagiocephaly. *J Craniofac Surg* 2000; 11: 177–83.

205. Aliberti F, Pittore L, Ruggiero C, *et al*. The treatment of the positional plagiocephaly with a new thermoplastic orthotic device. *Childs Nerv Sys* 2002; 18: 337–9.

206. Loveday BP, de Chalain TB. Active counterpositioning or orthotic device to treat positional plagiocephaly? *J Craniofac Surg* 2001; 12: 308–13.

207. Vles JS, Colla C, Weber JW, *et al*. Helmet versus nonhelmet treatment in nonsynostotic positional posterior plagiocephaly. *J Craniofac Surg* 2000; 11: 572–4.

208. Littlefield TR, Beals SP, Manwaring KH. Treatment of craniofacial asymmetry with dynamic orthotic cranioplasty. *J Craniofac Surg* 1998; 9: 11–19.

209. Vander Kolk CA, Carson BS. Labroid synostosis. *Clin Plast Surg* 1994; 21: 575–84.

210. Persing JA, Delashaw JB, Jane JA, Edgerton MT. Lambdoid synostosis: surgical considerations. *Plast Reconstr Surg* 1988; 81: 852–60.

211. Muakkassa KF, Hoffman HJ, Hinton DR, *et al*. Labroid synostosis. Part 2: Review of cases managed at the Hospital for Sick Children, 1972–1982. *J Neurosurg* 1984; 61: 340–7.

212. Thaller SR, Hoyt J, Boggan J. Surgical correction of unilateral lambdoid synostosis: occipital rotation flap. *J Craniofac Surg* 1992; 3: 12–19.

213. Kaiser G. The clinical significance of bilateral synostosis of the lambdoid suture and the usefulness of its treatment. *Childs Brain* 1984; 11: 87–98.

214. Zoller JE, Mischkowski RA, Speder B. Preliminary results of standardized occipital advancement in the treatment of lambdoid synostosis. *J Craniomaxillofac Surg* 2002; 30: 343–8.

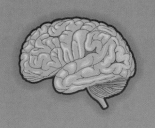

CHIARI MALFORMATIONS AND SYRINGOHYDROMYELIA

12

John C Wellons III, R Shane Tubbs, and W Jerry Oakes

INTRODUCTION

The Chiari malformations are a group of neuroanatomic and physiologic pathologic conditions described in the 1890s by Hans Chiari (1851–1916), an Austrian professor of pathology in Prague, Czechoslovakia. He detailed three degrees of hindbrain herniation (Chiari I, II, and III) and in a later publication added a fourth (Chiari IV) (Table 12.1).[1,2] In 1894, Julius A. Arnold (1835–1915), a professor of pathologic anatomy in Heidelburg, described a single myelodysplastic patient with hindbrain herniation.[3] Because of this single case report, Arnold's name has often been added to Chiari's when describing a Chiari II malformation (Arnold–Chiari malformation). However, this is considered unjustified, and Arnold's name is slowly fading from modern terminology.

Chiari III malformation rarely occurs and may be confused with an occipital encephalocele (Figure 12.1). In fact, only one case existed in Chiari's original description.[1] This malformation consists of a sac-like structure protruding from the upper cervical/occipital area and containing components of the brainstem and cerebellum. Other brain anomalies commonly seen with the Chiari II malformation may be present as well. Surgical intervention includes sac excision, replacement of the neural contents into the posterior fossa, dural and skin coverage, and cerebrospinal fluid (CSF) diversion if hydrocephalus develops.

Chiari IV malformation is characterized by severe cerebellar aplasia or hypoplasia and a small posterior fossa (Figure 12.2). Tentorial hypoplasia may be identified, but no hindbrain herniation exists, unlike the other three Chiari malformations. This has been removed from the Chiari classification scheme by most authors. These patients, despite a striking radiographic appearance, tend to appear amazingly well and may have only mild to moderate neurologic deficits.

Other varying degrees of hindbrain herniation exist. Recently, observations based on magnetic resonance imaging (MRI) have delineated two more classifications. Their names are highly descriptive of the anatomy but the malformations are not commonly diagnosed. Chiari 1.5 includes tonsillar herniation, as seen in Chiari

Table 12.1 Chiari malformations

Type I
Caudal descent of the cerebellar tonsils into the cervical spine
- rarely seen below C2
- not associated with myelomeningoceles
- hydrocephalus seen in < 10% of patients

Type II
Caudal descent of the cerebellar vermis and lower brainstem into the cervical spine
- commonly seen below C2
- multiple posterior fossa and cerebral anomalies associated with the hindbrain hernia, including:
  "beaking" of the dorsal midbrain, enlargement of the massa intermedia, medullary "kinking," and hypoplasia of the tentorium
- hydrocephalus almost always present
- very commonly seen in conjunction with myelomeningoceles

Type III
Protrusion of a sac from the craniocervical junction that contains portions of the cerebellum and brainstem
- commonly associated with hydrocephalus

Type IV
Severe hypoplasia or aplasia of the cerebellum associated with a diminutive posterior fossa

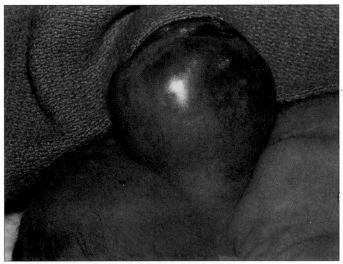

Figure 12.1 Neonate with a large cystic mass emanating from the craniocervical junction that contained both cerebellum and brainstem. This is a Chiari III malformation. On long-term follow-up this child was seen to have multiple severe neurologic deficits and developed hydrocephalus soon after closure of the lesion.

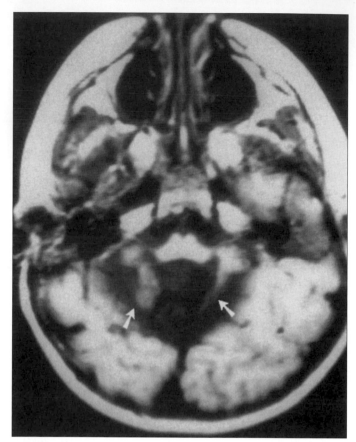

Figure 12.2 Sagittal MRI through the midline demonstrating minimal development of the cerebellum. Of note is the caudal displacement of the torcula (arrowhead). This child was evaluated for relatively mild coordination difficulty and is intellectually normal. The virtual absence of a cerebellum was truly surprising.

I malformation, associated with an elongated, caudally displaced brainstem and fourth ventricle, much like that seen in Chiari II malformation, thus the name Chiari 1.5, denoting a malformation half way between a Chiari I and II. Treatment options remain the same as in Chiari I.[4] A group of patients recognized and described only recently, comprises those with syringohydromyelia but with minimal to no findings of hindbrain herniation, informally referred to as Chiari 0. Although referred to as a Chiari malformation, there is no hindbrain malformation and this malformation also appears to be uncommon. However, because posterior fossa decompression (following an adequate exclusion of other etiologies of syringohydromyelia) has been noted to cause dramatic clinical and radiographic improvement, physiologically it responds to surgical intervention much like a Chiari I malformation, thus its name, "Chiari 0."[5]

CHIARI I

Patients with more than 3–5 mm of caudal displacement of the cerebellar tonsils inferior to the plane of the foramen magnum are generally considered to meet the radiologic criteria of a Chiari I malformation.[6] Up to 7 mm of tonsillar herniation has been considered normal in the past.[7] Pointed or "pegged" tonsillar tips and soft tissue "crowding" at the level of the foramen magnum are

Table 12.2 Radiographic criteria for Chiari I malformation

Caudal descent of the cerebellar tonsils > 3 mm below the plane of the foramen magnum
"Pegged" or pointed appearance of the tonsillar tips
Crowding of the subarachnoid space in the area of the craniocervical junction

also associated with asymmetric cerebellar tonsillar descent (Table 12.2, Figure 12.3). Craniocervical junction and basilar skull anomalies are seen in nearly 50% of patients with Chiari I malformations in select series.[8] Hydrocephalus has been noted in up to 10% of this population, and using MRI, syringohydromyelia has been reported in 50–75%.[7–12] Associated spinal anomalies include Klippel–Feil deformity, atlantoaxial assimilation, retroflexion of the dens (or odontoid process), and scoliosis.[7]

Many theories have been developed to explain Chiari malformations. Currently, the most appealing theory emphasizes the difficulty in rapidly equilibrating the CSF pressure wave seen during the Valsalva maneuver.[13] During this delay in achieving equilibrium, there is a vector of force out of the intracranial cavity (Figure 12.4). The prolonged intracranial hypertension relative to the intraspinal compartment may last several seconds or minutes. With time this force results in the downward migration of the cerebellar tonsils at the foramen magnum, causing impaction of these structures and resulting in obstruction of normal CSF flow between the posterior fossa and the cervical subarachnoid space. Conditions that impede the physiologic flow of CSF at the foramen of Magendie enhance the formation of the malformation. This could include arachnoid veils or septations in this region as well as adhesions. Alternatively, conditions that artificially lower the intraspinal pressure relative to the intracranial pressure (lumboperitoneal shunts) have been seen to "cause" the

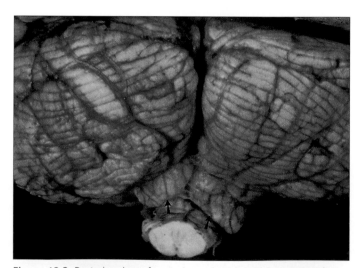

Figure 12.3 Posterior view of a specimen demonstrating asymmetric descent of the cerebellar tonsils (Chiari I malformation). The tonsils can be identified by their vertically oriented folia (arrows). This adult presented with downbeat nystagmus and difficulty with ambulation. There was no evidence of syringohydromyelia. She died abruptly of an unrelated cause prior to intervention for this lesion.

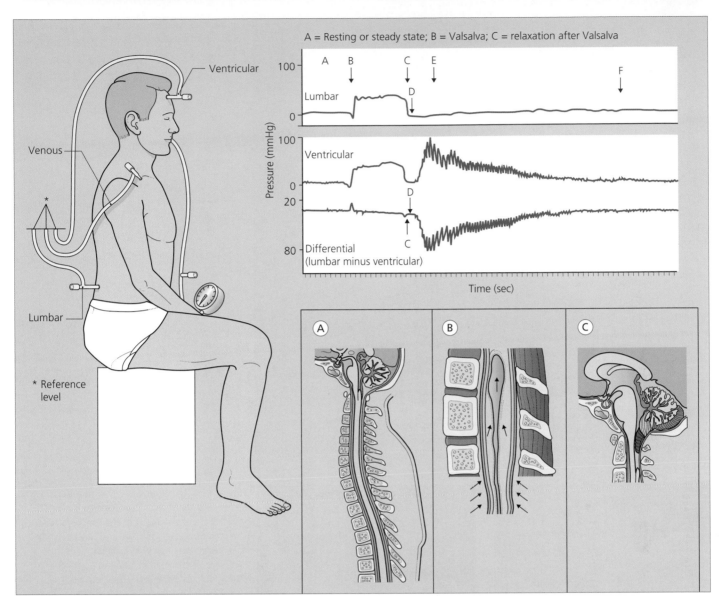

Figure 12.4 When ventricular and lumbar subarachnoid pressure are simultaneously monitored in a patient with a Chiari I malformation the pressures are the same in the resting state when calibrated against a reference (**A**). With Valsalva there is an abrupt rise of lumbar pressure (**B**) exceeding that seen in the ventricular system. With relaxation (**C**) the lumbar space has its pressure rapidly fall and return to the baseline. The ventricular pressure, on the other hand, cannot equilibrate, and sustained intracranial hypertension relative to the intraspinal compartment is maintained for several seconds to a few minutes. This vector of force is the pathophysiologic mechanism for the development of progressive displacement of the cerebellar tonsils into the cervical spine and the development of syringohydromyelia (after B. Williams).

Chiari I malformation with the subsequent development of syringohydromyelia.[14]

Initially considered an "adult" disease, the type I malformation is reported more frequently now in the pediatric population as a result of the widespread availability of detailed MRI. The clinical presentation of Chiari I malformation essentially falls into three categories (Figure 12.5). These three categories are:

1 signs or symptoms related to brainstem compression;
2 signs or symptoms associated with cerebellar compression; or
3 spinal cord dysfunction secondary to syringohydromyelia.

Most commonly, patients present with occipital or cervical pain that is nonradicular but frequently associated with dysesthesias in the C2 dermatome.[4] The neck pain or headache is frequently brought on by exertion or by coughing or sneezing (Valsalva-induced). Nonverbal children may relate their pain via irritability, crying, failure to thrive, or by the presence of opisthotonos.

The diagnosis can easily be confirmed with MRI. A standard protocol brain MRI allows direct sagittal as well as axial imaging demonstrating the posterior fossa abnormality. The presence and extent of syringohydromyelia should be determined by a cervical spine MRI (Figure 12.6). Computed tomography (CT) with intravenous contrast, ultrasonography, or other imaging modalities are not considered adequate for evaluation of the soft tissue of the craniocervical junction or the cervical spine. CT may further elucidate the bony abnormalities and plain films may assist in the

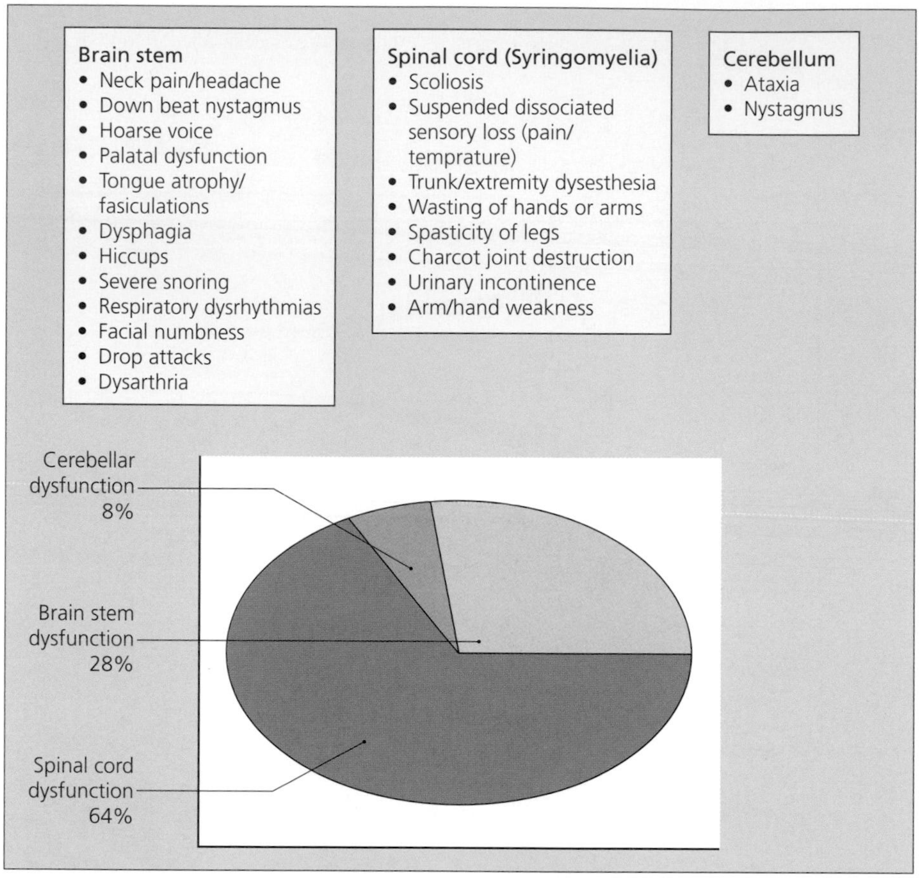

Brain stem
- Neck pain/headache
- Down beat nystagmus
- Hoarse voice
- Palatal dysfunction
- Tongue atrophy/ fasiculations
- Dysphagia
- Hiccups
- Severe snoring
- Respiratory dysrhythmias
- Facial numbness
- Drop attacks
- Dysarthria

Spinal cord (Syringomyelia)
- Scoliosis
- Suspended dissociated sensory loss (pain/ temprature)
- Trunk/extremity dysesthesia
- Wasting of hands or arms
- Spasticity of legs
- Charcot joint destruction
- Urinary incontinence
- Arm/hand weakness

Cerebellum
- Ataxia
- Nystagmus

Cerebellar dysfunction 8%

Brain stem dysfunction 28%

Spinal cord dysfunction 64%

Figure 12.5 Symptoms and signs of patients with Chiari I malformations.

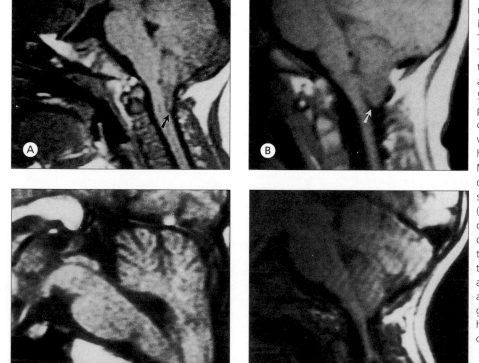

Figure 12.6 (A) Midsagittal MRI of a patient who meets all criteria for a Chiari I malformation, including caudal descent of the tonsils (arrow). The patient is asymptomatic and has no syrinx. This patient was followed expectantly for more than 4 years but did not develop any problem attributable to the lesion. (B) Midsagittal MRI of a 5-year-old with cough-induced neck and head pain as a result of caudal displacement of the cerebellar tonsils (arrow). His physical examination was normal. Following operative intervention the headaches completely disappeared. (C) Midsagittal MRI of a patient with significant caudal displacement of the cerebellar tonsils as well as significant ventral compression of the medulla (arrow). This patient should undergo decompression of the bone and soft tissues compromising the ventral brainstem through a transoral procedure rather than directing attention to the Chiari malformation. (D) Midsagittal MRI of a 5-year-old male presenting with very dysesthetic arms, spasticity, and marked difficulty with his gait. The Chiari I malformation is apparent, but a huge syrinx beginning just below C2 is also obvious (arrow).

evaluation of stability issues. Dynamic MRI (MRI-cine) has been used to evaluate CSF flow around the craniocervical junction.[15]

No medical treatment exists for the Chiari malformations. Numerous therapeutic paradigms exist (Figure 12.7) The first decision that must be made is whether the lesion is truly symptomatic. Observation is warranted in asymptomatic patients without an associated syrinx. In symptomatic patients or asymptomatic patients with syringomyelia, surgical intervention is recommended. The degree of brainstem compression and tonsillar herniation is taken into account as well. The vast majority of patients undergoing surgical treatment receive a posterior fossa decompression. In less than 10% of patients, hydrocephalus is associated with the Chiari I malformation, in which case a ventriculoperitoneal shunt should be the initial form of therapy. Similarly, symptomatic ventral compression out of proportion to dorsal compression requires a ventral decompression (i.e. transoral odontoid resection), especially in cases of myelopathy. The goal of the operation is to enlarge the posterior fossa and to re-create the cisterna magna, thereby permitting normal flow of CSF from the posterior fossa to the cervical subarachnoid space. In the majority of Chiari I patients with a syrinx, the syrinx decreases in size and does not require direct treatment because the posterior fossa decompression treats the underlying pathologic process causing the syringomyelia.

The surgical technique for a Chiari I decompression is similar to the exposure used for a posterior fossa tumor (Figure 12.8). The patient should be prone and the neck flexed. The incision extends from a point just below the inion to the spinous process of C2. An avascular plane between the paraspinous muscles is followed down to bone and a subperiosteal dissection is then performed. A moderate suboccipital craniectomy is followed by the removal of the posterior ring of C1. Some techniques advocate either closing now or opening the outer layer of the dura and then closing.[16,17] We open all layers of the dura and clip the opened arachnoid to the dural edge. Any arachnoid adhesions potentially obstructing the outflow of CSF from the foramen of Magendie are removed and the floor of the fourth ventricle is examined. A portion of the occipital pericranium is harvested through a separate incision and sewn to the dural edges as a dural augmentation graft, thereby enlarging the posterior fossa. The wound is closed in anatomic layers and the patient undergoes recovery with the head of the bed elevated.

The results of craniocervical decompression are encouraging in long-term follow-up.[18] Postoperative outcome is not age-based and early treatment tends toward better outcomes. Nearly 85% of patients will have relief of their head and neck pain.[8,19] The likelihood of decrease in the size of an associated syrinx is somewhat lower. However, the syrinx decreases in size or collapses in the majority, albeit not all, of the patients who undergo a well-performed posterior fossa decompression. Postoperative MRI has demonstrated relatively rapid resolution of syringohydromyelia in the majority of patients in many series.[10] If decompression fails to improve the symptoms or decrease the size of the syrinx in a 6-month period, a re-examination with MRI is indicated. In patients in which there remains anatomic or physiologic obstruction to normal CSF flow in the posterior fossa, consideration should

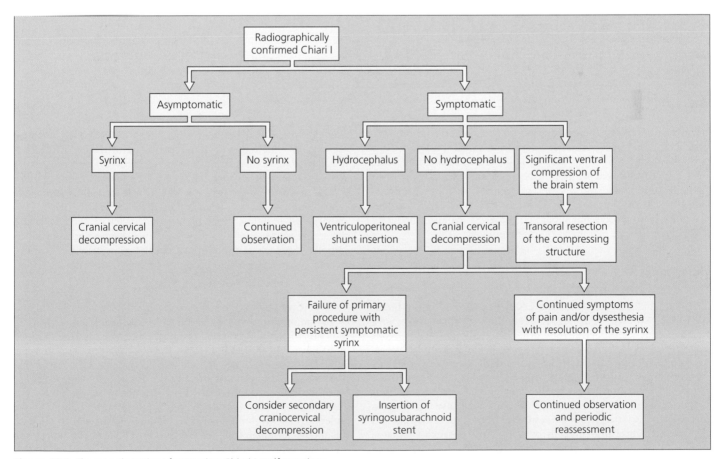

Figure 12.7 Therapeutic options for treating Chiari I malformations.

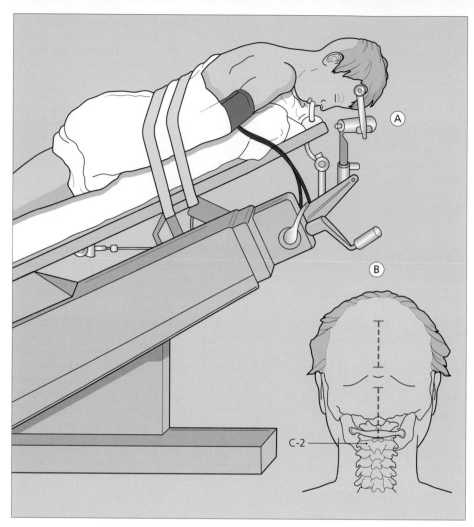

Figure 12.8 Operative position for Chiari decompression. **(A)** The operative field is maintained horizontally with the head flexed and held in a pin fixation device. **(B)** Preparation is made for a midline linear incision 2 cm below the external occipital protuberance and extending to the spinous process of C2. A 3-cm incision is made above the inion to harvest pericranium for grafting material.

C-2

be given to either a re-exploration of the posterior fossa with coagulation and/or resection of a cerebellar tonsil. Placement of a syringosubarachnoid shunt may be indicated in recalcitrant cases of syringomyelia that do not respond to an adequate posterior fossa decompression. Advanced symptoms of medullary dysfunction, muscle wasting, or dysesthesias in the trunk or extremities are unlikely to resolve but should not progress. Mild to moderate scoliosis has a high likelihood of improvement.

CHIARI II

The caudal displacement of the cerebellar vermis, lower brainstem, and fourth ventricle is seen almost exclusively with myelomeningoceles. Numerous other anomalies of the nervous system and its support structure are seen in various combinations. Luckënschädel (or abnormalities in the skull) decreases with age. Abnormalities of the cervical spine include the Klippel–Feil deformity, a malformation of the dens or the posterior arch of C1, or an enlarged cervical canal.[20] Of particular note for surgeons is the vertical straight sinus resulting from the low-lying and hypoplastic tentorium cerebelli, as well as the possibility of large venous lakes in the tentorium. Fenestrations may also be seen in the falx cerebri. Hydrocephalus occurs in approximately 90% of

patients with Chiari II malformations.[21] Colpocephaly may be present, in which the occipital horns and atria are disproportionally enlarged in relation to the remainder of the ventricular system. Diastematomyelia, which is a splitting of the spinal cord, is seen in up to 6% of patients with Chiari II malformation and syringohydromyelia has been reported to occur in between 20% and 95% of patients.[4,22] Numerous anomalies of the brain may occur. The more common malformations seen include partial or complete agenesis of the corpus callosum or septum pellucidum, an enlarged massa intermedia, tectal beaking, cerebellar inversion, absence of the falx cerebelli, and cervicomedullary kinking[23] (Table 12.3).

The pathophysiology of the malformation has been postulated to be similar to that of the Chiari I malformation, that is, a difficulty in equilibrating the dynamic CSF pulse pressure induced by Valsalva.[24] In the case of Chiari II, the presence of CSF pooling in or leaking from the myelomeningocele sac lowers the intraspinal pressure and the result is the ectopia of not only the cerebellar tonsils but the above-mentioned portions of the brainstem. Recent findings of reduced hindbrain herniation in some children who undergo fetal myelomeningocele closure would seem to support this theory, although long-term results are lacking.[25] However, the numerous other malformations may not be fully explained in this paradigm.

Table 12.3 Chiari II neuropathologic changes

"Beaking" of the dorsal midbrain through fusion of the superior and inferior colliculi

"Kinking" of the medulla

Enlargement of the massa intermedia

Hypoplasia of the tentorium and falx cerebri

Polygyria

Inversion of the cerebellum

Scalloping of the petrous ridges

Lückenschädel of the skull

Hydrocephalus

Similarly grouped as in the earlier section, the symptoms of Chiari II malformation are best considered according to the area demonstrating disturbed function: brainstem, cerebellar, or spinal cord dysfunction (Figure 12.9). Approximately 33% of these patients will develop some symptom of hindbrain herniation prior to the age of 5 years and outcome significantly worsens for presentation of these symptoms before 3 months of age.[4,7] Symptoms that may result in death if left untreated include stridor, apnea, and dysphagia resulting in aspiration, and are the leading cause of death in myelodysplastic patients.[26] Nystagmus may be the earliest sign of cerebellar dysfunction and the initial spinal cord symptoms (weakness, bowel and bladder dysfunction) are secondary to the inadequate formation of the lower spinal cord. It is important to note that spinal cord function can worsen during development and that ventriculoperitoneal shunt malfunction, syringohydromyelia formation, or spinal cord tethering must be ruled out and surgically dealt with if present. Scoliosis may also be present in this population and may be related to syringohydromyelia.[27]

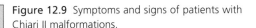

Figure 12.9 Symptoms and signs of patients with Chiari II malformations.

Brain stem
- Dysphagia, poor suck response
- Nasal vocalization, palatal weakness
- Aspiration pneumonia
- Gastrooesophageal reflux
- Tongue fasiculations/atrophy
- Opisthotonos
- Central apnea, especially during sleep
- Poor or weak cry
- Severe or prolonged breath-holding spells
- Inspiritory wheezing
- Nerve VI palsy
- Facial weakness
- Lack of response to insired CO_2
- Tracheal anaesthesia
- Depressed or absent gag response
- Prolonged hiccups

Spinal cord
- Upper extremity spasticity
- Persistent cortical thumbs
- Suspended dissociated sensory loss (pain/temperature)
- Upper extremity weakness and hand muscle wasting
- Scoliosis

Cerebellum
- Appendicular/truncal ataxia
- Nystagmus

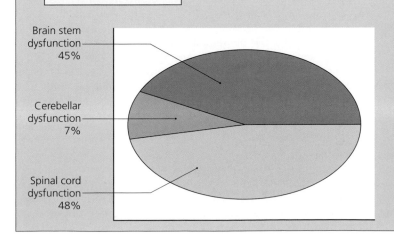

Brain stem dysfunction 45%

Cerebellar dysfunction 7%

Spinal cord dysfunction 48%

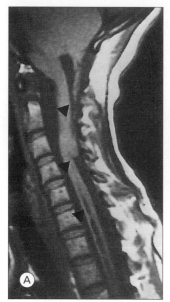
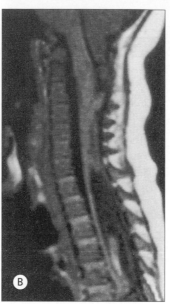
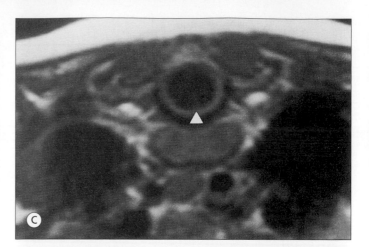
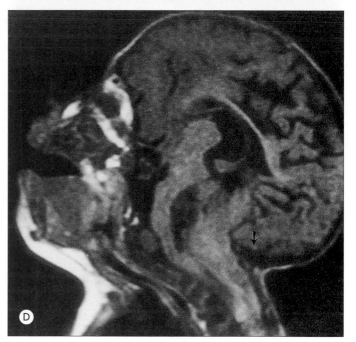

Figure 12.10 **(A)** Midsagittal MRI of the craniocervical junction in a patient with a Chiari II malformation. The brainstem and cerebellar vermis are caudally displaced. The choroid plexus (upper arrowhead) and medullary kink (middle arrowhead) are apparent. A moderate-sized syrinx (lower arrowhead) is also seen. **(B)** Midsagittal MRI of a patient with a Chiari II malformation. Again the medullary kink and caudally displaced vermis are apparent. The syrinx, however, is massively dilated in the lower cervical and upper thoracic regions. Interestingly, this patient's neurologic function was not seriously compromised with regard to hand function despite this massively dilated syrinx. **(C)** Axial MRI of the patient in **(B)**, showing a thin rim of cord tissue (arrowhead) surrounding a massively dilated syrinx. With time, serious compromise of motor and sensory function of the arms developed. **(D)** Severe Chiari II malformation with much of the brainstem and cerebellum displaced into the cervical spine. The torcula is positioned at the foramen magnum. The upper cervical spine is deviated markedly anteriorly, compromising the trachea and esophagus. The spine is widely bifid posteriorly.

MRI continues to be the imaging procedure of choice in these patients (Figure 12.10).[28] Indeed, the advent of MR technology enabled the identification of the associated developmental abnormalities mentioned previously. Plain dynamic cervical spine X-rays may assist with any question of instability just as plain thoracic and lumbar X-rays would help to follow the degree of scoliosis. Spinal cord syringes are best identified and followed with spinal MRI.

Adequate shunt function must be established prior to pursuing decompression of a symptomatic Chiari II malformation (Figure 12.11). This includes surgical inspection of the shunt and the presence of a ventricular catheter that is free of intraventricular adhesions. The number of Chiari II decompressions at our institution has decreased significantly following the establishment of this paradigm. Symptoms warranting intervention include inspiratory stridor, sleep apnea, recurrent aspiration pneumonia, opisthotonos, and progressive spasticity or ataxia.

When surgical decompression is elected, patients are positioned prone with the neck flexed. Unlike surgical decompression

of a Chiari I malformation, decompression of a Chiari II malformation rarely includes a suboccipital craniectomy. A laminectomy must be performed that includes the entire area of the displaced cerebellar vermis (Figures 12.12, 12.13). The dura is opened widely and the fourth ventricle is identified. Following the choroid plexus through the dense arachnoidal scarring will usually lead to the foramen of Magendie and the fourth ventricle. This is the crucial goal of the procedure. If any question exists as to the patency of the foramen, then a stent should be placed. The medullary kink, if present, must not be mistaken for the vermis, or the surgeon will end up dissecting into the brainstem. An expansion duraplasty is performed and the remainder of the wound is closed in layers.

Outcome following surgery is dependent on the severity of symptoms prior to intervention. Infants presenting with brainstem symptoms are less likely to have a significant improvement in their symptoms following decompression. Few studies exist regarding outcome, however, earlier intervention and fewer symptoms are thought to predict success.[29,30]

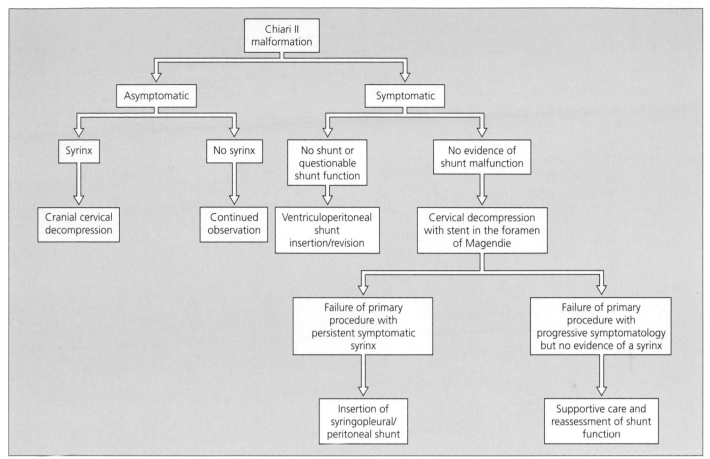

Figure 12.11 Therapeutic options for treating patients with Chiari II malformations.

SYRINGOHYDROMYELIA

Syringohydromyelia is a secondary process with many etiologies. The term "syringomyelia" has been used to describe any longitudinal fluid collection within the spinal cord. This term, however, refers to fluid collections outside the central canal. "Hydromyelia" refers to fluid collections enlarging the central canal. Combining the two words, "syringohydromyelia" better connotes this disease process and is considered to be more proper terminology. However, for the purposes of simplicity we have used the term "syringomyelia" or "syrinx" throughout this chapter to denote any fluid collection within the spinal cord. Known pathologic situations in which a syrinx may form include post-traumatic circumstances, or in association with Chiari malformations, neoplasms, arteriovenous malformations, arachnoiditis, or occult spinal dysraphism. Idiopathic syringohydromyelia also exists. The mechanism by which the fluid accumulates varies significantly and a useful informal system to classify syrinxes divides them into either communicating (Chiari, occult spinal dysraphism) or non-communicating (neoplasm, arteriovenous malformations, arachnoiditis, traumatic).

Fluid collections that begin in the ependyma-lined central canal (hydromyelia) may cause an outpouching in weak areas that can grow into the white matter of the cord (Figure 12.14). The absence of ependyma then enables the syrinx to enlarge with less constraint. Of note are the crossing fibers of the spinothalamic tract in the ventral white commissure that is particularly vulnerable to syrinx expansion.

Symptoms include loss of pain and temperature sensation in the arm or chest, diminished or absent deep tendon reflexes, and spasticity of the lower extremities. Longer-term findings include wasting of the intrinsic muscles of the hand and scoliosis. Dysesthetic pain in the chest and arms is a particularly poor prognostic indicator for postoperative relief of symptoms. Acute loss of neurologic function may occur with coughing or straining. When the Valsalva maneuver causes the epidural venous complex to expand, the cavity may be forced to dissect through white matter within the cord (Figure 12.15). This may result in symptomatic or asymptomatic enlargement of the syrinx.

MRI is the diagnostic procedure of choice in this condition (Figure 12.16). Unless a readily available etiology is seen on MRI (enhancing spinal tumor) or is known (history of trauma), an MRI of the craniocervical junction should be performed to evaluate for Chiari malformation. Up to 75% of patients with Chiari I malformations will have an associated syrinx identified on MRI.[7,8,10–12] Between 20% and 95% of patients with Chiari II malformations will have a syrinx seen on imaging.[4]

If symptoms are functionally significant or progressive, intervention should be considered, with the recommended procedure varying widely depending on the underlying condition (Figure

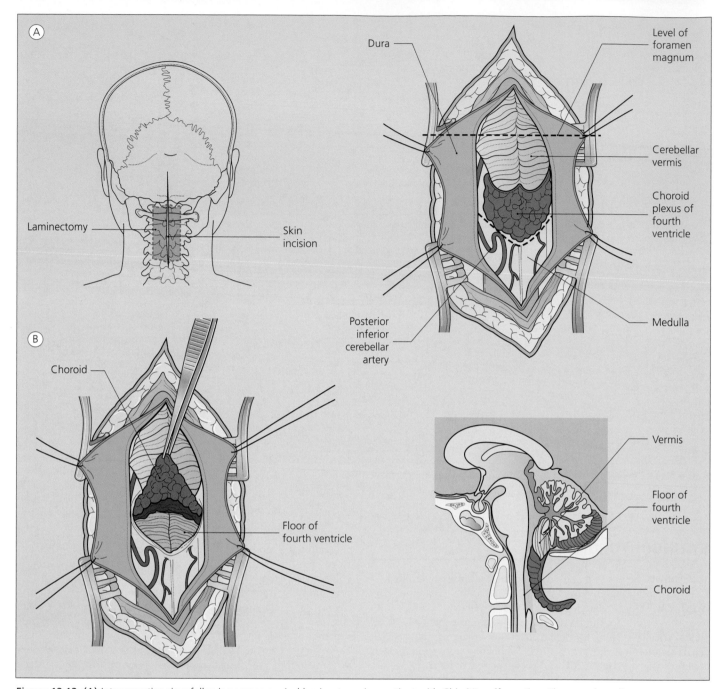

Figure 12.12 (A) Intraoperative view following upper cervical laminectomy in a patient with Chiari II malformation. The granular yellow-orange choroid plexus may be visualized through the arachnoid. The horizontal folia of the cerebellar vermis are apparent and the caudally displaced medulla and posterior inferior cerebellar artery immediately below the choroid plexus can also be seen. **(B)** With dissection of the thickened arachnoid in the area of the choroid plexus the avascular floor of the fourth ventricle can be visualized. A stent is placed through this opening to maintain its integrity.

12.17). No medical therapy exists for syringohydromyelia. If no alternative explanation for a surgically significant syrinx is identified, exploration of the craniocervical junction should be considered.[5,31] Follow-up MRI can readily evaluate residual or recurrent fluid. In the setting of a residual syrinx following a decompressed Chiari I malformation, the patient should return to the operating room and the posterior fossa should be explored for re-adhesion of the arachnoid at the outlet of the fourth ventricle.

It is common for a cerebellar tonsil to be either partially coagulated or resected sub-pially during the secondary procedure.

When operative therapy turns to stenting or shunting the syrinx, note that the arachnoid flow tends to be compromised in certain pathologic states (i.e. arachnoiditis, post-traumatic) and therefore the distal end of the shunt should be placed either in the pleural space or the peritoneum. If the distal end of a syrinx stent is placed in the intrathecal space, it is imperative that it be placed

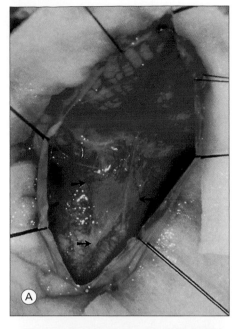

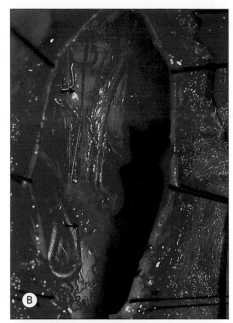

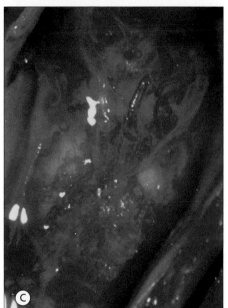

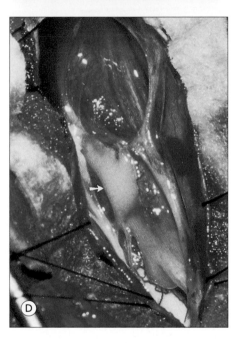

Figure 12.13 **(A)** Intraoperative view of a Chiari II malformation with the dura open. The cerebellar vermis is minimally displaced; however, the brainstem with its fourth ventricle is displaced well below the foramen magnum. The triangular appearance of the lower brainstem is apparent, with a veil over its opening (arrows). **(B)** Intraoperative view of a Chiari II malformation with the horizontal folia of the cerebellar vermis (upper arrow) and yellow-orange appearance of the choroid plexus (lower arrow) apparent. The redundant left posterior inferior cerebellar artery can also easily be seen lying on the dorsal aspect of the medulla. **(C)** Intraoperative intradural view of a Chiari II malformation with significant thickening of the arachnoid and neovascularity over the dorsal vermis and brainstem. In this patient the plane of dissection to allow opening of the foramen of Magendie is much less obvious. **(D)** Severe caudal displacement of the vermis and brainstem to the level of T4. The waxy avascular yellow appearance of the cerebellar vermis (arrows) is apparent. These tissues have been displaced to such a severe degree that they have become ischemic and gliotic.

in the subarachnoid space for absorption to take place properly. Re-establishment of a patent spinal canal and subarachnoid space may be undertaken in the setting of traumatic disruption through removal of bone fragments or bony realignment. This is made more difficult in the setting of a previous surgical fusion. Occasionally, syrinxes are multicompartmental and will require drainage at multiple sites. If the syrinx is the result of either arteriovenous malformations or tumor, primary treatment is directed at the appropriate pathology. Outcome is dependent on the degree of disability prior to intervention and the cause of the syrinx.

SUMMARY

Time and, when necessary, surgical intervention are needed to better elucidate the natural history of the hindbrain herniation syndromes known as the Chiari malformations. Numerous abnormalities of the nervous system may also be associated with them, and a unified theory has yet to be fully discerned. Syringohydromyelia continues to be closely tied in with these abnormalities at the craniocervical junction and also occurs in response to other pathological processes of the spinal cord.

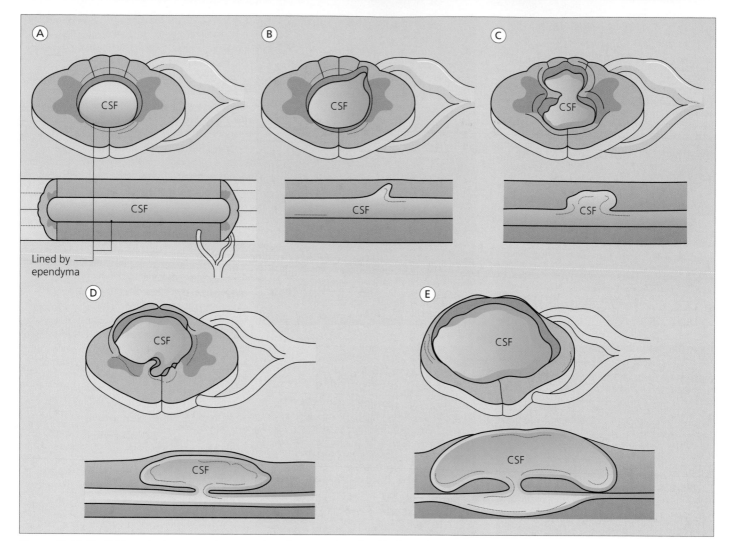

Figure 12.14 (A–E) Stages in the progressive expansion of an ependyma-lined hydromyelia to a larger cavity compressing the central canal. This large cavity has no ependymal lining and so could be termed a syrinx.

CLINICAL PEARLS (continued on p. 194)

(continued on p. 194)

- Chiari malformations are pathologic herniations of the hindbrain through the foramen magnum and into the cervical spinal canal. Chiari malformations are being recognized with increasing frequency because of the increased availability of MRI.

- Chiari I malformation represents downward herniation of the cerebellar tonsils into the cervical canal at least 3–5 mm on sagittal MRI. The impaction of the tonsils in the foramen magnum cause an anatomic and physiologic block of CSF which normally flows from the posterior fossa into the cervical subarachnoid space. The symptoms of Chiari I malformation commonly include headache or neck pain worsened by activity or Valsalva maneuver, or signs of brainstem compression. Syringomyelia and scoliosis may be

associated with Chiari I, and those patients often present with signs of spinal cord dysfunction.

- The most widely accepted treatment of Chiari I malformation is a posterior fossa decompression with a C1 laminectomy and dural augmentation graft. The goal of surgery is to enlarge the posterior fossa and permit normal flow of CSF from the posterior fossa to the cervical subarachnoid space. In the majority of patients, the symptoms of headache resolve and there is a concomitant collapse of the associated syrinx. Only rarely does the surgeon have to treat directly the associated syringomyelia.

- Chiari II malformation, which is a downward migration of the cerebellar vermis and brainstem through

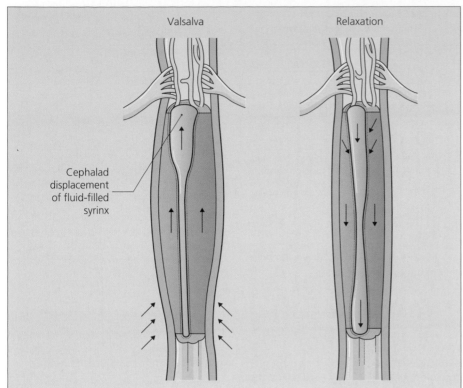

Valsalva

Relaxation

Cephalad displacement of fluid-filled syrinx

Figure 12.15 Increased intra-abdominal pressure caused by the Valsalva maneuver forces blood into the epidural venous complex. When the epidural veins are forcefully expanded against the enlarged cystic cord they may force the cyst to be displaced (usually cephalad). This sudden displacement with forceful coughing or sneezing may actually be associated with a significant worsening of the patient's neurologic condition.

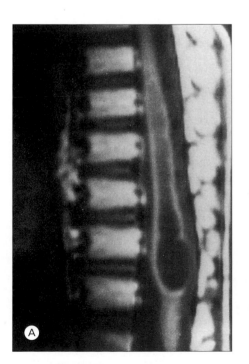

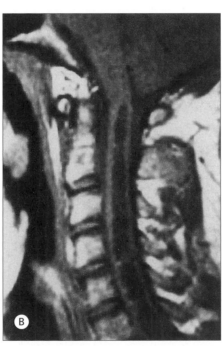

Figure 12.16 (A) Midsagittal MRI of a patient with occult spinal dysraphism including a tethered spinal cord and diastematomyelia without a fibrous septum. In the upper lumbar region a terminal syrinx can easily be appreciated. This patient was "asymptomatic" at this time. Following drainage of the syrinx, however, significant improvements in the patient's spontaneous gait and urinary stream were noted. **(B)** Patient who developed a traumatic thoracic fracture and post-traumatic syringomyelia that extends to the craniocervical junction. In this patient progressive weakness of the arms and hands was the primary clinical manifestation.

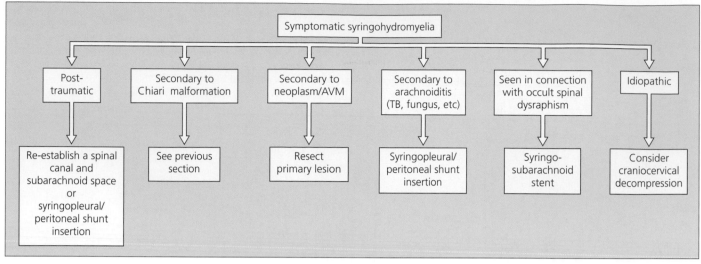

Figure 12.17 Therapeutic options for patients with symptomatic syringohydromyelia.

CLINICAL PEARLS, *cont'd*

the foramen magnum, is most commonly seen in patients with myelomeningocele. It is associated with hydrocephalus in 90% of the patients. Syringomyelia is also very common. In addition, on MRI, patients often have low-lying tentorium, tectal beaking, cervicomedullary kinks, agenesis of the corpus callosum, and other brain abnormalities. A small, but significant, number of patients will present with acute brainstem, cerebellar, or progressive spinal cord dysfunction. The initial step in this treatment should be the surgical establishment of a functioning shunt. If the symptoms progress or do not resolve in this setting, then a formal decompressive procedure may be required.

- Syringohydromyelia, or cavitation of the spinal cord, has many etiologies in addition to hindbrain herniation. Signs and symptoms of a syrinx include pain and temperature loss, reflex changes, or motor weakness. Treatment of the syrinx, when not the result of hindbrain herniation, often includes shunting of the syrinx into the peritoneum or pleura. The goal is to drain the syrinx and to re-establish a patent subarachnoid space.

REFERENCES

1. Chiari H. Uber Veranderungen des Kleinhirns infolge von Hydrocephalie des Grosshirns. *Dtsch Med Wochenshr* 1891; 17: 1172–5.
2. Chiari H. Uber Veranderungen des Kleinhirns, der Pons und der Medulla oblongata infolge von congenitaler Hydrocephalie des Grosshirns. *Denkschr Akad Wiss (Wien)* 1895; 63: 71–115.
3. Koehler PJ. Chiari's description of cerebellar ectopy (1891): with a summary of Cleland's and Arnold's contributions and some early observations of neural-tube defects. *J Neurosurg* 1991; 75: 823–6.
4. Iskandar B, Oakes W. Chiari malformation and syringomyelia. In: Albright L, Pollack I, Adelson P (eds). *Principles and Practice of Pediatric Neurosurgery*. New York, NY: Thieme; 1999: 165–87.
5. Iskandar BI, Hedlund GL, Grabb PA, Oakes WJ. The resolution of syringomyelia without hindbrain herniation after posterior fossa decompression. *J Neurosurg* 1998; 89: 212–16.
6. Aboulezz AO, Sartor K, Geyer CA, Gado MH. Position of cerebellar tonsils in the normal population and in patients with Chiari I malformation: a quantitative approach with MR imaging. *J Comput Assist Tomogr* 1985; 9: 1033–6.
7. Oakes WJ, Tubbs RS. Chiari malformations. In: Winn HR (ed.). *Youmans Neurological Surgery: A Comprehensive Guide to the Diagnosis and Management of Neurosurgical Problems*, 5th edn. Philadelphia, PA: W.B. Saunders; 1993.
8. Menezes AH. Chiari I malformations and hydromyelia complications. *Pediatr Neurosurg* 1991; 17: 146–54.
9. Logue V, Edwards MR. Syringomyelia and its surgical treatment—an analysis of 75 patients. *J Pediatr* 1991; 118: 567–9.
10. Batzdorf U. Chairi I malformation with syringomyelia. Evaluation of surgical therapy by magnetic resonance imaging. *J Neurosurg* 1988; 68: 726–30.
11. Cahan LD, Bentson JR. Consideration in the diagnosis and treatment of syringomyelia and Chiari malformation. *J Neurosurg* 1982; 57: 24–31.
12. Carmel PW, Markesbery WR. Early descriptions of the Arnold–Chiari malformation. The contribution of John Cleland. *J Neurosurg* 1972; 37: 543–7.
13. Williams B. Simultaneous cerebral and spinal fluid pressure recordings, II: cerebrospinal dissociation with lesions at the foramen magnum. *Acta Neurochir* 1981; 59: 123–42.
14. Welch K, Shillito J, Strand R, Fischer EG, Winston KR. Chiari I malformation—an acquired disorder? *J Neurosurg* 1981; 55: 604–9.

15. Armonda RA, Citrin CM, Foley KT, Ellenbogen RG. Quantitative cine-mode magnetic resonance imaging of Chiari I malformations: an analysis of cerebrospinal fluid dynamics. *Neurosurgery* 1994; 35: 214–223; discussion 223–4.

16. Haines SJ, Berger M. Current treatment of Chiari malformations types I and II: a survey of the Pediatric Section of the American Association of Neurological Surgeons. *Neurosurgery* 1991; 28: 353–7.

17. Isu T, Sasaki H, Takamura H, Kobayashi N. Foramen magnum decompression with removal of the outer layer of the dura as treatment of syringomyelia occurring with Chiari I malformation. *Neurosurgery* 1993; 33: 844–849; discussion 849–50.

18. Dyste GN, Menezes AH, VanGilder JC. Symptomatic Chiari malformations: an analysis of presentation, management, and long-term outcome. *J Neurosurg* 1989; 71: 159–68.

19. Nagib MG. An approach to symptomatic children (ages 4–14 years) with Chiari type I malformation. *Pediatr Neurosurg* 1994; 21: 31–5.

20. Curnes JT, Oakes WJ, Boyko OB. MR imaging of hindbrain deformity in Chiari II patients with and without symptoms of brainstem compression [see comments]. *Am J Neuroradiol* 1989; 10: 293–302.

21. Rauzzino M, Oakes WJ. Chiari II malformation and syringomyelia. *Neurosurg Clin N Am* 1995; 6: 293–309.

22. Emery JL, MacKenzie N. Medullo-cervical dislocation deformity (Chiari II deformity) related to neurospinal dysraphism (meningomyelocele). *Brain* 1973; 96: 155–62.

23. Tubbs RS, Dockery SE, Salter G, *et al.* Absence of the falx cerebelli in a Chiari II malformation. *Clin Anat* 2002; 15: 193–5.

24. Williams B. Cerebrospinal fluid pressure-gradients in spina bifida cystica, with special reference to the Arnold–Chiari malformation and aqueductal stenosis. *Dev Med Child Neurol Suppl.* 1975; 17: 138–50.

25. Tulipan N, Hernanz-Schulman M, Bruner J. Reduced hindbrain herniation after intrauterine myelomeningocele repair: A report of four cases. *Pediatr Neurosurg* 1988; 29: 274–8.

26. Davidson Ward SL, Nickerson BG, vanderHal A, Rodriguez AM, Jacobs RA, Keens TG. Absent hypoxic and hypercapneic arousal responses in children with myelomeningocele and apnea. *Pediatrics* 1986; 78: 44–50.

27. Hall PV, Lindseth RE, Campbell RL, Kalsbeck JE. Myelodysplasia and developmental scoliosis: a manifestation of syringomyelia. *Spine* 1976; 1: 48–56.

28. Curnes JT, Oakes WJ, Boyko OB. MR imaging of hindbrain deformity in Chiari II patients with and without symptoms of brainstem compression. *Am J Neuroradiol* 1989; 10: 293–302.

29. Pollack IF, Pang D, Albright AL, Krieger D. Outcome following hindbrain decompression of symptomatic Chiari malformations in children previously treated with myelomeningocele closure and shunts. *J Neurosurg* 1992; 77: 881–8.

30. Charney EB, Rorke LB, Sutton LN, Schut L. Management of Chiari II complications in infants with myelomeningocele. *J Pediatr* 1987; 111: 364–71.

31. Tubbs RS, Elton S, Grabb P, Dockery SE, Bartolucci AA, Oakes WJ. Analysis of the posterior fossa in children with the Chiari 0 malformation. *Neurosurgery* 2001; 48: 1050–5.

PATHOPHYSIOLOGY AND CLINICAL PRESENTATION

Cerebral blood flow and ischemic thresholds

Brain mass represents approximately 2% of body weight, but its circulation is endowed with 20% of the cardiac output and its energy requirements account for 20% of total body oxygen consumption (Figure 13.1).[1] These tremendous metabolic demands are required to maintain the high degree of order required for control of body functions and behavior. Among the brain's metabolic requirements are: (1) the synthesis and transport of substrates and macromolecules, including neuro-transmitters; (2) the maintenance of strict osmotic compartmentalization and integrity of cellular and support structures; and (3) the orderly execution of biochemical reactions involving various biomolecules. A substantial amount of energy in the brain is also required for heat production. Such heat is by no means "wasted," since its release is necessary for the unidirectional flow of various biochemical reactions (away from equilibrium) and the maintenance of an optimal temperature for enzymatic function.

To function metabolically, the brain needs a steady flow of oxygen and substrate delivered by the cerebral circulation.[1] *Ischemia* is the condition in which cerebral blood flow is not sufficient to maintain cerebral metabolic functions. Ischemia may

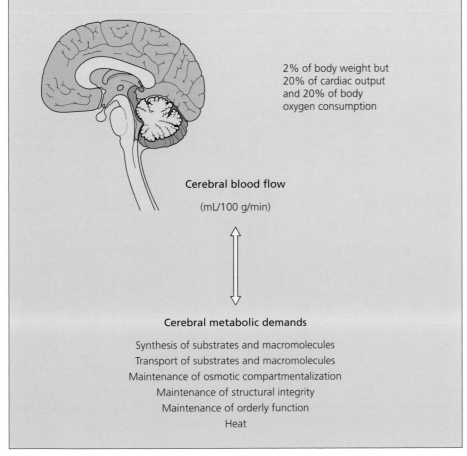

Figure 13.1 Blood flow and brain metabolic demands.

2% of body weight but 20% of cardiac output and 20% of body oxygen consumption

Cerebral blood flow

(mL/100 g/min)

Cerebral metabolic demands

Synthesis of substrates and macromolecules
Transport of substrates and macromolecules
Maintenance of osmotic compartmentalization
Maintenance of structural integrity
Maintenance of orderly function
Heat

be complete (absent cerebral blood flow) or incomplete (insufficient cerebral blood flow), global (affecting the whole brain) or focal (affecting a region of the brain). Regional cerebral blood flow (rCBF) is usually expressed in milliliters per 100 grams of brain tissue per minute (mL/100 g/min). Normal rCBF is typically in the range 50–60 mL/100 g/min, is greater in gray than in white matter, and may be higher during functional activation of individual brain regions.

Specific *ischemic thresholds* have been identified in humans and experimental animals (Figure 13.2).[2] Intact cellular structure and function are well maintained whenever the rCBF exceeds 20–25 mL/100 g/min. Below this threshold, there is impaired cellular function characterized by slowing and decreased amplitude of the electroencephalogram, disruption of evoked cortical responses, and degraded clinical function related to the particular region of the brain. Intact cellular structure appears to be maintained unless the rCBF drops below 5–10 mL/100 g/min. This threshold for tissue infarction depends not only on the the rCBF level but also on the duration of ischemia (see Figure 13.2). Higher ranges of rCBF may still result in tissue infarction, if they persist for long periods of time.[2]

This concept of ischemic thresholds accounts for the transient cerebral dysfunction without residual tissue infarction that is sometimes observed clinically. Also, it indicates that a region of the brain can be functionally impaired indefinitely without adequate rCBF but still remain structurally intact as long as it receives enough blood flow for cellular maintenance ("idling neurons").

Mechanisms of ischemia

Global brain ischemia is encountered with hemodynamic failure or cardiac arrest. Focal brain ischemia may result from a variety of mechanisms (Figure 13.3). Cardiogenic emboli may arise from dysfunctional valves or mural thrombi and lodge in the cerebral arteries, resulting in focal ischemia. Artery-to-artery embolism may result from atherosclerotic disease in large cerebral arteries, with platelet, calcific, or thrombotic emboli lodging in smaller arteries downstream. Embolic arterial occlusions typically result in infarction in the territory of the occluded artery. However, collateral circulation (see below) or fragmentation of the embolus (with reperfusion) can limit the size of such infarctions.

Occlusion of large cerebral arteries may cause thromboemboli to propagate in more distal vessels. Also, large-vessel occlusions can cause hemodynamic insufficiency in the watershed zones of the territory supplied by the occluded artery. Lastly, occlusion of small penetrating arteries can result in small infarctions within the territory of such deep penetrating vessels. These are known as lacunar infarctions.

The occlusion of a given cerebral artery does not always result in a predictable infarction. Collateral pathways (Figure 13.4) may redistribute the blood flow sufficiently to prevent infarction in particular regions of the brain.[3] The competence of the collateral pathways depends on individual vascular anatomy (collateral pathways may be atretic or particularly prominent in certain individuals) and on the chronicity of ischemia (certain collateral pathways may become more prominent with longer durations of chronic ischemia).

Major collateral pathways include the epicerebral leptomeningeal circulation (consisting of the network of small arteries in the subarachnoid space surrounding the brain), the anterior circle of Willis (anterior cerebral and communicating arteries), the posterior circle of Willis (posterior communicating artery), and the ophthalmic artery (allowing communication between the external and internal carotid circulations). Less prominent collateral pathways may be operative in pathologic situations of chronic ischemia. These include transdural, transcerebral (across the dura mater), cervical muscular collaterals, and a proliferation of deep cerebral arteries (often resembling a puff of smoke on angiography, hence the Japanese term "moyamoya collaterals").

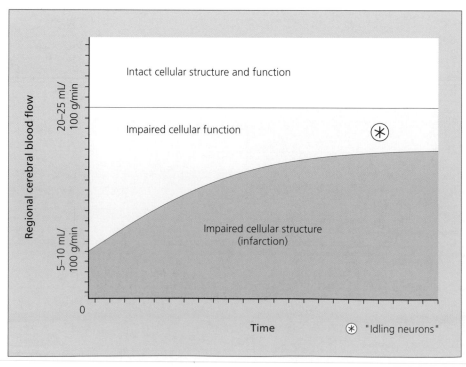

Figure 13.2 Cerebral blood flow and ischemic thresholds. Several lines of evidence from humans, primates and higher mammals demonstrate clear thresholds for impaired cellular function and tissue infarction. Such thresholds depend on the level of regional cerebral blood flow and also the duration of ischemia. Longer periods of hypoperfusion increase the likelihood of tissue infarction. This concept explains clinical observations of transient ischemia, and also the possibility of preserved but dysfunctional tissue in moderate ischemia ("idling neurons"). (Figure modified from reference 2.)

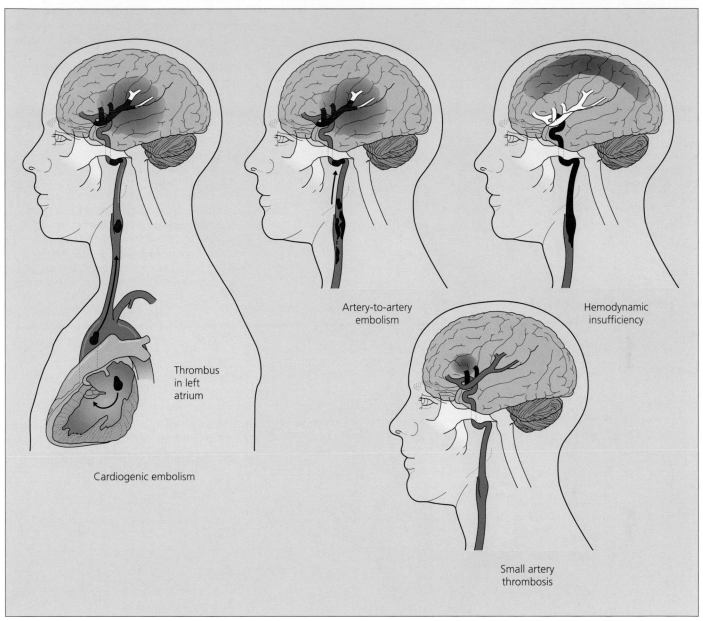

Figure 13.3 Mechanisms of focal ischemia. Cardiogenic embolism results from a variety of cardiac pathologies, including valvular disease, mural thrombus, and atrial myxoma, and can lead to the occlusion of cerebral arteries with resulting territorial infarctions. Artery-to-artery embolism involves platelet aggregates, thrombi, or fragments of atheroma originating in atherosclerotic large arteries and leads to occlusion of smaller cerebral arteries downstream with territorial infarctions. Hemodynamic insufficiency results from occluded large vessels and impaired collateral pathways, causing "watershed" infarctions. Small artery thrombosis is caused by occlusion of sclerotic small cerebral vessels with lacunar infarctions involving the respective territories of these deep arteries.

Clinical and pathologic spectrum

A wide spectrum of clinical manifestations and vascular and parenchymal pathologic changes are associated with brain ischemia (Table 13.1).

Clinical spectrum

Occlusive cerebrovascular disease may be totally asymptomatic or it may be accompanied by subtle clinical signs such as a cervical bruit (on auscultation). A cervical bruit is an index of systemic vasculopathy, including coronary and carotid occlusive disease, and is not a reliable herald of severe or clinically relevant carotid occlusive disease.

Transient (less than 24 hours) or reversible (less than 3 days) clinical symptoms of ischemia may include a temporary focal neurologic dysfunction in which there is complete clinical recovery between or following the spell(s). Transient ischemic attacks (TIAs) or reversible ischemic neurologic deficits (RINDs) affecting the carotid circulation include temporary focal paresis, dysphasia, focal sensory disturbance, or amaurosis fugax (transient monocular blindness). TIAs or RINDs affecting the vertebrobasilar circulation include crossed motor or sensory symptoms (affecting one side of the face and the contralateral half of the body), drop attacks (sudden falls), tinnitus, vertigo, diplopia,

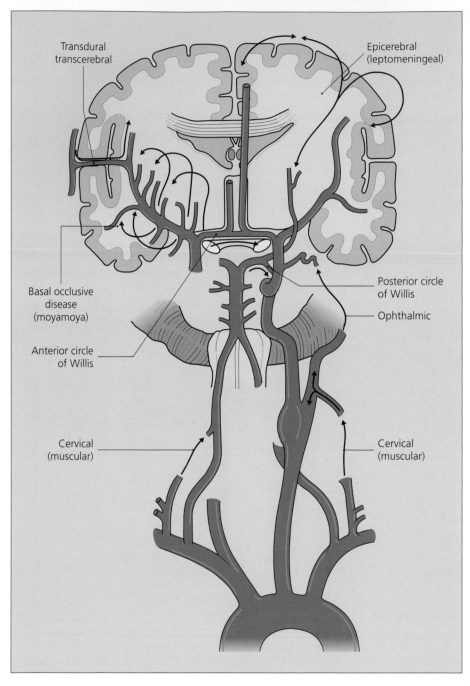

Figure 13.4 The collateral pathways. Collateral pathways allow redistribution of blood flow in the presence of arterial insufficiency, which prevents infarction in particular regions of the brain. Major collateral pathways include the epicerebral (leptomeningeal) collaterals (providing communication between various vascular territories), the anterior circle of Willis (providing communication between cerebral hemispheres), the posterior circle of Willis (providing communication between the vertebrobasilar and carotid circulations), and the ophthalmic collaterals (providing communication between the external carotid and internal carotid circulations). Less prominent collateral pathways may be operative in pathologic situations of chronic ischemia and include transdural transcerebral collaterals from the arteries of the dura mater, and basal occlusive collaterals (proliferation of arterial channels in the region of the perforating arteries).

dysarthria, dysphagia, or homonymous visual field disturbances. Such reversible symptoms may result from temporary cerebrovascular circulatory compromise (embolus with rapid fragmentation or transient hemodynamic insufficiency) or minute cerebral infarctions (with rapid recovery of clinical symptoms).

Ischemic stroke results in a permanent focal functional neurologic deficit referable to the region of the brain infarction. An ischemic infarct may be totally asymptomatic if it affects noneloquent regions of the brain. Subtle or reversible symptoms may occur with smaller infarctions. Minor stroke results in persistent residual symptoms that are not severely disabling (incomplete paresis, partial dysphasia, etc.). Major stroke typically results in profound multimodal neurologic deficits, such as hemiplegia, hemisensory deficit, hemineglect, and hemianopsia.

Possible cumulative effects of multiple infarctions are mental deterioration and cognitive decline. In general, the larger the area of parenchymal infarction the more prominent the clinical symptoms. However, the location of the infarction and other factors, including age and general medical condition, also play a role in the functional sequelae of stroke. Therefore, the clinical spectrum of symptomatic brain ischemia does not necessarily correspond to proportional parenchymal brain damage.

Vascular pathologic spectrum

As with brain infarction, a spectrum of vascular pathologies can cause brain ischemia.[3]

Cardiac disease can cause brain ischemia through a variety of mechanisms. Cardioembolic stroke may result from atrial

Table 13.1 Clinical and pathologic spectrum of brain ischemia

Clinical spectrum	Vascular pathologic spectrum	Parenchymal pathologic spectrum
Asymptomatic	Cardiopathies	Vascular disease without parenchymal damage
Transient ischemia	Large vessel atherostenosis	Arterial territorial infarction (complete or incomplete)
Reversible ischemia	Large vessel occlusion (atheromatous, thrombotic, or embolic)	Watershed infarction (cortical or periventricular)
Minor stroke		Lacunar infarction
Major stroke	Small vessel arteriosclerosis	Subcortical arteriosclerotic encephalomalacia
Multi-infarct state	Other arteriopathies	Cortical atrophy Binswanger's disease

fibrillation, atrial or ventricular mural thrombus, mural myxoma, and infected or noninfected valvular vegetations. Cardiac dysrhythmia or aortic stenosis may result in global cerebral ischemia or in the accentuation of focal cerebrovascular occlusive disease. There is also a noncausal association between coronary artery disease and cerebrovascular occlusive disease as both pathologic processes share many risk factors (see below).[4]

Large-vessel atherosclerotic disease preferentially affects the carotid bifurcation in the neck, but it may involve the intrapetrous and intracavernous carotid arteries or more distal cerebral arteries less frequently. Large-vessel atherosclerosis may be responsible for artery-to-artery embolism of calcific fragments, thrombi, or platelet aggregates originating at the atherosclerotic plaque. In addition, large-vessel atherosclerosis may result in thrombotic arterial occlusion with subsequent hemodynamic compromise (depending on collateral circulation), thrombotic propagation (beyond collateral pathways), or tail embolism from the fresh occluding thrombus.

Small-vessel arteriosclerosis may affect perforating branches of the cerebral arteries at the base of the brain. Pathology in these vessels typically consists of lipohyalinosis, which is strongly associated with long-standing arterial hypertension.

Other arteriopathies that may affect the cerebral circulation include congenital, inflammatory, and idiopathic arteriopathies. A peculiar form of basal idiopathic occlusive vasculopathy affects arteries at the circle of Willis and their branches, with secondary proliferation of collateral vessels at the base of the brain, simulating a puff of smoke on angiography and given the term "moyamoya" disease from the Japanese language.

Parenchymal pathologic spectrum[5]

As mentioned previously, occlusive cerebrovascular disease may be present without parenchymal damage or clinical symptoms. In other situations, it may result in complete arterial territorial infarction (typically a wedge-shaped infarction outlining the territory of a major cerebral artery). Such arterial territorial infarction is usually thromboembolic in etiology and implies occlusion of the major vessel and impairment of the collaterals to that territory.

An incomplete arterial territorial infarction may be present, depending on the pattern and competence of collateral pathways.

Watershed infarctions affect the most distal territory of vascular supply. Watershed territories include the border zone of supply of the anterior, middle, and/or posterior cerebral arteries (usually high over the cerebral convexity). Another watershed territory may exist in periventricular regions between the penetrating branches of cortical vessels and perforating arteries that arise at the base of the brain.

Lacunar infarction refers to a small cavitation necrosis in the brain, corresponding to the territory of a deep parenchymal vessel. They have been shown to occur with occlusion of lipohyalinotic perforating arteries. Lacunar-like ischemic cavitations also occur in the watershed territories (hemodynamic) or as a result of embolism.[5]

Other parenchymal changes secondary to ischemia include cortical atrophy, subcortical arteriosclerotic encephalomalacia (leukoaraiosis), and the multi-infarct state, including Binswanger's disease.

Natural history

The natural history of many cerebrovascular disease entities has been elucidated with the advent of reliable diagnostic techniques (see below). It has been convincingly demonstrated that transient, reversible, or other ischemic insults predispose the patient to further brain ischemia, including massive devastating stroke.[6] The precise pathophysiology of the ischemic event greatly influences the prognosis.[7] Of patients with TIA, 20% to 30% will sustain a major ischemic stroke in the same territory in the subsequent 3–5 years. Patients with severe preocclusive carotid stenosis and TIA appear to be at much higher risk of subsequent stroke (up to 30% per year), while patients with completed carotid occlusion and a flurry of TIAs (around the time of occlusion) are very unlikely to sustain delayed ischemic infarction in the same territory.

Carotid stenoses are not static lesions.[7,8] Once a diagnosis of carotid stenosis has been established, it is likely that the lesions will progress in more than 50% of cases over the subsequent 1 to 5 years. This progression may be accelerated by uncontrolled vascular risk factors (see below).

The most risky phase following symptomatic brain ischemia is immediately after the ischemic spell. Up to one third of patients with ischemic symptoms may suffer further neurologic deterioration during the same hospitalization.[6] Again, the pathophysiologic mechanism of ischemia will largely determine the likelihood of further symptoms. Several lines of evidence indicate that the most critical periods in the natural history of an arterial stenosis are immediately preceding and immediately following arterial occlusion.[5,7–10] Therefore, the most serious lesions are those that are preocclusive or have recently occluded. This is mostly related to the ominous prognosis of propagating thrombosis and thromboembolism.

Between 30 and 60% of major (disabling) strokes are preceded by a temporary or minor ischemic insult.[6] It is therefore cardinal to identify the pathophysiologic mechanism of ischemia even when there are only minor symptoms, since many patients have much to lose from subsequent infarction in the same territory. Also, minor symptoms are often misinterpreted by patients and misdiagnosed by physicians, and transient symptoms can be missed if they occur during sleep.[6] Asymptomatic disease cannot be ignored because ominous occlusive cerebrovascular disease can well occur in the absence of any overt clinical symptoms.[6,11] In fact, a substantial fraction of disabling infarctions are not preceded by symptoms.

DIAGNOSTIC STUDIES

Doppler ultrasonography

Noninvasive examination of the cerebral circulation has been made possible by ultrasound applications of the Doppler principle[12] (i.e. the frequency shift of echoed signals in relation to signals emitted by the instrument, thereby revealing the velocity of moving blood in the insonated artery). It is known that blood velocity increases substantially at and just beyond a stenotic lesion. In addition, B-mode ultrasonography allows visualization of arterial walls based on their relative density to ultrasound beams.

Duplex sonography allows real-time imaging of extracranial carotid arteries using B-mode scanning of the vessel wall with simultaneous Doppler information about intravascular blood velocity. The resulting reconstruction provides an accurate representation of arterial stenosis and its resulting hemodynamic impact. Duplex ultrasonography of extracranial carotid arteries is highly sensitive to stenotic changes in the carotid arteries. However, ulcerative lesions may be missed unless heavily calcified or associated with local hemodynamic changes. Also, an artery can be assumed to be obstructed when the external and internal arteries are superimposed in one plane or when there is severe preocclusive stenosis and sluggish antegrade flow.[12]

Transcranial Doppler ultrasonography uses a low-frequency probe for improved tissue penetration (2 MHz as opposed to 7–10 MHz for Doppler study of extracranial vessels). The majority of the skull is opaque to ultrasound signals except for the thin squamosal portion of the temporal bone (temporal window), the orbits (orbital window), and the foramen magnum. These three windows allow insonation of vessels leading to and arising from the circle of Willis. Directional flow in these vessels can be accurately evaluated using transcranial Doppler, thereby providing a noninvasive index of collateral pathways. Also, flow velocities in the intracranial vessels may indicate hyperdynamic flow states or focal stenoses. Lastly, transcranial Doppler has been used to detect embolism in the intracranial cerebral circulation.

Both extracranial and transcranial Doppler studies are strongly technician-dependent. They need to be interpreted in conjunction with other diagnostic studies to avoid errors. Ultrasound evaluation of the cervical carotid arteries is an excellent way to rule out large-vessel carotid occlusive disease in the presence of symptomatic brain ischemia. However, this method cannot reliably assess the precise severity and extent of stenosis and there will be significant errors in evaluating severe preocclusive stenosis.

Arteriography

Injecting radiographic contrast material into cerebral arteries provides an excellent view of large and small cerebral arteries and facilitates a survey of flow dynamics and collateral pathways into various vascular territories (Figure 13.5, 13.6). These studies reliably show stenotic lesions in vessels larger than 1–2 mm and can also reveal embolic sources, including luminal thrombi and ulcerations. A complete survey of the cerebral circulation allows evaluation of collateral pathways, including their patency and contribution to the particular pathophysiologic situation, and determines the presence of occlusive disease, which might affect the collateral pathways. Many centers currently perform arterial digital subtraction angiography, which provides excellent visualization of arterial anatomy using small catheters and low contrast volume, resulting in lower procedure-related morbidity than conventional angiographic techniques. Transfemoral retrograde arterial catheterization has all but eliminated complications related to direct puncture of cerebral arteries. Finally, newer flow-directed catheters allow superselective arteriography as well as selective injection of therapeutic agents into small arterial branches.

A typical angiographic study in a case of brain ischemia would include selective injection of both carotid circulations (with extracranial and intracranial views in at least two planes) as well as visualization of the aortic arch, the origin of the great vessels, and preferably a view of the posterior circulation (essential if posterior circulation ischemia is suspected). In the presence of an arterial lesion, a careful evaluation of the cerebral angiogram should estimate dynamic flow rate and patterns of collateral circulation and rule out pseudo-occlusion (the false angiographic appearance of an occlusion as a result of exceedingly low flow rates). Pseudo-occlusion is demonstrated by obtaining late views of the apparently occluded artery to show the faint appearance of sluggish antegrade flow. In the setting of arterial branch occlusions, upstream vessels should be closely examined for potential emboligenic sources (e.g. atherosclerotic ulcers).

Computed tomography

The advent of computed tomography (CT) scanning of the brain has revolutionized the diagnosis of brain ischemia.[13] A patient with acute ischemic insult will usually have a negative CT scan, thereby ruling out other structural pathology, including hemorrhage, as a cause of the symptoms. Within hours of the ischemic spell (longer for small regions of ischemia), the CT scan shows decreased density in the infarcted parenchyma. This becomes more evident and well demarcated by 24–48 hours. Upon intravenous contrast administration, there may be enhancement of the infarcted tissue, indicating breakdown of the blood–brain barrier. This is noticeable several days after the onset of ischemia and remains prominent for several weeks. Chronic cerebral infarctions do not reveal contrast enhancement and essentially consist of cavitated lesions filled with cerebrospinal fluid.

The location of cerebral infarction can often be correlated with clinical symptoms.[13,14] Also, the CT may reveal evidence of prior remote ischemic insults. The appearance of cerebral infarction on CT scan can suggest a probable pathophysiologic mechanism (Figure 13.7).[14] Small lacunar cavitations are usually the result of small-vessel occlusive disease, and rarely of hemodynamic ischemia or embolism. Large wedge-shaped infarctions suggest thromboembolism and territorial arterial infarction. Ill-defined infarctions at the borders of arterial territories (high convexity or periventricular regions) could suggest hemodynamic ischemia.[14]

Other changes on the CT scan may indicate chronic cerebrovascular disease. Focal sulcal atrophy may indicate chronic hemodynamic insufficiency. Also, radiolucencies in the periventricular regions have been associated with cerebrovascular disease risk factors and subtle dementia. These have been referred to as "leukoaraiosis" and can represent an index of brain parenchymal changes caused by chronic cerebrovascular disease.[15]

Magnetic resonance imaging

All ischemic lesions visible on CT scan are more sensitively visualized by magnetic resonance imaging (MRI). In addition, MRI can reveal evidence of parenchymal infarction several hours before a CT scan.[16] In patients with cerebrovascular disease many lesions that cannot be seen on the CT scan are evident on MRI. Some of these MRI lesions represent subtle infarctions missed by the

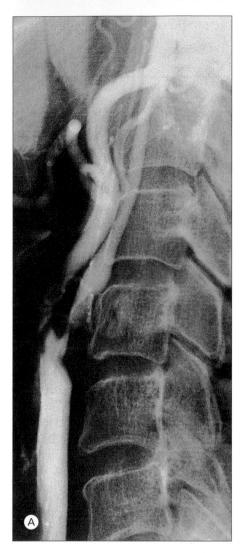

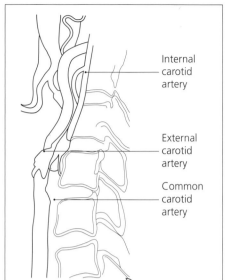

Internal
carotid
artery

External
carotid
artery

Common
carotid
artery

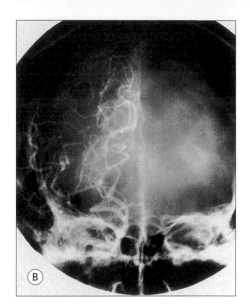

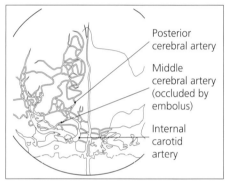

Posterior
cerebral artery

Middle
cerebral artery
(occluded by
embolus)

Internal
carotid
artery

Figure 13.5 Cerebral angiography. **(A)** Right common carotid arteriogram showing severe right internal carotid artery stenosis from atheroma at the carotid bifurcation. **(B)** Anteroposterior intracranial view of the same injection, revealing occlusion of the middle cerebral artery from embolism presumably originating from the atheroma upstream. The posterior cerebral artery fills from this same injection, indicating patency of the posterior circle of Willis.

CT scan; however, the majority correlate with the appearance of leukoaraiosis on the CT scan (Figure 13.8)[16,17] as well as various risk factors of cerebrovascular disease (including age). The lesions may indicate parenchymal brain changes caused by chronic cerebrovascular disease.[17]

More recently, flow imaging using MRI has enabled the cervical and intracranial vessels to be seen with a sensitivity, specificity, and spatial resolution exceeding that of ultrasound studies. This technique, magnetic resonance angiography, is in its infancy but may soon be perfected, replacing conventional angiography in certain situations. The more modern diffusion, perfusion, and spectroscopic imaging of MRI can reveal ischemic changes minutes after the onset of symptoms. These techniques are not yet widely available to the clinician.

Cerebral blood flow and metabolism

The above diagnostic methods do not provide a direct measure of rCBF or metabolism. Direct measurements can be useful in individual clinical situations when there is a difficult differential diagnosis or when therapeutic choices depend on, or are titrated against, cerebral blood flow and metabolic rates. It must be emphasized that this is rarely the case in routine clinical practice.[18]

The rCBF can be measured using the washout technique of inhaled or intravenously administered substances. This is the basis for various xenon rCBF measurements, including the CT technique that provides a quantified measure of rCBF with a tomographic spatial resolution of several millimeters.[19] The dynamic accumulation and/or washout of photon-emitting substances administered intravenously are the basis for single photon emission computed tomography (SPECT) (Figure 13.9). The regional cerebral metabolic rate of glucose and oxygen can be quantified tomographically using positron emission tomography (PET). These sophisticated and highly expensive instruments are available at few institutions and currently have limited clinical application. However, such instruments are powerful research tools that have significantly advanced our knowledge of pathophysiologic phenomena in brain ischemia.

PREVENTION AND MEDICAL MANAGEMENT

Risk factor modification

Several factors associated with a statistically increased risk of symptomatic brain ischemia[4] are age, essential hypertension, heart disease, and a prior history of symptomatic brain ischemia. Other

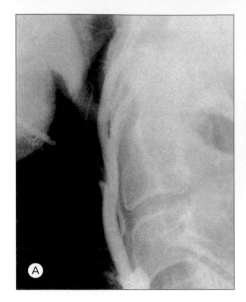
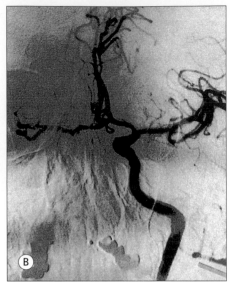
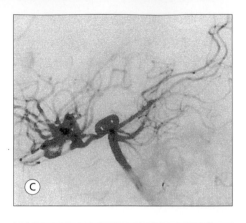
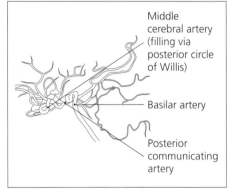
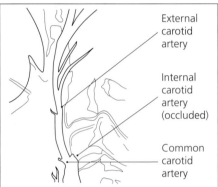
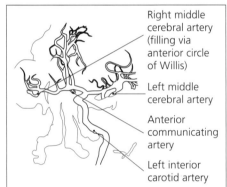

Figure 13.6 Cerebral angiography. **(A)** Right common carotid arteriogram injection revealing occlusion of the internal carotid artery just distal to its origin. **(B)** Anteroposterior intracranial (subtracted) view of the contralateral internal carotid artery injection showing filling of both cerebral hemispheres via a patent anterior circle of Willis. **(C)** Injection of the vertebrobasilar system (lateral view) in same case reveals filling of the right middle cerebral artery distribution via the posterior communicating artery, indicating patency of the posterior circle of Willis. This patient tolerated internal carotid artery occlusion without infarction and in view of excellent collateral filling is at low risk of subsequent brain ischemia in the same territory.

risk factors for stroke include diabetes, smoking, hyperlipemia, peripheral atherosclerotic occlusive disease, and the use of certain birth control pills. Controversy exists as to whether each of these factors independently increases the risk of stroke; clearly, many of these risks are interrelated.

Modification of risk factors (e.g. controlling arterial hypertension and discontinuing smoking) has been shown to alter the risk of subsequent stroke.[20] Risk factor modification may slow the progression of atherogenesis and alter hematologic and rheologic factors, lessening the risk of further ischemic insults. Risk factor modification alone will not reverse severe arterial stenosis and cannot *per se* eliminate all risk of subsequent stroke. However, it can be part of a comprehensive strategy of stroke prevention used in conjunction with other medical and surgical therapeutic options.

Medical therapy for stroke prevention

Antiplatelet therapy (usually aspirin 325–975 mg daily) has been shown to decrease the risk of ischemic stroke in several clinical settings,[21] an effect that seems more pronounced in males. But the risk of stroke is not altogether eliminated. In fact, given the pathophysiologic heterogeneity of stroke discussed previously, aspirin alone would not be expected to eradicate the risk of ischemic brain damage. Antiplatelet therapy can prevent the formation of mural fibrin-platelet clumps, which may play a role in retinal and cerebral emboli. Antiplatelet therapy can also inhibit the process of mural thrombosis in the heart and large vessels and improve blood flow characteristics in the cerebral microcirculation. More recently, aspirin has been shown to reduce (but not eliminate) the risk of cerebral embolism from atrial fibrillation.[22]

Anticoagulation therapy with heparin or warfarin inhibits the process of thrombosis and may prevent propagating thromboembolism when there is acute large-vessel occlusion and stroke-in-evolution.[21,23] Several clinical trials in progress address specific issues in various ischemic situations. A recently completed multi-institutional trial has demonstrated the effectiveness of warfarin therapy in the prevention of cerebral embolism from atrial fibrillation.[22] The beneficial effect of anticoagulation in this setting was far greater than the protection provided by antiplatelet therapy; however, the risks of anticoagulation therapy (especially prolonged anticoagulation) should be weighed against any proven

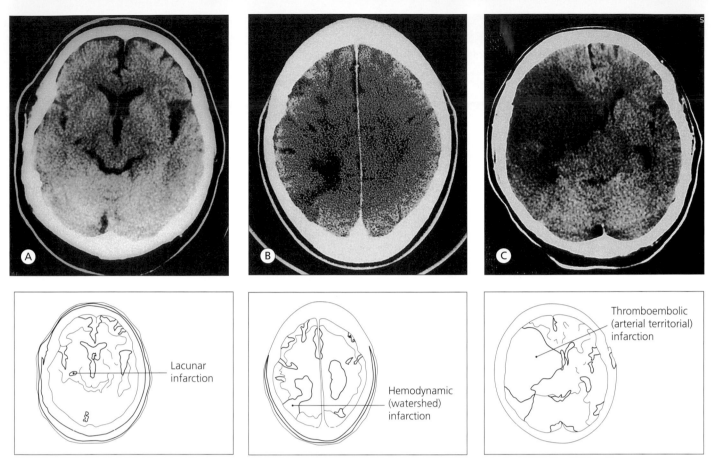

Figure 13.7 CT scan of cerebral infarction. **(A)** Lacunar infarction in the posterior limb of the internal capsule, presumed secondary to small-vessel disease; larger lacunar infarctions may also result from cerebral embolism. **(B)** Watershed infarction, presumably hemodynamic, in the territory bordering the middle cerebral and posterior cerebral arterial circulations. **(C)** Complete middle cerebral artery territorial infarction, presumed to be thromboembolic. Other embolic infarctions may result in partial arterial territorial parenchymal damage, depending on the size of the occluded branch, subsequent fragmentation of the embolus, and collateral pathways.

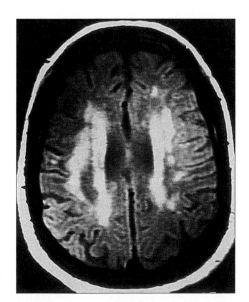

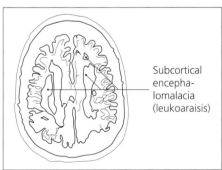

Figure 13.8 MRI in brain ischemia. This modality is highly sensitive to parenchymal changes of ischemia. In this case, there are multiple focal confluent regions of increased signal in the centrum semiovale and periventricular regions. These changes, typical of subcortical encephalomalacia (leukoaraiosis), correlate with age and cerebrovascular risk factors. These changes may be an index of parenchymal brain changes with chronic cerebrovascular disease.

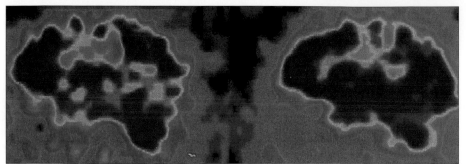

Figure 13.9 Single photon emission computed tomographic (SPECT) cerebral blood flow scan in a patient with carotid occlusion and frequent spells of hemiparesis but no evidence of infarction on CT or MRI scan. The parasagittal cuts demonstrate focal hypoperfusion in the watershed border zone between the territories of the anterior cerebral and middle cerebral arteries.

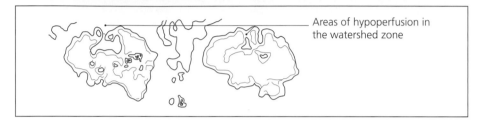

Areas of hypoperfusion in the watershed zone

or suspected benefits.[24] Risks of systemic or cerebral hemorrhage are in the range of 1–5% per year depending on the anticoagulation regimen and patient population. Anticoagulation is contraindicated when there is extensive brain infarction (high risk of hemorrhagic sequelae) or evidence of central nervous system or systemic bleeding. Chronic anticoagulation is contraindicated in unreliable or noncompliant patients and in those who are subject to frequent falls or trauma. Little consensus exists about the optimal regimen of anticoagulation for brain ischemia. There is no evidence that vigorous anticoagulation (beyond 1.5 to 2 times control values on clotting tests) provides any additional protection, yet it subjects the patient to increased hemorrhagic risk compared to lesser degrees of anticoagulation.

In summary, antiplatelet therapy is indicated in the presence of asymptomatic cerebrovascular disease and following TIA, RIND, or previous stroke. Antiplatelet therapy is not a substitute for other therapeutic intervention for cardiac disease or pre-occlusive large-vessel stenosis. Anticoagulation therapy may be useful in the setting of cardioembolism, preocclusive large-vessel stenosis (as a temporary measure or in patients who are not candidates for surgery), and in certain cases of stroke-in-evolution if there is suspicion of propagating thrombosis and thromboembolism. This therapy may also be indicated if hypercoagulability predisposes the patient to cerebral ischemia.

Management of acute brain ischemia

General medical measures are indicated in the management of each case of acute brain ischemia (Table 13.2). Whenever necessary, airway support must be established. There should be careful attention to hemodynamic and rheologic optimization, electrolyte balance, and nutritional maintenance. Deep vein thromboembolic and gastrointestinal bleeding prophylaxis and respiratory and physical therapy are indicated in all cases of major stroke and should be initiated as soon as possible.[25]

Regardless of the extent of clinical symptoms, diagnostic studies should be undertaken following immediate medical stabilization. Most clinicians agree that a TIA or RIND should be treated as a medical emergency until the possibility of serious impending progression has been eliminated. Initial diagnostic studies should include parenchymal neuroimaging (CT or MRI) and vascular evaluation. Duplex ultrasonography with or without transcranial Doppler examination or magnetic resonance angiography (where available) can be used as a screening measure. Cerebral angiography is performed whenever large-vessel disease has not been reliably ruled out by noninvasive studies or when the diagnosis or pathophysiologic mechanisms remain in question. A cardiac evaluation is performed in every case and should at least include an electrocardiogram and an echocardiogram. Patients with strongly suspected cardioembolism should probably be studied by transesophageal echocardiography because of its higher sensitivity. Patients considered for major surgical procedures should undergo a cardiology clearance, including a thorough evaluation of cardiac risks and possible coronary angiography.

Stroke is a powerful risk factor of subsequent myocardial infarction and cardiac death.

Therapy should be initiated to limit ischemic parenchymal damage and to prevent progressive ischemia. In all cases in which a significant region of tissue injury is suspected, consideration should be given to treating the patient with one or more regimens or agents that have been shown, in experimental and clinical studies, to reduce parenchymal damage from brain ischemia[26] (i.e. mannitol, dextran, hypertensive hypervolemic therapy, avoidance of hemoconcentration and, possibly, anticonvulsants and calcium channel blockers).

Therapy to prevent recurrent ischemia should be initiated according to suspected or demonstrated pathophysiologic mechanisms. The type of therapy depends on the nature and extent of vascular and parenchymal pathology. Such therapy may include antiplatelet drugs, anticoagulants, surgical intervention, and, possibly, endovascular therapy. Risk factor modification and long-term rehabilitation should be instituted in every case.[25]

SURGERY FOR EXTRACRANIAL CAROTID DISEASE

Indications

Convergent evidence from clinical registries, natural history studies, and at least two recent multi-institutional prospective

Table 13.2 Management of acute brain ischemia

General medical measures	Diagnostic studies	Therapy to limit parenchymal damage	Therapy to prevent recurrent ischemia
Airway support	Parenchymal neuroimaging	Mannitol	Antiplatelet therapy
Nutritional support	(CT or MRI)	Anticonvulsants (?)	Anticoagulant therapy
Electrolyte balance	Vascular evaluation (ultrasound, angiography)	Calcium-channel blockers (?)	Surgery
Hemodynamic optimization	Cardiac evaluation	Dextran (or related agents) (?)	Endovascular therapy (?)
Hemostatic optimization	Hemostatic optimization	Hypertensive therapy (?)	Risk factor modification
Rheologic optimization		Hypervolemic therapy (?)	
Deep-vein thromboembolic prophylaxis		Hemodilution (?)	
Gastrointestinal bleeding prophylaxis		Thrombolysis (?)	
Respiratory therapy			
Physical therapy			

Table 13.3 Carotid endarterectomy indications

Proven indication	Other possible indications	Possible contraindications
Severe (>70%) internal carotid artery cross-sectional stenosis* and previous ipsilateral cerebral or retinal ischemic symptoms	Less severe stenosis in presence of deep shaggy ulceration and definite attributable symptoms Preocclusive asymptomatic stenosis	Serious medical risk (consider regional anesthesia) Recent large parenchymal infarction

*Measured as angiographic vessel diameter at narrowest point, divided by normal distal vessel diameter beyond the atheromatous plaque.

randomized trials have demonstrated the effectiveness of carotid endarterectomy for stroke prevention in severe (greater than 70%) cervical internal carotid artery stenosis and previous ipsilateral cerebral or retinal ischemic symptoms. Carotid artery surgery in this setting has been shown to decrease significantly the risk of subsequent stroke compared to the best medical therapy alone.[27]

Other possible indications for carotid endarterectomy include less severe stenosis in the presence of deep shaggy ulceration and definite attributable symptoms and preocclusive asymptomatic stenosis (Table 13.3).[28] Possible contraindications to carotid endarterectomy include serious medical risk (consider regional anesthesia) and recent large parenchymal infarction (high risk of perfusion breakthrough and brain hemorrhage). Recent limited parenchymal infarction is not a contraindication to carotid endarterectomy.

Carotid artery surgery has also been used when the patient has acute carotid occlusion and minor stroke (thrombectomy and endarterectomy). External carotid endarterectomy is indicated for ipsilateral retinal or cerebral symptoms in the setting of chronic carotid occlusion and impaired external carotid collaterals (or ulcerated carotid bifurcation stump and proximal external carotid artery emboligenic sources).[28] These indications have not been thoroughly examined in scientific studies.

Carotid endarterectomy

The technique of carotid endarterectomy is illustrated in Figure 13.10. A cervical incision is made along the anterior border of the sternocleidomastoid muscle. Dissection then proceeds through the platysma layer and medial to the sternocleidomastoid muscle along its length (with interruption of the common facial and other bridging veins). The carotid sheath is entered medial to the internal jugular vein, exposing the distal common carotid artery and the proximal several centimeters of internal and external carotid arteries. The carotid body may be anesthetized to blunt hemodynamic instability during the remainder of the operation. Systemic anticoagulation is administered (typically 100 IU heparin/kg body weight) followed by temporary cross-clamping of the carotid bifurcation. An arteriotomy is performed at the distal common carotid artery and along the proximal internal carotid artery to a point just beyond the stenotic plaque. Endarterectomy is then performed in the subintimal plane, separating the plaque from the underlying arterial media. This portion of the operation is performed with technical precision so that all potential intimal flaps and sources of emboli are removed. The distal intima along the internal carotid artery is tacked down with carefully placed 7-0 vascular sutures unless it is absolutely adherent to the underlying vessel wall. The arteriotomy is closed with a continuous

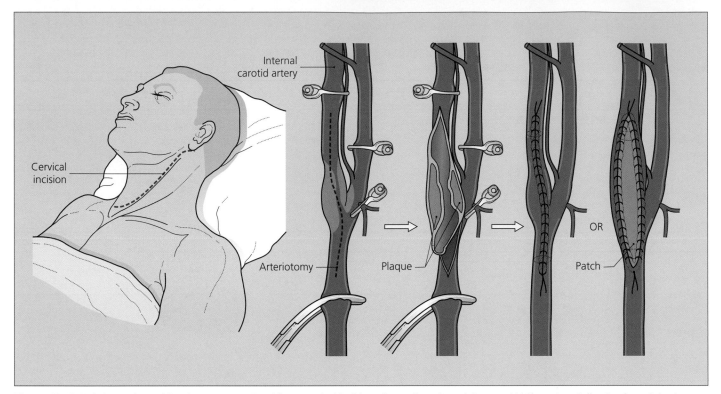

Figure 13.10 Technique of carotid endarterectomy. An oblique cervical incision allows dissection of the carotid bifurcation. Following heparinization, the arteries of the bifurcation are cross-clamped and an arteriotomy is performed. The plaque is dissected precisely in the subintimal plane, with a subsequent closure (primary or via patch reconstruction) of the arteriotomy. Other adjuvant technical aspects of the operation include intraoperative monitoring during cross-clamping, microsurgical technique allowing optimal lighting and magnification, patch angioplasty, shunting, and verification of patency.

5-0 or 6-0 vascular suture. A vein or synthetic patch may be incorporated in the arteriotomy closure to widen the vessel lumen.

The success of carotid endarterectomy clearly depends on the technical precision of the operation and the meticulous prevention of cerebral complications during the procedure. Anesthetic technique should maximize cerebral and cardiac protection, and intraoperative hypotension must be avoided, especially during carotid cross-clamping. Intraoperative monitoring using electro-encephalography, evoked potential monitoring, transcranial Doppler, cerebral blood flow, or other modalities enhances operative safety. Electroencephalography is widely used, and has been shown to be a reliable predictor of intraoperative brain ischemia.[28]

Technical adjuncts to this operation include meticulous hemo-static dissection and optimal illumination and magnification. The operating microscope enables neurosurgeons to pay meticulous attention to intimal flaps and arteriotomy closure. Luminal shunting may prevent hemodynamic cerebral insufficiency during carotid cross-clamping; however, it hinders visualization and tech-nical perfection of the endarterectomy itself and may increase the chance of intraoperative cerebral embolism. Selective shunting, indicated by electroencephalographic changes during carotid cross-clamping, allows selection of patients whose circulation requires a shunt (and enables an easier and technically superior operation), while sparing a shunt in the majority of patients.[28]

Patching during arteriotomy closure increases luminal diameter. It may decrease the likelihood of postoperative carotid occlusion[29] and carotid restenosis. Patching may increase the likelihood of suture line disruption and lengthen the duration of cross-clamping. Many surgeons use patch angioplasty in endarter-ectomies, except with large vessels and very focal stenoses.[29]

Many surgeons advocate intraoperative verification of arterial patency, which can be done using ultrasonography or intra-operative angiography. Reversal of anticoagulation is optional, and there are many theoretical arguments against it (the endarterec-tomized vessel is most thrombogenic in the first 90 minutes following carotid endarterectomy). However, this consideration must be balanced against the risk of bleeding from the arteriotomy and other sites. The majority of surgeons drain the wound but this too must be viewed in light of the overall hemostatic aspects of the dissection.

Outstanding results have been reported with carotid endar-terectomy whether or not one or more of the above technical adjuncts is used. The routine or selective use of most of the aforementioned modalities continues to be debated. However, the common denominator of operative success is careful anesthetic management and compulsive attention to the technical details of vascular repair.

Surgical results

A combination of judicious patient selection and superior surgical technique should ensure an operative mortality rate of less than 2% and stroke rate of less than 4%. This outcome has been consistently accomplished by experienced and well-trained surgeons in symptomatic and asymptomatic patients (morbidity rates are slightly higher in symptomatic cases). A preoperative grading of medical, angiographic, and neurologic risks may help one predict the surgical outcome. It is unlikely that the operation will provide a significant overall benefit unless the surgical team can achieve this standard of surgical performance. Carotid artery surgery should be used judiciously in conjunction with other medical treatment modalities and risk factor modification programs for optimal stroke prevention.

Carotid artery surgery helps prevent subsequent brain ischemia secondary to hemodynamic insufficiency, arterial embolism, or propagating thrombosis from the diseased artery. The surgery does not necessarily protect against other mechanisms of brain ischemia, and it does not eliminate the risk of subsequent stroke altogether.

The benefits of carotid artery surgery appear to be durable. Recurrent stenosis (50% narrowing) occurs at a rate of 5–10% per year following operation but is not always symptomatic.[30] Symptomatic brain ischemia attributable to a previously operated artery is rare and may be amenable to successful reoperation. The use of patch angioplasty, risk factor modification, and medical therapy may decrease the likelihood of symptomatic restenosis.[29,30]

NONATHEROSCLEROTIC CAROTID OCCLUSIVE DISEASE

Carotid occlusive disease can be documented in the absence of atherosclerotic risk factors. Fibromuscular dysplasia is a vasculopathy affecting multiple large and medium-sized arteries, including renal and carotid arteries.[31] When affecting the cervical carotid circulation, it may result in a bead-like, string-like, or pseudoaneurysmal appearance of the carotid artery. This may predispose the patient to carotid dissection or hemodynamic insufficiency.

Carotid dissection results from disruption of the intimal vascular plane, with blood flow partially directed in the sub-intimal, intramedial, or subadventitial plane.[32] Carotid dissection may occur spontaneously or following blunt trauma, and it has also been associated with fibromuscular dysplasia. The most frequent location of vessel disruption is at the level of the second vertebral body, usually well beyond the carotid bifurcation and just proximal to the carotid canal of the skull. It has been postulated that this location predisposes the artery to tethering against the bony lateral mass of the axis.

Carotid dissection can result in occlusion, near-occlusion, and/or intraluminal or subintimal thrombosis. In fact, the angiographic appearance of a tapered occlusion or stenosis of the internal carotid artery beyond a normal (nonatheromatous) bifurcation is nearly pathognomonic of dissection. Pseudo-aneurysmal outpouching may occur at the level of dissection.

Carotid dissection should be treated medically since surgical correction of the intimal flap is typically too risky (the dissection usually extends into the bony carotid canal). Anticoagulation therapy appears to provide excellent protection against thrombo-embolic complications and may enhance vascular healing.[32] If anticoagulation therapy is used, a large number of carotid dissections will heal, so angiographically the vessel returns to normal or near-normal appearance. A small number will undergo complete carotid occlusion, while the remainder will continue to show varying degrees of stenosis, irregularity, and aneurysmal appearance. Upon vascular healing and resolution of the severe stenotic appearance of a dissection, anticoagulation therapy may be converted to antiplatelet therapy, which is usually continued indefinitely.

VERTEBRAL ARTERY OCCLUSIVE DISEASE

Infarctions of the vertebrobasilar territory carry a grave prognosis, with acute mortality ranging between 20% and 30%. Nearly half of the patients suffer previous TIAs or minor strokes in the same distribution, while subsequent stroke occurs within 5 years in 26–35% of patients with vertebrobasilar TIA. This rate is comparable to that following TIAs in the carotid territory.[28]

Isolated stenosis at the origin of a single vertebral artery is usually well tolerated, and many patients remain asymptomatic despite the absence or occlusion of one vertebral artery. However, extracranial vertebral artery disease is not always benign. At autopsy more than half of posterior circulation infarctions are associated with extracranial occlusion or stenosis of a single vertebral artery. Less commonly, vertebrobasilar ischemia results from traumatic or spontaneous dissection of a vertebral artery, tethering by a fibrous cervical band, or extensive compression by an osteophyte. Occasionally, obstruction of the subclavian artery proximal to the origin of the vertebral artery will reverse flow in the vertebral artery and produce a steal of blood from the vertebral artery to the ipsilateral brachial artery. This subclavian steal is often asymptomatic and has rarely been convincingly associated with serious neurologic morbidity. While embolism occurs in certain patients, hemodynamic mechanisms are thought to be the major etiologic factors in vertebrobasilar ischemia. Propagating thrombosis from fresh occlusion of an artery also plays a role in cases with serious infarction.

No medical or surgical therapy has been demonstrated to be effective in preventing vertebrobasilar ischemia. As a result of the wide variety of possible mechanisms, it is not likely that a single modality will be beneficial in all cases. A rational therapeutic approach to the individual patient requires accurate delineation of pathophysiologic mechanisms. Antiplatelet therapy is likely to be effective when there are mild atherosclerotic plaques in the vertebrobasilar circulation with or without symptoms. Antiplatelet therapy is not likely to improve the hemodynamic consequences of severe stenosis or vascular occlusion. Antiplatelet therapy does not protect against vascular occlusion or propagating thrombosis. Anticoagulant therapy is indicated when there is severe hemodynamically significant stenosis or fresh luminal thrombosis and propagating thromboembolism.

Surgical intervention should be considered in situations of accessible focal stenoses of the vertebral artery, especially when contralateral vertebral artery occlusion is present.[28] The goals of surgical intervention in extracranial vertebral artery disease are to reverse hemodynamic compromise and eliminate embolic sources. Indications for surgery include persistent clinical symptoms of vertebrobasilar ischemia and angiographic evidence of hemo-dynamic compromise. Lesions without hemodynamic compromise are considered for surgery only after the failure of antiplatelet or anticoagulant therapy. Surgical options include vertebral artery transposition, vertebral endarterectomy, and other more specialized procedures.

Vertebral artery transposition is indicated in focal vertebral artery origin stenosis or in the rare situations of subclavian steal with demonstrated symptoms of vertebrobasilar ischemia. The goal of the operation is to transpose the vertebral artery (distal to stenotic segment) onto the common carotid artery in an end-to-side fashion. This results in vertebral artery flow arising from the common carotid artery, thereby bypassing the stenotic lesion (Figure 13.11). The operation is performed via a transverse incision 2 cm above the clavicle, and extending approximately

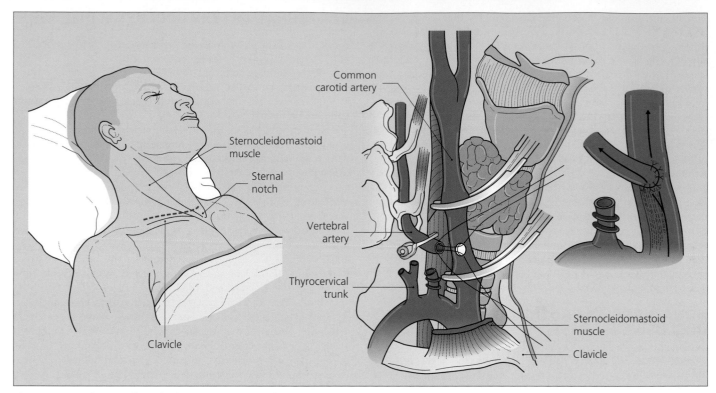

Figure 13.11 Technique of vertebral artery transposition for severe origin stenosis of the vertebral artery and hemodynamic insufficiency in the vertebrobasilar circulation. A transverse lateral cervical incision allows exposure of the vertebral artery and common carotid artery. The vertebral artery is transected just distal to the stenosis and transposed in an end-to-side fashion to the common carotid artery. This operation is also performed in rare cases of clearly symptomatic subclavian steal.

6–8 cm behind the anterior border of the sternocleidomastoid muscle. The sternocleidomastoid muscle is divided transversely and the carotid sheath is entered by retraction of the jugular vein. The common carotid artery is isolated and followed proximally to locate the subclavian artery. Then the vertebral artery is identified (usually 1–2 cm proximal to the origin of the thyrocervical trunk) and dissected from its origin at the subclavian artery to its point of entrance into the bony foramen transversarium. After full heparinization (see carotid endarterectomy), the origin of the vertebral artery is double clipped and the artery is transected just distal to the stenotic lesion. After microvascular preparation and tapering of the vessel end, it is transposed in an end-to-side fashion onto the nearby common carotid artery. The latter is cross-clamped for the duration of anastomosis, with monitoring undertaken as in carotid endarterectomy. End-to-side anastomosis is performed using a 7-0 suture under microsurgical magnification.

In various series the reported outcome of this procedure, including prevention of further symptomatic ischemia, is comparable to that of carotid endarterectomy.[28]

Other extracranial vertebral artery procedures include endarterectomy of a focal arterial segment, untethering of stenosing fibrous bands, or resection of compressing osteophytes. These procedures are performed via a direct approach, ensuring adequate surgical exposure for proximal and distal control on the vertebral artery.

INTRACRANIAL OCCLUSIVE DISEASE

Atherosclerotic occlusive disease may affect vessels that are inaccessible to direct extracranial endarterectomy. Such intracranial stenoses have a serious prognosis and are associated with a significant risk of subsequent stroke and myocardial infarction.[33] Extracranial-to-intracranial (EC–IC) bypass surgery in the setting of symptomatic stenoses has not been effective. In fact, there is a significant likelihood of a bypass converting a stenotic lesion into a symptomatic occlusion with disastrous consequences.[34] Intracranial arterial stenoses are best treated medically. Rare surgical options include extracranial endarterectomy of upstream tandem stenoses and EC–IC bypass after all medical therapy has failed and convincing hemodynamic compromise has been demonstrated (see below).

Occlusion of major cerebral arteries is associated with a significant risk of stroke at the time of vessel occlusion. Delayed ischemia is uncommon but may occur via a wide variety of mechanisms. These include thromboembolism via collateral pathways or progressive hemodynamic compromise because of impaired collaterals. Also, small-vessel disease may occur incidentally in the same territory as an occluded artery.[35]

Bypass surgery was designed to provide collateral blood flow to the territory of occluded or severely stenosed cerebral arteries. A large international cooperative study, however, failed to reveal any benefit of EC–IC bypass surgery in the setting of symptomatic arterial occlusions and inaccessible stenoses.[36] However, the study was not designed to assess, with statistical reliability, benefit or lack of benefit from the procedure in specific subgroups of patients. Two particular subgroups were not addressed: those for whom the best available medical therapy had failed and those with clearly documented hemodynamic compromise. (1) For patients for whom the best available medical therapy failed, over 50% of the patients admitted to the study did not have a trial on medical therapy and may have been less likely to benefit from additional revascularization than patients who had further brain ischemia despite antiplatelet therapy or anticoagulation. (2) For patients with clearly documented hemodynamic compromise, over one-third of the patients in the study had internal carotid artery occlusion without subsequent symptoms, while many others had hemodynamically insignificant lesions. Including all patients with brain ischemia without regard to the pathophysiologic mechanisms in each subgroup (i.e. including a large number of patients who by current understanding of the disease would not be candidates for the procedure) may have diluted the study. A limited number of patients who have clear hemodynamic compromise and/or for whom medical therapy has failed may benefit from the procedure, although the study was not designed to uncover benefit in these patients.[28,37]

There is a consensus among many cerebrovascular surgeons that a small group of patients with arterial occlusions, impaired collaterals, and demonstrated progressive ischemia despite anticoagulant therapy may benefit from revascularization surgery. Two strict criteria must be met to justify a bypass procedure in the era following the EC–IC bypass study: demonstrated hemodynamic compromise (impaired collaterals and preferably a confirmatory study demonstrating rCBF compromise) and failed maximal medical therapy.[28,37]

Several techniques provide a bypass graft between the extracranial and intracranial circulations,[28,37] including direct anastomoses of the superficial temporal artery to cortical branches of the middle cerebral artery. Also, long segments of high-flow grafts can be established between the cervical carotid arteries and more proximal segments of the middle cerebral artery. The preferred procedure currently performed at our institution interposes a reversed short segment of saphenous vein between the superficial temporal artery at the level of the zygoma (in an end-to-side fashion) to an M2 segment of the middle cerebral artery within the sylvian fissure (also in an end-to-side fashion) (Figure 13.12). This allows the creation of a high-flow conduit with high short-term and long-term patency rates and low operative morbidity.[28,37]

Other clinical situations in which an EC–IC bypass procedure might be considered include giant cerebral aneurysms not amenable to direct clipping and vascular reconstruction (where the parent vessel must be sacrificed), extensive brain tumors invading cerebral arteries, and progressive occlusive vasculopathies (including "moyamoya" disease). Bypass surgery in these cases is individualized according to the angiographic collateral pattern, rCBF measurements, and tolerance of temporary occlusion tests (which may be performed using intravascular balloons with the patient awake and anticoagulated).[38]

An EC–IC bypass procedure is rarely considered for progressively symptomatic intracranial vertebrobasilar occlusive disease that occurs despite anticoagulant therapy. In such instances, anastomosis of the occipital or superficial temporal artery may be

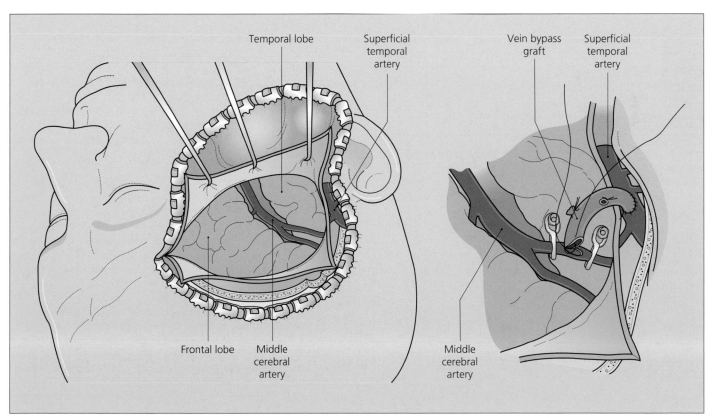

Figure 13.12 Superficial temporal artery-to-middle cerebral artery bypass technique. This is one of many possible technical methods of providing a bypass between the extracranial and intracranial circulations. The superficial temporal artery is exposed at the level of the zygomatic arch. A small pterional craniotomy is performed with splitting of the sylvian fissure, and exposure of the middle cerebral artery bifurcation. An interpositional vein bypass graft is then performed in an end-to-side fashion to both arteries. Other technical approaches for bypass include direct artery-to-artery end-to-side anastomosis, the use of more peripheral middle cerebral artery branches, and modifications of the technique for posterior circulation bypass.

CLINICAL PEARLS

- The brain requires 20% of the cardiac output to function normally. Cerebral blood flow below 20mL/100g/min can foretell an ischemic event. Transient ischemic attacks (TIAs) are ischemic events that reverse within 24 h; reversible ischemic neurologic deficits (RINDs) reverse in less than 3 days. Of all patients suffering a TIA, 20–30% will develop a stroke in the same territory within 5 years. Moreover, 30–60% of all strokes are preceded by a temporary or minor neurologic event.

- Brain ischemia can be caused by cardiac disease, large vessel disease, such as carotid atherosclerotic disease, small vessel disease associated with hypertension, or a variety of congenital, inflammatory, or idiopathic arteriopathies. Risk factors for stroke include increasing age, hypertension, diabetes, smoking, atherosclerotic disease, and certain drugs.

- There is a beneficial effect of anticoagulation with warfarin for prevention of stroke associated with atrial fibrillation. Antiplatelet therapy is indicated in patients with asymptomatic cerebrovascular disease and those suffering from TIAs, RINDs, or previous strokes. Multi-institutional trials have demonstrated the effectiveness of carotid endarterectomy for stroke prevention in severe (greater than 70%) carotid artery stenosis in patients with ipsilateral ischemic symptoms.

- Vertebral artery occlusive disease associated with infarction carries a grave prognosis. The acute mortality is between 20 and 30%. No medical or surgical therapy has been shown to be uniformly effective in preventing vertebrobasilar ischemia. Antiplatelet therapy may be indicated in patients with atherosclerotic disease but may not be effective in patients with severe stenosis. Anticoagulation may be indicated in patients with stenosis,or luminal thrombosis.

- The efficacy of extracranial to intracranial (EC–IC) bypass and endovascular stenting in cerebral ischemic disease has yet to be proven but ongoing studies are researching the safety and efficacy of such novel surgical therapies compared with medical therapy.

performed (directly or via an interpositional vein graft) to the posterior inferior cerebellar artery, anterior inferior cerebellar artery, superior cerebellar artery, or posterior cerebral artery, depending on the site of arterial stenosis and collateral pathways.[28]

CONCLUSION

Brain ischemia is the result of complex interactions between the brain parenchyma, vascular occlusive disease, and cerebral blood flow. Multiple pathophysiologic mechanisms are frequently operating, and interact closely to determine the eventual clinical prognosis. Therapeutic modalities include a variety of medical treatments and selected surgical procedures, which should be judiciously combined and/or individualized in each case, and which must be guided, whenever possible, by a rational analysis of pathophysiologic mechanisms and natural history. It is not likely that any single treatment will benefit all patients with brain ischemia. Further studies are likely to clarify the role of individual treatment modalities in the light of such pathophysiologic heterogeneity.

REFERENCES

1. Siesjo BK. *Brain Energy Metabolism*. New York, NY: John Wiley & Sons; 1978: 1–149.
2. Jones TH, Morawetz RB, Crowell RM, *et al*. Thresholds of focal cerebral ischemia in awake monkeys. *J Neurosurg* 1981; 54: 773–82.
3. Raichle MF. The pathophysiology of brain ischemia and infarction. *Clin Neurosurg* 1982; 29: 379–89.
4. Wolf PA, D'Agostino RB, Belanger AJ, *et al*. Probability of stroke: a risk profile from the Framingham Study. *Stroke* 1991; 22: 312–18.
5. Ringelstein EB, Zeumer H, Angelou D. The pathogenesis of strokes from internal carotid artery occlusion: diagnostic and therapeutical implications. *Stroke* 1983; 14: 867–75.
6. Toole JF. Transient ischemic attacks. In: Toole JF (ed.). *Cerebrovascular Disorders*. New York, NY: Raven Press; 1984: 101–16.
7. Bogousslavsky J, Despland PA, Regli F. Prognosis of high-risk patients with nonoperated symptomatic extracranial carotid tight stenosis. *Stroke* 1988; 19: 108–11.
8. Javid H, Ostermiller WE, Hengesh JW, *et al*. Natural history of carotid bifurcation atheroma. *Surgery* 1970; 67: 80–9.
9. Pessin MS, Hinton RC, Davis KR, *et al*. Mechanisms of acute stroke. *Ann Neurol* 1979; 6: 245–51.
10. Norrving B, Nilsson B. Carotid artery occlusion: acute symptoms and long-term prognosis. *Neurol Res* 1981; 3: 229–36.
11. Bogousslavsky J, Despland PA, Regli F. Asymptomatic tight stenosis of the internal carotid artery: long-term prognosis. *Neurology* 1986; 36: 861–3.
12. Smith R, Brown R, Martin J, *et al*. Noninvasive carotid artery testing: an expanding science. In: Wood JH (ed.). *Carotid Artery Surgery in Stroke*. Philadelphia, PA: Hanley and Belfus; 1989: 27–42.
13. Savoiardo M. CT scanning. In: Barnett HJM, Stein BM, Mohr JP, Yatsu FM (eds). *Stroke: Pathophysiology, Diagnosis and Management*. New York, NY: Churchill Livingstone; 1986: 189–219.
14. Wozard R. Watershed infarctions and computed tomography: a topographical study in cases with stenosis or occlusion of the carotid artery. *Neuroradiology* 1980; 19: 245–8.
15. Hachinski VC, Potter P, Merskey H. Leuko-araiosis. *Arch Neurol* 1987; 44: 21–3.
16. Awad IA, Modic M, Little JR, *et al*. Focal parenchymal lesions in transient ischemic attacks; correlation of CT and MRI. *Stroke* 1986; 17: 399–403.

17. Awad IA, Spetzler RF, Hodak JA, *et al*. Incidental subcortical lesions identified on MRI in the elderly, I: correlation with age and cerebrovascular risk factors. *Stroke* 1986; 17: 1084–9.

18. Yanagihara T, Wahner HW. Cerebral blood flow measurement in cerebrovascular occlusive disease. *Stroke* 1984; 15: 816–22.

19. Yonas H, Goode WF, Gur D, *et al*. Mapping central blood flow by xenon-enhanced computed tomography: clinical experience. *Radiology* 1984; 152: 435–42.

20. Hypertension Detection and Follow-up Program Cooperative Group. Five-year findings of the Hypertension Detection and Follow-up Program, III: reduction in stroke incidents among persons with high blood pressure. *JAMA* 1982; 247: 633–8.

21. Dykan ML. Anticoagulant and platelet antiaggregating therapy in stroke and threatened stroke. *Neurol Clin* 1983; 1: 223–42.

22. Kelly RE. Stroke prevention in Atrial Fibrillation Study – preliminary results. Presented at 16th International Joint Conference on Stroke and Cerebral Circulation; February 21, 1991; San Francisco, CA.

23. Putnam SF, Adams HB, Usefulness of heparin in initial management of patients with recent transient ischemic attacks. *Arch Neurol* 1985; 42: 960–2.

24. Levine M, Hirsch J. Hemorrhagic complications of long-term anticoagulant therapy for ischemic cerebral vascular disease. *Stroke* 1986; 17: 111–16.

25. Hachinski V, Norris JW. *The Acute Stroke*, Contemporary Neurology Series 27. Philadelphia, PA: FA Davis; 1985.

26. Siesjo BK, Wieloch T. Cerebral metabolism in ischemia: neurochemical basis for therapy. *Br J Anaesthiol* 1985; 57: 47–62.

27. NASCET Investigators. Clinical Alert. Benefit of carotid endarterectomy for patients with high grade stenosis of the internal carotid artery. Bethesda, MD: National Institute of Neurological Disorders and Stroke; February 25, 1991.

28. Spetzler RF, Nehls DG, Awad IA. Ischemia and infarction: surgical treatment. In: Toole JF (ed.). *Handbook of Clinical Neurology: Vascular Diseases, Part I*. New York, NY: Elsevier Science; 1989: 441–58.

29. Awad IA, Little JR. Patch angioplasty in carotid endarterectomy: advantages, concerns and controversies. *Stroke* 1989; 20: 417–22.

30. Clagett GP, Rich NM, McDonald PT, *et al*. Etiologic factors for recurrent carotid artery stenosis. *Surgery* 1983; 93: 913–18.

31. Olivi A, Tew JM, Van Loveran HR. Fibromuscular dysplasia. In: Wood JH (ed.). *Carotid Artery Surgery in Stroke. Neurosurgery: State of the Art Reviews*. Philadelphia, PA: Hanley and Belfus; 1989:193–200.

32. Hart RG, Easton JD. Dissections and trauma of cervico-cerebral arteries. In: Barnett HJM, Stein BM, Mohr JP, Yatsu FM (eds). *Stroke: Pathophysiology, Diagnosis, and Management*. New York, NY: Churchill Livingstone; 1986: 775–88.

33. Marzewski DJ, Furlan AJ, St Louis P, *et al*. Intracranial internal carotid artery stenosis: long-term prognosis. *Stroke* 1982; 13: 821–4.

34. Awad IA, Furlan AJ, Little JR. Changes in intracranial stenotic lesions after extracranial–intracranial bypass surgery. *J Neurosurg* 1984; 60: 771–6.

35. Furlan AJ, Whisnant JP, Baker HL. Long-term prognosis after carotid artery occlusion. *Neurology* 1980; 30: 986–8.

36. EC-IC Bypass Study Group. Failure of extracranial–intracranial arterial bypass to reduce the risk of ischemic stroke, results of an international randomized trial. *N Engl J Med* 1985; 313: 1191–200.

37. Awad IA, Spetzler RF. Extracranial–intracranial (EC–IC) bypass surgery: a critical analysis in light of the International Cooperative Study. *Neurosurgery* 1986; 19: 655–64.

38. Little JR, Rosenfeld J, Awad IA. Internal carotid artery occlusion for cavernous segment aneurysm. *Neurosurgery* 1989; 25: 398–404.

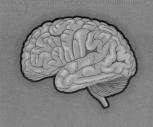

INTRACRANIAL ANEURYSM

14

H Hunt Batjer, James P Chandler, Christopher C Getch, Lance Gravely, and Bernard R Bendok

Intracranial aneurysmal disease encompasses a surprisingly broad spectrum of hemorrhagic and ischemic cerebrovascular entities. Clinical syndromes range from a completely silent and asymptomatic state to sudden death. This chapter provides an overview of the disease and discusses how to manage patients suffering from the various symptoms produced by aneurysms as well as some of the technical aspects of surgical treatment. While a number of types of aneurysm are known to occur on the intracranial vessels (including those that are atherosclerotic, tumor-related, infectious, and traumatic), the major thrust of this discussion is the most common type, the saccular or berry aneurysm.

EPIDEMIOLOGY

The actual incidence of aneurysms in the general population is difficult to estimate as autopsy series vary depending on the age of the individuals studied. It is clear, however, that the frequency with which aneurysms are detected increases with age.[1] The risk of developing aneurysms may differ among racial groups. Based on extrapolation from an autopsy series reported by McCormick and Acosta-Rua, it is likely that 10 to 15 million Americans harbor aneurysms,[1] an incidence of more than 5% of the adult population. Kassell and Drake's 1982 study estimated that in North America approximately 28 000 people a year suffer subarachnoid hemorrhage (SAH) from a ruptured aneurysm.[2] Sadly, fewer than 40% of patients so stricken return to functional life despite modern treatment.[2] To add to this catastrophic loss to society, the age of SAH patients (the mean age is approximately 50 years[2]) is considerably less than that of patients disabled from occlusive cerebrovascular disease. In addition to the large number of patients who suffer from a ruptured aneurysm, neurosurgeons frequently see patients who have developed neurologic deficits from intracranial mass effect because of enlarging aneurysms or who present with focal cerebral ischemic symptoms as a result of embolization from the lumen of large or giant aneurysms.

PATHOLOGY

The histology of cerebral arteries, particularly at points of bifurcation (either vestigial or persistent), is germane to the various theories of aneurysmal development. An outer layer of fibrous adventitia overlies the muscular media, which contributes most of the strength in maintaining vessel integrity. Deep to the media lies the intima, whose luminal surface is lined by a layer of endothelial cells. The internal elastic lamina separates the intima from the media, but the external elastic lamina present in extracranial vessels is absent in arteries (Figure 14.1).[3] Sekhar and Heros summarized the available histological data and noted that a number of congenital factors have been implicated in the pathogenesis of these lesions: medial defects, elastic defects, sites of origin of small vessels, and failure of branch involution. They suggest that acquired factors may also play a role, including degenerative changes, thinning of the media, inflammation, atherosclerosis, hypertension, and hemodynamic stress.[3]

It is likely that aneurysms arise from a complex multifactorial set of circumstances involving a congenital anatomic predisposition enhanced by local or systemic environmental factors that further weaken the arterial wall and lead to aneurysmal dilatation. The overwhelming majority of such lesions are found at the branching points of large subarachnoid conducting arteries, indicating that the point of bifurcation is an extremely vulnerable site. Evidence strongly supports the role played by hemodynamic stress in creating new aneurysms. De novo aneurysms commonly develop in the anterior communicating artery region several years following occlusion of one carotid artery.[4] Also seen are acute distension and fatal rupture of a distal basilar aneurysm after carotid ligation for giant cavernous aneurysms, an event precipitated by recruitment of retrograde flow through the posterior communicating artery.[5] In addition, regrowth of an imperfectly clipped aneurysm as a result of induced hypertension postoperatively has been noted.[6] A final point of supporting evidence can be found in patients harboring high-flow arteriovenous malformations: A higher than expected incidence of aneurysms, especially on feeding arteries, has been noted in this population, and often the aneurysms are in atypical distal sites close to the malformation (Figure 14.2).[7]

As an aneurysm enlarges, its complexity often increases in relation to its wall and to the efferent circulation. The wall of a large (12–25 mm) or giant (> 25 mm in diameter) aneurysm usually has regions of extremely tough hyalinized tissue as well as regions of extremely attenuated transparent tissue, a phenomenon that can complicate obliteration. Furthermore, efferent vessels are further displaced from the parent arterial trunk, often appearing to arise from the aneurysm itself (Figure 14.3). Dissection usually permits accurate reconstruction, although occasionally a large efferent branch actually arises from the fundus of the aneurysm itself.

Intracranial aneurysms have been associated with intracranial vascular malformations as well as other systemic conditions, such as coarctation of the aorta, polycystic kidney disease, extracranial fibromuscular dysplasia, Marfan syndrome, tuberous sclerosis, and Ehlers–Danlos syndrome.[8]

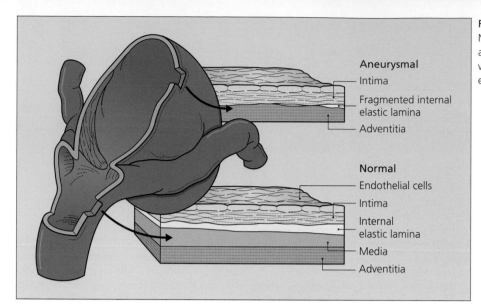

Figure 14.1 Histologic layers of cerebral arteries. Note the absence of media in the aneurysmal wall and the fragmented internal elastic lamina. The wall may be quite sclerotic in some areas and extremely thin in others.

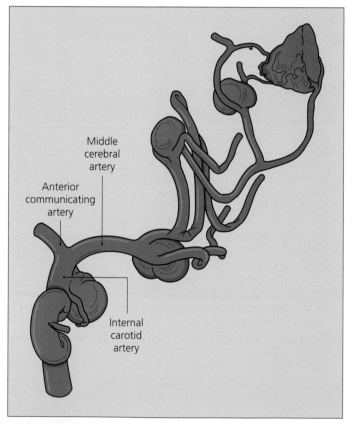

Figure 14.2 When high-flow situations complicate cerebral hemodynamics, such as an intracranial arteriovenous malformation, aneurysms are found with a relatively high frequency on feeding arteries and often in atypical distal sites.

NEUROLOGY

Symptoms

Few physicians would fail to diagnose accurately a 50-year-old woman who collapsed at home with the sudden onset of the worst headache of her life, subsequently vomited, briefly lost consciousness, and was noted to have subhyaloid ocular hemorrhages and a rigid neck. Unfortunately, for many patients this catastrophic episode of SAH sets in motion a cascade of neurologic events that ultimately prove fatal, even if rebleeding does not occur. For this reason, it is of paramount importance to identify premonitory symptoms that herald either sudden enlargement of an aneurysm or a minor leak. In most surgeons' experience, between 25% and 50% of patients give a history of a warning leak a few days or weeks prior to a major SAH.[8] While the symptoms of a warning leak can be distressingly mild, the sudden onset of headache (even if short-lived) or minor focal neurologic deficit should heighten the physician's suspicions. Diagnosis is usually difficult; consequently, a number of patients, sent home from the physician's office or emergency room and instructed to take analgesics, ultimately suffer catastrophic rebleeding episodes several days later.

A number of patients experience sentinel symptoms more consistent with acute distention or enlargement of the aneurysm. While the exact type of focal sign that develops depends on the aneurysmal site, the patient most commonly notes eye, facial, or head pain, visual loss, or double vision. The onset of a third cranial nerve palsy (Figure 14.4), particularly with a fixed dilated pupil, mandates diagnostic studies to rule out a posterior carotid wall aneurysm or a distal basilar aneurysm (Figure 14.5). Thus, the minimum diagnostic workup of a new third cranial nerve palsy includes computed tomography (CT) scan to rule out minor or frank SAH and an ipsilateral carotid and single vertebral arteriogram. Oculomotor palsy with pupillary sparing may be seen without a focal mass in patients with diabetes and hypertensive cerebrovascular disease.

The diagnostic workup of a patient presenting with classic SAH includes a CT scan without enhancement, which in the first few days after SAH detects blood in the subarachnoid, subdural, or interventricular spaces or within the brain parenchyma in over 95% of cases (Figure 14.6).[9,10] If the CT scan is negative and the history is extremely suggestive, the physician can elect to proceed with lumbar puncture to look for evidence of red blood cells or xanthochromia. Despite a negative CT scan, we often proceed with CT angiography or four-vessel digital subtraction angiography if the history is substantially suggestive. It is possible that a small

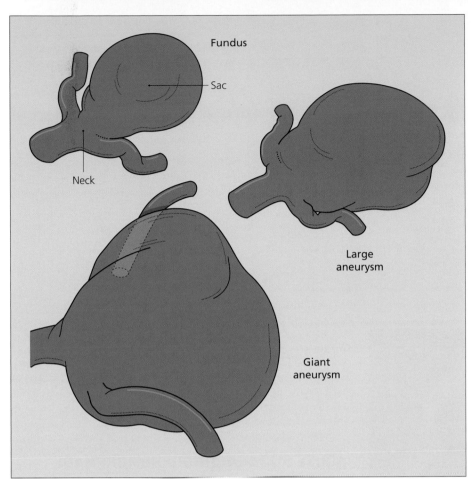

Figure 14.3 This figure depicts the potential evolution of a small aneurysm into a large and finally giant aneurysm. With each stage of enlargement, the efferent branches migrate farther out onto the sac itself.

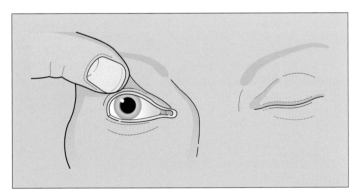

Figure 14.4 A patient with a third cranial nerve palsy will exhibit some or all of the following signs: ptosis, pupillary dilation, and inability to elevate, depress, or medially deviate (adduct) the eye. These findings (particularly pupillary dilation) strongly suggest focal mass effect.

Table 14.1 Subarachnoid hemorrhage grading scale

I	Alert, oriented, asymptomatic
II	Alert, oriented, headache, stiff neck
III	Lethargy or confusion, may have minor neurologic deficit (hemiparesis)
IV	Stupor or dense focal deficit (hemiplegia)
V	Comatose

Modified from Hunt and Hess.[11]

leakage of blood could be loculated around the aneurysmal fundus and not disseminate into the cerebrospinal fluid (CSF). When a patient is first evaluated several days after a suggestive headache, the CT is often negative because the blood is isodense with brain tissue. Definitive angiography is indicated in these cases – with or without supportive CSF findings.

The initial neurological examination is critical for determining the patient's fitness for early surgical intervention (see below) and for acquiring prognostic data. A variety of grading scales are used;

we continue to use the original Hunt–Hess scale with minor modifications (Table 14.1).[11] As seen in the original report by Hunt and Hess, morbidity and mortality clearly increase with each ascending category.[11]

As previously mentioned, aneurysms may slowly enlarge over time and become extremely large. The clinical signs and symptoms may mimic other conditions that result in local brain distortion or generalized elevations of intracranial pressure. A CT scan with and without enhancement detects the presence and location of such lesions and calcification in the wall. While the distribution of contrast material within the lesions may suggest intraluminal thrombosis, in our experience magnetic resonance imaging (MRI)

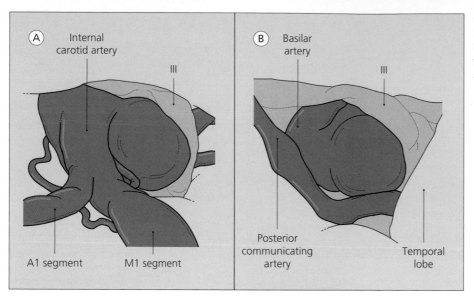

Ⓐ Internal carotid artery

III

A1 segment   M1 segment

Ⓑ Basilar artery

III

Posterior communicating artery

Temporal lobe

Figure 14.5 The presence of a third cranial nerve palsy (especially with pupillary involvement) may be the result of an ipsilateral posterior carotid wall aneurysm (**A**) or a distal basilar artery aneurysm (**B**).

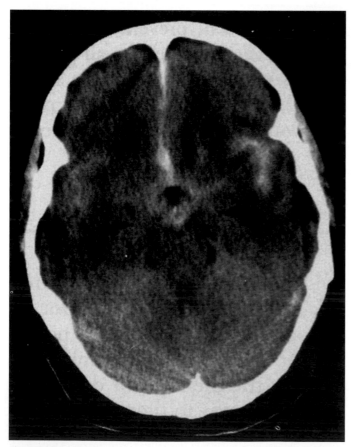

Figure 14.6 CT scan performed shortly after SAH reveals diffuse blood in the subarachnoid cisterns.

is considerably more helpful in this regard. These imaging studies should be followed by formal four-vessel diagnostic angiography to identify the afferent and efferent vessels involved and determine the presence of other aneurysms, because 15% of aneurysm patients harbor multiple lesions.

Patients with large aneurysms may develop a stuttering or progressive neurologic course as a result of embolization from within the lumen. CT, MRI, and angiography, as mentioned above, are important for locating and quantifying intraluminal debris as well as for determining whether significant infarction or brain edema is present, because these factors may affect the timing of intervention.

ACUTE SUBARACHNOID HEMORRHAGE

Natural history

To formulate rational treatment strategies for SAH, it is necessary to understand its natural history and common sequelae. For those surviving their initial hemorrhage, the peak risk of rebleeding occurs during the first 24–48 hours.[9,12,13] On the first day of SAH, there is a 4.1% risk of rebleeding, which decreases steadily until the third day when there is a 1.5% per day risk of rebleeding.[12] By day 14, a cumulative rebleeding incidence of 19% was noted in the Cooperative Aneurysm Study.[12] Six months following SAH, 50% of patients have re-bled and the long-term risk stabilizes at 3% per year.[13]

Complications

Symptomatic cerebral ischemia secondary to cerebral vasospasm peaks in onset between 7 and 10 days postSAH.[14–16] The risk of symptomatic vasospasm can be accurately predicted by the admission CT scan. Those with a thick clot within the subarachnoid cisterns have a much higher risk than those with thin layering.[17] Using modern and current medical and surgical technology to treat SAH, vasospasm is the leading cause of death and disability, accounting for 14% of poor outcomes while rebleeding accounts for only 7%.[9,16]

Hydrocephalus, either communicating or noncommunicating, frequently develops in the first few days after SAH and partly explains the "tight, swollen brain" frequently encountered when surgery is performed on acute conditions. In most patients this condition resolves with time and requires no specific therapy. In about 10% of patients permanent CSF diversion is necessary.

Medical complications

A multitude of medical complications may develop during the patient's acute illness. While it is beyond the scope of this chapter to deal thoroughly with each of these entities, brief mention will be made of the most common.

Pulmonary complications are not infrequent in SAH patients, particularly elderly individuals with pre-existing chronic obstructive lung disease. These patients, particularly those in poor neurologic grade, are often difficult to wean from ventilators postoperatively because of their abnormal pulmonary physiology and decreased level of consciousness. Pulmonary edema is occasionally evident on admission to the hospital. In our experience this phenomenon occurs more frequently in the severely neurologically injured (grades III, IV, V) patient. It is not known whether this condition represents "neurogenic" pulmonary edema or is secondary to acute cardiac dysfunction, but massive catecholamine release at the time of hemorrhage can damage the myocardium and pulmonary tissue. Thus, this surge is likely to contribute in a major way to postSAH pulmonary dysfunction. As a result of the frequent transient loss of consciousness associated with SAH, a moderate number of patients have aspiration pneumonitis shortly after admission. Occasionally this complication progresses to full blown adult respiratory distress syndrome with pulmonary failure.

Cardiac physiology is tightly linked to neurophysiology and most acute neurologic conditions are followed by various electrocardiogram (ECG) changes. The outpouring of catecholamines during SAH probably directly induces some subendocardial damage. Rarely, acute myocardial infarction and even cardiogenic shock accompany SAH, gravely complicating management. Most neurosurgeons consult a cardiologist to assist in the perioperative care of the patient when significant ECG changes are noted. Cardiac enzymes and echocardiography should be obtained immediately. These high-risk patients must be closely watched for malignant arrhythmias.

Electrolyte disturbances are quite common after SAH, especially hyponatremia. Doczi and colleagues noted a 10% incidence in anterior communicating aneurysm patients and only a 3% incidence in patients who bled from other sites.[18] Most authorities now believe that hyponatremia results from a neurologically induced salt-wasting state rather than inappropriate secretion of anti-diuretic hormone as was previously thought. It is critical to remember that these patients are volume-depleted and require fluid and electrolyte resuscitation rather than the fluid restriction in vogue in past years. Fluid restriction does not correct the volume or electrolyte abnormality and may precipitate symptomatic cerebral ischemia from vasospasm. Diabetes insipidus with progressive hypernatremia is frequently seen in comatose patients with lethal hemorrhages and massively elevated intracranial pressure. Much less frequently, this disorder can be seen in patients who have suprasellar giant aneurysms, are in good neurologic condition, but have hypothalamic injury from either hemorrhage or direct damage to hypothalamic tissue or relevant perforating arteries.

Infectious systemic complications are common because of the high incidence of patients who are on controlled ventilators and have catheters placed in their veins, arteries, and urinary bladder. Postoperative meningitis is uncommon but its presence signals the possibility of CSF leak into the frontal or ethmoid sinuses. Isolated organisms commonly inhabit the paranasal sinuses.

After SAH, venous thrombosis occurs in about 2% of patients and has been implicated in pulmonary embolism in 1%.[19] Our method of prevention includes TED hose and pneumatic compression devices for all patients in the intensive care unit, with early postoperative ambulation when possible. Our current practice involves prophylactic vena caval filters for high-risk patients. Table 14.2 summarizes the major medical and neurologic complications that may accompany SAH.

Table 14.2 Summary of major medical and neurologic complications of subarachnoid hemorrhage

Venous thromboembolism	Pulmonary failure
Infection	Hydrocephalus
Diabetes insipidus	Vasospasm
Syndrome of inappropriate anti-diuretic hormone secretion	Rebleed
Cardiac injury	Direct brain injury

TREATMENT

This section will provide a conceptual framework from which management strategies can be developed for the individual patient. It should be emphasized that no two patients are truly similar or have identical systemic physiology. Therefore, despite the plethora of diagnostic information, the most effective way to time intervention is by acquiring a critical, subjective "feel" for the patient's neurologic and systemic status. For the purposes of discussion, "good grade" will refer to Hunt–Hess grades I and II and grade III patients who are confused but have a normal level of consciousness. Specific emphasis will focus on surgical strategies with the clear recognition that endovascular strategies are critical to a comprehensive cerebrovascular team. Multidisciplinary evaluation and case selection reduce morbidity and mortality.

Since the peak incidence of rebleeding occurs within the first 48 hours posthemorrhage, the most effective strategy to minimize this risk is to secure the ruptured aneurysm as soon as possible. Unfortunately, many patients referred to neurosurgical centers arrive one or more days after the original SAH, thus treatment within the first 48 hours is not always possible. Second, it is not in the patient's best interest to undergo aneurysm surgery at night, when the surgeon is tired and the operating room staff (including the anesthesiology staff and scrub and circulating nurses) may be suboptimal. This heightened risk at "off-hours" times is also present in the endovascular suite. The heightened risk to the patient under these circumstances far outweighs the risk of rebleeding while waiting for the first elective surgical day, when the proper team is assembled. Third, not all aneurysms are alike; some require extensive retraction and dissection, which may not be tolerated well by the freshly injured brain. It is likely that patients in poor neurologic condition are often worsened by a hasty operation and would be better served by allowing the brain a few days to recover. In these situations, endovascular therapy is an attractive option even if only palliative. However, the cerebrovascular team should secure ruptured aneurysms prior to the onset of delayed ischemia from vasospasm because the most effective forms of therapy for vasospasm involve hypervolemia and hypertension, highly dangerous maneuvers when unsecured aneurysms are present. Therefore, in general we attempt to achieve

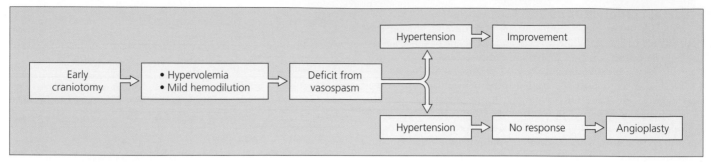

Figure 14.7 Prophylactic and therapeutic strategy for vasospasm at Northwestern University Medical School.

obliteration of the offending aneurysm prior to days 5 to 7, especially if the CT scan suggested a high likelihood of vasospasm. The entire issue of surgical timing, however, remains highly controversial.[2,9,12,20–22]

Antifibrinolytic therapy (ε-aminocaproic acid) became available more than 20 years ago. It provided great hope that patients with ruptured aneurysms could be prevented from rebleeding or that rebleeding could be delayed, allowing time for surgical intervention. The Cooperative Aneurysm Study found that the rebleeding rate at 14 days was 11.7% if antifibrinolytics were used and 19.4% if no antifibrinolytics were used. However, cerebral ischemia from vasospasm was more frequent if antifibrinolytics were used (32.4%) than if no antifibrinolytics were used (22.7%). Thus, the mortality rate of the two groups over the first month was identical.[23] We tend to use antifibrinolytic therapy in the poor-grade patient who clearly will not be an operative candidate for some time, despite the knowledge that we are increasing his risk of symptomatic vasospasm. The role of endovascular strategies in poor-grade patients is evolving and attractive, but results are ambiguous.

Symptomatic vasospasm is the leading cause of disability and death following SAH and, to date, eludes definitive treatment. While most known vasoactive compounds have been tried in this condition, very few modalities have lasting value. Kosnik and Hunt observed a striking response in patients with induced hypertension.[24] The use of pressors remains a mainstay of therapy. The efficacy and safety of pressors seems to be markedly enhanced by volume expansion, and the combination of hypervolemia and hypertension remains the most effective medical means of reversing these neurologic deficits.[25] One large series reported clinical response in 70% of patients treated in this way.[26] Complications have resulted, however, including systemic cardiopulmonary decompensation, conversion of ischemic infarction to hemorrhagic infarction, hematomas, progressing brain edema, and new aneurysms.[26–29] Calcium-channel blockers have been widely studied and used clinically during the 1980s, but convincing evidence of their efficacy has not been absolutely clarified in the literature. Angiographic arterial narrowing is not prevented nor reversed by these agents. Recently interventional techniques have become available that have significant value for medical failures in our unit;[30] one technique, transluminal angioplasty, has the potential durably to reverse arterial narrowing in the major cerebral conducting vessels.

Our current strategy for managing delayed ischemic complications involves mild to moderate volume expansion with crystalloid and colloid solutions, followed by early craniotomy or Gugliemi detachable coils to secure the ruptured aneurysm. We attempt to maintain this status through the period of maximal risk of vasospasm (days 5 to 10). Concurrently, we attempt to maximize blood rheologic properties to improve tissue perfusion by maintaining mild hemodilution (hematocrit 30–34). Should a focal neurologic deficit develop we immediately add a vasopressor (dopamine) and raise the systolic blood pressure up to the 200 mmHg range or until the deficit reverses. If this medical therapy fails to improve the patient's condition and the CT scan does not show obvious infarction, we proceed immediately with angiography with plans for angioplasty. To date, this protocol has been effective, and the incidence of virulent cases of vasospasm has clearly decreased over the past decade (Figure 14.7).

The ability temporarily to occlude cerebral arteries safely and reliably is of considerable value for two reasons. First, the frequent use of temporary clips to soften or "defuse" an aneurysm during final dissection and clipping has decreased the risk of premature intraoperative rupture. The occurrence of significant premature bleeding converts an orderly, precise microsurgical procedure into a stressful situation that may adversely affect the patient.[31] Second, many large and giant aneurysms, particularly those with calcific walls and mural thrombus, must be temporarily excluded from the cerebral circulation to allow definitive arterial reconstruction (Figure 14.8). Regrettably, this temporary interruption is prolonged in some cases, thus exceeding the ischemic threshold and leading to infarction.

Barbiturates are effective in protecting the brain from ischemic and hypoxic insults both experimentally and clinically.[32–34] This protective effect is probably caused by a substantially depressed cerebral metabolic rate, evidenced by the lack of electroencephalogram (EEG) activity. Unfortunately, some elderly patients – especially those with significant heart disease – may become significantly hypotensive at the dosage required for cerebral metabolic depression. This toxic effect substantially diminishes potential available collateral circulation during occlusion of a major cerebral vessel. Also, the prolonged anesthetic effect of high doses of a barbiturate can obscure important neurologic changes in the immediate postoperative period. For these reasons, we have used etomidate and other short-acting metabolic suppressants to accomplish brain protection without cardiotoxicity.[35] Before placing temporary arterial clips, our anesthesiologists ensure normotension and mild hypothermia (34°C), accomplish EEG burst suppression with an appropriate agent, and maintain EEG suppression throughout the duration of temporary arterial occlusion.

SURGICAL MANAGEMENT OF SPECIFIC ANEURYSMS

The following discussion, an overview of some general problems caused by aneurysms in various locations, illustrates the anatomic

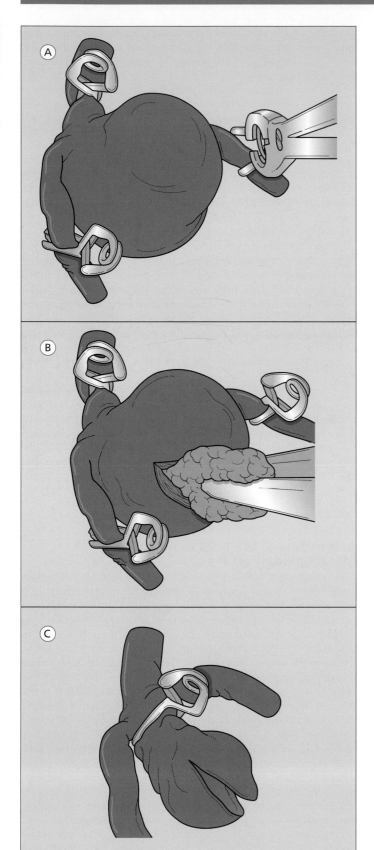

Figure 14.8 (A–C) Temporary arterial occlusion is often necessary in repairing complex large or giant aneurysms. Not infrequently, the aneurysm must be widely opened to allow evacuation of debris and thrombus before definitive clip reconstruction can be performed.

complexities and unique features found by the neurosurgeon treating these various lesions. We will not focus on endovascular techniques as they are considered elsewhere in this text. It is important to understand that generalities regarding the care of SAH patients are difficult to apply to the individual case. The treatment of aneurysmal disease has been remarkably aided by development of the surgical microscope; its ability to magnify and brilliantly illuminate very narrow exposures has had an incredible impact on neurosurgery in general and aneurysmal disease in particular. Tiny vessels that serve as end arteries for eloquent brain regions, including the brainstem and diencephalon, are simply not visible to the naked eye, but can now be safely and elegantly spared during the clip reconstruction of difficult aneurysms.

The pterional "frontotemporal" craniotomy

The pterional craniotomy is an extremely versatile procedure that has become fundamental to managing a variety of neoplastic, congenital, and vascular processes. Neurosurgeons must become intimately familiar with the advantages of this approach and its many modifications and develop an appreciation for the neurovascular anatomy viewed from this unusual perspective. In this exposure the anatomy is viewed in an oblique and inverted orientation. Fortunately, experience quickly renders the microanatomy viewed from this perspective familiar, predictable, and natural.

A key element of this operative approach is patient position. Careful attention to this basic first step facilitates exposure and allows complex procedures to be carried out through small bony windows, a limited dural opening, and with a minimum of cerebral cortex exposed. The Mayfield–Keys three-point skull fixation device should be employed in virtually all aneurysm procedures as it provides almost absolute head stability in the event of sudden patient movement or coughing during inadvertent emergence from anesthesia (Figure 14.9). In general, it is most convenient to apply the three-point fixation with two pins anteriorly contralateral to the planned exposure and one pin posterior to the planned surgical incision just above the mastoid region. After inserting the pins, the surgeon performs three distinct maneuvers to position the head optimally for the procedure.[36]

Rotation

The head is rotated toward the contralateral or nonoperated side to an angle determined by the target anatomic site. In general, when treating internal carotid or distal basilar artery aneurysms, minimal head rotation (20°) is employed because with further rotation the temporal lobe gravitationally migrates posteriorly and thus encroaches upon the operative field. Aneurysms of the middle cerebral artery bifurcation require somewhat more rotation (45°) to expose the sylvian fissure maximally for a convenient transsylvian dissection. For aneurysms of the anterior communicating artery, even more rotation is necessary (45° to 60°) to simplify the exposure of the medial gyrus rectus and interhemispheric fissure. In this dissection, temporal lobe encroachment does not limit exposure of the anterior communicating region because of its anterior location in the skull (Figure 14.10A).

Flexion

This subtle maneuver is designed to maintain a perpendicular relationship between the floor of the anterior cranial fossa and the long axis of the patient's body. The maneuver is accomplished by achieving the degree of desired rotation, then flexing the neck gently, bringing the chin toward the contralateral clavicle. Be

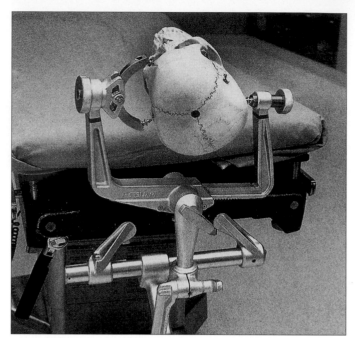

Figure 14.9 The Mayfield–Keys three-point skull fixation device provides optimal head stability so that inadvertent patient movement will not result in catastrophic injury to neural or vascular structures.

careful to avoid compromising cervical venous return. Successful accomplishment of this maneuver allows the seated surgeon comfortable access to the target region without awkwardly encroaching on the patient's ipsilateral shoulder (Figure 14.10B).

Extension "tilt"

When this critical manipulation is successful, the frontal lobe gravitationally falls away from the floor of the anterior cranial fossa. To minimize necessary retraction and optimally display the vascular structures at the skull base, the vertex of the skull is tilted inferiorly so the maxillary eminence rises superior to the brow (Figure 14.10C). After this final maneuver, the Mayfield device is secured to the operating table. With experience, the surgeon can literally see the vascular anatomy with its associated target aneurysm as the head is manipulated externally. Once the surgeon has this level of experience, measuring degrees of rotation and extension is unnecessary, and he or she simply positions the head for optimal exposure of the lesion.

Surgical technique

The surgical incision is begun about 1 cm anterior to the tragus at the level of the zygoma and extends superiorly immediately behind the hairline and gently curves anteriorly to the midline (Figure 14.11). Every attempt is made to keep the incision behind the hairline for cosmesis, although this can be difficult in a balding patient. Numerous options are available for reflecting the scalp flap, including an interfascial dissection described by Yasargil.[37,38] Perhaps the most widely used is an incision through the galea, temporalis fascia, and muscle to the bone, reflecting the scalp flap in a single layer (Figure 14.12). It is important to preserve the frontalis branch of the facial nerve and mobilization of the temporalis muscle anteriorly and inferiorly enough for the anatomic key to be well exposed. Certain surgical targets require aggressive

exposure of the temporal squama. While the craniotomy flap varies somewhat depending on the surgical target, in general a power craniotome is used to fashion a frontal temporal craniotomy by connecting three burr holes (Figure 14.13). Placing the posterior burr hole immediately inferior to the superior temporal line allows a cosmetic closure of the temporalis muscle over this bony defect. After the bone flap is removed, the anterior temporal bone is extracted with rongeurs as is the lateral third of the sphenoid ridge (Figure 14.14). Often it is necessary to remove the deepest portion of the sphenoid ridge with a power drill. The drill is also used to resect the inner table of the frontal bone medially; the resultant bony removal enables excellent access to the parasellar region with a minimum of frontal retraction. The dura mater is opened in a semilunar fashion and reflected over the sphenoid ridge to maximize cortical exposure (Figure 14.15).

After satisfactory exposure of the parasylvian region, the surgical microscope is brought into the field and the remainder of the procedure is accomplished with magnified vision. The initial brain retraction involves the progressive elevation of the posterior frontal cortex immediately anterior to the sylvian fissure from the sphenoid ridge (Figure 14.16). Keeping the sphenoid ridge as a directional indicator will ensure safe arrival at the carotid cistern. Once this cistern is reached, the optic nerve can be viewed medially through the arachnoid even after a brisk SAH (Figure 14.17).

At this point, either a microknife or microscissors is used to open sharply this dense arachnoid extending from the pre-chiasmatic region across the carotid cistern and laterally to dissect fully the medial aspect of the sylvian fissure (Figure 14.18). Once this arachnoid is fully dissected, the entire subarachnoid course of the carotid artery will be seen, including its bifurcation into the middle and anterior cerebral arteries. From this point, the principles of further dissection are governed by the specific aneurysmal site.

Aneurysms of the proximal carotid (paraclinoidal) artery

This interesting family of aneurysms arises from the most proximal intracranial segment of the internal carotid artery. It is not uncommon to see bilateral proximal carotid aneurysms, particularly in women. These aneurysms are often termed carotid-ophthalmic artery aneurysms, implying a distinct relationship to the origin of the ophthalmic branch. More commonly, however, the aneurysms arise some distance from the origin of the ophthalmic artery and occasionally have projections that make the ophthalmic artery unlikely as the site of origin. It is likely that the presence of a third group of proximal carotid aneurysms is simply the result of the hemodynamic stress of a sharp bend in the carotid artery as it leaves the cavernous sinus, which over time can weaken the vessel wall tissue. Regardless of their configuration, these aneurysms present several unique technical problems to the neurosurgeon. Their extremely proximal intracranial location makes the essential vascular principle of proximal control difficult if not impossible to achieve intracranially. Secondly, when these aneurysms reach significant size, they routinely attenuate the optic nerve traumatically and often cause associated visual neurologic deficit. This factor frequently mandates that the surgeon not only exclude the aneurysm from circulation but deflate it to decompress the optic nerve. This is difficult, particularly in large and giant aneurysms whose walls may be calcified. The multiple clips that aneurysms of this type require may distort or compress

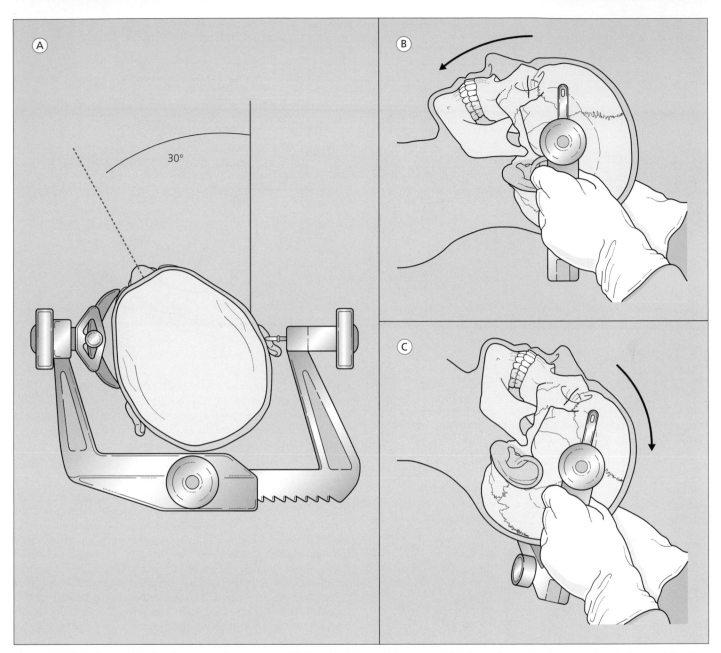

Figure 14.10 Patient positioning for pterional craniotomy. **(A)** Rotation. The head is elevated slightly relative to the thorax and rotated contralaterally by an extent dictated by the specific operative target (less rotation for carotid and basilar bifurcation aneurysms and more rotation for aneurysm of the middle cerebral artery or anterior communicating region). **(B)** Flexion. The neck should then be gently flexed, bringing the chin toward the contralateral clavicle. This subtle maneuver orients the floor of the anterior cranial fossa perpendicular to the long axis of the patient's body, maximizing the surgeon's access to the anatomic target without encroachment on the patient's ipsilateral shoulder. **(C)** Extension (tilt). While maintaining the previous elements of rotation and flexion, the vertex is tilted inferiorly so that the maxillary eminence rises superior to the brow. The degree of extension will vary somewhat with the target aneurysm (less for paraclinoidal aneurysms and more with distal basilar aneurysms).

the optic nerve. A third unique feature of this particular aneurysm is its relationship to the bony floor of the skull. The anterior clinoid process often hoods the lateral aspect of the carotid artery as it emerges from the roof of the cavernous sinus. The optic strut (the inferior bony aspect of the optic canal) can obscure the proximal neck of the aneurysm. After years of studying the proximal carotid anatomy, a unique anatomic point has emerged. While large sacs can distort each neurovascular structure, the

proximal (and healthy) carotid artery is *always* located at the lateral aspect of the optic canal. In many patients, the dural edge (falciform ligament) is generous and simple incision along the lateral aspect of the optic nerve permits exposure of the proximal carotid, ophthalmic artery origin, and proximal neck. This is especially true for carotid-ophthalmic aneurysms and superior hypophyseal variants. Lesions projecting laterally into the anterior clinoidal process itself and those arising in the carotid cave require

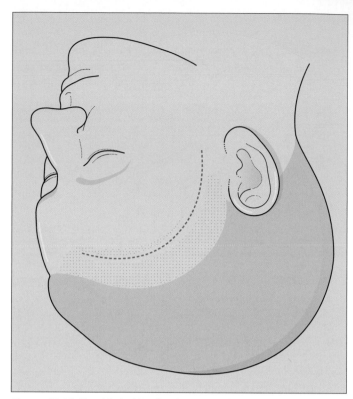

Figure 14.11 The skin incision for the pterional craniotomy extends from the zygoma to the midline, curving gently just posterior to the hairline.

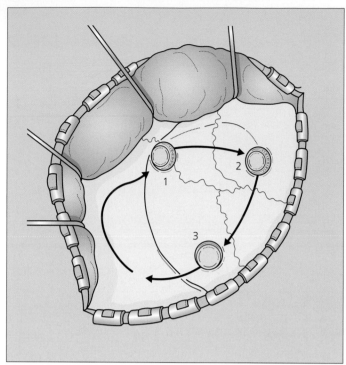

Figure 14.13 The pterional craniotomy is performed with power instruments so that three burr holes are placed, one at the anatomic key, one inferiorly on the temporal squama, and one posteriorly just inferior to the superior temporal line. The bone is cut as shown, exposing the frontal and temporal dura and the sphenoid ridge.

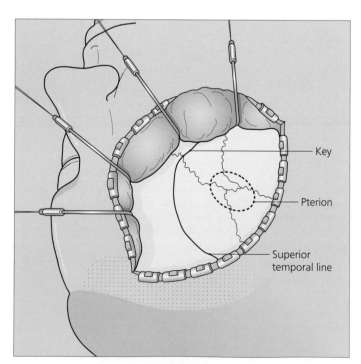

Figure 14.12 A commonly employed means of opening the scalp involves incision of the skin, galea, temporalis fascia, and muscle with reflexion of the resultant flap in a single layer.

aggressive bony resection of the anterior clinoid and optic strut.[36,39] Figure 14.19 illustrates the unique relationship of proximal carotid aneurysms to the optic nerve and skull base as well as a potential clipping solution after resecting a portion of the anterior clinoid process. In the majority of large and giant ruptured proximal carotid aneurysms, the patient is served well, in our opinion, by exposing the cervical internal carotid artery prior to initiating the craniotomy. This guarantees early proximal control should difficulties arise and facilitates temporary arterial occlusion, aneurysm decompression, and intraoperative angiography.

Aneurysms of the posterior carotid wall

Posterior carotid wall aneurysms include lesions arising immediately distal to the posterior communicating artery as well as those arising immediately distal to the anterior choroidal artery. Because these lesions are perhaps the most common intracranial aneurysms, most neurosurgeons quickly become familiar with the involved microanatomy and treat these lesions successfully in the majority of cases. Enlarging aneurysms at this site can become symptomatic prior to frank SAH by compression of the tentorial incisura, which produces pain, and of the third cranial nerve (see Figure 14.5). In our experience, early warning signs of some type are more frequently seen with aneurysms of the posterior carotid wall than with any other intracranial aneurysm. The relative simplicity of the anatomy of these aneurysms as well as the frequency with which they are exposed and treated should not induce a sense of complacency in the operating surgeon. The intimate association between the distal neck of the common

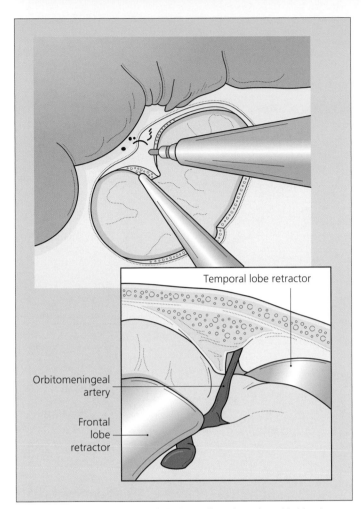

Figure 14.14 After removal of the bone flap, the sphenoid ridge is resected to the level of the orbitomeningeal artery. The inner table of the frontal bone can also be resected. This maneuver is particularly useful in exposing the anterior communicating region.

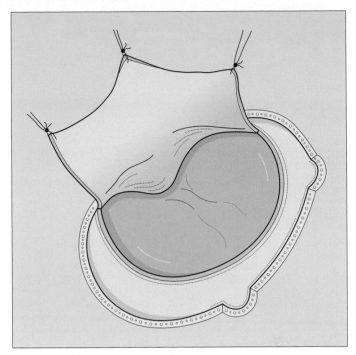

Figure 14.15 The dura is opened in a semilunar fashion and reflected with stay sutures.

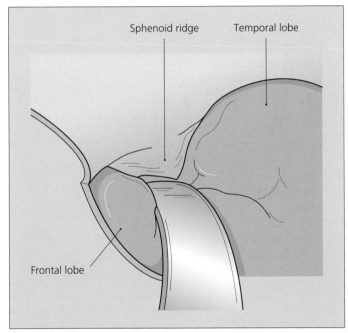

Figure 14.16 As the retractor is deepened medially, the posterior frontal cortex is elevated. Gently following the course of the sphenoid ridge helps keep the direction of retraction correct.

carotid-posterior communicating artery aneurysm to the anterior choroidal artery, together with the fragility of the anterior choroidal artery place it very much "in harm's way" (Figure 14.20). The anterior choroidal artery supplies the posterior limb of the internal capsule, the lentiform nucleus, the optic tract, the amygdala, and the choroid plexus of the temporal horn. Injuring it by aggressive dissection techniques or placing a small piece of cotton in the distal neck of the aneurysm to control minor intraoperative bleeding can result in profound and devastating neurologic deficit. It should be stressed that the distal course of the anterior choroidal as it travels posteriorly must be carefully freed from the aneurysmal fundus so the distal clip blade does not compromise this vital structure. The posterior communicating artery usually arises just proximal to the origin of a carotid posterior communicating artery aneurysm and every attempt should be made to preserve this vessel. Important anterior thalamo-perforating branches ramify from the posterior communicating artery. Occasionally patients have persistent fetal circulation in which the posterior cerebral artery originates from the carotid, and the P1 segment is nonexistent. This phenomenon can be discerned from the preoperative arteriogram and, when approaching the posterior carotid wall aneurysm, the neurosurgeon should

know whether or not the posterior cerebral artery is fetal. It is sometimes acceptable to include the posterior communicating artery in the clip, assuming the anterior thalamoperforators will be irrigated retrograde from the P1 segment off the basilar artery. Nevertheless, when possible, all components of the circle of Willis should be preserved, particularly in the SAH patient who may subsequently develop vasospasm and increase reliance on available

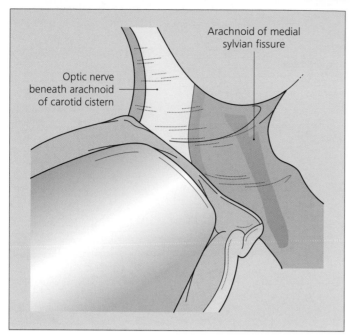

Figure 14.17 Safe arrival at the carotid cistern is heralded by visualization of the optic nerve through the arachnoid medially. The retractor is stabilized just lateral to the nerve so the arachnoid of the carotid cistern and medial sylvian fissure is placed on gentle stretch.

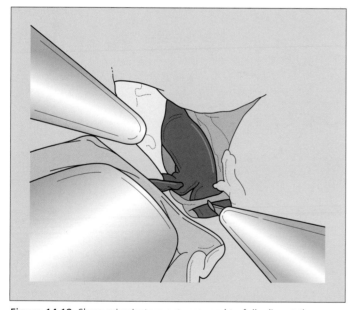

Figure 14.18 Sharp microinstruments are used to fully dissect the parasellar cisterns from the prechiasmatic cistern across the carotid cistern into the medial aspect of the sylvian fissure.

Figure 14.19 Proximal carotid (paraclinoidal) aneurysm. **(A)** These aneurysms often distort and attenuate the optic nerve and may have their proximal neck obscured by the dura covering the lateral aspect of the optic canal or by the bony anterior clinoidal process. Without securing proximal control in the neck or by endovascular means, it is obvious that true control of this aneurysm may be achieved intracranially only at some peril. **(B)** To resect the anterior clinoid process, a dural flap is fashioned and reflected over the fundus of the aneurysm. A high-speed drill is then used to remove as much bone as is necessary to expose the proximal neck of the aneurysm. **(C)** The specific clip placement chosen must not jeopardize the optic nerve or the patency of the internal carotid or the ophthalmic artery.

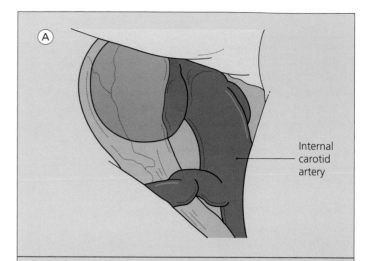

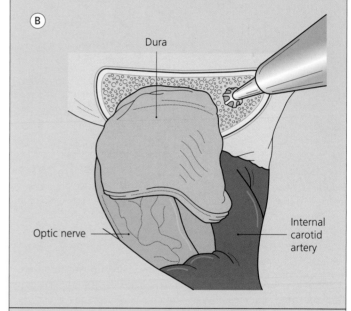

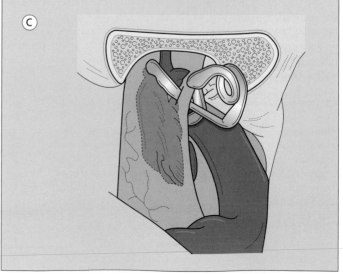

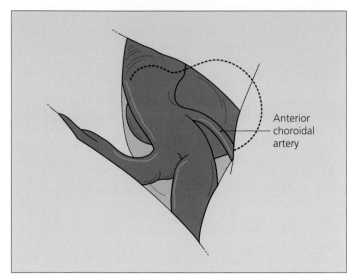

Figure 14.20 Posterior carotid wall aneurysm. Despite their frequency and relative simplicity, especially the ease of achieving early proximal control intracranially, the neurosurgeon should not be nonchalant or complacent. The anterior choroidal artery is in intimate relationship with the distal neck and simple retraction and mild compression can have devastating consequences.

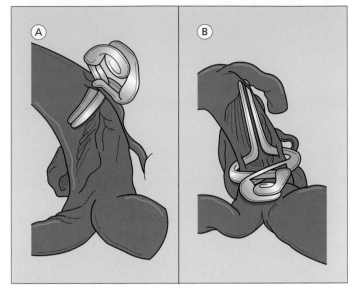

Figure 14.21 Alternatives for clipping posterior carotid wall aneurysms. **(A)** For small aneurysms, a direct clip placement perpendicular to the carotid artery is often the best alternative. **(B)** For larger aneurysms in this location, the degree of "gathering" of tissue by a perpendicular clip placement can jeopardize the carotid artery as well as apply serious shear stresses to the aneurysm neck during closure. The aperture clip allows blade closure parallel to the carotid artery, minimizing these deleterious events.

natural collateral pathways. The most common clip arrangement for a posterior communicating artery aneurysm is perpendicular to the carotid artery (Figure 14.21A). In relatively small aneurysms, the resultant degree of shortening of the carotid artery is trivial and thus acceptable. In larger broad-based aneurysms, clipping perpendicular to the carotid artery can substantially foreshorten, and even wrinkle, the carotid artery and impose shear forces on the fragile neck of the aneurysm during closure of the clip. The aperture clip originally developed by Drake[40,41] allows clip placement so the blades close parallel to the carotid artery, minimizing the shear forces (Figure 14.21B). Regardless of the clip chosen, it is critical to inspect the course of the anterior choroidal and posterior communicating arteries to ensure that these vessels have not been compromised.

For patients presenting with acute or chronic third nerve palsies, it has been our policy to evacuate the aneurysmal contents but not develop the dissection plane between the aneurysmal fundus and the third cranial nerve, to avoid further damage to this already diseased and fragile structure. Many neurosurgeons believe that eliminating the direct pulsations from the arterial tree does as much as any other maneuver to allow recovery of the nerve's function.

Aneurysms of the carotid bifurcation

Despite the fact that the intracranial carotid bifurcation is frequently tortuous and subject to continuous hemodynamic stress, it is a relatively rare site for aneurysmal development. Aneurysms of this region typically project superiorly and occasionally superoposteriorly. An occasional patient presents with a primarily intracerebral hemorrhage and a hematoma anterior and inferior to a classic putaminal hypertensive hemorrhage. These hematomas may be associated with a paucity of true subarachnoid blood. This CT picture in a non-hypertensive patient should immediately alert the clinician to the presence of an ominous vascular condition.

The operative exposure and definitive clipping of aneurysms at this site requires considerable dissection of the carotid cistern and the sphenoidal portion of the sylvian fissure. The proximity of the distal anterior choroidal artery and the infinite variability of the subarachnoid course of the medial lenticulostriate branches from the middle cerebral and anterior cerebral arteries explains the often intimate association of these vessels with the aneurysmal neck (Figure 14.22). Often, the recurrent artery is also intimate to the posterior neck. When the surgeon uses a clip with long blades, particularly in large and broad-based aneurysms of the carotid bifurcation, these penetrating vessels must be visible in the depths of the exposure.

There are two key aspects to surgical dissection: proximal control of the internal carotid artery in the carotid cistern must be achieved, and the sphenoidal portion of the sylvian fissure must be opened widely. As the dissection is carried more distally along the internal carotid, simultaneous extension of the sylvian dissection along the M1 segment from distal to proximal assures an atraumatic arrival at the carotid bifurcation and control of the afferent and efferent circulation. It is essential that the surgeon enter the operating room knowing whether the anterior communicating artery is patent. Sacrifice of the ipsilateral A1 segment is a valuable therapeutic option in difficult large and giant aneurysms as well as a life-saving maneuver in the event of an untimely intraoperative rupture. Knowing that the anterior communicating artery is patent enables definitive clipping, which incorporates the A1 segment if premature rupture develops (Figure 14.23).[36] A small clip can then be added to the A1 segment to insure against retrograde irrigation of the aneurysm. It should be emphasized that medial sylvian dissection is critical to minimize the degree of frontal lobe retraction required for the exposure of this particular aneurysm.

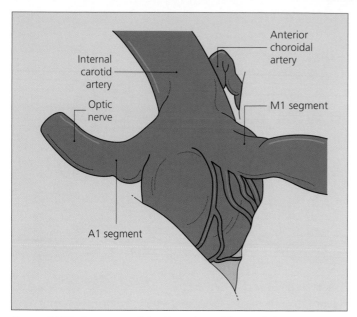

Figure 14.22 Aneurysms of the internal carotid artery bifurcation are frequently in intimate association with the distal course of the anterior choroidal artery as well as the medial lenticulostriate arteries arising from the middle and anterior cerebral arteries.

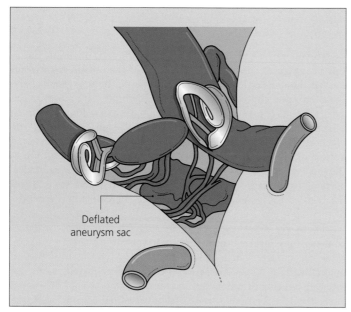

Figure 14.23 Carotid bifurcation aneurysm. If the anterior communicating artery is known to be patent, a valuable option for ceasing untimely intraoperative rupture is to incorporate the ipsilateral A1 segment into the definitive clipping, thus relying on the contralateral carotid to irrigate the anterior cerebral artery territory bilaterally.

Aneurysms of the middle cerebral artery bifurcation

Aneurysms of the middle cerebral artery bifurcation are quite common and hemorrhage from these lesions can produce several unique features. As aneurysms become relatively large at this site, they can erode through the lateral aspect of the sphenoidal portion of the sylvian fissure, occasionally causing hemorrhage directly into the subdural space. Acute subdural hematoma with relatively less blood directed into the subarachnoid space occurs in 5–10% of these patients. Knowledge of this phenomenon should alert the neurosurgeon evaluating a patient who had an unwitnessed motor vehicle accident and is found to have an acute subdural hematoma. It is possible that the hemorrhage caused a loss of consciousness, which precipitated the car accident. Additionally, the anatomy of the middle cerebral artery bifurcation just medial to the limen of insula allows aneurysmal growth to occur in the substance of the temporal lobe or invaginate the pia-arachnoid of the medial temporal lobe (Figure 14.24). When rupture occurs at the distal aspect of the fundus, a hematoma frequently develops primarily within the temporal lobe. This complication can be an acute life-threatening emergency simply because of mass effect from the hematoma. If a patient is found to have striking mass effect from a temporal hematoma after becoming immediately comatose or deteriorating upon arrival in the emergency room, he or she should not be evaluated as a standard SAH patient by the Hunt–Hess criteria. The surgeon should consider the patient to have a life-threatening mass and perform immediate surgical therapy to remove the hematoma and definitively clip the aneurysm. If possible, a diagnostic angiography should be obtained before exploring these lesions, although this can be deferred in the rapidly deteriorating patient.

Significant controversy exists in the neurosurgical community regarding the most appropriate means to dissect these aneurysms. Many surgeons prefer to isolate proximal control at the carotid cistern and dissect from proximal to distal through the sylvian fissure until the bifurcation is reached. This type of maneuver requires a significant amount of frontal lobe retraction but has the theoretical advantage of enabling early proximal control. Other surgeons advocate an approach through the temporal lobe itself; this type of superior temporal gyrus approach is especially useful

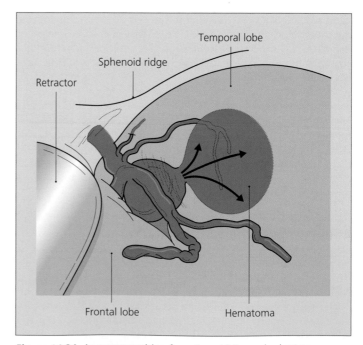

Figure 14.24 Aneurysms arising from the middle cerebral artery bifurcation often project into the medial aspect of the temporal lobe. Upon rupture, a hematoma may develop primarily within the temporal lobe itself and only minimally involve the subarachnoid space.

in patients with a temporal lobe hematoma. Nevertheless, it does require re-entry into the subarachnoid space as the region of the limen of insula is approached. In our opinion, the preferred approach to most lesions of the middle cerebral bifurcation (with the exception of those associated with large hematomas) lies in a direct transsylvian approach. The dissection is initiated through the lateral aspect of the sylvian fissure 2–3 cm from the sphenoid ridge (Figure 14.25). Dissection via this route allows the surgeon to stay within the subarachnoid space from the outset, minimizes the degree of brain tissue retraction necessary and, with experience, allows proximal control to be achieved safely. As the dissection deepens within the sylvian fissure, the small middle cerebral branches are dissected down to the M2 segments and, using knowledge of the aneurysmal anatomy and how it projects, a safe dissection plane (usually posterosuperiorly) is followed, until the M1 segment is clearly visualized, at which point proximal control is assured. On initial exposure, aneurysms at this site frequently appear to have substantially widened the true bifurcation region, with the M2 segments appearing to emerge from the aneurysmal fundus itself. These vessels should be dissected from the aneurysmal neck to the point at which definitive clip reconstruction can be accomplished.

Aneurysms of the anterior communicating artery

Aneurysms in the region of the anterior communicating artery are perhaps the most common cause of SAH and represent approximately 30% of all cases of SAH in the early Cooperative Aneurysm Study.[42] The anterior communicating artery, as well as the A1 segments of the anterior cerebral artery, are some of the most variable components of the circle of Willis and frequent

anomalies (i.e. irregularities in size, the tendency of one A1 segment to be dominant over the contralateral one, and fenestration, duplication, or triplication of the anterior communicating artery itself) are the rule rather than the exception. Each of these circumstances produces a hemodynamic predisposition to the development of aneurysms. In fact, most anterior communicating aneurysms arise from the junction of the dominant A1 segment with the anterior communicating artery. Hemorrhage from this region is only very rarely preceded by local signs of mass effect as aneurysms must be extremely large before neurologic symptoms manifest. Once hemorrhage occurs, the unique anatomic relationships predispose the individual to diffuse SAH, focal interhemispheric SAH, intraventricular hemorrhage (by rupture of the aneurysm up through the lamina terminalis into the anterior third ventricle), and intracerebral hemorrhage (typically a flame-shaped frontal lobe hematoma). When two or more of these patterns occur together, the study is virtually diagnostic of hemorrhage from an anterior communicating artery aneurysm.

Several points about the operative treatment of these patients deserve mention. In general the bony craniotomy should be carried somewhat more medially and inferiorly than the craniotomy designed for other lesions. This is because the anterior communicating complex is located slightly anterior to the carotid cistern. By enlarging the craniotomy to the midpupillary line and carrying the bony incision down to the brow (with every attempt made to avoid the frontal sinus), the surgeon has maximal flexibility in terms of instrument usage and will not be impeded by contacting bone. The microsurgical procedure is focused less on the medial sylvian fissure than on opening the carotid cistern, at which point a decision must be made either to isolate the A1 segment at the carotid bifurcation or to create a more medial exposure of this vessel. Considerable difference of opinion exists but, generally, mobilization of gyrus rectus from the optic nerve is thought to allow safe proximal dissection of the A1 segment without the additional brain retraction necessary to expose the carotid bifurcation (Figure 14.26). The A1 is then followed to the point at which it angles superiorly and heads into the interhemispheric fissure. Attention is then directed not to the anterior communicating artery, but to the contralateral A1 segment, which often enters the interhemispheric fissure at a mirror image site from the ipsilateral vessel (Figure 14.27). Once definitive proximal control has been obtained, the retractor is withdrawn by about 1–1.5 cm, allowing a small amount of gyrus rectus to herniate over the retractor blade, which immediately obscures the anterior communicating region. This tissue is aggressively resected with cautery and suction (Figure 14.28). The overlying veil of pia arachnoid is then opened sharply, allowing full definition of the ipsilateral A2 segment. Subsequent dissection is defined by the orientation of the aneurysm but must focus on the identification of the A2 segment on the contralateral side. Once this vessel is seen, definitive dissection of the anterior communicating artery and neck of the aneurysm is possible. Great care must be taken to avoid occluding perforating arteries that emanate from the posterior aspect of the anterior communicating artery in the clip (Figure 14.29). This technical error can produce serious psychological and hypothalamic sequelae.

Injury to these penetrating arteries, as well as inadvertent injury to the aneurysm and the major parent vasculature, can be avoided by a very thorough dissection in each case. All aspects of the complex, including both A1 and A2 segments and both sides of the anterior communicating artery, should always be seen and understood prior to definitive neck dissection and clipping.

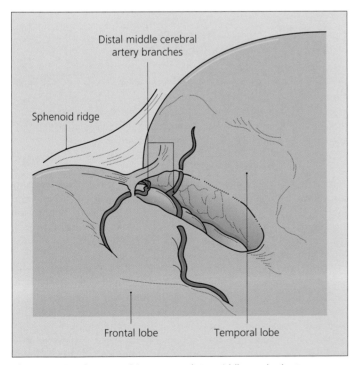

Figure 14.25 The transsylvian approach to middle cerebral artery bifurcation aneurysms minimizes brain retraction but defers achievement of proximal control until somewhat late in the dissection.

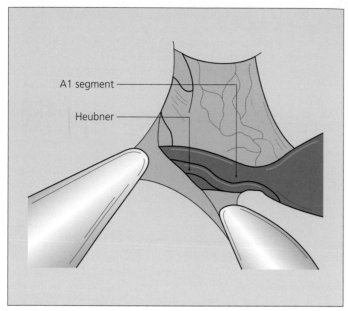

Figure 14.26 In approaching anterior communicating artery aneurysms, the additional brain retraction needed to isolate the origin of the A1 anterior cerebral segment at the carotid bifurcation can be avoided by dissecting the gyrus rectus from the optic nerve and tract. Deepening this plane will expose the A1 proximal to the anterior communicating artery.

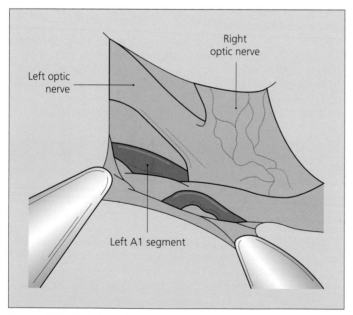

Figure 14.27 Isolation of the contralateral A1 segment completes acquisition of proximal control.

Aneurysms of the vertebral artery–posterior inferior cerebellar artery

Aneurysms of the proximal intracranial vertebral artery typically occur immediately distal to the origin of the posterior inferior cerebellar artery (PICA). This variety of posterior circulation aneurysm is second only to the distal basilar artery in frequency of occurrence. CT scanning following SAH often localizes the

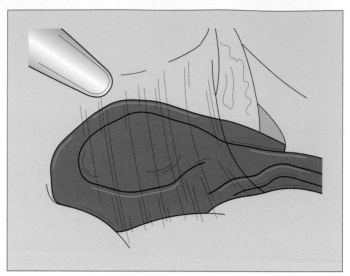

Figure 14.28 The gyrus rectus tissue immediately overlying the anterior communicating complex is aggressively resected leaving a layer of pia arachnoid obscuring the distal anterior cerebral branches (A1) and the aneurysm.

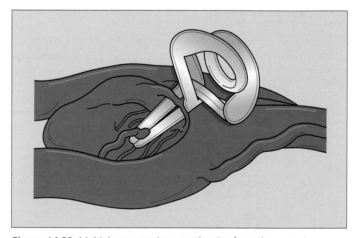

Figure 14.29 Multiple penetrating vessels arise from the posterior aspect of the anterior communicating artery. This schematic illustration shows that the use of excessive clip length and poor visibility behind the aneurysm can cause injury to these important vessels.

hemorrhage to the appropriate lateral aspect of the brainstem and sometimes a small portion of the hemorrhage will extend into the fourth ventricle (through the foramen of Luschka). Surgery of aneurysms in this region is complicated by the intimate relationship of the aneurysm to the brainstem and to the critical lower cranial nerves (cranial nerves IX, X, XI).

To expose this region, the patient can be positioned in the lateral position with a small roll or gel pad under the dependent axilla. The vertex is tipped slightly inferiorly and the chin is rotated approximately 10° toward the floor (Figure 14.30). This so-called "park-bench position" allows the seated surgeon comfortable access to the subarachnoid space lateral to the medulla. A craniotomy or craniectomy is performed that includes the foramen magnum and generously exposes the ipsilateral cerebellar hemisphere. The subarachnoid dissection begins in the cisterna magna, progressively elevating the cerebellar tonsil to

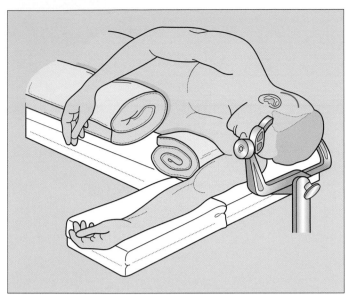

Figure 14.30 For exposure of vertebral-PICA aneurysms the patient is positioned laterally on the operating table with the vertex tilted slightly toward the floor with approximately 10° of rotation of the chin to the floor.

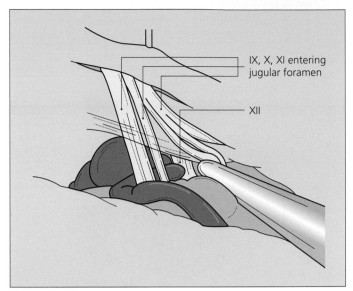

Figure 14.31 The typical vertebral-PICA aneurysm is dissected between the fibers of the lower cranial nerves, which exit at the jugular foramen.

allow identification of the vertebral artery proximal to the PICA origin. The fibers of the 10th cranial nerve are gently dissected and they usually separate, allowing adequate room for exposure between these fibers (Figure 14.31). Great care is used in dissection as undue trauma to these delicate fibers can result in vocal cord paralysis, a potential cause of dangerous postoperative aspiration. Fortunately, the vertebral artery typically travels almost due medially after the PICA origin, making it relatively protected, even from a blind clip application. When necessary, small groups of fibers of the 12th cranial nerve may be either sectioned or included in a difficult clip placement, a maneuver safer than the aggressive dissection necessary to free them completely; its use is associated with either no neurologic deficit or a trivial one.

Aneurysms of the vertebral confluens and lower basilar trunk

This group of extremely difficult aneurysms taxes the ingenuity of the most experienced vascular neurosurgeons because of the depth of exposure, the requirement for optimal exposure ventral to the brainstem, and the frequent need for innovative cranial base exposures which will be discussed below. The vertebral confluens is a unique arterial site in which two large vessels join to form a larger vessel. Taking the direction of normal flow into account, the previous discussion of pathophysiology of aneurysms suggests that aneurysmal dilatation would not occur at this site. Unfortunately, the anatomy of distal vertebral arteries and the lower basilar trunk only rarely occurs in the textbook configuration. Tremendous asymmetry between the sizes and lengths of the vertebral arteries can occur and the confluens itself can be extremely tortuous and, on occasion, located well into the cerebellar pontine angle. In addition, fenestrations of the lower basilar trunk are not uncommon in patients who develop aneurysms in these sites. Obviously, the anatomic anomalies that seem to predispose aneurysmal development also gravely complicate dissection in a very deep wound, which is often packed with fresh subarachnoid

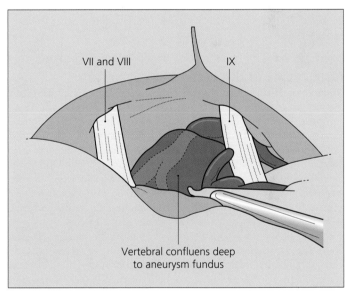

Figure 14.32 The region of the vertebral confluens is typically defined between the seventh and eighth cranial nerves superiorly and the ninth nerve inferiorly. The depth of exposure, relationship to the brainstem, and frequency of arterial anomalies make this a very difficult exposure.

blood. In general, lesions in this area are exposed through a lateral patient position and the early portion of the dissection is simply a continuation of what was previously described for vertebral-PICA aneurysms. Dissection is usually carried out between the fibers of the ninth cranial nerve below and the seventh and eighth cranial nerves above (Figure 14.32). Aneurysms of the lower basilar trunk are usually associated with the origin of the anterior inferior cerebellar artery and the sixth cranial nerve. Their exposure typically involves a cranial base approach, either by sectioning the tentorium from a subtemporal approach or by an exposure anterior to or through the sigmoid sinus. The variants of petrosal resections and their specific uses will be discussed in the next section.

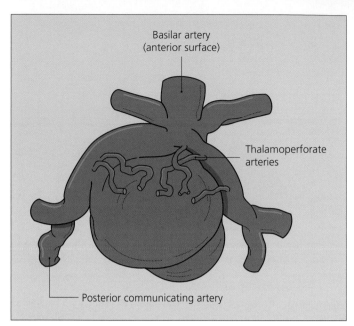

Figure 14.33 Aneurysms of the distal basilar artery must be treated with a precise awareness of the constant presence and infinite variability of the posterior thalamoperforating arteries supplying the mesencephalon and diencephalon.

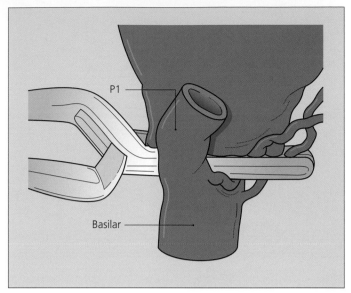

Figure 14.34 Clip applied to a basilar bifurcation aneurysm with inadvertent occlusion of thalamoperforating vessels. This error is almost always devastating to the patient.

Aneurysms of the distal basilar artery

Aneurysms arising from the basilar apex or immediately distal to the origin of the superior cerebellar arteries comprise the most common form of posterior circulation aneurysm. Definitive surgical treatment became possible significantly later than it did for other types of aneurysmal disease, and it reflects the outstanding contributions made by Professors Charles Drake and Gazi Yasargil.[37,38,40,41] Access to the distal basilar artery in the interpeduncular cistern, which requires deep exposure from any approach, is complicated by the myriad of vital perforating arteries arising from the posterior aspect of the distal basilar artery and both P1 segments (Figure 14.33).[43] Failure to design specific operative strategies to ensure preservation of these vessels invariably results in clip occlusion and an almost certain likelihood of the patient suffering mesencephalic or diencephalic infarction (Figure 14.34). Three specific operative approaches have been designed to expose and treat aneurysms of the distal basilar artery, each with advantages, disadvantages, and limitations.

Pterional (transsylvian) approach

The pterional approach, particularly with wide sylvian fissure dissection, is extremely versatile and used for many aneurysms of the distal basilar complex.[44] Wide dissection of the parasellar cisterns enables access to the interpeduncular cistern by one or multiple routes (Figure 14.35). The dissection plane and the approach can be developed lateral to the internal carotid artery wherein the posterior communicating artery is followed to the junction of the P1 and P2 segments of the posterior cerebral artery. The P1 is then followed proximally to isolate proximal control on the distal basilar artery. Similarly, a dissection plane can be developed medial to the carotid artery that separates the small perforating arteries to the hypothalamic region and optic tract, opening the membrane of Liliequist, thereby directly exposing the basilar trunk in the interpeduncular cistern. In particularly

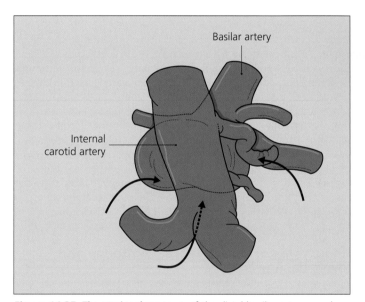

Figure 14.35 The pterional exposure of the distal basilar artery may be accomplished by an approach lateral to the internal carotid, medial to the internal carotid, or superior to the carotid bifurcation.

high basilar bifurcation aneurysms, it may be necessary to gain additional superior exposure by developing the plane immediately above the carotid bifurcation. This can be done by carefully dividing the arachnoidal fibers that bind together the small lenticulostriate vessels and, with patience, adequate separation of this tissue can be developed, allowing elevation of the optic tract with workable space within the interpeduncular cistern. In fact, regardless of the procedure, defining each of these planes minimizes the obscuring of vital anatomy by instruments placed in the exposure. Figure 14.36 illustrates a technique whereby a right-handed surgeon can approach the bifurcation region by using the microscope's line of sight medial to the carotid artery and passing the

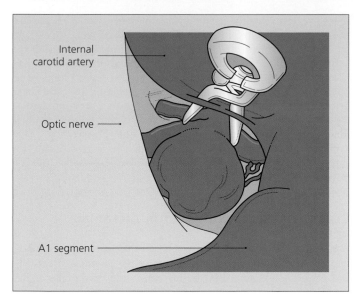

Figure 14.36 The surgeon can take advantage of the versatility of the pterional exposure by directing the microscope, and thus the line of sight, medial to the carotid artery and inserting the clip lateral and posterior to the carotid so the bulk of the clip and applier do not obscure the view.

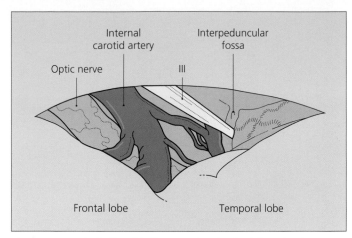

Figure 14.37 The half and half approach to basilar bifurcation improves access to the posteriorly located thalamoperforating arteries and improves illumination. The uncus is mobilized out of the tentorial incisura with a second retractor.

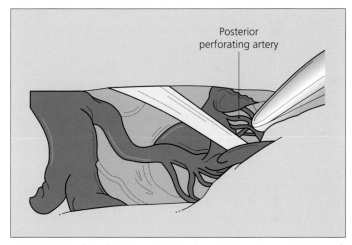

Figure 14.38 The subtemporal approach maximizes the surgical view of the thalamoperforating arteries while rendering the access to the contralateral posterior cerebral artery more difficult.

clip applier lateral to the carotid artery, minimizing the obscuring of this narrow space. This transsylvian exposure can be used to treat a wide variety of aneurysms in this location because it allows the surgeon a good view of the anatomy. It also enables exquisite access to the proximal basilar trunk and both P1 segments for definitive temporary occlusion with aneurysmal decompression, if necessary, to control intraoperative bleeding or facilitate the dissection of difficult large and giant lesions.

Half-and-half approach

Drake has described this modification of the pterional exposure to improve access to the posterior reaches of the interpeduncular cistern through a slightly more lateral viewpoint.[41] This approach involves rotating the head a bit more than in a direct transsylvian exposure and mobilizing the temporal lobe with superior and slightly lateral displacement of the uncus (Figure 14.37). In addition to the improved posterior exposure, this approach offers an improved view of the entire interpeduncular fossa. In many circumstances, it is a very desirable approach to plan from the outset of the procedure.

Subtemporal approach

The lateral view of the interpeduncular cistern, which was highly developed by Drake,[41] offers perhaps the ideal view of the vital perforators posterior to the aneurysmal fundus (Figure 14.38). For the typical superior projecting aneurysm, this viewpoint maximizes one's ability to salvage the perforating arteries, although the contralateral posterior cerebral artery is more difficult to see and quite difficult, if not impossible, to occlude temporarily. For a standard subtemporal clipping, however, the space anterior to the aneurysmal neck can usually be retracted gently so that the contralateral P1 segment with its initial anterior course can be definitively seen. Drake's innovation of the aperture or fenestrated clip has greatly simplified the subtemporal clipping of basilar bifurcation aneurysms such that the P1 segment and any

associated perforating arteries may be included in the fenestration (Figure 14.39).

Extended lateral approach

Over the past several years, a continued struggle with basilar apex aneurysms has resulted in the evolution in our center of a hybrid operative approach. If one thinks conceptually, both the transsylvian and subtemporal approaches have certain assets and liabilities. The transsylvian view has the advantage that all five involved vessels can be seen *enface*. In addition, the surgeon has immediate access to full trapping of the circulation at that site. The primary disadvantage of the transsylvian view is that there is relatively poor access to the posterior reaches of the interpeduncular cistern where the perforating vessels lie. The great advantage of the subtemporal view is that the lateral view facilitates exposure and dissection of the posteriorly located perforators. The primary disadvantage of this approach is that the exposure is narrow, and it is rare to have access to all appropriate vessels for a full trapping, should that be required.

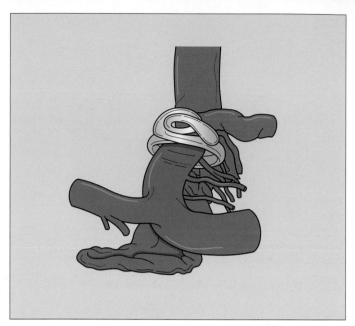

Figure 14.39 Aperture or fenestrated clips for subtemporal clipping of basilar bifurcation aneurysms have proven to be immensely valuable. The ipsilateral P1 segment with associated perforating arteries may be safely included in the fenestration.

The extended lateral blunt exposure is performed from the surgeon's dominant side. A traditional pterional craniotomy is performed, followed by a wide resection of the temporal squama and sphenoid ridge. The sylvian fissure is completely dissected, and the sphenoparietal venous drainage is detached from the floor of the middle cranial fossa. With complete sylvian dissection and gravitational assistance, the temporal lobe migrates posteriorly. The surgical dissection is focused not on the opticocarotid triangle nor on the posterior communicating artery corridor. Rather, this approach centers on the third cranial nerve. All attachments between the third nerve and the uncus are taken down, and as the exposure deepens, the uncus and all temporal lobe structures that have migrated into the incisura are elevated by a temporal lobe retractor. This maneuver gives the surgeon access to the tentorial incisura as far back as the cerebral peduncle. At that point, when performed from the surgeon's dominant side, excellent access to the direct lateral view (just as one would have with the sub-temporal approach) is accomplished. Therefore, the assets of each primary approach are capitalized upon (perforator exposure and access to the contralateral P1 and superior cerebral arteries) and the liabilities of both approaches are negated. The surgeon can dissect perforators to a true-lateral view and during clip application, with simple adjustments of the microscope, have access to the full benefits of the wide transsylvian view.

A final point should be mentioned that has greatly simplified clipping of these treacherous lesions. If one avoids the true surgical neck on the operated side and begins the dissection inferior to the P1 origin, the difficulty posed by the broad neck of these aneurysms and the constant finding that the aneurysm sac itself begins to develop well below the superior aspect of the P1 origin can be eliminated. The dissection when performed below the P1 origin allows the surgeon to roll the anatomy out of the interpeduncular fossa and work across the basilar trunk at a site where the distance to be traveled is considerably foreshortened.

Once one notes that the posterior thalamal perforates have changed course, the contralateral P1 contribution has been seen. An elegant strategy at that point involves the use of temporary occlusion for softening and the application of a very short fenestrated clip, allowing the ipsilateral P1 to reside in the fenestration. The purpose of the initial and primary clip is simply to gather the artery neck together and to close definitively the contralateral aspect of the neck. Once that is achieved, usually there is residual filling through the ipsilateral neck at the fenestration. This problem can be simply remedied by applying a traditional clip through the surgical neck to gather the tissue between the P1 origin and the end of the fenestration.

Cranial base exposures for intracranial aneurysms

In recent years, modifications to some of the previously described operative exposures have enabled neurosurgeons more effectively to treat complex aneurysms arising within the constraints of the cranial base. The broader exposure yielded by these procedures provides the surgeon with an enhanced view of the vascular anatomy with little to no need for brain retraction, and perhaps most importantly, additional working room. The exposures most beneficial to the neurovascular surgeon are detailed below.

Orbitozygomatic approach

The addition of an orbital or orbitozygomatic osteotomy to a standard pterional craniotomy should be considered with carotid wall, anterior communicating, and basilar quadrification aneurysms. The additional 10–15° of exposure this maneuver provides are invaluable in situations where a swollen, tense brain exists (Figure 14.40A).

Following a standard pterional craniotomy as described previously, dura overlying the orbital roof is stripped posteriorly toward the orbital apex, medial to the cribriform, and lateral to the dura of the superior orbital fissure. Periorbita is stripped from the superior and lateral walls of the orbit to a depth of approximately 3 cm. If the zygomatic process is to be included in the osteotomy, the full extent of the zygomatic arch is exposed prior to the reflexion of the temporalis muscle. Resection of the orbital zygomatic segment is best accomplished with a combination of reciprocating saw and osteotomes. The initial bone cuts are made with a reciprocating saw through the supraorbital ridge and frontal zygomatic process with the former being just lateral to the supraorbital foramen (Figure 14.40B). Narrow osteotomes complete the resection across the orbital roof, greater and lesser wing of the sphenoid bone. Once the masseter has been released from the inferior surface of the zygomatic arch, the piece may be removed *en bloc*. It is important to preserve at least 3 cm of the orbital roof and lateral wall so as to minimize the possibility of a postoperative pulsatile enophthalmos.

Perhaps the most important element to this exposure is the resection of the proximal lesser and greater wings of the sphenoid bone inclusive of the anterior clinoid process. This bony resection is particularly useful for ophthalmic and superior hypophyseal aneurysms. The post-clipping reconstruction is performed in a standard fashion with a micro-plating system and a hydroxyapatite compound or methylmethacrylate to fill in any bony defects.

Petrosal approach

The combined subtemporal, suboccipital, or petrosal approach provides the most direct access to aneurysms from the basilar

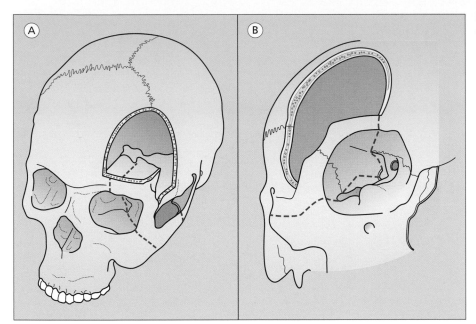

Figure 14.40 Demonstration of orbital **(A)** and orbitozygomatic **(B)** osteotomies.

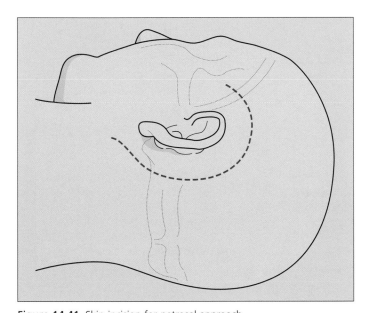

Figure 14.41 Skin incision for petrosal approach.

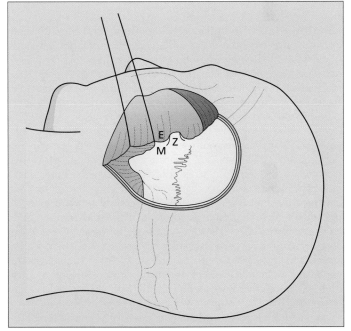

Figure 14.42 Exposure for mastoid (M), roof of zygoma (Z), and external auditory meatus (E).

apex to the vertebral basilar junction. Variations to this approach include a retrolabyrinthine exposure, a partial labyrinthectomy, a total labyrinthectomy, and a transcochlear resection with facial nerve mobilization. It is the retrolabyrinthine or partial labyrinthine exposure that is most favored at our institution as they are the only petrosal approaches which preserve hearing.

The patient is positioned supine with a shoulder roll ipsilateral to the side of the approach and the head is turned through 90° then gently extended toward the floor, and, if necessary, the shoulder is taped caudally. A curvilinear incision is made originating 2 cm superior and anterior to the ear and curved along a 2 cm posterior margin from the ear to a point 2 cm inferior to the

mastoid tip (Figure 14.41). The temporalis and occipital frontalis muscles are divided and reflected laterally with the scalp to expose the external auditory meatus centrally, the temporal zygomatic root rostrally, and the entire mastoid process posterior inferiorly (Figure 14.42). A mastoidectomy is performed with early identification and skeletonization of the transverse and sigmoid sinuses as far laterally as the jugular bulb (Figure 14.43). Care is taken to preserve the bony labyrinth, in situations where only a retrolabyrinthine, presigmoid exposure is necessary. With a partial labyrinthectomy, as many as five additional millimeters of room can be created, providing for several degrees of added maneuverability at the level of the petrous apex. This is accom-

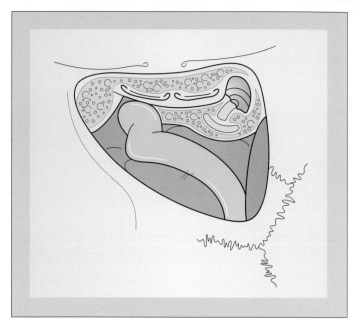

Figure 14.43 Mastoidectomy with exposure of sigmoid sinus, semi-auricular canals, and skeletonized seventh nerve.

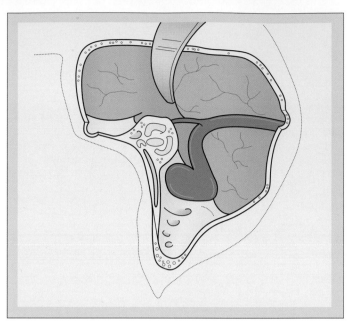

Figure 14.44 Full exposure with mastoidectomy, suboccipital, and subtemporal craniotomies.

plished with cautious drilling of the posterior and superior semi-circular canals to expose the underlying membranous labyrinth. Once identified, the exposed orifices are immediately waxed off. The horizontal semicircular canal is preserved. A completed mastoidectomy should yield exposure of tegmental and posterior fossa dura. This dural exposure facilitates the addition of a subtemporal and suboccipital craniotomy (Figure 14.44). The dural opening is typically presigmoid, originating just superior and anterior to the jugular bulb and directed toward the superior petrosal sinus. The sinus is ligated and the dural cut carried rostrally to the dura of the middle fossa, then the dura tented laterally. The tentorium is coagulated with the bipolar cautery and cut toward the incisura. Care then is exercised to avoid injury to the fourth nerve as it courses adjacent to the mid-brain en route to the tentorial edge. The tentorium can be partially excised or coagulated to enhance visualization. The mid-brain, clivus, basilar artery, and cranial nerves III to XII are clearly visible with this exposure. A modification of this approach to include a retro-sigmoid dural exposure with ligation of the non-dominant transverse sinus has been described; however, in our experience this maneuver creates an unacceptable risk of venous infarction.

After the aneurysm has been appropriately secured, a watertight dural closure should be attempted. A dural graft is often necessary. Mastoid air cells should be thoroughly waxed and fat should be placed in the mastoid defect. Lumbar spinal fluid drainage should be considered in situations where watertight dural closure cannot be achieved.

Far lateral transcondylar approach

Aneurysms of the vertebral artery distal to the posterior inferior cerebral artery up to the maximal origin of the anterior inferior cerebral arteries are comfortably accessible with a far lateral exposure. The addition of partial condylectomy gains access to the ventral brainstem. This approach requires that the patient be positioned in either a park-bench or three-quarter prone position as previously described. We favor a curvilinear incision, typically arising approximately 1 cm superior to the inion, curving laterally

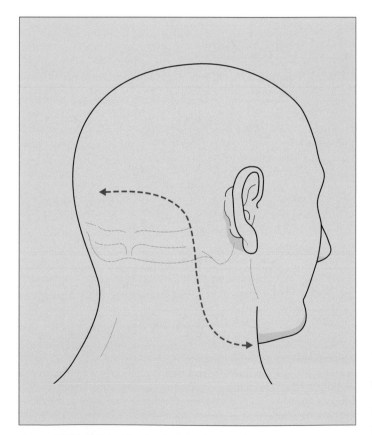

Figure 14.45 Skin incision for far lateral approach.

to 2 cm posterior to the ipsilateral ear, and continuing caudally to end 3 cm posterior inferior to the mastoid tip, just over to the mid-portion of the sternocleidomastoid muscle (Figure 14.45). The scalp and fascia are reflected medially to expose the under-lying intermixed fascia of the first-layer muscle group, which

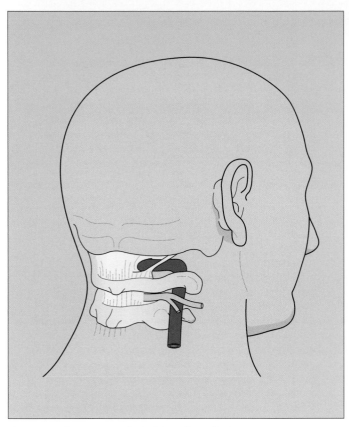

Figure 14.46 Exposure of C1, C2, and vertebral artery.

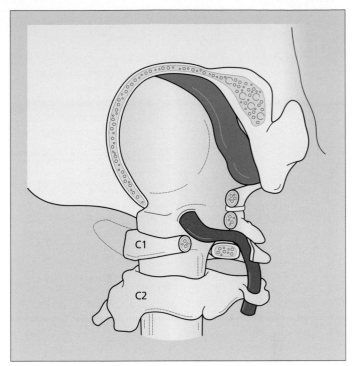

Figure 14.47 Mobilization of vertebral artery with condylectomy and craniotomy and C1 laminectomy with dural exposure.

includes the occipital frontalis, trapezius, and sternocleidomastoid muscles. These muscle layers are divided at their attachment to the superior nuchal line, the trapezius reflected inferomedially, and the sternocleidomastoid detached from the mastoid process and reflected inferolaterally. The spinalis capitis and semispinalis capitis are sequentially detached from the occiput. The occipital artery can be dissected free of longissimus capitis, and this muscle is caudally reflected from its attachment to the undersurface of the mastoid process. With these muscles reflected, the suboccipital triangle is brought into view. The triangle is composed of the recti and obliquus muscles. The superior oblique and inferior oblique can be followed laterally to their attachment to the C1 lateral mass and then should be detached. The lateral portion of C1 and C2 should be completely exposed. Within this exposed atloaxis interval, the vertebral artery encased in a rich venous network can be isolated (Figure 14.46). The dorsal ramus of the C2 nerve root is a reliable landmark for certain identification of the vertebral artery. Next, the rectus muscles are stripped from their attachments to the C1 ring and C2 spinous process to expose the inferior aspect of the occiput and the foramen magnum. The intervening atlo-occipital membrane is cleared to expose the underlying dura, and the lateral portion of the C1 arch is removed. Narrow bone longeurs are then utilized to skeletonize the foramen transversarium, and the vertebral artery is mobilized laterally to expose the atlo-occipital joint.

At this point, a burr hole is placed just caudal to the mastoid, and a suboccipital craniotomy is performed inclusive of the foramen magnum. With the vertebral artery isolated in a vessel loop, the atlo-occipital joint is drilled from medial to lateral, taking care to preserve at least 50% of the joint so as to not create

an instability and obviate a subsequent fusion procedure. The condylar vein will be encountered with drilling and can typically be controlled with bipolar cautery and bone wax. The landmark which typically signifies the completion of the condylectomy is the dense cortical bone encountered medially, which represents the posterolateral aspect of the hypoglossal canal.

With bone work complete, the vertebral artery is to its dural entry zone, and a linear incision preserving a cuff around this vertebral entry is performed. This approach should yield direct visualization of the clivus and will allow for the maximum degree of pre-pontine working room (Figure 14.47).

As with the other cranial base exposures described here, it is imperative to achieve watertight dural closure. One should not hesitate to utilize fat and alternative tissue grafts or lumbar drains if any doubts of the integrity of the dural closure exist.

CONCLUSION

Today, debate rages as to whether intracranial aneurysms when found to be small and asymptomatic should be treated at all. It is clear that many small aneurysms have a low risk of yearly rupture, but it should be kept in mind that should that rupture occur, major morbidity and mortality are to be expected. It is clear that many issues need to be carefully clarified with regard to natural history risk. Aneurysm morphology and neck to fundus ratios have a bearing on the physics of pulsatile flow within the fundus and are likely to affect the rupture rate. Daughter sacs and irregularities of the sac are often correlated with surgical inspection demonstrating marked attenuation of numerous areas of the sac itself. These factors should be studied carefully in terms of risk prediction.

Endovascular techniques have made major strides over the past decade and appear to have treatment risks equal or superior

CLINICAL PEARLS

- The incidence of intracranial aneurysms is difficult to estimate in the general population, but it is believed to affect about 5% of the population in North America. Of the people who suffer an aneurysmal rupture, fewer than 40% return to their previous lifestyle and function, and approximately 30% will die prior to reaching a hospital.

- The majority of cerebral aneurysms arise at branching points of large arteries. Hemodynamic stress may contribute to the development and continued growth of aneurysms. Intracranial aneurysms are also associated with polycystic kidney disease, coarctation of the aorta, Marfan syndrome, fibromuscular dysplasia, tuberous sclerosis and Ehlers–Danlos syndrome.

- Approximately 25–50% of all patients will have warning symptoms that herald the onset of a major subarachnoid hemorrhage (SAH). The work-up of a patient with a suspected SAH includes a history, examination and CT scan. If the scan is negative, but the suspicion of a bleed remains high, a lumbar puncture can be performed looking for evidence of red blood cells or their breakdown products. Angiography remains the gold standard for diagnosis of intracranial aneurysms.

- After a patient suffers a subarachnoid hemorrhage from an aneurysm, the risk of rebleeding is greatest on the first day (4.1%). By day 14, the cumulative rebleed incidence is 19%. Six months later 50% of patients have re-bled, but thereafter the long-term risk falls to approximately 3% per year. The risk of symptomatic cerebral ischemia from vasospasm peaks between 7 and 10 days postSAH, and remains the most significant cause of death and disability after a SAH, and one of the most formidable treatment challenges to the neurosurgeon.

- The treatment goal is to obliterate the ruptured aneurysm as soon as is safely possible followed by maximum treatment of symptomatic vasospasm. The treatment of symptomatic vasospasm includes hypervolemic, hypertensive therapy to vasodilate the affected arteries. Interventional endovascular vasodilatation has also been used successfully. Endovascular occlusion of cerebral aneurysms with coils has become an essential part of the armamentarium in the treatment of these dangerous lesions. The question of whether clipping or coiling an aneurysm is superior has yet to be answered; however, these are lesions that require an individualized approach depending on a multitude of factors. The patient is presumably best treated at centers in which highly experienced physicians in both endovascular and microvascular techniques cooperatively manage these challenging lesions.

to open surgical strategies. Debate continues regarding case selection. Contemporary endovascular strategies continue to suffer from efficacy issues and durability problems. Based on surgical experience over many decades, there is little evidence to suggest that anything less than precise and durable aneurysm obliteration provides significant long-term protection to the patient.[29,45–49]

Clearly, much work is left to be done in enhancing endovascular as well as microsurgical techniques. As these advances occur, careful study of the extremely heterogeneous nature of intracranial aneurysms must be carried out in a focused and non-shotgun fashion to answer specific questions. The question is not whether clipping or coiling is superior as a generality. In reality, these techniques are often synergistic and complementary. Surgical techniques can create a very narrow opening into a complex aneurysm that would permit easy access for coiling when that would not have been feasible originally. It is critical that all centers offering state of the art cerebrovascular medicine have robust and highly expert physicians in both endovascular and microvascular neurosurgery.

REFERENCES

1. McCormick WF, Acosta-Rua GJ. The size of intracranial saccular aneurysms: an autopsy study. *J Neurosurg* 1970; 33: 422–7.
2. Kassell NF, Drake CG. Timing of aneurysm surgery. *Neurosurgery* 1982; 10: 514–19.
3. Sekhar LN, Heros RC. Origin, growth, and rupture of saccular aneurysms: a review. *Neurosurgery* 1981; 8: 248–60.
4. Somach FM, Shenkin HA. Angiographic end results of carotid ligation in the treatment of carotid aneurysm. *J Neurosurg* 1966; 24: 966–74.
5. Batjer HH, Mickey BE, Samson D. Enlargement and rupture of distal basilar aneurysm following iatrogenic carotid occlusion. *Neurosurgery* 1987; 20: 624–8.
6. Adamson T, Batjer HH. Aneurysm recurrence associated with induced hypertension and hypervolemia. *Surg Neurol* 1988; 29: 57–61.
7. Batjer HH, Suss RA, Samson DS. Intracranial arteriovenous malformations associated with aneurysms. *Neurosurgery* 1986; 18: 29–35.
8. Weir B. *Aneurysms Affecting the Nervous System*. Baltimore, MD: Williams & Wilkins; 1987: 54–133.
9. Kassell NF, Torner JC. The International Cooperative Study on timing of aneurysm surgery: an update. *Stroke* 1984; 15: 566–70.
10. Adams HP, Kassell NF, Torner JC. Usefulness of computed tomography in predicting outcome after aneurysmal subarachnoid hemorrhage: a preliminary report of the Cooperative Aneurysm Study. *Neurology* 1985; 35: 1263–7.
11. Hunt WE, Hess RM. Surgical risk as related to time of intervention in the repair of intracranial aneurysms. *J Neurosurg* 1968; 28: 14–19.
12. Kassell NF, Torner JC. Aneurysmal rebleeding: a preliminary report from the Cooperative Aneurysm Study. *Neurosurgery* 1983; 13: 479–81.
13. Jane JA, Kassell NF, Torner JC, *et al.* The natural history of aneurysms and arteriovenous malformations. *J Neurosurg* 1985; 62: 321–3.

14. Weir B, Grace M, Hansen J, *et al*. Time course of vasospasm in man. *J Neurosurg* 1978; 48: 173–8.

15. Kwak R, Niizuma H, Takatsugu D, *et al*. Angiographic study of cerebral vasospasm following rupture of intracranial aneurysms, I: time of the appearance. *Surg Neurol* 1979; 11: 257–62.

16. Kassell NF, Sasaki T, Colohan ART, *et al*. Cerebral vasospasm following subarachnoid hemorrhage. *Stroke* 1985; 16: 562–72.

17. Fisher CM, Kistler JP, Davis JM. Relation of cerebral vasospasm to subarachnoid hemorrhage visualized by computerized tomographic scanning. *Neurosurgery* 1980; 6: 1–9.

18. Doczi T, Bende J, Huzka E, *et al*. Syndrome of inappropriate secretion of antidiuretic hormone after subarachnoid hemorrhage. *Neurosurgery* 1981; 9: 394–7.

19. Kassell NF, Boarini DJ. Perioperative care of the aneurysm patient. *Contemp Neurosurg* 1984; 6: 1–6.

20. Ljunggren B, Brandt L, Kagstrom E, *et al*. Results of early operations for ruptured aneurysms. *J Neurosurg* 1981; 54: 473–9.

21. Ljunggren B, Saveland H, Brandt L, *et al*. Early operation and overall outcome in aneurysmal subarachnoid hemorrhage. *J Neurosurg* 1985; 62: 547–51.

22. Winn HR, Newell DW, Mayberg MR, *et al*. Early surgical management of poor-grade patients with intracranial aneurysms. *Clin Neurosurg* 1990; 36: 289–98.

23. Kassell NF, Torner JC, Adams HP. Antifibrinolytic therapy in the acute period following aneurysmal subarachnoid hemorrhage: preliminary observations from the Cooperative Aneurysm Study. *J Neurosurg* 1984; 61: 225–30.

24. Kosnik EJ, Hunt WE. Postoperative hypertension in the management of patients with intracranial aneurysms. *J Neurosurg* 1976; 45: 148–54.

25. Finn SS, Stephenson SA, Miller CA, *et al*. Observations on the perioperative management of aneurysmal subarachnoid hemorrhage. *J Neurosurg* 1986; 65: 48–62.

26. Kassell NF, Peerless SJ, Durward QJ, *et al*. Treatment of ischemic deficits from vasospasm with intravascular volume expansion and induced arterial hypertension. *Neurosurgery* 1982; 11: 337–43.

27. Gentleman D, Johnston R. Postoperative extradural hematoma associated with induced hypertension. *Neurosurgery* 1985; 17: 105–6.

28. Terada T, Komai N, Hayashi S, *et al*. Hemorrhagic infarction after vasospasm due to ruptured cerebral aneurysm. *Neurosurgery* 1986; 18: 415–18.

29. Batjer HH, Samson DS. Causes of morbidity and mortality from surgery of aneurysms of the distal basilar artery. *Neurosurgery* 1989; 25: 904–16.

30. Higashida RT, Hieshima GB, Tsai FY, *et al*. Transluminal angioplasty of the vertebral and basilar artery. *AJNR* 1987; 8: 745–9.

31. Batjer HH, Samson DS. Intraoperative aneurysmal rupture: incidence, outcome, and suggestions for surgical management. *Neurosurgery* 1986; 18: 701–7.

32. Michenfelder JD, Theye RA. Cerebral protection by thiopental during hypoxia. *Anesthesiology* 1973; 39: 510–17.

33. Michenfelder JD, Milde JH. Influence of anesthetics on metabolic, functional and pathological responses to regional cerebral ischemia. *Stroke* 1975; 6: 405–10.

34. Michenfelder JD, Milde JH, Sundt TM Jr. Cerebral protection by barbiturate anesthesia. *Arch Neurol* 1976; 33: 345–50.

35. Batjer HH, Frankfurt AI, Purdy PD, *et al*. Use of etomidate, temporary arterial occlusion, and intraoperative angiography in large and giant cerebral aneurysm surgery. *J Neurosurg* 1988; 68: 234–40.

36. Samson DS, Batjer HH. *Intracranial Aneurysm Surgery: Techniques*. Mount Kisco, NY: Futura Publishing Co; 1990.

37. Yasargil MG. Operative anatomy. In: Yasargil MG (ed.). *Microneurosurgery*. Stuttgart: Georg Thieme Verlag; 1984; vol. 1: 5–168.

38. Yasargil MG. Pathological considerations. In: Yasargil MG (ed.). *Microneurosurgery*. Stuttgart: Georg Thieme Verlag; 1984; vol. 1: 279–349.

39. Heros RC, Nelson PB, Ojemann RG, *et al*. Large and giant paraclinoid aneurysms: surgical techniques, complications, and results. *Neurosurgery* 1983; 12: 153–63.

40. Drake CG. Giant intracranial aneurysms: experience with surgical treatment in 174 patients. *Clin Neurosurg* 1979; 26: 12–95.

41. Drake CG. The treatment of aneurysms of the posterior circulation. *Clin Neurosurg* 1979; 26: 96–144.

42. Locksley HB. Report on the Cooperative Study of Intracranial Aneurysm and Subarachnoid Hemorrhage, section V, part 1: natural history of subarachnoid hemorrhage, intracranial aneurysms and arteriovenous malformations: based on 6368 cases in the cooperative study. *J Neurosurg* 1966; 25: 219–39.

43. Grand W, Hopkins LN. The microsurgical anatomy of the basilar artery bifurcation. *Neurosurgery* 1977; 1: 128–31.

44. Samson DS, Hodosh RM, Clark WK. Microsurgical evaluation of the pterional approach to aneurysms of the distal basilar circulation. *Neurosurgery* 1978; 3: 135–41.

45. Drake CG, Vanderlinden RG. The late consequences of incomplete surgical treatment of cerebral aneurysms. *J Neurosurg* 1967; 27: 226–38.

46. Drake CG, Friedman AH, Peerless SJ. Failed aneurysm surgery: reoperation in 115 cases. *J Neurosurg* 1984; 61: 848–56.

47. Feuerberg I, Lindquist C, Lindqvist M, *et al*. Natural history of postoperative aneurysm rests. *J Neurosurg* 1987; 66: 30–4.

48. Todd NV, Tocher JL, Jones PA, *et al*. Outcome following aneurysm wrapping: a 10-year follow-up review of clipped and wrapped aneurysms. *J Neurosurg* 1989; 70: 841–6.

49. Lin T, Fox AJ, Drake CG. Regrowth of aneurysm sacs from residual neck following aneurysm clipping. *J Neurosurg* 1989; 70: 556–60.

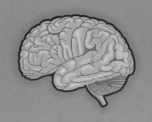

VASCULAR MALFORMATIONS AFFECTING THE NERVOUS SYSTEM

15

Andrew T Parsa and Robert A Solomon

HISTORICAL OVERVIEW

In their comprehensive review of historical developments in the treatment of vascular malformation Yasargil and colleagues give credit to William Hunter for providing many important early concepts[1] (Table 15.1). Hunter's descriptions of extracranial arteriovenous malformations (AVMs) documented in his 1762 monograph formed the basis for testing divergent theories regarding the physiology, pathology, and development of these lesions. Applying Hunter's teleological framework almost 100 years later, Rokitansky was the first comprehensively to describe angiomas of the intracranial cavity, speculating that these were in fact highly vascular tumors. Later in 1851 Virchow and others refined Rokitansky's description to include a rudimentary classification system of telangiectasias, and of venous, arterial, arteriovenous, and cystic angiomas. Virchow's work is particularly noteworthy because his extensive pathological studies determine

that only a small percentage of angiomas are neoplastic; and that the majority of these represent some type of congenital anomaly. D'Arcy Power described clinical correlation of the pathology defined by Virchow and his contemporaries in 1888, as did Steinhil three years later in 1891. D'Arcy Power's description of a 20-year-old man with right-sided hemiplegia and a left sylvian fissure AVM is an early model for anatomical localization of this disease process.[1]

From the 1890s to the 1930s as surgery for intracranial mass lesions increased so did descriptive reports of AVMs. The first well-documented successful excision of an intracranial AVM was performed in 1889. In this case Pean, a French general surgeon, operated on a 15-year-old boy who presented with left-sided seizures and a right-sided frontal–parietal lesion. Subsequently Cushing and Dandy in 1928 each described their individual series of 14 and 15 patients respectively.[2,3] In a later 1928 monograph entitled *Tumors Arising from the Blood-vessels of the Brain*,

Table 15.1 Historical milestones in understanding the pathogenesis and treatment of vascular malformations

Time frame	Contributor	Contribution
1792	Hunter	Wrote a monograph on vascular malformation
1850s	Rokitansky	First to describe angiomas of intracranial cavity
1851	Virchow	Rudimentary classification of malformations
Late 1880s	D'Arcy Power/Steinhil	Correlation of clinical features with location of AVM
1889	Pean	First attempt at surgical excision of a vascular malformation
Late 1920s	Cushing/Dandy	Described personal series of intracranial vascular malformations
1920s	Egaz Moniz	Introduction of cerebral angiography
1940s	Olivecrona and others	Larger series of angiographically documented vascular malformations
1950s	Lussenhop	Attempted therapeutic embolization of intracranial vessels
1960s	Yasargil, Donaghy	Development of microvascular neurosurgery
1960s	Leksell	Clinical use of stereotactic focused beam radiation therapy of selected intracranial targets
1990s	Contemporary authors	Elucidation of genomics of cavernous malformations

Cushing and Bailey summarized the expert opinions of their era in describing a group of lesions referred to as angiomatous malformations.[4] The authors elaborated upon standard principles that form the basis of our treatment strategies today including surgical ligation of feeding vessels, nidus removal, as well as radiation therapy and judicious observation. Their remarkably detailed anatomical, pathological, and surgical primer is a landmark treatise that foreshadowed many of the developments to follow in the 20th century.

There is no single historical event more important to the treatment of AVM patients than the development of intracerebral angiography. The application of angiography as a diagnostic tool serves as a logical milestone for classifying early experiences. The work of Cushing, Dandy, and Bailey described in the 1920s should be considered distinct from that of pioneers such as Olivecrona, Penfield, Eriksen, and Pilcher who collectively described, throughout the 1940s, the treatment of over a hundred AVM patients using pre-operative angiograms.[1] The relatively recent development of embolization and the advent of endovascular procedures represent additional treatment milestones. Fundamental developments in neuroimaging, such as the computed tomography (CT) scanner and magnetic resonance imaging (MRI), surgical tools such as the operating microscope, and adjuncts such as gamma-knife radiosurgery have also optimized outcomes for many AVM patients.

Currently we continue to make diagnostic and therapeutic advances in the treatment of patients with AVMs. Frameless stereotaxis and functional mapping have facilitated lesion localization while the endovascular field seems to become more refined on an annual basis. Despite these technical advances there currently remains a sub-population of patients for whom no treatment can be undertaken safely. It is these patients in particular who provide the historical impetus to develop more effective treatment modalities.

There are still no clear answers to many fundamental medical and scientific questions regarding AVMs. Yasargil and colleagues inform us that historical controversy has always existed for the pathogenesis, nomenclature, classification, diagnosis, and treatment of AVMs.[1] We would add to these topics the issue of AVM natural history. In the 21st century the medical staff charged with the care of AVM patients face the same questions addressed by early pioneers. Multidisciplinary paradigms of management are being applied as advances in evidence-based medicine raise the possibility of delineated optimal patient care. In this chapter we detail the clinical and scientific topics that have fostered more effective strategies for the treatment of AVM patients. In addition we include a review of several patients treated at our institution, exemplifying the multidisciplinary approach necessary for obtaining a favorable outcome.

PATHOLOGICAL CLASSIFICATION (Table 15.2)

Detailed descriptions of malformations are often confounded by the quality of the operative or post-mortem specimen. The propensity for these lesions to bleed as well as the dynamic nature of their growth can obscure pathological characteristics. Pre-operative treatment modalities such as embolization and radiation therapy can also alter the microscopic appearance of malformations. Despite these difficulties there are fundamental structures that define various malformations. Furthermore, these structural characteristics have a radiological correlate that can facilitate early diagnosis.

Table 15.2 Classification of vascular malformations

1 Capillary telangiectasias
2 Cavernous malformations
3 Venous malformations
4 Arteriovenous malformations

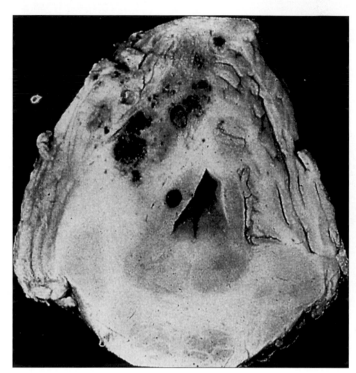

Figure 15.1 Autopsy specimen cross-section through level of the pons demonstrating capillary telangiectasia in cerebellar peduncle.

Capillary telangiectasias

Capillary telangiectasias are composed exclusively of small capillary-type blood vessels that resemble normal capillaries surrounded by parenchyma that is normal in appearance. They are typically less than 1 cm in diameter and occur most commonly in the pons. These lesions are usually found incidentally upon autopsy, and rarely have clinical sequelae such as bleeding or thrombosis (Figure 15.1). Capillary telangiectasias are being recognized with increasing frequency on MRI studies as new sequences are applied. These lesions enhance with contrast material but are otherwise undetectable on conventional MRI. A typical capillary telangiectasia lacks the hemosiderin rim of cavernous malformations and demonstrates increased susceptibility only on gradient echo images, likely because of contrast being dependent on blood oxygen levels.

Capillary telangiectasias are clinically significant because these lesions may represent earlier versions of cavernous malformations. In 1991 Rigamonti and colleagues reviewed the histories of 20 patients with cavernous malformations and analyzed the clinical, radiographic, and surgical-autopsy data associated with these lesions.[5] In some patients, multiple lesions, including cavernous malformations, capillary telangiectasias, and transitional forms between the two, were identified. Based on this analysis, they concluded that capillary telangiectasia and cavernous malformations represent two pathological extremes within the same vascular malformation category and proposed grouping them as a single entity. More recently this group has described the juxtaposition of a capillary telangiectasia, cavernous malformation, and developmental venous anomaly in the brainstem of a single patient.[6] Juxtaposition of these three different vascular lesions in the brainstem of an otherwise normal individual suggested that the lesions were related. It is now hypothesized that a developmental event disrupting local capillary–venous structures occurs in capillary telangiectasia, subsequently leading to the formation of cavernous malformations.[6] Capillary telangiectasias can also more rarely occur in association with AVMs.[7]

Cavernous malformations

Cavernous malformations are composed of cystic vascular spaces lined by a single layer of endothelial cells. These sinusoidal vessels form a compact mass with no intervening neural parenchyma. The lack of neural tissue is a characteristic historically used to distinguish cavernous malformations from capillary telangiectasias. Recent application of electron microscopy has revealed that endothelial cells within cavernous malformations lack tight junctions.[8]

Upon gross examination cavernous malformations are well-circumscribed focal areas of reddish-purple discoloration up to a few centimeters in size. Hemorrhage results in variable deposition of hemosiderin, reactive gliosis, and focal areas of calcification. The absence of direct arterial input makes it difficult to visualize these lesions on conventional angiography, however their appearance on MRI is very characteristic (Figure 15.2). Blood of varying ages in and around these lesions gives a stereotypical pattern of heterogeneity.

Venous malformations

Venous malformations have been described as the most common type of vascular malformation at autopsy.[1] These lesions are composed of anomalous veins separated by normal neural parenchyma. The malformations may be composed of a single, greatly dilated, tortuous vein or a number of smaller veins coalescing at a single point; there is never direct arterial input. Accordingly, these lesions have a characteristic appearance in the venous phase of an angiogram that is described as *caput medusae*. Venous malformations can also be visualized as linear signals in unusual locations during contrast-enhanced CT scans or conventional MRI scans (Figure 15.3). From a clinical perspective these lesions are considered benign and any hemorrhage associated with a venous malformation is usually secondary to a nearby cavernous malformation (Figure 15.4).

Arteriovenous malformations

The essence of AVM pathology is arterial shunting into draining veins without intervening capillaries. Several recent studies have delineated the nature of structures that facilitate this shunting using conventional histological methods,[9,10] as well as scanning electron microscopy.[11] In each of these reports shunting arterioles can be seen communicating directly with AVM core vessels. These pathological hallmarks have distinctive radiographic correlates that

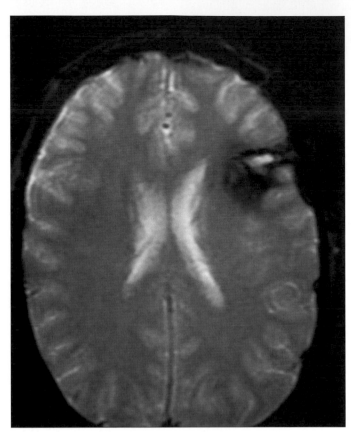

Figure 15.2 Gradient echo sequence axial MRI showing typical appearance of left frontal cavernous malformation.

span the spectrum of AVM pathology. Focal lesions may demonstrate a clear arterial supply of a tight nidus with pathognomonic early draining veins (Figure 15.5). Using contrast, characteristic angiographic features of diffuse lesions included multiple small arterial feeders, small ectatic vessels in the malformation itself, multiple small draining veins, and a diffuse, puddling appearance of the contrast dye.[12]

Most vascular channels within an AVM are venous in morphology, however transitional vessels are quite common. Vascular channels vary in accordance with the spectrum of pathology. A tightly compacted nidus without intervening neural parenchyma is characteristic of focal lesions, while diffuse lesions contain normal cerebral tissue between abnormal vessels.[12] Regardless of where they fall on this spectrum, the propensity for AVMs to bleed has a histologic and pathologic correlate. Microscopic areas of hemosiderin deposition and abnormal gliotic parenchyma can be identified even in patients who do not present after an ictal event. These microhemorrhages are followed by thrombosis and reparative fibrosis, which in turn lead to scar formation and calcification.

Other vascular lesions can be found in association with AVMs including venous and arterial aneurysms (Figure 15.6). Venous aneurysms do not typically have a clinicopathologic correlate, however there are important clinical implications and surgical considerations for AVM patients with an associated arterial aneurysm (Figure 15.7). These aneurysms have been classified as intranidal, flow-related, or unrelated to the AVM nidus.[13] In a recent review of 632 patients Redekop and colleagues found that intranidal aneurysms have a high correlation with hemorrhagic clinical presentation and a risk of bleeding during the follow-up

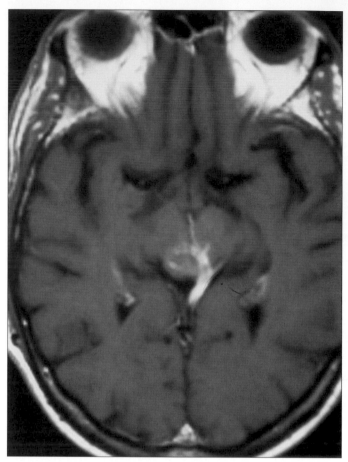

Figure 15.3 Contrast enhanced T1 MRI showing venous angioma arising from the dorsal aspect of the midbrain.

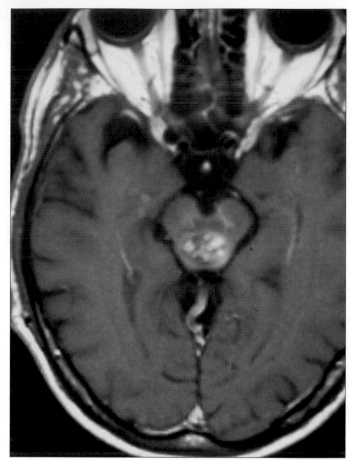

Figure 15.4 Lower section taken in same patient as Figure 15.3 showing associated cavernous malformation in the midbrain.

period that considerably exceeds what would occur in their absence.[13] Patients with flow-related aneurysms in association with an AVM may present with hemorrhage from either lesion. Aneurysms that arise on distal feeding arteries near the nidus have a high probability of regressing with substantial or curative AVM therapy. In a more recent analysis of AVM patients (240 treated for AVM and two for an aneurysm) feeding vessel pedicle aneurysms appeared to occur more frequently in conjunction with infratentorial AVMs.[14]

EMBRYOLOGY OF ARTERIOVENOUS MALFORMATIONS

There are several aspects of AVM morphological characteristics that resemble the anastomatic plexuses of developing vasculature in the embryo. These similarities have lead many investigators to speculate that there is a fundamental arrest of vascular development associated with the formation of AVMs.[15] Mullan and colleagues have attempted to correlate several clinical, anatomic, and angiographic features of lesions from AVM patients with known events in central nervous system vasculature development.[16] These authors hypothesize that AVMs begin during human embryonic development during the sequential formation and absorption of surface veins; mainly in the 40- to 80-mm length interval. Accordingly, discordance of vein formation and resorption can potentially result in predictable anomalies. Absence of the

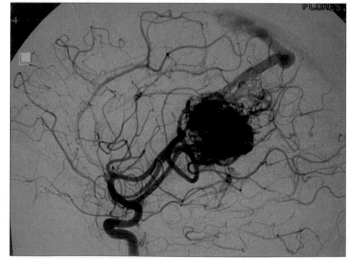

Figure 15.5 Typical angiographic appearance of an inferior frontal AVM with a tight nidus and early draining vein going up to the saggital sinus.

middle cerebral vein or its failure to communicate with the cavernous sinus in AVM patients may correlate with the late development of that vein embryologically; and to its even later connection to the cavernous sinus. Other circumstantial embryological correlates include the entry of the superior ophthalmic vein

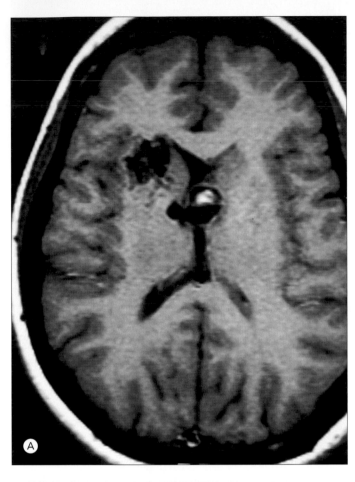

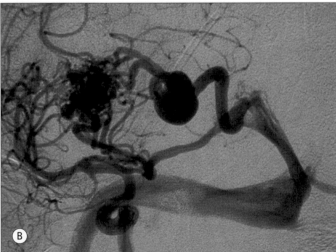

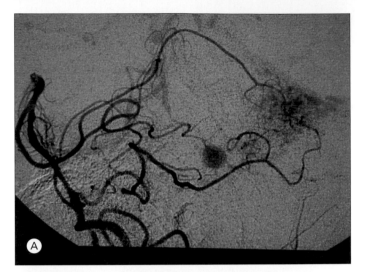

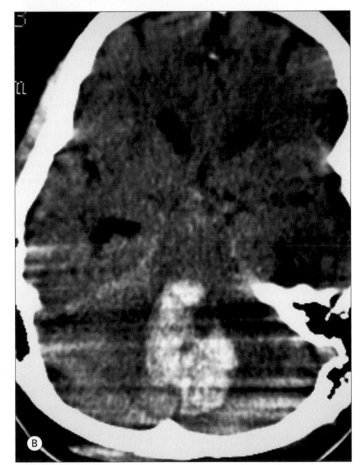

Figure 15.6 Patient with a right caudate AVM with a large venous aneurysm in the third ventricle. **(A)** Axial T1 MRI; **(B)** lateral carotid angiogram.

Figure 15.7 Patient with a cerebellar AVM presenting with vermian hemorrhage from a distal feeding artery aneurysm. **(A)** Lateral vertebral angiogram demonstrating proximal feeding artery aneurysm; **(B)** axial CT scan demonstrating vermian hemorrhage from aneurysm.

into the cavernous sinus through the inferior rather than the superior orbital fissure, the relative infrequency of middle cerebral vein backflow in the presence of an extensive cavernous fistula, and the relative infrequency of hemorrhage in relation to the inferior petrosal fistula.[16] Each of these findings is consistent with a relationship between the anomaly and older venous pathways.

The occurrence of hemorrhage in association with a superior petrosal sinus fistula and the failure of the superior petrosal sinus to connect to the cavernous sinus may also have an embryological correlate.[16] In addition, an insult at the time when the paired internal cerebral veins fuse into one channel could explain vein of Galen aneurysms and an absent or deformed straight sinus.

The view of Mullan and colleagues that specific embryological events are associated with AVM is supported by a number of clinical syndromes in children with AVMs.[17-19] These syndromes can range in severity and involvement of other organ systems. Hereditary hemorrhagic telangiectasia (HHT) is an autosomal dominant vascular dysplasia that can involve multiple organs.[19] Visceral involvement includes pulmonary, gastrointestinal, and cerebral AVMs, which have been reported predominantly in adults. Clinical evidence of an embryological etiology for AVMs also comes from anecdotal case reports that describe as yet unnamed syndromes. An example of this is the case of a 14-year-old boy with syndactyly of all limbs and intracranial dural AVM.[20] The coincidence of syndactyly and an AVM in this patient is consistent with a single common intrauterine insult occurring during the 2nd month of gestation. The differentiation of cerebral vessels *in utero* approximately matches the time frame for normal interdigital tissue regression at 5–7 weeks gestational age.

PHYSIOLOGY OF ARTERIOVENOUS MALFORMATIONS

The physiology of AVMs and surrounding brain can be influenced by many factors including size, location, associated vascular anomalies, and the presence of hemorrhage. Despite the great variety of attributes found among AVM patients there are some common principles that apply to each of these lesions. In their early review addressing the pathophysiology of cerebral ischemia accompanying AVM Spetzler and Selman describe several landmark papers that have lead to theoretical models of AVMs and facilitated our current understanding.[21] The key components to current models of AVM physiology include the feeding AVM artery, the surrounding brain normally perfused by this artery, and the arteriovenous shunt facilitated by the AVM.[22]

A basic theory of AVM physiology has been described by Spetzler to explain the phenomenon of ischemic related changes in the brain surrounding the AVM. As the arteriovenous shunt at the center of the AVM becomes more pronounced, flow occurs preferentially towards the arteriovenous shunt (i.e. the path of least resistance) resulting in a reduction of cerebral perfusion pressure in the vascular beds supplied by the feeding artery. This decrease in nutrient flow is directly proportional to the flow rate through the arteriovenous shunt, the length of the feeding vessel, and the local venous pressure. In a compensatory response normal cerebral autoregulation accommodates the reduced blood flow to the surrounding parenchyma by dilating nutrient arterioles. However, continuous exposure to low perfusion pressures may result in permanent dilatation of the nutrient arteries and permanent structural changes in the vasculature. Eventually these vascular beds, previously under normal autoregulation, regress into passive networks that are pressure dependent. Autonomic input can no longer dilate vasculature to facilitate increased flow, nor can autonomic input constrict these vessels if the relative pressure into the system suddenly increases. Ischemic changes occur when the capacity for compensatory vasodilatation is exceeded by the reduction in nutrient artery flow; which in turn is dependent upon the arteriovenous shunt at the core of the AVM.

Applying this model of ischemia, Spetzler has provided a possible explanation for bleeding in areas of brain surrounding a resected AVM.[22] The phenomenon of normal perfusion pressure breakthrough can occur after removal of an AVM and also relates to the loss of autonomic responses in chronically dilated vascular beds. Successful treatment of an AVM is defined as removal of the

arteriovenous shunt. When an arteriovenous shunt is obliterated the perfusion pressure of surrounding brain can increase from sub-normal to normal physiological values. Under non-pathological circumstances the autonomic response to this subtle increase in pressure would be to constrict feeding vessels. However, the chronic dilatation of the vascular beds precludes a normal response, resulting in hemorrhage and edema of the surrounding brain,[22] or even distant areas within the proximal arterial territory supplying the AVM.[23]

The complexity of AVM physiology has become more apparent as tools are developed to model variable flow rates and perfusion pressures.[24-26] Lo and others have described a bio-mathematical analysis of hemodynamic alterations in intracranial AVM based on fluid dynamic formulations of flow rates, cerebral perfusion pressure, intra-AVM pressure gradients, and hemodynamic resistances. Their model demonstrated that:

1. vascular steal is inversely proportional to the haemodynamic resistance of the AVM;
2. hemorrhage probability is related to the distribution of cerebral perfusion pressure across large thin-walled shunts;
3. normal reperfusion pressure after AVM obliteration is dependent on the ratio of resistance of surrounding vasculature versus any residual AVM; and
4. hyperemic complications post-treatment are likely to occur in high-flow AVMs that demonstrate steal.

In general, the findings from this mathematical model of AVM physiology reflect the clinical pathophysiology of AVM patients.[25]

As techniques evolve for measuring flow rates and pressures in and around AVMs,[27-30] mathematical and computer models of AVM physiology may have more of an impact. Other theories have examined the role of the venous circulation and the relationship to postoperative hyperemic complications. Al-Rodhan and collegues have proposed that edema and hemorrhage after AVM resection result from venous outflow obstruction. This process leads to passive hyperemia and engorgement of tissues, and stagnant flow in AVM feeding vessels.[31] Schaller and co-workers have suggested that postoperative hyperperfusion injury after AVM resection results from the unconstrained arterial inflow into cortical areas rendered ischemic by longstanding preoperative venous hypertension.[32,33]

No one theory completely explains all the pathophysiologic phenomena that have been observed with cerebral AVMs. Most likely there is some combination of preoperative steal and post-operative venous occlusion that leads to edema and hemorrhage in a small subset of patients after AVM resection.

ARTERIOVENOUS MALFORMATION MOLECULAR BIOLOGY

Genetic mutations associated with vascular malformations

Two fundamental approaches have been undertaken to identify genetic defects associated with vascular malformations: linkage analysis of patients and family members associated with hereditary disorders and molecular analysis of operative specimens for defective or missing gene products.

The first of these approaches has been applied most successfully in identifying a gene associated with familial cerebral cavernous malformations (CCMs).[34] Over the course of several years, investigators and clinicians have worked to establish the genetic pattern, location, and identity of genes associated with

CCM. Initially the recognition of unrelated Hispanic-American families in which CCMs segregated as an autosomal dominant trait established a genetic basis for this disease.[34,35] Linkage analysis subsequently identified locus heterogeneity, with disease genes for CCM at chromosomal regions 7q, 7p, and 3q.[36] Efforts that have focused on the 7q locus have identified mutations in the gene Krev Interaction Trapped 1 (krit1) in French and Hispanic-American families with CCM.[37–40] The krit1 gene was originally identified through its interaction with the Ras-family GTPase krev1/rap1a in a two-hybrid screen, inferring a role in GTPase signaling cascades. Collectively the data from linkage analysis suggest that aberrant Ras signaling pathways may be implicated in the development of cavernous malformations. To date, all mutations of the krit1 gene result in loss of function; which was recently confirmed in an analysis of four Hispanic-American families with CCM mapping to 7q.[38] In these families, the krit1 gene revealed a point mutation in exon 6 that predicts the substitution of a premature termination codon for glutamine at codon 248. The search for mutated genes that map to 7p and 3q is ongoing and will be facilitated by progress on the human genome project; as well as investigator consortiums that pool data from multiple families.

The second approach to identifying mutations in genes associated with AVM involves the molecular analysis of operative specimens for defective or missing gene products. As mentioned previously, HHT is an autosomal dominant vascular dysplasia that can involve multiple organs.[19] Most cases of HHT are caused by mutations in the endoglin gene on chromosome 9 (HHT type 1) or the activin receptor-like kinase 1 gene on chromosome 12 (HHT type 2), which leads to telangiectases and AVM of the skin, mucosa, and viscera. A logical hypothesis generated from these genetic studies is that these genes are missing or mutated in cerebral AVM specimens. However, this hypothesis may in fact be an oversimplification. Recently, Bourdeau and colleagues have demonstrated in HHT type 1 patients that the endoglin gene product is intact in AVM specimens.[41] When analyzed by immunostaining and densitometry, normal blood vessels of the brain and vessels adjacent to the AVM showed a 50% reduction in the endoglin : PECAM-1 ratio; suggesting that all blood vessels of HHT1 patients express reduced endoglin in situ and that AVMs are not attributed to a focal loss of endoglin. In the case of HHT1, molecular analysis of intraoperative specimens has demonstrated that the endoglin gene product is intact; providing the impetus to search for alternative genetic mutations.

ARTERIOVENOUS MALFORMATION EPIDEMIOLOGY

Determining the true epidemiology and natural history of AVMs has been confounded by the heterogeneity of divergent patient populations, and varying institutional bias towards treatment. Several recent literature reviews have sought to consolidate relevant retrospective and prospective studies in an effort to provide a consensus view. At our institution Berman and colleagues have attempted to determine the incidence and prevalence of AVM by critically reviewing the original sources from which these rates were derived.[42] Relevant original literature including autopsy series, the Cooperative Study of Intracranial Aneurysms and Subarachnoid Hemorrhage, related analyses, and other population-based studies were reviewed. The results of their analysis showed that many of the prevalence estimates (500–600 per 100 000 population) were based on autopsy data, a source that is inherently biased. Other estimates (140 per 100 000 population)

originated from an inappropriate analysis of data from the Cooperative Study. The most reliable information came from a population-based study of Olmsted County in Minnesota,[43] however, prevalence data specific to AVMs were not found in that study. Owing to variation in the detection rate of asymptomatic AVMs, Berman and colleagues contend that the most reliable estimate for the occurrence of the disease is the detection rate for symptomatic lesions: 0.94 per 100 000 person-years (95% confidence interval, 0.57–1.30 per 100 000 person-years). This figure is derived from a single population-based study, but it is supported by a re-analysis of other data sources.[43] The prevalence of detected, active (at risk) AVM disease is unknown, but it can be inferred from incidence data to be lower than 10.3 per 100 000 population.[42]

In a more recent review of the literature, Al-Shahi and Warlow concluded that there is very little accurate information about the frequency and clinical course of AVMs because the methods of most studies have been flawed, and AVMs tend to be treated once they are discovered.[44] Consolidation of the relevant literature for AVMs in adults yielded an incidence of AVMs at approximately 1 per 100 000 per year in unselected populations, and a point-prevalence in adults of approximately 18 per 100 000. Further analysis suggested that AVMs account for between 1 and 2% of all strokes, 3% of strokes in young adults, 9% of subarachnoid hemorrhages and that they are responsible for 4% of primary intracerebral hemorrhages overall (when not stratified by age); and up to 33% of primary intracerebral hemorrhages in young adults. With respect to clinical sequelae, Al-Shahi and Warlow concluded that at least 15% of people affected by AVMs are asymptomatic, about 20% present with seizures and for approximately 66% of them the dominant mode of presentation is with intracranial hemorrhage. The limited high-quality data available on prognosis suggest that long-term crude annual case fatality is 1–1.5%, the crude annual risk of first occurrence of hemorrhage from an unruptured AVM is approximately 2%, but the risk of recurrent hemorrhage may be as high as 18% in the first year, with uncertainty about the risk thereafter. For untreated AVMs, the annual risk of developing de novo seizures was determined to be 1%.[44]

One of the few prospective studies on AVMs was published by Ondra and colleagues in 1990.[45] The authors followed 166 unoperated symptomatic patients with AVMs of the brain. Follow-up data were obtained for 160 (96%) of the original population, with a mean follow-up period of 23.7 years. The rate of major rebleeding was 4.0% per year, and the mortality rate was 1.0% per year. At follow-up review, 23% of the series were dead from AVM hemorrhage. The combined rate of major morbidity and mortality was 2.7% per year. These annual rates remained essentially constant over the entire period of the study. Most significantly, the authors concluded that there was no difference in the incidence of rebleeding or death regardless of presentation with or without evidence of hemorrhage. The mean interval between initial presentation and subsequent hemorrhage was found to be 7.7 years.[45] Collectively, many of the questions regarding AVM natural history will remain unanswered until modern day prospective studies, such as the one reported by Ondra, are initiated.

ARTERIOVENOUS MALFORMATION CLINICAL PRESENTATION

Hemorrhage

Intracranial hemorrhage is by far the most frequent presenting symptom for patients with intracranial vascular malformations. Between 50 and 75% of patients have hemorrhages as the initial symptom related to an AVM (42, 43). These hemorrhages are most often intracerebral because of the location of AVMs within the parenchyma; and are often accompanied by secondary subarachnoid and intraventricular hemorrhage. Unlike hemorrhages associated with ruptured aneurysms, AVM subarachnoid blood comes from venous channels carrying blood with arterial pressure and is rarely associated with vasospasm. In general, patients with an AVM bleed survive and improve overtime as the intraparenchymal clot resolves. This is in stark contrast to patients with a ruptured aneurysm who have a high risk for rebleeding and/or vasospasm after their initial hemorrhage.

The clinical sequelae of a hemorrhage depends upon the location and extent of intracranial mass effect. Patients with hemorrhage in proximity to functional motor cortex may sustain contralateral hemiparesis or hemiplegia; whereas patients with hemorrhage in clinically silent areas of the brain (i.e. the right frontal lobe) may have no focal deficits. Headaches and seizures may also be associated with intracranial hemorrhage. Recurrent hemorrhages are usually separated by years and sometimes decades. As described previously, the prospective study of Ondra and colleagues suggests a 4% per year major rebleeding risk.

Seizures

Seizures are the second most common symptom associated with supratentorial intracranial vascular anomalies. Approximately 25–50% of all patients with AVMs present with a focal or generalized seizure, without obvious hemorrhage.[44] In general, epilepsy associated with intracranial vascular anomalies can be controlled with effective medical management. Accordingly the presence of a seizure disorder alone is not sufficient to warrant radical surgical treatment of an AVM or cavernous malformation. In some cases surgical treatment will diminish an associated seizure disorder, however often there is no improvement. Therefore, the selection of patients for surgical treatment should be based on the risk of future hemorrhage.

Headache

Headaches are a frequent problem in patients with AVMs but are rarely encountered in other vascular lesions without evidence of hemorrhage.[46,47] A headache disorder similar to classical migraine headaches has been described for AVM patients.[48] These headaches are usually unilateral and do not shift from side to side as seen in migraine headache patients. However, auras, visual symptomatology, and severe debilitating intermittent headaches have been described in patients with AVMs. Patients with lesions of the occipital lobe are especially prone to developing a migraine-like headache disorder.[47] More generalized headaches related to elevated venous pressures and stretching of venous sinuses and dura, have also been reported.[44] These headaches are less dramatic than those seen with the occipital lobe AVMs and are rarely of a debilitating nature.

Steal syndromes

A rare but important symptom associated with AVMs is related to the phenomenon of arterial steal.[49] This symptom is most relevant to a sub-group of patients who develop progressive neurological deficits without hemorrhage over many years in conjunction with high-flow AVMs. Although a definitive explanation for this problem is lacking,[50] the deficits that develop are most likely related to the cumulative effect of steal from normal perfusion of the surrounding brain by the AVM. As described previously, the phenomenon of normal perfusion pressure breakthrough may in fact be related to the physiologic environment created by chronic steal syndromes.

OPTIONS FOR TREATMENT

The choice of treatment for patients should consider risks attendant to each therapeutic option, as well as the natural history of the individual patient.[51] Therapeutic alternatives include the following either individually, or in combination:

1 operative resection or obliteration;
2 endovascular embolization; and
3 radiosurgery.

Judicious observation should always be a consideration, especially in patients who are high-risk because of medically related issues, or lesion size, location, and vascular anatomy.

In general, venous malformations and capillary telangiectasias do not require therapeutic intervention because of their relatively benign nature. Cavernous malformations are best left untreated when they are found incidentally;[52] however, if they present with a hemorrhage they should be considered for surgical resection.[53,54] Symptomatic cavernous malformations of the supratentorial compartment and spinal cord can often be excised and cured by surgery. Cavernous malformations of the cerebellum can also usually be readily excised when presenting with hemorrhage. In contrast, cavernous malformations of the brainstem are difficult to treat surgically without incurring significant morbidity.[55] Since the natural history shows that the risk of these lesions is low, only appropriate low-risk surgical procedures should be considered. High-risk surgery to remove deep capsular, basal ganglia, or brainstem malformations requires a clinical prodrome of progressive neurological decline and multiple hemorrhages.

The most important clinical decision-making with regard to vascular malformations is related to AVMs. The age of the patient, location of the AVM, size of the AVM, and vascular configuration are important factors that warrant consideration when making a decision about treatment.[51]

Surgical intervention

Surgical removal of an AVM is the most definitive treatment and offers the patient the best chance of an immediate cure. The presenting symptom of an AVM is probably the least important factor in deciding whether or not a patient should be subjected to an intracranial operation. The previously described natural history studies clearly demonstrate that even patients who present with nonhemorrhagic seizures and headaches are at significant risk for AVM-associated intracranial bleeding.[45] In general, the risk of operative intervention cannot be justified in asymptomatic patients over the age of 55 years. After this age the risks of surgery are about equal to the risk of allowing the lesions to develop naturally over the projected lifetime of the individual. Location is also critical. For example, AVMs located in areas such as the brainstem or basal ganglia should be treated surgically only in young patients who present with symptomatic hemorrhage and significant neurological disability.[56,57] Lesions located in the medial hemisphere also have a high degree of operative difficulty compared with other supratentorial lesions.[58] In contrast, malformations that are small, polar in location, and readily accessible can be treated surgically, even in older individuals.

The size and vascular configuration of the lesion formed the basis of a rudimentary classification system described by Spetzler and Martin in 1986.[59] In this system lesions are graded on the basis of size, pattern of venous drainage, and neurological eloquence of adjacent brain. All AVMs fall into one of six grades. Grade I malformations are small, superficial, and located in noneloquent cortex; Grade V lesions are large, deep, and situated in neurologically critical areas; and Grade VI lesions are essentially inoperable AVMs. Retrospective and prospective application of this grading scheme to a series of surgically excised AVMs has demonstrated correlation with the incidence of postoperative neurological complications.[59,60]

The Spetzler–Martin grading scale fails to address many aspects of surgical risk. A very important feature of AVMs that predicts complex surgery and high risk is the presence of a deep perforator supply to an AVM. When lenticulostriate and/or thalamoperforate vessels supply the malformation, critical brain areas must be violated to secure the arterial supply. Similarly, superficial AVMs that have an exclusively cortical arterial supply and cortical venous drainage, even when large and located in eloquent areas, can be safely excised. Therefore, the decision to resect is multifactorial. Ideally patients should be younger than 50 years and have small, cortically based lesions that present to the surface with primary cortical arterial supply and cortical venous drainage. Deep malformations, especially those with deep arterial and venous associations, are better treated conservatively or with stereotactic radiosurgery when appropriate.

Example case: arteriovenous malformation treated with embolization and surgical excision

A 28-year-old man presenting with a generalized seizure was found upon further work-up to have a 2.0 × 4.0 cm vascular malformation extending from the surface of the parietal lobe down to the atrium of the left lateral ventricle (Figure 15.8). The patient recovered to a normal neurological baseline and was treated with phenytoin for his seizure. He subsequently underwent a series of embolizations over a 1-month period. Arterial flow into the malformation was significantly reduced as shown in Figure 15.9. A craniotomy and wide dural opening revealed focal abnormalities on the brain surface overlying the malformation (Figure 15.10) facilitating localization of the lesion. A circumferential

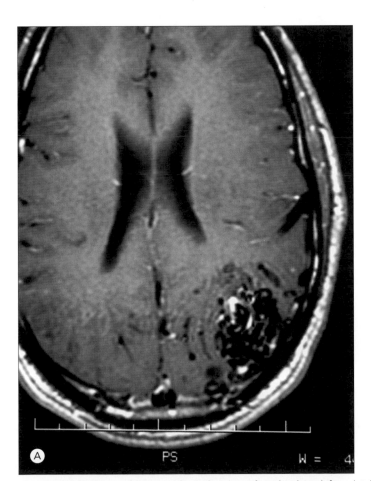

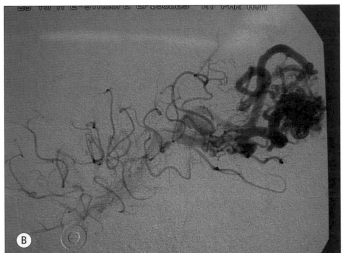

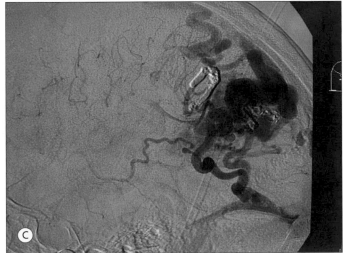

Figure 15.8 A 28-year-old man with single seizure found to have left parietal AVM. **(A)** T1 MRI showing left parietal AVM; **(B)** early arterial phase angiogram showing primarily middle cerebral artery supply to the malformation; **(C)** venous phase angiogram showing primary superficial cortical venous drainage of the malformation after partial arterial embolization.

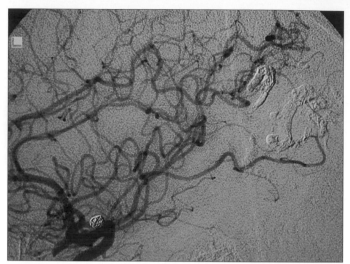

Figure 15.9 After extensive embolization treatment, there is only delayed partial filling of the malformation (same case as in Figure 15.8).

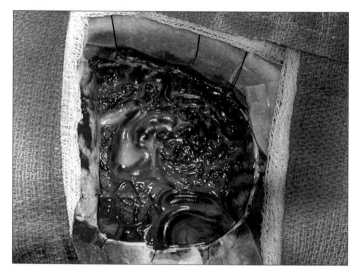

Figure 15.10 Operative photo of cortical surface before AVM resection (same case as in Figure 15.8).

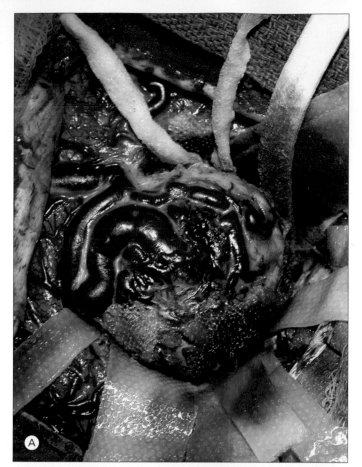

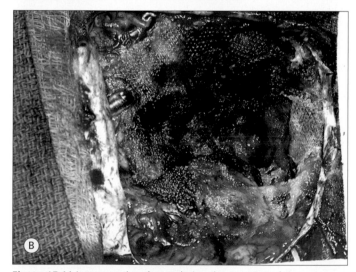

Figure 15.11 Intraoperative photos during the resection of the malformation. **(A)** After separation of the superficial parts of the malformation from surrounding brain; **(B)** appearance of the resection cavity after complete resection (same case as in Figure 15.8).

resection was undertaken to carefully remove the lesion en bloc (Figure 15.11). An immediate postoperative angiogram confirmed complete excision of the malformation and the patient sustained no postoperative complication. This case illustrates the value of preoperative embolization, and the technique of surgical resection.

Operative technique

The details of operative approaches to AVM lesions will vary significantly depending upon size, location, and vascular configuration. Several groups have described specific considerations regarding medial hemisphere,[58] basal ganglia,[57,61] posterior fossa,[62–64] and brainstem locations.[56,65,66] The reader is referred to these excellent reviews for technical details on the surgery of lesions in these specific areas. General considerations for operative technique include preoperative evaluation and preparation, intraoperative goals, and postoperative management.

Prior to surgery each patient should be thoroughly evaluated for coexisting medical conditions such as hypertension that may effect subsequent management. In addition, a complete radiological work-up should include high-quality angiograms and, when possible, MRI sequences that facilitate localization. The patient is prepared by achieving adequate anticonvulsant drug levels prior to surgery. Patients are at a higher risk for seizures following surgical

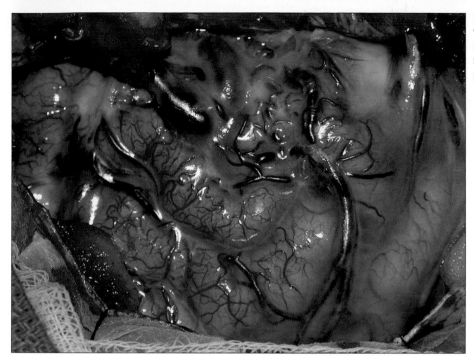

Figure 15.12 Surface of the brain demonstrating venous anatomy along the superior aspect of the right frontal lobe with the veins entering the superior saggital sinus along the top of the photograph.

resection, possibly secondary to changes in venous blood flow patterns.[67] Accordingly, it is essential to load patients preoperatively and to maintain adequate anticonvulsant drug levels in the immediate postoperative period.

In general, initial intraoperative goals of AVM surgery include lesion localization, exposure of relevant anatomy, and brain relaxation. Localization can be facilitated by correlation of anatomic landmarks with the lesion anatomy, or by means of stereotaxis. A wide craniotomy and dural opening are used to expose the relevant anatomy. When opening the dura it is important to avoid compromising any dura-based venous drainage of the lesion. Brain relaxation is accomplished by administration of mannitol, appropriate positioning of the patient's head above the heart, hyperventilation, and, occasionally, cerebrospinal fluid drainage via a spinal or intraventricular drain.

After an adequate exposure the next surgical goal is to localize the lesion within the surgical field. The arterialized distended veins of an AVM are the best surface landmark and can be correlated with the angiogram to pinpoint the location of arteries that often lie deeper (Figure 15.12). The bulk of the malformation may flare out under otherwise normal appearing cortex so that only the tip of the lesion is seen. After exposure of the malformation surface and thorough review of the angiogram, a circumscribing incision is made, avoiding normal cortex. Care should be taken during this stage of the surgery to avoid disturbing any major draining veins. Smaller vessels may be interrupted, but even with a major deep draining vein, the primary cortical vein should be left intact until much later in the operation. Nutrient arteries are usually found deep in the sulcus. They are cauterized, clipped, and divided, working circumferentially around the margins of the malformations. Thus, the entire cortical margin and subcortical surface of the malformation are circumscribed, avoiding the major veins while securing the arterial supply.

In general, bipolar cautery is used to secure arterial feeders. Some larger vessels will require clipping while smaller arteries can be cauterized and sectioned primarily. As deeper portions of the malformation are uncovered, a gliotic area surrounding the malformation can be separated from the normal white matter. This often affords an excellent plane of dissection that is aided by previous hemorrhages. However, deep areas of the malformation are sometimes supplied by numerous tiny penetrating vessels transversing the white matter, which can be extremely difficult to cauterize. It is these deep portions of the malformation that pose the greatest surgical challenge for hemostasis. Once the lesion has been circumferentially dissected, a test occlusion of the draining vein is undertaken to evaluate the effects of removing the vessel (Figure 15.13). In addition, the resection cavity should be finally inspected at systolic blood pressure above the patient's baseline pressure parameters.

Postoperative management

Following total removal of the AVM, the two most prevalent complications are hemorrhage and seizures.[44] In most instances clinically significant hemorrhage is the result of residual AVM secondary to incomplete excision. These hemorrhages typically occur within the first 12–24 hours postoperatively and will be associated with a clinical decline necessitating hematoma evacuation. Other causes of postoperative hemorrhage include insufficient occlusion of major arterial inputs, venous occlusion, and normal perfusion pressure breakthrough phenomena.[22] Maintenance of strict blood pressure parameters postoperatively is critical, as is formal documentation of complete removal of the AVM by means of a high-quality postoperative angiogram. We typically procure an angiogram immediately after the operation in a fully equipped angiogram suite. During this immediate postoperative period the patient is kept intubated and sedated, while the operating room and staff remain available in the event that residual AVM is found. In most institutions, the quality of the intraoperative angiography is not sufficient to evaluate fully the complex vascular changes often seen after AVM resection. The

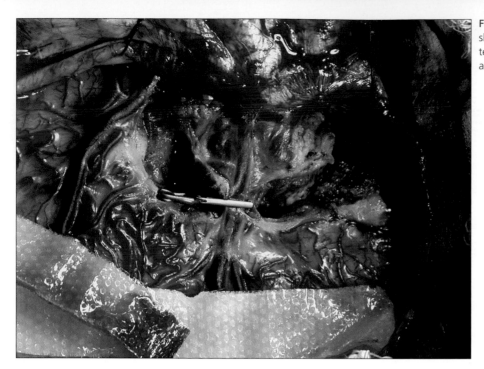

Figure 15.13 Same patient as in Figure 15.12 showing later stage in the resection with temporary clip on one of the involved veins to assess safety for permanent occlusion.

decision to resect additional cortical and white matter areas that contain abnormal vessels is crucial in terms of potential postoperative deficits. High-quality angiography is required to differentiate dysplastic vessels that will involute spontaneously from dangerous residual arteriovenous malformations (Figure 15.14).

Seizures may occur postoperatively even though adequate levels of anticonvulsants have been maintained before, during, and after the operation. If a seizure does occur postoperatively, control should be gained as rapidly as possible using standard multiple drug therapy. Once the patient is stabilized in the post-ictal period, a head CT should be obtained to document that there is no hematoma. Following surgery, 24 hours of ICU monitoring is sufficient in uncomplicated cases. Patients can then be rapidly tapered off dexamethasone, and they can begin ambulating. Seizure prophylaxis is generally advisable for approximately 6 months following uncomplicated surgery, but longer periods may be required in patients who develop postoperative seizures or in patients with a previous history of seizures. In these cases, anticonvulsant medication is continued for at least 1 year after the last seizure.

Embolization

Endovascular embolization is an important adjunct to the management of patients with AVM. The technology is rapidly improving in both safety and efficacy. In general, the procedure is facilitated by femoral arterial access and fluoroscopic guidance of a catheter into the feeding artery of an AVM. Subsequently embolic materials, such as wire coils, pellets, particulate slurries, or glue, are injected in a controlled fashion to occlude the arterial supply of the AVM.[68] Although embolization treatment can rarely completely annihilate an AVM, it is almost never appropriate to apply this modality as the sole treatment.[69–72] A partially treated AVM may be more likely to bleed than an untreated AVM; therefore endovascular treatment is not recommended unless

utilized as part of a multimodality plan geared towards total obliteration of the malformation.

In an optimal scenario embolization can successfully remove deep feeders to the malformation, greatly decreasing the risk of postoperative hemorrhage and associated morbidity. For large AVMs, the gradual occlusion of flow through the AVM greatly reduces the incidence of aterial and venous circulatory changes that lead to hyperemia and hemorrhage after surgical excision. In some instances, embolization treatment can reduce a large malformation down to a small size that may be amenable to radiosurgery.[69] The value of this approach has yet to be proven because recanalization in treated, but not excised, AVMs can occur.[73] The choice of whether to integrate embolization into the treatment plan is actively debated;[74] in part because the risks attendant on embolization may differ depending upon the experience of the interventional team. Independently assessed data on frequency, severity, and determinants of neurological deficits after endovascular treatment of AVM are scarce. Recently at our institution 233 consecutive AVM patients receiving one or more endovascular treatments (for a total of 545 procedures) were analyzed prospectively.[75] The Rankin Scale was used to assess neurological impairment before and after completed endovascular therapy. Demographic, clinical, and morphological predictors of treatment-related neurological deficits were identified using multivariate logistic regression models. The analysis assessed lesion characteristics such as AVM size, venous drainage pattern, and eloquence of AVM location. Mean follow-up time was 9.6 months (SD 18.1 months). Two hundred patients (86%) experienced no change in neurological status after treatment, and 33 patients (14%) showed treatment-related neurological deficits. Of the latter, five (2%) had persistent disabling deficits (Rankin score > 2), and two (1%) died. Increasing patient age, number of embolizations, and absence of a pretreatment neurological deficit were associated with new neurological deficits. None of the morphological AVM characteristics that were tested predicted

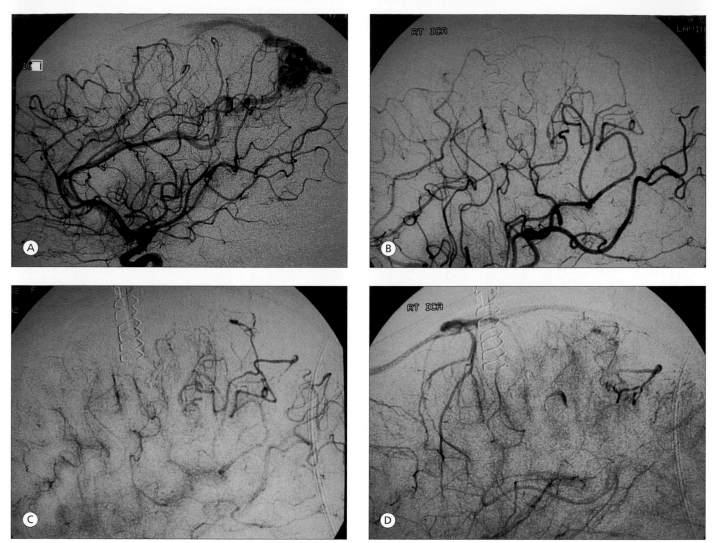

Figure 15.14 Patient with parietal AVM depicted in lateral carotid angiogram **(A)**; **(B)** early arterial phase of immediate postoperative angiogram, suggesting complete resection; **(C)** late arterial phase of the postoperative angiogram showing residual abnormal vessels that were supplying the AVM (note that there is no early draining vein); **(D)** venous phase of the angiogram showing persistence of the residual dysplastic arterial vessels suggesting slow flow. No abnormalities remained on 1 month follow-up angiogram.

treatment complications. From independent neurological assessment and prospective data collection, these findings suggest a low rate of disabling treatment complications after endovascular brain AVM treatment in high-volume centers.

Radiosurgery

Cushing and Bailey were among the first to describe radiation therapy for AVM patients.[4] Since their initial descriptions, great progress has been made with regard to improvements in target resolution and associated reduction in treatment morbidity.[76] The principles of stereotactic radiosurgery are based upon delivering high-energy radiation to a well-defined volume containing the nidus of the malformation. Gradual sclerosis of the blood vessels subsequently occurs, obliterating the AVM over a period of 1–2 years. Radiosurgery was first performed with a device called the gamma knife.[77] However, because this instrument is expensive and depends on high-energy cobalt sources it is not widely available. Proton beams and linear accelerators have been effectively used for radiosurgery because these high-energy radiation sources are more readily available and can be easily interfaced with standard CT and angiographically directed stereotactic equipment. Depending on several factors, including size and vascular characteristics, obliteration of an AVM seems to take 1–2 years following delivery of a therapeutic dose.[78] Regardless of the source utilized, radiosurgery is highly effective for AVMs < 2.0 cm in largest diameter, whereas larger malformations are less responsive.[79–81]

With proper dosimetry the immediate side-effects of radiosurgery have been moderate and limited to mild episodes of radiation necrosis.[82] However, the difficulty associated with treating patients with radiosurgery relates to the possibility of post-treatment hemorrhage. Because of the late onset of therapeutic effect, there is a definitive risk of hemorrhage after radiosurgery. The long-term side-effects of radiosurgery, as well as the risk of bleeding, have been studied by a number of different groups.[83–86] In particular, Flickinger and colleagues have been extremely prolific with respect to reporting their collective

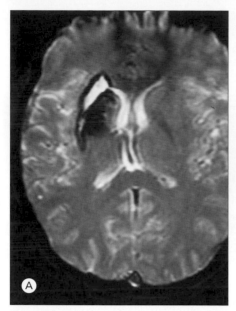 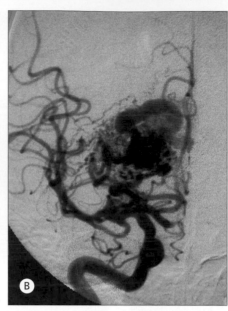 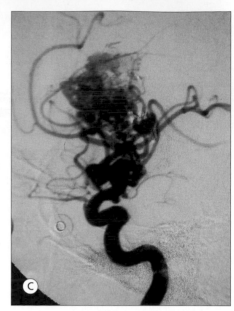

Figure 15.15 Pretreatment imaging studies of 33-year-old woman with basal ganglia hemorrhage as seen in axial MRI in **(A)**; **(B)** anteroposterior angiogram showing AVM of the caudate with deep venous drainage and lenticulostriate perforator supply; **(C)** lateral pretreatment angiogram.

experience using the gamma knife for the treatment of AVM patients. In a series of articles, starting in 1995 and running through to the present day, this group has described retrospective data with long-term follow-up on patients treated at their institution, as well as patients treated at other collaborative centers.[80,81,87–92] In 1999, a multi-institutional study of 102 AVM patients who developed neurological sequelae after radiosurgery was published.[87] These patients were derived from a pool of 1255 AVM patients treated with radiosurgery. Complications consisted of 80/102 patients with evidence of radiation injury to the brain parenchyma (seven also with cranial nerve deficits, 12 also with seizures, and five with cyst formation), 12/102 patients with isolated cranial neuropathies, and 10/102 patients with only new or worsened seizures. Severity was classified as minimal in 39 patients, mild in 40, disabling in 21, and fatal in two patients. Symptoms resolved completely in 42 patients for an actuarial resolution rate of 54% ± 7% at 3 years post-onset. Multivariate analysis identified significantly greater symptom resolution in patients with no prior history of hemorrhage ($P = 0.01$, 66% versus 41%), and in patients with symptoms of minimal severity: headache or seizure as the only sequelae of radiosurgery ($P < 0.0001$, 88% versus 34%). This large study demonstrates that the late sequelae of radiosurgery can manifest in various ways. However, further long-term studies of these problems are needed to take into account symptom severity and prior hemorrhage history. In addition, it will be important to weigh institutional bias towards treatment with respect to effects upon clinical decision-making.

Example case: basal ganglia AVM treated successfully with embolization and radiosurgery

A 33-year-old woman presented with sudden onset of severe headache and left-sided hemiplegia. Work-up at that time revealed a large hemorrhage in the right basal ganglia with an associated AVM fed mostly by the lenticulostriates on the right side (Figure 15.15). It occupies deep basal ganglia structures and drains by a large draining vein that goes up the superior sagittal

sinus. The patient underwent two stages of embolization and one treatment with radiosurgery. The location of the lesion in proximity to the right thalamus and internal capsule made this a very unfavorable lesion for surgical resection. MRI 1 year after treatment shows radiation injury in the region of the AVM (Figure 15.16). A follow-up angiogram 3 years after treatment of the AVM with radiosurgery revealed complete obliteration of the AVM (Figure 15.17).

CLINICAL PEARLS

- A review of the history of vascular malformations affecting the nervous system is instructive.

- Major classes of vascular malformations are: capillary telangiectasias, cavernous malformations, venous malformations, and arteriovenous malformations. Mixed lesions, of course, may occur.

- Vascular malformations develop early in embryonic life as a result of maldevelopment of vascular channels.

- In major vascular malformations, arteriovenous shunting occurs through the path of least resistance, bypassing the brain parenchyma, resulting in tissue ischemia. "Normal perfusion pressure breakthrough" may occur after AVM resection, resulting in edema and hemorrhage at the operative site.

- Distinct genetic mutations result in cavernous vascular malformations.

- Epidemiology and natural history of AVMs are subjects of controversy.

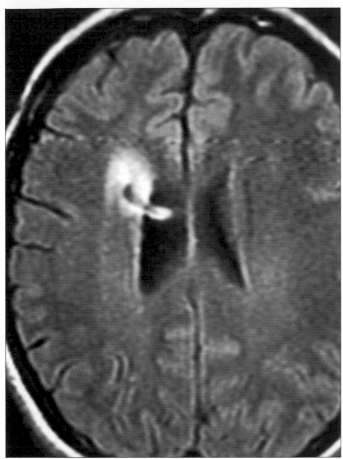

Figure 15.16 One year post gamma-knife treatment showing radiation injury in region of the AVM.

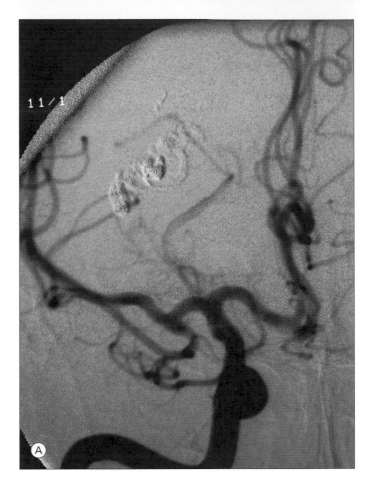

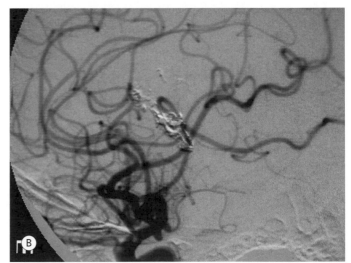

Figure 15.17 Three-year follow-up angiograms anteroposterior (A) and lateral (B) showing complete obliteration of the malformation.

CLINICAL PEARLS, cont'd

- Clinical presentation of vascular malformations include hemorrhage, seizures, headache, and steal syndromes.

- Treatment options include surgical resection, endovascular therapy, radiosurgery, or a judicious combination thereof.

SUMMARY

Great progress in the treatment of patients with vascular malformations has been achieved since Rokitansky's initial description of intracranial AVMs.[1] The prospective analysis of evidence-based clinical outcome data will be critical in accurately determining the long-term effect of many treatment modalities. The advent of endovascular techniques combined with advances in radiosurgery have provided important surgical adjuncts to the treatment of these difficult lesions. We look forward to the contributions of the clinicians and scientists who have combined efforts to understand the molecular and genetic etiology of these lesions.

REFERENCES

1. Yasargil MG. *Microneurosurgery*, Vol. 3A. New York: Thieme; 1984.
2. Cushing H. *The Harvey Cushing Collection of Books and Manuscripts*, Vol. 1. New Haven: Yale University Department of the History of Science and Medicine; 1943.
3. Dandy WE. *Selected Writings of Walter Dandy*, Vol. 1. Springfield: Thomas; 1957.

4. Cushing H, Bailey P. *Tumors Arising from Blood-vessels of the Brain*. Springfield: Charles C. Thomas Publishing; 1928: 9.

5. Rigamonti D, Johnson PC, Spetzler RF, Hadley MN, Drayer BP. Cavernous malformations and capillary telangiectasia: a spectrum within a single pathological entity. *Neurosurgery* 1991; 28: 60–4.

6. Clatterbuck RE, Elmaci I, Rigamonti D. The juxtaposition of a capillary telangiectasia, cavernous malformation, and developmental venous anomaly in the brainstem of a single patient: case report. *Neurosurgery* 2001; 49: 1246–50.

7. Awada A, Watson T, Obeid T. Cavernous angioma presenting as pregnancy-related seizures. *Epilepsia* 1997; 38: 844–6.

8. Wong JH, Awad IA, Kim JH. Ultrastructural pathological features of cerebrovascular malformations: a preliminary report. *Neurosurgery* 2000; 46: 1454–9.

9. Kida Y, Kobayashi T, Tanaka T, Mori Y, Hasegawa T, Kondoh T. Seizure control after radiosurgery on cerebral arteriovenous malformations. *J Clin Neurosci* 2000; 7 (Suppl. 1): 6–9.

10. Meng JS, Okeda R. Histopathological structure of the pial arteriovenous malformation in adults: observation by reconstruction of serial sections of four surgical specimens. *Acta Neuropathol (Berl)* 2001; 102: 63–8.

11. Yamada S, Liwnicz B, Lonser RR, Knierim D. Scanning electron microscopy of arteriovenous malformations. *Neurol Res* 1999; 21: 541–4.

12. Chin LS, Raffel C, Gonzalez-Gomez I, Giannotta SL, McComb JG. Diffuse arteriovenous malformations: a clinical, radiological, and pathological description. *Neurosurgery* 1992; 31: 863–868; discussion 868–9.

13. Redekop G, TerBrugge K, Montanera W, Willinsky R. Arterial aneurysms associated with cerebral arteriovenous malformations: classification, incidence, and risk of hemorrhage. *J Neurosurg* 1998; 89: 539–46.

14. Westphal M, Grzyska U. Clinical significance of pedicle aneurysms on feeding vessels, especially those located in infratentorial arteriovenous malformations. *J Neurosurg* 2000; 92: 995–1001.

15. Jellinger K. Vascular malformations of the central nervous system: a morphological overview. *Neurosurg Rev* 1986; 9: 177–216.

16. Mullan S, Mojtahedi S, Johnson DL, Macdonald RL. Embryological basis of some aspects of cerebral vascular fistulas and malformations. *J Neurosurg* 1996; 85: 1–8.

17. Kondziolka D, Humphreys RP, Hoffman HJ, Hendrick EB, Drake JM. Arteriovenous malformations of the brain in children: a forty year experience. *Can J Neurol Sci* 1992; 19: 40–5.

18. Di Rocco C, Tamburrini G, Rollo M. Cerebral arteriovenous malformations in children. *Acta Neurochir* 2000; 142: 145–56.

19. Morgan T, McDonald J, Anderson C, *et al*. Intracranial hemorrhage in infants and children with hereditary hemorrhagic telangiectasia (Osler–Weber–Rendu syndrome). *Pediatrics* 2002; 109: E12.

20. Sekhon LH, Morgan MK, Johnston IH. Syndactyly and intracranial arteriovenous malformation: case report. *Br J Neurosurg* 1994; 8: 377–80.

21. Spetzler RF, Selman. Pathophysiology of cerebral ischemia accompanying arteriovenous malformations. In: Wilson CB, Stein BM (eds). *Intracranial Arteriovenous Malformations*. Baltimore, MD: Williams & Wilkins: 1984: 24–31.

22. Spetzler RF, Hargraves RW, McCormick PW, Zabramski JM, Flom RA, Zimmerman RS. Relationship of perfusion pressure and size to risk of hemorrhage from arteriovenous malformations. *J Neurosurg* 1992; 76: 918–23.

23. Solomon RA, Michelsen WJ. Defective cerebrovascular autoregulation in regions proximal to arteriovenous malformations of the brain: a case report and topic review. *Neurosurgery* 1984; 14: 78–82.

24. Lo EH. A haemodynamic analysis of intracranial arteriovenous malformations. *Neurol Res* 1993; 15: 51–5.

25. Kader A, Young WL. The effects of intracranial arteriovenous malformations on cerebral hemodynamics. *Neurosurg Clin N Am* 1996; 7: 767–81.

26. Kailasnath P, Chaloupka JC. Mathematical modeling of AVM physiology using compartmental network analysis: theoretical considerations and preliminary in vivo validation using a previously developed animal model. *Neurol Res* 1996; 18: 361–6.

27. Kader A, Young WL, Massaro AR, *et al*. Transcranial Doppler changes during staged surgical resection of cerebral arteriovenous malformations: a report of three cases. *Surg Neurol* 1993; 39: 392–8.

28. Tsuchiya K, Katase S, Yoshino A, Hachiya J. MR digital subtraction angiography of cerebral arteriovenous malformations. *Am J Neuroradiol* 2000; 21: 707–11.

29. Uggowitzer MM, Kugler C, Riccabona M, *et al*. Cerebral arteriovenous malformations: diagnostic value of echo-enhanced transcranial Doppler sonography compared with angiography. *Am J Neuroradiol* 1999; 20: 101–6.

30. Manchola IF, De Salles AA, Foo TK, Ackerman RH, Candia GT, Kjellberg RN. Arteriovenous malformation hemodynamics: a transcranial Doppler study. *Neurosurgery* 1993; 33: 556–62; discussion 562.

31. Al-Rodhan NR, Sundt TM, Jr, Piepgras DG, Nichols DA, Rufenacht D, Stevens LN. Occlusive hyperemia: a theory for the hemodynamic complications following resection of intracerebral arteriovenous malformations. *J Neurosurg* 1993; 78:167–75.

32. Schaller C, Urbach H, Schramm J, Meyer B. Role of venous drainage in cerebral arteriovenous malformation surgery, as related to the development of postoperative hyperperfusion injury. *Neurosurgery* 2002; 51: 921–7; discussion 927–9.

33. Meyer B, Urbach H, Schaller C, Schramm J. Is stagnating flow in former feeding arteries an indication of cerebral hypoperfusion after resection of arteriovenous malformations? *J Neurosurg* 2001; 95: 36–43.

34. Gunel M, Awad IA, Finberg K, *et al*. A founder mutation as a cause of cerebral cavernous malformation in Hispanic Americans. *N Engl J Med* 1996; 334: 946–51.

35. Gunel M, Awad IA, Anson J, Lifton RP. Mapping a gene causing cerebral cavernous malformation to 7q11.2-q21. *Proc Natl Acad Sci USA* 1995; 92: 6620–4.

36. Gunel M, Awad IA, Finberg K, *et al*. Genetic heterogeneity of inherited cerebral cavernous malformation. *Neurosurgery* 1996; 38: 1265–71.

37. Zhang J, Clatterbuck RE, Rigamonti D, Dietz HC. Cloning of the murine Krit1 cDNA reveals novel mammalian 5' coding exons. *Genomics* 2000; 70: 392–5.

38. Zhang J, Clatterbuck RE, Rigamonti D, Dietz HC. Mutations in KRIT1 in familial cerebral cavernous malformations. *Neurosurgery* 2000; 46: 1272–1277; discussion 1277–9.

39. Verlaan DJ, Davenport WJ, Stefan H, Sure U, Siegel AM, Rouleau GA. Cerebral cavernous malformations: mutations in Krit1. *Neurology* 2002; 58: 853–7.

40. Notelet L, Chapon F, Khoury S, *et al*. Familial cavernous malformations in a large French kindred: mapping of the gene to the CCM1 locus on chromosome 7q. *J Neurol Neurosurg Psychiatr* 1997; 63: 40–5.

41. Bourdeau A, Cymerman U, Paquet ME, *et al*. Endoglin expression is reduced in normal vessels but still detectable in arteriovenous malformations of patients with hereditary hemorrhagic telangiectasia type 1. *Am J Pathol* 2000; 156: 911–23.

42. Berman MF, Sciacca RR, Pile-Spellman J, *et al*. The epidemiology of brain arteriovenous malformations. *Neurosurgery* 2000; 47: 389–96; discussion 397.

43. Brown RD, Jr, Wiebers DO, Torner JC, O'Fallon WM. Frequency of intracranial hemorrhage as a presenting symptom and subtype analysis: a population-based study of intracranial vascular malformations in Olmsted Country, Minnesota. *J Neurosurg* 1996; 85: 29–32.

44. Al-Shahi R, Warlow C. A systematic review of the frequency and prognosis of arteriovenous malformations of the brain in adults. *Brain* 2001; 124: 1900–26.

45. Ondra SL, Troupp H, George ED, Schwab K. The natural history of symptomatic arteriovenous malformations of the brain: a 24-year follow-up assessment. *J Neurosurg* 1990; 73: 387–91.

46. Gawel MJ, Willinsky RA, Krajewski A. Reversal of cluster headache side following treatment of arteriovenous malformation. *Headache* 1989; 29: 453–4.

47. Kupersmith MJ, Vargas ME, Yashar A, *et al*. Occipital arteriovenous malformations: visual disturbances and presentation. *Neurology* 1996; 46: 953–7.

48. Monteiro JM, Rosas MJ, Correia AP, Vaz AR. Migraine and intracranial vascular malformations. *Headache* 1993; 33: 563–5.

49. Sheth RD, Bodensteiner JB. Progressive neurologic impairment from an arteriovenous malformation vascular steal. *Pediatr Neurol* 1995; 13: 352–4.

50. Mast H, Mohr JP, Osipov A, *et al*. "Steal" is an unestablished mechanism for the clinical presentation of cerebral arteriovenous malformations. *Stroke* 1995; 26: 1215–20.

51. Mattle HP, Schroth G, Seiler RW. Dilemmas in the management of patients with arteriovenous malformations. *J Neurol* 2000; 247: 917–28.

52. Labauge P, Brunereau L, Laberge S, Houtteville JP. Prospective follow-up of 33 asymptomatic patients with familial cerebral cavernous malformations. *Neurology* 2001; 57: 1825–8.

53. Moriarity JL, Wetzel M, Clatterbuck RE, *et al*. The natural history of cavernous malformations: a prospective study of 68 patients. *Neurosurgery* 1999; 44: 1166–71; discussion 1172–3.

54. Zabramski JM, Wascher TM, Spetzler RF, *et al*. The natural history of familial cavernous malformations: results of an ongoing study. *J Neurosurg* 1994; 80: 422–32.

55. Kupersmith MJ, Kalish H, Epstein F, *et al*. Natural history of brainstem cavernous malformations. *Neurosurgery* 2001; 48: 47–53; discussion 53–44.

56. Solomon RA, Stein BM. Management of arteriovenous malformations of the brain stem. *J Neurosurg* 1986; 64: 857–64.

57. Solomon RA, Stein BM. Interhemispheric approach for the surgical removal of thalamocaudate arteriovenous malformations. *J Neurosurg* 1987; 66: 345–51.

58. Sisti MB, Kader A, Stein BM. Microsurgery for 67 intracranial arteriovenous malformations less than 3 cm in diameter. *J Neurosurg* 1993; 79: 653–60.

59. Spetzler RF, Martin NA. A proposed grading system for arteriovenous malformations. *J Neurosurg* 1986; 65: 476–83.

60. Hamilton MG, Spetzler RF. The prospective application of a grading system for arteriovenous malformations. *Neurosurgery* 1994; 34: 2–6; discussion 6–7.

61. Richling B, Bavinzski G. Arterio-venous malformations of the basal ganglia. Surgical versus endovascular treatment. *Acta Neurochir Suppl*. 1991; 53: 50–9.

62. Batjer H, Samson D. Arteriovenous malformations of the posterior fossa. Clinical presentation, diagnostic evaluation, and surgical treatment. *J Neurosurg* 1986; 64: 849–56.

63. Drake CG, Friedman AH, Peerless SJ. Posterior fossa arteriovenous malformations. *J Neurosurg* 1986; 64: 1–10.

64. George B, Celis-Lopez M, Kato T, Lot G. Arteriovenous malformations of the posterior fossa. *Acta Neurochir (Wien)* 1992; 116: 119–27.

65. Sisti MB, Stein BM. Arteriovenous malformations of the brain stem. *Neurosurg Clin N Am* 1993; 4: 497–505.

66. Lawton MT, Hamilton MG, Spetzler RF. Multimodality treatment of deep arteriovenous malformations: thalamus, basal ganglia, and brain stem. *Neurosurgery* 1995; 37: 29–35; discussion 35–6.

67. Piepgras DG, Sundt TM, Jr, Ragoowansi AT, Stevens L. Seizure outcome in patients with surgically treated cerebral arteriovenous malformations. *J Neurosurg* 1993; 78: 5–11.

68. Deveikis JP. Endovascular therapy of intracranial arteriovenous malformations. Materials and techniques. *Neuroimaging Clin N Am* 1998; 8: 401–24.

69. Henkes H, Nahser HC, Berg-Dammer E, Weber W, Lange S, Kuhne D. Endovascular therapy of brain AVMs prior to radiosurgery. *Neurol Res* 1998; 20: 479–92.

70. Marks MP, Lane B, Steinberg GK, *et al*. Endovascular treatment of cerebral arteriovenous malformations following radiosurgery. *Am J Neuroradiol* 1993; 14: 297–303; discussion 304–5.

71. Nakahara I, Taki W, Kikuchi H, *et al*. Endovascular treatment of aneurysms on the feeding arteries of intracranial arteriovenous malformations. *Neuroradiology* 1999; 41: 60–6.

72. Valavanis A, Yasargil MG. The endovascular treatment of brain arteriovenous malformations. *Adv Tech Stand Neurosurg* 1998; 24: 131–214.

73. Mizutani T, Tanaka H, Aruga T. Total recanalization of a spontaneously thrombosed arteriovenous malformation. Case report. *J Neurosurg* 1995; 82: 506–8.

74. Martin NA, Khanna R, Doberstein C, Bentson J. Therapeutic embolization of arteriovenous malformations: the case for and against. *Clin Neurosurg* 2000; 46: 295–318.

75. Hartmann A, Pile-Spellman J, Stapf C, *et al*. Risk of endovascular treatment of brain arteriovenous malformations. *Stroke* 2002; 33: 1816–20.

76. Ogilvy CS. Radiation therapy for arteriovenous malformations: a review. *Neurosurgery* 1990; 26: 725–35.

77. Massager N, Regis J, Kondziolka D, Njee T, Levivier M. Gamma knife radiosurgery for brainstem arteriovenous malformations: preliminary results. *J Neurosurg* 2000; 93 Suppl 3: 102–3.

78. Chang JH, Chang JW, Park YG, Chung SS. Factors related to complete occlusion of arteriovenous malformations after gamma knife radiosurgery. *J Neurosurg* 2000; 93 Suppl 3: 96–101.

79. Friedman WA, Bova FJ, Mendenhall WM. Linear accelerator radiosurgery for arteriovenous malformations: the relationship of size to outcome. *J Neurosurg* 1995; 82: 180–9.

80. Flickinger JC, Pollock BE, Kondziolka D, Lunsford LD. A dose-response analysis of arteriovenous malformation obliteration after radiosurgery. *Int J Radiat Oncol Biol Phys* 1996; 36: 873–9.

81. Flickinger JC, Kondziolka D, Maitz AH, Dade Lunsford L. An analysis of the dose-response for arteriovenous malformation radiosurgery and other factors affecting obliteration. *Radiother Oncol* 2002; 63: 347–54.

82. Werner-Wasik M, Rudoler S, Preston PE, *et al*. Immediate side effects of stereotactic radiotherapy and radiosurgery. *Int J Radiat Oncol Biol Phys* 1999; 43: 299–304.

83. Voges J, Treuer H, Lehrke R, *et al*. Risk analysis of LINAC radiosurgery in patients with arteriovenous malformation (AVM). *Acta Neurochir Suppl (Wien)* 1997; 68: 118–23.

84. Voges J, Treuer H, Sturm V, *et al*. Risk analysis of linear accelerator radiosurgery. *Int J Radiat Oncol Biol Phys* 1996; 36: 1055–63.

85. Naoi Y, Cho N, Miyauchi T, Iizuka Y, Maehara T, Katayama H.

Usefulness and problems of stereotactic radiosurgery using a linear accelerator. *Radiat Med* 1996; 14: 215–19.

86. Malone S, Raaphorst GP, Gray R, Girard A, Alsbeih G. Enhanced in vitro radiosensitivity of skin fibroblasts in two patients developing brain necrosis following AVM radiosurgery: a new risk factor with potential for a predictive assay. *Int J Radiat Oncol Biol Phys* 2000, 47: 185–9.

87. Flickinger JC, Kondziolka D, Lunsford LD, *et al*. A multi-institutional analysis of complication outcomes after arteriovenous malformation radiosurgery. *Int J Radiat Oncol Biol Phys* 1999; 44: 67–74.

88. Flickinger JC, Kondziolka D, Lunsford LD. Radiosurgery of benign lesions. *Semin Radiat Oncol* 1995; 5: 220–4.

89. Flickinger JC, Kondziolka D, Pollock BE, Maitz AH, Lunsford LD. Complications from arteriovenous malformation radiosurgery:

multivariate analysis and risk modeling. *Int J Radiat Oncol Biol Phys* 1997; 38: 485–90.

90. Flickinger JC, Kondziolka D, Maitz AH, Lunsford LD. Analysis of neurological sequelae from radiosurgery of arteriovenous malformations: how location affects outcome. *Int J Radiat Oncol Biol Phys* 1998; 40: 273–8.

91. Flickinger JC, Kondziolka D, Lunsford LD. Dose selection in stereotactic radiosurgery. *Neurosurg Clin N Am* 1999; 10: 271–80.

92. Flickinger JC, Kondziolka D, Lunsford LD, *et al*. Development of a model to predict permanent symptomatic postradiosurgery injury for arteriovenous malformation patients. Arteriovenous Malformation Radiosurgery Study Group. *Int J Radiat Oncol Biol Phys* 2000; 46: 1143–8.

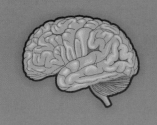

SPONTANEOUS INTRACEREBRAL HEMORRHAGE

16

Neil A Martin and Martin C Holland

Spontaneous intracerebral hemorrhage (ICH) is defined as bleeding into brain parenchyma without accompanying trauma. The impact of ICH on the general population can be fully grasped when viewed within the broader category of stroke, currently the leading cause of neurologic deficit in the world and the third leading cause of death in the United States (behind cancer and heart disease), accounting for 15% of all US deaths annually.[1] Significantly, ICH accounts for 10–17% of all strokes.[2–5] Moreover, the mortality for ICH is considerably higher than that for nonhemorrhagic or ischemic stroke (cerebral infarct) as seen in a study by the Machlachlan Acute Stroke Unit in Toronto. Of 1073 patients admitted with completed stroke, mortality at 30 days from supratentorial and infratentorial infarct was 15% and 18% respectively, compared to that for ICH which was 58% and 31% respectively.[6] Indeed, some studies quote a mortality figure as high as 90%.[7]

The incidence of stroke remains underreported because of the inherent shortcomings of epidemiologic, pathologic, and clinical studies. Even so, it is estimated that 500 000 people suffer a stroke each year, 150 000 of whom will die.[1] Moreover, with 2 000 000 stroke survivors requiring chronic care, the cost in terms of medical expense amounts to over 7 billion dollars annually,[8] not to mention the cost in terms of physical and emotional suffering. It should be mentioned, however, that the incidence of both stroke and ICH has declined at an annual rate of 1% per year since 1915, with an acceleration in the decline to over 5% per year since 1975, reflecting an improvement in both the prevention and treatment of stroke.[7]

PATHOPHYSIOLOGY

Spontaneous ICH results from an intracerebral arterial or, less frequently, venous rupture, which leads to the formation of an intraparenchymal hematoma. The hematoma expands following the path of least resistance, usually along white matter tracts, and occasionally dissects its way into the ventricular system. In time, the bleeding slows and eventually stops as increasing tissue pressure leads to tamponade of the rupture site. Neurologic deficit results from both direct tissue destruction and indirect compression of neural structures, usually in proportion to both the volume of the hematoma and its rate of expansion. A slowly expanding lesion, for example, tends to dissect along white matter tracts, leaving functional units intact, whereas a rapidly expanding lesion tears through tissue planes and severs axons, permanently disrupting neural function.

Intracranial hemorrhages may be classified according to their location (Figure 16.1). An *epidural hematoma* is usually the result of a meningeal artery tear in which blood accumulates between bone and dura mater. Because of its arterial origin, the hematoma grows under considerable pressure, often leading to herniation syndromes. A *subdural hematoma* may result when cerebral bridging veins tear or when a subarachnoid or intraparenchymal bleed extends into the subdural space through a tear in the arachnoid. A *subarachnoid hemorrhage* involves the accumulation of blood between the arachnoid and the pia mater; it is often the result of an aneurysmal rupture, although arteriovenous malformations or trauma figure often in this entity. An *intraventricular hemorrhage* may be arterial or venous, it may be isolated or extend from an intraparenchymal bleed, it often leads to obstructive hydrocephalus, and it usually has a poor prognosis. *Intraparenchymal hemorrhages* can occur at any site within the central nervous system, though some areas are more susceptible than others. Eighty per cent occur within the cerebral hemispheres while the remaining 20% are infratentorial. Of note, hypertensive bleeds occur in the deep gray matter (65%), pons (11%), and cerebellum (8%), whereas bleeds associated with other disorders are likely to be located in the subcortical white matter (45%), deep gray matter (36%), pons (10%), and cerebellum (3%).[2,9–11] Similarly, bleeds at any one particular location tend to be associated with certain conditions more than others (Figure 16.2). For example, *lobar bleeds* – found in the subcortical white matter – are often associated with tumors, vascular malformations, and cerebral amyloid angiopathy; *basal ganglia bleeds*, which may extend to include the internal capsule and thalamus, are often associated with hypertension as are *brainstem bleeds*, though these are usually much more serious. Finally, *cerebellar bleeds* tend to accompany tumors, vascular malformations, blood dyscrasias, and hypertension.[2,12]

ETIOLOGY

By far the most important risk factor associated with ICH is hypertension, with 40–60% of all ICH patients found to have this disorder. Aneurysms (20%), vascular malformations (5–7%), coagulopathies (5–7%), and tumors (1–11%), as well as hemorrhagic infarcts, cerebral amyloid angiopathy, and drug reactions, account for the remaining major etiologies of ICH (Figure 16.3).[2,11]

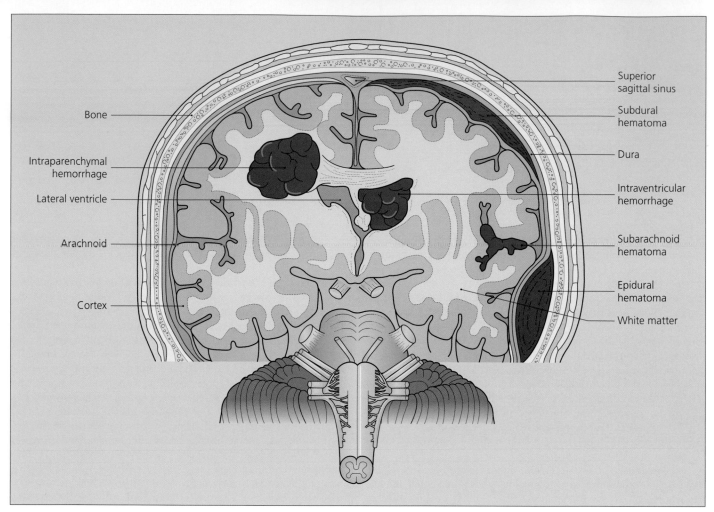

Figure 16.1 Types of intracranial hemorrhage.

Hypertension

As previously noted, it has been established that patients who have chronic hypertension are predisposed to ICH. Compared to hemorrhages from other causes, this type of bleed is more frequently associated with a fatal outcome, reflecting both its high incidence and its tendency to occur in critical locations. To review, the most common location for hypertensive bleeds is the basal ganglia, followed by the pons and cerebellum, regions that are variously supplied by the lenticulostriate branches off the middle cerebral artery or the paramedian branches off the basilar artery. There has been much research on the mechanism leading to hemorrhage in such cases. For many years it was assumed that hypertensive bleeds were the result of rupture of the miliary aneurysms described by Charcot and Bouchard in 1868, as these were frequently seen on the perforating arteries of the basal ganglia and pons of hypertensive patients, which, as previously noted, are common sites of hemorrhage in these patients (Figure 16.3A). Later investigations, however, have shown these to be pseudoaneurysms, that is, small collections of extravasated blood covered by a thin fibrin layer,[13,14] presumably the result of an aborted or limited arterial rupture. Microscopic studies have since demonstrated changes in the walls of the lenticulostriates and paramedian arteries of hypertensive patients (alternately called "lipohyalinosis," "fibrinohyalinosis," or "angionecrosis"), which are

characterized by the deposition of fat cells as well as a fibrin-like material within the media of the affected vessels (see Figure 16.3A). Furthermore, these changes are often seen closer to the bleeding site than are miliary aneurysms and are now considered the primary lesion leading to arterial wall weakness and subsequent rupture.[11,14] That these vessels are affected more than others may reflect the fact that they are small arterial twigs branching directly off major arteries (e.g. middle cerebral or basilar). As such, they are subjected to much higher pressures than the similar-sized cortical vessels that lie at the end of a multiple series of arterial splits, each of which lowers intraluminal pressure, thus affording these smaller vessels some measure of protection against the effects of systemic hypertension.

A great deal of controversy remains regarding the role of miliary aneurysms in hypertensive bleeds. Regardless of this, hypertension remains the major risk factor in the development of fatal or disabling ICH.

Nonhypertensive intracerebral hemorrhage

There are a number of conditions that are statistically less important than hypertension but are nonetheless the etiology of a significant number of spontaneous ICHs: aneurysms (20%), vascular malformations (5–7%), coagulopathies (5–7%), and

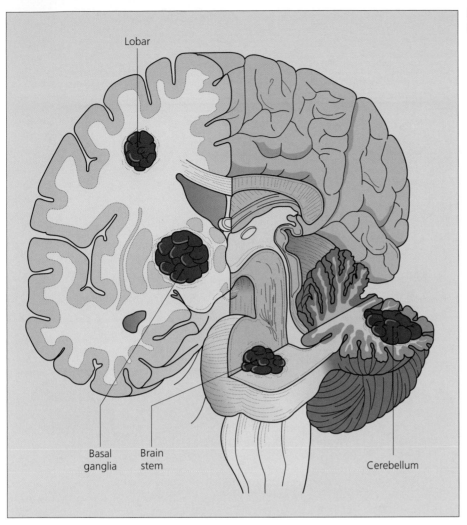

Figure 16.2 Locations of intraparenchymal hemorrhage.

tumors (1–11%) are the most common, with cerebral amyloid angiopathy, hemorrhagic infarcts, and drug-induced hemorrhages, among others, making up a small percentage of cases.[2,11]

Aneurysms

Aneurysms are saccular or fusiform arterial deformities, the result of dissection and protrusion of the intima through a structural defect in an artery's muscular layer, whose underlying cause may be embolic, neoplastic, traumatic, or atherosclerotic. Most aneurysms, however, are the so-called berry aneurysms whose etiology is probably a combination of congenital, hereditary, and acquired factors.

BERRY ANEURYSMS Berry aneurysms (Figure 16.3B) are typically found at the bi- or trifurcations of major cerebral arteries – usually those forming the circle of Willis – and may be associated with inherited disorders such as Ehlers–Danlos syndrome or other diseases that weaken the media of cerebral arteries. Similarly, a tumor, vascular malformation, or any other process that alters cerebral hemodynamics by increasing arterial blood flow or raising intraluminal hydrostatic pressure may eventually lead to the formation of an aneurysm. There is a general disagreement over the exact process of aneurysm formation, however. One school of thought proposes that a congenital defect in the muscular layer

leads to aneurysmal dilatation of arteries. A second claims that the primary lesion is the damage that normally occurs over time to the lamina elastica interna, with some people being more affected than others. A third, holding a somewhat middle ground, states that both congenital and acquired processes are needed for an aneurysm to form. Especially susceptible to degenerative changes are the arterial branch points, where the normal near-laminar flow of blood gives way to high turbulence, creating higher-than-normal pressure points against the arterial wall. In time, the aneurysm may enlarge and rupture, spilling blood into the subarachnoid space, often with accompanying ICH. In particularly violent ruptures, the hematoma may either dissect its way into the ventricular system or rip the arachnoid forming a subdural hematoma.

Since berry aneurysms tend to occur in the large arteries at the base of the brain and posterior fossa, the neural structures at greatest risk for damage are the diencephalon and brainstem; when these structures are injured, the outcome may be fatal. The prevalence of ICH after berry aneurysm rupture has not been well established, though 5–25% of operative reports and 50–100% of autopsy reports indicate the presence of ICH after aneurysmal rupture.[15] This is significant to the neurosurgeon because the presence as well as location of the hematoma may alter the need, timing, and approach of surgery.

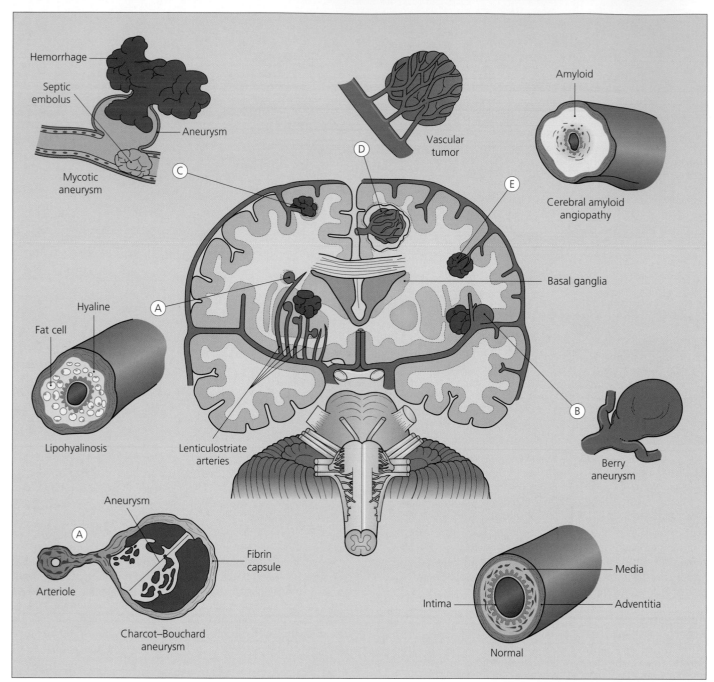

Figure 16.3 The major causes of ICH, the principal locations at which they present, and detailed morphologic or histologic features associated with the process. A normal vessel has an intima composed of a single layer of epithelial cells surrounded by a layer of smooth muscle and elastic tissue, both of which are enveloped by the adventitia, a thick layer of collagenous connective tissue. **(A)** Bleeds caused by hypertension occur in the basal ganglia and brainstem. Typical histologic changes are the formation of Charcot–Bouchard or miliary aneurysms as well as "lipohyalinosis" with deposition of hyaline and fat cells within the arterial wall. **(B)** Berry aneurysms form at the bi- or trifurcations of arteries and usually lead to subarachnoid hemorrhage, although they may rupture into the brain parenchyma. **(C)** When a septic embolus lodges in and infects a cortical arteriole, its wall weakens and a mycotic aneurysm forms, which may bleed, usually into the subcortical white matter. **(D)** Hemorrhage tends to occur at the periphery of tumors such as glioblastomas, melanomas, and bronchogenic carcinomas. **(E)** Cerebral amyloid angiopathy is characterized by weakening of the vessel as a result of deposition of amyloid within the media and adventitia and should be suspected in the elderly patient, especially when hypertension is not present.

MYCOTIC ANEURYSMS Mycotic aneurysms usually form in the smaller cortical arteries when septic emboli lodge in the vessel, extend their infection (usually bacterial, not fungal, despite the name) through the arterial wall, and damage the media; this sets the stage for subsequent aneurysmal dilatation and rupture (Figure 16.3C). This is usually seen in the setting of subacute bacterial endocarditis, where up to 17% of patients develop cerebral emboli.[16] On occasion, the aneurysm forms a thrombus, and if the infection has been adequately treated, no further intervention is needed. If the aneurysm continues to enlarge, however, it should be surgically clipped and resected to prevent rupture and continued infection.

NEOPLASTIC ANEURYSMS Arterial invasion by a tumor rarely leads to muscular weakness and subsequent aneurysmal formation. On the rare occasion that one does form, it may require clipping with or without concomitant tumor removal.

ATHEROSCLEROTIC ANEURYSMS These usually occur in the setting of severe atherosclerosis with accompanying hypertension. The vertebrobasilar system is usually involved and rupture is extremely rare.

Vascular malformations

There are four basic types of vascular malformations. The most common and most significant clinically is the arteriovenous malformation, a congenital vascular anomaly consisting of a tangle of vessels fed by one or more arteries and draining directly into the venous circulation without the benefit of intervening capillaries to decrease venous blood flow and pressure (Figure 16.4A). Much less important are the cavernous and venous angiomas (Figure 16.4B), which consist of large anomalous venous channels within the deep white matter. Cavernous angiomas differ from venous angiomas in that the latter contain normal brain tissue within their confines whereas the former have none. Also less important are

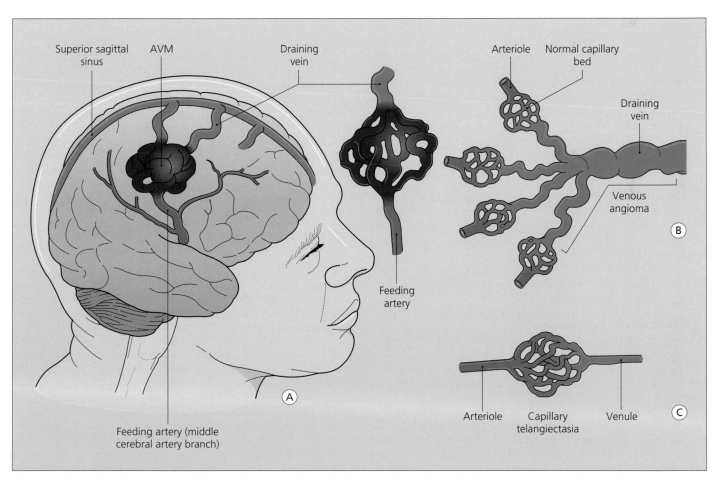

Figure 16.4 Vascular malformations. **(A)** The arteriovenous malformation is depicted here in a typical location within the brain. It is fed by a branch from the middle cerebral artery and its major draining vein is emptying into the superior sagittal sinus. In the simplified version of the arteriovenous malformation note that the arterial system drains directly into the venous system without an intervening capillary bed, which would normally reduce the pressure on the venous side. **(B)** In the venous malformation, a series of normal capillary beds drain into several abnormally dilated venous channels, all of which meet at a common draining vein, forming the typical caput medusae of the venous angioma. **(C)** Capillary telangiectasias consist of a series of dilated capillaries that lack normal elastic tissue, thus making them more susceptible to hemorrhage.

the capillary telangiectasias (Figure 16.4C), small, capillary-like vessels mostly found in the brainstem and cerebellum. These last three entities are of dubious clinical significance, though the telangiectasias, because of their location, may cause severe neurologic deficits if they hemorrhage.

Arteriovenous malformations, on the other hand, are notorious for bleeding; over one-half of them present as a hemorrhage. ICH accounts for 60% of cases, subarachnoid hemorrhage for 30%, and intraventricular hemorrhage for less than 10%.[17] These bleeds are arteriovenous; as such they are less violent than aneurysmal ruptures and the accompanying neurologic deficits, usually focal, are more slowly progressive. Hemorrhage tends to occur during the second to fourth decade of life compared to hypertensive or aneurysmal bleeds, which occur in an older population.

Interventional radiographic embolization of these lesions has made their surgical removal considerably safer and occasionally unnecessary, thus paving the way for better and safer treatment of these vascular abnormalities.

Coagulopathies

Approximately 5–7% of ICH cases are caused by an underlying coagulopathy.[2] Systemic disorders such as leukemia, thrombocytopenia, and liver and renal failure, as well as anticoagulation therapy with warfarin, aspirin, or dipyridamole, account for the majority of cases. Significantly, ICH is the primary complication of anticoagulation therapy, with approximately 2% of all such patients developing bleeds.[18] These types of hemorrhage tend to occur in cortical and subcortical regions, especially in the cerebellum, and usually follow a protracted course. In most cases, the underlying coagulopathy must be corrected prior to surgical evacuation of the hematoma unless the patient's life is in immediate danger. Most of these bleeds, however, can be followed with serial tomographic studies and tend to resolve once the underlying coagulopathy is corrected.

Tumors

Massive hemorrhage into a tumor is a rare event; in most studies only about 1% of tumors develop bleeds.[18] These occur mostly in malignant neoplasms, either primary, such as glioblastoma multiforme, or metastatic, especially bronchogenic carcinoma and malignant melanoma (see Figure 16.3D). Reports of bleeds into oligodendrogliomas, choroid plexus papillomas, choriocarcinomas, and even benign meningiomas are found in the literature though these are indeed rare.

Cerebral amyloid angiopathy

Cerebral amyloid angiopathy is a rare cause of ICH. It must, however, be suspected in the elderly patient with no history of hypertension. It is characterized by the deposition of amyloid in the media and adventitia of medium-sized hemispheric arteries (see Figure 16.3E).

It is estimated that during the seventh decade of life 10% of the population develops cerebral amyloid angiopathy, and by age 90 the incidence increases to 60%. Of note, this entity may account for as much as 30% of senile dementia, and it may be one of the major etiologic factors of spontaneous ICH in the elderly.[18]

The typical clinical picture is one of multiple, recurrent subcortical lobar bleeds. These can be asymptomatic or massive, leading to acute neurologic deterioration and death. The diagnosis is one of exclusion and may be confirmed on biopsy or necropsy when other more common etiologies have been excluded.

Hemorrhagic infarcts

Hemorrhagic infarcts occur when an area of infarction – the result of a recent thromboembolic event – is reperfused with blood that then leaks into brain tissue through broken down, necrotic vessel walls. Patients on anticoagulation therapy can have particularly severe courses, as is occasionally seen in the patient who, while taking warfarin after artificial valve replacement, develops valvular infectious or thrombotic vegetations and subsequent cardioembolic events. Managing these patients is particularly difficult. To prevent further bleeding one must correct the patient's coagulopathy. This, however, increases the patient's risk of developing further embolic events. These hemorrhages tend to be multicentric, are usually found in the subcortical white matter, and often extend into the cortex or, occasionally, subarachnoid space. They are often treated conservatively and may be followed closely with serial computed tomography (CT) scans of the head.

Drugs

Both legal and illegal drugs can cause spontaneous ICH. The agents most likely to cause bleeds are the amphetamines, although others (e.g. cocaine, pseudoephedrine, and heroin) have also been associated with ICH. Two basic mechanisms for this exist: (1) a pharmacologically-induced rise in blood pressure leads to arterial rupture similar to that seen in the hypertensive patient and (2) an intravenous injection of a nonsterile substance leads to a condition known as necrotizing angiitis, which is characterized by chronic damage to the smaller cortical vessels, causing arterial wall degeneration and bleeding if the intraluminal pressure exceeds arterial wall strength. The hemorrhages tend to be subcortical in location and are usually preceded by a hypertensive crisis that occasionally occurs without a known precipitating factor.

ICH has also been associated with chronic alcoholism and is often seen as petechial hemorrhage of the mamillary bodies. This, however, is thought to be more the result of cirrhosis of the liver and the accompanying coagulopathy of liver disease than a primary effect on the cerebral vasculature.

SIGNS AND SYMPTOMS

ICH has a wide range of presentations, from asymptomatic or transient ischemic attack-like to coma or death, each determined by the size and location of the hemorrhage. Early diagnosis of ICH can be extremely difficult without the help of modern radiographic studies such as CT or magnetic resonance imaging (MRI), since the majority of patients present in the manner of cerebral infarct patients – hemiplegia is found in up to 95% of cases, stupor or drowsiness in 45–50% of cases, and coma in approximately 30% of cases. Other findings, which depend primarily on the location of the bleed, include headache, nausea, vomiting, seizures, cranial nerve deficits, ataxia, and aphasia. Overall, about one-third of patients present with maximal deficits at onset while the remaining two-thirds have a gradual presentation of symptoms and smooth progression of deficits over minutes or hours. It is diagnostically useful to know that there is never a regression of symptoms in the acute phase of ICH; thus a bleed can be effectively ruled out as a cause of stroke if symptom regression occurs. Other signs of ICH that help distinguish it from cerebral infarct are bilaterality of symptoms, persistent headache with nuchal rigidity, and neural deficits that localize over the distribution of two or more major arteries. Autonomic changes with vomiting and a rapid deterioration in neurologic status may suggest extension of the hemorrhage into the ventricular system.

In the days and weeks following the bleed, the patient's clinical course largely depends on several factors, the most important of which is the amount and location of permanent tissue loss occurring during the initial event. Other important prognostic factors include the patient's age, severity of neurologic deficits on the initial examination, the presence or absence of intraventricular hemorrhage, and/or obstructive hydrocephalus as well as the ensuing amount of cerebral edema, its subsequent impact on intracranial pressure, and its potential for causing a herniation syndrome. Systemic disorders such as hypertension and diabetes mellitus as well as individual organ dysfunction (i.e. cardiac, pulmonary, or renal) have an indirect yet significant impact on survival during the subacute period (2–4 weeks postictus), whereas central nervous system complications such as hydrocephalus and edema tend to influence the early clinical course.[10]

As mentioned above, the location of the bleed largely determines the observed neurologic deficits (Figure 16.5). Basal ganglia and thalamic bleeds, for example, present as massive hemiplegia, with thalamic bleeds occasionally including a hemisensory loss. Cortical hemorrhages are often accompanied by seizures as well as *focal neurologic deficits* (see Figure 16.5A) as

local tissue damage secondary to the hemorrhage disrupts fiber tracts and causes symptoms referable to the area involved. Thus a patient presenting with a small hemorrhage in the posterior limb of the right internal capsule would likely exhibit contralateral (left) hemiplegia and possibly hemianesthesia if the thalamus were involved as well. Posterior fossa lesions are often accompanied by nausea, vomiting, decreased mentation, and hydrocephalus as well as cranial nerve deficits, plegia, paresis, autonomic abnormalities, and anesthesia from brainstem bleeds or ataxia, nystagmus, and dysmetria from cerebellar involvement. The extension of hemorrhage into the ventricular system is particularly important as it is associated with a high mortality (65–75% of all fatal hypertensive bleeds), autonomic abnormalities, neurologic deficits whose severity is out of proportion to the size of the bleed, as well as a decreased level of consciousness and the development of obstructive hydrocephalus.[18] *Hydrocephalus* is often associated with posterior fossa lesions or intraventricular hemorrhages which block ventricular outflow channels (see Figure 16.5B). *Herniation* is usually the result of a significant increase in intracranial pressure either from a hematoma swelling or hydrocephalus. Figure 16.5C shows transtentorial uncal herniation as a result of a massive right hemispheric bleed. This situation is a neurosurgical emergency and requires immediate intervention directed at relieving the increased pressure – evacuating the hematoma in this case.

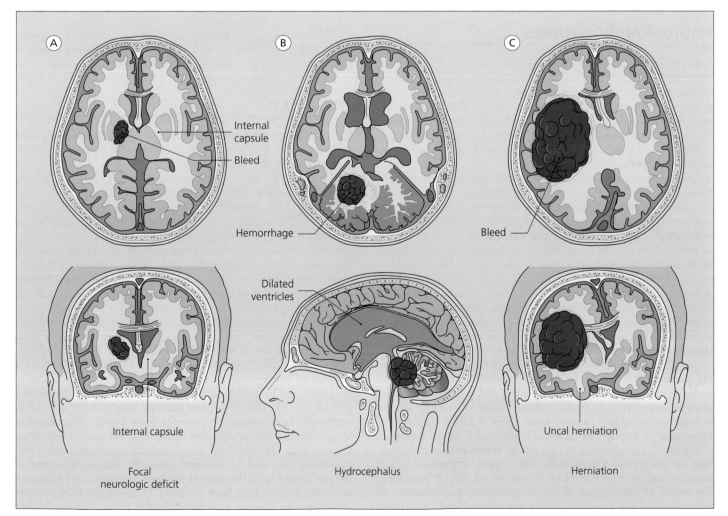

Figure 16.5 Effects of intracerebral hemorrhage.

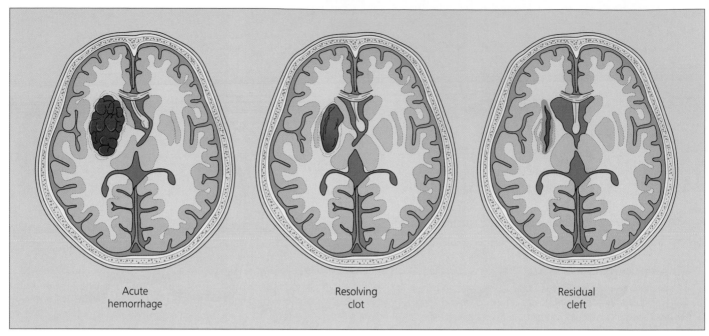

| Acute hemorrhage | Resolving clot | Residual cleft |

Figure 16.8 Spontaneous resolution of an ICH. The natural history of an ICH is characterized by liquefaction of both the clot and necrotic brain tissue with ensuing reabsorption of both.

CLINICAL PEARLS

- Intracranial hemorrhage (ICH) accounts for over 10% of all strokes. Stroke is the third leading cause of death in the USA and the main cause of neurologic deficit in the world.

- Spontaneous ICH results from intracranial artery or, less commonly, venous rupture. The most common risk factor is hypertension (40–60%), followed by aneurysms, vascular malformations, coagulapathies, angiopathies, drugs, and tumors.

- Cerebral amyloid angiopathy, although a rare cause of ICH, should be suspected in elderly patients who may have no history of hypertension. About 10% of all people who reach 70 have this angiopathy. This figure rises to 60% by the ninth decade of life.

- Two-thirds of patients with an ICH have a gradual onset of symptoms, whereas one-third present with maximal deficits immediately. ICH can be treated medically or surgically. Medical therapy is aimed at treating the underlying hypertension and/or coagulopathy. However, if the patient rapidly deteriorates or needs immediate alleviation of rising intracranial pressure, surgical evacuation of the hemorrhage should be considered.

- The prognosis for ICH depends on the location and severity of the bleed and the age/condition of the patient. Brainstem and diencephalic bleeds have a poorer prognosis than those in the cerebral hemisphere.

The prognosis of ICH depends on several factors. Location and size of hemorrhage are of primary importance. They are closely followed by the patient's age, development and severity of post-hemorrhagic complications such as cerebral edema, hydrocephalus, and herniation syndromes, as well as systemic disorders, including pulmonary emboli, myocardial infarcts, and pneumonia.

In general, brainstem and diencephalic bleeds herald a poor prognosis, especially if intraventricular hemorrhage is present, and every effort should be made to treat these patients aggressively early in their clinical course, if any chance for recovery exists.

REFERENCES

1. Kuller LH. Incidence, rates of stroke in the 80s. *Stroke* 1989; 20: 841–3.
2. Cahill DW, Ducker TB. Spontaneous intracerebral hemorrhage. In: Weiss MH, *et al.* (eds). *Clinical Neurosurgery: Proceedings of the CNS, Los Angeles, 1981*. Baltimore: Williams & Wilkins; 1982; 29: 722–79.
3. Kurtzke JF. *Epidemiology of Cerebrovascular Disease*. Berlin: Springer-Verlag; 1969.

4. Mohr JP, Caplan LR, Melski JW, *et al*. The Harvard Cooperative Stroke Registry: a prospective registry. *Neurology* 1978; 28: 754.

5. Toole JF, Patel AN. *Cerebrovascular Disorders*, 2nd edn. New York, NY: McGraw-Hill; 1967.

6. Chambers BR, *et al*. Prognostic profiles in acute stroke. In: Hachinski V, Norris JW (eds). *The Acute Stroke, Contemporary Neurology Series* 27. Philadelphia, PA: FA Davis Company; 1985: 245–58.

7. Wolf PA, Kannel WB, *et al*. Epidemiology of stroke in North America. In: Barnett HJM, Mohr JP, Stein BM, Yatsu FM (eds). *Stroke: Pathophysiology, Diagnosis, and Management*. New York, NY: Churchill Livingstone; 1986: 19–29.

8. Weinfeld FD (ed.). The national survey of stroke. *Stroke* 1981; 12(suppl): 1–71.

9. Freytag E. Fatal hypertensive intracerebral hematomas: a survey of the pathological anatomy of 393 cases. *J Neurol Neurosurg Psychiatr* 1968; 31: 616.

10. Hachinski V, Norris JW. *The Acute Stroke, Contemporary Neurology Series* 27. Philadelphia, PA: FA Davis Company; 1985.

11. Kase CS, Mohr JP. General features of intracerebral hemorrhage. In: Barnett HJM, Stein BM, Mohr JP, Yatsu FM (eds). *Stroke: Pathophysiology, Diagnosis, and Management*. New York, NY: Churchill Livingstone; 1986: 497–523.

12. Kase CS, Robinson RK, *et al*. Anticoagulant-related intracerebral hemorrhage. *Neurology* 1985; 35: 943.

13. Fisher CM. Cerebral miliary aneurysms in hypertension. *Am J Pathol* 1972; 66: 313.

14. Okizaki H. *Fundamentals of Neuropathology: Morphologic Basis of Neurologic Disorders*, 2nd edn. New York, NY: Igaku-Shoin; 1989.

15. Fox JL. *Intracranial Aneurysms*. New York, NY: Springer-Verlag; 1983.

16. Mohr JP, Kistler JP, *et al*. Intracranial aneurysms. In: Barnett HJM, Mohr JP, Stein BM, Yatsu FM (eds). *Stroke: Pathophysiology, Diagnosis, and Management*. New York, NY: Churchill Livingstone; 1986: 643–77.

17. Mohr JP, Tatemichi TK, *et al*. Vascular malformations of the brain. In: Barnett HJM, Mohr JP, Stein BM, Yatsu FM (eds). *Stroke: Pathophysiology, Diagnosis, and Management*. New York, NY: Churchill Livingstone; 1986: 679–705.

18. Castel JP, Kissel P. Spontaneous intracerebral and infratentorial hemorrhage. In: Youmans J (ed.). *Neurological Surgery*, 3rd edn. Philadelphia, PA: WB Saunders Co; 1990: 1890–917.

Table 17.1 Complications of neuroendovascular surgery

Local
Hematoma
Pseudoaneurysm
Distal embolus
Dissection
Occlusion
Tissue necrosis
Vasospasm

Systemic
Contrast reaction
Renal failure
Pulmonary edema
Pulmonary embolization
Myocardial infarction
Postembolic syndrome

Neurologic
Stroke
Transient ischemic attack
Dissection
Vessel occlusion
Convulsion
Intracerebral hemorrhage
Subarachnoid hemorrhage
Normal perfusion pressure breakthrough
Microembolic load
Device failure or device glued to vessel
Cranial nerve palsy

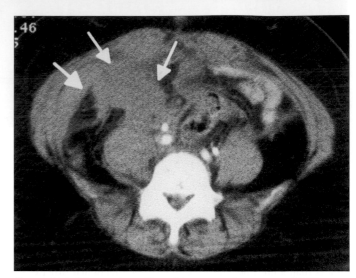

Figure 17.1 A large retroperitoneal hematoma is seen on axial CT following a transfemoral intervention in which thrombolysis was performed with heparinization. The arrows indicate areas of hemorrhage extending from the abdominal wall to the retroperitoneal space.

PERI- AND POST-PROCEDURAL CONSIDERATIONS

The majority of neuroendovascular procedures are performed using local anesthesia with intravenous sedative hypnotics and analgesics.[2] As a result of the potential for respiratory compromise with intravenous sedatives and analgesics, constant monitoring of oxygen saturation and respiratory rate is performed. Intravenous access is maintained. Most patients have been *non per os* beginning the evening before and are mildly dehydrated. It is preferable to administer intravenous fluid prior to infusing intra-arterial contrast. In addition, diabetic patients on the oral hypoglycemic metformin hydrochloride (glucophage) must not restart their oral agents for 2 days following administration of intra-arterial contrast because of an elevated risk for renal failure. Patient's renal function is tested 48 hours post-procedure and oral metformin is re-initiated if studies are normal. Systolic blood pressure is monitored at 3-minute intervals throughout the procedure. Constant monitoring of heart rate is performed, as is serial monitoring of neurologic status.

Cerebral angiography is low-risk, but not risk-free. Complications can be viewed as neurologic, systemic, or local (Table 17.1). The overall risk of permanent neurologic injury during angiography is approximately 0.07% and of nonneurologic complication is 0.6% (Figure 17.1).[3]

The role of anticoagulation and antiplatelet therapies has been recognized in the prevention of thromboembolic complications during and after neuroendovascular procedures. Most of the data have been derived from the cardiac literature through prospective randomized trials.[4]

CATHETERS AND ARTERIAL ACCESS

The arterial system can be accessed through radial, brachial, cervical, and femoral approaches, as well as by selective arterial cut-down. However, the femoral approach has been shown to be safe and reliable over time. Other approaches are indicated only in select circumstances when transfemoral access is not possible. The femoral artery is located over the medial aspect of the femoral head. The inguinal ligament is approximated by a line drawn between the anterior superior iliac spine and the pubic tubercle. It serves as the division between the leg and abdomen. An arterial puncture above the inguinal ligament runs the risk of creating a retroperitoneal hematoma, which is a potentially life-threatening complication. The appropriate puncture point is two finger-breadths (2–3 cm) below the inguinal ligament. The femoral artery lies medial to the femoral nerve and lateral to the femoral vein. The artery is localized by placing two fingers over the pulse, one proximal and one distal. The skin between the fingers and the subcutaneous tissues are anesthetized. A small stab wound is made with a no. 11 blade scalpel and a single-wall puncture needle is used to access the artery. The needle is advanced until the pulsations of the artery can be felt against the tip of the needle. The needle is passed through the outer wall of the femoral artery. Endoluminal placement is verified by the ready return of arterial blood and a J-wire is passed through the needle and into the artery. The needle is removed, and a sheath is placed over the wire and into the artery. The sheath consists of a hydrophilic sheath and obturator. The obturator has a tapered end and fits within the sheath, allowing it to pass easily over the wire into the vessel. Once the sheath and obturator have been introduced into the vessel, the obturator is removed. Sheaths minimize trauma to the artery and allow better transmission of torque to catheters for manipulation. In addition, they facilitate the rapid exchange of catheters and are hemostatic. We connect sheaths to a continuous heparinized saline flush to prevent back bleeding and thrombus formation. We utilize 5-French sheaths for diagnostic work and 6-French sheaths for most interventional procedures.

Endovascular procedures fall into two categories: diagnostic and therapeutic. Catheters come in numerous shapes and sizes. Diagnostic catheters are used for rapid infusion of contrast. The catheters have preshaped tips with a wide variety of configurations. Guide catheters are used during therapeutic interventions. They are transit catheters with large inner lumens through which a working catheter (microcatheter) or device for deployment is passed in a co-axial fashion to more distal pathology. Catheters are passed over wires to achieve distal access to a vessel. For example, a guidewire is placed within a catheter and is manipulated out of its distal end and into the region of interest. The guidewire is then stabilized by placing it under gentle tension or slight backward force as the catheter is pushed over the wire. This maneuver is repeated time and time again whether using diagnostic, guide, or microcatheters to achieve access to a vascular distribution.

The microcatheter is the workhorse of any embolization. Coated with proprietary hydrophilic coatings, they are made for achieving access to distal vascular beds. Both over-the-wire catheters and flow-directed catheters are used. Flow-directed catheters have a fairly stiff body and distally are graduated in stiffness to a very "floppy" tip, which can be directed by blood flow. They are extremely useful for arteriovenous malformation (AVM) embolization. Such catheters can also be used over-the-wire with newer microwires designed specifically for use with flow-directed catheters to achieve distal access to AVMs. Microcatheters are passed over microwires that generally range in size from 0.008" to 0.018". Microcatheter and microwire diameters are measured in hundredths of inches, diagnostic and guide catheters are measured in French, and most balloons, transit devices, coils, and stents are measured in millimeters. It helps to remember that 1 French = 0.3 mm = 0.012".

Thromboembolic complications are among the most significant complications of endovascular work. Thus, guide catheters and microcatheters are flushed with heparinized saline at all times during a procedure. Heparin, 5000 IU/l of saline, is attached to all interventional catheters, i.e. guide catheters and microcatheters. Sheaths are attached to flushes containing 2000 IU heparin/l.

NEUROENDOVASCULAR INTERVENTIONS

Some of the techniques used in neuroendovascular surgery include balloons for temporary and permanent parent-vessel occlusion; angioplasty for vaso-occlusive disease; embolic agents for treating tumors, aneurysms, and AVMs; pharmacologic infusions for vasospasm and stroke; and stents for endoluminal reconstruction of vessels.

Temporary and permanent balloon occlusion

Temporary balloon occlusion (BTO) involves inflation of a non-detachable endovascular balloon in a vessel to determine whether the patient can tolerate occlusion or sacrifice of the vessel. The information gleaned from BTO is used to determine the need for revascularization. In such cases, an extracranial to intracranial bypass can be planned in advance. Patients are fully anticoagulated and activated clotting times (ACTs) are measured every 15 minutes to maintain an ACT of > 300 seconds. While electro-

encephalography (EEG), somatosensory potentials (SSEP), and transcranial Doppler (TCD) have been used to extend the usefulness of awake BTO.[5–7] We perform awake BTO with a hypotensive challenge. Following an initial period of 20 minutes of BTO at normotensive levels, nipride is infused to achieve a drop of approximately 30% of mean arterial blood pressure for approximately 20 minutes.[8,9] If patients become symptomatic at any time, the balloon is deflated and the procedure is terminated. In children who are unable to co-operate fully, BTO is performed under general anesthesia and CT perfusion is performed.[10] CT perfusion predicts acute supratentorial ischemia with 91–93% sensitivity.[11]

If the vessel is to be occluded, options include the use of a detachable balloon or placement of endovascular coils. Detachable balloons are loaded on a catheter, floated into place, and inflated. The catheter is then withdrawn, leaving the balloon in place. Risks associated with balloons include balloon embolization, vessel rupture, stroke, thromboemboli, and subacute ischemia.

Endovascular embolizations

Embolic agents in neuroendovascular surgery are varied and wide-ranging. In general, particulate and cytotoxic agents are used for tumor embolizations, glues are used for high-flow lesions such as fistulae and arteriovenous malformations, and detachable coils are used to treat aneurysms. Of course, combinations of embolic agents may be used in the treatment of many vascular malformations.

Tumor embolizations

Patients chosen for tumor embolization are selected on an individual basis. The role of preoperative embolization is to reduce blood supply. In patients with lesions that are difficult to access surgically or in those patients of poor medical grade, embolization can be used to control tumor growth through serial treatments which result in tumor necrosis. Conceptually, it is easiest to think in terms of blood supply to an individual tumor to determine its suitability for embolization. Tumors that receive their blood supply from the external carotid artery are inherently safer to embolize than those which rely on intracranial vessels for their blood supply (referred to as pial supply). Extracranial–intracranial anastomoses are a source of potential communication between extracranial and intracranial blood vessels. Failure to recognize these natural communications can result in potentially devastating complications during embolization procedures if the agent courses from the extracranial to the intracranial compartment. The typical anastomoses are listed in Table 17.2.

Blood supply to tumors can be considered as pial (intracranial blood vessels), extracranial (arising from the external carotid or other brachiocephalic vessels), or mixed (both). Tumors with a "mixed" intracranial–extracranial supply will frequently have a "punched-out"-appearing vascular blush during the capillary or venous phase of selective angiography. These tumors pose a risk for inadvertent embolization of normal tissue if embolization is too aggressive and the joint blood supply is not recognized. Generally, tumors with external carotid artery supply are well suited to embolization, whereas those with pial supply are not embolized (Figure 17.2). Protective embolization refers to the planned embolization of a normal arterial branch to embolize a pathologic branch. For example, the intentional occlusion of an intercostal artery may be performed during the embolization of a spinal tumor. The tissue of the embolized normal vessel is fed by

Table 17.2 Dangerous extracranial to intracranial anastomoses

Vessel	Anastomoses
Internal maxillary artery	Ophthalmic artery
Superficial temporal artery	Ophthalmic artery
Middle meningeal artery	Petrous internal carotid artery Ophthalmic artery
Ascending pharyngeal artery	Meningohypophyseal trunk Petrous internal carotid artery Middle meningeal artery
Posterior auricular artery	Cervical vertebral artery Occipital artery
Occipital artery	Posterior auricular artery Vertebral artery Ascending cervical artery Deep cervical artery
Ascending cervical artery	Vertebral artery Occipital artery

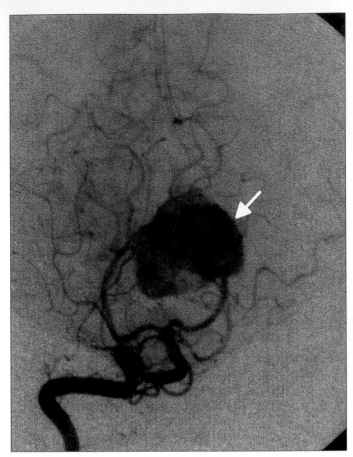

Figure 17.2 A right anteroposterior vertebral artery angiogram reveals an intra-axial tumor supplied by branches of the superior cerebellar arteries bilaterally. The lesion exhibits a profound "tumor blush" during the late arterial phase (arrow).

collateral anastomoses, and the embolic agent now flows only to the diseased tissue.

Tumor embolization occurs in a manner similar to other neuroendovascular procedures. A guide catheter is placed within the parent vessel leading to the pathology. Mild systemic heparinization is achieved and a microcatheter and microwire are prepared for accessing the vessels leading to the lesion. In the case of meningiomas, access with a suitable microcatheter can proceed to within millimeters of the tumor through the middle meningeal artery. Once distal access has been achieved, the embolic agent is prepared. The most common agent in use today is polyvinyl alcohol particles. Ranging in prepared sizes, from between 49 and 150 μm to over 500 μm in diameter, the particle size can be tailored to the lesion. Other agents include absolute ethanol (a cytotoxic agent), collagen preparations, silk, coils, and embolic glues. Smaller particles penetrate further into a vascular bed, resulting in actual necrosis as they provide an impediment to collateral revascularization. Larger particles (150–250 μm) do not provide regions of necrosis within the tumor bed. When using smaller particles, a delay of 3–10 days between tumor embolization and surgery maximizes tumor necrosis.[12] Particles are mixed in a 50 : 50 solution of contrast and heparinized saline. The mixture is infused by hand under constant fluoroscopic guidance (Figure 17.3A,B). Constant monitoring allows the surgeon to gauge the flow within the vessel by observing contrast washout following each gentle infusion. As flow in the target vessel diminishes as a result of the filling of the vascular bed by the embolic agent, reflux near the catheter tip will occur. This is the endpoint of the procedure. Reflux proximal to the catheter tip can lead to embolization of normal vascular beds through adjacent normal arterial branches.

Arteriovenous malformations

AVMs are complex vascular lesions thought to arise between the 4th and 8th weeks of gestation. The primary features of an AVM

are direct connections between arteries and veins, without a capillary bed. There is no normal brain tissue within an AVM. The overall incidence of AVM is 1/100 000 (0.001%) and the average patient presents during the fifth decade of life.[13] The majority of AVMs present with headache, seizures, or hemorrhage.

Intracranial hemorrhage is the most common presenting complaint, followed by seizure and headache.[14,15] As the number of MRI studies of the brain continues to increase, larger numbers of asymptomatic or headache-associated AVMs are likely to be found. The risk of re-hemorrhage from an AVM has been evaluated using both meta-analysis and population-based cohorts. The average yearly risk of hemorrhage ranges from 2 to 4%. It is believed that smaller AVMs tend to present more often with hemorrhage, whereas larger AVMs present with seizures.[16,17]

Management options for AVMs include observation, surgery, focused radiation, and endovascular embolization. In general, multimodality treatment approaches offer greater success than any one therapy alone.[18] Endovascular treatment is considered adjunctive treatment, as complete obliteration of an AVM nidus is possible in fewer than 20% of cases.[19,20] AVM embolization is utilized to diminish the overall size of a lesion and make it more amenable to gamma-knife therapy; or, it is used before surgery, to embolize deep feeding vessels that may not be readily accessible at surgery or to treat large feeding arteries to diminish overall blood loss. AVM embolization has been shown to limit blood loss and shorten

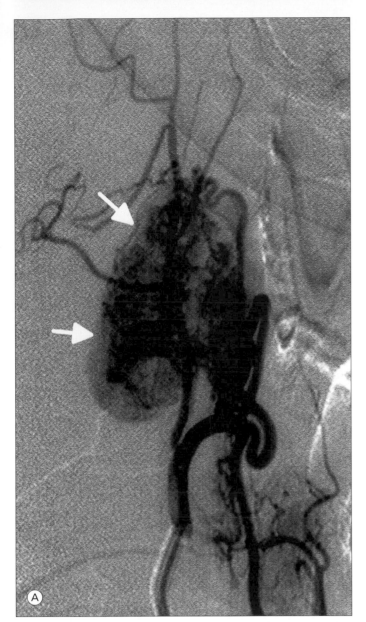

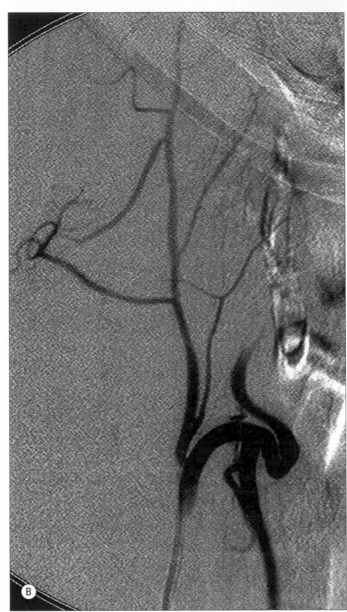

Figure 17.3 Anteroposterior views of a thyrocervical artery angiogram revealing the tumor blush (arrows) of an extracranial cervical tumor **(A)**. Following polyvinyl-alcohol-particle embolization **(B)** the tumor blush is gone and the normal vasculature remains.

operative time (Figure 17.4A–C).[21,22] Palliative embolization is performed in cases in which an AVM is a source of ischemia and in which functional deficits occur because of steal from surrounding normal parenchyma. Endovascular embolization can in many cases halt the progression of neurologic deterioration by diminishing the shunting of blood through the AVM and thereby increasing perfusion to normal brain. In addition, lesions with significant symptoms of headache may benefit from embolization of any dural feeding vessels.[23] As with any therapy, the goal is to maximize patient benefit and minimize patient risk.

Technically, the embolization of AVMs is similar to other endovascular interventions. Femoral artery access is obtained, adequate anticoagulation is achieved, and a guide catheter is placed into the appropriate parent vessel in the neck and a microcatheter is chosen. Ideally, the nidus of an AVM is catheterized and embolized. The nidus is the region of arteriovenous shunting. Arteries which directly supply an AVM can be successfully embolized with minimal morbidity, whereas vessels which indirectly supply an AVM and primarily supply normal brain tissue (en-passage vessels) are high-risk for embolization because of their dual role. Other high-risk features of AVMs include deep venous drainage, outflow compromise, i.e. venous stenosis or thrombosis, and location in eloquent cortex. While AVMs have traditionally been embolized with a bevy of materials, currently, only a few agents and materials are used. Metallic coils made of platinum or stainless steel, with or without fibers, are sometimes used to slow the flow through an arteriovenous fistula. Coils are made in a number of lengths and configurations and can be injected or delivered through microcatheters directly into the AVM. Absolute ethanol is a sclerosing agent that causes protein denaturation,

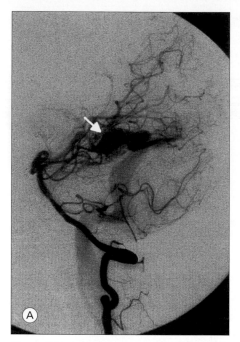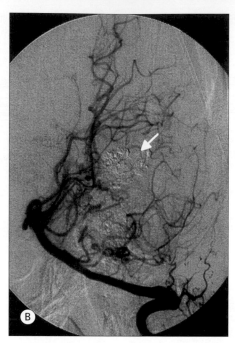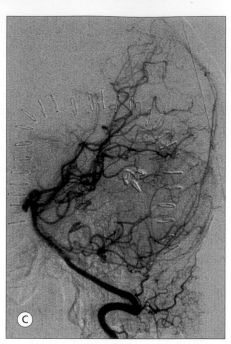

Figure 17.4 Lateral views, vertebral artery angiogram, of a small tentorial AVM prior to embolization, after embolization, and following surgical removal. **(A)** The AVM is seen during the arterial phase of the angiogram with early venous drainage to the transverse sinus (arrow). Following preoperative embolization **(B)**, the AVM is almost completely embolized. Embolic agent (NBCA) is seen within the AVM (arrow). Following surgery **(C)** the AVM has been removed and normal vessels and venous drainage are noted. Two aneurysm clips are noted within the surgical field.

cytotoxic cell death and irreversible damage to the intimal lining of blood vessels. It is used on a limited basis by most endovascular specialists.[24] Polyvinyl alcohol particles are rarely used today in AVM embolization because of their inherent complications and lack of permanence. They have been implicated in pulmonary embolization, and increases in AVM intranidal pressure, making hemorrhage more likely.[25] Used for nearly 25 years, N-butyl-2-cyanoacrylate (NBCA) was recently approved for use in AVM embolization by the Food and Drug Administration. NBCA is mixed in varying proportions with a lipid vehicle (ethiodol) depending on the flow characteristics of the lesion being treated. NBCA rapidly polymerizes upon contact with ionic solutions. To prevent polymerization within the microcatheter, dextrose solution is infused to fill the catheter with nonionic solution prior to infusing the NBCA. NBCA can penetrate deeply into an AVM nidus. However, it is a difficult embolic agent to use and requires significant experience.

Dural arteriovenous fistulas

Dural arteriovenous fistulas and malformations (DAVF) are thought to occur secondary to sinus thrombosis. The fistula occurs during recanalization of the sinus. Intradural veins develop alternative sites for drainage. Symptoms are related to arterial steal and to venous hypertension. Many dural AVFs do not require treatment. DAVFs are divided into benign and aggressive lesions. Benign lesions cause symptoms such as pulsatile tinnitus, increased intracranial pressure or ocular complaints without vision changes. Aggressive lesions typically are heralded by intracranial hemorrhage, seizures, and progressive neurologic deficit. The behavior of a DAVF is almost always predicated on its venous drainage.[26,27] Aggressive lesions tend to have intradural venous drainage, Galenic drainage, variceal or aneurysmal dilatations, or stenoses of

intradural veins. Patients presenting with intracranial hemorrhage should be treated as soon as possible as they have an increased risk for repeated hemorrhage.[27,28] Patients with benign lesions should be followed over time as lesions can progress to more aggressive types. However, they can also spontaneously regress.

Treatment of DAVFs is aimed at symptomatic relief. For aggressive lesions, the plan is for complete exclusion of the malformation (Figure 17.5A,B). Approaches to DAVFs have included surgical skeletonization of the sinus, radiation therapy, transarterial embolization, transvenous embolization, compression therapy, observation, or a combination of modalities. The principle of successful treatment is obliteration of the venous outflow of the fistula. Occlusion of the venous side of a fistula is generally performed in a manner similar to accessing the arterial side of an intracranial malformation. The sinus/fistula is occluded with a combination of coils and NBCA through superselective placement of a microcatheter. In some cases, it is possible to catheterize the arterial side of a lesion selectively and embolize to the venous side with NBCA. This effectively excludes the lesion from the circulation. Recent reports of transvenous approaches have been highly successful, clinically curing up to 96% of patients.[29] Arguably, most patients should be first evaluated for an endovascular approach for treatment of their DAVF.

Spinal arteriovenous malformations

Spinal arteriovenous malformations and fistulas are complex lesions ranging from simple arteriovenous fistulas to large complex malformations involving both the spinal cord and vertebrae. The lesions are categorized as types I–IV. Type I AVMs are actually dural arteriovenous fistulas which typically cause symptoms such as vague pain and progressive myelopathy because of venous congestion. Type IA AVMs are supplied by a single arterial fistula

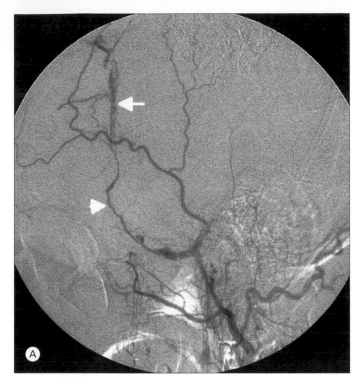
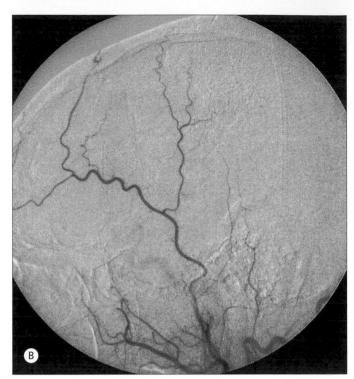

Figure 17.5 (A,B) A right external carotid artery angiogram (lateral view) in a patient presenting with subarachnoid hemorrhage and intracerebral hemorrhage. The arrowhead points to the middle meningeal artery (MMA). The arrow denotes the venous side of the MMA–venous fistula. Following bilateral MMA embolization with NBCA, the arteriovenous fistula is no longer evident. Cerebral angiography 1 year later revealed no evidence of residual fistula.

(Figure 17.6A,B), Type IB lesions have two or more fistulas. Type II AVMs are similar to intracranial AVMs, as they are intramedullary with a compact nidus. Type III AVMs are large complex, intra- and extramedullary lesions that may involve the vertebrae and surrounding tissues. Type IV lesions are intradural extramedullary AVFs and are further subdivided A–C.[30,31] Endovascular treatment of these lesions is generally adjunctive to surgery. The goals are similar to those of intracranial lesions, namely, to improve function, halt progressive neurologic decline, minimize blood loss preoperatively, and, in certain cases, to cure fistulas. Spinal interventions require a co-axial system just as intracranial lesions do. Because of the relatively small size of spinal segmental vessels, most work is performed through a 5-F guide catheter or in some cases a 5-F diagnostic catheter serves as a guide. A microcatheter and microwire are used to access the lesion. AVMs are treated with NBCA embolization.

Intracranial aneurysms

Improved endovascular techniques, devices with hydrophilic coatings, and anticoagulation have had profound influences on the endovascular treatment of intracranial aneurysms. The current debate regarding the most appropriate role for surgery versus endovascular therapy for patients with unruptured and ruptured aneurysms is beyond the scope of this chapter. The decision to treat a given aneurysm surgically or with endovascular techniques must be performed on an individual case-by-case basis. General guidelines used in our practice and their rationale will be presented.

Poor surgical outcomes in patients with ruptured aneurysms are associated with older age, severe medical co-morbidities, poor Hunt–Hess grade, posterior circulation aneurysms, and surgery during the period of onset of vasospasm.[32] In such patients, aneurysms amenable to endovascular coiling should logically be considered for therapy if they possess characteristics suitable for an endovascular approach. Traditionally, a fundus to neck ratio of 2 : 1 with a diameter at least as great in the smallest dimension as the smallest endovascular coil diameter (2 mm) is reasonable to coil. Issues important to endovascular occlusion are significantly different from those for open surgery. The ability to have a "working view" in which the vessels adjacent to the aneurysm are seen relative to the aneurysm coils to ensure patency is of critical importance. The inability to visualize adequately the adjacent vasculature is an indication for open surgery. Aneurysm location is otherwise of minimal concern as almost any lesion can be accessed with a microcatheter. Other appropriate indications for endovascular occlusion include: a second ipsilateral aneurysm not addressed at the initial operation, patients with multiple aneurysms and an unknown site of rupture, incompletely clipped aneurysms, coincident vasospasm, and patients requiring anticoagulation.

The microcoils used to embolize aneurysms are made from wound platinum (Figure 17.7A,B). There are many different manufacturers of coils today. However, all coils share a basic construct. A stiff, pushable wire is connected to the coil at a detachment zone. The detachment zones are typically proprietary. Some of the mechanisms for detachment include electrolysis, hydraulic detachment, or a simple unscrewing of the push wire

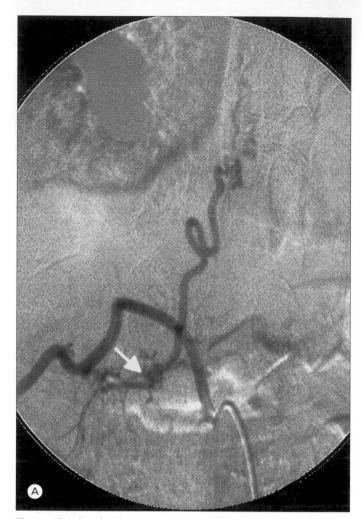
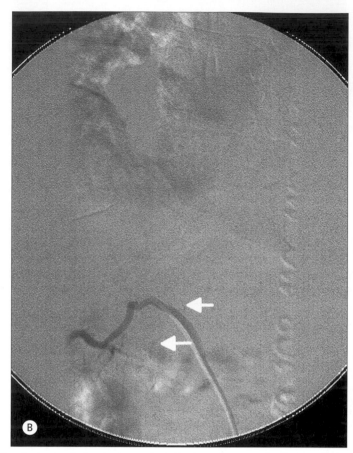

Figure 17.6 (A, B) Following selective injection of the right L2 segmental artery (anteroposterior view), a radiculodural arteriovenous fistula is marked by the arrow (Type I AVF). Retrograde spinal venous engorgement is noted extending rostrally from the fistula. **(B)** The fistula and proximal venous component of the lesion have been embolized with NBCA. The normal radiculodural arterial supply is now revealed (arrows).

from the coil. Coils come in a variety of diameters and lengths. They are chosen to fill an aneurysm from largest to smallest, as though one were constructing layers of an onion from the outside to the middle. Coils come in varying stiffnesses, diameters, lengths, and configurations, including three-dimensional, and two-dimensional constructs.

Aneurysm embolization is performed in most cases under general anesthesia. Similar to other procedures, access to the cranial vessels is obtained as close to the skull base as possible with a guide catheter. Aneurysms are coiled with patients fully anticoagulated.[4] Protamine sulfate is immediately available to reverse heparin anticoagulation as necessary. A microcatheter designed specifically for aneurysm coiling is prepared. These catheters have two marker bands. One band is at the distal end of the catheter and the second aligns with a marker on the coil corresponding to delivery of the coil-detachment zone to the catheter aneurysm junction. First, the microwire is carefully negotiated into the aneurysm, followed by gentle delivery of the catheter over-the-wire into the aneurysm. Using digital subtraction angiography, the aneurysm is measured and an appropriate coil is chosen. Coils are delivered sequentially, with angiographic runs performed following placement of each coil, but prior to detachment. Coils that

prolapse into the parent vessel lumen or fail to deploy in a stable configuration are gently retrieved into the microcatheter and redeployed into the aneurysm. Following placement of the final coil, angiographic images are obtained. Patients are returned to the intensive-care unit following completion of embolization.

Stroke thrombolysis

Stroke is the third leading cause of death and the number one cause of adult disability in the United States. Over 700 000 people will have a new or repeat stroke in the United States every year. To gain a perspective on the public-health issues associated with stroke, it should be noted that more than 50% of the cost of caring for a stroke survivor is borne more than 2 years after the initial stroke. With a progressively aging population and a stroke risk which doubles every 10 years after the age of 55,[33,34] the role of endovascular therapies will continue to expand. However, while significant advances in the prevention and treatment of acute stroke have been made, practitioners to date have had limited success in the treatment of acute stroke.

The majority of strokes are thromboembolic in nature. This patient group stands to benefit from intravenous or intra-arterial

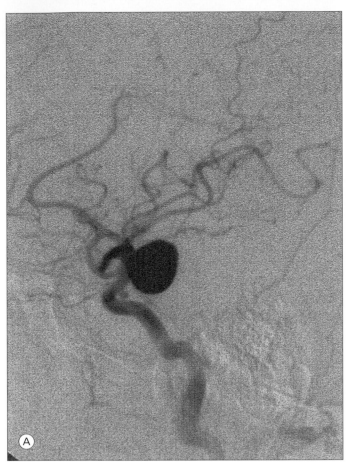 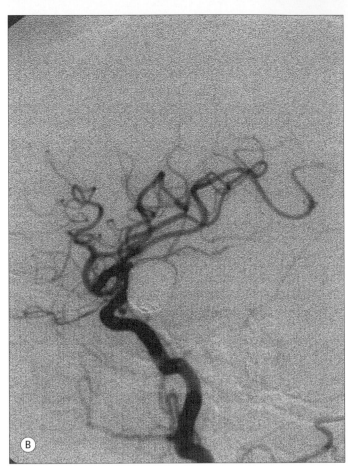

Figure 17.7 (A, B) An elderly woman presented with subarachnoid hemorrhage. Right common carotid artery angiography (lateral view) shows a large supraclinoid internal carotid artery aneurysm. As a result of the large neck size, the aneurysm was embolized with detachable microcoils using balloon assistance. Following embolization **(B)** the aneurysm has been excluded from the circulation and the internal carotid artery remains patent.

thrombolysis. Intravenous administration of recombinant tissue plasminogen activator (rt-PA) has been shown to benefit those patients presenting within 3 hours of their initial symptomology[35] as shown by improved outcome at 3 months relative to controls. Patients who present outside the 3-hour window, but within 6 hours are candidates for intra-arterial thrombolysis. The PROACT (Prelyse in acute cerebral thromboemolism) II trial showed the effectiveness of rt-PA in the treatment of acute thromboembolic stroke involving the middle cerebral artery.[36] A screening CT examination of the brain is performed. If CT examination of the brain does not show evidence of ischemia or intracerebral hemorrhage, the patient proceeds to emergent cerebral angiography and possible intra-arterial thrombolysis. A number of medical co-morbidities are contraindications to intra-arterial thrombolysis, including recent major surgery, recent intracerebral hemorrhage, a history of gastrointestinal hemorrhage, and any other significant medical co-morbidities predisposing to hemorrhagic diasthesis.

An emergent screening angiogram is performed using local anesthetic and intravenous sedation. A 6-F sheath is placed within the femoral artery to provide adequate access for use of a guide catheter and microcatheter as necessary. The first vessel catheterized corresponds to the most likely symptomatic territory, i.e. the right common carotid artery would be catheterized in a patient with left-sided hemiplegia. Once the occluded vessel has been identified, an exchange-length wire is passed through the diagnostic catheter and the diagnostic catheter is exchanged for a guide catheter. As with all interventions, all catheters and sheaths are flushed with heparinized saline (5 IU cm^3). A microcatheter of at least 0.014" internal diameter is chosen. Utilizing digital subtraction angiography and road-mapping, the microcatheter is delivered over-the-wire to the occluded vessel. The microwire is passed through the clot and into the distal vessel, followed by the microcatheter. In our practice, time permitting, most patients undergo rapid sequence intubation, induction of general anesthesia and pentobarbital drip for brain protection. We believe this permits control of the patients' airway, minimizes motion, and allows control of ventilation and oxygenation (Figure 17.8A,B). A microcatheter angiographic run is performed to verify placement of the microcatheter distal to the site of occlusion. Approximately 2–3 mg of rt-PA is infused distal to the occlusion. Following this, the catheter is pulled into the region of the occlusion and an additional 5–6 mg is infused slowly into the clot. The catheter is then pulled proximal to the lesion and additional rt-PA is infused. Following infusion, serial angiography is performed to check the patency of the vessel. Generally, no more than 0.5 mg/kg rt-PA is administered intra-arterially. Adjuvant technical maneuvers during stroke thrombolysis include angioplasty of the clot, wire mani-

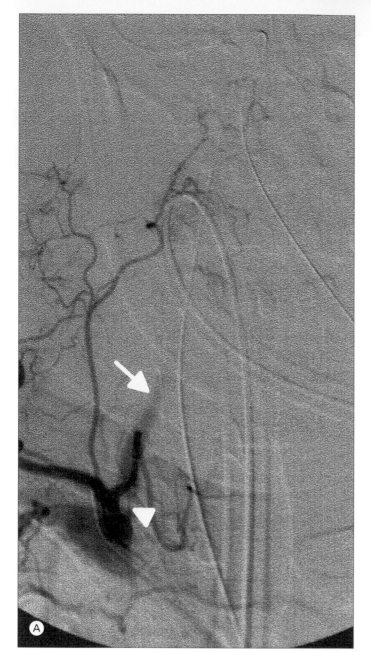

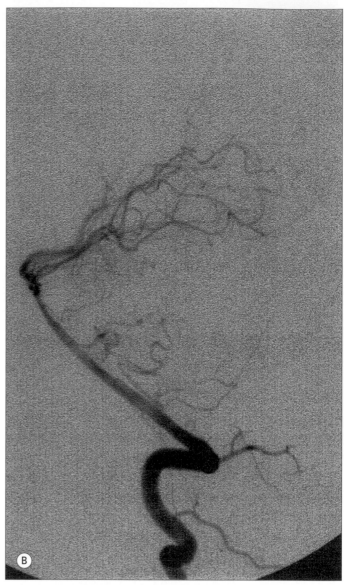

Figure 17.8 (A, B) A middle-aged man presented with symptoms of progressive brainstem dysfunction and ultimate coma. **(A)** An anteroposterior subclavian artery injection shows slow flow in the right vertebral artery (VA; arrow) and a severe right VA origin stenosis (arrowhead). Following endoluminal stent placement at the VA origin, recombinant tissue plasminogen activator thrombolysis, basilar artery stent placement, and infusion of a IIB/IIIA inhibitor, the vertebrobasilar circulation is re-established as seen following selective right VA angiography (lateral) **(B)**.

pulation, and occasionally stent placement in regions of inflow stenosis, i.e. the vertebral artery origin or the common carotid artery.[37] Occasionally, salvage therapy with a glycoprotein IIB/IIIA inhibitor is performed to lyse platelet-mediated subacute thrombosis resistant to thrombolysis with rt-PA.[38]

Angioplasty and papaverine for vasospasm

In spite of maximal medical therapy, delayed ischemic neurological deficit occurs in 20–30% of patients following aneurysmal subarachnoid hemorrhage. Symptomatic cerebral vasospasm is the delayed onset of arterial narrowing and occurs in as many as 20–30% of all patients suffering from aneurysmal subarachnoid hemorrhage.[39] Up to 7% of patients will die from subarachnoid-hemorrhage-related vasospasm and another 7% will suffer severe deficits secondary to vasospasm. Up to 40% of patients with delayed ischemic neurological deficit will develop ischemic infarctions.[40] The degree of spasm is related to the amount and length of time blood is in contact with the outside of the vessel. Breakdown products of hemoglobin have been implicated as probable causative agents of spasm. Immediate CT and cerebral angiography (in the absence of stroke on CT) are indicated when-

Table 17.3 Indications for intracranial angioplasty

Post-subarachnoid hemorrhage vasospasm
Hemodynamically significant stenosis
Pre- or post-stent dilatation

Table 17.4 Indications and contraindications for carotid artery stenting

Indications
Contralateral central nerve palsy
High carotid bifurcation
Post-radiation stenosis
Contralateral occlusion
Previous carotid endarterectomy with restenosis
Tandem lesion
Severe coronary artery disease

Contraindications
NASCET-eligible
Long lesion
Recent stroke
Intraluminal thrombus
Profound tortuosity

ever a patient has developed a progressive or acute change in neurologic status which fails to improve with medical therapy (Triple H therapy – hypervolemia, hemodilution, and hypertension).[41] While vasospasm can also be diagnosed with noninvasive modalities, such as transcranial Doppler, it is unable to predict severe angiographic vasospasm reliably in up to 50% of patients.[42] Treatment of arterial vasospasm involves microcatheter infusion of papaverine or balloon angioplasty. Infusion of intra-arterial papaverine is typically for treatment of small-vessel disease distal to the middle cerebral artery bifurcation, the A1/A2 junction, and the P1/P2 junction. Papaverine is considered a short-term solution (less than 24 hours). Balloon angioplasty is durable and the effect is immediate (Table 17.3).[43–45]

Angioplasty is performed under general anesthesia because of an increased risk of vessel rupture in awake patients with vasospasm. Angioplasty requires placement of a guide catheter through which the balloon is manipulated. Balloons are chosen to effect coverage of the vessel length to minimize the number of manipulations and are undersized by at least 0.5 mm to prevent overdistension of the target vessel. Others use graduated balloons from small to larger to minimize the risk of vessel rupture.[46] Patients are fully anticoagulated throughout the procedure. Angioplasty is performed within the major vessels of the circle of Willis, including the intracranial internal carotid artery, the M1 segment of the middle cerebral artery, the A1 segments, the dominant vertebral artery, the basilar artery, and occasionally the P1 segments of the posterior cerebral arteries. In spite of its immediate angiographic and clinical effects, the long-term benefits of angioplasty relative to outcome have yet to be proven.[47]

Extracranial and intracranial stenting for atherosclerotic disease

Carotid atherosclerotic disease

The role of carotid endarterectomy has been defined by multi-center trials for both symptomatic and asymptomatic carotid disease.[48,49] The patients selected for carotid endarterectomy in these trials were a highly selected group which in most cases excluded high-risk patients. High-risk patients are defined as those with liver, heart, kidney, or lung failure; cancer, cardiac valve disease, recent myocardial infarction or angina, previous carotid endarterectomy (CEA); and progressive neurologic deficit. Controlled trials of carotid stenting are currently being performed in these high-risk groups. It should be noted that carotid stenting is an unapproved procedure when performed outside clinical trials using devices not approved for carotid deployment. However, in spite of this, there are patients who benefit from carotid stenting. Arguably, patients should be considered candidates for carotid artery stenting when they have 70% or greater stenosis and a contralateral cranial nerve palsy, a surgically inaccessible carotid bifurcation (C2 or above), post-radiation stenosis, contralateral occlusion, a previous CEA with restenosis (Figure 17.9A,B),

tandem lesions, or severe coronary artery disease.[48,50–53] From the global Carotid Artery Stent Registry, the 30-day major and minor stroke risk and procedure-related death rate following carotid stenting is 4.77%. This compares favorably to carotid endarterectomy.[54] Currently, patients meeting the criteria set forth in the North American Symptomatic Carotid Endarterectomy Surgery Trial (NASCET), should undergo CEA. However, those patients deemed high risk (not meeting NASCET entry criteria) should be evaluated on an individual basis relative to local expertise in CEA versus carotid artery stenting (Table 17.4).

Patients presenting for carotid artery stenting undergo a full medical work-up as outlined previously. Three days prior to their procedure, an antiplatelet regimen consisting of clopidogrel (75 mg) and aspirin (325 mg) is initiated.[55] Patients are positioned supine and access is obtained with a 6-F sheath. Full systemic heparinization is achieved and verified by ACT. A diagnostic catheter is advanced into the target common carotid artery (Figure 17.10, 1). Using road-mapping, the catheter is advanced over-the-wire into the external carotid artery and the wire used to manipulate the diagnostic catheter is removed (Figure 17.10, 2, 3). A stiff, exchange-length wire is then placed into the external carotid artery and the diagnostic catheter is removed (Figure 17.10, 4–6). At this time, the previously placed sheath is also removed and a 6-F 90-cm sheath with an obturator is advanced over the wire and into the common carotid artery proximal to the carotid bifurcation (Figure 17.10, 7, 8). The obturator and wire are removed (Figure 17.10, 9, 10). As always, the sheath is continuously flushed with heparinized saline. Working views are obtained by performing angiography through the sheath. A working view shows the lesion, separates the external carotid from the internal carotid arteries, and provides bony landmarks for later stent deployment. Measurements are generated from digital subtraction angiographic images of the lesion. Lesion length, as well as the width of the internal and common carotid arteries, are obtained. An exchange-length microwire is advanced across the lesion and predilatation of the stenosis is performed with an angioplasty balloon (Figure 17.10, 11–13). Anecdotal evidence suggests that a longer length of dilatation may prevent in-stent stenosis. A self-expanding stent is chosen and oversized by approximately 1 mm relative to the common carotid artery. If the lesion is entirely within the internal carotid artery, the stent is sized

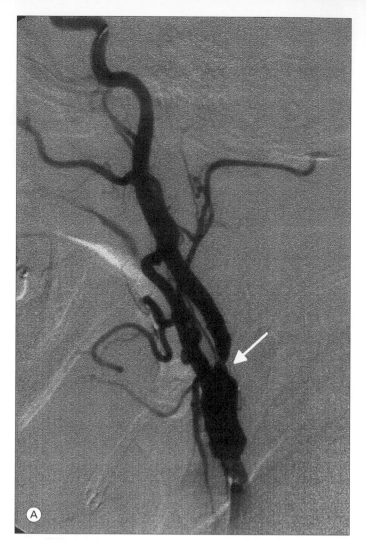
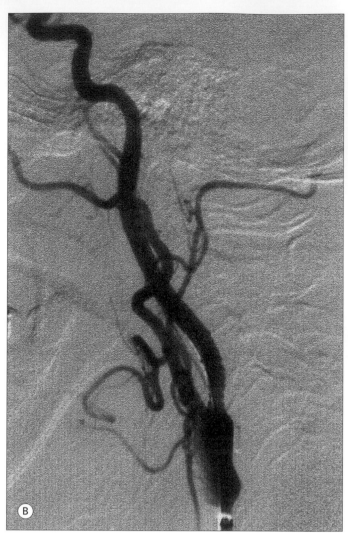

Figure 17.9 (A, B) A lateral left CCA angiogram showing a severe carotid stenosis (arrow) in an elderly woman 2 years following carotid endarterectomy. The patient presented with hemispheric transient ischemic attacks. Following placement of an endoluminal stent, the native luminal diameter has been re-established **(B)**.

1 mm over target artery diameter. It is important to cover the entire length of the lesion (Figure 17.10, 14–17). Crossing the external carotid origin is not a source of morbidity. Postdilatation is performed using a balloon sized to the diameter of the internal carotid artery (Figure 17.10, 18, 19). We usually base this on the diameter of the distal stent within the internal carotid artery. Following postdilatation, the angioplasty balloon is removed and a post-stent-placement angiographic run is obtained. Hemodynamic instability is a common occurrence during carotid angioplasty and stent placement is manifested by occasional episodes of aystole and hypotension. These are readily treated by deflation of the angioplasty balloon and small doses of atropine. Occasionally, pressors are necessary to augment blood pressure, which may remain diminished for several days following manipulation of the carotid baroreceptors.[56]

Vertebral artery atherosclerotic disease

Vertebrobasilar insufficiency is manifested by at least two of the following: (1) bilateral hemianopsia, (2) dysarthria, (3) diplopia, (4) gait ataxia, (5) bilateral motor or sensory complaints, and (6) dysmetria.[57] Numerous surgical procedures have been devised to treat extracranial and intracranial sources of vertebrobasilar disease. However, the definitive role of surgery has never been shown relative to extracranial vertebrobasilar disease and intervention is reserved for those patients who have failed medical therapies.[58–60] Surgical approaches are often technically demanding and associated with potential morbidity. Vertebral artery atherosclerotic disease occurs most commonly at the origin of the vertebral artery, a region readily accessible to endovascular intervention. Early reports suggest that vertebral artery origin stenting may be both safe and efficacious.[61–63]

Technically, the performance of vertebral artery stenting differs little from that of carotid artery stenting. Following adequate preoperative antiplatelet therapy, access to the femoral artery is obtained and intravenous heparin is administered to achieve an ACT of approximately 250–300 seconds. A 6-F guide catheter is placed within the subclavian artery and an exchange-length microwire is advanced across the vertebral artery origin lesion and stabilized in the distal vertebral artery (Figure 17.11A,B). A balloon expandable stent of appropriate diameter and length is chosen. Stents are sized to the normal vertebral artery diameter. The coronary stent is advanced across the lesion and gently pulled

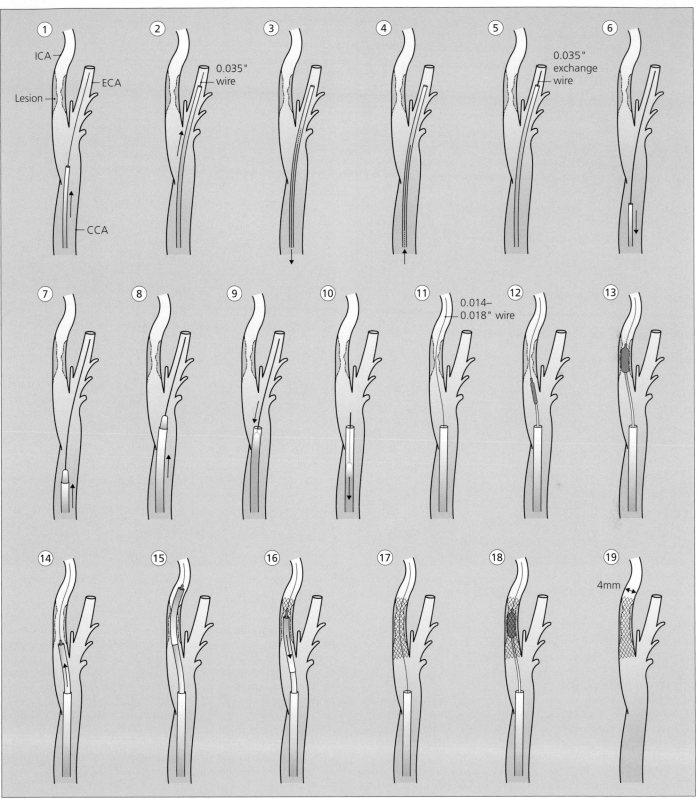

Figure 17.10 Placement of a carotid stent. (1) A lesion is seen in the internal carotid artery (ICA). The diagnostic catheter is in the common carotid artery (CCA), the guidewire is manipulated into the external carotid artery (ECA). (2) The diagnostic catheter is passed over-the-wire into the ECA. (3) The diagnostic guidewire is removed. (4), (5) A stiff, exchange-length wire is passed into the ECA through the diagnostic catheter. (6) The diagnostic catheter is removed. (7), (8) The sheath and obturator are passed over-the-wire into the CCA. (9), (10) The obturator and exchange-length wire are removed. (11) A microwire is manipulated across the lesion into the distal ICA proximal to the skullbase. (12), (13) An angioplasty balloon is advanced across the lesion and inflated. (14) The angioplasty balloon is removed. (15) The self-expanding stent is advanced over-the-wire, across the lesion. (16) Following positioning, the stent is unsheathed. (17) The stent deployment is complete. (18) Post-stent angioplasty is performed to remove any remaining area of in-stent stenosis. (19) Final view showing the carotid following stent-assisted angioplasty.

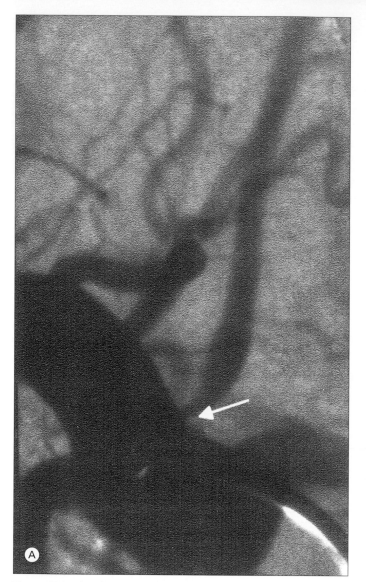

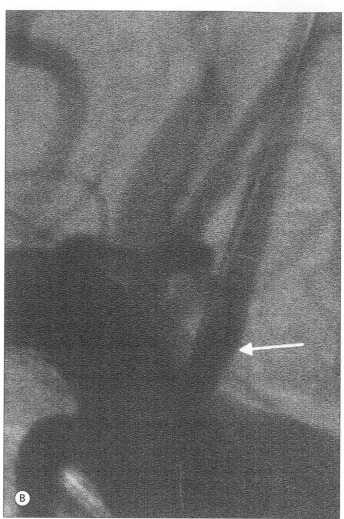

Figure 17.11 (A, B) A severe vertebral artery origin stenosis is noted on anteroposterior right subclavian artery angiography **(A)** (arrow). Following placement of an endoluminal coronary stent **(B)** the native luminal diameter is re-established (arrow).

back to bridge slightly the vertebral artery/subclavian junction. The stent is deployed at nominal pressures. Following stent placement, patients are maintained on antiplatelet therapy indefinitely.

Intracranial stenting

Intracranial stenting is not commonly performed. However, increasingly, patients refractory to medical management are referred for endovascular treatment. Recently, several small series have published the results associated with intracranial stenoses. Because of the difficulty of delivering relatively stiff coronary devices safely into the intracranial circulation, the role of intracranial stenting has been limited. Serious complications such as periprocedural death and brainstem stroke range from 0 to 36%.[64,65] Other complications have included in-stent stenosis, pseudoaneurysm formation, dissection, surgery for access-site-related complications, and hemiparesis. Stents have been delivered within the vertebrobasilar system and as far as the middle cerebral artery M1 segment.[64–68] Deployment of an intracranial stent is performed in a manner similar to stent placement

in the vertebral circulation (Figure 17.12A,B). An exchange-length transit wire is negotiated into the intracranial circulation using a microcatheter, followed by placement of the stent either primarily or after initial angioplasty. The ability to deliver an intracranial stent in the anterior cerebral circulation is determined by the morphology of the carotid as it passes through the skull base. In the vertebrobasilar system, the tortuosity of the vertebral artery often determines the ability to deliver a device into the skull. The ultimate role of intracranial stenting in the treatment of atherosclerotic disease has yet to be determined. It is currently reserved for patients in whom medical therapy has failed.

DISCUSSION

Endovascular therapies have improved rapidly in the last decade. Improvements in imaging, microcatheters, the development of compliant navigable stents and angioplasty balloons have led to steady increases in the number of patients successfully treated

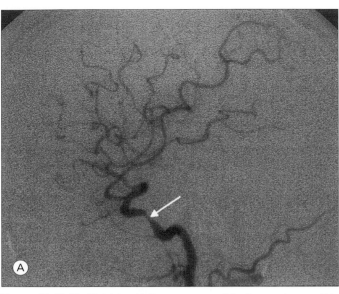
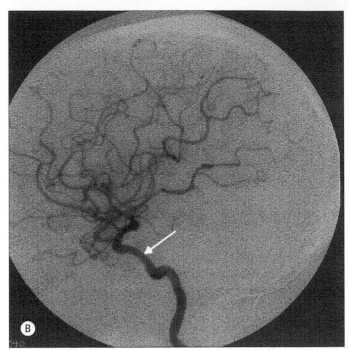

Figure 17.12 (A, B) A lateral left common carotid artery angiogram (A), shows a severe intracranial stenosis (arrow) in a man with crescendo transient ischemic attacks in spite of anticoagulation with warfarin. Following placement of an intracranial stent (arrow) (B) the normal internal carotid artery diameter has been re-established and the patient's symptoms resolved.

CLINICAL PEARLS

- Technical complications are a rare cause of morbidity, greater morbidity is caused by unrecognized comorbidities, i.e., contrast reaction, renal insufficiency, suboptimal anticoagulation, cardiac insufficiency.

- Retroperitoneal hematoma should be considered in any case in which unexplained fluctuations in blood pressure or heart rate occur.

- Protective embolization should be considered in any situation in which selective catheterization of an extracranial pathologic arterial branch cannot be achieved.

- Endovascular embolization of large "inoperable" arteriovenous malformations and arteriovenous fistulas should be considered to slow or halt the progression of neurologic deficit secondary to vascular "steal."

- Endovascular treatment of aneurysms is dependent on the morphology of the aneurysm neck and the ability to generate a "working" view which shows the aneurysm neck clearly delineated from the surrounding vessels.

- An aneurysm treated by endovascular means requires a period of regular follow-up to ensure that the lesion has not recurred.

- The decision to utilize intra-arterial recombinant tissue plasminogen activator must be made with consideration of the patient's neurologic deficit at presentation versus the likelihood of a good recovery without treatment. Patients with minimal neurologic deficit should not be considered for IA rT-PA.

- Intracranial angioplasty with semicompliant balloons of no greater diameter than the parent vessel is indicated for patients with hemodynamically significant lesions of the intracranial circulation.

- Carotid artery stenting is indicated for patients with high-risk surgical lesions. However, those patients with long lesions, a free thrombus, or difficult to negotiate anatomy are high-risk for endovascular treatment.

with endovascular techniques. In many cases, endovascular techniques have supplanted open surgery as the preferred means of therapy. The role of endovascular surgery will continue to expand as we search for minimally invasive, efficacious therapies that minimize morbidity and mortality.

REFERENCES

1. Higashida RT, Hopkins LN, Berenstein A, et al. Program requirements for residency/fellowship education in neuroendovascular surgery/interventional radiology: a special report on graduate medical education. Am J Neuroradiol 2000; 21: 1153–9.
2. Qureshi AI, Suri MF, Khan J, et al. Endovascular treatment of intracranial aneurysms by using Guglielmi detachable coils in awake patients: safety and feasibility. J Neurosurg 2001; 94: 880–95.
3. Cloft HJ, Joseph GJ, Dion JE. Risk of cerebral angiography in patients with subarachnoid hemorrhage, cerebral aneurysm, and arteriovenous malformation: a meta-analysis. Stroke 1999; 30: 317–20.
4. Qureshi AI, Luft AR, Sharma M, et al. Prevention and treatment of thromboembolic and ischemic complications associated with endovascular procedures: Part II – Clinical aspects and recommendations. Neurosurgery 2000; 46: 1360–76.
5. Dorfler A, Wanke I, Wiedemayer H, et al. Endovascular treatment of a giant aneursym of the internal carotid artery in a child with visual loss: case report. Neuropediatrics 2000; 31: 151–4.
6. Friedmann WA, Chadwick GM, Verhoeven FJ, et al. Monitoring of somatosensory evoked potentials during surgery of the middle cerebral artery aneurysms. Neurosurgery 1991; 29: 83–8.
7. Taki W, Nishi S, Yamashita K, et al. Selection and combination of various endovascular techniques in the treatment of giant aneurysms. J Neurosurg 1992; 77: 37–42.
8. Anon V, Aymard A, Gobin Y. Balloon occlusion of the internal carotid artery in 40 cases of giant intracavernous aneurysms: technical aspects, cerebral monitoring, and results. Neuroradiology 1992; 34: 245–51.
9. Nimi Y, Berenstein A, Setton A, et al. Occlusion of the internal carotid artery based on a simple tolerance test. Intervent Neuroradiol 1996; 2: 289–96.
10. Perez-Arjona A, DelProposto Z, Sehgal V, et al. New techniques in cerebral imaging. Neurol Res 2002; 24(S1): S17–S26.
11. Mayer TE, Hamann GF, Baranczyk J, et al. Dynamic CT perfusion imaging of acute stroke. Am J Neuroradiol 2000; 21: 1441–9.
12. Wakhloo AK, Juefngling FD, Van Velthoven V, et al. Extended preoperative polyvinyl alcohol microembolization of intracranial meningiomas: assessment of two embolization techniques. Am J Neuroradiol 1993; 14: 583–6.
13. Berman MF, Sciacca RR, Spellman JP, et al. The epidemiology of brain arteriovenous malformations. Neurosurgery 2000; 47:389–397.
14. Fisher WS. Intracranial vascular malformations: clinical presentations. In: Batjer HH, Caplan LR, Friberg L, et al. (eds), Cerebrovascular Disease. Philadelphia: Lippincott-Raven; 1997: 657–67.
15. Troupp H, Marttila I, Halonen V. Arteriovenous malformations of the brain. Prognosis without operation. Acta Neurochir (Wein) 1970; 22: 125–8.
16. Ondra SL, Troupp H, George ED, et al. The natural history of symptomatic arteriovenous malformations of the brain: a 24-year follow-up assessment. J Neurosurg 1990; 73: 387–91.
17. Wilkins, RH. Natural history of intracranial vascular malformations: a review. Neurosurgery 1985; 16: 421–30.
18. Smith KA, Shetter A, Speiser B, et al. Angiographic follow-up in 37 patients after radiosurgery for cerebral arteriovenous

19. Deruty R, Pelissou GI, Morel C, et al. Reflections on the management of cerebral arteriovenous malformations. Surg Neurol 1998; 50: 245–55.
20. Gobin YP, Laurent A, Merienne L, et al. Treatment of brain arteriovenous malformations by embolization and radiosurgery. J Neurosurg 1996; 85: 19–28.
21. Nussbaum ES, Heros RC, Camarata PJ. Surgical treatment of intracranial arteriovenous malformation with an analysis of cost-effectiveness. Clin Neurosurg 1995; 42: 348–69.
22. DeMeritt JS, Pile-Spellman J, Mast H, et al. Outcome analysis of preoperative embolization with N-butyl cyanoacrylate in cerebral arteriovenous malformations. Am J Neuroradiol 1995; 16: 1801–7.
23. Al-Yamany M, Terbrugge K, Willinsky R, et al. Palliative embolization of brain arteriovenous malformation presenting with progressive neurological deficit. Intervent Neuroradiol 2000; 6: 177–83.
24. Yakes WF, Krauth L, Ecklund J, et al. Ethanol endovascular management of brain arteriovenous malformations: initial results. Neurosurgery 1997; 40: 1152–4.
25. Choi IS. Embolization of Intracranial and Spinal Tumors. Neurosurgical Topics. Rolling Meadows, IL: AANS Publications; 1995: 263–77.
26. Mullan S, Johnson DL. Combined sagittal and lateral sinus dural fistulae occlusion. J Neurosurg 1995; 82: 159–65.
27. Awad IA, Little JR, Akarawi WP, et al. Intracranial dural arteriovenous malformations: factors predisposing to an aggressive neurological course. J Neurosurg 1990; 72: 839–50.
28. Duffau H, Lopes M, Janosevic V, et al. Early rebleeding from intracranial dural arteriovenous fistulas: report of 20 cases and review of the literature. J Neurosurg 1999; 90: 78–84.
29. Roy D, Raymond J. The role of transvenous embolization in the treatment of intracranial dural arteriovenous fistulas. Neurosurgery 1997; 40: 1133–41.
30. Djindjian M, Djindjian R, Rey A, et al. Intradural extramedullary spinal arterio-venous malformations fed by the anterior spinal artery. Surg Neurol 1977; 8: 85–93.
31. Anson JA, Spetzler RF. Interventional neuroradiology for spinal pathology. Clin Neurosurg 1992; 39: 388–417.
32. Kassell NF, Torner JC, Jane JA, et al. The international cooperative study on the timing of aneurysm surgery. Part 2: surgical results. J Neurosurg 1990; 73: 37–47.
33. Taylor TN, Davis PH, Torner JC, et al. Lifetime cost of stroke in the United States. Stroke 1996; 27: 1459–66.
34. Kaste M, Fogelholm R, Rissanen A. Economic burden of stroke and the evaluation of new therapies. Public Health 1998; 112: 103–12.
35. Anonymous. Tissue plasminogen activator for acute ischemic stroke. The National Institute of Neurological Disorders and Stroke rt-PA Stroke Study Group. N Engl J Med 1995; 333: 1581–7.
36. Furlan A, Higashida R, Wechsler L, et al. Intraarterial prourokinase for acute ischemic stroke. The PROACT II study: A randomized controlled trial. Prolyse in acute cerebral thromboembolism. JAMA 1999; 2822: 2003–11.
37. Ringer AJ, Qureshi AI, Fessler RD, et al. Angioplasty of intracranial occlusion resistant to thrombolysis in acute stroke. Neurosurgery 2001; 48: 1282–8.
38. Ringer AJ, Tomsick TA. Developments in endovascular therapy for acute ischemic stroke. Neurol Res 2002; 24(S1): S43–6.
39. Kassell NF, Sasaki T, Colohan AR, et al. Cerebral vasospasm following aneurysmal subarachnoid hemorrhage. Stroke 1985; 16: 562–72.
40. Martin NA, Saver J. Intensive care management of subarachnoid hemorrhage, ischemic stroke, hemorrhagic stroke. Clin Neurosurg 1997; 45: 101–12.

41. Awad IA, Carter LP, Spetzler RF, et al. Clinical vasospasm after subarachnoid hemorrhage: response to hypervolemic hemodilution and arterial hypertension. Stroke 1987; 18: 365–72.

42. Vora YY, Suarez-Almazor M, et al. The role of transcranial Doppler in the diagnosis of cerebral vasospasm following subarachnoid hemorrhage. Neurosurgery 1999; 44: 1237–47.

43. Elliott JP, Newell DW, Lam DJ, et al. Comparison of balloon angioplasty and papaverine infusion for the treatment of vasospasm following aneurysmal subarachnoid hemorrhage. J Neurosurg 1998; 88: 277–84.

44. Barnwell SL, Higashida RT, Halbach VV, et al. Transluminal angioplasty of intracerebral vessels for cerebral arterial spasm: reversal of neurological deficits after delayed treatment. Neurosurgery 1989; 25: 424–9.

45. Bejjani GK, Bank WO, Olan WJ, et al. The efficacy and safety of angioplasty for cerebral vasospasm after subarachnoid hemorrhage. Neurosurgery 1998; 42: 510–17.

46. Song JK, Elliott JP, Eskridge JM. Neuroradiologic diagnosis and treatment of vasospasm. Neuroimaging Clin N Am 1997; 7: 819–35.

47. Polin RS, Coenen VM, Hansen CA, et al. Efficacy of transluminal angioplasty for the management of symptomatic cerebral vasospasm following aneurysmal subarachnoid hemorrhage. J Neurosurg 2000; 92: 284–90.

48. Barnett HJM, Taylor DW, Eliasziw M, et al. for the North American Symptomatic Carotid Endarterectomy Trial Collaborators. Benefit of carotid endarterectomy in patients with symptomatic moderate or severe stenosis. N Engl J Med 1998; 339: 1415–25.

49. Executive Committee for the Asymptomatic Carotid Atherosclerosis Study. Endarterectomy for asymptomatic carotid artery stenosis. JAMA 1995; 273: 1421–8.

50. Mericle RA, Kim SH, Lanzino G, et al. Carotid artery angioplasty and use of stents in high-risk patients with contralateral occlusions. J Neurosurg 1999; 90: 1031–6.

51. Kim SH, Mericle RA, Lanzino G, et al. Carotid angioplasty and stent placement in patients with tandem stenoses1995. Neurosurgery 1998; 43: 708 (abstract).

52. Lopes DK, Mericle RA, Lanzino G, et al. Carotid angioplasty and stenting before coronary artery bypass grafting. Neurosurgery 1998; 43: 686 (abstract).

53. Moore WS, Barnett HJM, Beebe HG, et al. AHA Medical/Scientific Statement Special Report: Guidelines for Carotid Endarterectomy. A multidisciplinary consensus statement from the Ad Hoc Committee, American Heart Association. Stroke 1995; 26: 188–201.

54. Wholey M. Global Carotid Artery Stent Registry: updated results. Carotid Intervent 1999; 1: 94–6.

55. Fessler RD, Guterman LR, Hopkins LN. Carotid artery stenosis: medical, surgical, and endovascular approaches. Tech Vasc Interv Radiol 2000; 3: 71–4.

56. Vitek JJ, Roubin GS, New G, et al. Carotid stenting. Tech Vasc Interv Radiol 2000; 3: 75–85.

57. Whisnant JP, Cartlidge NA, Elveback LR. Carotid and vertebral-basilar transient ischemic attacks: effect of anticoagulants, hypertension, and cardiac disorders on survival and stroke occurrence – a population study. Ann Neurol 1978; 3: 107–15.

58. Allen GS, Cohen RJ, Preziosi TJ. Microsurgical endarterectomy of the intracranial vertebral artery for vertebrobasilar transient ischemic attacks. Surgical correction of lesions affecting the second portion of the vertebral artery. Neurosurgery 1981; 8: 56–9.

59. Ausman JI, Diaz FG, los Reyes RA, et al. Posterior circulation revascularization. Superficial temporal artery to superior cerebellar artery anastomosis. J Neurosurg 1982; 56: 766–76.

60. Berguer R, Morasch MD, Kline RA. A review of 100 consecutive reconstructions of the distal vertebral artery for embolic and hemodynamic disease. J Vasc Surg 1998; 27: 852–9.

61. Chastain HD II, Campbell MS, Iyer S, et al. Extracranial vertebral artery stent placement: in-hospital and follow-up results. J Neurosurg 1999; 91: 547–52.

62. Fessler RD, Wakhloo AJ, Lanzino G, et al. Stent placement for vertebral artery occlusive disease: preliminary clinical experience. Neurosurg Focus 1998; 5: 15.

63. Fessler RD, Wakhloo AJ, Lanzino G, et al. Transradial approach for vertebral artery stenting: technical case report. Neurosurgery 2000; 6: 1524–8.

64. Levy EI, Hanel RA, Bendok BR, et al. Staged stent-assisted angioplasty for symptomatic intracranial vertebrobasilar stenosis. J Neurosurg 2002; 97: 1294–301.

65. Levy EI, Horwitz MB, Koebbe CJ, et al. Transluminal stent-assisted angioplasty of the intracranial vertebrobasilar system for medically refractory, posterior circulation ischemia: early results. Neurosurgery 2001; 48: 1215–21.

66. Gomez CR, Misra VK, Campbell MS, et al. Elective stenting of symptomatic middle cerebral artery stenosis. Am J Neuroradiol 2000; 21: 971–3.

67. Barakate MS, Snook KL, Harrington TJ, et al. Angioplasty and stenting in the posterior cerebral circulation. J Endovasc Ther 2001; 8: 558–64.

68. Sam Shin Y, Yon Kim S, Young Bang O, et al. Early experiences of elective stenting for symptomatic stenosis of the M1 segment of the middle cerebral artery: reports of three cases and review of the literature. J Clin Neurosci 2003; 10: 53–9.

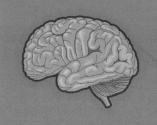

THE MULTIPLY INJURED PATIENT

18

Jack E Wilberger

Neurosurgeons are frequently faced with diagnosing and treating head and spine injuries in multitraumatized patients. The neurosurgeon may function as a member of a coordinated trauma team or direct general surgeons and other subspecialists in the management of multitrauma patients. Head and spinal/spinal cord injuries rarely occur in isolation; the incidence of associated injuries is well known (Figure 18.1).[1–3] In addition, the impact of associated injuries and subsequent pathophysiologic derangements, such as hypoxia and hypotension, on the morbidity and mortality from head injury have been clearly delineated.

Multitraumatized patients are assessed and treatment priorities are established based on the nature of the injuries and the stability of vital signs. Familiarity with assessment and management protocols for multitrauma patients gives the neurosurgeon a better appreciation of the interrelationships in multisystem injury, enabling him or her to plan an effective sequence of diagnostic testing and treatment of the associated head and/or spine injury.

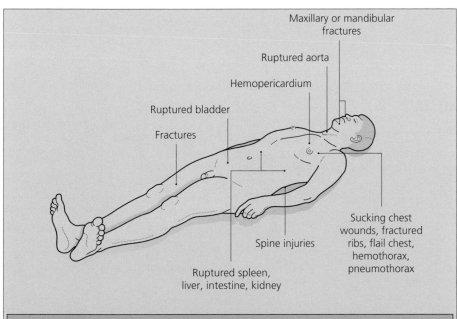

Figure 18.1 Multiple system injuries associated with head and spinal cord injury.

Maxillary or mandibular fractures

Ruptured aorta

Hemopericardium

Ruptured bladder

Fractures

Sucking chest wounds, fractured ribs, flail chest, hemothorax, pneumothorax

Spine injuries

Ruptured spleen, liver, intestine, kidney

Multisystem injury		
	Head injury	Spinal cord injury
Pulmonary	78%	10.5%
Musculoskeletal	43%	18%
Abdominal	53%	2.5%
Cardiovascular	3%	1.5%
Endocrine	23%	
Spine	6%	
Head		16%

Figure 18.2 Trauma management protocol – American College of Surgeons Advanced Trauma Life Support.

Primary survey

Airway:
    airway maintenance
        with C-spine control

Breathing

Circulation:
    hemorrhage control

Disability

Exposure:
    remove all clothes
        for examination

Resuscitation

Ventilate/oxygenate

Shock management

NG/urinary catheters

Operating room

Uncontrollable shock

Life-threatening injuries

Secondary survey

Complete system-by-system examination

Radiographs (chest, C-spine)

Peritoneal lavage

CT scan

Complete radiographs

Definitive care

ASSESSMENT OF THE MULTITRAUMA PATIENT

Multitraumatized patients require continual reassessment to establish treatment priorities. Most trauma protocols involve a rapid primary assessment of the patient, resuscitation of vital signs, a more detailed secondary assessment, and initiation of definitive care (Figure 18.2).[4]

The primary assessment of the multitrauma patient has three main goals: establishment and protection of the airway, ventilation, and maintenance or restoration of normal hemodynamic parameters. However, immediately life-threatening injuries – cardiac tamponade, tension pneumothorax, exsanguinating hemorrhage – may require operative intervention after securing airway control but before further assessment.

Airway obstruction may manifest itself in a variety of ways – inability to speak (laryngeal injury), stridor, or abnormal upper airway sounds, such as snoring, gurgling, or gargling. Hypoxia and/or hypercarbia from airway obstruction may result in agitation, combativeness, or obtundation. The most common causes of airway obstruction – prolapse of the tongue, foreign bodies, retained secretions, blood – are easiest to alleviate with such maneuvers as the chin lift, jaw thrust, suctioning, and oropharyngeal or nasopharyngeal airways (Figure 18.3). It must be kept in mind that airway obstruction is not only an acute phenomenon but may also be progressive and recurrent. Thus these maneuvers may need to be repeated frequently. If they are primarily or secondarily unsuccessful, airway control must be established by intubation. Endotracheal intubation – orally or nasally – is generally the preferred route. While intubation is being initiated, ventilation of the patient continues to be of paramount importance. Prolonged attempts at intubation should be accompanied by concomitant intermittent ventilation.

In some patients, such as those with massive facial fractures, laryngeal fractures, or tracheal obstruction, endotracheal intubation may be technically impossible. Inability to intubate demands creation of a surgical airway. Surgical cricothyroidotomy appears to provide the quickest and safest route to definitive airway control (Figure 18.4). Emergency tracheostomy has been largely abandoned because of its time-consuming nature and tendency to cause excessive blood loss.

Once the airway is securely established and maintained, adequate ventilation must be provided. Positive pressure breathing techniques supplemented by 100% oxygen are the surest means to this end.

Injured patients who present in shock are near death; thus it is vitally important to recognize shock in the multitrauma patient and to identify rapidly its probable cause. Bleeding may be external and controllable by applying direct pressure over lacerations or open extremity fractures. However, in the blunt trauma victim bleeding is just as likely to be internal, within the retroperitoneum, abdomen, or thorax, and thus occult and not directly controllable.

There is a graded physiologic response to hemorrhage based on the volume of blood loss and compensatory mechanisms that may prevent a significant fall in blood pressure until over 30% of

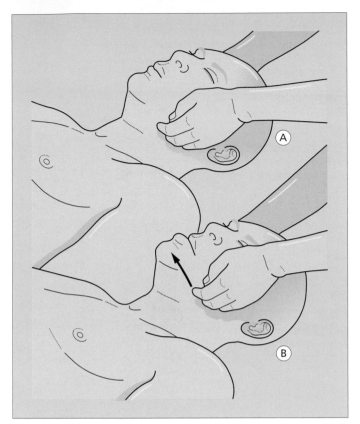

Figure 18.3 Airway management techniques in the unconscious patient. The jaw thrust maneuver is shown.

blood volume is lost (Table 18.1). The earliest signs of shock are tachycardia and cutaneous vasoconstriction, not hypotension. A mean arterial pressure of 65–70 mmHg (80–90 mmHg systolic) is the goal in maintaining adequate organ perfusion. Palpating the pulse may indicate systolic blood pressure – the presence of a radial pulse indicates a systolic pressure greater than 80, a femoral pulse indicates one greater than 70, and a carotid pulse indicates a systolic pressure greater than 60.

The first step in fluid resuscitation is establishing vascular access. A large bore 14- to 16-gauge catheter in the peripheral veins is preferable, but saphenous or femoral vein cut-down is an acceptable alternative. Central lines are generally reserved for monitoring rather than initial resuscitation because they are potentially complicated by pneumothorax, hydrothorax, air embolism, or infection.

Fluid resuscitation is generally initiated with isotonic electrolyte solutions (Ringer's lactate, normal saline). Such solutions effectively increase intravascular volume immediately, while over time correcting interstitial fluid deficits.[5] If a 1–2 litre isotonic fluid bolus (20 mL/kg in children) does not stabilize vital signs, blood replacement should be initiated. Fully cross-matched blood is preferable; however, this is usually too time-consuming in the acute setting. Thus most early transfusions use type-specific or type O packed cells. Recently, considerable interest has arisen over the use of hypertonic solutions (3% saline) in trauma resuscitation because of the small volume required and the rapid restoration of arterial pressure. Holcroft and colleagues reported significant improvement in patient survival when hypertonic solutions were used in resuscitation during transport.[6]

Isotonic fluid and/or blood may now be replaced at very high infusion rates (up to 1 L/min) using a variety of rapid infusion

Table 18.1 Estimated fluid and blood requirements* (based on patient's initial presentation)

	Class I	Class II	Class III	Class IV
Blood loss (mL)	up to 750	750–1500	1500–2000	2000 or more
Blood loss (%blood volume)	up to 15%	15–30%	30–40%	40% or more
Pulse rate	< 100	> 100	> 120	≥ 140
Blood pressure	normal	normal	decreased	decreased
Pulse pressure (mmHg)	normal or increased	decreased	decreased	decreased
Capillary blanch test	normal	positive	positive	positive
Respiratory rate	14–20	20–30	30–40	> 35
Urine output (mL/hour)	≥ 30	20–30	5–15	negligible
Central nervous system mental status	slightly anxious	mildly anxious	anxious and confused	confused–lethargic
Fluid replacement (3:1 rule)	crystalloid	crystalloid	crystalloid + blood	crystalloid + blood

*For a 70-kg male.
Reproduced with permission from the American College of Surgeons Committee on Trauma.
Advanced Trauma Life Support Course Instruction Manual, 1985: 185.

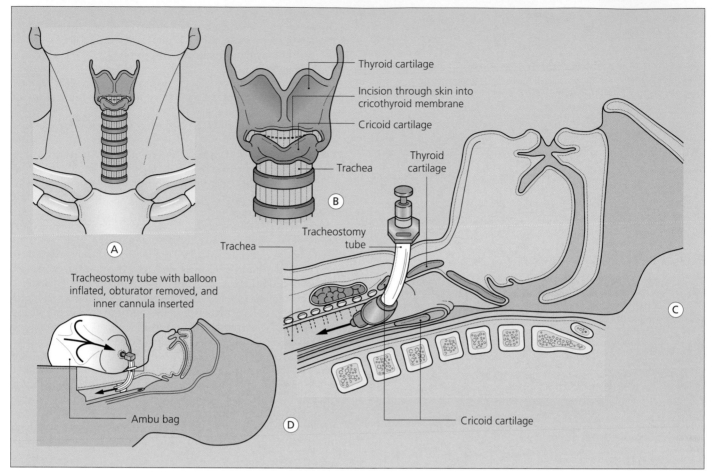

Figure 18.4 (A–D) Surgical technique of cricothyroidotomy. (Modified with permission from the American College of Surgeons Committee on Trauma. *Advanced Trauma Life Support Course Instruction Manual* 1985: 176.)

devices. Such rapid replacement may, however, predispose the patient to problems such as hypothermia, coagulopathy, or fluid overload. Thus all replacement fluids should be warmed prior to administration. If more than 10 units of blood must be replaced, platelets should also be given to reduce the risk of dilutional coagulopathy.

The pneumatic antishock garment is frequently used during transport and resuscitation of the multitraumatized patient to assist in blood pressure control (Figure 18.5). It sustains blood pressure by increasing total peripheral resistance. However, the garment is not a substitute for and should not delay adequate volume replacement. The pneumatic antishock garment has been particularly useful in splinting and hemorrhage control for pelvic and multiple lower extremity fractures. It may also help in tamponading soft tissue hemorrhage in the lower half of the body. Because of its effects on the circulatory system, the pneumatic antishock garment is contraindicated in patients whose injuries are complicated by myocardial infarction, congestive heart failure, or pulmonary edema.

When there is a transient or minimal response to initial fluid resuscitation a variety of reasons must be considered. The two primary concerns are that fluid loss was greater than initially estimated or that significant blood loss is continuing. The former requires a readjustment in fluid replacement calculations, the latter demands immediate surgical intervention. Other possible

etiologies for continued or recurrent hypotension include ventilation problems, cardiogenic shock, acute massive gastric distention, diabetic acidosis, hypoadrenalism, and neurogenic shock.

In neurogenic or vasomotor spinal shock a significant drop in blood pressure is related to an underlying spinal cord injury. The hypotension results from sympathetic vascular denervation with subsequent vasodilatation producing a shock-like picture. In the patient who is multiply injured it is sometimes difficult to determine whether the low blood pressure is secondary to associated blood loss or related to the spinal injury. With spinal vasomotor shock, fluid resuscitation is often ineffective because of the abnormal vascular tone, and vasopressors may be necessary for adequate restoration of normal blood pressure (Table 18.2).

The final components of the primary survey are a mini-neurologic examination and complete exposure of the patient to allow adequate examination of all body areas for obvious injury. At this stage the neurologic examination is generally limited to determining if the patient is awake and alert, and appropriately or inappropriately responsive to stimuli or unconscious.

The secondary survey begins when the patient is satisfactorily stabilized, the primary assessment is completed, and fluid resuscitation is progressing. This survey involves an in-depth examination of all body systems – head/neck, chest, abdomen, extremities – as well as important diagnostic studies such as radiographs, peritoneal lavage, and laboratory studies.

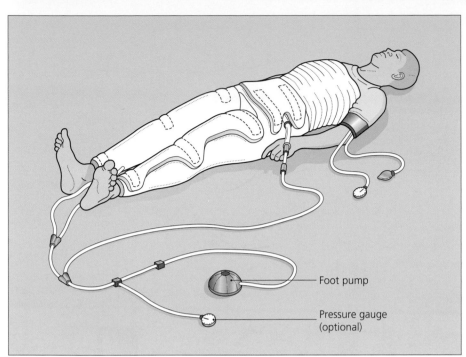

Figure 18.5 Pneumatic antishock garment.

Foot pump

Pressure gauge
(optional)

Examination of the head and neck aims to clarify intracranial injuries using the Glasgow Coma Score as well as to identify penetrating wounds and closed maxillofacial injuries. The chest is examined visually for penetrating and/or sucking wounds and flail segments and by auscultation for absent or diminished breath sounds and distant heart sounds. Immediate closed tube thoracostomy is indicated for penetrating wounds or pneumo- or hemothorax (Figure 18.6). For pneumothorax the optimal chest tube is placed in the second intercostal space, midclavicular line, and directed superiorly and anteriorly. For penetrating wounds and hemothorax the tube is placed in the seventh or eighth intercostal space, midaxillary line, and directed posteriorly and inferiorly. Two tubes may be appropriate for combined injuries. After placement the tube must be continually monitored for blood loss. If more than 1500 mL of blood is already in the chest or blood loss continues at a rate exceeding 200 mL/hour, thoracotomy is indicated.

Immediate pericardiocentesis is indicated if cardiac tamponade is suspected because the patient has a penetrating injury in the vicinity of the heart, a distended neck vein, and/or muffled heart sounds.

The abdomen is first inspected for evidence of penetrating injury (e.g. gunshot or stab wounds); given the high incidence of associated intra-abdominal injury, exploratory laparotomy is virtually always indicated. The traditional findings of intra-abdominal injury include pain, guarding, rigidity, and loss of bowel sounds. However, in up to 20% of alert patients the abdominal examination may be misleading after blunt trauma. Thus the ancillary diagnostic tests, such as peritoneal lavage and abdominal computed tomography (CT) scanning (discussed later), are often of primary importance in determining the presence or absence of intra-abdominal injury.

Extremity trauma is present in up to 80% of multitrauma patients but is rarely life-threatening. Splinting is usually accomplished in the prehospital treatment phase. Examination is directed to identifying and protecting open fractures and dislocations, and determining if there are associated vascular or neurologic injuries. Traumatic amputations, bilateral femoral shaft fractures, and major pelvic fractures demand increased attention and often rapid intervention because they are potentially life-threatening.

The secondary survey is completed with a full neurologic evaluation to determine the degree and extent of any associated head or spinal cord injuries and the necessity for skull X-rays, spine radiographs, CT scan, or magnetic resonance imaging (MRI) studies.

In any multiply injured patient tetanus prophylaxis must be considered. The need for tetanus immunization depends on the patient's immunization status and the risk of the wound. Immunization status is often not elicitable and many patients must be treated prophylactically (Table 18.3).

The trauma management protocol is completed when definitive care has been instituted for each organ system injury. However, trauma is not necessarily a static process. As one problem is addressed another may surface, or underlying medical problems may assume increasing importance. As an example, sepsis and organ failure are the most common causes of late death from trauma. Therefore, a high index of suspicion must be maintained, the trauma patient must be constantly re-evaluated, and diagnostic or treatment approaches should be readjusted to ensure optimal chance for recovery.

Table 18.2 Clinical differentiation of hemorrhagic versus neurogenic shock

	Hemorrhagic shock	Neurogenic shock
Pulse	tachycardia	bradycardia
Skin	cool, clammy	dry, warm
Mental status	altered	normal
Urine output	low	normal

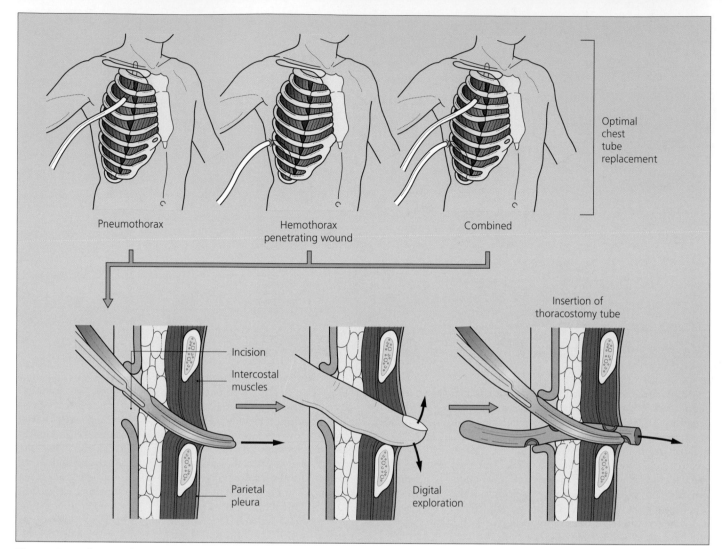

Pneumothorax

Hemothorax
penetrating wound

Combined

Optimal
chest
tube
replacement

Insertion of
thoracostomy tube

Incision

Intercostal
muscles

Parietal
pleura

Digital
exploration

Figure 18.6 Technique of closed tube thoracostomy.

TRAUMA SCORING SYSTEMS

A basic understanding of the systems for scoring trauma severity is important when dealing with multitrauma patients. The Glasgow Coma Score is a widely accepted scoring system used to quantify head injury severity, guide treatment, and give preliminary prognostic information. Similar scoring systems have been developed for the multitrauma patient. Most are based on the Abbreviated Injury Scale (AIS), which provides a numerical score to each injured system based on severity. The higher the score, the more likely it is that the patient will die. However, a simple arithmetic relationship does not exist. The Injury Severity Score (ISS) is derived from the AIS by summing the squares of the AIS values. The ISS has been shown to correlate not only with mortality but also with the length of hospital stay and the degree of permanent disability, provided the patient's age is taken into account.[7] Two major criticisms of the ISS are that it gives inadequate weight to associated head injuries and that it requires detailed identification of anatomic injury, which is usually only accurately determined after definitive management has occurred.

The Trauma Score was developed to overcome these problems by measuring the physiologic state (i.e. the cardiovascular, respiratory, and central nervous systems) of the patient immediately after injury (Table 18.4).[8] The Trauma Score is appropriate for both assessment and trauma triage, and can be applied at the scene of the injury. Experience has demonstrated that patients likely to benefit from prompt diagnosis and timely definitive care at a trauma center have scores of twelve or less at the scene of injury.

More recently a system known as ASCOT has been evaluated as a more sensitive descriptor of multisystem injury. ASCOT separates severe head, thoracic, and abdominal injuries from other injuries in an attempt to provide better information for triage, treatment, and prognosis after trauma.

HYPOXIA, HYPOTENSION, AND NEUROLOGIC INJURY

The interrelationships of multisystem and neurologic injury are nowhere more clearly defined than they are regarding hypoxia and/or hypotension (Figure 18.7). Recognition and prevention

Table 18.3 Tetanus prophylaxis of the injured patient

History of tetanus immunization (no. of doses)	Clean, minor wounds		Tetanus-prone wounds	
	TD*	TIG	TD*	TIG[†]
Uncertain	yes	no	yes	yes
0–1	yes	no	yes	yes
2	yes	no	yes	no[‡]
3 or more	no[§]	no	no[¶]	no

TD, tetanus–diphtheria toxoid; TIG, tetanus immune globulin.
* For individuals less than 7 years old, DTP (diptheria, pertussis, tetanus; DT, if pertussis vaccine is contraindicated) is preferred to tetanus toxoid alone. For individuals 7 years old and older, TD is preferred to tetanus toxoid alone.
[†]When TIG and TD are given concurrently, separate syringes and separate sites should be used.
[‡]Yes, if wound is more than 24 hours old.
[§]Yes, if more than 10 years since last dose.
[¶]Yes, if more than 5 years since last dose. (More frequent boosters are not needed and can accentuate side-effects.)
Reproduced with permission from the American College of Surgeons Committee on Trauma. *Advanced Trauma Life Support Course Instruction Manual*, 1985: 277.

Table 18.4 Trauma score

	Points/score
Respiratory rate	
≥36/min	2
25–35/min	3
10–24/min	4
0–9/min	1
None	0
Respiratory expansion	
Normal	1
Shallow	0
Retractive	0
Systolic blood pressure	
≥90 mm Hg	4
70–89 mm Hg	3
50–69 mm Hg	2
0–49 mm Hg	1
No pulse	0
Capillary return	
Normal	2
Delayed	1
None	0
Glasgow Coma Score (GCS)	
Eye opening	
Spontaneous	4
To voice	3
To pain	2
None	1
Verbal response	
Oriented	5
Confused	4
Inappropriate words	3
Incomprehensible words	2
None	1
Motor response	
Obeys command	6
Localizes pain	5
Withdraw (pain)	4
Flexion (pain)	3
Extension (pain)	2
None	1
Total Glasgow Coma Score points	**Score**
14–15	5
11–13	4
8–10	3
5–7	2
3–4	1
Total	1–16

or treatment of associated hypoxia and hypotension in the multitraumatized, neurologically injured patient are of paramount importance. Miller and colleagues were among the first, in 1978, to point out the magnitude of the problem.[9] In 100 consecutive severely head-injured patients on initial emergency room evaluation, 13% were hypotensive (systolic blood pressure < 95 mmHg) and 30% were hypoxic (P_{O_2} < 65 mmHg). Five years later pilot data from 581 comatose head-injured patients in the National Coma Data Bank found almost 20% to be hypoxic (P_{O_2} < 60 mmHg) and 31% to be hypotensive (systolic blood pressure < 90 mmHg) before definitive hospital treatment.

The increased morbidity and mortality in hypoxic/hypotensive head-injured patients has been clearly established. As early as 1977 Rose and co-workers found a 54% incidence of these factors in a group of patients who "talked and died."[10] Gildenberg and Makela found a correlation between time from head injury to intubation and outcome.[11] Similarly, the National Coma Data Bank found a 20% incidence of hypoxia in head-injured patients with a good outcome while 45% of patients with vegetative/dead outcomes had been hypoxic.[2] It has also been found that there may be an association between hypoxia and a greater incidence of increased intracranial pressure.[12] Many studies have also shown an association between acute hypotension and poor outcome after head injury.[2,3,10]

The clinical effects of superimposed hypoxia and/or hypotension on the spinal cord injury patient have not been as clearly delineated. However, it is known from research data that hypoxia and ischemia are important in the propagation of further neuronal damage after spinal cord injury.[13]

THE NEUROLOGICALLY INJURED MULTITRAUMATIZED PATIENT

The multitraumatized neurologically injured patient may present particular difficulties in assessment and management. Specific questions often raised in this regard include airway protection and maintenance in association with potential spine injury; fluid resuscitation in the head-injured patient; abdominal evaluation in the unconscious or spinal cord injury patient; and timing of CT/MRI during initial evaluation and resuscitation.

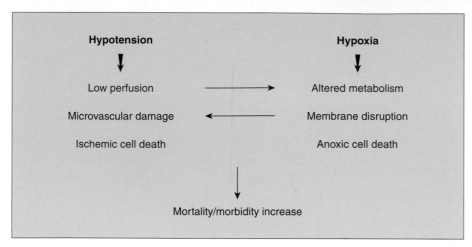

Hypotension

Hypoxia

Low perfusion   ⟶   Altered metabolism

Microvascular damage   ⟵   Membrane disruption

Ischemic cell death   Anoxic cell death

Mortality/morbidity increase

Figure 18.7 Secondary insults to the injured brain.

Airway protection and maintenance

Avoiding head/neck hyperextension and hyperflexion is essential to airway control in patients with potential spine injuries. Upper airway obstruction is generally simply relieved by removing foreign debris or using chin lift or jaw thrust maneuvers that do not require any movement of the neck. However, if airway patency cannot be maintained, intubation is necessary. The safest intubation route in this situation is via the nasotracheal route with the neck in a neutral position. Head stabilization with manual in-line traction should be provided by an experienced member of the trauma team. Fiberoptic endotracheal intubation can also be accomplished safely in this setting; however, it may be too time consuming in the multitrauma patient. If a surgical airway must be provided, a cricothyroidotomy is generally the safest and most reliable way to proceed.

An associated issue is that of the risk of passing nasal tubes (nasotracheal or nasogastric) in multitrauma patients suspected of having a significant basilar skull fracture. There have been several dramatic reports of intracranial penetration of such tubes through areas of major bony disruption in the frontal fossa. In patients with routine basilar skull fractures who have either no or minimal evidence of cerebrospinal fluid leakage there appears to be negligible risk in passing nasal tubes. However, in those patients with marked cerebrospinal fluid rhinorrhea, significant bony disruption should be suspected and strong consideration given to using the oral route for all tubes.

However, with life-threatening airway problems, re-establishment and protection of the airway by any means should take precedence over concerns of spinal alignment or basilar skull disruption.

Fluid resuscitation

There has been longstanding caution over the "excessive" fluid resuscitation of patients with head injury based on concerns about promoting cerebral edema formation and subsequent intracranial hypertension. Hypotension arising from brain injury is a terminal event resulting from brainstem failure. Thus hypotension in the head-injured patient is most often due to volume loss, which requires adequate fluid resuscitation to restore an optimal level of cerebral perfusion. Restoration of adequate cerebral perfusion may in itself result in significant neurologic improvement.

There are few systematic studies of the effects of fluid resuscitation on the outcome of head injury in the multitraumatized patient.[14] One study from Kings County Hospital in New York attempted to correlate intracranial pressure changes with aggressive fluid resuscitation (a mean of 5 L fluid resuscitation per patient) in a consecutive series of multitraumatized patients with associated head injury. No patient had a rise in intracranial pressure greater than 2 mmH$_2$O or a deterioration in neurologic examination during continuous infusion or bolus fluid therapy.[15] Thus the benefits of adequate fluid resuscitation, regardless of the total volume needed for stable blood pressure, may outweigh the potential disadvantages in the head-injured patient.

There is increasing interest in the use of hypertonic saline and dextran in trauma resuscitation. A 7.5% NaCl/12% dextran-70 solution significantly improved cardiac output over traditional resuscitation fluids.[16] It has been suggested that this regimen has a high plasma oncotic pressure that shifts extracellular fluid into the plasma space. Caution, however, is warranted when using this treatment in head-injured patients. While the 7.5% saline/dextran is superior to Ringer's lactate, with significantly less fluid infused early in resuscitation, the beneficial effects are not sustained and cerebral blood flow decreases 24 hours after injury.[17]

Mannitol is an ancillary method of fluid resuscitation in the head-injured patient. The hyperosmolar effect of osmotic diuretics, such as mannitol, causes transient increases in intravascular volume. However, as diuresis is induced, marked hypotension may be precipitated in the marginally compensated or resuscitated multitrauma victim. Thus osmotic diuretics must be used judiciously in the multitrauma patient lest the potential beneficial effects on lowering intracranial pressure be offset by subsequent hypotension and inadequate cerebral perfusion.

Abdominal evaluation

Abdominal assessment after blunt trauma may be quite difficult and is often misleading in the multitrauma patient. Signs and symptoms of injury may not become apparent for hours or days. With associated head injury and unconsciousness or spinal cord injury and lack of sensation, the abdominal evaluation becomes treacherous.

Generally the physical examination guides a diagnosis of acute abdominal injury. However, when the physical examination cannot

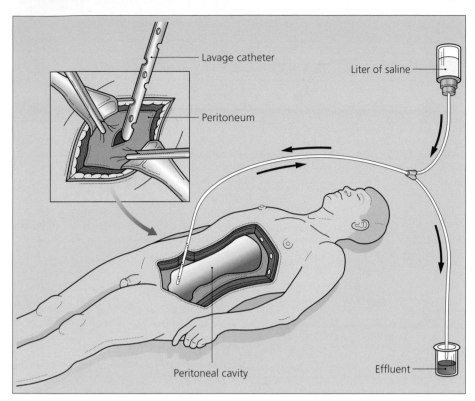

Figure 18.8 Surgical technique of open peritoneal lavage.

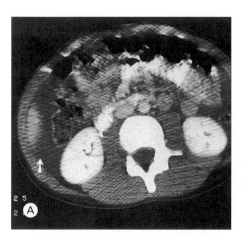

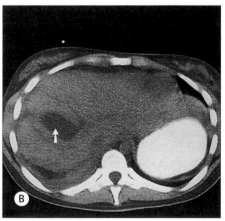

Figure 18.9 Abdominal CT scans posttrauma demonstrating **(A)** the presence of blood within the peritoneal cavity (arrows) and **(B)** a liver laceration (arrow).

be relied upon, ancillary studies come into play. The two most frequently used are peritoneal lavage and abdominal CT scanning. Such tests are indicated as primary evaluations in unconscious patients, patients with cervical and thoracic spinal cord injury, and patients with unexplained shock.

Peritoneal lavage has proven quite reliable, with a 1–2% false-negative/false-positive rate over a wide variety of published studies.[18–20] There are numerous techniques for peritoneal lavage, but the safest is incising down to the peritoneum and introducing a large lavage catheter into the peritoneal cavity under direct vision (Figure 18.8). A liter of saline is then introduced and the resultant effluent is analyzed. Accepted parameters as heralds of significant intra-abdominal injury are a red blood cell count greater than 100 000/mm^3, white blood cell count greater than 500/mm^3, spun hematocrit greater than 2, or the presence of bile, bacteria,

or fecal material. A negative peritoneal lavage, however, does not rule out possible retroperitoneal injury.

Abdominal CT scans are becoming popular in the evaluation of stable patients suspected of harboring abdominal injury and may provide more specific and sensitive information regarding the degree and extent of specific organ injury (Figure 18.9).[21–23]

Timing of CT/MRI in initial evaluation and resuscitation

CT may be critical in managing the head injury patient, and MRI is assuming greater importance in assessing acute spinal cord injury; however, the sequencing of these tests raises difficult questions in the multitrauma patient. Concerns arise over placing the patient in a relatively inaccessible location where vital signs

CLINICAL PEARLS

- The ABC of management in the multiply injured patient includes: a) establishment and protection of the airway; b) ensuring adequate ventilation; and c) maintenance or restoration of the circulation and hemodynamic parameters.

- Trauma protocols involve a rapid assessment of the injuries, followed by resuscitation of the vital signs, then a secondary survey to obtain details on the injuries, followed by definitive treatment of the injuries.

- In hypovolemic shock, fluid resuscitation is performed with isotonic electrolyte solutions such as saline or Ringer's solution. In neurogenic or vasomotor shock, the blood pressure can drop despite fluid resuscitation due to an underlying spinal cord injury. In those patients a vasopressor may be need to restore normal blood pressure.

- In general, hemodynamically unstable multitrauma patients require immediate treatment of their shock, only then to be followed by a CT scan of the head or ICP monitoring. The benefits of adequate fluid resuscitation and the avoidance of ischemia and hypoxia far outweigh the risks of damage or elevation of ICP in multitrauma patients with an associated head injury.

cannot be fully monitored. A trauma-oriented CT scan of the head may take less than 10 minutes, while a spinal MRI may take up to 1 hour. During a CT scan it is possible to monitor the ECG and blood pressure; however, during MRI only the ECG can be monitored continuously.

In general a hemodynamically unstable patient should not be subjected to CT or MRI. The extreme example of this is patients who require immediate operative intervention – thoracotomy or laparotomy – for uncontrollable shock before assessment or treatment of an associated head or spine injury can be accomplished. Such situations are generally accompanied by marked hypotension that in and of itself renders the neurologic examination invalid. In such a setting, if there is strong suspicion of associated severe head injury based on information from the accident scene, one of two actions may be considered: the making of emergency burr holes or the monitoring and treatment of intracranial pressure during the operation.[24] If the burr holes indicate a significant extra-axial mass, simultaneous craniotomy can be undertaken. However, intracranial surgery in the midst of an emergency thoracotomy or laparotomy may prove technically quite difficult. The alternative, establishing intracranial pressure monitoring, is for the most part more easily accomplished, allowing initiation of appropriate medical therapy as indicated. Regardless of the action chosen, a CT scan can then be performed at the end of the operation or when the patient is felt to be hemodynamically stable.

REFERENCES

1. Bracken MB, Shepard MJ, Collins WF, et al. A randomized, controlled trial of methylprednisolone or naloxane in the treatment of acute spinal cord injury. N Engl J Med 1990; 322: 1405–11.
2. Eisenberg HM, Cayard C, Papanicolaou FF, et al. The effects of three potentially preventable complications on outcome after severe closed head injury. In: Ishal S, Nagai H, Brock M (eds). Intracranial Pressure V. Tokyo: Springer Verlag; 1983; 549–53.
3. Klauber MR, Toutant SM, Marshall LF. A model for predicting delayed intracranial hypertension following severe head injury. J Neurosurg 1984; 61: 695–9.
4. Commitee on Trauma. Advanced Trauma Life Support. Chicago, IL: American College of Surgeons; 1985.
5. Velanovich V. Crystalloid vs. colloid resuscitation: a meta-analysis of mortality. Surgery 1989; 105: 65–70.
6. Holcroft J, Vassar M, et al. 3% saline and 7% dextran-70 in the resuscitation of severely injured patients. Ann Surg 1987; 206: 279–85.
7. Baker SP, O'Neill B, Haddon W, Long WB. The injury severity score: a method for describing patients with multiple injuries and evaluating emergency care. J Trauma 1974; 14: 187–96.
8. HR, Sacco WJ, Commazzo AJ, et al. Trauma score. Crit Care Med 1981; 9: 672–6.
9. Miller JD, Corales RL, Sweet RC, et al. Early insults to the injured brain. JAMA 1978; 240: 439–42.
10. Rose J, Balronen S, Jennett B. Avoidable factors contributing to death after head injury. Br Med J 1977; 21: 615–18.
11. Gildenberg PL, Mekela ME. The effect of early intubation and ventilation on outcome following head trauma. In: Dacey RG, Winn RR, et al. (eds). Trauma of the Central Nervous System. New York, NY: Raven Press; 1985.
12. Harr FL. Incidence and significance of early hypoxia in head-injured patients. American Association of Neurological Surgery Abstract Book; 1981.
13. Senter HJ, Venes JL. Altered blood flow and secondary injury in experimental spinal cord trauma. J Neurosurg 1978; 49: 569–78.
14. Gunnar W, Jonasson O, et al. Head injury and hemorrhagic shock: studies of the blood–brain barrier and intracranial pressure after resuscitation with normal saline solution, 3% saline solution and dextran-40. Surgery 1988; 103: 398–405.
15. Maltz S, Scalea T, Duncan A, et al. Fluid resuscitation in the head-injured patient. American Association for the Surgery of Trauma Abstract Book; 1989.
16. Halvorsen L, Gunther RA, Holcroft JW. Dose–response characteristics of hypertonic saline dextran solutions. Surg Forum 1990; 41: 30–4.
17. Walsh J, Zhuang J, Shackford SR. Fluid resuscitation of focal brain injury and shock. Surg Forum 1990; 41: 56–9.
18. Fisher RP, Beverlin BC, Engrav LH, et al. Diagnostic peritoneal lavage: 14 years and 2,568 patients later. Am J Surg 1978; 136: 701–4.
19. Powell DC, Bivins BA, Bell RM. Diagnostic peritoneal lavage. Surg Gynecol Obstet 1982; 155: 257–64.

20. Thal ER, Shires GT. Pertoneal lavage in blunt abdominal trauma. *Am J Surg* 1973; 125: 64–9.

21. Federle LP, Crass RA, Jeffrey RB, Trunkey DD. Computed tomography in blunt abdominal trauma. *Arch Surg* 1982; 17: 645.

22. Federle MP, Goldberg HI, Kaiser JA, *et al*. Evaluation of abdominal trauma by computed tomography. *Radiology* 1981; 138: 637–44.

23. Marx JA, Moore EE, Jorden RC, Eule J. Limitations of computed tomography in the evaluation of abdominal trauma. *J Trauma* 1985; 25: 933–7.

24. Wilberger JE. Emergency burr holes: current role in neurosurgical acute care. In: Mangiardi JR (ed.). *Topics in Emergency Medicine* 1990; 11: 69–75.

CLOSED HEAD INJURY

19

Raj K Narayan and Suzanne Kempisty

Head injury is arguably the most common cranial condition that neurosurgeons deal with and, unlike certain other clinical entities, it is likely to remain primarily under our purview for the foreseeable future. Contrary to popular belief, major strides have been made over the past three decades in reducing the mortality and morbidity from head injury. While controlled and strictly comparable data are hard to come by, well-documented series have demonstrated declining mortality from severe head injury: from 50% in 1970 to around 36% in the 1980s and possibly even lower currently. Although this is hard to prove conclusively, the most probable cause for this dramatic improvement in results is the wider availability and better application of emergency medical services and critical-care methodologies.

The first evidence-based guidelines for the management of traumatic brain injured patients were published in 1995,[1] with an updated version published in 2000.[2] Also in 2000, the Cochrane Library published a series of reviews that provided evidence-based standards and guidelines for the management of traumatic brain injured patients.[3–5] Evidence-based guidelines for the management of penetrating head injury have also been recently published.[6]

The essential element of such intensive care is to maintain an optimal milieu in the injured brain to facilitate healing and to prevent secondary injury to the damaged neurons (Figure 19.1). Most importantly, this means providing the brain with adequate oxygen and avoiding hyponatremia and hyperglycemia. Of these, the first priority is the maintenance of oxygenation. Unfortunately, this is also the most difficult to achieve, since several factors conspire against it, including mass lesions with elevated intracranial pressure (ICP), reduced blood pressure, and hypoxia

secondary to pulmonary complications. Hence, these occurrences need to be monitored constantly and treated early.

While better critical care and physiological management have proven to be valuable, pharmacological interventions have yet to be proven effective in the clinical setting. Despite promising results in animal models, clinical studies to date have not generated drug treatments with proven benefit.[7]

CLASSIFICATION

While head injuries could be classified in several different ways, the most practical categorizations are based on mechanism, severity, and morphology (Figure 19.2).

Mechanism

Although the words "closed" and "penetrating" are widely used to describe types of head injuries, they are not mutually exclusive. For example, a depressed skull fracture could be assigned to either of these two categories, depending on the depth and severity of the bony injury. For practical purposes, the term *closed head injury* is usually associated with auto accidents, falls, and assaults, while *penetrating head injury* is most often associated with gunshot wounds and stab injuries. Penetrating head injuries are dealt with in Chapter 20.

Severity

Prior to 1974, different authors used various terms to describe patients with head injury, making it virtually impossible to compare groups of patients from different centers. In 1974, Teasdale and Jennett,[8] by identifying the clinical signs that predicted outcome most reliably and that seemed to have the least inter-observer variation, designed what has come to be known as the Glasgow Coma Scale (GCS). The introduction of the GCS (Table 19.1) brought some degree of uniformity into the head injury literature.[8] This scale has gained widespread use for the description of patients with head injuries and has also been adopted for the description of patients with altered levels of consciousness due to other causes.

Jennett and Teasdale defined coma as the inability to obey commands, to utter words, and to open the eyes.[9] A patient needs to meet all three aspects of this definition to be classified as comatose. In a series of 2000 patients with severe head injury, these authors observed 4% who did not speak but could obey commands and another 4% who uttered words but did not obey.

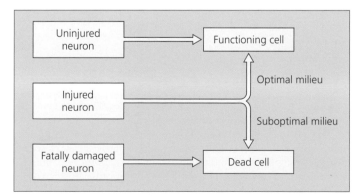

Figure 19.1 An optimal milieu must be maintained for healing in the injured brain.

Figure 19.2 Classification of head injury.

By mechanism			
	Closed	High velocity (auto accidents)	
		Low velocity (falls, assault)	
	Penetrating	Gunshot wounds	
		Other open injuries	

By severity	
Mild: GCS 14–15	
Moderate: GCS 9–13	
Severe: GCS 8 or less, comatose	

By morphology			
Skull fractures	Vault	Linear or stellate	
		Depressed or nondepressed	
	Basilar	With/without CSF leak	
		With/without nerve VII palsy	
Intracranial lesions	Focal	Epidural	
		Subdural	
		Intracerebral	
	Diffuse	Mild concussion	
		Classic concussion	
		Diffuse axonal injury	

Among patients who could neither obey nor speak, 16% opened their eyes and were therefore judged not to be in coma. Patients who open their eyes spontaneously, obey commands, and are oriented score a total of 15 points, whereas flaccid patients who do not open their eyes or talk score the minimum of 3 points. No single score within the range of 3 to 15 forms the cut-off point for coma. However, 90% of all patients with a score of 8 or less, and none of those with a score of 9 or more, are found to be in coma according to the preceding definition. Therefore, for all practical purposes, a GCS score of 8 or less has become the generally accepted definition of a comatose patient.

The distinction between patients with severe head injury and those with mild to moderate injury is thus fairly clear. However, distinguishing between mild and moderate head injury is more of a problem.[10] Somewhat arbitrarily, head-injured patients with a GCS score of 9 to 13 have been categorized as "moderate," and those with a GCS score of 14 or 15 have been designated "mild." Eighty per cent of head injuries are categorized as mild, 10% as

Table 19.1 The Glasgow Coma Scale (GCS)	
Eye opening (E)	
Spontaneous	4
To call	3
To pain	2
None	1
Motor response (M)	
Obeys commands	6
Localizes pain	5
Normal flexion (withdrawal)	4
Abnormal flexion (decorticate)	3
Extension (decerebrate)	2
None (flaccid)	1
Verbal response (V)	
Oriented	5
Confused conversation	4
Inappropriate words	3
Incomprehensible sounds	2
None	1

GCS sum score = (E + M + V); best possible score = 15; worst possible score = 3.

moderate, and 10% as severe. Williams and colleagues reported that the neurobehavioral deficits in patients with mild head injury (GCS 14 or 15) and an intracranial lesion on initial computed tomography (CT) scan were similar to those in patients with moderate head injury (GCS 9 to 13), while patients with mild head injury uncomplicated by an intracranial lesion on CT scan did significantly better.[11]

Morphology

The advent of CT scanning has revolutionized the classification and management of head injury. Thus, although certain patients who are rapidly deteriorating may be taken to surgery without a CT scan, the vast majority of severely injured patients should have the benefit of a CT scan before surgical intervention. Furthermore, frequent follow-up CT scans are essential because the morphologic picture in head injury often undergoes a remarkable evolution

over the first few hours, days, and even weeks after the injury. Morphologically, head injuries may be broadly classified into two types: skull fractures and intracranial lesions.

SKULL FRACTURES

In current practice in developed countries, CT scans are the imaging study of choice and plain skull films are obtained infrequently. Skull fractures may be seen in the cranial vault or skull base, may be linear or stellate, and may be depressed or nondepressed (Figure 19.3). Basal skull fractures are harder to document on plain X-ray films and usually require CT scanning with bone-window settings for identification. The clinical signs of a basal skull fracture include cerebrospinal fluid (CSF) leakage from the nose (rhinorrhea) or ear (otorrhea), blood behind the eardrum (hemotympanum), brusing behind the ear (postauricular ecchymoses or Battle's signs), bruising around the eyes (periorbital ecchymoses or racoon eyes). The presence of these clinical signs should increase the index of suspicion and help in the identification of a basal skull fracture. Most require no treatment, but persistent CSF leakage may require placement of a lumbar drain or operative repair.

A depressed skull fracture may cause pressure on the brain. As a general guideline, fragments depressed more than the thickness of the skull require elevation. Open or compound skull fractures have a direct communication between the scalp laceration and the cerebral surface because the dura is torn. These require early surgical repair. Outcome after a depressed skull fracture is based on the severity of the underlying injury to the brain.

A linear vault fracture increases the risk of intracranial hematoma. For this reason, the detection of a skull fracture on plain skull radiograph always calls for a CT scan of the head and generally warrants admission to the hospital for observation.

INTRACRANIAL LESIONS

Intracranial lesions may be classified as focal or diffuse, although these two forms of injury frequently coexist. Focal lesions include epidural hematomas, subdural hematomas, and contusions (or intracerebral hematomas). Diffuse brain injuries, in general, have

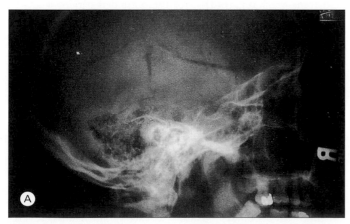
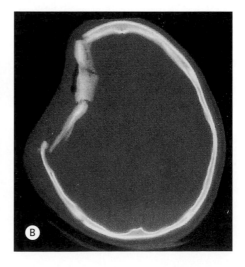

Figure 19.3 **(A)** Linear skull fracture and **(B)** depressed skull fracture.

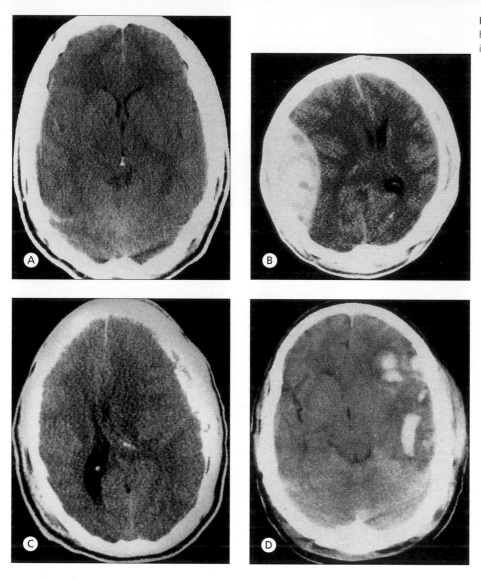

Figure 19.4 (A) Diffuse brain injury; **(B)** epidural hematoma; **(C)** subdural hematoma; and **(D)** intracerebral hematoma.

relatively normal appearing CT scans (Figure 19.4A) but manifest an altered sensorium or even deep coma. The cellular basis of diffuse brain injury has become much clearer in recent years.

Epidural hematomas

Epidural hematomas (Figure 19.4B) are located outside the dura but within the skull. They are most often located in the temporal or temporoparietal region and classically result from tearing of the middle meningeal vessels. While these clots are usually thought to be arterial in origin, they may be secondary to venous bleeding in at least one-third of cases. Occasionally, an epidural hematoma may result from torn venous sinuses, particularly in the parieto-occipital region or posterior fossa.

Epidural hematomas are relatively uncommon, occurring in 0.5% of all head-injured patients and in 9% of those who are comatose. If treated early, the prognosis is usually excellent because the damage to the underlying brain is usually limited. Outcome is directly related to the status of the patient before

surgery. For patients not in coma, the mortality from epidural hematoma approximates 0%, for the obtunded patient it is 9%, and for patients in a coma the mortality is 20%.

Subdural hematomas

Subdural hematomas (Figure 19.4C) are much more common than epidural hematomas (approximately 30% of severe head injuries). They occur most frequently from a tearing of bridging veins between the cerebral cortex and the draining sinuses. However, they can also be associated with lacerations of the brain surface or substance. A skull fracture may or may not be present.

The brain damage underlying acute subdural hematomas results from direct pressure caused by the hematoma, brain swelling and increased intracranial pressure, or diffuse axonal injury as a result of mechanical distortion of the brain parenchyma. The injury in patients with subdural hematoma is usually much more severe, and the prognosis is much worse, than for epidural hematomas. The mortality in a general series may be around 60% but can be lowered by very rapid surgical intervention and aggressive medical management.[12]

Contusions and intracerebral hematomas

Pure cerebral contusions are fairly common. Their frequency has become much more apparent as the quality and number of CT scans have increased. Furthermore, contusions of the brain are almost always seen in association with subdural hematomas. The vast majority of contusions occur in the frontal and temporal lobes, although they can occur at almost any site, including the cerebellum and brainstem. The distinction between contusions and traumatic intracerebral hematomas remains somewhat ill-defined. The classic "salt-and-pepper" lesion is clearly a contusion, while a large hematoma clearly is not (Figure 19.4D). However, there is a gray zone, and contusions can, over a period of hours or days, evolve into intracerebral hematomas. Management of the intracerebral hematoma is dependent on the neurological status of the patient. Rapid surgical evacuation decompression is recommended if there is a significant mass effect (generally, a 5 mm or greater actual midline shift).

Diffuse injuries

Diffuse brain injuries form a continuum of progressively severe brain damage caused by increasing amounts of acceleration–deceleration injury to the brain. In its pure form, diffuse brain injury is the most common type of head injury.

A mild concussion is an injury in which consciousness is preserved, but there is a noticeable degree of temporary neurologic dysfunction. These injuries are exceedingly common and, because of their mild degree, are often not brought to medical attention. The mildest form of concussion results in transient confusion and disorientation without amnesia. This syndrome is usually completely reversible and is associated with no major sequelae. Slightly greater injury causes confusion with both retrograde and post-traumatic amnesia.

A classic cerebral concussion is that post-traumatic state which results in loss of consciousness. This condition is always accompanied by some degree of retrograde and post-traumatic amnesia, and the length of post-traumatic amnesia is a good measure of the severity of the injury. The loss of consciousness is transient and reversible. The patient has returned to full consciousness by 6 hours, although it is usually much sooner. While the great majority of patients with classic cerebral concussion have no sequelae other than amnesia for the events relating to the injury, some patients may have more long-lasting, although sometimes subtle, neurologic deficits.

Diffuse axonal injury is the term used to describe a prolonged post-traumatic state in which there is loss of consciousness from the time of injury that continues beyond 6 hours. This phenomenon may further be broken down into mild, moderate, and severe categories.[13] Severe diffuse axonal injury usually occurs in vehicular accidents, comprising about 36% of all patients with diffuse axonal injury. These patients are rendered deeply comatose and remain so for prolonged periods of time. They often demonstrate evidence of decortication or decerebration (motor posturing) and often remain severely disabled, if they survive. These patients often exhibit autonomic dysfunctions such as hypertension, hyperhidrosis, and hyperpyrexia, and were previously thought to have primary brainstem injury. It is now believed that diffuse axonal injury throughout the brain is the more common pathologic basis.

EVALUATION

Mild head injury

Approximately 80% of patients presenting to the emergency room with head injury fall under the category of mild head injury. These patients are awake but may be amnesic for events surrounding the injury, with a GCS score of 14 or 15. There may be a history of brief loss of consciousness, which is usually difficult to confirm. The issue is often confounded by alcohol or other intoxicants.

Most patients with mild head injury make uneventful recoveries, albeit often with some neurologic sequelae. However, about 3% of patients deteriorate unexpectedly, and can become neurologically devastated if the decline in mental status is not noticed early.[14] How can a physician guard against such an occurrence? The classic struggle between "cost-effective" and the "best possible" management is clearly evident here, and practice varies in different centers.

In 1999, a Task force on Mild Traumatic Brain Injury was devised under the support of the European Federation of Neurological Societies. The efforts of the task force produced the recommendations for the management of Mild Traumatic Brain Injury.

The classification of Mild Traumatic Brain Injury is based on the admission GCS score, duration of loss of consciousness, and post-traumatic amnesia, as well as neurological findings and risk factors for intracranial complications. The task force developed a scheme (Figure 19.5) to guide initial management with respect to ancillary investigation, hospital admission, observation, and follow-up.[15]

In the head-injured patient, skull X-ray films may be examined for the following features: linear or depressed skull fractures, position of the pineal gland if calcified, air–fluid levels in the sinuses, pneumocephalus, facial fractures, and foreign bodies. The routine ordering of skull X-rays in patients with minor head injury has come under some criticism. Studies comparing skull radiography with CT have shown a low sensitivity and specificity of the presence of a skull fracture on skull radiographs for intracranial hemorrhage.[16] A meta-analysis confirmed that skull radiography is of little value in the clinical assessment of Mild Traumatic Brain Injury.[17]

CT is considered the gold standard for the detection of intracranial abnormalities after Mild Traumatic Brain Injury. CT is recommended for those with loss of consciousness and/or post-traumatic amnesia and is considered mandatory in all patients with GCS scores of 13 or 14, or the presence of risk factors.

The cervical spine and other parts must be X-rayed if there is any pain or tenderness. Non-narcotic analgesics such as acetaminophen are preferred, although codeine may be used if there is an associated painful injury. Tetanus toxoid must be administered if there are any associated open wounds. Routine blood tests are usually not necessary if there are no systemic injuries. A blood alcohol level and urine toxic screen can be useful both for diagnostic and for medicolegal purposes.

Moderate head injury

Patients with moderate head injury constitute approximately 10% of head injury patients seen in the emergency room. They are still able to follow simple commands but are usually confused or somnolent and may have focal neurologic deficits such as a hemiparesis. Approximately 10% of these patients will deteriorate and lapse into coma. Therefore, they should be managed as for severely head-injured patients, although they are not routinely intubated (Figure 19.6).

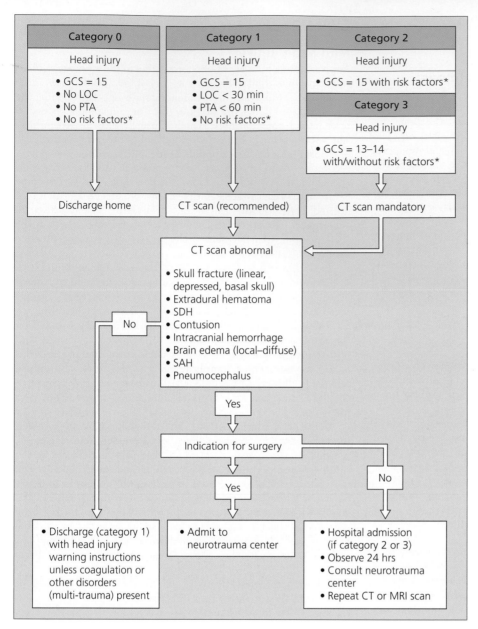

Figure 19.5 Algorithm for management of mild head injury. *Risk factors include: ambiguous accident history, continued post-traumatic amnesia, retrograde amnesia > 30 min, clinical signs of skull fracture, headache, vomiting, focal neurologic deficit, seizure, age < 2 years and > 60 years, coagulation disorder, or high-energy (speed) accident.

On admission to the emergency room, a brief history is obtained and cardiopulmonary stability is ensured prior to neurologic assessment. A CT scan of the head is obtained in all moderately head-injured patients. In a review of 341 patients with a GCS of 9 to 12, 40% of cases had an abnormal initial CT scan and 8% required surgery.[18] The patient is admitted for observation even if the CT scan is normal. If the patient improves neurologically and a follow-up CT scan of the head shows no surgical mass lesion, he or she may be discharged from the hospital over the next few days. On the other hand, if the patient lapses into coma, the management principles described for severe head injury are adopted.

Severe head injury

Severely head-injured patients are those who are unable to follow simple commands even after cardiopulmonary stabilization.

Although this definition includes a wide spectrum of brain injury, it identifies the patients who are at greatest risk of suffering significant morbidity and mortality. We believe that in such patients a "wait and see" approach can be disastrous and that prompt diagnosis and treatment are of the utmost importance (Table 19.2).[12,19,20]

MANAGEMENT OF SEVERELY HEAD-INJURED PATIENTS

Cardiopulmonary stabilization

Brain injury is often adversely affected by secondary insults. In a study of 100 consecutive patients with severe brain injury evaluated on arrival in the emergency room, 30% were hypoxemic (P_{O_2} < 65 mmHg), 13% were hypotensive (systolic blood pressure < 95 mmHg), and 12% were anemic (hematocrit

Definition
The patient may be confused or somnolent but is still able to follow simple commands (GCS 9–13)
Initial work-up
Same as for mild head injury, except that baseline blood work (CBC, Chem 7, PT/PTT) may be obtained
CT scan of the head is advisable in all cases
Admission for observation is the safest option, even if the CT scan is normal
After admission
Frequent neurologic checks
Follow-up CT scan if condition deteriorates or preferably prior to discharge

If patient improves (90%)	If patient deteriorates (10%)
Discharge when stable	If the patient stops following simple commands, repeat CT scan and manage per severe head injury protocol
Follow-up clinic	

Figure 19.6 Algorithm for management of moderate head injury.

< 30%).[21] It has subsequently been demonstrated that hypotension at admission (systolic blood pressure < 90 mmHg) is one of three factors in severe head injury with a normal CT scan (the other two being age over 40 years and motor posturing) that, when noted at admission, are associated with subsequent ICP elevation.[22] High ICP is in turn associated with poorer outcome. Subsequent analyses have also confirmed a strong association between hypotension and worse outcomes in patients with severe head injury.[23] It is imperative, therefore, that cardiopulmonary stabilization be achieved rapidly.

Airway

A frequent concomitant of severe concussion is transient respiratory arrest. Prolonged apnea may often be the cause of "immediate" death at the scene of an accident. If artificial respiration can be instituted immediately, a good outcome is possible.[24] Apnea, atelectasis, aspiration, and adult respiratory distress syndrome are frequently associated with severe head injury, and by far the most important aspect of the immediate management of these patients is the establishment of a reliable airway. *Severely head-injured patients should be intubated early.* One hundred per cent oxygen is then used for ventilation until blood gases can be checked and appropriate adjustments of the F_1O_2 made. There is little danger of oxygen toxicity if 100% oxygen is used for less than 48–72 hours.

Blood pressure

Hypotension and hypoxia are the principal enemies of the head-injured patient. It has been shown that the presence of hypotension (systolic blood pressure < 90 mmHg) in severely head-injured patients increases the mortality rate from 27% to 50%.[25] Furthermore, it was found that 35% of patients arriving at major trauma centers are hypotensive. While the airway is being established, another group of emergency room personnel should be checking the patient's pulse and blood pressure and taking steps to obtain venous access.

If the patient is hypotensive, it is vital to restore normal blood pressure as soon as possible. Hypotension is usually not the result of the brain injury itself, except in the terminal stages when medullary failure supervenes. Far more commonly, hypotension is a marker of severe blood loss, which may be either "overt" or "occult," or possibly both. One must also consider associated spinal cord injury (with quadriplegia or paraplegia), cardiac contusion or tamponade, and tension pneumothorax as possible causes. While efforts are in progress to determine the cause of the hypotension, volume replacement should be initiated.

The importance of routine abdominal paracentesis in the hypotensive comatose patient has been demonstrated.[26] Either high-resolution rapid CT scan or ultrasound is an acceptable option. It must be emphasized that *a patient's neurologic examination is meaningless as long as he or she is hypotensive.* Time after time, we have seen hypotensive patients who are unresponsive to any form of stimulation revert to a near-normal neurologic examination soon after normal blood pressure has been restored.

Catheters

A Foley catheter (16 to 18 Fr for average adults) should be carefully inserted and a urine sample should be sent for urinalysis and toxic screen (when appropriate). Gross hematuria suggests renal injury and is an indication for an abdominal CT scan and an emergency intravenous pyelogram. Mild hematuria may be secondary to traumatic catheterization, renal contusion, or, rarely, to a dissecting aortic aneurysm. Special attention must be paid to maintaining accurate records of fluid intake and output, especially in children and the elderly. In addition to ensuring fluid balance, such records help assess blood loss and monitor renal perfusion.

A nasogastric tube, preferably a Salem sump (double-lumen plastic catheter), should be inserted and connected to a wall suction unit. Potential, albeit rare, complications of this procedure, such

Table 19.2 Initial management of severe head injury

Definition
The patient is unable to follow even a simple command because of impaired consciousness

Management
History
Age of patient and type and time of accident
Drug or alcohol intake
Neurologic progression
Progression of vital signs
Vomiting, aspiration, anoxia, or seizures
Past medical history, including medications and allergies

Cardiopulmonary stabilization
Airway: intubate early
Blood pressure: normalize promptly using normal saline or blood
Catheters: Foley, nasogastric tube
Diagnostic films: cervical spine, chest, skull, abdomen, pelvis, extremities

General examination

Emergency measures for associated injuries
Tracheostomy
Chest tubes
Neck stabilization: hard collar, Gardner–Wells tongs, traction
Abdominal paracentesis

Neurologic examination
Eye opening
Motor response
Verbal response
Pupillary light reaction
Oculocephalics (doll's eye)
Oculovestibulars (caloric)

Therapeutic agents
Sodium bicarbonate, phenytoin, mannitol, hyperventilation

Diagnostic tests
CT scan, MRI scan, air ventriculogram, or angiogram (in descending order of preference)

as intracranial passage of the tube secondary to a basal skull fracture, must be kept in mind. In patients with anterior basal skull fractures it is probably wise to pass the tube under direct vision with a laryngoscope or to pass it through the mouth.

Diagnostic radiographs

As soon as the preliminary steps towards cardiopulmonary stabilization have been taken, diagnostic radiographs should be obtained.

Cervical spine films (cross-table lateral and anteroposterior) or full cervical spine CT scan are the first to be taken in the severely traumatized patient and must be read by a knowledgeable reader before the patient's neck can be moved. Features to look for in this study are loss of alignment of the vertebral bodies, bony fractures or compressions, loss of alignment of the facet joints, and prevertebral soft tissue swelling (more than 5 mm opposite the C3 vertebral body is significant). Every effort must be made to visualize the lower cervical levels (C6–T1); these are often obscured by the shoulders, especially in heavy-set patients. On plain films, fracture–subluxations at these levels may be overlooked if the films are not repeated with caudal traction on both arms and greater X-ray penetration (Figure 19.7). If these maneuvers also fail, a "swimmer's view" lateral film can be obtained. If any of these films show any of the abnormalities listed above, the neck must remain immobilized in a hard collar (Philadelphia) pending further studies (high-resolution CT scan). Cervical spine CT is indicated for the unconscious patient with suspicious or inadequate cervical radiographs and with all cervical fractures or suspected fractures on initial plain films. There are several studies that have demonstrated the value of the full CT scan, with saggital and coronal reconstructions, for the exclusion of significant spinal injury.[27] Widening, slippage or rotational abnormalities of the cervical vertebrae suggest soft tissue injury. An absence of such signs appears to exclude significant instability. Additional modalities, such as magnetic resonance imaging (MRI), can also be employed, although these are not generally used as initial studies.

The chest film is useful in ruling out endotracheal tube malposition, pneumothorax, hemothorax, lung contusion, hemoperi-

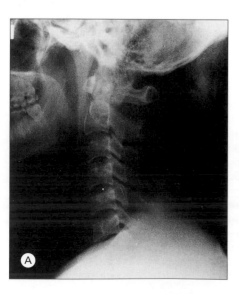 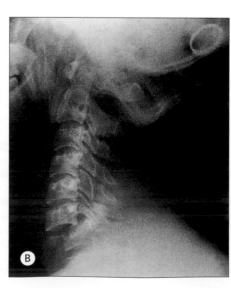

Figure 19.7 (A) The lower cervical spine is obscured by the shoulders. **(B)** Traction on the shoulders reveals a fracture-subluxation at C6–C7.

cardium, rib fractures, thoracic spine fractures, and other thoracic pathology that may have a bearing on patient management.

Although skull films (anteroposterior and lateral) have been overshadowed by CT scanning, they can be helpful in identifying maxillofacial injuries, depressed skull fractures, and penetrating injuries. The presence of intracranial air (pneumocephalus) or of an air–fluid level in one of the sinuses can alert the clinician to a basal skull fracture that might otherwise have gone undetected.

A single anteroposterior abdominal film (kidney, ureter, and bladder; KUB) is usually taken in trauma patients. This may help identify large retroperitoneal hematomas, lumbosacral spine fractures, distended viscera, and possibly subdiaphragmatic air.

Anteroposterior and lateral pelvic films are usually obtained, looking for pelvic injuries which may be the site of significant blood loss. The extremities may be studied whenever indicated to rule out fractures or subluxations.

General examination

During the process of cardiopulmonary stabilization, the clinician conducts a rapid general examination looking for other injuries. In one series of severely, head-injured patients, more than 50% had additional major systemic injuries requiring care by other specialists (Table 19.3).[21] One must check for head and neck, thoracic, abdominal, pelvic, and spinal injuries, and injuries involving extremities.

Neurologic examination

As soon as the patient's cardiopulmonary status has been stabilized, a rapid and directed neurologic examination is performed (Table 19.4). Although various factors may confound an accurate evaluation of the patient's neurologic state (e.g. hypotension, hypoxia, intoxication, sedation, or paralytic agents), valuable data can nevertheless be obtained. If a patient demonstrates variable responses to stimulation, or if the response on each side is different, the best response appears to be a more accurate prognostic indicator than the worst response. To follow trends in an individual patient's progress, however, it is better to report both the best and the worst responses. In other words, the right-side and left-side motor responses should be recorded separately. As the pain stimuli applied by different examiners are often variable, deep nail-bed pressure may be used as a standard stimulus.

One should not limit the examination to the GCS. Other important data in the initial assessment of patients with impaired consciousness are the patient's age, vital signs, pupillary response, and eye movements.[28] The GCS provides a simple grading of the arousal and functional capacity of the cerebral cortex, while the pupillary responses and eye movements serve as measures of brainstem function. Advanced age, hypotension, and hypoxia all adversely affect outcome. Indeed, there is considerable interplay between all these factors in determining the ultimate outcome in the severely head-injured patient.

Pupils

Careful observation of pupil size and response to light is important during the initial examination (Table 19.5). A well-known early sign of temporal lobe herniation is mild dilatation of the pupil and a sluggish pupillary light response. Compression or distortion of the oculomotor nerve during tentorial–uncal herniation impairs the function of the parasympathetic axons that transmit efferent signals for pupillary constriction, resulting in mild pupillary

Table 19.3 Systemic injuries in 100 patients with severe head injury	
Type of injury	Incidence (%)
Long-bone or pelvic fracture	32
Maxillary or mandibular fracture	22
Major chest injury	23
Abdominal visceral injury	7
Spinal injury	2

Adapted from Miller JD, Sweet RC, Narayan RK, Becker DP. Early insults to the injured brain. *JAMA* 1978; 240: 439–442.[21]

Table 19.4 Initial neurologic examination in head injury
Glasgow Coma Score
Pupillary response to light
Eye movements
Oculocephalic (doll's eye)
Oculovestibular (caloric)
Motor power
Gross sensory examination

dilatation. Sometimes, bilateral miotic pupils (1–3 mm) can occur in the early stages of herniation as a result of compromise of the pupillomotor sympathetic pathways originating in the hypothalamus, permitting a predominance of parasympathetic tone and pupillary constriction. In either instance, continued herniation causes increasing dilatation of the pupil and paralysis of its light response. With full mydriasis (8–9-mm pupil), ptosis and paresis of the medial rectus and other ocular muscles innervated by the oculomotor nerve appear. A bright light is always necessary to determine pupillary light responses. A magnifying lens such as the +20-diopter lens on a standard ophthalmoscope is helpful in distinguishing between a weak and an absent pupillary light reaction, especially if the pupil is small. A computerized pupillometer is currently undergoing clinical testing.[29]

Recognition of additional pupillary disorders that can occur in an unconscious patient is useful in the examination of the patient with head trauma (see Chapter 5). Disruption of the afferent arc of the pupillary light reflex within the optic nerve is detected by the swinging flashlight test. As the flashlight is swung from the normal eye to the injured eye, injury to the optic nerve is indicated by a paradoxic response of the pupil: dilatation rather than constriction. This paradoxic pupillary dilatation is termed an afferent pupillary defect or Marcus Gunn pupil, and in the absence of opacification of the ocular media it is unequivocal evidence of optic nerve injury.

Bilaterally small pupils suggest that the patient has used certain drugs, particularly opiates, or has one of several metabolic encephalopathies, or a destructive lesion of the pons. In these conditions pupillary light responses can usually be seen with a

Table 19.5 Interpretation of pupillary findings in head injury patients

Pupillary size	Light response	Interpretation
Unilaterally dilated	Sluggish or fixed	Nerve III compression secondary to tentorial herniation
Bilaterally dilated	Sluggish or fixed	Inadequate brain perfusion Bilateral nerve III palsy
Unilaterally dilated	Cross-reactive (Marcus Gunn)	Optic nerve injury
Bilaterally miotic	May be difficult to determine	Drugs (opiates) Metabolic encephalopathy Pontine lesion
Unilaterally miotic	Preserved	Injured sympathetic pathway (e.g. carotid sheath injury)

magnifying lens. Unilateral Horner's pupil is seen occasionally with brainstem lesions, but in the trauma patient attention should be given to the possibility of a disrupted efferent sympathetic pathway at the apex of the lung, base of the neck, or ipsilateral carotid sheath. Midposition pupils with variable light responses can be observed in all stages of coma. Traumatic oculomotor nerve injury is the diagnosis in patients with a history of a dilated pupil from the onset of injury, an improving level of consciousness, and appropriate ocular muscle weakness. A mydriatic pupil (6 mm or more) occurs occasionally with direct trauma to the globe of the eye. This traumatic mydriasis is usually unilateral and is not accompanied by ocular muscle paresis. Finally, bilaterally dilated and fixed pupils in patients with head injury may be the result of inadequate cerebral vascular perfusion caused by hypotension secondary to blood loss or elevation of intracranial pressure to a degree that impairs cerebral blood flow. Return of the pupillary response may occur promptly after the restoration of blood flow, if the period of inadequate perfusion has not been too long.

Eye movements
Ocular movements are an important index of the functional activity that is present within the brainstem reticular formation. If the patient is sufficiently alert to follow simple commands, a full range of eye movements is easily obtained and the integrity of the entire ocular motor system within the brainstem can be confirmed. In states of depressed consciousness, voluntary eye movement is lost and there may be dysfunction of the neural structures activating eye movements. In these instances, oculocephalic or oculovestibular responses are used to determine the presence or absence of an eye-movement disorder (see Chapter 5). If a neck fracture has been excluded, function of the pontine gaze center is quickly ascertained by the oculocephalic maneuver.

The oculovestibular response can be tested with ice water and only a small expenditure of time. Obstructions within the external auditory canal due to blood or cerumen must be removed, and ocular movement may be limited in patients with orbital edema. In alert patients, cold caloric stimulation causes fast-phase nystagmus in the direction opposite to the tonic eye deviation. The mnemonic "COWS" (cold opposite, warm same) refers to this phenomenon. However, in comatose patients, functional suppression of the reticular activating system is reflected by the absence of nystagmus in response to caloric stimulation, so that

only the tonic eye deviation is seen (cold same). Thus, irrigation with cold water in a comatose patient causes ipsilateral deviation of the eyes toward the stimulated side.

While oculocephalic and caloric testing is being performed, infranuclear, internuclear, and supranuclear ocular motility disorders are recognizable. A destructive lesion of a frontal or pontine gaze center results in tonic overaction of the opposite frontal-pontine axis for horizontal eye movement. This overaction results in ipsilateral deviation of the eyes with frontal lobe lesions, and contralateral gaze deviation with pontine lesions.

Third and sixth nerve palsies are generally not difficult to recognize in patients with head injury. Fourth nerve palsies cannot ordinarily be identified in coma because of the select action of the superior oblique muscle. In alert and recovering patients, however, superior oblique paresis causes troublesome double vision, especially with downward and inward gaze. Head tilt opposite the side of the paretic muscle lessens the diplopia, while ipsilateral tilt of the head increases it. Internuclear ophthalmoplegia is suggested by select adduction paresis without additional involvement of the pupil, lid, or vertical muscles innervated by the third nerve. This ophthalmoplegia results from disruption of the ipsilateral medial longitudinal fasciculus that connects the oculomotor subnucleus for medial rectus neurons to the contralateral horizontal gaze center. Either bilateral or unilateral internuclear ophthalmoplegia may be seen, depending on the extent of the brainstem trauma.

Motor function
The basic examination is completed by a gross test of motor strength, since severely head-injured patients are not sufficiently responsive for such a determination to be reliably made. Each extremity is examined and graded on the internationally used scale shown in Table 19.6.

Diagnostic procedures
As soon as a patient's cardiorespiratory condition has been stabilized and a preliminary neurologic examination completed, it behooves the physician to rule out the presence of an intracranial mass lesion. The patient is by this time intubated, often paralyzed with a paralytic agent, and on mechanical ventilation. This prevents the patient from straining and moving around, thus avoiding intracranial pressure surges and greatly enhancing the

Table 19.6 Motor function scale	
Normal power	5
Moderate weakness	4
Severe weakness (antigravity)	3
Severe weakness (not antigravity)	2
Trace movement	1
No movement	0

quality of the diagnostic studies. Needless to say, CT scanning has rendered all other diagnostic tests virtually obsolete. However, other tests have to be used in certain instances either to substitute for CT scanning or, as in the case of angiography, to obtain certain supplemental data.

Computed tomography

CT scanning is clearly the procedure of choice in the evaluation of the head-injured patient and has probably significantly improved outcome after head injury.[30] It is strongly recommended that an emergency CT scan be obtained as soon as possible (preferably within half an hour) after admission with a severe head injury. Centers dealing with a large number of such patients must make arrangements to have CT technicians in the hospital on a 24-hour basis, or within easy accessibility in an emergency. CT scans should also be repeated whenever there is a change in the patient's clinical status or an unexplained rise in intracranial pressure.

In a prospective study of CT scan abnormalities in 207 severely head-injured patients, we found the initial CT scan to be normal in 30% of cases. The remaining 70% of patients had CT scan abnormalities: low-density lesions in 10%, high-density nonsurgical lesions in 19%, and high-density lesions requiring surgery in 41%.[19]

Edema is seen on CT as a zone of low density associated with mass effect on the adjacent ventricles reflected as compression, distortion, and displacement of the ventricular system. The edema may be focal, multifocal, or diffuse. With diffuse cerebral edema it may be hard to appreciate the lower density since no area of normal brain density is available for comparison. In such cases there is usually bilateral ventricular compression which may be so gross that the ventricular system is not seen, especially in children. The picture of diffuse brain swelling on CT can be secondary to edema or vascular engorgement (hyperaemia).

Cerebral contusions are seen as nonhomogeneous areas of high density, often interspersed with areas of low density ("salt and pepper" appearance). The CT appearance results from multiple small areas of hemorrhage within the brain substance, associated with areas of edema (see Figure 19.4D). The margin is usually poorly defined. A mass effect is often seen, although this may be minimal. Depending on the extent of hemorrhage, the degree of edema, and the time course, a contusion may appear predominantly dense or lucent.

Although it is not always possible to differentiate between subdural and epidural hematomas on CT, the latter are typically biconvex or lenticular in shape, because the close attachment of the dura to the inner table of the skull prevents the hematoma from spreading (see Figure 19.4B). Approximately 20% of patients with an extracerebral hematoma have blood in both the epidural and subdural spaces at operation or autopsy. Since there is little chance of epidural blood mixing with CSF, these lesions appear as uniformly dense collections and are rarely isodense. However, they may develop in a delayed fashion, especially after evacuation of a contralateral "balancing" lesion.

The typical subdural hematoma is more diffuse than an epidural hematoma and has a concave inner margin that follows the surface of the brain (see Figure 19.4C). The distinction between acute, subacute, and chronic lesions is somewhat arbitrary. However, most acute subdural hematomas are hyperdense, most subacute lesions are isodense or of mixed density, and most chronic hematomas are hypodense as compared with brain tissue. Effacement of the cerebral sulci over the convexity and distortion of the ipsilateral lateral ventricle may suggest the presence of an isodense hematoma.

Traumatic intracerebral hematomas are usually located in the frontal and anterior temporal lobes, although they can occur in virtually any area. The majority of hematomas develop immediately after the injury, but delayed lesions are often noted, usually within the first week. They are high-density lesions and are usually surrounded by zones of low density caused by edema. Traumatic hematomas are more often multiple than hematomas from other causes.

Traumatic intraventricular hemorrhage was previously believed to have a uniformly poor prognosis but this is no longer considered true. It is frequently associated with parenchymal hemorrhage. The blood becomes isodense relatively rapidly and often disappears completely within a couple of weeks. A ventriculostomy is placed in the less bloody ventricle and CSF drainage is used to reduce pressure and drain away the blood.

Acute obstructive hydrocephalus may develop secondary to a posterior fossa hematoma that obstructs the ventricular pathways. However, delayed hydrocephalus is far more common, occurring in about 6% of patients with severe head injury. This communicating hydrocephalus results from blood in the subarachnoid space and is often evident by the 14th day after injury, although it can certainly become evident later.

Acute ischemic infarction appears as a low-density area compared with the adjacent brain. The infarction may be detectable on CT scan within 24 hours of onset and over 60% are clearly seen by 7 days. Contrast enhancement improves the diagnostic yield by nearly 15%, and MRI is even more sensitive.

Ventriculography

Before the advent of CT scanning, air ventriculography and angiography were the most important emergency radiologic tests for evaluating comatose head-injured patients. The former was favored because of the rapidity with which it could be obtained, even though the latter could provide more information. However, ventriculography is almost never used anymore if CT scanning is available.

Angiography

Angiography may be undertaken in the acutely head-injured patient when CT scanning is not available, when vascular injury is suspected, or when the findings on CT are not consistent with the patient's neurologic status. Traumatic carotid artery dissection may present with Horner syndrome, dysphasia, hemiparesis, obtundation, and monoparesis. When an isodense subdural hematoma is suspected, its presence can usually be confirmed by altering the CT window setting with a contrast-enhanced study, or with an MRI.

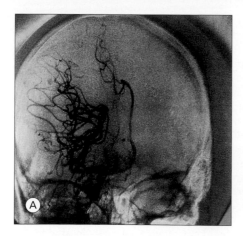
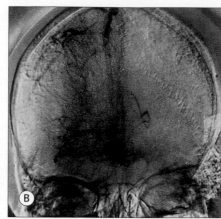

Figure 19.8 Angiograms showing severe mass effect secondary to a right acute subdural hematoma. **(A)** Arterial phase: the middle cerebral branches are displaced towards the midline and the pericallosal artery is markedly shifted across the midline because of subfalcine herniation. **(B)** Venous phase: the internal cerebral vein is shifted 2 cm towards the left.

Supratentorial mass lesions usually cause a contralateral shift of the anterior cerebral artery and the internal cerebral vein (Figure 19.8). The latter, being closer to the midpoint of the cranium, is less affected by rotation of the film – a common problem because of rotation of the head to either side. Although displacement of the vessels does not provide any features differentiating between parenchymal swelling and hematomas, a study of the pattern can help localize the lesion. Frontal lesions cause a bowing of the anterior cerebral artery, the so called "rounded shift," with limited displacement, if any, of the internal cerebral vein. Parietal lesions tend to cause a "square shift" of the anterior cerebral artery, primarily as a result of widening of the unyielding falx cerebri posteriorly, and the internal cerebral vein is more markedly displaced. Temporal lobe lesions result in medial displacement of the internal carotid artery bifurcation and a characteristic upward displacement of the middle cerebral artery group. Extra-axial mass lesions usually appear as avascular areas on angiography. The classic appearance of an extra-axial hematoma on the AP view consists of a clear gap between the inner table of the skull and the small vessels on the surface of the brain as seen in the venous phase.

Infratentorial mass lesions are difficult to detect angiographically, and vertebral injections are rarely undertaken for this purpose. Transtentorial herniation is seen on anteroposterior and lateral carotid angiograms as marked stretching of the anterior choroidal artery as a result of medial uncal displacement. If the posterior communicating arteries are visible, these will also be seen to be stretched and sometimes compressed against the posterior clinoid processes. The posterior cerebral arteries are inferiorly displaced on lateral view and are seen to be medially displaced along with both superior cerebellar arteries on anteroposterior view due to hippocampal gyrus herniation.

Intracranial pressure

Since the early 1970s, there has been an increasing interest in ICP monitoring and control (see Chapter 4). This has been associated with progressive evolution of related technology. However, the intraventricular catheter (or ventriculostomy) remains the most widely used and most useful device for measuring ICP and helping in its control and for maintaining cerebral perfusion pressure.[31,32]

Cerebral perfusion pressure (CPP) is the mean arterial blood pressure minus intracranial pressure. Since cerebral ischemia may be the single most important secondary effect affecting outcome following severe traumatic brain injury, it is useful to follow cerebral perfusion pressure rather than intracranial pressure

alone.[33] The Guidelines have recommended maintaining CPP at a minimum of 60 mmHg to possibly help in the avoidance of both global and regional ischemia. It is certainly possible that too great a CPP may also have a deleterious effect.

Head injury is the most common indication for ICP monitoring. As a general rule, patients who can follow simple commands need not be monitored and may satisfactorily be followed clinically. In patients who are unable to follow simple commands and have an abnormal CT scan, the incidence of intracranial hypertension is high (53–63%), and monitoring is warranted.[22] Severely head-injured patients with normal CT scans generally have a lower incidence of hypertension (approximately 13%) unless they have two or more of the following adverse features at admission: systolic blood pressure < 90 mmHg, unilateral or bilateral motor posturing, or age over 40 years. In the presence of these adverse features, the incidence of intracranial hypertension even in patients with normal CT scans is as high as those with abnormal CT scans on admission.[22] Compression or absence of basal cisterns has also been associated with intracranial hypertension.[34]

Normal ICP in a relaxed or paralyzed patient who is neither hypotensive nor hypercarbic is 10 mmHg (136 mmH$_2$O) or less. While pressures in the range of 10 to 20 mmHg (136–272 mmH$_2$O) may occur with moderate disturbances of intracranial volumes, pressures greater than these herald an intracranial hematoma, diffuse brain swelling, or both.

Most dangerous traumatic intracranial mass lesions shift the midline 5 mm or more. This is invariably associated with an elevated ICP unless a CSF leak is present. Significant temporal lobe lesions may cause only a minimal shift of the midline, but the ICP may be elevated and the third ventricle, if seen, will often be shifted more than the lateral ventricles. If there is little or no midline shift, the ICP is elevated, and the patient is not hypercarbic, then either there are bilateral mass lesions or there is serious diffuse brain swelling.

When intracranial pressure demonstrates an upward trend, certain basic items should be checked. The neck should be in a neutral position to facilitate venous drainage. In most cases, having the head end of the bed elevated approximately 30° is useful.[35] The calibration of the system must be checked, and one should confirm that the transducer is level with the foramen of Monro. If the patient is fighting the ventilator, he or she should be sedated or chemically paralyzed. If these measures are not adequate, various methods exist to reduce the ICP, including ventricular drainage, mannitol, and hyperventilation (see Chapter 4).

New technology now allows one to monitor cerebral oxygenation, via the LICOX CMP System. The purpose of this triple-lumen bolt system is to provide additional data including brain tissue oxygenation ($P_{BT}O_2$), temperature, as well as ICP in patients where cerebral hypoxia and/or ischemia are a concern. Normal brain tissue oxygen pressure is > 30 mmHg (range 25–50 mmHg) with ischemia reported at ranges less than 8–12 mmHg and cell death at < 5 mmHg.[36] Since the duration and severity of cerebral tissue hypoxia correlates with unfavorable outcomes in severe traumatic brain injury, this could prove a valuable tool in treatment management and possibly in predicting outcome. The monitor is able to indicate cerebral tissue perfusion status local to the sensor placement, although local brain oxygen levels may not reflect what is happening in the rest of the brain.

GUIDELINES FOR TREATMENT

It is difficult to lay down hard and fast rules regarding the management of a disease as diverse as head injury. The primary aim to treatment is to prevent secondary damage to an already injured brain. Nevertheless, in 1995 a document was developed by the Brain Trauma Foundation that established treatment protocols for the management of traumatic brain injury.[1,2] This document was the result of a joint effort between The Brain Trauma Foundation and The American Association of Neurological Surgeons. A panel of expert neurosurgeons with specific interests in the care of patients with severe head injury examined the available data on traumatic brain injury. Recommendations of care were formulated relying on scientific evidence rather than expert opinion. The recommendations were classified as Standards, Guidelines, or Options. Standards are accepted principles that reflect a high degree of clinical certainty, Guidelines represent a strategy that reflects moderate clinical certainty, and Options are strategies for which the clinical certainty is unclear. Table 19.7 presents an outline of these recommendations.[1,2]

Medical therapy

Anticonvulsants

The role of prophylactic anticonvulsants in patients with severe head injury has been more clearly defined with the advent of the published Guidelines. Post-traumatic seizures are classified as "early" occurring within 7 days of injury or "late," occurring more than 7 days after the injury.[38,39] It is desirable to prevent early and late seizure activity; although, these medications have been associated with adverse and neurobehavioral ill-effects. The classic study by Jennett[40] found post-traumatic epilepsy to occur in about 5% of all patients admitted to the hospital with closed head injuries and in 15% of those with severe head injuries. Three main factors were found to be linked to a high incidence of late epilepsy: early seizures occurring within the first week, an intracranial hematoma, or a depressed skull fracture. While certain earlier studies were unable to show significant benefit of prophylactically administered anticonvulsants, a double-blind study of 404 severely head-injured patients, who were randomized to receive phenytoin or placebo beginning within 24 hours of injury and continuing for 1 year, found that phenytoin reduced the incidence of seizures in the first week after injury but not thereafter.[41] This study appears to justify stopping prophylactic convulsants after the first week in most cases. In patients who have had a seizure, anticonvulsants are continued for at least a year.

Mannitol

Mannitol is widely used to reduce ICP (see Chapter 4) and its use is recommended by the Guidelines in the management of intracranial hypertension. The commonly used preparation is a 20% solution. The most widely accepted regimen is 0.25–1 g/kg given intravenously as a bolus. Serum osmolality should not generally be allowed to go much above 320 mOsm/L, if possible, to avoid systemic acidosis and renal failure. There is clinical and laboratory evidence to suggest that long-term, repeated use of mannitol can worsen brain edema and hence reverse the initial beneficial effect.[14]

Furosemide

Furosemide (Lasix) has been used alone and in conjunction with mannitol in the treatment of raised ICP. It has been shown that diuresis can be enhanced by the combined use of these agents with more pronounced and consistent brain shrinkage. A dose of 0.3–0.5 mg/kg of furosemide given intravenously is reasonable.

Barbiturates

Several studies have studied the protective effect of barbiturates on the brain in cerebral anoxia and ischemia. It has also been documented that barbiturates are effective in reducing ICP.[42] Although it is unclear whether barbiturates improve outcome from severe head injury, it is clear that pentobarbital is one of the few options available in patients with refractory intracranial hypertension (see Chapter 4). This drug should not be used in the presence of hypotension; in fact, the outcome in hypotensive patients who are put into pentobarbital coma is worse than in controls. Furthermore, hypotension is often associated with the use of this agent. Great care should be taken to maintain adequate cerebral perfusion pressure during the use of barbiturates.

Steroids

While steroids are clearly useful in reducing the edema associated with brain tumors, their value in head injury is not clear. In fact, most studies to date have not demonstrated any beneficial effect associated with steroids in terms of either ICP control or improved outcome from severe head injury. Furthermore, there is some evidence that steroids may have a deleterious effect on metabolism in these patients. It is possible that very high doses of particular steroids may have a beneficial effect in certain subsets of head-injured patients. However, currently available steroids in standard dose regimens have not proven to be valuable in severe head injury.

Surgical therapy

Indications for surgery

An important reason for operating on a mass lesion is a midline shift of 5 mm or more. Such a shift may be demonstrated by CT scan, occasionally by angiography, or ventriculography. Most epidural, subdural, or intracerebral hematomas associated with a midline shift of 5 mm or more are surgically evacuated. In a patient who has a small hematoma causing less than 5 mm shift and is alert and neurologically intact, a conservative approach is justified. However, the patient may deteriorate, and very close observation is vital. Should there be any change in mental status, a repeat CT scan should be obtained immediately.

Our policy is to operate on all comatose patients with an intracranial mass lesion and 5 mm or more of midline shift unless they are brain-dead. This policy is based on evidence that some patients

Table 19.7 Recommended standards, guidelines and options in the care of the head-injured patient

	Standard	Guideline	Option
Trauma systems and the neurosurgeon	Insufficient data	All regions in the USA should have an organized trauma care system	As delineated in the American College of Surgeons Committee on Trauma Resources for Optimal Care of the Injured Patient: 1993, neurosurgeons should have an organized and responsive system of care.[37] Neurosurgeons should initiate neurotrauma care planning (prehospital management and triage), maintain call schedules, review trauma care records for quality improvement, and participate in trauma education
Brain-specific treatments during initial resuscitation	Insufficient data	Insufficient data	The first priority is complete and physiologic resuscitation. No specific treatments should be directed at intracranial hypertension in the absence of signs of transtentorial herniation or progressive neurologic deterioration not attributable to extracranial explanation. If present, the physician should treat aggressively with rapid hyperventiliation and mannitol under conditions of adequate volume recuscitation
Resuscitation of blood pressure and oxygenation	Insufficient data	Hypotension (SBP < 90 mmHg) or hypoxia (apnea or cyanosis in the field or a P_aO_2 < 60 mmHg) must be scrupulously avoided, if possible, or corrected immediately	The mean arterial pressure should be maintained above 90 mmHg throughout the patient's course to attempt to maintain cerebral perfusion pressure (CPP) > 60 mmHg
Indications for intracranial pressure monitoring	Insufficient data	Intracranial pressure (ICP) monitoring is appropriate in patients with severe head injury with an abnormal CT scan such as hematomas, contusions, edema, or compressed basal cisterns. ICP monitoring is appropriate in patients with severe head injury with a normal CT scan if two or more of the following features are noted at admission: age over 40 years, unilateral or bilateral motor posturing, SBP < 90 mmHg. ICP monitoring is not routinely indicated in patients with mild or moderate head injury. However, a physician may choose to monitor ICP in certain conscious patients with traumatic mass lesions	
Intracranial pressure treatment threshold	Insufficient data	ICP treatment should be initiated at an upper threshold of 20–25 mmHg	Interpretation and treatment of ICP based on any threshold should be corroborated by frequent clinical examination and cerebral perfusion pressure
Cerebral perfusion pressure	Insufficient data	Insufficient data	Cerebral perfusion pressure should be maintained at a minimum of 60 mmHg
Hyperventilation	In the absence of increased ICP, chronic prolonged hyperventilation therapy (P_aCO_2 of 25 mm Hg or less) should be avoided	The use of prophylactic hyperventilation (P_aCO_2 < 35 mmHg) therapy during the first 24 hours after severe traumatic brain injury should be avoided because it can compromise cerebral perfusion at a time when cerebral blood flow is reduced	Hyperventilation therapy may be necessary for brief periods when there is acute neurologic deterioration or for longer periods if there is intracranial hypertension refractory to sedation, chemical paralysis, CSF drainage, and osmotic diuretics. Jugular venous oxygen saturation (S_jO_2), arterial–jugular venous oxygen content Differences (AV_dO_2), and cerebral blood flow monitoring may help to identify cerebral ischemia if hyperventilation, resulting in P_aCO_2 values less than 30 mmHg, is necessary

Continued

Table 19.7, *cont'd.*

	Standard	Guideline	Option
Mannitol	Insufficient data	Mannitol is effective for control of raised ICP after severe head injury. Limited data suggest that intermittent bolus doses may be more effective than continuous infusion. Effective doses range from 0.25 g to 1 g/kg body weight	The indication for use prior to ICP monitoring are signs of transtentorial herniation or progressive neurological deterioration not attributable to systemic pathology. (However, hypovolemia should be avoided by fluid replacement)
Barbiturates	Insufficient data	High-dose barbiturate therapy may be considered in hemodynamically stable salvageable severe head injury patients with intracranial hypertension refractory to maximal medical and surgical ICP lowing therapy	
Glucocorticoids	The use of glucocorticoids is not recommended for improving outcome or reducing ICP in patients with severe head injury	None	None
Nutrition	Insufficient data	Replace 140% of resting metabolism expenditure in non-paralyzed patients and 100% resting metabolism expenditure in paralyzed patients using enteral or parenteral formulae containing at least 15% of calories as protein by the 7th day after injury	The preferable option is use of jejunal feeding by gastrojejunostomy due to ease of use and avoidance of gastric intolerance
Anti-seizure prophylaxis	Prophylactic use of phenytoin, carbamazepine, or phenobarbital is not recommended post-traumatic seizures	None	It is recommended as a treatment option that anti-convulsants may be used to prevent early post-traumatic seizures in patients at high risk for seizures following head injury. Phenytoin and carbamazepine have been demonstrated to be effective in preventing early post-traumatic seizures. However, the available evidence does not indicate that prevention of early post-traumatic seizure improves outcome following head injury

with bilaterally nonreactive pupils, impaired oculocephalic responses, and decerebrate posturing can nevertheless make a good recovery. In one series, three of 19 such patients who were treated maximally ended up in the "good" or "moderately disabled" category, despite the foreboding constellation of signs.[43]

The management of brain contusions is somewhat less clearcut. Galbraith and Teasdale,[44] in their series of 26 patients with acute traumatic intracranial hematomas who were managed without surgery, found that all patients with ICP greater than 30 mmHg eventually deteriorated and required surgery. In contrast, only one patient with ICP less than 20 mmHg deteriorated. Patients in the 20–30 mmHg range were about evenly divided between the surgical and nonsurgical groups.

We have recently analyzed our experience with 130 head-injured patients with pure contusions who were managed with CT scanning and ICP monitoring as needed.[45] This study showed that patients with brain contusions who could follow commands at admission did not require ICP monitoring and, as a rule, did well with simple observation. However, those who could not follow

commands (in the absence of a focal lesion in the speech area) often had intracranial hypertension and needed to have their ICP monitored. The majority of these patients who had a midline shift of 5 mm or more required surgery.

It has been demonstrated conclusively that patients with a large (over 30 mL) temporal lobe hematoma have a much greater risk of developing tentorial herniation than those with a frontal or parietooccipital lesion.[46] The bias should therefore tilt towards early surgery in such cases.

Once a decision has been made as to whether the patient is a surgical candidate or not, he or she is promptly moved to the operating room or to the neurosurgical intensive care unit, respectively. If the patient is harboring a mass lesion, mannitol (1–2 g/kg) should be administered en route to the operating room. In addition, the patient can be hyperventilated briefly to achieve an arterial P_{CO_2} of 25–30 mmHg. As in all the maneuvers undertaken thus far, time is of the essence. The sooner the mass lesion is evacuated, the better the possibility of a good recovery.[12] If, on the other hand, no surgical lesion is found, the patient is carefully monitored in the NICU, both clinically and with various physiologic parameters, notably ICP recordings and serial CT scans. Any rise in ICP above 20 mmHg which cannot be readily explained and reversed or any deterioration in neurologic status warrants prompt repetition of the CT scan followed by appropriate corrective measures.

Since there is great concern about increased ICP as a result of a mass lesion, the anesthetic agents that are used in head-injured patients preferably should not increase the ICP. Nitrous oxide has only a slight vasodilatory effect and generally does not cause a significant ICP increase. It is therefore considered a good agent for use in the head-injured patient. A commonly used combination is nitrous oxide with oxygen, intravenous muscle relaxant, and thiopental. Hyperventilation and mannitol prior to and during induction can blunt the vasodilatory effect and limit intracranial hypertension to some degree while the cranium is being opened. If, during surgery, malignant brain swelling occurs that is refractory to hyperventilation and mannitol, pentobarbital in large doses (5–10 mg/kg) should be used. This agent can cause hypotension, especially in hypovolemic patients, and should therefore be used with caution.

SUBDURAL HEMATOMAS Acute subdural hematomas may result from bleeding from lacerated brain, ruptured cortical vessels, or an avulsed bridging vein. The most common sites for brain injury are the inferior frontal lobes and the anterior temporal lobes. In the surgical management of subdural hematomas, a large fronto-temporoparietal questionmark-shaped incision is recommended. This allows the surgeon to deal with bleeding near the midline as well as to debride effectively parts of the frontal, temporal, and parietal lobes as needed. If the patient is deteriorating rapidly, a quick temporal decompression can be performed via a small craniectomy before opening up the rest of the flap. This maneuver could reduce the probability of tentorial herniation. A generous subtemporal craniectomy may be useful in postoperative intra-cranial pressure control. The role of decompressive craniotomy with removal of the bone flap and creation of a dural pouch to allow brain swelling is currently being examined.

EPIDURAL HEMATOMAS Epidural hematomas are most often located in the temporal region and often result from tearing of the middle meningeal vessels due to a temporal bone fracture. Venous epidural hematomas may occur as a result of a skull fracture or an associated venous sinus injury. These tend to be smaller and usually have a more benign course. Such hematomas often present several hours or days after the initial injury and can be managed nonsurgically. However, usually an epidural hematoma represents a surgical emergency and should be evacuated as rapidly as possible. Every effort should be made to relieve the pressure as soon as possible. A more localized craniotomy flap is warranted for epidural hematomas.

CONTUSIONS/INTRACEREBRAL HEMATOMAS Contusions are most often located in the anterior and inferior frontal lobes as well as the anterior temporal lobes. Quite commonly, the CT appearance of a contusion evolves over several days so that what are initially small "salt and pepper" lesions coalesce to form hematomas. This phenomenon is also termed delayed traumatic intracerebral hematoma. Patients who are awake and alert but demonstrate cerebral contusions can be managed without surgery in the vast majority of cases.[45] However, patients who are comatose and have a significant midline shift usually need surgery.

Between these two extremes, there are patients who demonstrate alterations in levels of consciousness or focal neurologic deficits; in these, the decision to undertake surgical debridement is not always easy. As a general rule, debridement of the left frontal and temporal lobes is undertaken more reluctantly because the speech area is on this side.

DEPRESSED SKULL FRACTURES A skull fracture is considered significantly depressed if the outer table of the skull lies below the level of the inner table of the surrounding bone. Sometimes such depression may not be evident on plain X-rays, but it is usually seen clearly on the CT scan. Most closed depressed fractures occur in young children and may be of the pingpong ball variety. Surgery may be undertaken in such cases for cosmetic reasons or because of brain compression. In compound depressed fractures, the wounds are often dirty and contaminated. Hair, skin, or other foreign debris may be insinuated between the depressed bone fragments. Therefore, except in the simplest of injuries, the use of the operating room for the closure of such wounds is recommended.

VENOUS SINUS INJURIES Injuries of the major venous sinuses are among the most difficult problems a neurosurgeon has to face. As a general rule, ligation of the anterior third of the superior sagittal sinus is tolerated well; ligation of the posterior third is most likely to produce massive venous infarction of the brain. Ligation of the middle third of the superior sagittal sinus has somewhat unpredictable effects. A dominant transverse sinus usually cannot be safely ligated. While the use of shunts in the repair of these major sinuses has been often described, in our experience simple pressure with the use of hemostatic agents is much more practical in the majority of cases.

POSTERIOR FOSSA HEMATOMAS Posterior fossa hematomas, fortunately, are less common than supratentorial hematomas. In general, an aggressive surgical approach is recommended for most of these lesions because the patient can deteriorate very rapidly. Because it generally takes longer to expose the posterior fossa and because the brainstem structures are likely to suffer irreversible damage from a shorter period of compression, the surgeon does not have much leeway in terms of time.

PROGNOSIS

The Glasgow Outcome Scale (GOS) has been widely accepted as a standard means of describing outcome in head injury patients. This is a simple five-point scale (Table 19.8).[47] These categories are sometimes lumped together as either favorable outcomes (G, MD) or unfavorable outcomes (SD, V, or D). Post-traumatic amnesia is a fairly good prognostic indicator of outcome. First described by Russel in 1932, post-traumatic amnesia is defined as the duration of time from the point of injury until the patient has continuous memory of ongoing events. In most cases, the retrospective measurement of post-traumatic amnesia is unreliable. Therefore, Harvey Levin developed the Galveston Orientation and Amnesia Test (GOAT) to provide an objective reliable measurement of post-traumatic amnesia. The duration of post-traumatic amnesia has proven to be highly correlated with ultimate functional outcomes.[48]

Several statistical studies have reported the use of various prognostic indicators for predicting outcome in severe head injury.

Table 19.8 Glasgow Outcome Scale (GOS)

Good recovery (G)	Patient returns to preinjury level of function
Moderately disabled (MD)	Patient has neurologic deficits but is able to look after self
Severely disabled (SD)	Patient is unable to look after self
Vegetative (V)	No evidence of higher mental function
Dead (D)	

CLINICAL PEARLS

- The first priority in treating the head-injured patient is prompt physiologic resuscitation – restoration of blood pressure, oxygenation, and ventilation.

- Episodes of hypotension and/or hypoxia greatly increase morbidity and mortality after severe head injury; therefore even a single episode should be avoided if possible.

- Available literature indicates that glucocorticoids do not lower ICP or improve outcome in severely head-injured patients; therefore the routine use of steroids is not recommended.

- Mannitol is effective in reducing intracranial hypertension but is not to be used as a prophylactic treatment.

- Since cerebral ischemia may be the single most important secondary event affecting outcome following severe traumatic brain injury; maintaining the cerebral perfusion pressure greater than 60 mmHg may help avoid both global and regional ischemia. However, pushing the cerebral perfusion pressure much higher may have undesirable adverse effects.

- Chronic prophylactic hyperventilation should be avoided during the first 5 days after a severe traumatic brain injury, and particularly during the first 24 hours. Prophylactic hyperventilation therapy further reduces cerebral blood flow and thus has been associated with poorer outcomes.

Because of unexpected medical and surgical complications and the inherent unpredictability of disease, there is no absolutely unfailing prediction system. Based on experience with a large group of patients, an algorithm has been developed for approximate expected outcomes associated with certain prognostic features.[49] An attempt to predict mortality with 100% certainty appeared to work in one center.[50] However, when this system was applied to other patient populations, some patients who were predicted to die based on this scale instead survived.[51]

This highlights the difficulty in making foolproof predictions of outcome in patients with head injury. Nevertheless, certain broad predictions can be made based on the patient's initial examination and this can be valuable in counselling the family.

REFERENCES

1. Bullock R, Chestnut RM, Clifton G, et al. Guidelines for the management of severe head injury. *J Neurotrauma* 1996; 13: 641–734.
2. Bullock R, Chestnut RM, Clifton G, et al. Guidelines for the management of severe head injury. *J Neurotrauma* 2000; 17: 449–627.
3. Alderson P, Roberts I. Corticosteroids for acute traumatic brain injury. *Cochrane Database Syst Rev* 2000; 2: CD000196.
4. Roberts I. Barbiturates for acute traumatic brain injury. *Cochrane Database Syst Rev* 2000; 2: CD000033.
5. Schierhout G, Roberts I. Mannitol for acute traumatic brain injury. *Cochrane Database Syst Rev* 2000; 2: CD001049.
6. Guidelines for the management of penetrating brain injury. *J Trauma* 2001; 51: S3–S15.
7. Narayan RK, Michel ME, Ansell B, et al. Clinical trials in head injury. *J Neurotrauma* 2002; 19: 503–57.
8. Teasdale G, Jennett B. Assessment of coma and impaired consciousness. *Lancet* 1974; 2: 81–4.
9. Jennett B, Teasdale G. Assessment of impaired consciousness. In: Plum F (ed.). *Management of Head Injuries*. Philadelphia, PA: FA Davis Co.; 1981: 77–93.
10. Miller JD. Minor, moderate and severe head injury. *Neurosurg Rev* 1986; 9: 135–9.
11. Williams DH, Levin HS, Eisenberg HM. Mild head injury classification. *Neurosurgery* 1990; 27: 422–8.
12. Seelig JM, Becker DP, Miller JD, et al. Traumatic acute subdural hematoma: major mortality reduction in comatose patients treated within four hours. *JAMA* 1981; 304: 1511–18.
13. Gennarelli TA. Cerebral concussion and diffuse brain injuries. In: Cooper PR (ed.), *Head Injury*, 2nd edn. Baltimore: Williams & Wilkins; 1987: 108–24.
14. Dacey RG, Alves WM, Rimel RW, et al. Neurosurgical complications after apparently minor head injury—assessment of risk in a series of 610 patients. *J Neurosurg* 1986; 65: 203–10.
15. Vos PE, Battistin L, Birbamer G, et al. EFNS guideline on mild traumatic brain injury: report of an EFNS task force. *Euro J Neurol* 2002; 9: 207–19.
16. Borczuk P. Predictors of intra cranial injury in patients with mild head trauma. *Ann Emergency Med* 1995; 25: 731–6.
17. Hofman PA, Nelelemans P, Kemerink, GJ, Wilmink JT. Value of radiological diagnosis of skull fracture in management of mild head injury: meta-analysis. *J Neurol Neurosurg Psychiatr* 2000; 68: 416–22.
18. Stein SC, Ross SE. Moderate head injury: a guide to initial management. *J Neurosurg* 1992; 77: 562–4.
19. Stone JL, Lowe RJ, Jonasson O, et al. Acute subdural hematoma: direct admission to a trauma center yields improved results. *J Trauma* 1986; 26: 445–50.
20. Miller JD, Butterworth JF, Gudeman SK, et al. Further experience in the management of severe head injury. *J Neurosurg* 1981; 54: 289–99.
21. Miller JD, Sweet RC, Narayan RK, Becker DP. Early insults to the injured brain. *JAMA* 1978; 240: 439–442.
22. Narayan RK, Kishore PRS, Becker DP, et al. Intracranial pressure: to monitor or not to monitor? A review of our experience with severe head injury. *J Neurosurg* 1982; 56: 650–9.

23. Chestnut RM, Ghajar J, Maas AIL, *et al*. Early indicators of prognosis in severe traumatic brain injury. *J Neurotrauma* 2000; 17: 557–90.

24. Levine JE, Becker DP. Reversal of incipient brain death from head injury apnea at the scene of accidents. *N Engl J Med* 1979; 301: 109.

25. Chestnut RM, Marshall LF, Klauber MR, *et al*. Analysis of the role of secondary brain injury in determining outcome from severe head injury. *Presented at the Annual Meeting of the American Association of Neurological Surgeons*; 1990; Nashville, TN.

26. Butterworth JF, Maull KI, Miller JD, *et al*. Detection of occult abdominal trauma in patients with severe head injuries. *Lancet* 1980; 2: 759–62.

27. Schenarts PJ, Diaz J, Kaiser C *et al*. Prospective comparison of admission computed tomographic scan and plain films of the upper cervical spine in trauma patients with altered mental status. *J Trauma* 2001; 51: 663–8.

28. Narayan RK, Greenberg RP, Miller JD, *et al*. Improved confidence of outcome prediction in severe head injury: a comparative analysis of the clinical examination, MEPs, CT scanning and ICP. *J Neurosurg* 1981; 54: 751–62.

29. Taylor WR, Chen JW, Meltzer H, *et al*. Quantitative pupillometry, a new technology: normative data and preliminary observations in patients with acute head injury. Technical note. *J Neurosurg* 2003; 98: 205–13.

30. Wester K, Aas-Aune G, Skretting P, Syversen A. Management of acute head injuries in a Norwegian county: effects of introducing CT scanning in a local hospital. *J Trauma* 1989; 29: 238–41.

31. Feldman Z, Narayan RK. Intracranial pressure monitoring: techniques and pitfalls. In: Cooper PR, (ed.), *Head Injury*, 3rd edn. Philadelphia: Williams & Wilkins; 1993: 247–74.

32. Rosner MJ, Daughton S. Cerebral perfusion pressure management in head injury. *J Trauma* 1990; 30: 933–941.

33. Miller JD. Head injury and brain ischemia – implications for therapy. *Br J Anesth* 1995; 57: 120–30.

34. Marshall LF, Marshall SB, Klauber MR, *et al*. A new classification of head injury based on computerized tomography. *J Neurosurg* 1991; 75(suppl.): S14–S20.

35. Feldman Z, Kanter MJ, Robertson CS, *et al*. Effect of head elevation on intracranial pressure, cerebral perfusion pressure and cerebral blood flow in head-injured patients. *J Neurosurg* 1992; 76: 207–11.

36. Van Santbrink, H, Maas AI, Avezaat CJ. Continuous monitoring of partial pressure of brain tissue oxygen in patients with severe head injury. *Neurosurgery* 1996; 38: 21–31.

37. American College of Surgeons Committee on Trauma. *Resources for Optimal Care of the Injured Patient*. Chicago: American College of Surgeons; 1993.

38. Temkin NR, Dikmen SS, Winn HR. Postraumatic seizures. *Neurosurg Clin North Am* 1991; 2: 425–35.

39. Yablon SA. Posttraumatic seizures. *Arch Phys Med Rehabil* 1993; 74: 983–1001.

40. Jennett B. *Epilepsy After Nonmissile Head Injuries*, 2nd edn. London: Heinemann; 1975.

41. Temkin NR, Dikmen SS, Wilensky AJ, Keihm J, Chabal S, Winn HR. A randomized, double-blind study of phenytoin for the prevention of post-traumatic seizures. *N Engl J Med* 1990; 323: 497–502.

42. Eisenberg HM, Frankowski RF, Contant CF, Marshall LF, Walker MD. High-dose barbiturates control elevated intracranial pressure in patients with severe head injury. *J Neurosurg* 1988; 69: 15–23.

43. Becker DP, Miller JD, Ward JD, *et al*. The outcome from severe head injury with early diagnosis and intensive management. *J Neurosurg* 1977; 47: 491–502.

44. Galbraith S, Teasdale G. Predicting the need for operation in the patient with an occult traumatic intracranial hematoma. *J Neurosurg* 1981; 55: 75–81.

45. Sheinberg MA, Kanter MJ, Robertson CS, Contant CF, Narayan RK, Grossman RG. Continuous monitoring of jugular venous oxygen saturation in head-injured patients. *J Neurosurg* 1992; 76: 212–17.

46. Andrews BT, Chiles BW, Olsen WL, Pitts LH. The effect of intracerebral hematoma location on the risk of brain-stem compression and on clinical outcome. *J Neurosurg* 1988; 69: 518–22.

47. Jennett B, Bond M. Assessment of outcome after severe brain damage: a practical scale. *Lancet* 1975; 1: 480–4.

48. Levin HR *et al*. Posttraumatic amnesia as apredictor of outcome after severe closed head injury. Prospective assessment. *Arch Neurol* 1996; 8: 782–91.

49. Choi SC, Muizelaar JP, Barnes TY, Young HF. Prediction tree for severely head injured patients. *J Neurosurg* 1991; 75: 251–5.

50. Gibson RM, Stephenson GC. Aggressive management of severe closed head trauma: time for reappraisal. *Lancet* 1989; 2(8659): 369–71.

51. Feldman Z, Contant CF, Robertson CS, Narayan RK, Grossman RG. Evaluation of the Leeds prognostic score for severe head injury. *Lancet* 1991; 337: 1451–3.

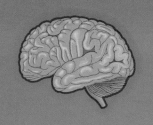

GUNSHOT WOUNDS OF THE HEAD

20

James Ecklund, Geoffrey SF Ling, and Setti S Rengachary

Firearm-related deaths are the second leading cause of deaths due to trauma. In the western world the USA has the highest frequency of firearm-related deaths. Handguns are the firearms most frequently used in fatal injuries in civilian trauma. The economic impact of firearm-related injuries is enormous. The annual incidence of firearm-related head injury deaths in the USA is 2.4/100 000 or approximately 6000 deaths per year.[1] Firearms are used by those responsible in 58% of homicides and 57% of suicides.[2] We have learned a great deal about gunshot wounds and their management from military experience gained during times of war, when a large number of firearm-related casualties are treated in a short period of time. Unfortunately over the last several decades civilian gunshot wounds have risen in prevalence. It is therefore critically important for military and civilian neurosurgeons to understand the concepts surrounding wound ballistics, mechanisms of injury, pathophysiology and the appropriate management of gunshot wounds to the head. Most recently guidelines on the management and prognosis of penetrating brain injury have been published and will be referred to, as appropriate, throughout this chapter.

FIREARMS AND BALLISTICS

A firearm is any weapon that uses an explosive powder charge to propel a projectile. Firearms are classified based on their size, their muzzle velocity and the type of projectile fired. Handguns in general are defined as a firearm operated by one hand. They tend to have lower muzzle velocity and much shorter barrels than rifles. Shotguns can deliver either a single projectile or multiple pellets, which have a large collective mass. Handguns and most rifles are further classified by the caliber of the weapon. Caliber is defined as the internal diameter of the barrel, and thus represents the widest diameter of the bullet. It may be expressed in millimeters, as in a 9-mm handgun, or in inches, as in a .22 rifle or .44 magnum. Magnum refers to a load with extra powder, which thereby imparts more velocity to the projectile.[3]

Shotguns are designated by gage instead of caliber. Gage is defined as the least number of balls made from 1 lb (454 g) of lead that will still fit in the barrel. In other words, the lead ball that would fit in a 12-gage barrel weighs 1/12th of a pound. Therefore a 12-gage shotgun has a larger barrel than a 20-gage shotgun. There are many types of shells, ranging from nine pellets per shell, as in number 00, to 2385 pellets per shell as in number 12.

Ballistics refers to the study of the motions of projectiles in flight; wound ballistics refers to the study of the projectile when it enters tissues. Ballistics relies on several factors, including kinetic energy, mass, velocity, shape of the projectile and fragmentation potential. When a bullet leaves the muzzle of a weapon, it has a certain velocity. Low-velocity weapons or firearms have muzzle velocities less than 1000 feet per second (300 m/s) and are seen in most handguns, with the exception of magnum loads. For example a .45 automatic has a muzzle velocity of 869 feet per second (260 m/s). Compare this with the 7.62-mm rifle, which has a muzzle velocity of 2830 feet per second (850 m/s). As a projectile travels to its target its velocity will decrease secondary to the friction of air resistance. This ability to overcome air resistance is expressed in the ballistic coefficient, which is different for different projectiles. The equation for ballistic coefficient includes a form factor, which relates to the shape. The sharper the nose of the bullet the less the velocity will be decreased because the projectile will experience less air resistance; the rounder the nose of the bullet or more irregular the shape, such as with shrapnel, the greater the effect of air resistance and the greater the subsequent velocity deterioration.[4,5] An example of the effects of this air resistance can be seen in the US Military M16A1 rifle which has a muzzle velocity of 3150 feet per second. At 300 yards (270 m) this muzzle velocity is decreased to 2186 feet per second and at 1000 yards (900 m) its velocity is 835 feet per second (945, 655 and 250 m/s, respectively).

Most barrels are grooved to impart some spin on a bullet as it departs the firearm (Figure 20.1). This spin stabilizes the bullet and helps to limit other behaviors of the bullet in flight, such as precession which is circular rotation around the center of the mass in a spiral fashion, and nutation, which is rotation in small circles forming a rosette pattern.[6] When the projectile ultimately strikes tissue its kinetic energy is transferred based on the equation $^1/_2 \, mv^2$ (where m is mass and v is velocity). If the projectile causes a perforating injury that goes through and through, the equation is modified to include the entry velocity minus the exit velocity. High-velocity projectiles create a complex wounding pattern. Upon impact a sonic shock wave is produced which is very brief (microseconds) and does not contribute substantially to tissue destruction. As the projectile penetrates brain tissue it crushes the tissue in its path, creating a permanent tract of tissue injury. In high-velocity injuries a temporary cavitation effect also occurs, which is a velocity-related phenomenon. This temporary cavity results from the transmission of kinetic injury where the surrounding tissue is rapidly compressed tangentially from the primary track. After the cavity expands to its maximum size it starts to collapse under negative pressure and can suck in external debris. This cavity will then undergo smaller expansions and contractions of diminishing amplitude. In relatively inelastic tissue, such as the brain, this results in a tract of injury up to

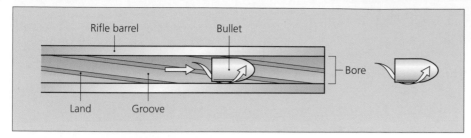

Figure 20.1 Spin stabilization of the bullet. As the bullet passes through the barrel, rifling imparts a rotary spin to the bullet. The spinning of the bullet lends stability to its flight and increases its total energy. The spinning process also adds a distinctive mark to the bullet sheath, which can be used to identify the weapon.

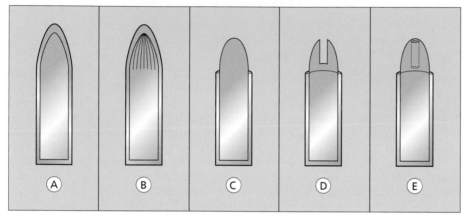

Figure 20.2 Varieties of bullets. **(A)** Fully jacketed military bullet. **(B)** Dumdum bullet. This is radially scored to weaken the tip so that it will mushroom upon impact. **(C)** Partially jacketed "soft point" bullet. The lead tip is unjacketed so that it will mushroom upon impact. **(D)** Hollow-point bullet. The forward end of the bullet is blunt and hollowed out to facilitate mushrooming. **(E)** Devastator bullet. Like **(D)**, but it has a canister filled with an explosive within the hollow tip of the bullet. This explodes upon impact, further increasing damage to the bullet tip. If the canister does not explode, the surgeon or pathologist retrieving the bullet from the tissue is at personal risk.

10–20 times the size of the projectile. The motion of the projectile in the tissue, or yaw, also affects the morphology of the temporary cavity. Yaw is deviation of the bullet in its longitudinal access from the straight line of flight. As the projectile rotates 90°, the primary track of tissue destruction increases based on the length of the projectile. This will impart greater kinetic energy directed tangentially and the size of the secondary cavity increases. This concept also explains why exit wounds are generally larger than entrance wounds in perforating injuries.[7]

The fragmentation potential of a bullet also relates to its wounding potential. Projectiles can deform or fragment on contact. Most civilian bullets are partially jacketed to ensure quick killing of the game during hunting. On impact the tip will mushroom and impart more kinetic injury causing more tissue destruction, a larger temporary cavity, and more likely early death. The Hague Convention of 1899 and the subsequent Geneva Convention require all military bullets to be fully jacketed to help limit the fragmentation potential. Irregularities in the jacket have also been used to enhance deformation. An example is the dumdum bullet, named after a village in India where they were first manufactured by the British. In contemporary civilian use the bullet is frequently only partially jacketed, leaving the tip uncovered. Hollow-point bullets are unjacketed with the addition of a hollow or blunt nose tip to enhance the efficiency of the mushrooming effect upon contact. An extreme version of this concept is the devastator bullet, which has a secondary explosive, generally made of lead azide, in the hollow tip, that is designed to explode upon impact (Figure 20.2). These are very unstable rounds and can frequently malfunction.[8] If the round does not explode on impact the surgeon or pathologist retrieving the bullet from the tissue can be at personal risk. In the event that devastator bullets are suspected precautions should include the use of rubber-tipped instruments, special protective clothing on a limited surgical team and avoidance of any use of ultrasound guidance or electrocoagulation.[9]

Wound ballistics for shotguns varies depending upon whether the shotgun is fired from close or long range. At long range the shotgun pellets scatter and act in an identical manner to multiple individual projectiles, with kinetic energy imparted separately by each pellet hitting the target. At close range the entire charge hits the target and acts similarly to a single missile with kinetic energy equivalent to a high-velocity projectile, with extensive fragmentation potential (Figure 20.3).

CLASSIFICATION OF MISSILE WOUNDS TO THE HEAD

One of the first classifications of penetrating head injuries was made by Cushing during his experience in World War I (Table 20.1). This was subsequently refined by Matson in World War II and remains remarkably similar to that still in use today.[10] When a projectile strikes the head it may create a tangential wound, a penetrating wound, or a perforating wound. One must also be aware of the potential for intracranial ricochet of projectiles and the possible careening of projectiles inside the skull and around the brain[11] (Figure 20.4).

Tangential wounds

Tangential wounds generally occur when a missile strikes the head at an oblique angle and grazes the skull. It may travel in the subgaleal space and exit through or remain in the scalp. In addition to the scalp laceration, the projectile can cause varying degrees of damage to the skull, meninges and underlying cortex. Linear depressed skull fractures may be present. Injuries to underlying vessels can produce epidural or subdural hematomas. An area of cortical contusion also frequently underlies the fracture. The clinical presentation may include seizures, or a focal motor, sensory, or speech deficit. In some situations the neurological deficit may be much worse than expected from the clinical

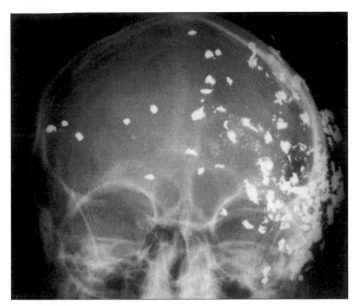

Figure 20.3 Shotgun blast at close range.

presence of an extra-axial hematoma or mass effect and the extent of cortical injury. Conservative treatment with local wound care is generally followed in the absence of an extra-cerebral hematoma, cerebrospinal fluid (CSF) leakage, or complex depressed skull fracture.

Penetrating wound

Depending on the velocity of the projectile, the bullet's energy may be spent on penetrating the skull, leaving only enough kinetic energy to pass partially through the brain substance (Figure 20.5). Some of the energy will be absorbed by the skull, and skull fragments are capable of producing secondary projectiles. It is not uncommon to find multiple bone or bullet fragments driven into the brain substance. Impact with the skull also enhances the fragmentation and yaw of the round. When bullets strike more perpendicular they are more likely to penetrate the skull than bullets that strike more tangentially. Penetrating wounds can cause localized brain contusions, lacerations, or hematomas. Pseudoaneurysms or arteriovenous fistula development can also occur, especially when the tract is near the skull base or sylvian fissure.

In some instances after the bullet has gone through the skull and through the brain substance it may hit the inner table of the opposite side of the calverium and ricochet, with re-entry of the bullet into the brain tissue causing further damage. Therefore, the neurosurgeon should recognize that correlation of an entrance wound and plain X-ray data alone may be deceiving because plain films cannot assess for the presence of an intracranial ricochet. A CT scan, however, will show the exact bullet track. In rare

examination of the wound. In most instances, however, the neurological deficit is minimal. Tangential gunshot wounds carry a better prognosis than any other type of gunshot wound to the head. Computed tomography (CT) scan will allow a good assessment of the degree of skull fracture and cortical contusion. The surgical management of these patients will depend on the

Table 20.1 Classification of craniocerebral injuries by Cushing[19] and Matson[10]

CUSHING (World War I)		MATSON (World War II)	
Grade	Description	Grade	Description
I	Scalp lacerations, skull intact	I	Scalp wound
II	Skull fractures, dura intact	II	Skull fracture, dura intact
III	Depressed skull fracture and dural laceration	III	Skull fracture with dural/brain penetration A: Gutter-type (grazing) – in-driven bone with no missile fragments B: Penetrating – missile fragments in brain C: Perforating – through and through
IV	In-driven bone fragments	IV	Complicating factors: A: Ventricular penetration B: Fractures of orbit or sinus C: Injury of dural sinus D: Intracerebral hematoma
V	Penetrating wound with projectile lodged		
VI	Wounds penetrating ventricles with: A: Bone fragments B: Projectile		
VII	Wounds involving : A: Orbitonasal region B: Auropetrosal region		
VIII	Perforating wounds		
IX	Bursting skull fracture, extensive cerebral contusion		

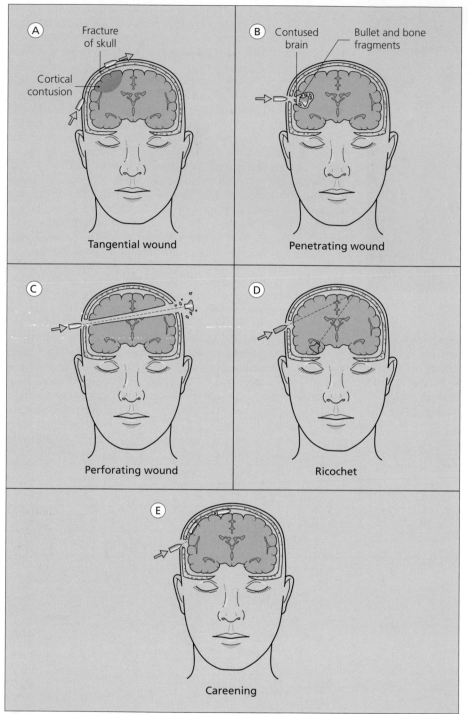

Figure 20.4 Varieties of missile wounds to the head. **(A)** Tangential wound. The bullet grazes the skull but does not penetrate it. There may be a depressed fracture of the skull. The presence of cortical contusion is a hallmark of this type of injury. Tangential wounds carry the best prognosis because they result in limited brain injury. **(B)** Penetrating wound. The skull is penetrated, but the bullet does not have enough energy left to penetrate the entire brain. **(C)** Perforating wound. The bullet goes through the entire head, causing devastating injury as a result of cavitation. This type of wound carries the worst prognosis. **(D)** Ricochet. The bullet strikes the opposite inner table of the skull and reflects back into the brain causing further damage. **(E)** Careening. The bullet hugs the inner table of the skull and may cause major venous sinus injury.

instances, bullets can also migrate in a delayed manner, especially if near a ventricular system or a non-fragmented round[12,13] (Figure 20.6). If a significant delay occurs between the initial radiographic studies and surgical intervention, a repeat film may be considered.

Another unusual event is careening of the bullet. After the bullet has penetrated the outer and inner tables of the skull it may change direction as it encounters the dura and travel along the inner table of the skull. This is an unusual occurrence, however intracranial hematomas and injury to major venous sinuses may be seen with this injury.

Perforating wounds

Perforating wounds are generally the most devastating missile injury to the head (Figure 20.7). They require a higher velocity missile than a simple penetrating wound. The wound entry is generally smaller than the exit wound because of the secondary cavitation which is usually several times larger than the diameter of the bullet. Since these wounds tend to be higher velocity than the penetrating wounds they tend to cause a larger temporary cavitation. This cavitation in both penetrating and perforating wounds can cause widespread punctate hemorrhages and rupture

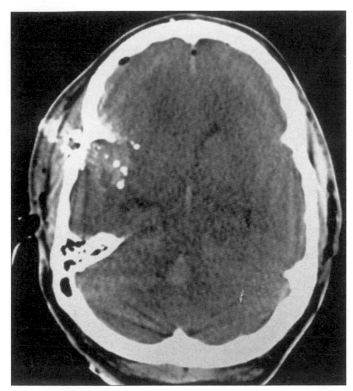

Figure 20.5 Example of a penetrating wound.

MANAGEMENT OF PATIENTS WITH GUNSHOT WOUNDS TO THE BRAIN

Initial assessment and care

Upon the patient's arrival at the emergency department initial efforts are directed toward maintaining an adequate airway, especially in those patients who have gunshot wounds through the face and mandible. A patent airway is maintained by either an oral airway or an endotracheal tube depending on the clinical situation. Respiratory support with a ventilator may also be necessary. Circulatory support should be instituted as appropriate with volume and/or pharmacologic blood pressure support, with euvolemia being the goal.

A quick history is obtained from the patient's relatives or law enforcement officers with emphasis on the circumstances of the incident, such as whether the gunshot was suicidal, accidental, or homicidal. Suicidal attempts are known to correlate with a higher mortality.[14,15] The age of the patient is also important; an increase in age correlates with an increase of mortality after penetrating brain injury. The caliber of the weapon, independent of velocity at the time of impact, is not useful in prognosis. However, the type of firearm and the range at which the patient was shot can be important factors in that the velocity and mass together can give an approximation of the total kinetic injury imparted to the brain.[15]

Concurrent with obtaining the history a brief clinical assessment is made. The entrance and exit wounds if present are inspected (Figure 20.8). Powder stippling near the entrance wound indicates an injury at close range. Bulky absorbent dressings are applied as a preliminary measure and a quick neurological evaluation is made. This includes assessment of consciousness, pupillary size and reaction, brainstem reflexes (such as vestibular–ocular, corneal and gag reflexes), and the presence of spontaneous respirations. Motor activity is assessed as well, to determine whether the patient has spontaneous purposeful movements, decorticate, decerebrate, or flaccid limbs. It is well known that a low Glasgow Coma Scale correlates with higher mortality and an unfavorable outcome. Hypotension and hypoxia are both associated with increased mortality, and the presence of bilateral fixed and dilated pupils is highly predictive of mortality. In addition to the routine laboratory work-up, one should screen for

of cell membranes far from the bullet tract. Even if the primary injury by the missile is to the cerebral hemispheres, temporary cavitation may cause membrane dysfunction as far away as the brainstem, causing acute apnea and cardiorespiratory failure. After this initial transient rise in intracranial pressure from the secondary cavitation, delayed increases in intracranial pressure (ICP) occurs as a result of contusions, hematomas and progressive edema. The kinetic injury transmitted through the brain by the explosive temporary cavitation may also be sufficient to cause multiple basilar fractures in the skull remote from the entry point.

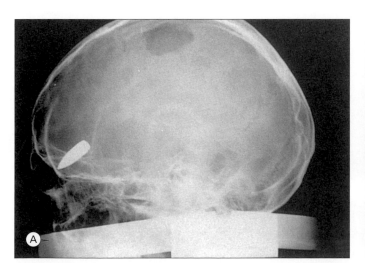

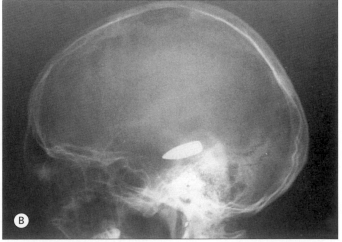

Figure 20.6 Spontaneous migration of an intracranial bullet. (A) A fully jacketed, undeformed bullet is located in the frontal pole of the brain. (B) The bullet has spontaneously migrated to the temporal area, due to gravitational forces causing it to sink within the brain substance.

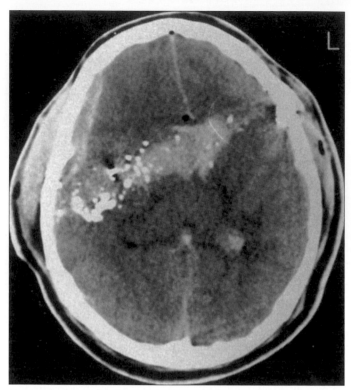

Figure 20.7 Example of a perforating wound.

disseminated intravascular coagulopathy (DIC). The pulpy contused brain tissue releases thromboplastin, and many patients may manifest features of DIC. It is also known that the presence of coagulopathy on admission is associated with increased mortality, particularly at lower levels of the Glasgow Coma Scale.[15] At the end of the clinical assessment plain radiographs of the skull in the anteroposterior and lateral views are taken, unless a non-contrast CT scan is immediately available.

Imaging

Radiologic imaging of patients with missile wounds to the head is crucial in planning the clinical management and determining the prognosis. While plain radiographs of the skull can easily be obtained in the emergency room and often provide considerable information about the missile and the tract, they can be misleading in the presence of an intracranial ricochet. An estimation of caliber may also be made from plain films. However, fragmentation of the bullet may prevent precise determination of the caliber and the knowledge of caliber alone independent of velocity estimations can be misleading as to the true kinetic energy imparted.

CT scans tends to be the primary radiologic assessment tool for missile wounds to the head. A noncontrast CT scan with bone windows should be performed as part of the emergency room evaluation. Much important information can be obtained from the CT. The precise location of the bullet or bullet fragments, including any additional bony fragments along the bullet track or in secondary tracks, can be determined. Bone fragments are usually distinguished from bullet fragments by the lack of scatter on CT (Figure 20.9). The true tract of injury can be identified on CT scans, including any richochet. The greatest advantage of CT scanning is the ability to identify and locate precisely hematomas,

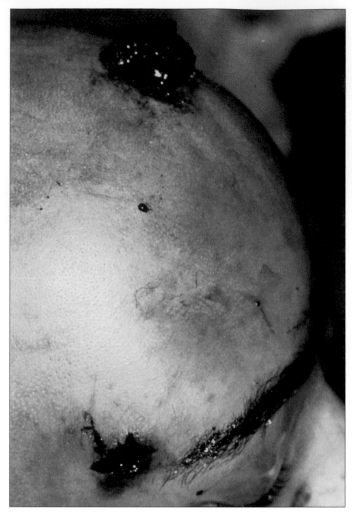

Figure 20.8 Self-inflicted gunshot wound with suicidal intent. The patient was right-handed. The wound of entry is in the right temporal region behind the eye. Note the small area of powder burn immediately below the wound of entry. There is considerable periorbital swelling. The exit wound is near the midline vertex. Note that the wound of exit is much larger than the wound of entry.

contusions and mass effect. Intracranial bleeding results from transection of various dural or parenchymal vessels in the bullet's path, which may result in epidural, subdural, parenchymal, or intraventricular hematomas (Figure 20.10). On rare occasions a hematoma may be found far from the damage in an area opposite the wound of entry. Since no other diagnostic test gives this extensive information, the CT scan assumes a role of primary practical importance.

Evidence that CT also provides prognostic value has recently been published in the *Guidelines for the Management of Penetrating Brain Injury*.[15] It has been shown that bihemispheric lesions relate to an increased mortality and that multi-lobar injuries are strongly associated with mortality when compared with unilobar injuries. Injuries with intraventricular hemorrhage and injuries with cisternal effacement also have an increased mortality rate. Interestingly, there is no established relationship between midline shift or large contusions and mortality, however the presence of midline shift does have important implications for the surgical management of these patients.

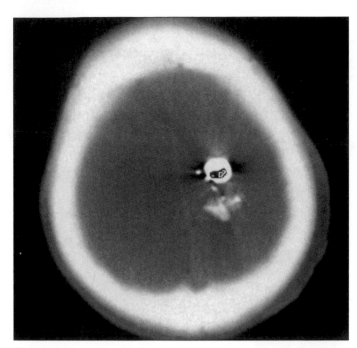

Figure 20.9 CT scan of the head with bone windows in a patient with a gunshot wound. There are in-driven bullet and bone fragments. The bone fragments can be distinguished from bullet fragments by the lack of scatter.

CT scanning does have some limitations. It does not always correlate with the true extent of damage, in that physiologic damage and dysfunction may occur remote from the tract. Metallic artifacts and scatter can also compromise image quality.

Angiography should be considered in gunshot wounds to the head when a vascular injury is suspected. Patients that have an increased risk of vascular injury include those with a wound trajectory through or near the sylvian fissure, supraclinoid carotid, basilar cisterns, or a major venus sinus. Also, the development of an otherwise unexplained subarachnoid hemorrhage or delayed hematoma should also prompt the consideration of a vascular injury necessitating the need for angiography.[15,16]

Magnetic residence imaging (MRI) should probably be avoided and is not recommended in the acute management of gunshot wounds to the head. Ferromagnetic materials within fragments can rotate and move in response to the magnetic field causing additional injury. Although many bullet fragments will have no ferromagnetic properties, there is great variation and MRIs in general should be avoided.

Medical and ICP management

The first decision made on the level of aggression of both medical and surgical management of a patient with a gunshot wound to the head must take into account the prognostic implications of the clinical and historical data discussed in the preceding sections. No absolute criteria regarding aggressive management can be given since no single prognostic factor is absolute. One must take into account all the historical, clinical and radiographic information in addition to the patient's desires, or the families' perception of the patient's desires, to each individual case. Grahm has published some guidelines he found prudent based on his management of 100 gunshot wound victims in a civilian setting.[17] His guidance relies very heavily on the initial presenting Glasgow Coma Scale and CT scan findings. According to Grahm et al., any patient with a Glasgow Coma Scale above 7 should be treated aggressively. Any patient with a post-resuscitative Glasgow Coma Scale of 3–5, and the absence of a large hematoma causing mass effect, should be considered for conservative management because of the almost assured poor prognosis despite aggressive measures. Based on prognostic considerations, those with Glasgow Coma Scale scores of 5–7 should also be considered for conservative management in the presence of a multilobular dominant injury or a transventricular wound tract.

After the decision has been made to manage the patient aggressively, ICP monitoring should be considered when the clinician is unable to assess the neurologic examination accurately. In general this implies a Glasgow Coma Scale of 7 or less. Management of ICP should probably follow the guidelines published for the management of severe head injury, which includes maintaining ICP below 20 and cerebral perfusion pressure above 60. Broad spectrum antibiotics are recommended in gunshot wounds to the head. It is commonly believed that because bullets assume high temperatures a bullet will be sterile when it strikes the target. Both clinical and experimental observations have indicated that this is not the case. The most common source of contamination is the patient's skin, hair, or clothing; in addition the external air maybe sucked into the wound during the temporary cavitation, along with dirt and skin flora, resulting in bacterial contamination in the depths of the wound.

Anti-seizure medications are also recommended to prevent posttraumatic seizures. Similar to closed head injuries prophylactic treatment with anti-convulsives beyond the first week after gunshot wound to the head has not been shown to prevent the development of new seizures.

CSF leaks should also be vigorously managed. CSF leaks are correlated with a much higher incidence of infection and subsequently a poorer outcome. Leaks at the site of entry and exit site require surgical closure of the skin and dura. More remote CSF leaks from basal skull fractures or air sinus penetration require either direct surgical repair or CSF diversion when appropriate.[15,18]

Surgical management

As mentioned previously, a CSF leak, especially in orbito-facial cranial wounds, a Glasgow Coma Scale score of 8 or higher, and the presence of a significant hematoma regardless of poor Glasgow Coma Scale score are definite indications for surgical intervention. Because the extent of brain debridement has been a subject of debate, we will refer to the history of this issue in some detail. In World War I Harvey Cushing reduced operative mortality of penetrating brain injury from 56% to 28% in 3 months by aggressively and meticulously debriding all devitalized tissue, removing all visualized bone and metal fragments, and emphasizing good closures.[19] In World War II the operative mortality was further reduced to 14.5% through the use of antibiotics and better availability of blood. In the Korean conflict, the surgical mortality dropped to 10%. During this conflict we also learned the importance of early surgical assessment in the treatment of clinically significant hematomas. Six months into the conflict neurosurgeons were placed in the combat zone. The number of patients in whom hematomas where found during surgery rose to 41%, compared with 7% during the first 6 months when operative intervention was delayed by transportation out of the combat zone. After World War II and the Korean War a number of studies

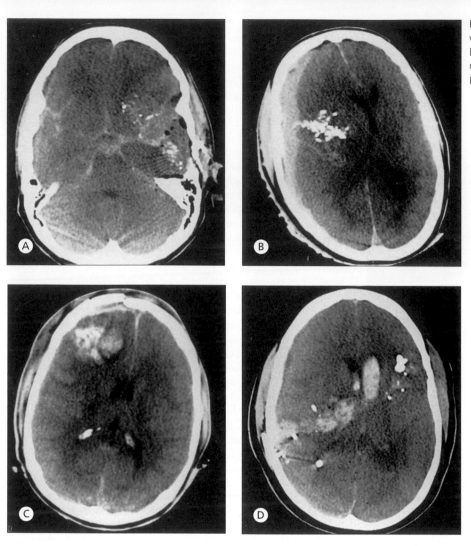

Figure 20.10 Intracranial bleeding from gunshot wounds to the head. **(A)** Subarachnoid hemorrhage. **(B)** Subdural hematoma. **(C)** Confluent intracerebral hematoma. **(D)** Intraventricular hematoma.

were published which implied that postoperative infections and abscesses were the result of inadequate debridement. This prompted a more aggressive approach during the Vietnam War, when every attempt was made to remove all in-driven bone and metal fragments and devitalized tissues were aggressively debrided. If further evaluation at higher echelon hospitals revealed bone or metal fragments, the patients were subjected to second and sometimes third operative debridements.[20] Long-term evaluation of these patients through the Vietnam Head Injury Study indicated that their was no significant difference in the rates of infection and posttraumatic seizures in patients regardless of the persistence of intracranial bone or metal fragments. This observation has led to a more conservative approach in more recent conflicts. In the Israeli–Lebanese conflict, systematic analysis of patients who survived gunshots wounds to the head indicated that debridement of the bullet tract should be limited to removal of easily accessible fragments and fragments removable by gentle irrigation. Aggressive attempts at retracting and resecting brain tissue to access deeply in-driven fragments does not appear warranted.[21] Thus the most recent war experienced forms the benchmark that is followed in most civilian gunshot wounds today. The recent *Guidelines for the Management of Penetrating Brain Injury* acknowledged that the treatment of small entrance bullet wounds by local wound care and closure when the scalp is not devitalized and there is no significant intracranial pathology is a reasonable option for management. Treatment of more extensive wounds that have no viable scalp, bone, or dura may require more extensive debridement before primary closure through a craniotomy or craniectomy. The evacuation of hematomas with significant mass affect and the removal of devitalized brain tissue and safely accessible bone fragments is recommended. However, routine removal of distant bone and metal fragments is not recommended. Also aggressive surgical debridement of the missile tract in the absence of mass effect is not recommended. If an open air sinus injury occurs, such as in orbito-facial cranial wounds, a more aggressive surgical approach with repair of the dura is indicated to achieve primary repair and to prevent CSF leakage. In addition, a high suspicion for vascular complications should be maintained in patients with an orbito-facial injury or delayed hematoma. When a traumatic intracranial aneurysm or a traumatic arteriovenous fistula is identified treatment by appropriate surgical or endovascular means is recommended.[15]

CONCLUSION

The management of gunshot wounds to the head requires a firm understanding of the wounding mechanisms, prognostic indicators, clinical evaluation, medical and surgical intervention and potential complications. These patients should be treated through standard advanced trauma life support (ATLS) protocols and should undergo an early CT scan of the brain. If aggressive intervention is decided upon, based on prognostic and family considerations, antibiotic and anti-convulsant treatment and aggressive ICP management should be instituted. Surgical intervention should be performed on patients with significant hematomas with mass effect, orbital facial wounds, wounds with CSF leakage and in wounds with significantly devitalized scalp and tissue. Local wound management can be considered in patients without significant hematomas or devitalized scalp.

CLINICAL PEARLS

- Post resuscitation neurologic status and CT findings will determine aggressiveness of treatment.

- Broad spectrum antibiotics, anticonvulsants, ICP control less than 20-25, and CPP greater than 60 should be maintained.

- CSF Leaks lead to increased infectious complications should be aggressively treated.

- Angiography should be performed when the wound tract crosses sylvian fissure, vessels at base of skull, major veous sinuses, or for delayed hemorrhage.

- Extent of wound debridement is dictated by presence of hematomas with mass effect and amount of devitalized tissue.

REFERENCES

1. Trask TW, Narayan RK. Civilian penetrating head injury. In: Narayan RK, Wilberger JE, Povlishock JT (eds). *Neurotrauma*. New York: McGraw-Hill; 1996: 869–87.
2. Kaufman HH, Schwab K, Salazar AM. A national survey of neurosurgical care for penetrating head injury. *Surg Neurol* 1991; 36: 370–7.
3. Barach E, Tomlanovich M, Nowak R. Ballistics: a pathophysiologic examination of the wounding mechanisms of firearms: Part I. *J Trauma* 1986; 26: 225–35.
4. Ordog GJ, Wasserberger J, Subramanian B. Wound ballistics: theory and practice. *Ann Emerg Med* 1984;13:1113–22.
5. Adams DB. Wound ballistics: a review. *Milit Med* 1982; 147: 831–5.
6. Hopkinson DA, Marshall TK. Firearm injuries. *Br J Surg* 1967; 54: 344–53.
7. Fackler ML, Malinowski JA. The wound profile: a visual method for quantifying gunshot wound components. *J Trauma* 1885; 25: 522–9.
8. Sykes LN, Champion HR, Fouty WJ. Dumdums, hollow-points, and devastators: techniques designed to increase wounding potential of bullets. *J Trauma* 1988; 28: 618–23.
9. Rosenberg WS, Harsh IV GR. Penetrating wounds of the head. In Wilkens RH, Rengachary SS (eds). *Neurosurgery*. New York: McGraw-Hill; 1996: 2813–20.
10. Knightly JJ, Pullliam MW. Military head injuries. In: Narayan RK, Wilberger JE, Povlishock JT (eds). *Neurotrauma*. New York: McGraw-Hill; 1996: 891–902.
11. Bakay L. Missile injuries of brain. *NY State J Med* 1982; 3: 313–19.
12. Rengachary SS, Carey M, Templer J. The sinking bullet. *Neurosurgery* 1992; 30: 291–5.
13. Rapp LG, Arce CA, McKenzie R, *et al*. Incidence of intracranial bullet fragment migration. *Neurol Res* 1999; 21: 475–80
14. Selden BS, Goodman JM, Cordell W, Rodman GH. Outcome of self-inflicted gunshot wounds of the brain. *Ann Emerg Med* 1988; 17: 247–53.
15. Aarabi B, Alden TD, Chestnut RM, *et al*. Management and prognosis of penetrating brain injury. *J Trauma* 2001; 51(suppl.): S1–86.
16. Amirjamshidi A, Rahmat H, Abbassioun K. Traumatic aneurysms and arteriovenous fistulas of intracranial vessels associated with penetrating head injuries occuring during war: principles and pitfalls in diagnosis and management. *J Neurosurg* 1996; 84: 769–80.
17. Grahm TW, Williams FC, Harrington T, Spetzler RF. Civilian gunshot wounds to the head: a prospective study. *Neurosurgery* 1990; 27: 696–700.
18. Meirowsky AM, Caveness WF, Dillon JD, *et al*. Cerebrospinal fluid fistulas complicating missile wounds of the brain. *J Neurosurg* 1981; 54: 44–8.
19. Cushing H. Notes on penetrating wounds of the brain. *Br Med J* 1918; 1: 221–6.
20. Carey ME, Young HF, Mathis JL. The neurosurgical treatment of craniocerebral missile wounds in Vietnam. *Surg Gynecol Obstet* 1972; 135: 386–90.
21. Brandvold B, Levi L, Feinsod M, George E. Penetrating craniocerebral injuries in the Israeli involvement in the Lebanese conflict, 1982–1985. *J Neurosurg* 1990; 72: 15–21.

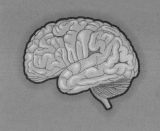

TRAUMATIC SKULL AND FACIAL FRACTURES

21

Fred H Geisler and Paul N Manson

SKULL FRACTURES

Skull fractures are classified in three ways: by pattern (linear, comminuted, depressed), by anatomic location (vault convexity, base), and by skin integrity (open, closed).

The pattern of a skull fracture is affected by two factors. The first factor is the force of impact. A linear fracture results first at a point of weakness when the skull structure fails to undergo further elastic deformation as a response to impact; the fracture typically starts at the point of weakness in response to the maximal stress (the point of weakness is often remote from the actual impact point) and extends to the point of impact. A comminuted fracture results when the impact force is sufficient to break the bone into multiple pieces under the point of impact and further through areas of weakness. Comminution absorbs the force of the injury. With even larger impact energies, the comminuted pieces can be driven inward to create a depressed fracture and may penetrate the dura and cortical surface of the brain.

The second factor is the ratio of the impact force to the impact area. If the impact, even one of high energy, is dispersed over a large area, as in a blunt head injury to an individual wearing a motorcycle helmet, it often produces no skull fracture, even though the brain may be severely injured. Parenthetically, it should be noted that some helmets, by the efficiency of their very force-transferring protection, have created basal skull fractures by transferred energy absorbed from protection of the vault and face transmitted through the mandible to the skull base. However, if the impact, even one of low energy, is concentrated in a small area, such as from a hammer blow, it often produces a small depressed fracture with multiple linear skull fractures radiating from the site of impact.

The location of a skull fracture is classified by its geography in two distinct areas: the skull convexity (generally termed "skull vault fracture") or the base of the skull (generally termed "basilar fracture"). Any of the two areas can occur singly or in combination. The pattern may also become more comminuted with increasing energy forces. A skull fracture can be further classified as "open" or "closed" by the presence or absence, respectively, of an overlying scalp laceration. In addition, a fracture extending into the skull base with violation of the paranasal sinuses or middle ear structures is also considered an "open" fracture.

Linear skull fractures

A linear skull fracture is a single fracture line that goes through the entire thickness of the skull.

Diagnosis

Although it is generally accepted that clinical indications for radiologic examination include loss of consciousness, retrograde amnesia, discharge from nose or ear, eardrum discoloration or hemotympanum, positive Babinski's reflex, or cranial nerve abnormalities, controversy exists (based on a cost–benefit analysis) regarding the use of plain X-rays to diagnose linear skull fractures. The patient's eventual neurologic outcome depends largely on the brain injury, rather than on the presence of a fracture *per se*. However, for a few patients radiologic examination may make a crucial difference. For example, a linear fracture crossing the path of the middle meningeal artery in even a mild head injury indicates risk for late neurologic deterioration from an epidural hematoma. Furthermore, computed tomography (CT) scans of the skull may detect depressed fractures, puncture wounds, and intracranial foreign objects that might otherwise elude physical examination. In practice a CT scan should be obtained in most cases, however, plain skull radiographs usually add little information. Medico-legally, it is usually best to obtain a CT scan, especially if the patient is an equivocal historian or if there is evidence of a cognitive issue or indication of a significant force of injury.

Management

Linear skull fractures require no stabilization or exploration when the scalp is closed, and when there is no evidence of epidural hematoma or underlying dural or cortical injury. Even when a scalp laceration is present, very seldom is surgical exploration with bone removal necessary. Exceptions would include a machete injury to the skull producing a linear skull fracture with underlying dural laceration and brain damage. The skull fracture does, however, show that significant head trauma has occurred, and a careful assessment of the brain, facial structures, and cervical spine is required. Open linear fractures are debrided of foreign material, devitalized soft tissue and bone fragments; the damaged soft tissue at the edges of the laceration is excised to bleeding tissue and the laceration is closed after thorough cleansing. If there is insufficient vascularized soft tissue present to permit excision of the contused devitalized tissue, a rotation flap and skin graft to the donor area may have to be considered.

Growing skull fracture in children

A rare complication after linear skull fracture in young children (usually less than 2 years) is a growing skull defect at the fracture site. In these cases the dura is torn under the linear skull fracture. The pathogenesis is thought to be an expanding pouch of arachnoid passing through the torn dura and skull fracture, acting as a one-way valve that traps cerebrospinal fluid (CSF) and causes pressure erosion of the fracture edges to enlarge the fracture; alternatively the growth of the brain, which produces pulsating spreading tensile pressure forces on the edges of an unrepaired dural laceration, may also cause a skull defect to enlarge. The brain may sometimes herniate through the skull defect, causing a new neurologic deficit. These lesions are surgically repaired with closure of the dura, and perhaps replacement or repair of the bone defect.

Comminuted fractures

A comminuted fracture occurs when multiple linear fractures radiate from the point of impact. Some of the fracture lines may involve the suture lines (diastatic fracture) or may stop at them. Around the point of impact there may be free fragments of bone.

Diagnosis

Diagnosis is made on skull radiographs and CT of the head with bone windows.

Management

If the skin is closed and no depression of bone fragments greater than the thickness of the skull is demonstrated on CT,

management is as for linear skull fractures. However, in many of these cases surgery is performed for the underlying intracranial pathology, such as an epidural hematoma (Figure 21.1). After the intracranial pathology has been corrected, the bone fragments are primarily replaced as a cranioplasty after cleansing. If the skin is open and free bone fragments are present, cleansing or debridement of the contaminated fragments and soft tissue is performed before dural and scalp closures (Figure 21.2).

Depressed skull fractures

In a depressed skull fracture, the greatest bone depression can occur at the interface of fracture and intact skull or near the center of the fracture if several fragments are displaced inward. Impacted fractures are wedged into position by blocked bone edges.

Diagnosis

Many patients with depressed skull fractures experience initial loss of consciousness and neurologic damage. However, 25% of patients experience neither loss of consciousness nor neurologic deficit and another 25% experience only brief loss of consciousness. Although the diagnosis of a depressed skull fracture is often indicated on routine skull radiographs by an area of double density

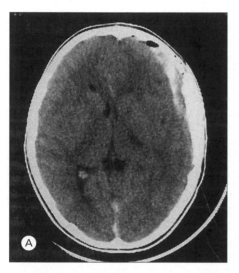
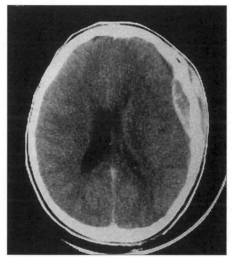

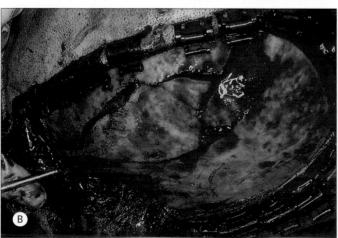
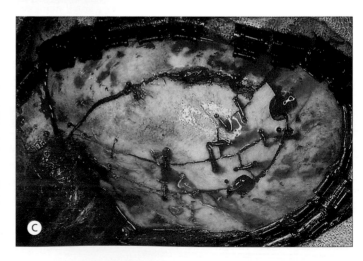

Figure 21.1 Comminuted, minimally depressed open skull fracture with underlying epidural hematoma. **(A)** CT scan through the center of the depressed region. Note the small amount of air at the anterior edge of the epidural hematoma. **(B)** Intraoperative view of the depressed bone before elevation. **(C)** The bone was removed, sutured together, and replaced as a cranioplasty. The epidural hematoma was removed after the bone fragments had been removed.

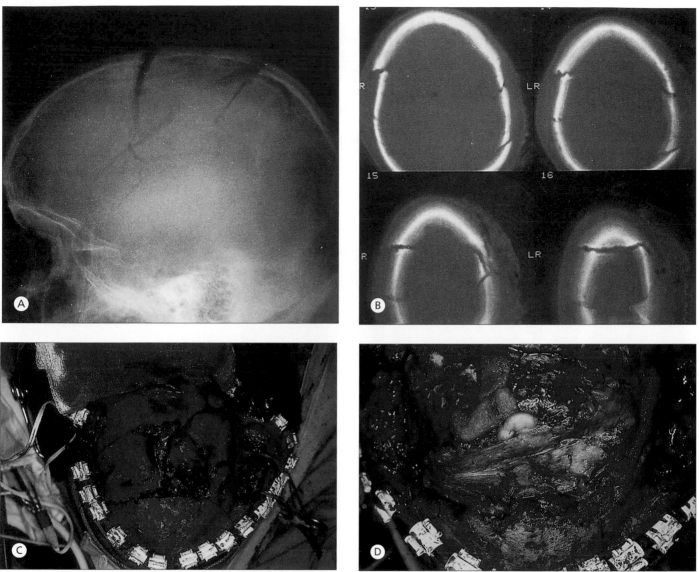

Figure 21.2 Comminuted skull fracture involving a diastatic fracture of both coronal sutures and additional fractures of the frontal and parietal bone bilaterally. In this case the skin was open and CSF was coming from the wound. **(A)** Lateral radiograph demonstrating the comminuted fracture. **(B)** CT scan with bone windows near the top of the head showing the comminuted fracture. **(C)** Intraoperative view of the fracture after the scalp was opened by extending the scalp laceration. **(D)** After the bone fragments were removed or debrided to expose the dural edges, a fascia lata graft was used to obtain the dural closure seen in this view.

(overlying bone fragments) or by multiple or circular fractures, the full extent and depth of injury are rarely appreciated without a CT scan. Physical examination is difficult because of scalp mobility and swelling. Scalp mobility can result in nonalignment of the scalp laceration and skull fracture; normal skull under a scalp laceration does not exclude a depressed fracture 1 or 2 cm from one edge of the laceration. Furthermore, traumatic swelling of the scalp minimizes the palpable and visual appearance of the step-off at the bony edges, preventing accurate clinical assessment of the extent of skull deformity for the first few days.

CT is the diagnostic method of choice. When image display windows are adjusted to optimize bony detail, they display the position, extent, and number of fractures, as well as the presence and depth of depression. With the imaging windows set to optimize intracranial contents, the same CT scan also allows

assessment of the underlying brain for contusion or hematoma, small bone fragments, or foreign bodies, as well as other traumatic intracranial pathology. Occasionally, coronal CT images through fractures near the vertex of the head or extending into the skull base are used to supplement the standard CT images, because the depth of a depression is more accurately measured on CT images perpendicular to the depression.

Management

Combined therapy of depressed fractures of the cranial vault extending to involve the frontal sinus or facial bones is covered in the sections on facial fractures. When a depressed skull fracture on the convexity also includes facial fractures, the intracranial injury is typically repaired first with removal of intracerebral hematoma and repair of dural laceration if present (Figures 21.3, 21.4).

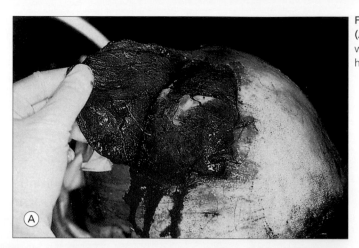

Figure 21.3 Open frontal and facial fracture. (A) View of frontal skull fracture under the wound. (B) CT scan showing the epidural hematoma under this open skull fracture.

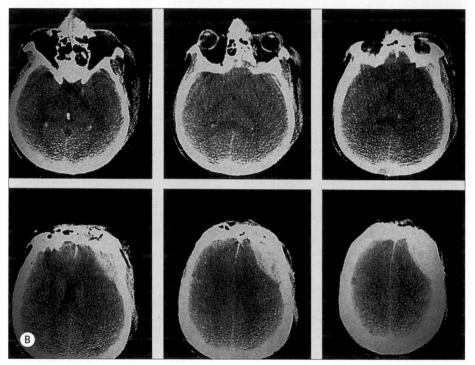

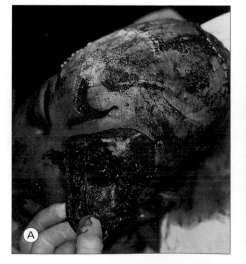
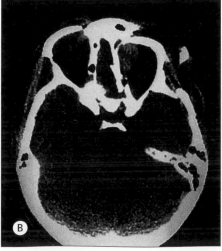

Figure 21.4 Open depressed skull fracture involving the frontal bone with extensive fractures and displacement of bones of the orbit and ethmoid region. (A) Presenting scalp laceration. (B) CT scan at the level of the orbit demonstrating extensive orbital and ethmoid fractures with displacement of the bony facial structures.

Although a focal neurologic deficit from the cortex directly under a depressed skull fracture is occasionally improved by elevation of the bone fragments (presumably by increasing local cortical blood flow), elevation usually produces no neurologic change, implying that impact produces the major cortical damage responsible for the brain deficit. The brain dysfunction usually undergoes a neurologic recovery phase of several weeks to months, similar to that after a stroke or a head injury without a depressed fracture. Likewise, the incidence of epilepsy after a depressed skull fracture is determined by the cortical damage at the time of impact. Therefore, the treatment of depressed skull fractures is based not on initiating neurologic recovery or preventing epilepsy but rather on correcting cosmetic deformity and preventing infection.

In closed depressed fractures, the indication for surgery is usually cosmetic, with the procedure performed on an elective basis in the first few days after the trauma, once the patient is cleared for elective anesthesia. The greatest cosmetic deformity occurs in the forehead. Exploration is more urgent for a large closed depressed fracture when the radiologic appearance suggests dural laceration, brain penetration, simultaneous frontal sinus fracture, mass effect, or underlying hematoma. The hematoma is evacuated, the dura is repaired, and the bone fragments are replaced and held in position with small plates and screws.

A compound depressed fracture is a neurosurgical emergency because of the risk of bacterial infection of the cranial cavity. The initial surgery is performed within 24 hours and usually within the first 12 hours. The major objectives are: removal of contaminated bone fragments and foreign material; debridement of devitalized scalp, dura, and brain; provision of a watertight closure of the dura. Often, foreign material or hair wedged between bone fragments cannot be seen through the overlying scalp incision, so simple wound irrigation and closure may be inadequate for debridement of foreign material. Dural closure is essential to prevent CSF leaks from the wound and brain herniation into the fracture area. Dural closure also prevents intracranial spread of infection from a scalp wound. Reconstruction of the calvarium is performed during the initial surgery if considered safe; otherwise, a cranial defect is left and the cosmetic repair is performed later. The major reasons to consider deferred calvarial reconstruction are to shorten additional anesthesia and blood loss by major head injury or multitrauma, especially with hemorrhage, gross contamination of wounds where the bone fragments cannot be adequately cleaned, and a delay of more than 24 hours for the initial surgery.

The scalp laceration associated with a compound depressed skull fracture is usually stellate and may contain areas of contused/devitalized tissue. These areas require debridement to normal vascularized scalp to allow prompt healing and prevent breakdown of the scalp covering the fracture site. Scalp breakdown can sometimes be treated locally and frequently will require early flap coverage. If early flap coverage is not successful, the replaced cranial bone may require debridement of any dead or necrotic bone or portion of the skin flap, flap rotation, and delayed cranioplasty will be required in stages.

Depressed fractures over dural sinuses

Depressed skull fractures over a venous sinus require special handling. Surgical elevation of these fractures may involve massive blood loss if a depressed fragment has been plugging a sinus tear. There are two strategies for management. The fracture can be carefully elevated, attempting to gain control of the venous sinus as soon as possible, preparing for significant transfusion requirements. If the fracture site is not grossly contaminated with foreign material, or will not cause a major cosmetic or functional deformity, or not cause intracranial hypertension secondary to sinus occlusion, such fractures are managed with scalp debridement alone and massive irrigation, followed by serial CT scans for signs of brain abscess for at least a year. A delayed cranioplasty may then be required.

Basilar skull fractures

Fractures of the base of the skull occur in 3.5–24% of head-injured patients. This wide variation results from differences in study populations and the difficulty in obtaining radiographic verification of the fractures. Linear fractures in the skull base carry a risk of meningitis, whereas this risk is extremely low in fractures of the convexity unless the scalp, bone, and dura are all violated. The dura is easily torn in a basal skull fracture; this places the subarachnoid space in direct contact with the paranasal sinuses or middle ear structures, providing a pathway for infection. For example, a persistent fistula allows a continuous CSF leak and bacterial colonization of the meninges will eventually develop.

Petrous bone fractures can be either longitudinal or transverse, relative to the long axis of the petrous pyramid. Longitudinal fractures are more common and usually involve the tympanic membrane or external ear canal, thereby producing otorrhea. Transverse fractures result from higher-energy impacts and can damage middle ear ossicules or the facial nerve. These fractures occur with or in continuity with linear, comminuted, or depressed skull fractures and not infrequently are large linear extensions of vault fractures, crossing the base of the anterior and middle cranial fossa (Figure 21.5).

Diagnosis

Clinical signs of basal skull fractures include bilateral periorbital ecchymoses (spectacle hematoma) (Figure 21.6), anosmia, or CSF rhinorrhea for anterior skull base fractures, as well as hemotympanum, blood in the external auditory canal, VIIth or VIIIth nerve palsies, ecchymosis over the mastoids (Battle's sign), or CSF otorrhea for temporal bone fractures (Figure 21.7). Frequently,

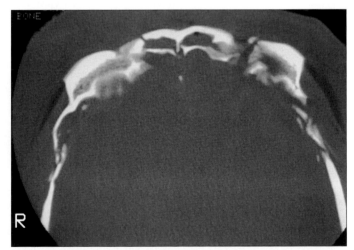

Figure 21.5 A type III frontobasilar fracture involves both the lateral and the center segment of the anterior skull.

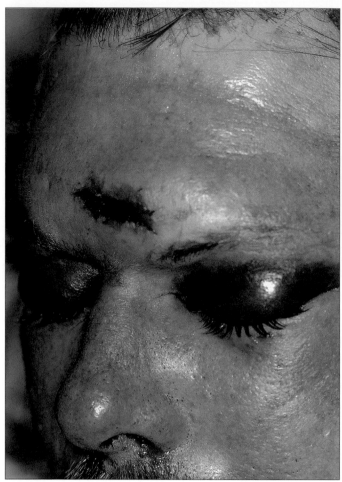

Figure 21.6 A bilateral spectacle hematoma from an open frontal sinus anterior skull base fracture.

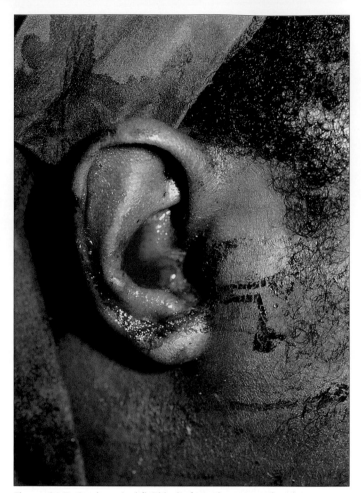

Figure 21.7 Cerebrospinal fluid leaks from the ear canal and a hematoma is visible in the postauricular area. These are signs of a fracture at the junction of the middle and posterior cranial fossa.

the CSF leak is first detected several days or weeks after the trauma. This delay often occurs because the CSF leak was hidden in bloody nasal discharge from facial fractures or, less frequently, is the result of delayed development of hydrocephalus with rupture of the arachnoid at the fracture site. A larger clear ring surrounding a central blood-tinged clot when a few drops of bloody discharge are placed on a paper towel indicates that CSF is probably mixed with the blood. This sign (the "double ring") (Figure 21.8) can also be noted on the patient's pillow during rounds.

Basal skull fracture with CSF rhinorrhea is common after head injury and has an estimated incidence in the United States of 150 000 cases per year. A clear, watery nasal discharge containing glucose indicates CSF rhinorrhea. An intermittent CSF leak from the paranasal sinuses can often be demonstrated by having the patient sit on the edge of the bed with the head close to the knees for 2 minutes and watching for clear fluid to drip from the nose.

Management

How a basal skull fracture is managed usually depends on whether a CSF leak is present. A patient with a basal skull fracture but no leak is observed for 2 to 3 days. During this time repeated checks for rhinorrhea and otorrhea are made to verify the absence of a CSF leak. Otorrhea is more likely than rhinorrhea to resolve

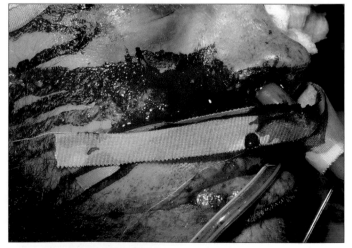

Figure 21.8 Brain and cerebrospinal fluid (CSF) leak from the nose after an extensive anterior skull base fracture. The adhesive tape on the endotracheal tube shows the "double ring" sign – a clearer blood-stained fluid (CSF) around a darker center (blood).

spontaneously. Because antibiotics are not effective in preventing meningitis and may select for resistant organisms if an infection occurs, prophylactic antibiotics are not used on a prolonged basis in patients with basal skull fractures. An exception is when definitive closure of a leak is performed.

A CSF leak is managed initially by observing the amount of leakage and monitoring for signs of infection: change in temperature, mental status, or white blood cell count. Radiographic or imaging studies may provide the area and size of the defect, which may contribute information on the likelihood of spontaneous closure. Most traumatic CSF leaks resolve spontaneously within the first week. If the leak persists beyond 5 to 7 days, lumbar taps are performed daily for 3 days, removing 30–50 mL of spinal fluid each time.

If spinal taps fail to stop the leak, spinal drainage can be used for 72 hours with the patient in a 30° head-up position. Should pneumocephalus develop during the course of CSF drainage, the drainage procedure is terminated and the dural leak is surgically closed. CSF leaks refractory to spinal fluid drainage require surgical closure; the exact site of the leak is determined pre-operatively from a CT scan with water-soluble intrathecal contrast, or from a nuclear cisternogram with nasal pledgets for small or questionable leaks. CT of the base of the skull can provide additional details of the pattern and size of the bone spicules in the fracture.

CSF otorrhea usually occurs through a fracture in the petrous bone with perforation of the tympanic membrane, although it can occasionally take place through a laceration of the external canal via fractured mastoid air cells. If the tympanic membrane remains intact, CSF that has gained access to the middle ear can flow through the eustachian tube and present as rhinorrhea. In these cases the CT scan typically images a fracture in the temporal bone and fluid in the mastoid air cells and middle ear. Blood from the ear canal or a tympanic canal laceration may also be caused by a temporomandibular joint injury or dislocation, either of which may produce some of the same symptoms (bloody fluid from the ear canal).

A patient with CSF otorrhea often presents with hearing loss or blood in the external ear canal. Irrigation and probing of the ear in cases of suspected otorrhea are not indicated initially because they increase the risk of infection. Such a patient is managed by placing a loose-fitting sterile gauze pad over the ear; the pad is changed every nursing shift and saved as an indicator of the amount of drainage from the ear. Most cases of otorrhea stop spontaneously within the first few days. A detailed auditory and vestibular examination is performed initially and 6 to 8 weeks after trauma to diagnose abnormalities and determine treatment progress or sequence.

Patients with basilar skull fracture who have immediate complete facial nerve paralysis and temporal bone fracture are considered for high-dose steroid treatment or surgical exploration to decompress or graft the nerve. Patients with delayed onset of the facial paralysis, or those who initially have only facial paresis are treated with steroids and observed, because some spontaneous recovery usually occurs.

MAXILLOFACIAL INJURIES

Skull and maxillofacial fractures often coexist after head trauma. For instance, fractures of the frontal bone or basilar skull commonly extend into the orbit, and midfacial fractures frequently accompany frontal skull, frontal sinus, or orbital fractures. In addition, fractures through the skull into the nasal sinuses can cause dural lacerations with CSF leak and/or pneumocephalus. When maxillofacial injury is suspected on physical examination, a CT scan of the face is the most useful diagnostic test and should be obtained at the time of the initial radiographic survey. CT scans should consist of bone and soft tissue windows and axial and coronal sections.

Assessment

The events of the injury should be ascertained and a complete history of the accident or injury should be recorded as described by the emergency medical technician, patient, or family members. A thorough facial physical examination is performed in sequence, concentrating on functional deficits in areas of injury. Consultations from specific specialists, such as an ophthalmologist, are also obtained. Cranial nerve abnormalities may also accompany facial fractures; oculomotor deficit, facial sensory deficit, or visual deficit are some common symptoms.

Soft-tissue injury implies the possibility of damage to deeper structures, which should be presumed until appropriate examination rules it out. Localized hematomas can be aspirated or removed to facilitate healing. Hematomas are usually diffuse, and not amenable to aspiration. Lacerations should be carefully debrided and repaired after damage to bones and deep soft-tissue structures has been excluded.

The facial bones should be examined in a methodical sequence from top to bottom. Symptoms that imply bony injury include soft-tissue injury (contusion, laceration, hematoma), bone movement, crepitation, localized tenderness, discomfort, numbness in the distribution of a cranial sensory nerve, paralysis in the distribution of a cranial motor nerve, malocclusion, visual acuity disturbance, diplopia, facial deformity or asymmetry, intraoral lacerations, fractured or avulsed teeth, air in soft tissues, and bleeding from the nose or mouth. The examiner should palpate the symmetry of the facial bones, comparing both sides. In some cases reference to old photographs can aid in documenting a pre-existing facial deformity or in establishing a change from a previous appearance. Dental malalignment (malocclusion) is an index of bone or tooth fracture, edema, or temporomandibular joint injury.

Facial sensation is noted in the supraorbital, supratrochlear, infratrochlear, infraorbital, and mental nerve regions of the trigeminal nerve distribution for both pin and light touch sensation. Diminished sensation in the distribution of a specific sensory nerve indicates injury from transection, impact, or continued compression of the nerve as the result of a fracture. The facial nerve is tested by comparing facial expression bilaterally. Extraocular movements and pupil response are compared, evaluating symmetry, pupil size, and the speed of pupil reaction bilaterally to both direct and consensual responses to light.

Emergency treatment is immediately directed towards life-threatening events such as airway obstruction or major hemorrhage from the scalp or face. During this phase, aspiration is usually prevented and the airway is maintained by orotracheal intubation, although occasionally an emergency tracheostomy is required. The stability of the cervical spine is assessed in every patient with head trauma during this phase.

The early management of maxillofacial injuries is based on clinical examination and facial CT scans (Figure 21.9). Both soft-tissue and bone windows are necessary on the CT scan to evaluate

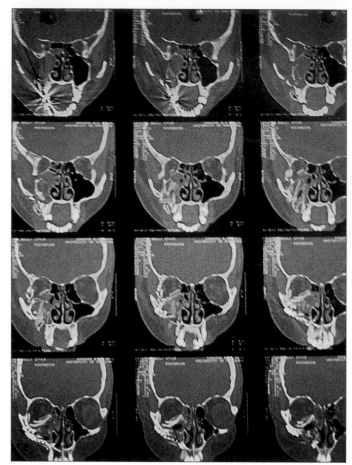

Figure 21.9 Two-dimensional facial CT scans are essential in facial fracture evaluation. They can be obtained rapidly after the CT evaluation of the brain. Axial and coronal windows should be obtained through the entire area of injury. Here, coronal CT scans demonstrate reduction of a zygomatic fracture by plate and screw fixation and orbital floor bone grafting.

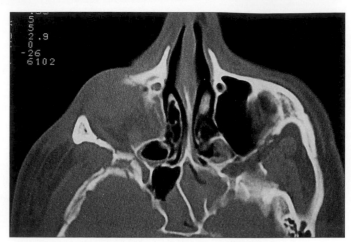

Figure 21.10 Axial window of an orbital fracture. The globe is prolapsing into the floor defect.

the brain and orbit fully. Axial (Figure 21.10) and coronal CT scans (direct or reformatted) are crucial to reveal details of fractures of the middle third of the orbit. Coronal sections (Figure 21.11) begin with the nasal pyramid and continue posteriorly through the orbital apex. Axial scans begin at the superior aspect of the skull and progress through the brain with standard axial brain imaging. The size and spacing of the cuts at the level of the frontal sinus must be reduced to 2 or 3 mm to obtain detail in the frontal sinus and orbit down to the maxillary alveolus. When a mandible fracture is suspected, the axial CT scanning is continued through the entire mandible and temporomandibular joints, visualizing both the horizontal and vertical portions. Although three-dimensional reconstruction with shading (Figure 21.12) adds spatial information, it does not provide the detail of two-dimensional axial and coronal images. In some cases, special reconstructions, as one performed in the longitudinal axis of the optic nerve in orbital injury, provide additional information (Figure 21.13).

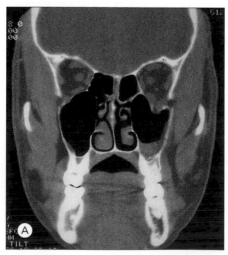
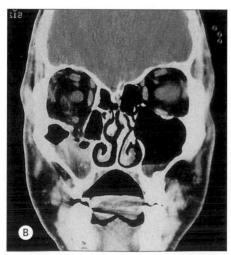
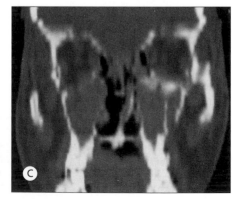

Figure 21.11 Direct coronal windows are preferable for evaluation of the orbit, sinuses, and palate. Both soft-tissue (A) and bone (B) windows should be obtained for the orbit. Two blow-out fractures are seen. In (A) the inferior meatus muscle is adjacent to the fracture. In (B) soft tissue windows clearly show the inferior meatus muscle adjacent to the fracture. (C) Reformatted images may be obtained where the direct coronal image is not possible. Their clarity depends on thin axial cuts.

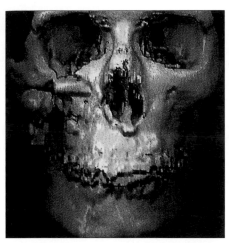

Figure 21.12 Three-dimensional CT scans add spatial perspective, but they do not replace two-dimensional CT scans and are not essential for reconstruction. A depressed zygomatic and orbital fracture is seen.

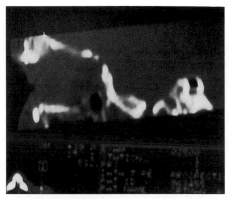

Figure 21.13 CT scans can be taken in the longitudinal axis of the optic nerve. Here, they provide information essential for the reconstruction of the orbital floor. Posteriorly, the intact orbit is visualized. Anteriorly, and in the middle orbital section, the broken rim fragments are visualized. Soft tissue may be herniated into the bone gap.

Associated conditions

Respiratory obstruction

Facial injuries can impair breathing in several ways. Fractured or avulsed teeth, broken dentures or bridgework, and foreign objects displaced into the airway must be removed. Facial fracture segments may be sufficiently displaced to compromise the airway. In addition, facial bleeding can contribute to aspiration and respiratory obstruction. Patients with combinations of burns and fractures of the upper and lower jaws, fractures of the nose, maxilla, and mandible, or fractures of the mandible that result in significant bleeding into the floor of mouth and neck all may have respiratory obstruction. Noisy respiration, stridor, hoarseness, drooling, inability to swallow or handle oral secretions, sternal retraction, and cyanosis all herald impending death from respiratory obstruction and immediate intubation or tracheostomy is therefore required. The use of plate and screw fixation for facial fracture reduction has allowed intermaxillary fixation to be discontinued postoperatively for many patients. Tracheostomy can often be avoided with the use of rigid fixation.

Profuse hemorrhage

Cutaneous bleeding that accompanies facial lacerations is usually controlled with digital pressure, which allows precise identification of the bleeding vessel for control with ligature. Blind probing in facial tissue or unselective ligature placement can damage branches of the facial nerve and should be avoided.

Bleeding from closed maxillofacial injuries usually results from fractures involving the sinuses. Bleeding from the nose (epistaxis) occurs with nasal, zygomatic, orbital, frontal sinus, nasoethmoidal, maxillary, and cranial base fractures. Although profuse nasopharyngeal hemorrhage usually accompanies Le Fort maxillary fractures, epistaxis is a nonspecific indication of many kinds of midfacial fractures. Usually the hemorrhage is self limiting. Several maneuvers usually control this hemorrhage when required, including an anteroposterior nasal pack, manual repositioning of the maxilla, and the application of intermaxillary fixation (rest position of the maxilla), or an external facial compression (Barton) dressing.

If profuse nasopharyngeal hemorrhage from closed fractures does not respond to the above measures, arterial embolization or arterial ligation can be performed. An angiogram is usually obtained to determine the major area of bleeding. In Le Fort fractures this usually involves branches of the internal maxillary artery. This artery can be embolized or selectively ligated directly through the back wall of the maxillary sinus, or arterial ligations of the external carotid and superficial temporal (both) arteries on the ipsilateral side usually reduces the bleeding substantially. Arterial ligation is rarely necessary.

Because bleeding abnormalities are noted early in patients with concomitant cerebral and facial fractures, replacement of depleted coagulation factors is based on the frequent assessment of coagulation factors in hemorrhaging patients. Because aspiration of blood, saliva, and gastric contents frequently accompanies maxillofacial injuries and can obstruct respiration, endotracheal intubation or tracheostomy is the definitive treatment.

Coma and brain injury

Coma or unconsciousness should not prevent or delay the treatment of facial fractures; many patients with facial fractures are in coma for several weeks before waking up. In patients with maxillofacial fractures, neurologic deficits from frontal lobe symptoms may be subtle or absent despite contusions imaged on brain CT scans. Confusion, somnolence, personality change, irritability, and difficulty in thinking are some of the symptoms of frontal brain contusion.

In patients with Glasgow Coma Scale scores of 14 or less, and especially when traumatic brain abnormality is visualized on CT scan, an intracranial pressure monitoring device may be employed in those patients who require anesthesia. An intracranial ventricular pressure monitor is used in the operating room during the facial repair, thus allowing optimal modification of the anesthesia and guidance in patients with multiple injuries.

Facial fracture classification by anatomic region

The treatment, and thus the description, of maxillofacial fractures are organized by anatomic region (Figure 21.14). The frontal bone region includes the frontal bone, the supraorbital rims bilaterally, and the frontal sinus (Figure 21.15). The upper midface region includes the zygomas laterally, the internal orbital area, and the nasoethmoidal area centrally. The lower midface consists of the

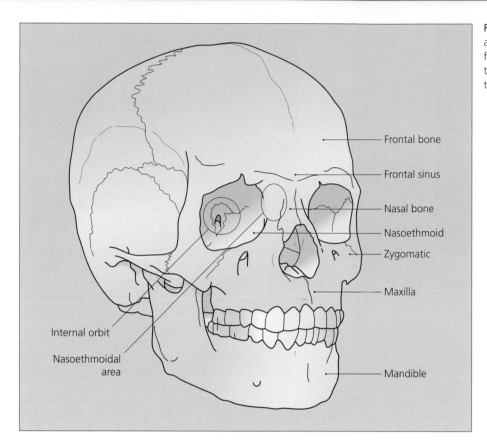

Internal orbit

Nasoethmoidal
area

Frontal bone

Frontal sinus

Nasal bone

Nasoethmoid

Zygomatic

Maxilla

Mandible

Figure 21.14 The anatomic regions of the face are shown. They include the frontal bone, the frontal sinus, the nose, the nasoethmoidal area, the zygoma, the internal orbit, the maxilla, and the mandible.

maxillary alveolus. The mandible consists of the horizontal portion containing the teeth and the vertical portion that includes the angle, ramus, coronoid and condylar processes. The pattern and displacement of the fractures in each anatomic region determines treatment. Orbital fractures are classified by their position on the orbital rim and by their involvement of the internal section of the orbit. Orbital rim fractures are divided into the supraorbital region, the nasoethmoidal region medially, and the zygomatic region inferolaterally (Figure 21.16). The internal orbit consists of the orbital floor, the lateral orbit, the medial (ethmoidal) orbit, and the orbital roof. Maxillary fractures are classified according to the pattern of Le Fort, based on the fracture's location.

Fractures of the frontal bone and supraorbital area

Fractures of the frontal bone area frequently extend into the orbital roof, frontal sinus and nose. A fracture in this area implies the possibility of injury to the dura and to the frontal brain. CSF rhinorrhea and pneumocephalus may be present.

Because of its strength the frontal bone is involved in only 5% to 10% of all facial fractures. Fractures that simultaneously involve the cranium and the orbit are high-energy injuries, and soft-tissue damage is more severe. Major injuries to the brain and the cervical spine frequently accompany these fractures, and contusion of the forebrain and orbital contents is routine.

The frontal and ethmoid sinuses render the frontal bone more vulnerable to injury and infection. Each major segment of the frontal sinus (generally two) has a "duct" (usually a broad ostium) that communicates with the upper portion of the nose. Sinus injury may therefore result in duct obstruction after fracture, mucosal edema, or damage (Figure 21.17). A cyst-like structure called a *mucocele* (obstructed mucous cyst) sometimes follows

mucosal injury; depending on its size, it may erode bone and penetrate into the orbit or intracranial cavity. Surgery at a later time is necessary to remedy either of these conditions, as symptoms of pain and sinusitis will persist. Since the posterior wall of the frontal sinus is in contact with the dura, any infection in that area represents an extradural abscess. Posterior wall fractures of the frontal sinus are often accompanied by dural tears. Many of these tears extend along the anterior basilar frontal region of the skull to cause a CSF leak or pneumocephalus. A small CSF leak is often masked by epistaxis in the early days after facial injury. When fractures in the posterior wall of the frontal sinus or the anterior base of the skull are noted, a CSF leak should be suspected.

Fractures of the frontal bone commonly extend to or involve the cranial sutures or other regions. When the fracture extends into the supraorbital region, the bone is usually depressed downward and posteriorly, compressing the orbital contents and producing a downward and forward dislocation of the globe (Figure 21.18). With more limited injuries, linear frontal skull fractures may extend into the orbit and along the cranial base. These fractures can create a CSF leak or obstruct sinus drainage by virtue of edema or bone displacement. As fracture patterns become more complex and severe, more bone displacement occurs. The anterior base of the skull and the roofs of the orbits become comminuted, and linear fractures extend from the anterior through the middle cranial fossa. The anterior and middle sections of the orbit displace, absorbing energy, and linear fractures extend from the displaced bone through the posterior portion of the orbit and into the middle cranial fossa. These fractures can account for basilar CSF leaks, pituitary disturbances, and dizziness from involvement of the temporal bone and vestibular structures.

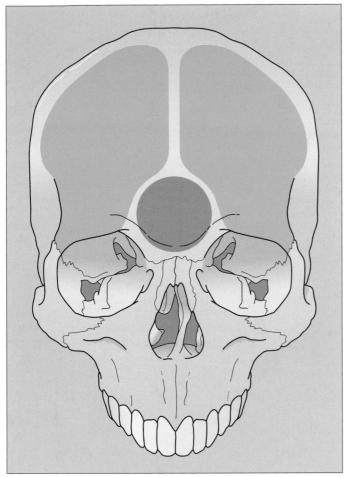

Figure 21.15 The divisions of the frontal bone are shaded. They include the central (frontal sinus) area (blue) and, laterally, the frontotemporo-orbital region (green), which extends to the coronal suture. Fractures often involve two of the three areas of the frontal skull.

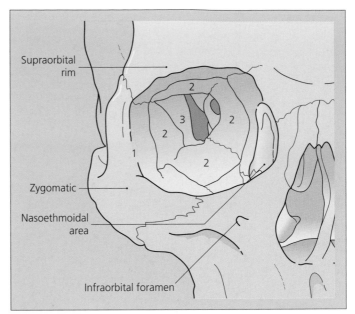

Figure 21.16 The orbit consists of three sections from anterior to posterior: (1) the thick rim anteriorly; (2) the thin middle section; and (3) the thick posterior third of the orbit. The posterior portion of the orbit represents the cranial base. The orbital rim can be conceptualized in three regions: superiorly, the supraorbital rim; inferiorly and laterally, the zygomatic region; medially, the nasoethmoidal area.

DIAGNOSIS The most common clinical signs of fractures of the frontal bone are an overlying bruise or hematoma and, less often, a laceration of the brow or the central forehead over the frontal sinus (Figure 21.19). CT scans occasionally show a posterior wall fracture of the frontal sinus without an accompanying anterior wall fracture. Fractures of the orbit usually result in palpebral and subconjunctival hematomas. A step deformity or irregularity in the orbital rim may be appreciated on palpation, but swelling may obscure the irregularity. If periorbital swelling is severe, complete ptosis exists. If the lid cannot be opened voluntarily, it should be opened manually to inspect the globe for integrity. Visual acuity should be assessed and extraocular muscle motion should be evaluated.

Evaluation of the visual system is critical. Supraorbital fractures, for example, represent 10% of all periorbital fractures but account for 30% of serious eye injuries. The most common serious injuries to the globe are rupture, retinal detachment, and vitreous or anterior chamber hemorrhage. The presence of globe injury modifies fracture treatment by severely limiting manipulation; avoidance of any pressure on the globe may take precedence over bone reconstruction. Visual acuity and pupil response are documented before and after any surgical treatment using a Rosenbaum pocket visual screening card. If this is not possible, the pupil response to light is evaluated both directly and consensually. Inability to move the globe into a particular field of gaze indicates either a cranial nerve palsy or local interference with an extraocular muscle secondary to contusion, local nerve injury, or incarceration of an extraocular muscle.

Fractures of the roof of the orbit usually produce a temporary paresis of the levator muscle that results in post-traumatic ptosis. This palsy may persist for months; no treatment to elevate the lid further is indicated until all chance for spontaneous recovery has been permitted (at least 6 months). Partial or complete spontaneous recovery usually occurs. The superior rectus muscle is usually undamaged in fractures of the superior orbit, but occasionally paresis occurs and mimics incarceration of the inferior rectus muscle (failure to elevate the globe). These conditions are differentiated by the combination of radiographic evaluation, forced-duction testing, and formal eye muscle evaluation. Entrapment of the levator and superior rectus muscles rarely occurs in orbital roof fractures.

Supraorbital fractures are usually displaced inward and downward (see Figure 21.18), producing a forward and downward displacement of the globe. The globe occasionally bulges forward so that the eyelids cannot close completely. In such cases urgent facial fracture reduction is required to protect the cornea. Fractures of the orbital roof may have a linear extension that enters the superior orbital fissure or optic foramen. Visual acuity is affected if the optic nerve is compressed by a displaced fracture fragment or by edema or nerve shearing, in which case the direct pupil response to light on the injured side is slower than the direct pupil response on the other side. Superior orbital fissure syndrome may also be present, consisting of palsy of extraocular muscle motion (cranial nerves III, IV, VI), ptosis, global proptosis, and anesthesia in the first division of the trigeminal nerve (the ipsilateral forehead). Patients may experience numbness in the

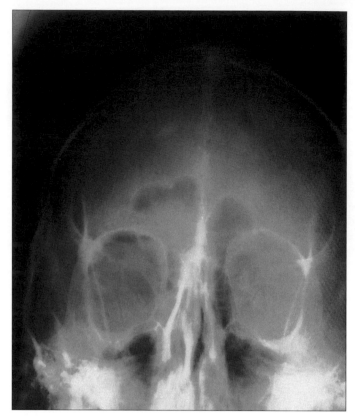

Figure 21.17 A fracture and frontal sinus duct obstruction are visible on this plain film. A mucocele might have a similar appearance.

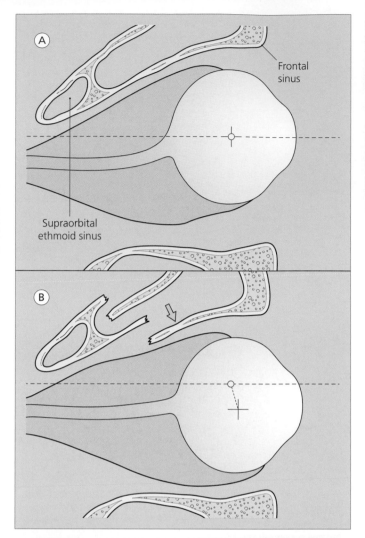

distribution of the supraorbital and supratrochlear nerves, which is usually transient, although lacerations in the area frequently divide the nerve, producing permanent numbness.

MANAGEMENT Displacement of more than 4 or 5 mm produces a depression or a change in globe position; release of the pressure on the globe or the nerves may improve function. Open skull fractures require debridement, repair of dural lacerations, evacuation of epidural hematomas, and appropriate surgical procedures for frontal lobe injury. Bone fragments are cleaned of mucosa and debris, and antiseptic irrigation is used. The frontal skull can be reconstructed primarily by linking the bone fragments with interfragment wires or plate and screw fixation and stabilizing the pieces securely (Figure 21.20) at their periphery with junctional rigid fixation.

Frontal sinus fractures

Fractures of the frontal sinus may involve the anterior wall, the posterior wall, or both. Fractures that obstruct the nasofrontal duct must be treated on a functional basis. Fractures that depress only the anterior wall of the frontal sinus are repaired for esthetic reasons. The symptoms of a frontal sinus fracture are usually localized bruising, hematoma, or laceration; the fracture often extends into the orbit, producing both palpebral and subconjunctival hematomas.

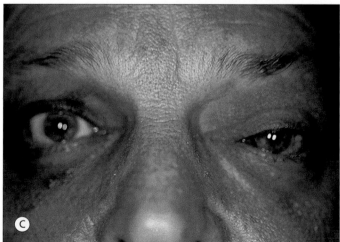

Figure 21.18 In a supraorbital fracture, posterior and inferior displacement of the superior orbital rim produces downward and forward dislocation of the globe. **(A)** The normal configuration of the superior orbit. **(B)** Dislocation of the superior orbital rim and globe displacement. **(C)** A patient with a displaced supraorbital fracture producing inferior globe displacement.

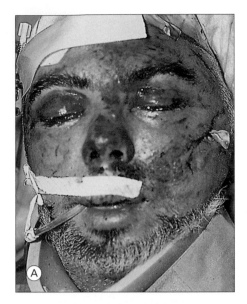

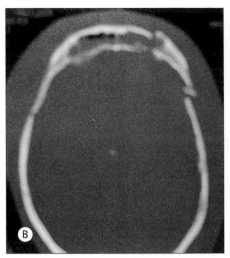

Figure 21.19 **(A)** A patient with a frontal and supraorbital fracture. **(B)** CT scan demonstrating fracture displacement.

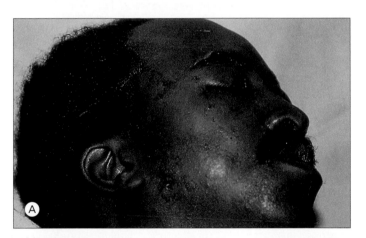

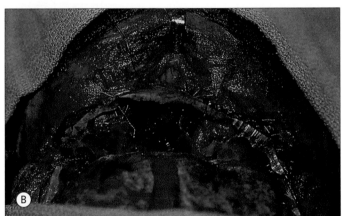

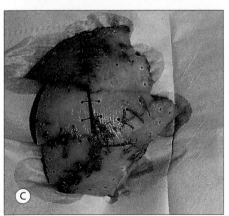

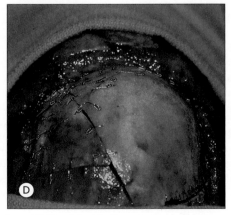

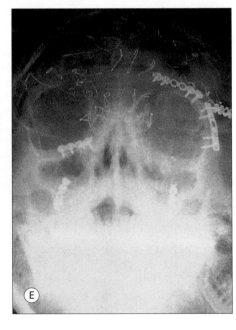

Figure 21.20 **(A)** A patient with a supraorbital fracture. **(B)** The defect in the anterior cranial base after removal of fractured bone. **(C)** The bone has been cleansed and debrided and the small fragments wired together on a back table while neurosurgery was in progress. **(D,E)** The bone is in place now, linked with interfragment wires. It will be stablized with rigid fixation to intact bone at its periphery.

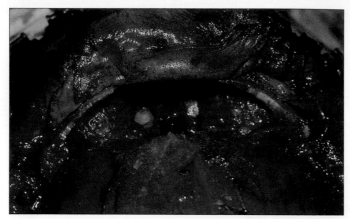

Figure 21.21 The nasofrontal duct should be plugged with several layers of bone graft. Bone provides strong stuctural material to close the opening between the intracranial cavity and the nose. Muscle and fascia deteriorate rapidly and do not provide stability.

DIAGNOSIS Frontal sinus fractures are diagnosed on CT scan with fracture through the front wall, back wall, or both walls. Displacement of bone at the posterior wall usually indicates an underlying dural laceration.

MANAGEMENT Localized fractures of the anterior wall are managed by returning the fragments to the proper position and debriding devitalized mucosa. If the nasofrontal duct is intact, fluid will flow freely into the nose; replaced bone fragments are stabilized with interfragment wires or plate and screw fixation. If the posterior wall is involved, the integrity of the dura is usually assessed by direct inspection at operation. Significant fractures of the anterior and posterior walls are best managed by intracranial exposure and debridement of small bone fragments. If the posterior wall of the sinus has been removed, the sinus should be "cranialized" by completely removing the mucosa and plugging the nasofrontal duct with several layers of bone grafts. A sheet bone graft is placed over the bone plugs and over the involved ethmoid sinuses (Figure 21.21). Any involved sinus must be debrided to minimize infection and delayed mucocele formation because obstruction of an ethmoid sinus produces an orbital or epidural abscess. The anterior wall of the frontal sinus is then reconstructed. Complete removal of sinus mucosa requires mucosal stripping and light burring of the bone fragments to which the mucosa was attached.

Less involved frontal sinus fractures may be managed by sinus obliteration. When fractures compromise nasal frontal duct function, all sinus mucosa should be removed and the walls of the sinus should be thoroughly burred to bleeding bone. The nasofrontal duct is then plugged with several layers of bone plugs taken from the calvaria, and the remainder of the sinus is filled with bone shavings (Figure 21.22). Alternatively (and less desirably), the sinus cavity can be left unfilled after the insertion of the bone plugs; obliteration will slowly occur by osteoneogenesis, which consists of proliferation of bone, granulation, and scar tissue. Osteoneogenesis is less reliable than bone graft obliteration. Unfortunately, regrowth of frontal sinus mucosa may occasionally occur, or the development of a cyst in a lacerated area of mucosa may produce a mucocele. Surgical intervention may be required for infection or erosion of the cyst into adjacent structures.

Orbital fractures

The supraorbital rims are weakened centrally by the presence of the frontal sinus. The supraorbital rim extends to join the temporal bone and the zygoma (see Figure 21.16). The orbit cavity itself has three sections (Figure 21.16), the rim, the middle and the posterior orbit. The midsection of the orbit can be divided into four regions (Figure 21.23), and the rim into three sections. Fractures occur first in the thin bone of the middle third of the orbit, then in the rim.

A blow to the lateral aspect of the upper face can fracture both the supraorbital rim and the zygoma. Cranio-orbital injuries call for both neurosurgery and orbital reconstruction. Zygomatic fractures usually extend from the junction medially with the maxilla at the infraorbital rim through the inferior and lateral orbit. Medially, the fracture often involves the canal for the infraorbital nerve, which is located 8–10 mm inferior to the lower orbital rim, parallel to the medial aspect of the cornea. A fracture here produces numbness in the infraorbital nerve distribution.

The nasoethmoidal orbital region represents the medial rim and medial wall of the orbit (see Figure 21.24). Posteriorly, the ethmoid air cells weaken the nasoethmoidal region, one of the thinnest portions of the orbital wall. Fractures involving the medial orbital rim displace the bone bearing the attachment of the medial canthal tendon posteriorly and laterally, which may also block the lacrimal system, resulting in tearing. Displacement of the medial orbital rim or the infraorbital rim and floor of the orbit alters the medial attachment of the eyelids and the suspensory ligaments of the globe, permitting globe and canthal ligament dystopia and telecanthus, which can be detected on physical examination.

The orbital roof is composed of the greater and lesser wings of the sphenoid. It separates the anterior cranial fossa from the orbital contents. Medially, at the frontal sinus, the orbital roof thins, becoming almost transparent. The attachment of the superior oblique tendon immediately behind the rim is often a separate small fragment in fractures. Diplopia produced by interference with superior oblique function is difficult to remedy. The surgeon must be aware of this attachment and avoid injury by making dissection wholly subperiosteal. The frontal sinus is extremely variable in size and shape; asymmetry is the rule. It does not develop until the teenage years and thus is absent in the pediatric trauma victim.

The medial wall of the orbit is formed by the thin orbital plate of the ethmoid bone. This bone is reinforced by septa within the ethmoid sinus, which gives it some additional strength (Figure 21.24). The lateral wall of the orbit consists of the orbital process of the malar bone anteriorly and the greater wing of the sphenoid posteriorly (Figure 21.25). The zygomaticosphenoid suture is involved in all zygoma fractures. Its broad surface forms an excellent area for confirmation of proper zygomatic alignment. With more comminuted orbital fractures, displacement of multiple walls of the orbit contributes to dramatic orbital deformity. Because soft-tissue orbital deformity is not entirely reversible with secondary corrections, the emphasis is on immediate definitive reconstruction.

The lateral canthal ligament attaches with the lateral aspect of the eyelids to the zygoma at Whitnall's tubercle, which is a shallow bulge in the internal aspect of the lateral orbital rim about 10 mm inferior to the zygomaticofrontal suture. The anterior limb

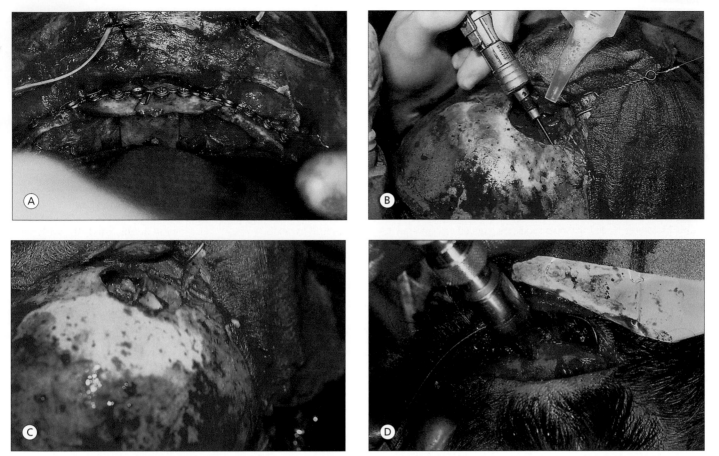

Figure 21.22 **(A)** A sheet bone graft should be laid across the plugged frontal sinus ducts to cover previously cleansed and debrided fractures involving the cranial base and ethmoidal sinuses. This layer is not watertight but begins to develop its own partition between the intracrinal cavity and the nose. **(B)** In cases where the sinus cavity is to be obliterated, the mucosa is thoroughly removed. The walls of the sinus should be burred lightly to eliminate areas where mucosa extends along the veins in the wall of the sinus cavity. After nasofrontal duct obliteration with bone plugs, the sinus cavity can be obliterated with particulate bone graft **(C)** taken from the parietal area with a craniotome **(D)**.

of the lateral canthal tendon is continuous with the galea, and the posterior limb joins the lateral extension of the levator tendon and Lockwood's suspensory ligament in its attachment to Whitnall's tubercle (Figure 21.26). The extraocular muscles travel close to the orbital walls in the posterior half of the orbit. In the anterior half, they are protected from orbital wall fractures only by a thin cushion of extramuscular cone fat. Thin "muscular check ligaments" extend from the extraocular muscles diffusely to the orbital walls (Figure 21.27). These ligaments, described by Leo Koorneef, diffusely interconnect the soft tissue of the orbit to provide structural continuity among all the orbital tissues, such as fat, muscle, periosteum, and globe. This interconnection of all orbital soft tissue is why diplopia (extraocular muscle restriction) occurs if a particular section of orbital fat is restricted by being caught in a fracture. The entrapped fat and ligament system, in the absence of extraocular muscle restriction, may cause diplopia.

The orbital floor is one of the weakest portions of the orbit. There is an initial concave section of the inferior orbit immediately behind the inferior orbital rim, and then a convex constriction. This complex orbital anatomy must be recreated when reconstructing the orbit. Because the complex curves of bone in relation to the soft tissue determine globe position (Figure 21.28), it is extremely important to mimic the exact curvature of the middle portion of the orbit and the position of the orbital rim. The concave roof must be reconstructed in its exact arching anatomic position or the globe will be displaced inferolaterally.

The posterior third of the orbit contains the optic foramen, the superior orbital fissure, and the posterior aspect of the inferior orbital fissure. The superior orbital fissure is bounded by the greater and lesser wings of the sphenoid (Figure 21.29). Linear fractures are commonly seen in the posterior portion of the orbit; however, displacement of bone is less common here. Usually, the anterior and middle sections displace, acting as a "shock absorber," protecting the posterior orbit from severe displacement.

The inferior orbital fissure separates the orbital floor from the lateral orbital wall. It contains veins, the infraorbital artery and nerve, and the zygomaticofacial nerve.

DIAGNOSIS A mobile or absent orbital roof may produce a pulsating exophthalmos in which cerebral pulsations are transmitted to the globe and its adnexal structures. This is corrected by reconstruction of the roof, separating the orbit from the intracranial contents with a bone graft (partition).

Fractures involving the orbital roof and middle cranial fossa may sometimes create a communication (carotid–cavernous sinus fistula) between the carotid artery and the cavernous sinus. A traumatic carotid–cavernous fistula is usually accompanied by severe visual and cranial nerve disturbances. Marked chemosis,

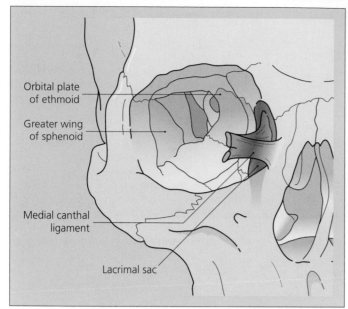

Figure 21.23 The midsection of the orbit is conceptualized in four regions: laterally, the orbital process of the zygoma and the greater wing of the sphenoid; inferiorly, the orbital floor; medially, the lamina papyracea of ethmoid bone; and superiorly, the orbital roof. The posterior third of the orbit contains the superior orbital fissure, the posterior portion of the inferior orbital fissure, and the optic foramen. The medial canthal ligament surrounds the lacrimal sac. A groove for the lacrimal sac is present immediately behind the orbital rim. The medial canthal ligament consists of anterior, superior, and posterior limbs.

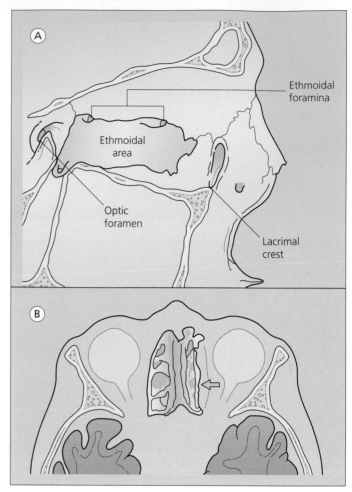

Figure 21.24 (A) The medial wall is the thinnest bone of the orbit but, reinforced by septa within the ethmoid sinus, is stronger than its thickness implies. The anterior and posterior ethmoidal foramina, located towards the upper portion of the medial orbital wall, are on the same level as the optic canal. These neurovascular foramina can be used as landmarks to direct the surgeon in his protection of the optic nerve. **(B)** Fractures of the ethmoid frequently show symmetric compression. Reconstruction involves bone grafting to the normal contour.

globe prominence, extraocular muscle palsy, and blindness are usually present. The fistula is confirmed by arteriography; attempts to obliterate it involve intravascular radiographic techniques.

The most common reason for a visual acuity deficit after trauma is optic nerve injury. Shearing, contusion, or compression may be involved. These injuries may occur with or without demonstrated fractures of the optic canal. If vision is lost at the moment of impact, decompression of an optic canal fracture usually does not increase the chance of visual recovery. In most cases, steroids (spinal cord doses) are given. However, if bone fragments that compromise the optic canal are demonstrated, or if a fluctuating or worsening partial visual deficit is seen, then decompression should be considered. Immediately after an optic nerve injury the optic disc usually looks normal. A patient may present with a Marcus Gunn pupil, in which the reaction to consensual constriction is present but the reaction to direct stimulus is reduced. Swinging a light from one globe to the other demonstrates pupillary dilatation in the affected eye (Figure 21.30).

Atrophy of the optic disk does not appear until 1 month after an optic nerve is injured, so it cannot be used as an acute indication of optic nerve damage. If vision is initially present after an injury and then deteriorates, swelling from hemorrhage and edema may be compromising the optic canal and compressing the optic nerve. Surgical and/or medical (high-dose steroids) decompression are indicated on an emergency basis for most of the nerve injuries. Some feel that optic nerve injury with no light perception should be treated with canal decompression, but the prognosis for this injury is poor no matter what is done.

MANAGEMENT Specific treatment of the orbital fractures and their interrelation with other facial fractures are covered in other sections.

Nasoethmoid orbital fractures

The nasoethmoid orbital fracture consists (in its simplest form) of injury to one or both frontal processes of the maxilla (medial orbital rims) and their attached canthal ligaments and the nose. The frontal process of the maxilla is the lower two thirds of the medial orbital rim. When this is fractured, the medial canthal ligament is displaced because of its attachment to the fractured bone segment. Nasoethmoid fractures often extend to adjacent areas, including the supraorbital region, the frontal sinus, the inferior orbit, the medial internal orbit, and the floor of the orbit.

These injuries, which may cause significant long-term deformity, especially telecanthus and enophthalmos, are often initially obscured by swelling. Patients usually present with bleeding from the nose, a nasal dislocation, and bilateral periorbital and sub-

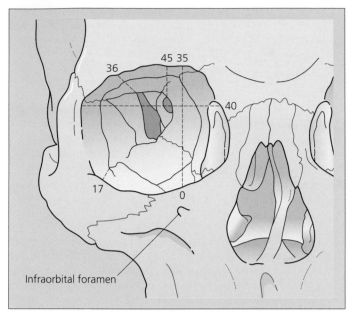

Figure 21.25 The lateral wall of the orbit. Often, the anterior portion of the greater wing of the sphenoid fractures and is involved in expansion of the orbital cavity. The distances of various structures from the rim are shown.

conjunctival hematomas (Figure 21.31). The nasal deformity consists of depression of the nasal dorsum, foreshortening of the nose, with an increased angle between the columella and the lip. Severe dislocation of the septum and a nasal septal perforation are often present. Forty per cent of nasoethmoid fractures are unilateral, and because of their proximity to the frontal sinus and the dura, a CSF leak may be present. Nasoethmoid fractures produce tearing by compromising the drainage of the lacrimal system as it passes through the maxilla. On palpation, pain and tenderness are found over the frontal process of the maxilla and the palpating finger, inserted deeply over the medial canthal ligament, discloses bony crepitus, movement, and tenderness. Telecanthus may be present if the medial orbital rim fracture

fragment has been dislocated laterally, in which case the palpebral fissure narrows.

DIAGNOSIS The presence of a nasoethmoid fracture can be determined by a bimanual examination (Figure 21.32). A palpating finger is placed deeply over the canthal ligament opposite a clamp placed intranasally, and the "central" (canthal ligament containing) bone fragment is moved between the finger and clamp.

On CT scan, fractures surround the lower two-thirds of the medial orbital rim. Medial and inferior internal orbital fractures are present, and the inferior orbital rim, piriform aperture, nose, and internal angular process of the frontal bone at the glabella are fractured.

Lacrimal system injury should be suspected in lacerations of the medial portion of the eyelids. The lacrimal system may also be compromised by fractures involving the bone surrounding the nasolacrimal duct. If the lacrimal system is transected, fluid emerges from a laceration on irrigation of the system with saline.

MANAGEMENT Nasoethmoid orbital fractures require a definitive open reduction consisting of interfragment wiring and plate and screw fixation of the assembled fragments. In some situations, this can be accomplished through a laceration or local incision; otherwise, a broad exposure must be provided by a coronal incision (Figure 21.33), bilateral lower eyelid and gingival buccal sulcus incisions. Usually, the surgeon is careful to avoid detaching the canthal ligament from the bone during fracture reduction. If the canthal ligament is detached, it must be reattached after assembly of the bone fragments to the proper area of the medial orbital rim. A separate set of transnasal wires, again passed posterior and superior to the lacrimal fossa through the nose, connects the canthal ligament to the bone in its proper position (Figure 21.34) after the bone reduction. Contoured bone grafts are used to reconstruct the medial and inferior internal orbit (Figure 21.35). Long, straight bone grafts are used to provide contour and to add dorsal height to the nose. These bone grafts are taken from either the calvarium, the iliac crest or a split rib.

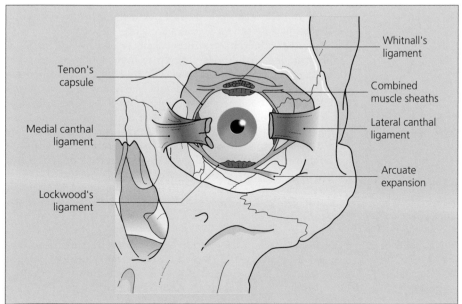

Figure 21.26 The fascial sling for globe support. The globe has been removed. Medially and laterally, the medial and lateral canthal ligaments provide attachments for structures that provide anterior globe support. Indicated are Lockwood's ligament, supporting the globe inferiorly, the medial and lateral canthal ligaments, and behind them, medial and lateral check ligaments. Superiorly, Whitnall's ligament is present. The combined muscle sheaths also attach to the globe and provide a relative sling for fat and globe support. These ligaments and their sheaths join to Tenon's capsule.

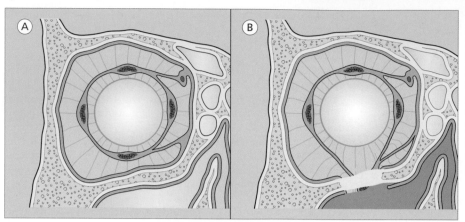

Figure 21.27 Entrapment of the fine ligament system described by Leo Koorneef may produce limitation of extraocular motion. **(A)** The normal system of ligaments that diffusely connect the bony walls of the orbit to the extraocular muscles and the globe. **(B)** An orbital floor fracture has trapped fat and its interconnecting ligaments in the fracture site. Ocular motility may be impaired by impingement of this fine ligament system. (After Koorneef L. Current concepts in the management of blow-out fractures. *Ann Plast Surg* 1982; 9: 185–99.)

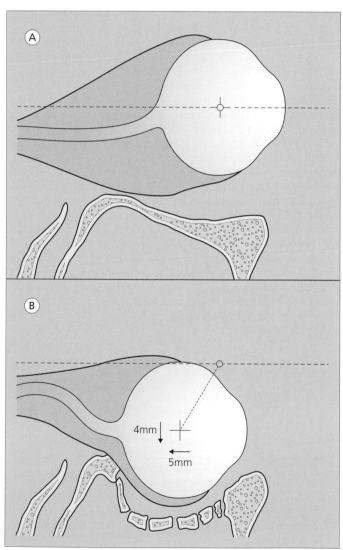

Figure 21.28 The curves of the orbit in the longitudinal axis of the optic nerve. The normal configuration (top) and the usual configuration in enophthalmos (bottom) of the orbital floor are indicated. An intact ledge of bone is present in the posterior orbit and provides a guide for floor reconstruction. First, the orbital rim should be properly positioned. The intact posterior ledge of bone provides a scaffold for bone support between the rim and posterior orbit. The soft tissue prolapsing into the maxillary sinus must be elevated, restoring globe position.

If a fracture compromises the lacrimal system, replacement of bone into its normal position is the initial treatment. If the lacrimal system is transected, a direct repair of lacrimal canalicular transection is performed with fine sutures under magnification over fine tubes (0.025 in; 0.6 mm). Both the upper and lower puncta should be intubated and the tubes should be brought into the nose through the nasolacrimal canal. They should remain in place for several months to splint the repair.

Fractures of the orbital floor

The bony orbital space is a modified cone or pyramid. Fractures of the inferior portion of the orbital floor often extend 30–35 mm behind the rim. The infraorbital nerve weakens the orbital floor. Fractures of the rim and floor damage the function of the nerve, producing hypesthesia of the upper lip, ipsilateral nose, and anterior maxillary teeth.

The most frequent fracture of the internal orbit is the blow-out fracture, which is usually confined to the floor and the lower portion of the medial wall (Figure 21.36). A depressed fracture of this section of the orbit allows the orbital tissue to be displaced downward into the maxillary and ethmoid sinuses. Medial, inferior, and posterior dislocation of the globe occurs. If fat is trapped in the fracture, it may interfere with the motion of the globe because of the internal ligament system of the orbital soft tissue (Figure 21.36). Alternatively, the inferior rectus muscle may be directly trapped in a small fracture, leading to restriction and possibly absolute incarceration of globe movement.

Patients with orbital fractures usually present with a history of a blunt injury to the orbit. They may have double vision when looking either upward or downward. Extraocular range of motion may be limited. Periorbital and subconjunctival hematomas are present, as is numbness in the infraorbital nerve distribution. It is imperative that the globe be examined; the possibility of hyphema, retinal detachment, or globe rupture exists with any fracture involving the orbit. The possible presence of an intraorbital foreign body should always be considered. Orbital fractures are accompanied in 10–15% of cases by a globe injury. The visual system and globe are evaluated by visual acuity, visual fields, funduscopic examination, extraocular motion, and intraocular pressure.

DIAGNOSIS When an inferior orbital floor fracture is accompanied by diplopia, the "forced-duction" test is used to confirm incarceration of orbital soft tissues in the fracture site. Absence of rotation on attempted movement with globe rotation documents muscle or extraocular system tissue restriction. A

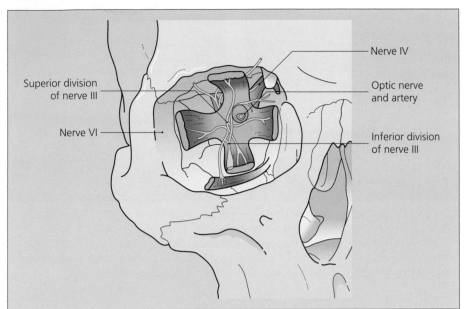

Figure 21.29 The contents of the superior orbital fissure include cranial nerves III, IV, and VI, the ophthalmic division of (trigeminal) cranial nerve V, and vascular structures. The optic foramen is contained within the lesser wings of the sphenoid and admits the optic nerve and ophthalmic artery.

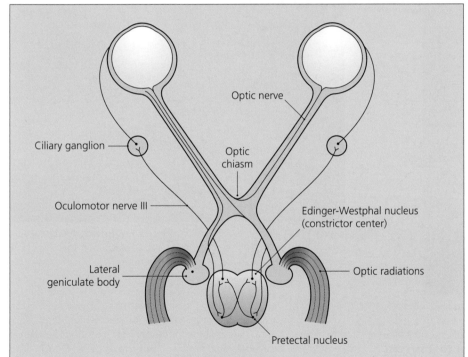

Figure 21.30 The normal pupil reflex pathway and the relation to the Marcus Gunn pupil. In the normal eye, light striking the retina produces an impulse in the optic nerve that travels to the pretectal nucleus, both Edinger–Westphal nuclei, via nerve III to the ciliary ganglion and pupillary constrictor muscles. In lesions involving the retina or optic nerve back to the chiasm, a light in the unaffected eye produces consensual constriction of the pupil of the affected eye, but a light in the affected eye produces a paradoxic dilatation of the affected pupil. (After Jabaley ME, Lerman M, Saunders HJ. Ocular injuries and orbital fractures: a review of 199 cases. *Plast Reconstr Surg* 1975; 56: 410.)

"force-generation" test provides additional information by demonstrating "pull" generated by extraocular muscles when the globe is held by forceps and rotation is attempted. Involuntary globe entrapment tethering soft tissue occurs most frequently with small orbital fractures. Enlargement of the orbital volume is generally produced by large fractures; globe dystopia and enophthalmos are the result of significant orbital cavity enlargement.

Enophthalmos denotes the backward dislocation of the globe into the orbit (Figure 21.37). Large fractures of the orbital floor allow the orbital soft tissue to prolapse backward, downward, and medially, resulting in a loss of globe support and a change in globe position. The anterior position of the globe on physical examination, is best compared by assessing the patient from an inferior view (Figure 21.38) or with Hertel exophthalmometry. The trauma of the injury may produce fat atrophy, which contributes to globe malposition. Acutely, periorbital injuries produce hemorrhage and edema. Initially, proptosis or exophthalmos appears. Acute enophthalmos is unusual and indicates a dramatic enlargement in the orbit. If the globe prolapses away from the lids, lubrication of the cornea cannot be accomplished; this is an urgent indication for orbital wall repair. Enophthalmos is usually accompanied by

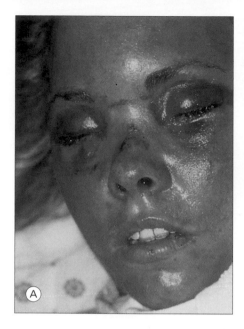

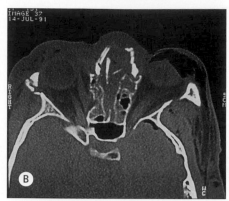

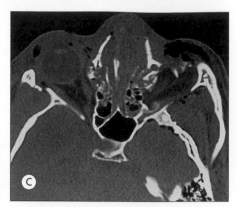

Figure 21.31 (A) In most patients with nasoethmoidal fractures, severe mid-facial injury is obvious. Bilateral periorbital hematomas are routine. Here, the nose has literally been driven into the mid-face and is depressed along its dorsum with foreshortening of the length (increased angle between the lip and columella). **(B,C)** CT scans of a nasoethmoidal orbital fracture demonstrate comminution of the entire medial orbit and nose.

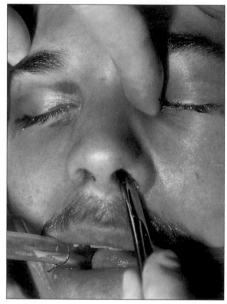

Figure 21.32 The bimanual examination is performed by placing a clamp inside the nose with its tip immediately adjacent to the attachment of the canthal ligament on the frontal process of the maxilla. It is important that the clamp *not be* placed beneath nasal bones or a false-positive diagnosis of a nasoethmoidal fracture will be obtained. A palpating finger is placed externally deeply over the canthal ligament. If the frontal process of the maxilla can be moved between the clamp and the palpating finger, a nasoethmoidal fracture is present. Mobility requires surgical reduction.

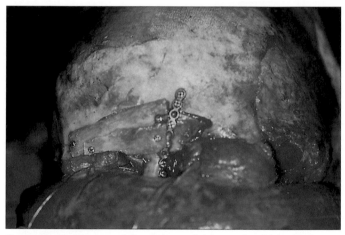

Figure 21.33 Exposure of the entire medial (nasoethmoidal orbital) section is provided by a coronal incision with dissection of the supraorbital area, orbital roofs, and lateral orbit.

inferior displacement (globe dystopia). Posterior displacement of the globe produces a supratarsal hollow and ptosis of the upper eyelid.

MANAGEMENT In many cases, the symptoms of a small internal orbital fracture resolve substantially within a short period. Frequently, double vision is the result of muscular contusion and resolves with observation. Surgery is usually indicated for double vision only when it occurs in a functional field of gaze and is the result of incarceration of the muscle or the ligament system. There are thus two indications for surgery for blow-out fractures: muscle or ligament entrapment, confirmed by CT scan and forced-duction examination, and enlargement of the orbit sufficient to produce enophthalmos. This generally requires more than 2 cm^2 of orbital floor involvement, with displacement of more than 3–4 mm. The size of the fracture can be accurately estimated on CT scans. The orbit should be reconstructed by bone grafts placed over the edges of the orbital defect so as to support the orbital contents (Figure 21.35).

Le Fort maxillary fractures
Fractures of the maxilla involve not only the lower maxilla but often the entire midfacial region. These fractures are termed Le Fort maxillary fractures after the classification used by René Le Fort (Figure 21.39) who described the three "great lines of weakness" of the maxilla through which fractures commonly occur.

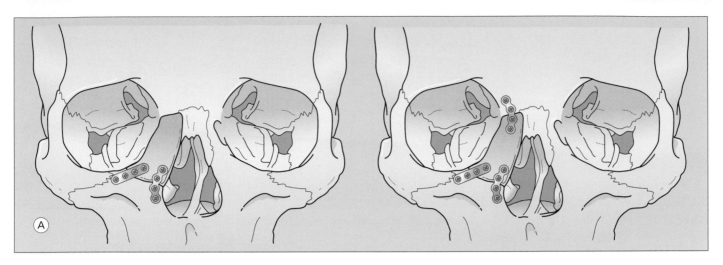

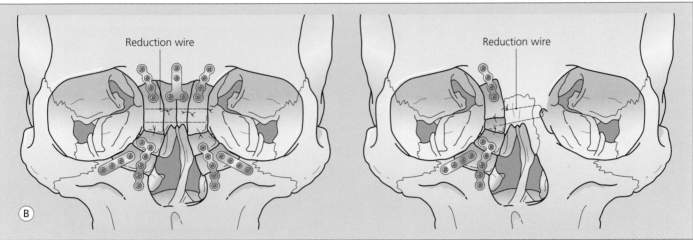

Figure 21.34 (A) Treatment of a simple nasoethmoidal orbital fracture by plate and screw fixation. Noncomminuted fractures can be treated in this fashion. **(B)** Comminuted fractures require thorough connection of all fragments with interfragment wires. The essential step in the treatment of a nasoethmoidal orbital fracture is to pass a wire between both medial orbital rim segments. This wire is passed transnasally posterior and superior to the lacrimal fossa.

DIAGNOSIS In 10% of Le Fort fractures the maxillary alveolus is split, usually in a sagittal (longitudinal) direction (Figure 21.40), increasing instability and making preservation of normal occlusion a challenge. Lower maxillary fractures are diagnosed by malocclusion and maxillary mobility. Upper maxillary fractures are diagnosed by maxillary mobility, malocclusion, periorbital hematomas, nasopharyngeal bleeding, pain, and the symptoms of zygomatic, orbital, and nasoethmoidal fractures. Examination for maxillary mobility is essential to confirm the presence of a Le Fort fracture. The maxilla should be grasped with one hand while the head is stabilized with the other. The level at which the mobility occurs indicates the level of the Le Fort fracture. Multiple level fractures may be seen in the same patient. Occasionally, Le Fort fractures are not mobile; they may be either impacted or incomplete.

MANAGEMENT The principal treatment of Le Fort fractures is intermaxillary fixation with the maxilla in occlusion with the mandible. Initial stabilization is generally accomplished by ligating arch bars to the upper and lower teeth and connecting the maxillary and mandibular arch bars with intermaxillary wires.

Fracture sites at the various levels of the midface (as defined by CT scans) are aligned, and then the nasofrontal and zygomaticomaxillary buttresses (Figure 21.41) are reconstructed with direct plate and screw fixation. This eliminates or decreases the need for intermaxillary fixation postoperatively.

A Le Fort I fracture is treated by placing the patient in intermaxillary fixation, exposing the four Le Fort I level buttresses, reducing the fracture, and using direct plate and screw fixation over the buttress fractures. (Figure 21.42). Bone grafts should span bone gaps of more than 3–5 mm.

Le Fort II fractures are treated by placing the patient in intermaxillary fixation. The fracture fragments are aligned with interfragment wires and stabilized with direct plate and screw fixation (Figure 21.43). Orbital floor defects are spanned with bone grafts, or perhaps with alloplastic implants for smaller defects. If rigid fixation is used, intermaxillary fixation is discontinued early postoperatively. Normal occlusion must be confirmed carefully for a 4- to 12-week period postoperatively. Patients with intermaxillary fixation require a liquid diet and should be placed on a soft diet when it is discontinued. The upper nose may need direct fixation through a coronal incision, and the

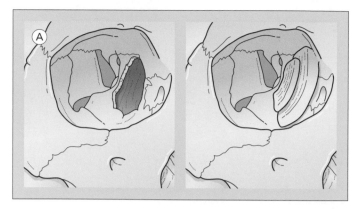
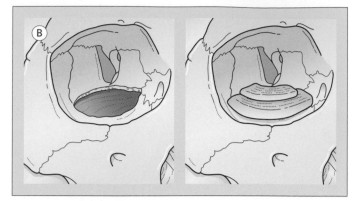

Figure 21.35 The usual internal orbital fractures involving the orbital floor **(A)** and the medial orbital wall **(B)**. Bone grafts can be used to restore internal orbital integrity.

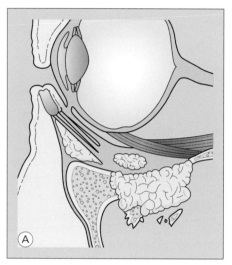
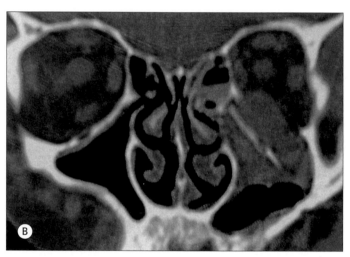

Figure 21.36 (A,B) An orbital blow-out fracture involving the thin portion of the orbital floor. Fat and its interconnecting fascia are trapped among the blow-out fracture fragments and limit the excursion of the inferior oblique and inferior rectus muscles. Diplopia may be present from muscle restriction in either up or down gaze.

lower orbital rims are reduced through bilateral lower eyelid incisions.

Le Fort III fractures are treated with surgical approaches to zygomatic, nasoethmoidal, and orbital floor fractures and to the Le Fort I level (Figure 21.44). Again, fragments are initially aligned with interfragment wires and stabilized with plate and screw fixation. A sagittal fracture of the maxilla is directly reduced through the palatal laceration or incision with plate and screw fixation. A small plate is also placed at the piriform aperture to unite the two maxillary segments. In some cases, an acrylic splint is placed in the palatal vault to adjust further the occlusal relationships. A "panfacial fracture" (Le Fort fractures, plus fractures of the nasoethmoidal and mandibular areas) is shown repaired with plate and screw fixation (Figure 21.44B). The mandible subcondylar and symphysis fractures were stabilized prior to the Le Fort fracture.

Fractures of the nose
A fracture of the nose may involve the cartilaginous nasal septum, the bony septum, and/or the bony nasal pyramid or the upper or lower lateral cartilages.

DIAGNOSIS Two types of dislocations occur in nasal fractures (Figure 21.45): posterior dislocation (shortening or flattening of the nose, resulting in a wider nasal bridge) and lateral dislocation (deviated nose). Any patient with a nasal fracture should have the nasal airway inspected. If a significant hematoma exists along the septum, it should be drained to prevent cartilage necrosis. Patients with nasal fractures usually have swelling over the external surface of the nose. A small laceration is often the clue to the presence of a fracture. Pain, crepitation, and periorbital ecchymosis are often present. The most reliable sign of a nasal fracture is epistaxis. Radiographic evaluation of the nose is best performed with a CT scan, which can confirm the nasal fracture and also rule out the possibility of adjacent fractures.

MANAGEMENT The treatment of nasal fractures involves reduction under local or general anesthesia. The septum is replaced into its proper position with Asch forceps. The nasal bones are first outfractured by levering the nasal bone outward to complete the fracture, which effectively releases incomplete components of the fracture, and then they are digitally returned to their proper positions. Antibiotic-impregnated nasal packing

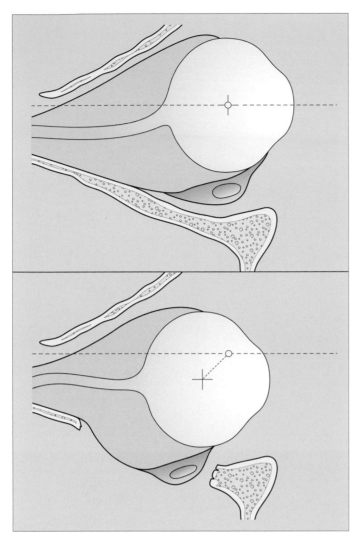

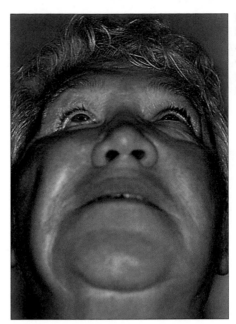

Figure 21.38
Enophthalmos is most accurately assessed by comparison of globe position from an inferior perspective.

Figure 21.37 The orbit's enlargement allows displacement of the globe backward and downward to produce enophthalmos.

supports the reduction of the nasal septum, completed by mechanical displacement and minimizes bleeding. An external splint is placed over the nasal pyramid to protect it during the healing period. It should be removed after 1 week. Nasal fractures frequently display residual mild deformity after this initial closed management. If the airway remains compromised by a deviated septum, a formal septal resection to improve respiratory symptoms may be performed after 3–6 months. Residual deformity of the nasal pyramid requires late osteotomy of the nose (rhinoplasty).

Fractures of the zygoma

The zygoma forms the lateral and inferior portion of the orbit and supports the lateral areas of the upper mid-face (Figure 21.46). The prominent position of the zygoma makes it a frequent recipient of traumatic dislocation. A fracture usually involves the entire zygoma, but may less commonly involve the zygomatic arch alone, which produces a minimal depression in the lateral cheek. Depression of the zygomatic arch may interfere with movement of the coronoid process of the mandible, a symptom requiring reduc-

tion. Since zygomatic fractures involve the lateral and inferior internal walls of the orbit, they may produce ocular symptoms that require treatment.

DIAGNOSIS The symptoms of zygomatic fractures are shown in Figure 21.47. The lateral canthus, which attaches to the frontal process of the zygoma, may be dislocated inferiorly, producing an antimongoloid slant to the palpebral fissure. Either swelling or dislocation of the zygoma may interfere with motion of the coronoid process by producing a mild temporary interference with occlusion. Hematomas are observed in the cheek, periorbital area, and mouth. Orbital symptoms produced by the fractures include diplopia, ocular dystopia, and eyelid dislocation. Palpation of the orbital rim may demonstrate a step deformity or depression. Palpation of the malar eminence, when compared with the normal side, demonstrates retrusion. With a medially dislocated zygomatic fracture, the orbital volume may be constricted, resulting in exophthalmos. With laterally or inferiorly dislocated zygomatic fractures, the orbital volume increases, and enophthalmos occurs.

Zygomatic fractures should be evaluated with axial and coronal CT scans including soft tissue and bone windows for evaluation of the orbital soft tissue and its relation to the fracture.

MANAGEMENT Treatment of fractures of the zygoma involves reduction, accomplished through lower eyelid and gingival buccal sulcus incisions, and immobilization with interfragment wires stabilized with plate and screw fixation. Thin bone grafts may be required to replace damaged sections of the zygomatic buttress, inferior rim and/or the walls of the orbit. If the zygomatic arch is laterally dislocated, a coronal incision must be used when reducing it. The coronal incision or an upper lid incision exposes the frontal process of the zygoma.

Initially, dislocated fragments of the zygoma are repositioned and aligned by drilling holes adjacent to the fractures and linking the fragments with small interfragment wires. The fracture fragments are held in initial position while rigid internal fixation is performed using small plates and screws (Figure 21.48). If the

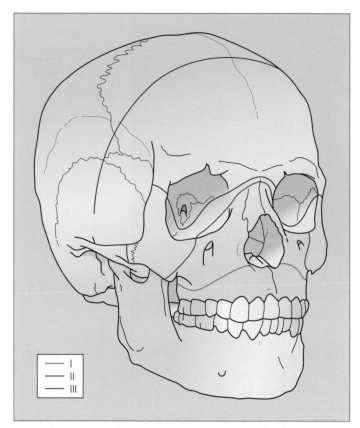

Figure 21.39 Le Fort fractures. Le Fort, on the basis of cadaver experiments, identified thinner areas of the midfacial skeleton that fracture more commonly. Often, combinations of fractures are seen. The Le Fort I fracture travels horizontally across the base of the piriform aperture, separating the lower portion of the maxillary sinuses from the upper midfacial skeleton. In the Le Fort II injury, a pyramidal lower facial segment is separated from the upper cranial facial skeleton. The fracture travels laterally through the Le Fort I, through the inferior orbital rims medially, and through either the cartilaginous portion of the nose or the nasofrontal junction centrally. In the Le Fort III injury, the cranium is separated from the midfacial skeleton through the internal orbital margins of the zygoma. The fracture begins at the zygomaticofrontal suture, extends down the junction of the greater wing of the sphenoid with the orbital process of the zygoma, crosses the orbital floor to travel up the medial orbital wall, comminutes the nasoethmoid region and the nasofrontal junction, and similarly transects the contralateral orbit. In practice, it is usual to see the Le Fort fracture level higher on one side than the other. Commonly, Le Fort III superior level injuries on one side occur with a Le Fort II superior level injury on the other.

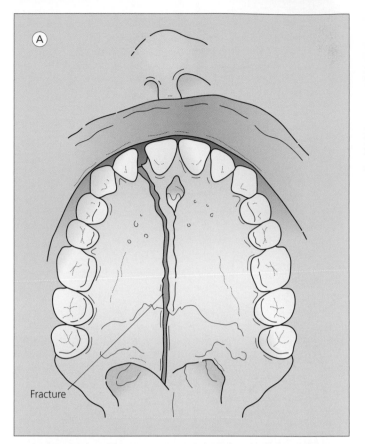

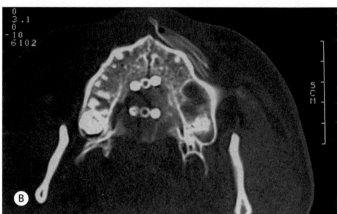

Figure 21.40 (A) Sagittal fracture of the maxilla. **(B)** Open reduction and internal fixation using small plates and screws is being performed in the roof of the mouth for this sagittal fracture of the palate.

lateral canthus is detached in the reduction, it should be replaced after bone assembly.

For an isolated, medially dislocated fracture of the zygomatic arch, whether isolated or occurring simultaneously with other fractures of the zygoma, a small incision can be made in the temporal hair and the "Gillies' approach" used to elevate the zygomatic arch into its proper position. An elevator is placed beneath the temporal fascia, sliding it under the arch, and the zygomatic arch is levered into its proper position.

Fractures of the mandible

The mandibular fracture is a common facial injury because the mandible's prominent position renders it susceptible to trauma. Mandibular fractures are often multiple and a second mandibular fracture should be suspected if a single fracture is identified. Mandibular fractures may be classified as closed or open; most mandibular fractures are open intraorally, especially those in the horizontal (tooth bearing) mandible. Mandibular fractures frequently occur in structurally weak portions of the mandible,

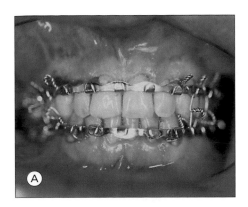

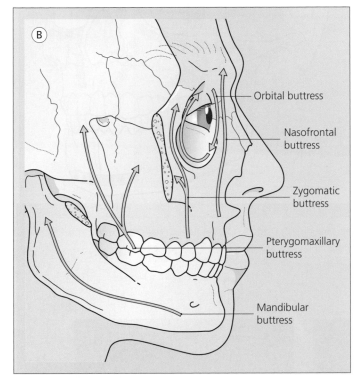

Orbital buttress

Nasofrontal buttress

Zygomatic buttress

Pterygomaxillary buttress

Mandibular buttress

Figure 21.41 **(A)** The treatment of a Le Fort fracture begins with intermaxillary fixation. **(B)** The internal buttress system of the maxilla must be restored by assembling the fragments and stabilizing them with interfragment plate and screw fixation. Here anterior, middle, and posterior maxillary buttresses are seen. The anterior and posterior buttresses are stabilized with rigid fixation, and the posterior buttress by intermaxillary fixation to an intact mandible.

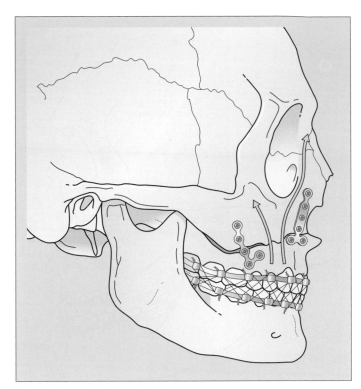

Figure 21.42 Diagram of Le Fort I fracture treatment.

such as the subcondylar region, the region of the angle, or the cuspid region (Figure 21.49). The edentulous mandible most commonly fractures in the body and angle region followed by the subcondylar area.

DIAGNOSIS The diagnosis of a mandibular fracture is suggested by malocclusion, pain, swelling, tenderness, crepitus, fractured teeth, gaps or discrepancies in the level of the dentition, asymmetry of the dental arch, presence of intraoral lacerations, broken or loose teeth, or numbness in the distribution of the mental nerve. An odor is frequently present. Fractured, missing, or dislocated teeth are frequently seen. An "open bite" occurs if the fracture sufficiently dislocates a segment of jaw so that the

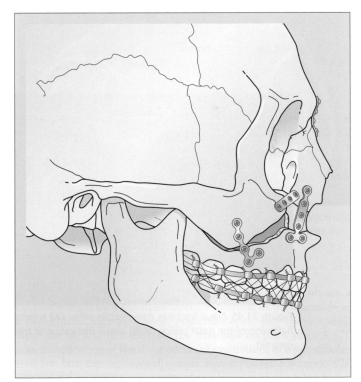

Figure 21.43 Diagram of Le Fort II fracture treatment.

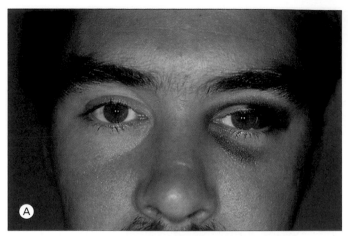
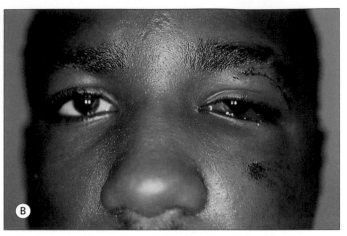

Figure 21.47 (A,B) The symptoms of zygomatic fractures almost always include the combination of periorbital and subconjunctival hematomas. Posterior displacement of the malar eminence, a palpable step deformity in the orbital rim, and numbness in the distribution of the infraorbital nerve are frequently present. Bleeding from the ipsilateral nose occurs if the fracture extends into the ipsilateral maxillary sinus. The congested swollen conjunctiva in **(B)** is a warning of retinobulbar hematoma and possible globe injury.

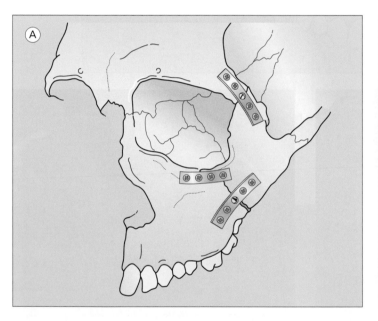
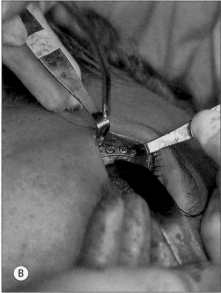
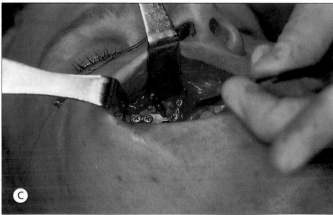
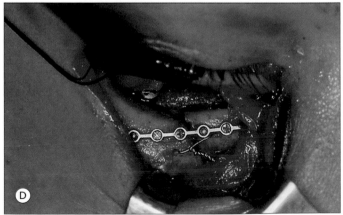

Figure 21.48 (A) Diagram of an open reduction and internal fixation of the zygoma. **(B)** A strong midface plate is placed at the zygomaticofrontal suture and a thinner microsystem plate at the inferior orbital rim. **(C)** Depending on the comminution of the fracture, the surgeon may need to plate the zygomaticomaxillary buttress or the zygomatic arch **(D)**.

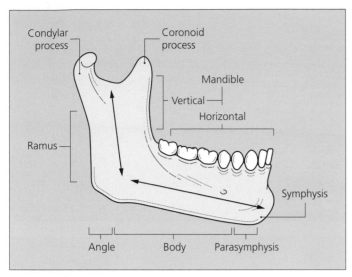

Figure 21.49 Parts of the mandible.

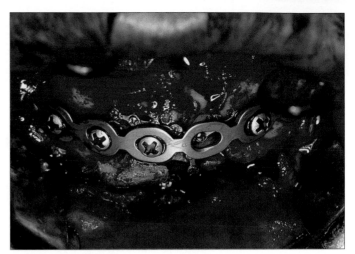

Figure 21.51 Rigid fixation in a mandibular fracture utilizes small and large plates for stabilization of all of the segments.

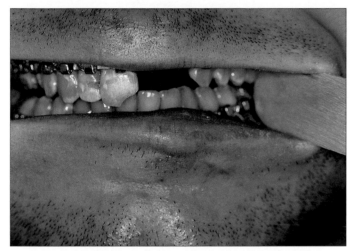

Figure 21.50 "Open bite" after mandibular fracture treatment. The front teeth cannot be brought into full occlusion because displaced posterior aspects of the mandible block its full motion.

teeth into occlusion (Figure 21.51). In some cases an acrylic splint can be applied to the teeth temporarily to align them. Some fractures are treated with intermaxillary fixation alone for 4–6 weeks after "closed reduction." For displaced fractures in both the horizontal and vertical portions of the mandible, direct open reduction of the fracture with plate and screw fixation is the preferred treatment. A plate is placed along the inferior border of the mandible, avoiding the mental nerve and tooth roots (Figure 21.52). At least two screws are placed to each side of the fracture in stable bone.

The angle region may be treated intraorally, with an intraoral incision, or, for more comminuted fractures, extraorally, with an incision in the upper neck in the hyoid crease or retromandibular area. Fractures of the condyle that require open reduction are treated with a preauricular approach, protecting the facial nerve. Mandibular fractures may be prone to complications such as nonunion, delayed union, and infection. Antibiotics are generally indicated at the time of the fracture reduction.

Facial fractures in children

Less than 5% of all facial fractures occur in children; of that 5%, most occur in those over 5 years of age. The bones of children are less brittle than those of adults, and they displace without fracture in many cases. If fractured, healing of the bone progresses more rapidly than in adults. Sinuses are small and therefore do not weaken the bony structure. The treatment of fractures in the upper face of a child follows the same principles described for adults. The emphasis is on early or immediate treatment because healing occurs rapidly. It may be difficult to reduce a Le Fort fracture after even 1 week. Intermaxillary fixation is often difficult to apply in children because of mixed dentition and inadequate root structure of the teeth and the shape of the crowns, which produces difficulty in ligating teeth. Arch bars may have to be supported by the use of piriform aperture wires, circum-mandibular wires, or suspension wires for stabilization. The application of acrylic splints can facilitate reduction. The use of miniature plate and screw fixation systems in children is preferred. The long-term efficacy of resorbable plates in pediatric facial fractures has yet to be defined. Healing times are shorter in children. Because of the prominence of the frontal skull in children, frontal skull and supraorbital fractures are frequent. Orbital floor fractures are not frequent because of the different situations of the maxillary sinus. The frontal sinus is absent.

Healing times are generally significantly reduced in children. One tends to minimize the use of fixation materials, which will remain, because of their role in growth reduction (5%).

SUGGESTED READING

Skull fractures

Bakay L, Glasauer FE. *Head Injury*. Boston: Little, Brown; 1980.

Becker DP, Gade GF, Young HF, Feuerman TF. Diagnosis and treatment of head injury in adults. In: Youmans JR (ed.), *Neurological Surgery*, 3rd edn. Philadelphia: WB Saunders Co.; 1990: 2017–148.

Cooper PR. Skull fracture and traumatic cerebrospinal fluid fistulas. In: Cooper PR (ed.), *Head Injury*, 2nd edn. Baltimore: Williams & Wilkins; 1987: 89–107.

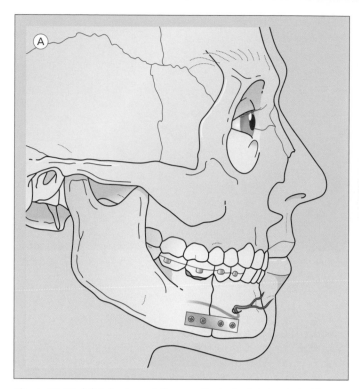

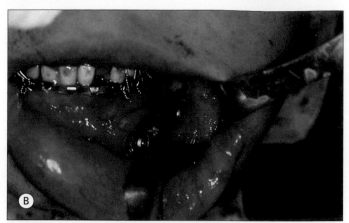

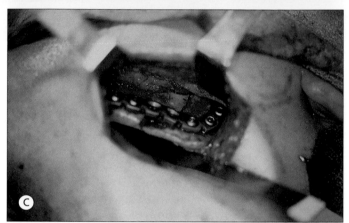

Figure 21.52 **(A)** A fracture of the mandibular body is treated with a compression plate along the inferior border of the mandible. **(B)** An intraoral exposure is used for plate and screw fixation of a fracture of the mandibular symphysis. **(C)** Plate and screw fixation of a mandibular angle fracture.

CLINICAL PEARLS

● Linear skull fractures do not require stabilization or treatment when the scalp is closed. Depressed skull fractures may need exploration depending on the extent of the injury to the underlying brain, frontal sinus or facial bones. Closed depressed fractures are usually repaired for cosmetic reasons. Compound depressed skull fractures with brain involvement are often neurosurgical emergencies. It becomes an emergency to treat the underlying brain injury, perform a water tight closure of the dura, and debride the devitalized scalp.

● Growing skull fractures, although rare, can occur in children under 2 years of age, and require surgical repair. If there is a tear in the dura after trauma, the pressure of the brain pulsations in a growing brain may enlarge the fracture and dural opening. The brain can herniated through this skull defect causing a pulsatile mass under the scalp.

● Basilar skull fractures may present with periorbital eccchymoses, hemotympanum or eccymosis over the mastoid. The management of these fractures is usually conservative unless a CSF leak is present. Many traumatic CSF leaks will spontaneously resolve in a week. Those that do not may be managed by CSF drainage, or in some cases surgical repair to avoid infection, once the location of the leak is identified.

● Frontal sinus fractures can be diagnosed on CT and are managed differently depending on whether the frontal or posterior wall is disrupted. Orbital fractures are managed based on the extent of the injury to the globe, optic nerve and orbital contents. Patients with a fluctuating or worsening exam will require decompression of their optic nerve and globe. There are two indications for surgery of orbital "blow out" fractures: muscle or ligament entrapment or enophthalmus (backward dislocation of the globe) caused by prolapse of the orbital contents through the fracture. Le Fort fractures are often injuries to the entire midface region. Their surgical management depends on the extent and stability of the maxillary fracture.

Eisenburg HM, Briner RP. Late complications of head injury. In: McLaurin RL, Venes JL, Schut L, Epstein F (eds), *Pediatric Neurosurgery*, 2nd edn. Philadelphia: WB Saunders Co.; 1989: 290–7.

Geisler FH, Greenberg J. Management of the acute head-injury patient. In: Salcman M (ed.), *Neurologic Emergencies*, 2nd edn. New York: Raven Press; 1990: 135–65.

Geisler FH, Salcman M. The head injury patient. In: Siegel JH (ed.), *Trauma—Emergency Surgery & Critical Care*. New York: Churchill Livingstone; 1987: 919–46.

Gudeman SK, Young HF, Miller JD, Ward JD, Becker DP. Indications for operative treatment and operative technique in closed head injury. In: Becker DP, Gudeman SK (eds), *Textbook of Head Injury*. Philadelphia: WB Saunders Co.; 1989: 138–81.

Jennett B, Teasdale G. *Management of Head Injuries*. Philadelphia: FA Davis, Co.; 1981.

Mealey J Jr. Skull fractures. In: McLaurin RL, Venes JL, Schut L, Epstein F (eds), *Pediatric Neurosurgery*, 2nd edn. Philadelphia: WB Saunders Co.; 1989: 263–70.

Thomas LM. Skull fractures. In: Wilkins RH, Rengachary SS (eds), *Neurosurgery*. New York: McGraw-Hill; 1985; vol. 2: 1623–6.

Tyson GW. *Head Injury Management for Providers of Emergency Care*. Baltimore: Williams & Wilkins; 1987.

Wilberger J, Chen DA. The skull and meninges. *Neurosurg Clin North Am* 1991; 2: 341–50.

Maxillofacial fractures

Adekeye EO, Ord RA. Giant frontal sinus mucocele. *J Maxillofac Surg* 1984; 12: 184.

Anderson RL. The medial canthal tendon branches out. *Arch Ophthalmol* 1977; 95: 2051.

Anderson RL, Panje WR, Gross CE. Optic nerve blindness following blunt forehead trauma. *Ophthalmology* 1982; 89: 445.

Angle EH. Classification of malocclusion. *Dent Cosmos* 1989; 41: 240.

Barton FE, Berry WL. Evaluation of the acutely injured orbit. In: Aston SJ, Hornblass A, Meltzer MA, Rees TD (eds), *Third International Symposium of Plastic and Reconstructive Surgery of the Eye and Adnexa*. Baltimore: Williams & Wilkins; 1982: 34.

Burstein F, Cohen S, Hudgins R, Boydston W. Frontal basilar trauma: classification and treatment. *Plast Reconstr Surg* 1997; 99: 1314.

Champy M, Lodde JP, Schmidt R, Jaeger JH, Muster D. Mandibular osteosynthesis by miniature screwed plates via a buccal approach. *J Maxillofac Surg* 1978; 6: 14.

Chen, Y-R., Fischer, D.M.: Discussion of: Blindness as a complication of LeFort osteotomies: the role of atypical fracture patterns and distortion of the optic canal. By Girotto J, Davidson J, Wheatley M, *et al*. *Plast Reconstr Surg* 1998; 102: 1422–3.

Clark N, Birely B, Manson PN, *et al*. High-energy ballistic and avulsive facial injuries: classification, patterns, and an algorithm for primary reconstruction. *Plast Reconstr Surg* 1996; 98: 583–601.

Converse JM, Firmin F, Wood-Smith D, Friedland JA. The conjunctival approach in orbital fractures. *Plast Reconstr Surg* 1973; 52: 656.

Converse JM, Smith B. Enophthalmos and diplopia in fracture of the orbital floor. *Br J Plast Surg* 1957; 9: 265.

Converse JM, Smith B. Blowout fracture of the floor of the orbit. *Trans Am Acad Ophthalmol Otolaryngol* 1960; 64: 676.

Converse JM, Smith B. Naso-orbital fractures (symposium: midfacial fractures). *Trans Am Acad Ophthalmol Otolaryngol* 1963; 67: 622.

Crawley W, Manson P. *Problems and Complications in Cranioplasty in Craniomaxillofacial Trauma, Perspectives in Plastic Surgery*. Philadelphia: Lippincott; 1991: 458–65.

Donald PJ, Ettin M. The safety of frontal sinus fat obliteration when sinus walls are missing. *Laryngoscope* 1986; 96: 190.

Dufresne C, Manson P, Iliff N. Early and late complications of orbital fractures. *Semin Ophthalmol* 1989; 4: 176–90.

Erling B, Iliff N, Robertson B, Manson P. "Footprints" of the globe: a practical look at the mechanism of orbital blowout fracture, with a revisit to the work of Raymond Pfeiffer. *Plast Reconstr Surg* 1999; 103: 1313–16.

Ferre J, Bordvre P, Huet P, Favre A. Usefulness of the galeal flap in treatment of intensive frontal bone defects: a study of 14 patients. *J Craniofac Surg* 1995; 6: 164–9.

Fiala TG, Novelline RA, Yaremchuk MC. Comparison of CT imaging artifact from craniomaxillofacial internal fixation devices. *Plast Reconstr Surg* 1993; 92: 1227–32.

Fiala TG, Paige TG, Davis TL, Campbell T, Rosen BS, Yaremchuk M. Comparison of artifact from craniomaxillofacial internal fixation devices: magnetic resonance imaging. *Plast Reconstr Surg* 1994; 93: 725–31.

Fujino T. Experimental "blowout fracture" of the orbit. *Plast Reconstr Surg* 1974; 54: 81.

Fukado Y. Results in 400 cases of surgical decompression of the optic nerve. In: Bleeker GM, *et al*. (eds), *Proceedings of Second International Symposium on Orbital Disorders*. Basel: Karger; 1975.

Girotto J, Gamble B, Robertson B, *et al*. Blindness following reduction of facial fractures. *Plast Reconstr Surg* 1998; 102: 1821–34.

Girotto J, Makenzie E, Fowler C, Redett R, Robertson B, Manson P. Long term physical impairment and functional outcomes following complex facial fractures. *Plast Reconstr Surg* 2001; 108: 312–28.

Gruss J. Complex craniofacial trauma: evolution of management: a trauma unit's experience. *J Trauma* 1990; 30: 377.

Gruss J. Advances in craniofacial fracture repair. *Scand J Plast Reconstr Hand Surg (Suppl.)* 1995; 27: 67–81.

Gruss JS, Hurwitz JJ, Nik NA, Kassel EE. The pattern and incidence of nasolacrimal injury in nasoethmoidal orbital fractures: the role of delayed assessment and dacryocystorhinostomy. *Br J Plast Surg* 1985; 38: 116.

Gruss JS, MacKinnon SE, Kassel E, Cooper PW. The role of primary bone grafting in complex craniomaxillofacial trauma. *Plast Reconstr Surg* 1985; 75: 17.

Gruss JS, Pollock RS, Phillips JH, Antonyshyn O. Combined injuries of the cranium and face. *Br J Plast Surg* 1989; 42: 385–98.

Gruss JS, Van-Wyck L, Phillips JH, *et al*. The importance of the zygomatic arch in complex midfacial fracture repair and correction of post traumatic orbito-zygomatic deformities. *Plast Reconstr Surg* 1990; 85: 878–90.

Hendler N, Viernstein M, Schallenberger C, Long D. Group therapy with chronic pain patients. *Psychosomatics* 1987; 22: 333.

Hendler H. The anatomy and psychopharmacology of chronic pain. *J Clin Psychiatr* 1982; 43: 15.

Hendrickson M, Clark N, Manson P. Sagittal fractures of the maxilla: classification and treatment. *Plast Reconstr Surg* 1998; 101: 319–32.

Iliff N, Manson P, Katz J, Rever L, Yaremchuk M. Mechanisms of extraocular muscle injury in orbital fractures. *Plast Reconstr Surg* 1999; 103: 787–99.

Jackson IT, Pellett C, Smith JM. The skull as a bone graft donor site. *Ann Plast Surg* 1983; 11: 527.

Jacobs JB, Perky MS. Traumatic pneumocephalus. *Laryngoscope* 1980; 90: 515.

Jones LT. An anatomical approach to problems of the "eyelids and lacrimal apparatus". *Arch Ophthalmol* 1961; 66: 111.

Kim LH, Lam LK, Moore MH, Trott JA, David DJ. Associated injuries in facial fractures: review of 839 patients. *Br J Plast Surg* 1993; 46: 65.

Kline RM, Wolfe SA. Complications associated with the harvesting of cranial bone grafts. *Plast Reconstr Surg* 1995; 95: 5.

Koorneef L. *Spatial Aspects of the Orbital Musculofibrous Tissue in Man: A New Anatomical and Histological Approach.* Amsterdam: Swets & Zeitlinger, BV; 1977.

Lessel S. Indirect optic nerve trauma. *Arch Opthalmol* 1989; 107: 382–6.

Manson PN. Some thoughts on the classification and treatment of Le Fort fractures. *Ann Plast Surg* 1986; 17: 356.

Manson PN. Facial bone healing and grafts: a review of clinical physiology. *Clin Plast Surg* 1994; 21: 331–48.

Manson P, Carson B. Commentary: growing skull fractures. *J Craniofacial Surg* 1995; 6: 111.

Manson PN, Shack RB, Leonard LG, Su CT, Hoopes JE. Sagittal fractures of the maxilla and palate. *Plast Reconstr Surg.* 1983; 72: 484.

Manson PN, Crawley WA, Yaremchuck MJ, Rochman GM, Hoopes JE, French JH. Midface fractures: advantages of immediate extended open reduction and bone grafting. *Plast Reconstr Surg* 1985; 76: 1.

Manson PN, Cifford CM, Su CT, Iliff NT, Morgan R. Mechanisms of global support and post traumatic enophthalmos, I: the anatomy of the ligament sling and its relation to intramuscular cone orbital fat. *Plast Reconstr Surg* 1986; 77: 193.

Manson PN, Crawley WA, Hoopes JE. Frontal cranioplasty: risk factors and choice of cranial vault reconstructive material. *Plast Reconstr Surg* 1986; 76: 888.

Manson PN, Grivas A, Rosenbaum A, Vannier M, Zinreich J, Iliff N. Studies on enophthalmos, II: the measurement of orbital injuries and their treatment by quantitative computed tomography. *Plast Reconstr Surg* 1986; 77: 203.

Manson P, Iliff N, Vander Kolk C, Yaremchuk M, Mirvis S. Rigid fixation of orbital fractures. *Plast Reconstr Surg* 1990; 86: 1103–9.

Manson P, Markowitz B, Mirvis S, Dunham M, Yaremchuk M. Toward CT-based facial fracture treatment. *Plast Reconstr Surg* 1990; 85: 202–12.

Manson P, Clark N, Robertson B, *et al.* Subunit principles in midface fractures: the importance of sagittal buttresses, soft tissue reductions and sequencing treatment of segmental fractures. *Plast Reconstr Surg* 1999; 103: 1287–306.

Manson P, Iliff N, Robertson B. The hope offered by early surgical treatment to those patients whose blowout fractures demonstrate tight muscle restriction or true muscle incarceration. *Plast Reconstr Surg* 2002; 109: 490–5.

Markowitz B, Manson P. Discussion: fronto basilar trauma: classification and treatment. *Plast Reconstr Surg* 1997; 99: 1322–3.

Markowitz B, Manson P, Sargent L, *et al.* Management of the medial canthal tendon in nasoethmoid orbital fractures: the importance of the central fragment in treatment and classification. *Plast Reconstr Surg* 1991; 87: 843–53.

Markowitz B, Manson P, Yaremchuk M, Glassman D, Kawamoto H. High-energy orbital dislocations: The possibility of traumatic hypertelorism. *Plast Reconstr Surg* 1991; 88: 20–9.

McKinnon CA, David DJ, Cooter RD. Blindness and severe visual impairment in facial fractures: an 11 year review. *Br J Plast Surg* 2002; 55: 1–7.

Merville L. Multiple dislocations of the facial skeleton. *J Maxillofac Surg* 1979; 2: 187.

Milauskas AT, Fueger GF. Serious ocular complications associated with blow-out fractures of the orbit. *Am J Ophthalmol* 1966; 62: 670.

Millman AL, Della Rocca RC, Spector S, Leipeskind, Messina A. Steroids and orbital blowout fractures–A new systematic concept in medical management and surgical decision making. *Adv Opthalmol Plast Reconstr Surg* 1987; 6: 291–301.

Pensler J, McCarthy JG. The calvarial donor site: an anatomic study in cadavers. *Plast Reconst Surg* 1985; 75: 648.

Phillips J, Gruss J, Wells M. Periorbital suspension of lower eyelid and cheek following subcilliary exposures of facial fractures. *Plast Reconstr Surg* 1991; 88: 145.

Putterman AM, Stevens T, Urist MJ. Nonsurgical management of blow-out fractures of the orbital floor. *Am J Ophthalmol* 1974; 77: 232.

Raflo GT. Blow-in and blow-out fractures of the orbit: clinical correlations and proposed mechanisms. *Ophthalmic Surg* 1984; 15: 114.

Rish BL, Dillon JD, Meirowsky AM, *et al.* Cranioplasty: a review of 1030 cases of penetrating head injury. *Neurosurgery* 1979; 4: 381.

Robertson B, Manson P. The importance of serial debridement and second look procedures in high-energy ballistic and avulsive facial injuries. *Operat Techn Plast Reconstr Surg* 1998; 5: 236–46.

Rumelt MB, Ernest JT. Isolated blowout fracture of the medial orbital wall with medial rectus muscle entrapment. *Am J Ophthalmol* 1972; 73: 451.

Sofferman RA, Danielson PA, Quatela V, Reed RR. Retrospective analysis of surgically treated Le Fort fractures. *Arch Otolaryngol* 1983; 109: 446.

Stranc MF, Robertson GA. A classification of injuries of the nasal skeleton. *Ann Plast Surg* 1979; 2: 468.

Vondra J. *Fractures of the Base of the Skull.* London: Iliffe Books; 1965.

Wolfe SA. Application of craniofacial surgical precepts following trauma and tumour removal. *J Maxillofac Surg* 1982; 10: 212.

Zide BM, McCarthy JG. The medial canthus revisited—an anatomical basis for canthopexy. *Ann Plast Surg* 1983; 11: 1.

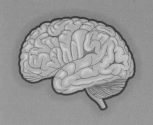

TRAUMATIC INTRACRANIAL HEMATOMAS

22

Marcelo Vilela and G Alexander West

INTRODUCTION

Traumatic intracranial hematomas are localized collections of blood that are directly related to the primary forces (impact, acceleration) and secondary factors that can play a role in head injury, such as coagulopathy, alcohol intake, cocaine abuse, hypotension, rupture of traumatic intracranial aneurysms, and decompression of the brain following removal of the hematoma.[1]

Post-traumatic intracranial hematomas are most frequently classified according to their location and mechanism of formation:[1]

- epidural hematoma;
- subdural hematoma;
- cerebral contusion;
- intraparenchymal hemorrhage.

ACUTE EPIDURAL HEMATOMA

The epidural hematoma (EDH) is a collection of blood between the skull and the dura mater. It is caused by a ruptured artery or vein in the epidural space as a result of a fracture of the skull at the moment of the impact in 60–90% of cases. In children fractures are less common.[1]

The clot enlarges because of the hydrostatic force of the blood from the ruptured vessel stripping the dura from the bone. The most common scenario is a fracture of the temporal bone causing a tear in the middle meningeal artery.

The clinical manifestations occur as a result of compression and displacement of brain tissue and the resulting increase in intracranial pressure. With increasing size of the EDH, the patient is more likely to become symptomatic. The neurological presentation varies according to the size, location and time course of the hematoma. Most commonly, patients with an acute EDH become symptomatic in less than 24 hours, with 60–75% under 12 hours. Often their neurological status can decrease very suddenly. Rarely, an EDH can enlarge slowly and become symptomatic days after the injury.[1]

The "lucid interval" is more commonly seen with EDH, although it can also occur with other intracranial lesions. It refers to an initial brief period of loss of consciousness (concussion) with recovery that is then followed by a progressive deterioration of the level of consciousness, often accompanied by hemiparesis. The presentation is variable and patients may be fully awake or obtunded when seen in the emergency room. Patients may also arrive in the emergency room unconscious because of an associated diffuse axonal injury, associated intracerebral hemorrhage, or drug intoxication.

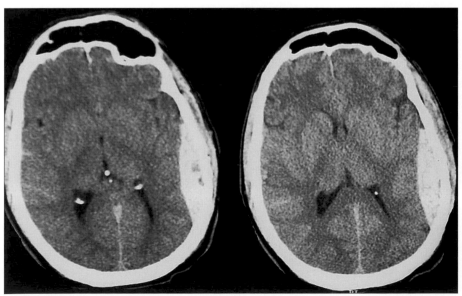

Figure 22.1 CT scans of a 42-year-old man hit by a hard object on the head. A left acute epidural hematoma over the temporoparietal region can be seen. There is a mass effect with mild compression of the ipsilateral ventricle. Note its typical biconvex configuration.

In the case where the EDH enlarges rapidly and is left untreated, signs of transtentorial herniation such as coma, dilation of ipsilateral or bilateral pupils, neurogenic hyperventilation and extensor posturing, and eventually, flaccidity and apnea, occur.

The diagnosis of an EDH is established by the presence of the typical biconvex lens-shaped hematoma adjacent to the skull, displacing the brain. The most common location is the temporo-parietal region. The presence of mass effect and midline shift depends on the size of the clot (Figures 22.1, 22.2).

Commonly, a ruptured vein causes an EDH and the pressure is not enough to cause a large clot. The patient can usually be managed conservatively if clinically indicated.

Epidural hematomas in the posterior fossa or temporal region are especially dangerous and should be managed nonoperatively only if they are small, the patient is in a very good neurological condition, and can be followed very closely both clinically and with frequent CT scans.

Operative management will also depend on several factors such as age, neurological status, time elapsed since the injury, presence of localizing signs, size and location of the hematoma and enlargement of the clot on serial computed tomography (CT) scans.[1] Clots larger than 15 mm in thickness, with volume greater than 25 cm^3 or with associated compressed basal cisterns and midline shift should be evacuated.[2,3]

A craniotomy that exposes the clot in its entirety is preferable to ensure complete removal and hemostasis, and to prevent reaccumulation of the clot by placing several tack-up sutures. Prognosis depends mainly on the initial neurological status and the presence of associated lesions.[1]

ACUTE SUBDURAL HEMATOMA

An acute subdural hematoma (ASDH) is characterized by an accumulation of blood between the dura mater and the arachnoid layer within 72 hours of injury. In elderly patients they are most commonly seen after falls, especially in the face of anticoagulation and alcohol abuse. In young patients it is usually caused by high-speed motor vehicle accidents and assaults. In children, one should suspect child abuse (shaken baby syndrome) and

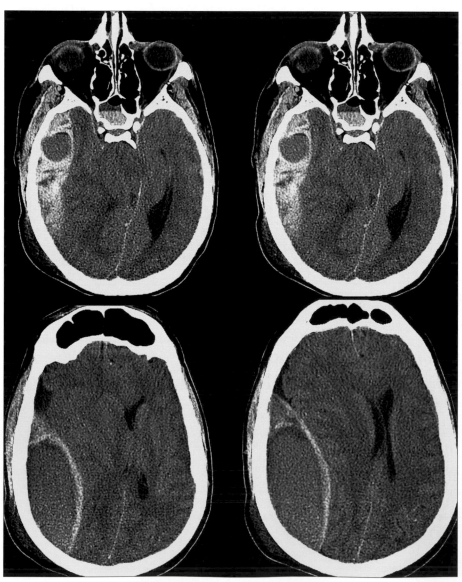

Figure 22.2 CT scans of a 34-year-old man show a right hyperacute epidural hematoma a few hours after he was assaulted. Note the presence of hypodense, non-clotted blood. No coagulopathy was present, which indicates that it is an active, recent bleeding. He underwent emergency craniotomy and made a full recovery, despite a preoperative Glasgow Coma Scale of 3 and dilated fixed pupils.

funduscopic examination should be carried out to look for retinal hemorrhages.

Most often ASDHs are caused by the rupture of bridging veins that traverse the subdural space. The inertial forces (acceleration–deceleration) at the moment of the injury usually are of short impact and abrupt angular acceleration and therefore occur at the periphery of the brain. This explains the rupture of parasagital veins.[4] The ASDH is usually accompanied by ipsilateral hemispheric brain swelling which contributes to the severity of the clinical picture.

Patients with an ASDH are usually comatose, with the ipsilateral pupil dilated, hemiparesis on the contralateral side and often extensor posturing. Occasionally there is hemiparesis ipsilateral to the hematoma, indicating compression of the opposite cerebral peduncle against the edge of the tentorium (Kernohan's notch).

Diagnosis of an ASDH is established by visualizing the crescentic hematoma extending over the fronto-temporo-parietal regions, commonly with mass effect, herniation of the uncus, midline shift, associated brain swelling, effacement of basal cisterns and dilatation of the contralateral temporal horn (Figure 22.3).

Management of patients with an ASDH depends on multiple factors. Patients with a Glasgow Coma Score (GCS) of 13 or higher, absence of associated intracerebral hemorrhage, contusions, edema or effacement of basal cisterns, midline shift less than 10 mm, and hematoma volume less than 25 cm³ can be initially managed conservatively.[2,3]

In patients with low GCS scores and/or evidence of herniation and high intracranial pressure, surgery should be performed as an emergency. A large craniotomy using a question-mark incision should be performed, exposing the frontal, temporal, and parietal lobes. The dura mater is opened and the clot evacuated.

Cruz and colleagues showed in a randomized trial that pre-operative administration of high doses of mannitol to patients with ASDH decreases postoperative brain swelling and intracranial pressures, and improves abnormal pupillary widening and cerebral extraction of oxygen.[5] Several authors support the idea of performing a decompressive craniectomy for ASDH associated with brain swelling.[2,5–7] In this context, after the hematoma is evacuated the brain is covered with either pericranium or dural substitutes such as bovine pericardium. The dura mater is left open, the bone flap is not replaced and the scalp is closed in the usual fashion. Advocates of this technique claim marked improvements in the intracranial pressures, better resolution of

the midline shift and early return of patent basal cisterns.[2,6,7]

Patients who are flaccid, with both pupils fixed and dilated will most likely not recover because devastating brain injury has already occurred. Patients over 65 years old and patients who are operated on more than 4 hours after the injury also have a very high mortality.[2,8] The overall mortality for ASDH is higher than 50% in most series.[1]

CHRONIC SUBDURAL HEMATOMA

By definition a chronic subdural hematoma (CSDH) is a subdural hematoma that is older than 3 weeks. Formation of a CSDH is thought to occur after an initial bleeding in the subdural space, which is usually asymptomatic. The acute blood may resolve completely, it may enlarge and develop into a subacute SDH causing symptoms, or it may liquefy and continue to enlarge, developing into a CSDH. In the case of progressive development of a CSDH, expansion of the subdural space occurs, which leads to further bleeding as a result of rupture of small bridging veins. With time, usually 1–3 weeks, membranes develop and tend to contain or compartmentalize the hematoma.[1]

Most commonly a CSDH is caused by a minor head trauma or fall, often not remembered by the patient or relatives. Bilateral clots are seen in about 20% of cases.[1] Risk factors are old age, alcohol abuse, seizures, cerebrospinal fluid shunts, anticoagulation, and patients at risk for falls.[1]

Common presenting symptoms are headaches, nausea, vomiting, hemiparesis, sensory deficits, language disturbances, gait problems, transient-ischemic-attack-like symptoms, and decreased consciousness.

CT scans will show a hypo- or isodense fluid collection over the frontoparietal region, often with significant mass effect and midline shift. It is common to see small acute clots mixed with the chronic collection. The hematoma usually achieves a large size before becoming symptomatic because of the slow growth (Figure 22.4).

Optimal surgical management is somewhat controversial. Traditionally, the operative technique for symptomatic patients involves placing burr holes or twist drills, one in the frontal and the other in the parietal region. The subdural space is irrigated gently, but thoroughly with saline until the fluid, which has a motor oil appearance, comes out clear. The patient is kept flat in

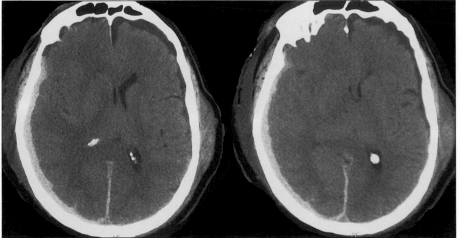

Figure 22.3 CT scans of a 60-year-old man who sustained a fall and had this right acute subdural hematoma. Note the midline shift, mass effect and compression of the third ventricle.

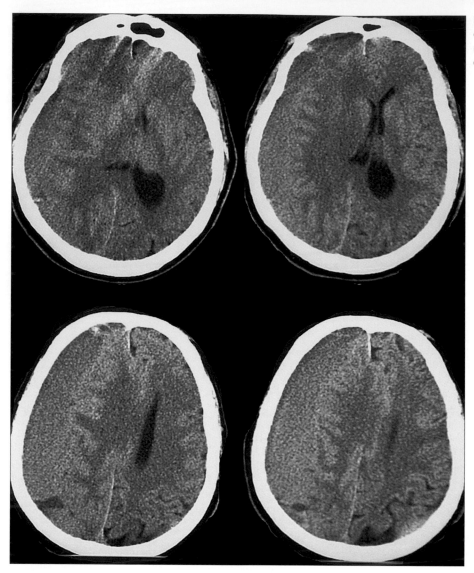

Figure 22.4 CT scans showing a large isodense chronic subdural hematoma extending over the right frontal-temporal-parietal region with mass effect and midline shift.

bed for 24–48 hours to allow re-expansion of the brain. Recent reports suggest that a single burr hole and a closed external drainage system offer the best results.[9]

The CSDH may re-accumulate and a second or third drainage may be necessary. In cases of multiple recurrences, a craniotomy or a craniectomy may be performed with drainage of the clot and removal of membranes.[1]

CEREBRAL CONTUSIONS

A brain contusion is a common consequence of head injury and is defined as scattered hemorrhages involving the cortex and adjacent white matter. Contusions occur predominantly in the basal frontal and temporal lobes, although they can also occur in other lobes of the brain and the cerebellum (Figure 22.5).[3]

The anterior and middle fossa have bony prominences that predispose these lobes to injury. At the moment of the trauma, the inertial forces move the brain against these bony indentations and rupture of small cortical and subcortical vessels occurs. "Coup" contusions occur on the same side as the impact and "counter-coup" contusions occur on the opposite side.

Contusions can enlarge after a significant period of time has elapsed and it is very important to repeat the imaging studies a few hours after the initial CT scan. Alcoholic patients are at particular risk because of frequent falls and abnormal coagulation pathways.

Presentation is variable and in part depends on the nature of the trauma and associated injuries. Some patients sustain small contusions after a minor fall or assault and have a favorable neurological course. Others have large contusions at the frontal or temporal lobes, with associated mass effect and midline shift. Interestingly, the mass effect and swelling can become more pronounced during the first 2 weeks because of the development of swelling around the contused brain.[1]

Large temporal contusions are often associated with local pressure and herniation of the uncus, which can occur even with normal intracranial pressures.[1] Sometimes an extensive temporal lobe contusion is associated with an ipsilateral ASDH and can be quite devastating; the so-called "burst temporal lobe" (Figure 22.6).

Large bifrontal contusions are commonly associated with central herniation and high intracranial pressures, characteristically with effacement of the basal cisterns, small lateral ventricles,

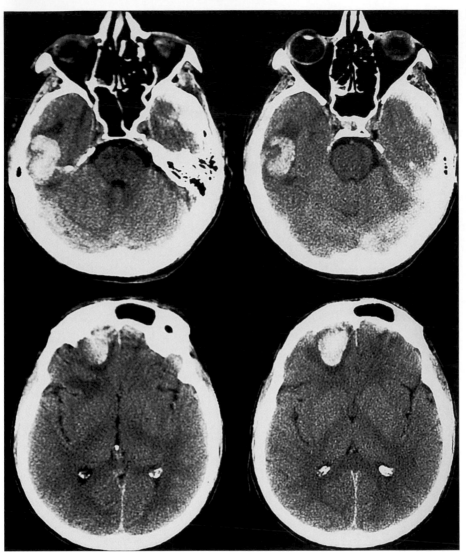

Figure 22.5 CT scans of an alcoholic patient who sustained a fall and developed small temporal and frontal contusions. Note patent basal cisterns and sylvian fissures, absence of mass effect and midline shift.

disappearance of the third ventricle, and progressive decrease in the level of consciousness (Figure 22.7).

The neurological status of the patient, location of the contusion, presence or absence of basal cisterns and ventricles on imaging studies, and intracranial pressures will dictate treatment of patients with cerebral contusions. Patients that are awake and following commands with no significant neurological deficits can often be managed conservatively, even when there are multiple contusions. Obtunded or comatose patients with significant contusions and mass effect or midline shift may benefit from a craniotomy and removal of the contused brain tissue.[1] Temporal lobe contusions on the dominant hemisphere with mass effect and midline shift can be managed with a decompressive craniectomy, only without removal of the lesion or brain tissue to preserve brain tissue that may be viable.

Patients with bifrontal contusions, effacement of basal cisterns and mildly elevated intracranial pressures can be initially managed conservatively using mannitol, mild-moderate hyperventilation guided by F_IO_2 measurements, hypertonic saline and deep sedation. When conservative measures fail and there is evidence of worsening of neurological status, CT scans and uncontrollable

intracranial pressure, a bifrontal decompressive craniectomy may be an option (Figure 22.8).[6,7]

INTRAPARENCHYMAL HEMATOMA

Intraparenchymal hematoma is defined as confluent, homogeneous areas of hemorrhage that occur inside the brain parenchyma. They are seen most commonly in the frontal and temporal regions, can be multiple in 20% of cases, are usually round-shaped and occur in the white and gray matter. Other locations are the corpus callosum, periventricular region, and basal ganglia.[1]

In contrast to contusions, traumatic intraparenchymal hematoma is not thought to be a result of brain parenchyma impacting against the skull base. The mechanism is usually acceleration–deceleration with "shearing" of perforating vessels for deep located hemorrhages and cortical and subcortical vessels for superficially located ones.[4]

Clinically, patients are often encountered with a depressed level of consciousness, reflecting the high-energy and severity of the injury.

CT scans of the head show one or more localized and non-

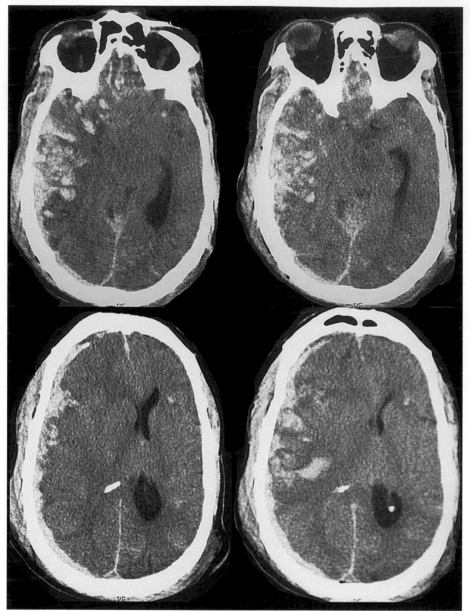

Figure 22.6 "Burst temporal lobe." CT scans of an alcoholic patient who sustained a fall. Multiple scattered temporal lobe contusions associated with an acute subdural hematoma. Note the midline shift, contralateral dilatation of the temporal horn, marked mass effect, distortion of the brainstem and absence of basal cisterns, indicating transtentorial herniation

contiguous hematoma, quite often deep in location (Figure 22.8A, left panel). After several hours, lesions that were not present initially or were just punctate hemorrhages can also enlarge and can be depicted on subsequent follow-up CT scans, the so-called delayed intracerebral hemorrhages.[1,3,7] Edema can be seen around the periphery of the hematoma after a few days, which aggravates the mass effect.[1]

Patients who have evidence of a decreasing level of consciousness and evidence of mass effect or shift from a superficially located clot may benefit from a craniotomy and evacuation of the hematoma. Hematoma in the temporal lobe can cause herniation even in the presence of normal intracranial pressures and must be watched closely when treated nonoperatively.[1] Patients with frontal hemorrhages who are initially managed nonoperatively are especially prone to early failure and have a higher chance of requiring delayed surgical decompression.[3] Deep hematoma located in the basal ganglia and/or corpus callosum are often not suitable for safe evacuation.[1]

Patients with high-energy-induced multiple hematomas and evidence of high intracranial pressure pose a significant problem. When there is one clot that is larger than the others surgery can be directed at evacuating the large clot.[7] When the clots are uniform in size and there is evidence of central herniation with small ventricles and effaced basal cisterns, management should be directed at controlling the intracranial pressure. A bifrontal decompressive craniectomy is an option for malignant intracranial hypertension or when conservative measures fail (Figure 22.8).[2,7]

Prognosis of patients with traumatic brain injury and intracerebral hematoma is related to initial neurological status, location of the hemorrhages, presence of diffuse axonal injury, and intracranial hypertension.[1,7]

This chapter contains material from the first edition, and we are grateful to the author of that chapter for his contribution.

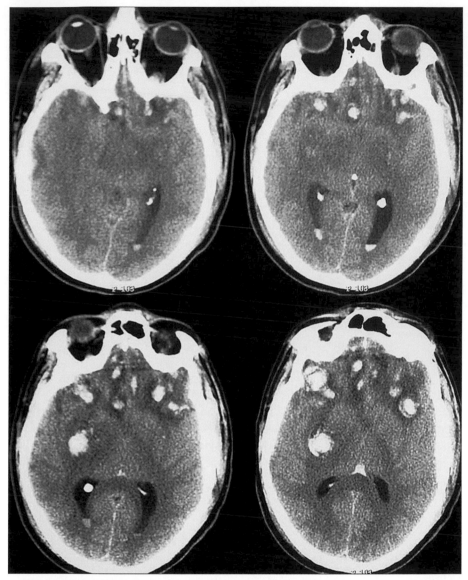

Figure 22.7 CT scans of a patient who was involved in a motor vehicle accident and sustained bifrontal contusions and a right basal ganglia hemorrhage. Note the extensive mass effect with compression of the lateral ventricles, absent third ventricle and effacement of the basal cisterns but no midline shift, indicating central herniation.

CLINICAL PEARLS

- Traumatic brain injury (TBI) continues to be an enormous public health problem, despite major advances in modern medicine. The annual incidence of TBI in the United States is estimated to be 180–220 cases per 100 000 population. As many as 10–30% of these injuries are fatal. Most patients with TBI (75–80%) have mild head injuries; the remaining injuries are divided equally between the moderate and severe categories. The cost to society is enormous, which includes both the in-patient and post-hospital care. Many of the severe, and also of the moderate, TBI cases have traumatic hematomas which require neurosurgical expertise.

- Traumatic intracranial hematomas are localized collections of blood that are directly related to the primary forces (impact, acceleration) and secondary factors that can play a role in head injury such as coagulopathy, alcohol intake, cocaine abuse, hypotension, rupture of traumatic intracranial aneurysms,

and decompression of the brain following removal of hematomas.

- Post-traumatic intracranial hematomas are usually classified according to their location and mechanism of formation. The hematomas are classified as (1) epidural hematoma, (2) subdural hematoma, (3) cerebral contusion, and (4) intraparenchymal hemorrhage. It is essential to understand the distinctive features of each type of injury, from the causal mechanisms to the distinct radiologic appearance on CT and MRI.

- Treatment of patients with each type of traumatic hematoma will depend on a number of variables. Most often operative management will also depend on several factors such as age, neurological status, time elapsed since the injury, presence of localizing signs, size and location of the hematoma and enlargement of the clot on serial CT scans, and intracranial pressure.

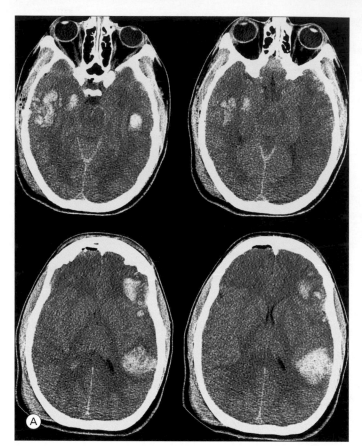
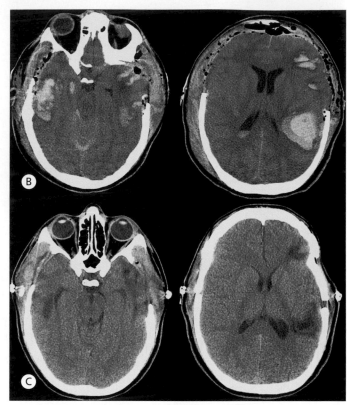

Figure 22.8 CT scans of an 18-year-old male who was hit by a train. **(A)** CT scans at admission show left frontal and bitemporal contusions and a left temporal intracerebral hemorrhage, with effacement of basal cisterns and ventricular compression. Initial intracranial pressure in the emergency room was 60 mmHg. **(B)** Immediate postoperative scans after an emergent decompressive bifrontal-bitemporal craniectomy was performed. There is improvement of the ventricle size but still some compression of the brainstem. **(C)** A cranioplasty was performed 6 months later. The patient made a full recovery and was back in school.

REFERENCES

1. Samudrala S, Cooper PR. Traumatic intracranial hematomas. In: Wilkins RH, Rengachary SS (eds). *Neurosurgery*, 2nd edn. New York: McGraw-Hill; 1985: 2797–807.
2. Munch E, Horn P, Schurer L, Piepgras A, Paul T, Schmiedek P. Management of severe traumatic brain injury by decompressive craniectomy. *Neurosurgery* 2000; 47: 315–22.
3. Patel NY, Hoyt DB, Nakaji P, *et al.* Traumatic brain injury: patterns of failure of nonoperative management. *J Trauma* 2000; 48: 367–74.
4. Genarelli TA, Meaney DF. Mechanisms of primary head injury, In: Wilkins RH, Rengachary SS (eds). *Neurosurgery*, 2nd edn. New York: McGraw-Hill; 1985: 2611–21.
5. Cruz J, Minoja G, Okuchi K. Improving clinical outcomes from acute subdural hematomas with the emergency preoperative administraton of high doses of manitol: a randomized trial. *Neurosurgery* 2001; 49: 864–71.
6. Guerra WKW, Gaab MR, Dietz H, Mueller JU, Piek J, Fritsch MJ. Surgical decompression for traumatic brain swelling: indications and results. *J Neurosurg* 1999; 90:187–96.
7. Caroli M, Locatelli M, Campanella R, Balbi S, Martinelli F, Arienta C. Multiple intracranial lesions in head injury. Clinical considerations, prognostic factors, management and results in 95 patients. *Surg Neurol* 2001; 56: 82–8.
8. Sakas DE, Bullock MR, Teasdale GM. One year outcome following craniotomy for traumatic hematoma in patients with fixed dilated pupils. *J Neurosurg* 1995; 82: 961–5.
9. Williams GR, Baskaya MK, Menendez J, Polin R, Willis B, Nanda A. Burr-hole versus twist drill drainage for the evacuation of chronic subdural haematoma: a comparison of clinical results. *J Clin Neurosci* 2001; 8: 551–4.

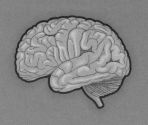

INJURIES TO THE CERVICAL SPINE

23

Ehud Mendel, Stephen J Hentschel, and Bernard H Guiot

INTRODUCTION

The cervical spine, being the most mobile portion of the spine, is the most common site of spinal injuries. The relative involvement of different spinal levels in injury is shown in Table 23.1. An estimated 12 000–14 000 spinal cord injuries occur each year out of the total of 200 000 traumatic spinal column injuries in the United States.[1–6] Nearly 10 000 patients will die each year as a result of an injury to the spinal cord.[5,7–10]

The most frequent age group to suffer an injury to the spinal cord is 15–30-year-olds, motor vehicle accidents, falls, and sports being the most common mechanisms of injury.[2,5,11–13] The cause of spinal injury varies with age, and particularly sex, with males being three to four times as likely to sustain an injury as females. Age is also a determinant of the type of spinal injury as children less than 4 years of age have fewer vertebral injuries than adults.[14] The injuries in this young pediatric population tend to occur between the occiput and C2, representing 40% of all pediatric spine injuries, whereas only 20% of adult spinal injuries occur in this location.[1,14–16] Anatomic differences of the pediatric spine include ligamentous laxity, increased mobility, incompletely ossified and wedge-shaped vertebral bodies, shallow and horizontal facet joints, and underdeveloped neck muscles when compared with adults.[14,15] Subluxation injuries without fracture and spinal cord injuries without radiographic abnormality (SCIWORA) are much less common in adults and are more likely to occur in younger patients.[14,15,17]

NEUROLOGIC INJURY

Up to 15% of patients sustaining a spinal injury secondary to trauma will sustain a neurologic injury as a result.[5,13] Injuries to the cervical spine, in particular, result in a much higher incidence of injury to the spinal cord than any other spinal level. The incidence of spinal cord injury ranges from 2% to nearly 100% of cervical spine injuries, depending on the cervical level involved, with an incidence of 40–60% overall (Table 23.2).[1,2,5,7–11,18,19] The incidence of spinal cord injury with cervical fracture is likely to be underestimated as some patients may die prior to medical attention. This is particularly true for atlanto-occipital dislocations, where 25% of patients may die as a result of respiratory arrest prior to evaluation.[4,5,13]

The level and mechanism of the spinal injury, the force involved, as well as the age and medical status of the patient, have important influences on the extent of neurological injury following trauma. In particular, conditions such as ankylosing spondylitis or Down syndrome, which have a significant effect on the relative rigidity (or laxity) of the spinal column, may predispose to neurological injury.[5,13] In addition, the status of the patient following spinal injury can influence neurologic injury, mainly through the deleterious effect of hypotension or hypoxia.[3,5,12,13]

IMAGING

A simple cross-table lateral is usually the first image of the cervical spine to be obtained following trauma. A swimmer's view may be required as it is necessary to image from the skull base to the top

Table 23.1 Incidence of adult cervical spine injuries

Level of Injury	Incidence
Cervical	60%
Thoracic	8%
Thoracolumbar	20%
Lumbar	10%
Sacral	2%

Table 23.2 Cervical spine injury and neurologic deficit

Level	Incidence of neurologic deficit
Atlanto-occipital dislocation	100%
Atlas	1%–2%
Axis	10%
C3–T1	6%
Unilateral cervical facet dislocation	60%
Bilateral cervical facet dislocation	100%

of the T1 vertebral body (Figure 23.1).[5,13,20] This combination of lateral X-rays has an 85% sensitivity and a negative predictive value of 97% for fracture.[20,21] An open-mouth odontoid view should be utilized to assess the C1–2 vertebrae and articulations and is particularly valuable for assessment of the odontoid process (Figure 23.2). If an open-mouth view cannot be obtained for whatever reason, the pillar (oblique) view can be utilized to demonstrate the odontoid process. The anteroposterior view is often ignored by inexperienced clinicians but can identify injuries with a rotatory component, such as unilateral facet dislocations, that may not be readily apparent on lateral films. With the use of the anteroposterior, lateral, and open-mouth odontoid views, the sensitivity and negative predictive values of the series are 92% and 99%, respectively.[20–22] Adding oblique views to the standard series does not increase the sensitivity.[23]

Computed tomography (CT) is particularly useful for evaluating the occipitocervical and the cervicothoracic junctions, however the routine use of CT in the trauma setting is difficult to recommend as there have been no direct comparisons with plain X-ray.[24,25] Areas identified as possible pathology on the plain radiographs should be further investigated with CT imaging with fine sections through the suspicious area (Figure 23.3).[13,20] Reconstructions in the sagittal and coronal planes may be helpful in further defining the nature of the injury (Figure 23.4).[20] Determining the level of pathology may be difficult in SCIWORA patients and in these cases, the neurologic examination is critical in evaluating the appropriate level to be studied.[14] As approximately 10% of patients with a cervical spine fracture have a second associated, noncontiguous vertebral column fracture, a complete radiographic assessment of the whole spinal column is warranted.[5,13] The exception to early CT after the initial lateral radiographs is the patient with an obvious facet fracture–dislocation injury.[18] These patients may benefit from early reduction of the fracture and realignment of the cervical spine. This will be discussed in a following section.

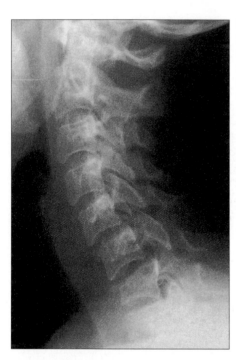

Figure 23.1 It is important to include the whole cervical spine and T1 in the radiographic assessment. This is an example of a C7 fracture and C6–7 subluxation with facet lock that could have been missed on an inadequate X-ray.

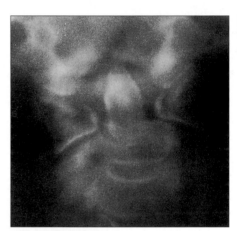

Figure 23.2 Odontoid fracture revealed on an open-mouth view.

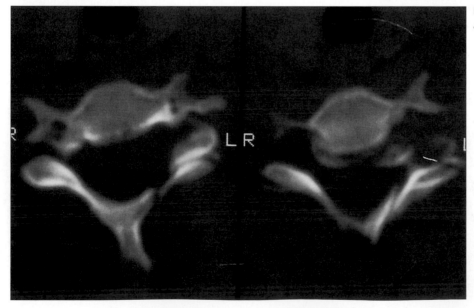

Figure 23.3 Fracture of the C4 body, lateral mass, and lamina, as seen on CT.

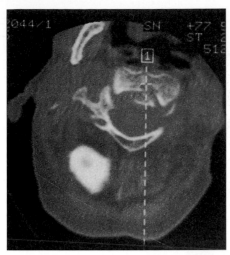

Figure 23.4 A C2 fracture identified on sagittal reconstruction (arrows).

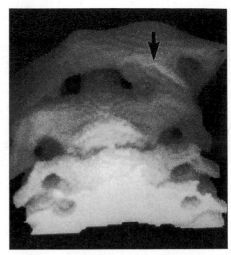

Figure 23.5 Three-dimensional CT study demonstrating a C1–2 rotational subluxation (arrow).

Issues regarding the appropriate use of X-rays in asymptomatic trauma patients have been raised for financial, resource allocation, and ionizing radiation concerns.[26] Trauma patients who meet the following criteria do not require X-ray evaluation of the cervical spine:

1 normal neurologic examination and a Glasgow Coma Scale (GCS) of 15, with no delayed or inappropriate responses;
2 not intoxicated;
3 no neck pain or midline tenderness;
4 no significant distracting injury such as long-bone fracture or visceral injury.[27]

Symptomatic patients who do not meet the above criteria should undergo a full radiographic assessment of the cervical spine.

Adjunctive imaging techniques, such as dynamic flexion and extension radiographs, myelography, angiography, and magnetic resonance imaging (MRI), may assist in the evaluation of the trauma patient, depending on the individual patient's circumstances.[28–30] Despite the potential utility of these other techniques, CT scanning should occur prior to obtaining dynamic or potentially time-consuming imaging modalities. CT myelography may be used to image the relationship of the bony elements to the neural elements and is more accurate than MRI in defining bony anatomy. However, now that MRI is readily available and non-invasive, CT myelography has been reserved for patients who either cannot tolerate an MRI or who have a pacemaker or ferromagnetic aneurysm clips and thus cannot receive an MRI. Three-dimensional CT can be useful in the evaluation of complex cervical spine fractures and particularly in operative planning (Figure 23.5).[30]

MRI is an extremely useful tool in the assessment of a patient with a cervical spine injury and may identify injuries, such as disc herniations, not seen on plain X-ray or CT scanning. A longitudinal assessment of the spine and spinal cord is provided with MRI, as are views in the axial, sagittal, and coronal planes (Figure 23.6).[5,9,13,20,31–33] MRI may be the only imaging modality on which an abnormality is found in patients with SCIWORA, as ligaments, soft tissues, and neural elements can be imaged with superior detail. In addition, hematomas within the spinal canal will not be identified on plain X-ray or may even be missed on CT, but are readily identified on MRI.[9,32,34] A proper MRI requires a co-operative patient and nonferromagnetic immobilization devices. It

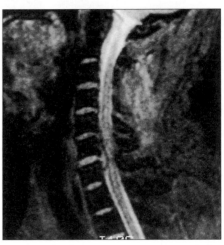

Figure 23.6 Traumatic disc herniation at C6–7 as revealed on MRI.

is often difficult to perform on combative patients and on those who require mechanical ventilation or close hemodynamic or cardiac monitoring, which is commonly the case in trauma patients.[18,20]

In the case of cervical trauma but no demonstrable fracture or dislocation injury on the initial standard cervical spine X-rays and CT studies, flexion and extension lateral cervical spine views are important additions to the radiographic assessment. Dynamic flexion–extension views may determine the presence of subluxation injuries or abnormal ligamentous laxity in patients who have persistent post-traumatic neck pain.[5,13] In the obtunded or unconscious patient, flexion and extension may be performed under fluoroscopy and may detect a previously unrecognized injury in approximately 1% of patients, although the clinical significance of this is not certain.[35,36] Fluoroscopy is probably only indicated in patients with high-risk injuries such as high-speed motor vehicle accidents, falls over 3 m, major associated injuries, or vehicle crashes involving a death at the scene, as low-risk injuries have only a 0.2% incidence of cervical spine injury.[37] MRI can be performed in flexion and extension, a technique that may be useful in identifying positional subluxation or compression of the cervical spinal cord.[20,32,33]

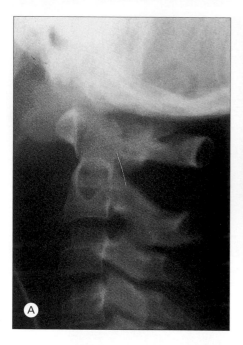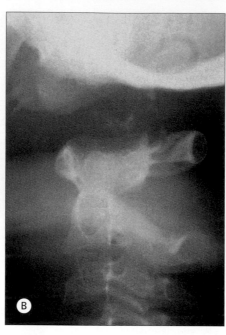

Figure 23.7 (A,B) Traumatic cranial–cervical dislocation.

MANAGEMENT

General principles

The clinician must maintain a high index of suspicion for potential spinal injury in all trauma patients. Proper immobilization must be maintained until the presence (or absence) of a spinal fracture or instability is determined. Immobilization of the head and neck is of the utmost importance during the resuscitation, triage, and radiographic evaluation phases of the trauma patient.[4,13] As 10% of patients may develop the first onset of signs of cervical spinal cord injury during the early evaluation phases following trauma, continued immobilization of the head and neck must be performed until a spinal fracture has been definitively excluded.[4,5] Fractures of the vertebrae of the cervical spine, fracture–subluxations, and isolated subluxations are the most common types of injuries to occur.[1,3,5,8,12,13,18] The unique anatomy and range of motion of the upper cervical spine creates a predisposition to a variety of fracture types.

Recently, guidelines for managing patients with cervical spine injuries have been prepared.[38] The recommendations of these guidelines are reflected in the following sections on management.

Atlanto-occipital dislocation

There is a high incidence of neurologic morbidity and even mortality with cranial–cervical disruption injuries, with many patients dying of severe brainstem injury or respiratory arrest at the scene.[34,39–41] These injuries are uncommon and are the result of massive traumatic flexion and distraction forces. Survivors may have multiple lower cranial nerve palsies or be severely impaired. However, up to 20% of survivors with this type of injury have a favorable functional outcome if prompt therapy and immobilization are instituted (Figure 23.7).[34,39–43] A useful classification describes anterior (type I), longitudinal (type II), and posterior (type III) dislocation, based on the movement of the occiput with respect to the cervical spine.[44]

These surviving patients who sustain cranial–cervical dislocation injuries should be evaluated with CT myelography or preferably MRI to evaluate for potential compression of the brainstem or upper cervical spinal cord. The use of traction is controversial in these patients and is associated with a 10% incidence of neurologic worsening.[45] External immobilization alone is ineffective as nearly 30% will experience neurologic deterioration or fail to achieve spinal stability.[45–47] Effective surgical stabilization of these patients requires open reduction and internal fixation (ORIF) from the occiput to C3 or C4.[34,39–41] This may be accomplished by fixation with one of several types of instrumentation (Figure 23.8), and must be supplemented by allograft or autogenic bone to provide for long-term stability.

Occipital condyle fractures

These injuries may be difficult to visualize on X-ray and thus have been underdiagnosed in the past. With increased use of CT scanning of the occipitocervical junction in the evaluation of the trauma patient, these injuries are recognized with increased frequency. They have been estimated to occur in 1–3% of cases of blunt craniocervical trauma.[48,49] High-risk patients, such as those experiencing a significant loss of consciousness, abnormalities of the lower cranial nerves, or those with high-energy injuries, should undergo CT of the craniocervical junction. Type I fractures (axial load and comminuted fractures) and type II fractures (extension of a skull-base fracture) are generally considered stable if isolated. Thus, symptomatic treatment is indicated and may include external immobilization in a collar.[50] Type III injuries (avulsion of a condylar fragment by the alar ligament) may be unstable and require rigid external immobilization in a collar or halo or even ORIF, if other injuries such as atlanto-axial instability are present.[50] Patients not treated may develop lower cranial nerve palsies, which still have a significant chance of resolving with immobilization.[51]

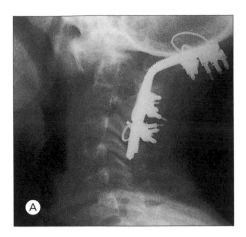
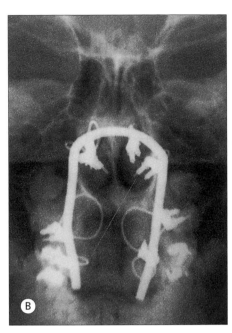

Figure 23.8 Lateral **(A)** and anteroposterior **(B)** views of cranial–cervical stabilization utilizing a contoured Steinmann pin.

Atlas fractures

The first cervical vertebra bridges the gap between the cranium and the rest of the cervical spine, making it vulnerable to a number of different fracture patterns. Fractures of the atlas account for approximately 5% of all cervical spinal injuries.[4,52] Injuries to C1 may occur in isolation but 40% are associated with fractures of C2.[13,53,54] While the Jefferson fracture, a four-part ring fracture, is the most frequent fracture pattern of C1, there are many other variants (Figure 23.9). Unilateral ring or lateral mass fractures may also occur when rotational or lateral flexion, as well as axial loads become part of the fracture mechanism.[4,13,52,55]

Most commonly, atlas fractures are treated nonoperatively. Spence found that the amount of lateral mass (of C1 with respect to C2) displacement is important in deciding upon appropriate therapy. The combined sum of the lateral mass displacement of C1 on C2 predicts the integrity of the transverse atlantoaxial ligament and thus predicts stability. He showed that if the combined sum of the displacement is 6.9 mm or greater, then it is likely that the transverse ligament is ruptured and the fracture is unstable.[52] Isolated atlas fractures with less than 6.9 mm can be adequately treated with a rigid collar, however fractures with greater than 6.9 mm displacement require halo immobilization.[54] The management scheme is highly effective, however it is not perfect as there are some fractures with less than 6.9 mm displacement that fail to heal properly with halo immobilization. This has caused some authors to recommend ORIF of all atlas fractures that have evidence of transverse ligament disruption on MRI.[31] Isolated anterior or posterior arch fractures can be effectively treated in a collar. Lateral mass fractures can typically be managed in a collar unless there is significant comminution, in which halo immobilization may be required for 8–12 weeks.[56]

Axis fractures

The axis is the largest of the cervical vertebrae and fractures of C2 account for 18% of all cervical spine traumatic injuries.[4,11,13,16,18,52,57] Odontoid process fractures are the most common C2 fracture, representing approximately 60% of

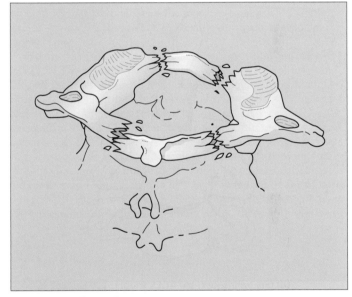

Figure 23.9 Jefferson fracture.

fractures at this level. The Anderson–D'Alonzo classification of odontoid fractures considers types I–III (Table 23.3).[58] Type I odontoid fractures are the rarest, while type II are the most common (Figure 23.10). Type III odontoid fractures (Figure 23.11) represent one-third of all odontoid fractures.[4,11,13]

Bilateral fractures of the pars interarticularis, or hangman's fractures, represent 4% of all cervical spine fractures and 20% of all axis fracture injuries.[4,11,13,16,59] As a result of a spacious spinal canal at this level, there is a low rate of neurological injury associated with this fracture pattern.[60] In the classification of Effendi, there are nondisplaced fractures (type I), fractures where the anterior fragment is displaced (type II), and fractures where the anterior fragment is in a flexed position and there is a C2–3 facet dislocation (type III) (Figure 23.12).[61]

facet dislocations have an 80% incidence.[18] Of particular importance, most injuries with unilateral dislocations are root injuries, while the most common neurological injury with bilateral facet dislocations is a complete spinal cord injury.

In designing the optimum regimen for management of patients with C4–T1 spinal injuries, it is important to consider the following factors: the mechanism of injury, the injury type, the extent of the neurological deficit, and the type of pathology present, such as hematoma, bone fragments, or disc material that may be intruding upon the spinal cord.[4,5,13,28,52,84,85] These injuries can be classified according to the system proposed by Allen and Ferguson that includes distraction/flexion (including facet dislocation), compression/flexion/vertical compression, extension, and subluxation injuries.[86]

General management principles of spinal cord injury apply for subaxial cervical spinal injuries as well. Specifically, C3–T1 fracture or subluxations should undergo early reduction and realignment as well as operative decompression of injuries with nonreducible compression of the spinal cord, especially for patients with incomplete spinal cord injuries. Patients with undisplaced vertebral body fractures or isolated posterior element fractures will heal with external immobilization alone. Facet dislocations that have been successfully reduced will heal with nonoperative immobilization if there is an associated facet fracture rather than a pure ligamentous injury. If the fracture or subluxation cannot be reduced by closed manipulation, ORIF is required, again more urgently if the patient has an incomplete neurological injury. ORIF is also indicated for patients who have failed to heal with external immobilization alone. Patients with pure ligamentous injuries should be considered for primary ORIF as the likelihood of healing with surgery is small.

The chosen surgical approach for patients with subaxial spinal injuries must take into account the potential need for decompression of the spinal cord or spinal roots, as well as the need for stabilization and fusion.[4,5,13,28,84,85] In general, anterior pathology is approached anteriorly and posterior pathology is approached posteriorly, although this may not always be the case. Posterior reconstructions may include sublaminar wires, spinous process wiring, lateral mass plates, or pedicle screws (usually only for C7 and T1), and must be augmented by a bony fusion.[4,28,87,88] Ventral stabilization can be performed following corpectomy and/or discectomy with an interbody graft and anterior plate (Figure 23.15).[4,85]

Nearly one-third of patients with facet dislocation injuries fail initial closed reduction.[18] One-third of patients will fail to maintain alignment with external immobilization alone, with pure ligamentous disruption being a predictor of failure.[18,89] Anterior or posterior stabilization procedures have a high chance of successful fusion, with only 2–5% of cases with postoperative instability.[90–94] Indications for surgical therapy include nonreducible spinal cord compression with deficit, ligamentous injury with facet instability, kyphosis ≥ 15°, vertebral body compression ≥ 40%, and subluxation ≥ 20%.[95]

Overall, cervical vertebral compression injuries have a 5% incidence of instability when treated with external immobilization alone.[90,96] Fractures of the extension type have an incidence of instability that may be as high as 24%, while those that are of the subluxation type may even have a somewhat higher incidence than that.

Cervical spinal cord injuries

While some patients suffer devastating spinal cord injuries at the time of the initial injury and have fixed neurological deficits, others suffer incomplete spinal cord injuries and have much to lose if hypoxia and hypotension are not treated aggressively. Signs of a complete spinal cord injury associated with neurogenic shock indicate a poor prognosis for recovery of neurological function.[18] Other factors that may be associated with the extent of neurological deficits include the force of the initial injury, the presence of continued spinal cord compression by bone, disc, or hematoma, and the presence of an irreducible spinal deformity. The use of high-dose steroids in the setting of spinal cord injury previously was considered to be standard, however the utility of the protocol has come under serious criticism recently and a detailed discussion is beyond the scope of this chapter.[97–99]

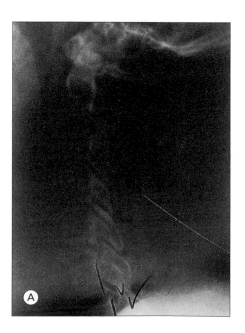
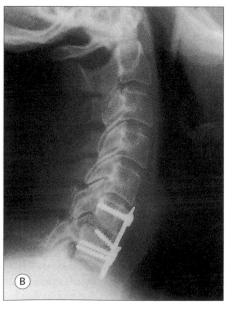

Figure 23.15 (A) Preoperative and **(B)** postoperative X-rays of a patient with a fracture dislocation injury at C6–7 following anterior C6–7 discectomy, interbody fusion, and anterior cervical plating.

Some authors have stated that the neurological outcome following cervical spinal cord injury may be optimized by initial attempts at closed reduction followed by rigid external immobilization.[13,18] Early closed reduction of these injuries with cranial–cervical traction offers the possibility of recovery of neurological function in select patients, particularly those patients with incomplete neurological injuries.[18] There is an 80% success rate with these maneuvers, a 1% chance of permanent neurological injury, and a 2–4% chance of transient neurological change.[100] There are only two well-documented cases in the literature that ascribe neurological injury during reduction manoeuvres to a herniated disc.[101,102] The presence of a herniated disc, which may be found in 46% of cases on the pre-reduction MRI, does not predict neurological outcome.[102,103] Thus, pre-reduction MRI does not increase the safety of the procedure and may delay therapy.[100] The timing of cervical spinal cord decompression appears to be important with respect to subsequent recovery of neurological function in certain patients, particularly those with central cord syndrome because of focal anterior pathology. These patients may benefit from early surgery and stabilization, although there are no randomized controlled trials to confirm this.[104–106]

There is a small subset of adult patients who have signs of a spinal cord injury, but who have no fracture or subluxation demonstrable on X-ray or CT. This is much more common in children and has been called the syndrome of spinal cord injury without radiographic abnormality (SCIWORA).[107] The presentation may be delayed by up to 4 days, and caution must be emphasized in managing children who initially present with mild neurological dysfunction, even though they may be currently neurologically normal as there have been reports of children initially cleared of spinal column pathology who have subsequently returned with signs of spinal cord injury.[15,17,107,108] These patients, as in all patients with spinal cord injury, must be properly immobilized and evaluated with CT, MRI, and flexion–extension X-rays. There is some evidence that somatosensory evoked potentials are useful in identifying the extent of injury, as well as in prognostication of expected neurological recovery.[14,15,17] Poor prognostic indicators include a complete neurological injury and age less than 4 years.[14,17] There is some evidence to suggest that MRI may be able to predict outcome, with a normal scan being predictive of an excellent neurological outcome.[109] Appropriate therapy includes rigid immobilization in a collar, restriction from activities that may result in further injury, and follow-up examination that should include flexion and extension views. Current recommendations are for 12 weeks in a hard cervical collar followed by another 12 weeks of restricted activity, although this may be difficult to accomplish in children.[110] Several investigators have described delayed SCIWORA injuries and/or recurrent spinal cord injuries among patients who presented with SCIWORA injuries but recovered and were cleared of vertebral column pathology on their initial hospital evaluation. No patient with SCIWORA has been noted to later develop spinal instability.

CONCLUSIONS

The cervical spine is the most common site of traumatic spinal column injuries. Patients suffering spinal cord injuries present with a variable extent of quadriparesis. If the level of injury is high enough, ventilatory drive may be poor so as to require mechanical ventilation. Therapy should be individualized for the patient and the specific type of injury and may appropriately include operative and nonoperative management, depending on the circumstances.

CLINICAL PEARLS

- The cervical spine is the most mobile portion of the spine and as such is quite vulnerable to traumatic injury.

- Neurological deficits are unfortunately very common and occur in 40–60% of patients.

- Conceptually, the cervical spine is made up of two regions, namely the craniocervical junction (C0–C2) and the subaxial spine (C3–C7).

- Injuries can be described as bony, ligamentous, or a combination of both according to various classification schemes. The type of injury dictates the mode of repair, which may consist of open or closed reduction, followed by external immobilization or internal stabilization and fusion. Spinal cord decompression may also be required.

This chapter contains material from the first edition, and we are grateful to the author of that chapter for his contribution.

REFERENCES

1. Bohlman H. Acute fractures and dislocations of the cervical spine: an analysis of three hundred hospitalized patients and review of the literature. *J Bone Joint Surg* 1979; 61A: 1119–42.
2. Bohlman H, Boada E. Fractures and dislocations of the lower cervical spine. In: Cervical Spine Research Society (ed.). *The Cervical Spines*. Philadelphia: Lippincott; 1983: 232–67.
3. Heiden J, Weiss M, Rosenberg A, Apuzzo M, Kurze T. Management of cervical spinal cord trauma in southern California. *J Neurosurg* 1975; 43: 732–6.
4. Sonntag V, Hadley M. Management of nonodontoid upper cervical spine injuries. In: Cooper P (ed.). *Management of Posttraumatic Spinal Instability: Neurosurgical Topics*. Rolling Meadows, IL: AANS Publications; 1990: 99–109.
5. Weiss J. Mid- and lower cervical spine injuries. In: Wilkins R (ed.). *Neurosurgery*. New York: McGraw-Hill; 1985: 1708–15.
6. Joint Section on Disorders of the Spine and Peripheral Nerves of the American Association of Neurological Surgeons and the Congress of Neurological Surgeons. Guidelines for the management of acute cervical spine and spinal cord injuries. Ch. 3. *Neurosurgery* 2002; 50: S21–9.
7. Harris P, Karmi M, McClemont E, Matlhoko D, Paul K. The prognosis of patients sustaining severe cervical spine injury (C2–C7 inclusive). *Paraplegia* 1980; 18: 324–30.
8. Heiden J, Weiss M. Cervical spine injuries with and without neurological deficit, I. *Contemp Neurosurg* 1980; 2: 1–6.
9. Mesard L, Carmody A, Mannarino E, Ruge D. Survival after spinal cord trauma: a life table analysis. *Archiv Neurol* 1978; 35: 78–83.
10. Riggins R, Kraus J. The risk of neurologic damage with fractures of the vertebrae. *Trauma* 1977; 17: 126–33.
11. Hadley M, Dickman C, Browner C, Sonntag V. Acute axis fractures: a review of 229 cases. *J Neurosurg* 1989; 71: 642–7.

12. Reiss S, Raque G, Jr, Shields C, Garretson H. Cervical spine fractures with major associated trauma. *Neurosurgery* 1986; 18: 327–30.

13. Sonntag V, Hadley M. Management of upper cervical spinal instability. In: Wilkins R (ed.) *Neurosurgery Update*. New York: McGraw-Hill; 1991: 222–3.

14. Hadley M, Zabramski J, Browner C, Rekate H, Sonntag V. Pediatric spinal trauma: a review of 122 cases of spinal cord and vertebral column injuries. *J Neurosurg* 1988; 68: 18–24.

15. Ruge J, Sinson G, McLone D, Cerullo L. Pediatric spinal injury: the very young. *J Neurosurg* 1988; 68: 25–30.

16. Schneider R. High cervical spine injuries. In: Wilkins R (ed.). *Neurosurgery*. New York: McGraw-Hill; 1985: 1701–8.

17. Pollack I, Pang D, Sclabassi R. Recurrent spinal cord injury without radiographic abnormalities in children. *J Neurosurg* 1988; 69: 177–82.

18. Hadley M, Fitzpatrick B, Browner C, Sonntag V. Facet fracture-dislocation injuries of the cervical spine. *Neurosurgery* 1992; 30: 661–6.

19. Gehweiler J, Jr, Clark W, Schaaf R, Powers B, Miller M. Cervical spine trauma: the common combined conditions. *Radiology* 1979; 130: 77–86.

20. Cohen W. Imaging and determination of posttraumatic spinal instability. In: Cooper P (ed.). *Management of Posttraumatic Spinal Instability: Neurosurgical Topics*. Rolling Meadows, IL: AANS Publications; 1990: 19–35.

21. Ross S, Schwab C, David E, Delong W, Born C. Clearing the cervical spine: initial radiologic evaluation. *J Trauma* 1987; 27: 1055–60.

22. Hoffman J, Mower W, Wolfson A, Todd K, Zucker M. Validity of a set of clinical criteria to rule out injury to the cervical spine in patients with blunt trauma: National Emergency X-Radiographic Utilization Study Group. *N Engl J Med* 2000; 343: 94–9.

23. Freemyer B, Knopp R, Piche J, Wales L, Williams J. Comparison of five-view and three view cervical spine series in the evaluation of patients with cervical trauma. *Ann Emergency Med* 1989; 18: 818–21.

24. Nunez D, Jr., Zuluaga A, Fuentes-Bernardo D, Rivas L, Beccera J. Cervical spine trauma: how much more do we learn by routinely using helical CT? *Radiographics* 1996; 16: 1318–21.

25. Berne J, Velmahos G, El-Tawil Q, *et al*. Value of complete cervical helical computed tomographic scanning in identifying cervical spine injury in the unevaluable blunt trauma patients with multiple injuries. *J Trauma* 1999; 47: 896–903.

26. Mirvis S, Diaconis J, Chirico P, Reiner B, Joslyn J, Militello P. Protocol driven radiologic evaluation of suspected cervical spine injury. *Radiology* 1989; 170: 831–4.

27. Joint Section on Disorders of the Spine and Peripheral Nerves of the American Association of Neurological Surgeons and the Congress of Neurological Surgeons. Guidelines for the management of acute cervical spine and spinal cord injuries. Ch. 4. *Neurosurgery* 2002; 50: S30–5.

28. Cooper P, Cohen W, Rosiello A, Koslow M. Posterior stabilization of cervical spine fractures and subluxations using plates and screws. *Neurosurgery* 1988; 23: 300–6.

29. Allen R, Perot PJ, Gudemna S. Evaluation of acute nonpenetrating cervical spinal cord injuries with CT metrizamide myelography. *J Neurosurg* 1985; 63: 510–20.

30. Hadley M, Sonntag V, Amos M, Hodak J, Lopez L. Three-dimensional computed tomography in the diagnosis of vertebral column pathological conditions. *Neurosurgery* 1987; 21: 186–92.

31. Dickman C, Mamourian A, Sonntag V, Drayer B. Magnetic resonance imaging of the transverse atlantal ligament for the evaluation of atlantoaxial instability. *J Neurosurg* 1991; 75: 221–7.

32. Chakers D, Flickinger F, Bresnahan J, Beattie M, Weiss K, Miller C. MR imaging of acute spinal cord trauma. *Am J Neuroradiol* 1987; 8: 5–10.

33. Pech P, Kilgore D, Pojunas K, Haughton V. Cervical spine fractures: CT detection. *Radiology* 1985; 63: 510–20.

34. Dickman C, Douglas R, Sonntag V. Occipitocervical fusion: posterior stabilization of the craniovertebral junction and upper cervical spine. *BNI Quarterly* 1991; 7: 2–13.

35. Davis J, Parks S, Detlefs C, GG W, Williams J, Smith R. Clearing the cervical spine in obtunded patients: the use of dynamic fluoroscopy. *J Trauma* 1995; 39: 435–8.

36. Ajani A, Cooper D, Scheinkestel C, Laidlaw J, Tuxen D. Optimal assessment of cervical spine trauma in critically ill patients: a prospective evaluation. *Anaesth Intensive Care* 1998; 26: 487–91.

37. Hanson J, Blackmore C, Mann F, Wilson A. Cervical spine injury: a clinical decision rule to identify high risk patients for helical CT scanning. *Am J Roentgenol* 2000; 174: 713–17.

38. Joint Section on Disorders of the Spine and Peripheral Nerves of the American Association of Neurological Surgeons and the Congress of Neurological Surgeons. Guidelines for the management of acute cervical spine and spinal cord injuries. *Neurosurgery* 2002; 50 (Suppl.).

39. Bools J, Rosem B. Traumatic atlantoccipital dislocation: two cases with survival. *Am J Neuroradiol* 1986; 7: 901–4.

40. Menezes A, VanGilder J, Graf C, McDonnell D. Craniocervical abnormalities: a comprehensive surgical approach. *J Neurosurg* 1980; 53: 444–5.

41. Ransford A, Crockard H, Pozo J, Thomas N, Nelson I. Craniocervical instability treated by contoured loop fixation. *J Bone Joint Surg* 1986; 68B: 173–7.

42. Joint Section on Disorders of the Spine and Peripheral Nerves of the American Association of Neurological Surgeons and the Congress of Neurological Surgeons. Guidelines for the management of acute cervical spine and spinal cord injuries. Ch. 14. *Neurosurgery* 2002; 50: S105–13.

43. Menezes A, Muhonen M. Management of occipito-cervical instability. In: Cooper P (ed.). *Management of Posttraumatic Spinal Instability: Neurosurgical Topics*. Rolling Meadows, IL: AANS Publications; 1990: 65–74.

44. Treynalis V, Marano G, Dunker R, Kaufman H. Traumatic atlanto-occipital dislocation: case report. *J Neurosurg* 1986; 65: 863–70.

45. Dickman C, Papadopoulos S, Sonntag V, Spetzler R, Rekate H, Drabier J. Traumatic occipitoatlantal dislocations. *J Spinal Disord* 1993; 6: 300–13.

46. Nischal K, Chumas P, Sparrow O. Prolonged survival after atlanto-occipital dislocation: two case reports and review. *Br J Neurosurg* 1993; 7: 677–82.

47. Kaufman R, Dunbar J, Botsford J, McLaurin R. Traumatic longitudinal atlanto-occipital distraction injuries in children. *Am J Neuroradiol* 1982; 3: 415–19.

48. Noble E, Smoker W. The forgotten condyle: the appearance, morphology, and classification of occipital condyle fractures. *Am J Neuroradiol* 1996; 17: 507–13.

49. Leone A, Cerase A, Colosimo C, Lauro L, Puca A, Marano P. Occipital condyle fractures: a review. *Radiology* 2000; 216: 635–44.

50. Joint Section on Disorders of the Spine and Peripheral Nerves of the American Association of Neurological Surgeons and the Congress of Neurological Surgeons. Guidelines for the management of acute cervical spine and spinal cord injuries. Ch. 15. *Neurosurgery* 2002; 50: S114–S119.

51. Legros B, Fournier P, Chiaroni P, Ritz O, Fusciardi J. Basal fracture of the skull and lower (IX, X, XI, XII) cranial nerves palsy: four case

reports including two fractures of the occipital condyle – a literature review. *J Trauma* 2000; 48: 342–8.

52. Spence K, Decker S, Sell K. Bursting atlantal fracture associated with rupture of the transverse ligament. *J Bone Joint Surg* 1970; 52A: 543–9.

53. Dickman C, Hadley M, Browner C, Sonntag V. Neurosurgical management of acute atlas-axis combination fractures: a review of 25 cases. *J Neurosurg* 1989; 70: 45–9.

54. Hadley M, Dickman C, Browner C, Sonntag V. Acute traumatic atlas fractures: management and long-term outcome. *Neurosurgery* 1988; 23: 31–5.

55. Keene G, Hone M, Sage M. Atlas fracture: demonstration using computerized tomography. *J Bone Joint Surg* 1978; 60A: 1106–7.

56. Joint Section on Disorders of the Spine and Peripheral Nerves of the American Association of Neurological Surgeons and the Congress of Neurological Surgeons. Guidelines for the management of acute cervical spine and spinal cord injuries. Ch. 16. *Neurosurgery* 2002; 50: S120–4.

57. Clark C, Apuzzo M. The evaluation and management of trauma to the odontoid process. In: Cooper P (ed.) *Management of Posttraumatic Spinal Instability: Neurosurgical Topics*. Rolling Meadows, IL: AANS Publications; 1990: 77–94.

58. Anderson L, D'Alonzo R. Fractures of the odontoid process of the axis. *J Bone Joint Surg* 1974; 56A: 1663–74.

59. Ryan M, Henderson J. The epidemiology of fractures and fracture-dislocations of the cervical spine. *Injury* 1992; 23: 38–40.

60. Mollan R, Watt P. Hangman's fracture. *Injury* 1982; 14: 265–7.

61. Effendi B, Roy D, Cornish B, Dussault R, Laurin C. Fractures of the ring of the atlas: a classification based on the analysis of 131 cases. *J Bone Joint Surg* 1981; 63B: 319–27.

62. Hadley M, Browner C, Sonntag V. Miscellaneous fractures of the second cervical vertebra. *BNI Quarterly* 1985; 1: 34–9.

63. Benzel E, Hart B, Ball P, Baldwin N, Orrison W, Espinosa M. Fractures of the C2 vertebral body. *J Neurosurg* 1994; 81: 206–12.

64. Fujimura Y, Nishi Y, Kobayashi K. Classification and treatment of axis body fractures. *J Orthopaed Trauma* 1996; 10: 536–40.

65. Greene K, Dickman C, Marciano F, Drabier J, Hadley M, Sonntag V. Acute axis fractures: analysis of management and outcome in 340 consecutive cases. *Spine* 1997; 22: 1843–52.

66. Lennarson P, Mostafavi H, Treynalis V, Walters B. Management of type II dens fractures: a case-control study. *Spine* 2000; 25: 1234–7.

67. Hadley M, Browner C, Liu S, Sonntag V. New subtype of acute odontoid fractures (type IIA). *Neurosurgery* 1988; 22: 67–71.

68. Verheggen R, Jansen J. Hangman's fracture: arguments in favor of surgical therapy for type II and III according to Edwards and Levine. *Surgical Neurol* 1998; 49: 253–62.

69. Joint Section on Disorders of the Spine and Peripheral Nerves of the American Association of Neurological Surgeons and the Congress of Neurological Surgeons. Guidelines for the management of acute cervical spine and spinal cord injuries. Ch. 17. *Neurosurgery* 2002; 50: S125–39.

70. Borne G, Bedou G, Pinaudeau M. Treatment of pedicular fractures of the axis: a clinical study and screw fixation technique. *J Neurosurg* 1984; 60: 88–93.

71. Gleizes V, Jacquot F, Signoret F, Feron J. Combined injuries in the upper cervical spine: clinical and epidemiological data over a 14 year period. *Eur Spine J* 2000; 9: 386–92.

72. Coyne T, Fehlings M, Wallace M, Bernstein M, Tator C. C1-C2 posterior cervical fusion: long-term evaluation of results and efficacy. *Neurosurgery* 1995; 37: 688–93.

73. Guiot B, Fessler R. Complex atlantoaxial fractures. *J Neurosurg* 1999; 91 (Suppl. 2): 139–43.

74. Montesano P, Anderson P, Schlehr F, Thalgott J, Lowrey G. Odontoid fractures treated by anterior odontoid screw fixation. *Spine* 1991; 16(Suppl. 3): S33–S37.

75. Geisler F, Cheng C, Poka A, Brumback R. Anterior screw fixation of posteriorly displaced type II odontoid fractures. *Neurosurgery* 1989; 25: 130–6.

76. Brant-Zawadzki M, Miller E, Federle M. CT in the elevation of spine trauma. *Am J Roentgenol* 1981; 136: 369–75.

77. Jenkins J, Coric D, Branch C, Jr. A clinical comparison of one- and two-screw odontoid fixation. *J Neurosurg* 1998; 89: 366–70.

78. Matsui H, Imada K, Tsuji H. Radiographic classification of os odontoideum and its clinical significance. *Spine* 1997; 22: 1706–9.

79. Stevens J, Chong W, Barber C, Kendall B, Crockard H. A new appraisal of abnormalities of the odontoid process associated with atlantoaxial subluxation and neurological disability. *Brain* 1994; 117: 133–48.

80. Morgan M, Onofrio B, Bender C. Familial os odontoideum: case report. *J Neurosurg* 1989; 70: 636–9.

81. Spierings E, Braakman R. The management of os odontoideum: analysis of 37 cases. *J Bone Joint Surg* 1982; 64B: 422–8.

82. Joint Section on Disorders of the Spine and Peripheral Nerves of the American Association of Neurological Surgeons and the Congress of Neurological Surgeons. Guidelines for the management of acute cervical spine and spinal cord injuries. Ch. 19. *Neurosurgery* 2002; 50: S148–55.

83. Dai L, Yuan W, Ni B, Jai L. Os odontoideum: etiology, diagnosis, and management. *Surgical Neurol* 2000; 53: 106–9.

84. Sonntag V, Hadley M. Nonoperative management of cervical spine injuries. *Clin Neurosurg* 1988; 34: 630–49.

85. Caspar W, Barbier D, Klara P. Anterior cervical fusion and Caspar plate stabilization for cervical trauma. *Neurosurgery* 1989; 25: 491–502.

86. Allen B, Ferguson R, Lehmann T, O'Brien R. A mechanistic classification of closed, indirect fractures and dislocations of the lower cervical spine. *Spine* 1982; 7: 1–27.

87. Roy-Camille R, Saillant G, Mazel C. Internal fixation of the unstable cervical spine by a posterior osteosynthesis with plates and screws. In: Cervical Spine Research Society (ed.). *Cervical Spine*. Philadelphia: JB Lippincott; 1989: 390–6.

88. Cherney W, Sonntag V, Douglas R. Lateral mass posterior plating and facet fusion for cervical spine instability. *BNI Quarterly* 1991; 7: 2–11.

89. Halliday A, Henderson B, Hart B, Benzel E. The management of unilateral lateral mass/facet fractures of the subaxial cervical spine: the use of magnetic resonance imaging to predict instability. *Spine* 1997; 22: 2614–21.

90. Bucholz R, Cheung K. Halo vest versus spinal fusion for cervical injury: evidence from an outcome study. *J Neurosurg* 1989; 70: 884–92.

91. Fehlings M, Cooper P, Errico T. Posterior plates in the management of cervical instability: long-term results in 44 patients. *J Neurosurg* 1994; 81: 341–9.

92. Maiman D, Barolat G, Larson S. Management of bilateral locked facets in the cervical spine. *Neurosurgery* 1986; 18: 542–7.

93. Rockswold G, Bergman T, Ford S. Halo immobilization and surgical fusion: relative indications and effectiveness in the treatment of 140 cervical spine injuries. *J Trauma* 1990; 30: 893–8.

94. Wolf A, Levi L, Mirvis S, *et al*. Operative management of bilateral facet dislocation. *J Neurosurg* 1991; 75: 883–90.

95. Joint Section on Disorders of the Spine and Peripheral Nerves of the American Association of Neurological Surgeons and the

Congress of Neurological Surgeons. Guidelines for the management of acute cervical spine and spinal cord injuries. Ch. 20. *Neurosurgery* 2002; 50: S156–S165.

96. Lind B, Sihlbom H, Nordwall A. Halo-vest treatment of unstable traumatic cervical spine injuries. *Spine* 1988; 13: 425–32.

97. Joint Section on Disorders of the Spine and Peripheral Nerves of the American Association of Neurological Surgeons and the Congress of Neurological Surgeons. Guidelines for the management of acute cervical spine and spinal cord injuries. Ch. 9. *Neurosurgery* 2002; 50: S63–S72.

98. Hurlbert R. Methylprenisolone for acute spinal cord injury: an inappropriate standard of care. *J Neurosurg* 2000; 93 (Suppl. 1): 1–7.

99. Hugenholtz H, Cass D, Dvorak M, *et al*. High-dose methylprednisolone for acute closed spinal cord injury – only a treatment option. *Can J Neurol Sci* 2002; 29: 227–35.

100. Joint Section on Disorders of the Spine and Peripheral Nerves of the American Association of Neurological Surgeons and the Congress of Neurological Surgeons. Guidelines for the management of acute cervical spine and spinal cord injuries. Ch. 6. *Neurosurgery* 2002; 50: S44–50.

101. Olerud C, Jonsson H, Jr. Compression of the cervical spinal cord after reduction of fracture dislocations: report of 2 cases. *Acta Orthopaed Scand* 1991; 62: 599–601.

102. Grant G, Mirza S, Chapman J, *et al*. Risk of early closed reduction in cervical spine subluxation injuries. *Journal of Neurosurgery* 1999; 90 (Suppl. 1): 13–18.

103. Vaccaro A, Falatyn S, Flanders A, Balderston R, Northrup B, Cotler J. Magnetic resonance evaluation of the intebral disc, spinal ligaments, and spinal cord before and after closed traction-reduction of cervical spine dislocations. *Spine* 1999; 24: 1210–17.

104. Dai L, Jia L. Central cord injury complicating acute cervical disc herniation in acute spinal cord trauma. *Spine* 2000; 25: 331–6.

105. Chen T, Dickman C, Eleraky M, Sonntag V. The role of decompression for acute incomplete cervical spinal cord injury in cervical spondylosis. *Spine* 1998; 23: 2398–403.

106. Chen T, Lee S, Lui T, *et al*. Efficacy of surgical treatment in traumatic central cord syndrome. *Surg Neurol* 1997; 48: 435–41.

107. Pang D, Wilberger J. Spinal cord injury without radiographic abnormalities in children. *J Neurosurg* 1982; 57: 114–29.

108. Hamilton M, Myles S. Pediatric spinal injury: review of 174 hospital admissions. *J Neurosurg* 1992; 77: 18–24.

109. Grabb P, Pang D. Magnetic resonance imaging in the evaluation of spinal cord injury without radiographic abnormality in children. *Neurosurgery* 1994; 35: 406–14.

110. Pang D, Pollack I. Spinal cord injury without radiographic abnormality in children: the SCIWORA syndrome. *J Trauma* 1989; 57: 114–29.

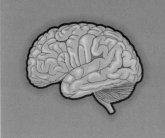

THORACOLUMBAR SPINE FRACTURES

24

Daniel R Fassett and Andrew T Dailey

Fractures of the thoracolumbar spine are a common entity seen by neurosurgeons and orthopedic surgeons. The biomechanics of the thoracolumbar spine make this area prone to traumatic injury. It is estimated that as many as 50 000 fractures of the spinal column occur each year in the United States, with the thoracolumbar junction being the second most common location for injury behind the lower cervical spine.[1]

BIOMECHANICS

The thoracolumbar junction is a zone of structural and functional transition, which makes it vulnerable to injury. This transition zone, between the rigid thoracic vertebral column and the relatively mobile lumbar column, creates a fulcrum at the thoraco-lumbar junction (Figure 24.1). In addition, the joining of the kyphotic thoracic spine with the lordotic lumbar spine places the thoracolumbar junction under maximal stress as a result of transfer of energy from the thoracic spine to the thoracolumbar junction.[2] For these reasons, the majority of fractures in the thoracic and lumbar spine occur at the thoracolumbar junction, with as many as 75% of fractures occurring between T12 and L2.[3–7]

RISK OF NEUROLOGICAL INJURY

Thoracolumbar fractures are associated with neurological injury in up to 48% of cases.[2,8,9] Of all patients with thoracic or lumbar fractures, approximately 19% suffer complete neurologic deficit, 26% have incomplete deficits, and 55% are neurologically intact.[10] Injuries to the spinal column at or above T12 (above the conus) are associated with higher risk of complete injuries, whereas incomplete deficits are more common below L1 (at the cauda equina).[10]

CLINICAL EVALUATION

The most important concern with any spinal fracture is the potential for neurological injury. Spinal precautions should be initiated immediately in all trauma to prevent iatrogenic neurological injury with unstable fractures. Patients with neurologic insult may be considered for corticosteroids following the national

acute spinal cord injury study (NASCIS) guidelines. Aggressive fluid resuscitation and maintenance of blood pressure have also been linked to recovery after spinal cord injury.[11] After adequate clinical and radiographic evaluation, spinal precautions may be cleared in patients without fractures.

Physical examination should start with visual inspection and palpation of the back. Widening between spinous processes can indicate posterior column involvement and step-offs indicate a translation injury. Ecchymosis and other cutaneous findings can help conceptualize the mechanism of injury and the likely spectrum of fractures that may be encountered. After general examination, an in-depth neurological examination should be performed. With the spinal cord transitioning from the conus medullaris to the cauda equina at the thoracolumbar junction, the clinical picture can be quite complex, with mixed upper and lower motor neuron signs. A thorough motor, sensory, reflex, rectal, and urinary examination should be performed to elucidate completely the nature of the neurological injury. Sacral sparing, which is the presence of preserved perianal sensation and voluntary anal contraction in the setting of an otherwise complete neurological deficit, should be evaluated in detail. Sacral sparing is significant as it marks an incomplete spinal cord injury with greater potential for recovery than a complete injury.[2,12]

RADIOGRAPHIC EXAMINATION

All patients with a clinical suspicion of spine injury, whether it be a neurologically intact patient with back pain or a non-responsive patient with a significant mechanism for injury, should be evaluated with, as a minimum, anteroposterior and lateral radiographs. Plain X-rays are useful in diagnosing compression injuries of the vertebral body and fractures of transverse and spinous processes. However, plain films alone may not provide adequate evaluation of ligamentous or bony injuries in the posterior column.[8] In patients with a high suspicion of injury, computed tomography (CT) imaging may be useful in diagnosing occult injury missed on plain films and further characterizing fractures.

For patients with neurological deficits, CT and magnetic resonance imaging (MRI) are useful in characterizing fractures, degree of spinal canal compromise, soft-tissue injury, and neural element injury. Sagittal and coronal CT reconstructions are especially useful to help visualize the abnormal anatomy and provide a clear idea of the fracture's classification.

Early surgical decompression is almost uniformly advocated in patients with incomplete neurological injuries and canal compromise.[23] The literature regarding the association of neurological deficit and degree of canal compromise is inconclusive, with some studies showing a correlation,[9,10,16] and others showing no correlation.[24] If there truly is an association between canal compromise and neurological status, it appears to be greatest with lesions at the conus and cauda equina.[10] In patients with complete neurological injuries or in neurologically intact patients, surgery may be delayed to allow time to consider the overall clinical picture.

Late neurological injury as a result of progressive deformity and neural element compression is of clinical concern but is very rare. In neurologically intact patients with retropulsed fragments, spontaneous remodeling will reduce the amount of canal compromise and the risk of neurological decline appears to be very low with conservative management according to many series.[25,26] However, caution should be exercised when considering the literature regarding conservative treatment of thoracolumbar fractures as there is a significant bias of treating less severe fractures with non-operative measures.

In terms of the potential for progressive kyphosis, controversy exists over which fracture patterns are unstable and require surgical stabilization. In general, the Comprehensive Classification system ranks fractures with increasing risk of instability. As one progresses from Type A fractures to Type B and C fractures, the risk of progressive kyphosis and the need for surgical intervention increases. The clinical significance of kyphosis with regard to long-term back pain is also uncertain. Some studies[10,25] have shown a correlation between kyphosis and pain, with a kyphosis greater than 30° having a higher degree of pain. However, many other studies[5,25,27] have shown no correlation between kyphotic deformity and long-term clinical outcome with regard to pain or work status. Although kyphosis can be corrected by surgery, the kyphotic correction is often not durable, especially with short-segment posterior instrumentation.[5,18] Between 60% and 70% of the kyphosis correction with short-segment posterior instrumentation will be lost within 1 year.[5,28] Anterior stabilization tends to have better maintenance of the kyphosis correction than posterior instrumentation.[29]

Management of burst fractures is very controversial, with some surgeons recommending a period of bed rest followed by rigid orthosis and others being more aggressive, with surgical intervention depending on the nature of the fracture. General indications for operative intervention in burst fractures include:

1 loss of anterior body height by 50% or more;
2 kyphotic angulation greater than 25%;
3 retropulsed fragments that cause greater than 50% canal compromise; and
4 three-column injury.[2,4,27,30–42,43]

In terms of surgical technique, great debate exists regarding the optimum surgical approach for surgical stabilization of unstable burst fractures with regard to anterior, posterior, or combined anterior–posterior approaches. All surgeons are comfortable with the posterior approach to the spine, while the anterior approach is more technically demanding. Posterior approaches have evolved from long fusions with hooks and Harrington rods that typically involved at least two segments above and below the fracture to short-segment instrumentation with transpedicular screws involving just one segment above and below the lesion. Short-segment instrumentation (Figure 24.4) has the benefit of incorporating fewer motion segments and biomechanical studies

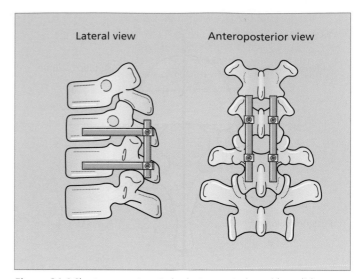

Figure 24.4 Short-segment posterior instrumentation with pedicle screws.

have shown that transpedicular screws are a more rigid construct than posterior distraction instrumentation like Harrington rods.[28,44] Drawbacks of posterior instrumentation include the inability to decompress anterior pathologies directly, the possible increased rate of hardware failure,[29] and the loss of the kyphosis correction.[5,10] Advocates of posterior surgery argue that posterior distraction techniques can often reduce anterior retropulsed fragments if the posterior longitudinal ligament is intact.[9,45] However, in most instances the reduction of retropulsed fragments is not complete. For some injuries posterior instrumentation will provide adequate stabilization for the patient to progress to solid fusion with a low morbidity.

Although anterior surgery (Figure 24.5) is more technically demanding, it has the advantage of directly treating the anterior and middle columns. Benefits of anterior surgery include direct decompression of the neural elements with the potential for better neurological recovery,[7,10,23,43,46] and restoration of the anterior and middle columns, which provides a more stable construct[28,47] with decreased hardware failure and preservation of kyphotic correction.[23,27,29,43,46] Combined anterior and posterior approaches may be of value in severe three-column injuries (AO Type C) or in situations of questionable bone strength (such as osteoporosis).

In summary, each fracture should be treated on an individual basis with regard to its potential for neurological recovery and requirements for stabilization. Thoracolumbar spine surgeons should be adept at both anterior and posterior approaches to have the flexibility to treat any fracture by the optimum approach.

This chapter contains material from the first edition, and we are grateful to the authors of that chapter for their contribution.

REFERENCES

1. Vaccaro AR, Silber JS. Post-traumatic spinal deformity. *Spine* 2001; 26 (24 Suppl.): S111–118.
2. Knightly JJ, Sonntag VKH. Thoracolumbar fractures. In: Menezes A, Sonntag V (eds). *Principles of Spinal Surgery.* New York: McGraw-Hill; 1996: 919–49.

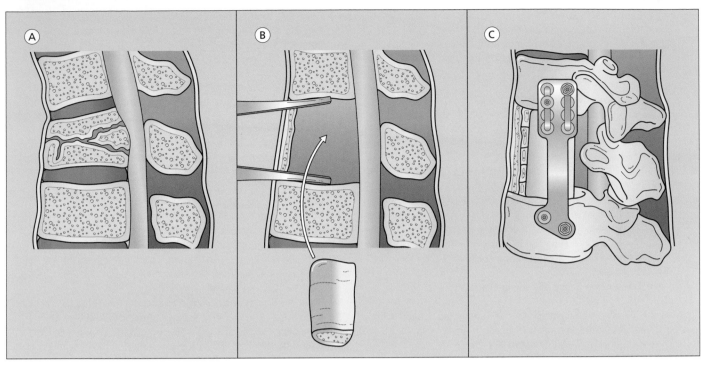

Figure 24.5 Anterior corpectomy with fusion and hardware.

CLINICAL PEARLS

- The thoracolumbar junction is a zone of structural and functional transition, susceptible to injury.

- Thoracic injuries are more likely to result in neurologic damage than lower lumbar injuries.

- Although controversial, high-dose intravenous methylprednisolone therapy is initiated; spinal injury precautions are taken during transfers.

- The back is inspected and palpated; motor, sensory, and reflex changes are noted paying special attention to sacral sparing.

- Appropriate imaging modalities (X-rays, CT, MRI) are utilized.

- There are several classification schemes for thoracolumbar fractures. A modified comprehensive classification is the most current but is cumbersome to follow in practice. A three-column concept forms a good basis for assessing stability and determining the need for surgical intervention.

- Treatment options include activity restriction, bracing, and surgical intervention. Common indications for surgical intervention are neurologic deficit from compression, and deformity (actual or potential).

- Anterior, posterior, and combined approaches for surgical decompression and stabilization are available. The choice depends largely upon the treating surgeon's experience, philosophy, and familiarity with the techniques.

3. Frankel HC, Hancock DO, Hyslop G, et al. The value of postural reduction in the initial management of closed injuries of the spine with paraplegia or tetraplegia. *Paraplegia* 1969; 7: 179–92.
4. Mumford J, Weinstein JN, Spratt KF, Goel VK. Thoracolumbar burst fractures: the clinical efficacy and outcome of nonoperative management. *Spine* 1993; 18: 955–70.
5. Knop C, Fabian HF, Bastian L, Blauth M. Late results of thoracolumbar fractures after posterior instrumentation and transpedicular bone grafting. *Spine* 2001; 26: 88–99.
6. Oner FC, Ramos LMP, Sinmermacher RKJ, et al. Classification of thoracic and lumbar spine fractures: problems of reproducibility. *Eur Spine J* 2002; 11: 235–45.

7. Bradford DS, McBride GG. Surgical management of thoracolumbar spine fractures with incomplete neurologic deficits. *Clin Orthoped Rel Res* 1987; 218: 201–15.
8. Leferink VJM, Veldhuis EFM, Zimmerman KW, et al. Classificational problems in ligamentary distraction type vertebral fractures: 30% of all B-type fractures are initially unrecognized. *Eur Spine J* 2002; 11: 246–50.
9. Kim NM, Lee HM, Chun IM. Neurologic injury and recovery in patients with burst fracture of the thoracolumbar spine. *Spine* 1999; 24: 290–4.
10. Gertzbein SD. Scoliosis Research Society: Multicenter Spine Fracture Study. *Spine* 1992; 17: 529–540.

11. Vale FL, Burns J, Jackson AB, Hadley MN. Combined medical and surgical treatment after acute spinal cord injury: results of a prospective pilot study to assess the merits of aggressive medical resuscitation and blood pressure management. *Spine* 1997; 87: 239–46.

12. Schrader SC, Sloan TB, Toleikis JR. Detection of sacral sparing in acute spinal cord injury. *Spine* 1987; 12: 533–5.

13. Holdsworth F. Fractures, dislocations, and fracture-dislocations of the spine. *J Bone Joint Surg (Am)* 1970; 53A: 1534–59.

14. Holdsworth F. Fractures, dislocations, and fracture-dislocations of the spine. *J Bone Joint Surg (Am)* 1963; 45B: 6–20.

15. Whitesides TE. Traumatic kyphosis of the thoracolumbar spine. *Clin Orthopaed Rel Res* 1977; 128: 78–92.

16. Denis F. The three column spine and its significance in the classification of acute thoracolumbar spinal injuries. *Spine* 1983; 8: 817–31.

17. McAfee PC, Yuan HA, Fredrickson BE, Lubicky JP. The value of computed tomography in thoracolumbar fractures. *J Bone Joint Surg* 1983; 65A: 461–73.

18. Chance GQ. Note on a type of flexion fracture of the spine. *Br J Radiol* 1948; 21: 452–3.

19. Magerl F, Harms J, Gertzbein SD, Aebi M. A new classification of spinal fractures (abstr). *Presented at American Academy of Orthopedic Surgeons, Vail, Colorado 1989*.

20. Magerl F, Harms J, Gertzbein SD, Aebi M. A comprehensive classification of thoracic and lumbar injuries. *Eur Spine J* 1994; 3: 184–201.

21. Gertzbein SD. Spine update classification of thoracic and lumbar fractures. *Spine* 1994; 19: 626–8.

22. Neumann P, Wang Y, Karrholm J, et al. Determination of the inter-spinous process distance in the lumbar spine. Evaluation of reference population to facilitate detection of severe trauma. *Eur Spine J* 1999; 8: 272–8.

23. McAfee CP, Bohlmann HH, Yuan HA. Anterior decompression of traumatic thoracolumbar fractures with incomplete neurological deficit using a retroperitoneal approach. *J Bone Joint Surg* 1985; 67-A(1): 89–103.

24. Gertzbein SD, Court-Brown CM, Marks P, et al. Neurological outcome following surgery for spinal fractures. *Spine* 1988; 13: 892–5.

25. Shen WJ, Liv TJ, Shen YS. Nonoperative treatment versus posterior fixation for thoracolumbar junction burst fractures without neurological deficit. *Spine* 2001; 26: 1038–45.

26. Cantor JB, Lebwohl NH, Garvey T, Eismont FJ. Nonoperative management of stable thoracolumbar burst fractures with early ambulation and bracing. *Spine* 1993; 18: 971–6.

27. Okuyama K, Abe E, Chuba M, et al. Outcome of anterior decompression and stabilization for thoracolumbar unstable burst fractures in the absense of neurological deficits. *Spine* 1996; 21: 620–5.

28. Lim TH, An HS, Hong JH, et al. Biomechanical evaluation of anterior and posterior fixations in an unstable calf spine model. *Spine* 1997; 22: 261–6.

29. Parker JW, Lane JR, Karaikovic EE, Gaines RW. Successful short-segment instrumentation and fusion for thoracolumbar spine fractures. *Spine* 2000; 25: 1157–69.

30. Bohler L. *The Treatment of Fractures*, 5th edn. New York: Grune & Stratton; 1956: 330.

31. Brown GA. Bone resorption in the canal following a thoracolumbar fracture with displaced diaphyseal fragment. *Iowa Orthoped J* 1989; 9: 69–71.

32. Denis F, Armstrong GW, Searls K, Matta L. Acute thoracolumbar burst fractures in the absence of neurological deficit: a comparison between operative and nonoperative treatment. *Clin Orthoped Rel Res* 1984; 189: 142–9.

33. Dewald RL. Burst fractures of the thoracic and lumbar spine. *Clin Orthoped Rel Res* 1984; 189: 150–61.

34. Dunn HK. Anterior spine stabilization and decompression for thoracolumbar injuries. *Orthoped Clinics North Am* 1986; 17: 113–19.

35. Ferguson RL, Allen BL. An algorithm for the treatment of unstable thoracolumbar fractures. *Orthoped Clinics North Am* 1986; 17: 105–12.

36. Garfin SR. Thoracolumbar spine trauma. In: Poss R (ed.), *Orthopedic Knowledge Update 3*. Park Ridge, IL: American Academy of Orthopedic Surgeons; 1990: 425–40.

37. Jacobs RR, Casey MP. Surgical management of thoracolumbar spinal injuries. *Clin Orthoped Rel Res* 1984; 189: 22–35.

38. Kostuik JP. Anterior fixation for fractures of the thoracic and lumbar spine with or without neurologic involvement. *Clin Orthoped Rel Res* 1984; 189: 103–15.

39. Kropinger WJ, Frederickson BE, Mino DE, Yuan HA. Conservative treatment of fractures of the thoracic and lumbar spine. *Orthoped Clinics North Am* 1986; 17: 161–70.

40. Roy-Camille R, Saillant G, Mazel C. Plating of thoracic, thoracolumbar and lumbar injuries with pedicle screw plates. *Orthoped Clinics North Am* 1986; 17: 105–12.

41. Weitzman G. Treatment of stable thoracolumbar spine compression fractures by early ambulation. *Clin Orthoped Rel Res* 1971; 76: 116–22.

42. Willen J, Lindahl S, Nordwall A. Unstable thoracolumbar fractures: a comparitive clinical study of conservative treatment and Harrington instrumentation. *Spine* 1985; 10: 111–22.

43. Carl AL, Tranmer BI, Sachs BL. Anterolateral dynamized instrumentation and fusion for unstable thoracolumbar and lumbar burst fractures. *Spine* 1997; 22: 686–90.

44. Gurwitz GS, Dawson JM, McNamara MJ, et al. Biomechanical analysis of three surgical approaches for lumbar burst fractures using short-segment instrumentation. *Spine* 1993; 18: 977–82.

45. Esses SI, Botsford DJ, Kostvik JP. Evaluation of surgical treatment for burst fractures. *Spine* 1990; 15: 667–73.

46. McGuire RA. Spinal trauma: the role of anterior surgery in the treatment of thoracolumbar fractures. *Orthopedics* 1997; 20: 959–62.

47. Shono Y, McAfee PC, Cunningham BW. Experimental study of thoracolumbar burst fractures. *Spine* 1994; 19: 1711–22.

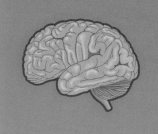

ACUTE NERVE INJURIES

25

Allan J Belzberg

Much of the knowledge for the management of peripheral nerve injuries has come from treating war injuries. Recent advances in instrumentation and microscopic surgical techniques have improved the prognosis of major peripheral nerve injuries. Challenges for the neurosurgeon in managing peripheral nerve injuries include deciding whether surgery is required, when to operate, and which injuries to repair for the best functional outcome.

It is useful to review the meaning of certain terms. *Neurotization* refers to the ingrowth of axons into tissue such as a distal nerve stump or a motor end plate in a muscle, which can occur spontaneously after injury to or surgical repair of a nerve. A *neurorrhaphy* is the joining together or *coapting*, usually by suture, of the two parts of a divided nerve to enable neurotization; if the nerve ends do not easily come together interpositional nerve grafts may be required. *Nerve transfer* refers to the transposition of freshly cut normal nerve to the distal stump of the injured nerve; it is used when the proximal stump of the injured nerve can no longer provide useful re-innervation (e.g. nerve root avulsion from the spinal cord). The term *anastomosis* should not be used for nerve repair since it refers to the union of hollow tubes.

ANATOMY

The structure of a peripheral nerve is constant regardless of the location in the body. It consists of nerve fibers, fasciculi, connective tissue, blood vessels, lymphatics, and nervi nervorum (Figure 25.1). Within an individual peripheral nerve the fascicular pattern changes along its course as a result of plexus formation along the course of the nerve and fibers coursing between fascicles. In a proximal nerve, fibers destined for skin are mixed with fibers destined for muscle. More distally, the sensory and motor fibers are segregated into separate fascicles.

RESPONSE TO INJURY

A peripheral nerve responds to injury in a predictable manner regardless of the etiology of the injury.

Neuronal response

Nerve injury leads to chromatolysis – swelling and displacement of the Nissl substance to the periphery of the cell – in the cell body. The closer the injury is to the spinal cord, the more hypertrophic the changes. Specific molecules help the neurons that have sustained an injury to survive. Trophic factors, such as nerve

growth factor, are taken from the terminal target tissue by the axon and transported retrograde to the neuronal cell body where they support gene regulation and promote survival of the neuron. The regenerating axons seek out sources of growth factors. Chemotactic factors may guide the growing axon sprouts for re-innervation of their target.

Axonal response

When an axon is divided, wallerian degeneration (changes in the distal nerve) occurs. The axon and myelin distal to the injury degenerate and are removed by phagocytic cells. Empty endoneurial tubes within the perineurium of the distal nerve remain. The proximal axons sprout new branches that, in the right environment, grow across the area of damage and enter the distal endoneurial tubes. The endoneurial tubes then direct the growing axons to peripheral targets. Schwann cells eventually move into the tubes to remyelinate the sprouting axons. If the sprouting axons do not reach a distal endoneurial tube or the tube has been replaced by fibrosis, the sprouts will form a local tangle or neuroma.

Muscle response

When a muscle loses its nervous innervation it degenerates. By 3 weeks postinjury, the beginnings of muscle fibrosis are reflected in histologic changes in the muscle. The fibrosis will gradually replace the muscle and by 2 years often only scar tissue is present. The muscle must be re-innervated within approximately 18 months of the injury to provide a functional outcome. Proximal nerve lesions are therefore at more risk of poor outcome because of the increased time required for axonal regeneration to reach target muscle.

Signs of acute muscle degeneration on electromyographic (EMG) examination include spontaneous muscle activity, fibrillations, and denervation potentials. The EMG changes occur only after wallerian degeneration and therefore take 1–2 weeks from the time of injury to appear. The first EMG is most often performed between 10 days and 2 weeks from the time of injury. An EMG performed within days of an injury will be normal, even if a severe injury to the nerve has occurred.

CLASSIFICATION OF INJURIES

In 1943 Seddon introduced a classification of nerve injury based on three types of nerve fiber injury.[1] Physiologic disruption is termed *neuropraxia*, axonal disruption is termed *axonotemesis*,

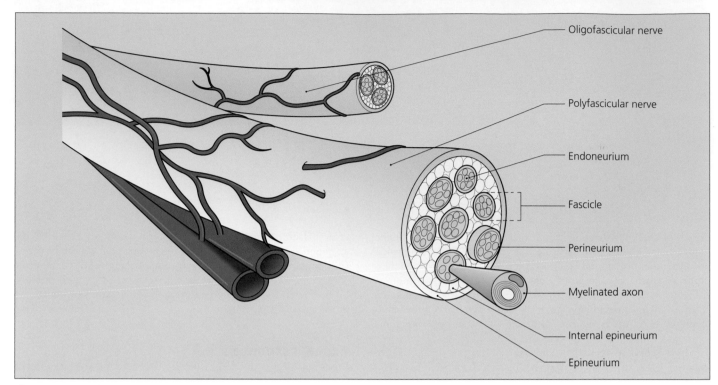

Figure 25.1 Peripheral nerve anatomy: epineurium, perineurium, endoneurium, oligofascicular nerve, polyfascicular nerve.

and division of the nerve trunk is termed *neuronotemesis*. This was followed by the Sunderland classification based on five degrees of increasing anatomic severity of injury (Table 25.1).[2] Pure grades of injury probably do not exist; the severity of most injuries occurs along a continuum.

SUNDERLAND CLASSIFICATION

First-degree injury

A grade I injury represents a reversible local conduction block at the site of injury. Symptoms and signs are variable and when mild may consist of paresis or sensory disturbance. A more severe injury may produce paralysis and/or complete sensory loss. Electrical studies demonstrate local conduction block abnormalities only at the site of injury. The pathology, consisting of local demyelination, is reversible. The injury does not require surgical intervention. Signs of recovery can begin within hours but may require several weeks.

Table 25.1 Sunderland classification of nerve injury

Classification	Description
Grade I	Loss of axonal conduction
Grade II	Loss of axonal continuity
Grade III	Loss of axonal and endoneurial continuity
Grade IV	Loss of perineurial continuity with fascicular disruption
Grade V	Loss of continuity of entire nerve trunk

Second-degree injury

In a grade II injury there is loss of continuity of the axons. Symptoms and signs consist of a dense sensory and motor loss distal to the lesion. The myelin, which is axon-dependent, degenerates but the endoneurial sheath and supporting elements, including perineurium, are preserved. The intact endoneurial tubes provide a guide for axonal regeneration, and the prognosis for a functional recovery is excellent. The axons can be expected to regenerate at a rate of approximately 1 mm/day.

After sufficient time for axonal growth to occur across the lesion, electrical studies can be used to confirm action potential conduction across the lesion. This is most accurate when performed intraoperatively. If a second-degree injury is confirmed, the lesion should not be surgically resected. An external neurolysis may be indicated to remove extensive scarring, but internal neurolysis is avoided as it will lessen the chance of a functional recovery.

Third-degree injury

In a grade III injury there is damage to the axons, degeneration of myelin, and loss of endoneurial tubes. Symptoms and signs consist of a dense sensory and motor loss. The perineurium is preserved, but because of the loss of the endoneurial tubes there is no guidance for regenerating axons. There is often intrafascicular bleeding, edema, and ischemia leading to fibrosis.

Recovery depends on the degree to which intrafascicular fibrosis prevents axonal regeneration into distal endoneurial tubes. When severe, little recovery can be expected. Spontaneous recovery of some function occurs if axons are able to cross the lesion and re-innervate distal targets. A third-degree injury will rarely recover to more than 60–80% of normal function. Surgical intervention such as nerve grafting is required only in severe third-degree injuries.

Fourth-degree injury

In a grade IV injury, the epineurium holds the nerve together but the internal anatomy, including the axon, endoneurial tube, and perineurium, is disrupted. The fascicular pattern is lost and regenerating axons cannot reach their targets. Electrical studies show no evidence of conduction across the lesion even after several months. Surgical intervention with nerve grafting is required for a functional recovery.

Fifth-degree injury

In a grade V lesion, there is loss of continuity of the nerve trunk. A grade V injury is commonly seen in laceration injuries but can also occur with severe stretch injury. The proximal nerve sprouts axons, but because of the discontinuity with the distal nerve, the sprouts tangle and form a neuroma. This injury requires surgical repair for a functional recovery.

MECHANISM OF INJURY

Laceration

Common causes of nerve lacerations are knife and glass injuries. The lesion may be a complete transection (grade V) or a partial laceration. In clean, sharp lacerations, the nerve should be repaired acutely. An experienced surgeon should perform the surgery once the patient's other injuries are stabilized. Waiting a few days to perform the repair while stabilizing other injuries or assembling a skilled surgical team will not affect the outcome.

Focal contusion

A focal contusion can produce a variety of injuries often within the same nerve. It is commonly seen in missile injuries such as gunshot wounds. Symptoms and signs are variable depending on the degree of injury. When contusion to the nerve occurs, often some resection of the two ends for a variable distance is required to allow a neurorrhaphy of viable nerve. If a large gap is produced, nerve grafting will be required. When a contusion to the nerve is suspected, repair should be delayed, allowing the extent of pathology to become apparent.

Stretch/traction injury

Traction is a common mechanism of injury in which the nerve may remain in continuity, but severe internal disruption occurs. The area of pathology can be local or spread over a large distance. Focal traction injuries, such as intraoperative retraction injury, have a good prognosis for functional recovery. Severe traction injuries, such as brachial plexus injury secondary to motorcycle injury, often require extensive nerve grafting. Common traction injuries are outlined in Table 25.2.

Measurement is made beginning at the injury site and moving distal to the first muscle innervated by the nerve. The time required for re-innervation is predicted using an estimated axonal regeneration rate of 1 mm/day. If there is failure to show evidence of re-innervation of the most proximal muscle at the expected time, either by clinical examination or by electrical examination,

surgical exploration is indicated. In most instances surgery should not be delayed beyond 3–4 months.

Compression

The extent of nerve damage in compression injuries correlates with the duration and degree of nerve compression. Compressing a nerve also compromises blood flow; therefore it is unclear to what extent physical deformation versus local ischemia forms the basis of the pathology.

Mild compression is associated with changes in paranodal myelin, invagination of myelin, and segmental demyelination. More severe compression produces wallerian degeneration. The symptoms and signs, and the need for surgical intervention, will depend on the severity of injury.

Common acute nerve injuries secondary to compression ischemia include "Saturday night palsy," which involves the radial nerve, nerve injury secondary to compression from a plaster cast, and compression from increased pressure in a fascial compartment.

Drug injection injury

Nearly any drug injected into a nerve can cause damage. The pathology often involves intraneural neuritis. The sciatic and radial nerves are the most commonly involved, often with iatrogenic injury. If there is no evidence of recovery at the predicted time, given the axonal regeneration rate of 1 mm/day, surgical intervention is indicated. A neuroma in continuity is a common finding at surgery. Determining the need for resection and grafting of a neuroma in continuity requires the skills of an experienced peripheral nerve surgeon.

Electrical injury

This injury occurs on contact with high-tension wire. Diffuse muscle and nerve damage is common, often requiring extensive resection and nerve grafting for functional recovery.

CLINICAL ASSESSMENT

To manage a peripheral nerve injury the physician must first determine the location and extent of nerve injury. The clinical history, physical examination, and laboratory investigations often allow an accurate assessment of the peripheral nerve injury. The physical examination includes testing of all muscles innervated by

Table 25.2 Stretch injuries	
Nerve	**Etiology**
Brachial plexus	Motorcycle accident
Upper or lower brachial plexus	Birth injury
Axillary nerve	Shoulder dislocation
Radial nerve	Humerus fracture
Common peroneal nerve	Head of fibula fracture

the injured nerve. All modalities of sensory function are tested, with special attention given to the area supplied solely by the injured nerve (autonomous zone). An EMG is first performed 2 weeks after injury. If the EMG remains normal 2 weeks after injury then there has not been axonal injury and a Sunderland grade I lesion is present with full recovery expected. Axonal injury with consequent denervation of muscle is associated with spontaneous activity on the EMG. A Sunderland grade II or higher lesion is present and axonal regeneration is required for recovery. The EMG is more sensitive than physical examination for signs of muscle re-innervation, and it should be repeated when axonal regeneration is expected to have reached the most proximal muscle, to confirm spontaneous regeneration of the nerve. A general approach to management of a peripheral nerve injury is seen in Figure 25.2.

The presence or absence of a sensory nerve conduction potential can be used to determine if a lesion is likely to be proximal or distal to the dorsal root ganglion (DRG). The peripheral sensory nerve cell body is located in the DRG. A lesion proximal to the DRG, such as a brachial plexus avulsion from the spinal cord, will usually not disconnect the peripheral axon from the cell body. No wallerian degeneration occurs in the sensory portion of the peripheral nerve and the sensory conduction potential remains intact. If, however, the lesion is distal to the DRG, there is sensory axonal wallerian degeneration and loss of the sensory conduction action potential.

The neurosurgeon must determine if there is avulsion of the roots from the spinal cord. This is important because with avulsion there is no spontaneous recovery. Physical examination shows decreased or absent power in all muscles innervated by the avulsed root. If only one root is avulsed, some power is often present, as most muscles are supplied by more than one root. Sensory loss occurs in a dermatomal distribution. Dense sensory loss occurs only in the autonomous zone, which may be quite small if only one root is avulsed. The presence of a Horner syndrome often indicates avulsion of T1 in brachial plexus injury. A myelogram followed by computed tomography (CT) or magnetic resonance imaging (MRI) that demonstrates the presence of pseudo-

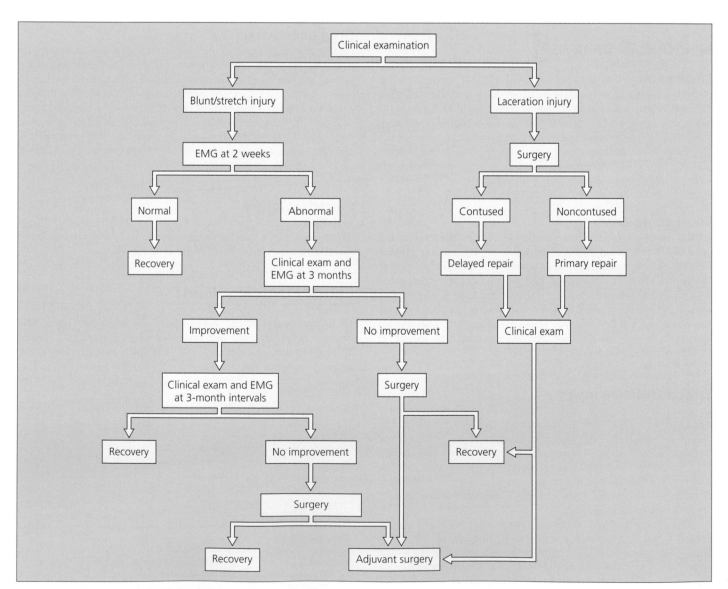

Figure 25.2 Management of peripheral nerve injuries.

meningoceles suggests that root avulsion has occurred. Injuries of sufficient violence to result in avulsion injury often result in a mixed lesion (proximal and distal to the DRG) and thus sensory nerve action potentials may be absent.

Ectopic mechanosensitivity can be used to assess growth of a nerve. Tapping the regenerating axons of the nerve will produce a paresthesia felt in the distribution normally innervated by the nerve (Tinel's sign). The Tinel's sign should move distally 1 mm/ day in accordance with the advancing axonal growth cone. Failure of the Tinel's sign to progress at the expected rate suggests the need for surgical exploration.

Some injuries can progress during the initial 12 hours after injury. Loss of function after 24 hours requires immediate assessment. Pathology such as a hematoma, compartment syndrome, or pseudoaneurysm may require urgent surgical intervention.

SURGICAL REPAIR

Surgical repair is used to restore continuity between proximal and distal axons, without which functional recovery will not occur. A direct suture repair using an epineurally placed suture is the preferred method. Under certain circumstances, such as a very distal lesion with separation of sensory and motor fascicles, a fascicular repair is indicated. If a gap occurs between the nerve ends it may not be possible to bring the nerve ends into close proximity for repair without undue tension at the suture site. An interpositional graft using harvested peripheral nerve from the patient is then used to bridge the gap.

Technical considerations

The goals of surgical repair are to appose healthy nerve ends without tension on the suture line and to align the fascicles, allowing appropriate re-innervation of target organs. Failure to achieve either goal leads to a nonfunctional outcome. If more than two 10-0 nylon epineural sutures are required to maintain approximation of the nerve ends, unacceptable tension is probably present. Tension will stimulate formation of excessive scar at the repair site, blocking growth of axons.

It is crucial that the operative set-up include microinstruments, such as jewelers' forceps, used to manipulate the nerve without producing tissue damage (Figure 25.3). Adequate illumination and magnification are also essential.

Correct positioning and draping of the patient allows freedom for manipulation of the joints to provide increased length of nerve for repair, adequate exposure to see movement of joints with nerve stimulation, and placement of a tourniquet to provide a bloodless field. Operating in a bloodless field facilitates dissection during nerve exploration. The surgical exposure progresses from normal anatomy to the area of injury.

Once the nerve is exposed proximally, electrical stimulation can help determine if there has been any recovery of motor function, which should suggest a good prognosis for spontaneous recovery. (When intraoperative electrical studies are performed, the tourniquet should be deflated to prevent confounding results secondary to ischemia.) The distal portion of the nerve is exposed and then the lesion is exposed. If a Sunderland grade V lesion is seen, surgical repair is performed.

When a neuroma in continuity is encountered several methods are employed to determine whether resection is necessary. An experienced surgeon can approximate the extent of internal fibrosis by palpating the neuroma. A firm neuroma implies extensive intraneural fibrosis with poor prognosis for functional recovery. An internal neurolysis performed with the operating microscope permits examination of the neuronal topography and amount of fibrosis but also places a regenerating nerve at great risk of damage.

Intraoperative electrophysiologic measurements can help clarify the nature of the lesion (Figure 25.4). A stimulating electrode placed on the nerve proximal to the lesion and a recording electrode placed on the nerve distal to the lesion record a compound nerve action potential. A compound nerve action potential recorded across the lesion indicates a good prognosis for spontaneous recovery so that only an external neurolysis is required. Failure to conduct across the lesion after sufficient time for spontaneous regeneration has elapsed indicates the need for resection and the likelihood of the need for grafting. When there is partial injury to a nerve, an internal neurolysis enables individual

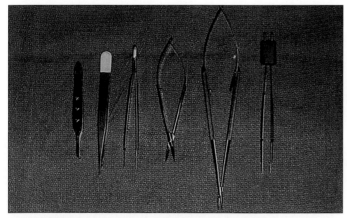

Figure 25.3 Microinstruments, including microbipolar tips, microneedleholder, microscissors, and a selection of jewelers' forceps.

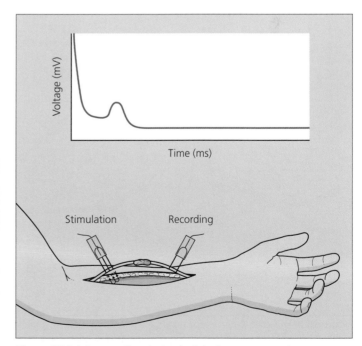

Figure 25.4 Intraoperative electrophysiologic measurements.

fascicles to be tested to determine which ones need to be repaired.

Tension on a suture line is associated with a poor surgical outcome. Several techniques are available to lengthen the nerve without creating tension. Maximal length is obtained by dissecting the nerve beyond the distal and proximal joints. The nerve can be mobilized for a length at least 50 times its diameter without risk of producing ischemia because of the nerve's longitudinal blood supply. Further length can be gained by splitting muscle branches from the main trunk. Other techniques for gaining length include flexion of the adjacent joint, nerve transposition (ulnar nerve at elbow), and bone removal (fibular head for peroneal nerve).

End-to-end repairs are the most common type of surgical repairs. Suture placement is either epineurial or perineurial, depending on whether the suture passes through epineurium or perineurium (Figure 25.5). Fine suture of 10-0 nylon is used to avoid excessive fibrosis. The more sutures placed, the greater the likelihood of producing fibrosis and interfering with axonal regeneration. Recently, the use of tissue glue (fibrin product) for coapting nerves has gained popularity. This greatly reduces surgical time and is particularly useful when the nerve repair does not span a joint, which lessens the need for strength at the repair site. Studies of the use of grouped fascicular repair versus epineurial repair have failed to demonstrate the advantage of fascicular repair.

A nerve injury often extends for a variable distance proximal and distal along the nerve. Once the nerve ends have been trimmed back to a normal-appearing fascicular pattern, a gap may occur that necessitates grafting (Figure 25.6). If a gap still remains after the various mobilization techniques described above have been utilized, then a nerve graft is the preferred method for avoiding tension on the suture line of a repair. Common donor nerves for graft material include sural nerve, medial antebrachial cutaneous nerve, and the superficial radial nerve of the arm (Table 25.3). Veins have also been used to provide a conduit with some success.

Table 25.3 Donor nerve graft

Donor nerve	Length
Medial cutaneous antebrachial	8–10 cm
Lateral cutaneous antebrachial	10–12 cm
Superficial radial sensory	10–12 cm
Dorsal cutaneous branch of ulnar	4–6 cm
Sural	20–35 cm

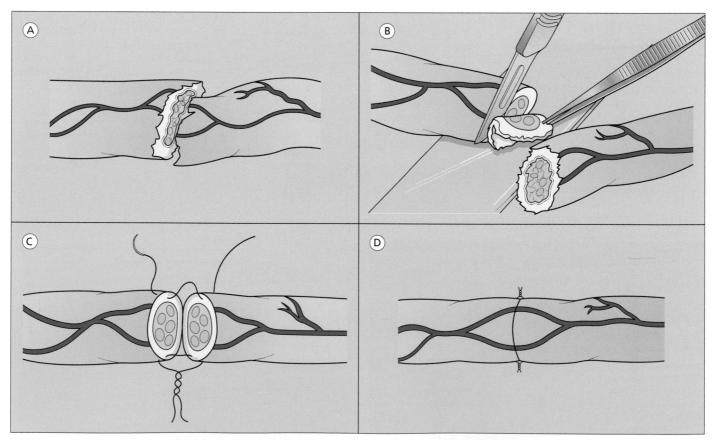

Figure 25.5 End-to-end nerve repair. **(A)** Laceration often results in minimal damage at the severed nerve edges. **(B)** The nerve end is resected back until a healthy fascicular pattern is seen. **(C)** One or two epineurial sutures are used to secure the ends. Visual clues such as surface vessels are used to allow accurate alignment.

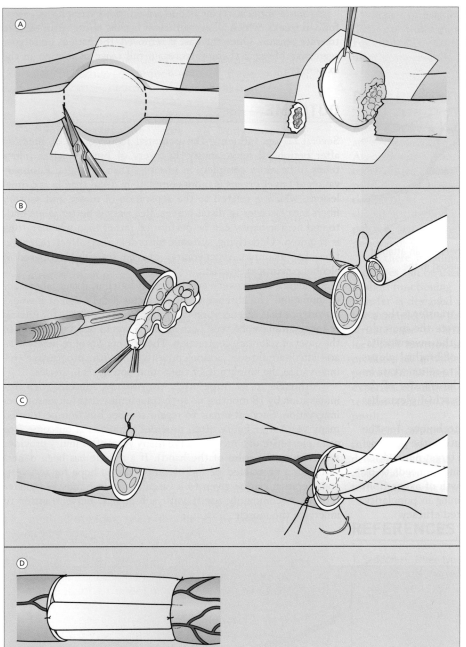

Figure 25.6 Nerve grafting. **(A)** A neuroma in continuity is resected. **(B)** The nerve ends are resected back to a healthy appearing fascicular pattern, leaving a large gap between the ends. **(C)** Grafts are placed and secured with epineurial sutures. **(D)** Grafting is completed.

Alternatives to autologous grafts include allografts with subsequent immunosuppression. These remain experimental. For short gaps, often in the digits of the hand, various artificial conduits have been developed, some resorbable and some impregnated with growth factors.

Grafts are revascularized from the recipient bed by small vessels. Small-diameter grafts are preferred because they are quickly revascularized. The center of a thick graft will be revascularized more slowly than the center of a thin graft and is a limiting factor on graft diameter. Several grafts may be required to form a cable whose cross-sectional area is equal to that of the nerve to be grafted (Figure 25.7). In general, one tries to target the graft to a distal target as this allows for more directed recovery.

For example, a graft from the C5 root may be directed at the musculocutaneous nerve rather than the upper trunk.

In certain instances, interfascicular grafting is performed (Figure 25.8). This technique is often used to repair distal injuries in which motor and sensory fascicles have separated. Performing interfascicular grafting is time-consuming and has not been associated with a significantly better outcome in most situations.

Nerve transfers are performed to restore lost function when suture or nerve graft is not possible. An uninjured nerve is divided, and the proximal stump is used to supply the damaged distal stump of another nerve. The conversion of the donor nerve to a new function depends on its capacity to integrate the proprioceptive messages from the re-innervated area. Some refer to this form

ENTRAPMENT NEUROPATHIES

26

Setti S Rengachary

Certain peripheral nerves, whether they are motor, sensory, or of mixed type, as they pass through their normal anatomic path in the extremities, course through narrow, constrained areas. Under certain circumstances, the nerves are susceptible to extrinsic compression at these sites.[1-3] Such a phenomenon is generically termed *entrapment neuropathy*.[4-6] Entrapment of nerves generally occurs as they pass beside a joint, such as the elbow, wrist, or hip. Although compression may occur elsewhere, it is uncommon in other areas of the extremities. This, along with the fact that entrapment neuropathy seldom occurs in the head or trunk, suggests that repetitive motion is a major factor that precipitates entrapment in an anatomically constrained segment.

Two types of anatomic constraints predispose to entrapment neuropathy. The first type (Figure 26.1A) is a fibro-osseous tunnel. The space available for the nerve within the tunnel becomes constricted either because the contents of the tunnel become larger or hypertrophic, as when a patient with tenosynovitis has carpal tunnel syndrome, or because the walls of the tunnel encroach upon the tunnel's lumen, as when fractured fragments of a carpal bone displace into the carpal canal. Compression of a nerve in a tunnel is an example of *static* compression. The second type (Figure 26.1B) involves *dynamic* compression of the nerve as it passes through a fibrotendinous arcade. The nerve is flanked by two bellies of a muscle that under static conditions do not compress the nerve. When they contract, however, they cause a shutter-like closure of the arcade, compressing the nerve. For example, this can occur at the arcade of Frohse in the supinator muscle, the two heads of the flexor carpi ulnaris at the entrance to the cubital tunnel, or the two heads of flexor digitorum sublimis forming the "sublimis bridge."

PATHOLOGY OF NERVE COMPRESSION[7]

The pathophysiologic changes following nerve compression[8-21] are dependent on the degree, rate and duration of compression. Loss of function of the nerve as a result of compression is manifested clinically by motor paralysis, paresthesia, or numbness. In physiologic terms, mild and brief compression produces a transient and reversible conduction block within the nerve. Sustained compression over a long period causes structural changes. Not all components of the nerve are equally susceptible to a given degree of compression. Nerve fibers that have a greater amount of epineurium compared to the nerve fascicles are less susceptible

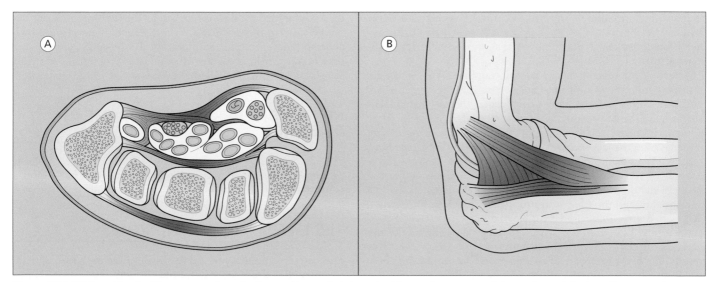

Figure 26.1 (A) Example of a fibro-osseous tunnel—the carpal tunnel at the wrist. The median nerve and the tendons of the long flexor muscles are the main contents of the tunnel. **(B)** Example of fibrotendinous arcade—the cubital canal at the elbow. The ulnar nerve enters the fibroaponeurotic arcade formed by the two heads of the flexor carpi ulnaris.

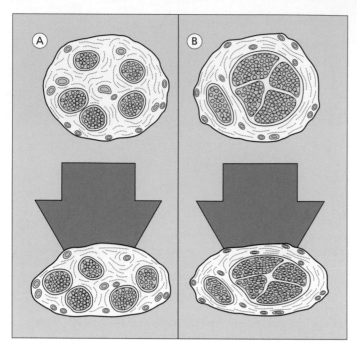

Figure 26.2 Nerves having a greater amount of epineurium (**A**) are less susceptible to compression than those having scanty epineurium (**B**).

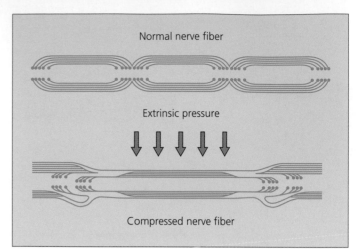

Figure 26.3 Telescoping of myelin sheath with acute and severe nerve compression.

to compression than those with larger fascicles and scanty epineurium (Figure 26.2). Also, within a given nerve, not all fibers undergo degenerative changes to the same extent. The superficially located fibers tend to bear the brunt of the compression, while the central fibers are relatively spared. Large, heavily myelinated fibers subserving light touch and motor function are more sensitive to compressive changes than unmyelinated fibers subserving pain sensation.

Impediment to microvascular flow appears to be a major factor in the pathophysiology of nerve impingement.[7] Capillary blanching and venular obstruction herald progressive compression. This leads to nerve ischemia, which in turn leads to endothelial impairment and progressive edema; the edema compounds the ischemia and swelling of the nerve. Critical swelling of a nerve within the constraints of its surroundings may lead to further nerve compression, a phenomenon that can be called a mini-compartmental syndrome.

Nerve compression blocks axonal transport. The antegrade transport from the nerve cell to the axon towards the synapse can be divided into fast and slow components; the fast component carries the membrane-associated materials and the slow components carry the cytoskeletal proteins. Nerve compression impedes both the fast and slow components of the antegrade flow, resulting in a swelling of the nerve proximal to the compression as a result of the damming up of the moving axoplasm within the fibers. Thus the distribution of cytoskeletal elements, axolemma constituents, and the transmitter substances required for synaptic conduction are all impaired by a block of antegrade flow. Retrograde axonal flow from the synaptic level to the cell body of the nerve is similarly blocked by compression of the nerve. This results in a loss of transfer of neuronotropic factors to the nerve cell body. The impairment of retrograde axonal transport results in certain changes in the nerve cell body comparable to those that occur after peripheral nerve section (wallerian degeneration). Thus, changes noted in the cell body are an eccentric nucleus,

dispersion of Nissl substance (chromatolysis), and a decrease in nuclear and whole cell volumes. The overall result of the impediment to axoplasmic flow is impaired membrane permeability and conduction block.

With acute and severe compression one observes a characteristic sequential invagination or telescoping of the myelin sheath (Figure 26.3). The polarity of invagination is reversed at the edges of the compression. With chronic compression, segmental demyelination occurs within the compressed segments, accounting for the slowing of conduction velocity of the nerve. In the early phases, the nerve fibers distal to the compression show normal morphology. With sustained compression, axolysis occurs within the compressed segment, leading to distal Wallerian degeneration.

DOUBLE CRUSH SYNDROME

If a nerve is compressed proximally, its distal part is more susceptible to compression than a normal nerve would be, because the antegrade axonal flow is blocked by the first compression. In a similar manner, if there is distal compression, the nerve cell body undergoes degeneration more quickly if a second compression is present proximally, because of impediment of retrograde flow. This latter syndrome is called a reverse double crush syndrome.[22]

NERVE COMPRESSION SYNDROME IN DIABETICS

Patients with diabetic neuropathy are more susceptible to compression, presumably because of accumulation of sorbitol, a metabolite of glucose, and the formation of endoneurial edema.

THE ENTRAPMENT SYNDROMES

The entrapment sites, the nerves involved at each site, and the corresponding syndromes are listed in Table 26.1. This chapter will cover the three most common entrapment syndromes; carpal tunnel syndrome, cubital tunnel syndrome and meralgia paresthetica.

Table 26.1 Entrapment syndromes

Location	Nerve entrapped	Compressing element	Clinical syndrome
Supracondylar region	Median nerve	Ligament of Struthers or supracondylar spur	High median entrapment neuropathy
Elbow	Median nerve	Bicipital aponeurosis (lacertus fibrosus), hypertrophic pronator teres muscle, or tendinous arch of flexor digitorum sublimis (the "sublimis bridge")	Pronator syndrome
Forearm	Anterior interosseous nerve	Variable anatomic abnormalities such as fibrous bands arising from pronator teres or flexor digitorum sublimis muscles; often no anatomic abnormalities may be demonstrated	Anterior interosseous nerve syndrome
Wrist	Median nerve	Carpal canal or element of its contents	Carpal tunnel syndrome
Elbow	Ulnar nerve	Variable: most commonly the fascial band binding the two heads of the flexor carpi ulnaris	Cubital tunnel syndrome, tardy ulnar palsy
Wrist	Ulnar nerve	Guyon's canal	Guyon's canal syndrome
Forearm	Posterior interosseous nerve	Arcade of Frohse	Posterior interosseous nerve entrapment syndrome
Forearm	Posterior interosseous nerve	Variable	Resistant "tennis elbow," radial tunnel syndrome
Forearm	Superficial radial nerve	Variable commonly extrinsic compression or trauma; sometimes the deep fascia of the forearm between the extensor carpi radialis longus and brevis	Superficial radial nerve syndrome
Neck	Brachial plexus	Cervical rib or fibrous band or scalenus anterior muscle	Thoracic outlet syndrome
Hip	Lateral femoral cutaneous nerve	Inguinal ligament and associated fasciae	Meralgia paresthetica
Knee	Peroneal nerve	Variable	Peroneal neuropathy
Ankle	Posterior tibial nerve	Tarsal tunnel	Tarsal tunnel syndrome
Shoulder	Suprascapular nerve	Suprascapular notch/foramen	Suprascapular nerve entrapment
Thigh	Saphenous nerve	Deep fascia roofing Hunter's canal	Saphenous nerve entrapment

Carpal tunnel syndrome[23]

The carpal tunnel syndrome[47] is the most common entrapment neuropathy encountered in clinical practice. It results from compression of the distal median nerve within the carpal tunnel, located in the proximal part of the palm of the hand.[44] The carpal tunnel is bounded dorsally by the carpal bones and ventrally by the transverse carpal ligament. The carpal bones form a shallow trough that is converted into a tunnel by the carpal ligament. The contents of the tunnel are the median nerve and tendons of the long flexor muscles (see Figure 26.1A). Any lesion affecting the synovial sheath tends to compromise the cross-sectional diameter of the carpal canal and may induce compressive neuropathy. Recent studies that include magnetic resonance imaging (MRI) and computed tomography (CT) scans show that patients with carpal tunnel syndrome tend to have small carpal canals. The small size of the carpal canal, measured by the decrease in its cross-sectional diameter, is a congenital or developmental phenomenon. Its small size in women may account for their higher incidence of carpal tunnel syndrome.

Clinical features[45]

Women are more commonly affected than men, by a ratio of seven to three. Most patients are middle-aged at the onset of symptoms. The predominant symptom is an aching, burning, tingling, numb sensation in the hand, ordinarily in the lateral half of the hand and the outer three or four digits. Frequently there may be an aching pain in the proximal forearm or even in the arm up to the shoulder. Typically patients wake up at night with increased pain, and they may shake their hand to obtain relief. Very frequently the symptoms are bilateral. In late stages patients complain of a weakness in the grip and tend to drop things.

In the early stages of the syndrome, at which time most patients are seen in the contemporary practice, there are few objective findings. Two mechanical tests can be performed. A Tinel's sign may be elicited by lightly tapping over the median nerve at the wrist crease, which results in a tingling in the distribution of the median nerve if positive. Phalen's test consists of asking the patient to flex the wrist to 90° for about 60 seconds, which will precipitate paresthesia in the distribution of the median nerve if positive. Neither of these tests is conclusive. Perception of light touch or pin prick in the tips of the fingers in the median nerve distribution may be impaired. In advanced cases there may be atrophy of the thenar muscles, especially in the abductor pollicis brevis.

There are several local and systemic risk factors that precipitate the symptoms of carpal tunnel syndrome (Table 26.2).

Diagnosis

The most important diagnostic tests are electromyography and study of nerve conduction velocity. The earliest and most significant finding is the prolongation of sensory latency. The sensory evoked response will show diminution of amplitude and may even be absent. Motor latency abnormalities occur late in the course of the disease. Needle electromyography may show loss of motor unit potentials and the presence of denervation potentials in the median-innervated muscles in the thenar eminence.

Table 26.2 Risk factors in the pathogenesis of carpal tunnel syndrome

Local factors	Systemic factors
Increased volume of the contents of the carpal canal	**Increased susceptibility of nerves to pressure**
Hypertrophic tenosynovitis	Alcoholic or diabetic polyneuropathy
Masses: neurofibroma, hemangioma, lipoma, ganglion cyst, gouty tophus, xanthoma	Hereditary neuropathy with liability to pressure palsies
Anomalous muscles and tendons	Amyloidosis
Persistent median artery with or without thrombosis, aneurysm, arteriovenous malformation	Proximal lesions of the median nerve ("double crush" syndrome)
Acute palmar space infections	Other polyneuropathies
Hemorrhage	
	Factors unique to women
Reduction in the capacity of the carpal canal	Pregnancy and lactation
Congenitally small carpal canal	Menstrual cycles
Idiopathic or familial thickening of the transverse carpal ligament	Contraceptive pills
Malunion or callus following	Menopause
Colles' fracture or fracture of the carpal bones	Toxic shock syndrome
Unreduced dislocations of the wrist or intercarpal joints	Eclampsia
Improper immobilization of the wrist ("cotton loader position")	**Other hormonal factors**
Compression by cast	Myxedema
Exostoses	Acromegaly
	Other systemic factors
Other local factors	Obesity
Burns at the wrist	Raynaud's disease
Long-term hemodialysis	Athetoid-dystonic cerebral palsy
	Inflammatory and autoimmune disorders
	Rheumatoid arthritis
	Dermatomyositis
	Scleroderma
	Polymyalgia rheumatica
	Metabolic disorders
	Mucopolysaccharidoses
	Mucolipidoses
	Amyloidosis
	Chondrocalcinosis
	Gout

Treatment

In early cases with minimal symptoms or in individuals in whom the syndrome is expected to be transient, conservative treatment should be instituted. This consists of a wrist splint at night and anti-inflammatory drugs. Injection of local anesthesia and steroids around the median nerve may be beneficial, but accidental injection directly into the nerve may result in annoying paresthesias in the distribution of the median nerve.

Surgical therapy is indicated when conservative measures fail. The surgical procedure can be performed by either the open method or an endoscopic technique. The steps in the surgical sectioning of the transverse carpal ligament are shown in Figure 26.4. Usually local or regional anesthesia (Bier block) is used. General anesthesia may be used if the patient is extremely nervous.

Endoscopic section of the carpal ligament has recently been introduced. The advantages are that the postoperative recovery period is shorter, a sensitive scar in the palm of the hand is avoided, and the structural integrity of the carpal tunnel mechanism is minimally disturbed. However, there is a greater risk of injury to the ulnar artery and to the sensory branch of the median nerve serving the middle and ring fingers.

Cubital tunnel syndrome

The cubital tunnel syndrome[48–71] results from entrapment of the ulnar nerve at the elbow. The cubital tunnel is located on the medial side of the elbow joint. It is a fibro-osseous tunnel that is roofed by the aponeurotic attachment of the two heads of the flexor carpi ulnaris and a tough fascial band that bridges these two heads (see Figure 26.1B). The floor is formed by the medial ligament of the elbow joint. During flexion of the elbow, the volume of the cubital tunnel decreases; the reverse happens in extension. This is because the points of attachment of the flexor carpi ulnaris, that is, the medial epicondyle and the olecranon process, are farthest apart during flexion. Thus, there is more tension on the fascial band between these two heads, which increases the pressure on the cubital tunnel.

Clinical features

The major presenting symptoms are weakness and atrophy of the intrinsic muscles of the hand and tingling and numbness in the medial two fingers. The onset of symptoms is generally insidious. Men are affected three times more commonly than women. An obvious etiologic factor, such as an old, healed, supracondylar fracture, a ganglion cyst of the elbow, or synovitis, is sometimes evident. In the majority of instances, however, there is no apparent cause. The presence of a rare anomalous muscle, anconeus epitrochlearis, is an uncommon cause.

On objective testing there is weakness of the ulnar-innervated muscles in the hand, including the palmaris brevis, abductor digiti quinti, opponens digiti quinti, flexor digiti quinti, adductor pollicis, the medial two lumbricals, and all of the interossei. The flexor carpi ulnar is generally not affected because the fibers that subserve the motor innervation are thought to be very deep within the nerve and thus less susceptible to compression than the more superficial fibers to the intrinsic muscles.

Froment's sign is elicited by asking the patient to grasp a piece of cardboard between the index finger and thumb against resistance. In patients with weakness of the adductor pollicis there will be flexion of the first interphalangeal joint and the thumb.

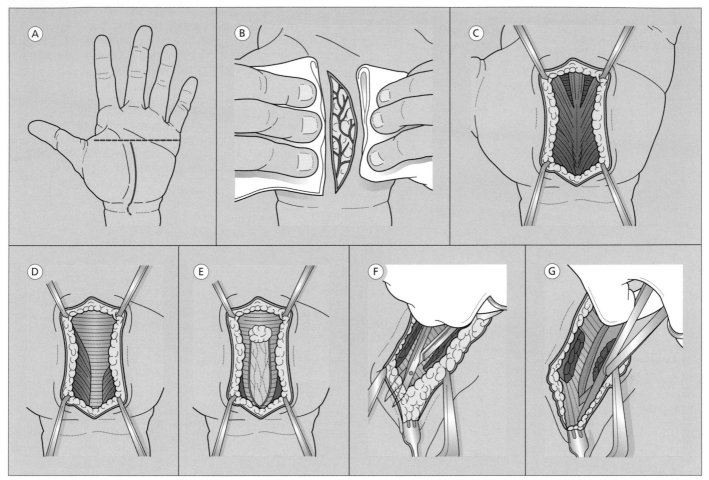

Figure 26.4 (A) The skin incision extends from the wrist crease to a point in the midpalm in line with the fully extended thumb (horizontal interrupted line). An optional extension may be carried out in the distal forearm (curvilinear interrupted line) to facilitate exposure of the proximal part of transverse carpal ligament and the distal part of the deep fascia of the forearm. Note that the main skin incision is not in the palmar skin crease but just medial to it. **(B)** Protrusion of exuberant palmar subcutaneous fat after the skin incision is made. **(C)** Exposure of the palmar aponeurosis. **(D)** Exposure of the transverse carpal ligament after midline section and retraction of the palmar aponeurosis. The distal margin of the transverse carpal ligament can faintly be seen blending with the deep fascia of the palm. The proximal part of the transverse carpal ligament is covered by the hypothenar and thenar muscles. In many instances (not shown in this illustration) they may meet and interdigitate in the midline, blocking the transverse carpal ligament from view. **(E)** About 80% of the transverse carpal ligament has been divided, exposing the median nerve. Note the constant fat globule superficial to the median nerve at the distal end of the exposure. **(F)** Proximal skin is undermined with retraction to facilitate exposure of the proximal part of the transverse carpal ligament. **(G)** Section of the most proximal part of the transverse carpal ligament and the distal deep fascia of the forearm.

Diagnosis

The characteristic electrodiagnostic finding is a delay in the conduction velocity in the ulnar nerve across the elbow. The sensory latency is prolonged, and the amplitude of the motor response in the abductor digiti minimi is decreased. A needle examination of the ulnar-innervated muscles may show denervation potentials.

Tardy ulnar paralysis should be differentiated from lesions in the spinal cord affecting the C8, T1 segments, such as syringomyelia, spinal cord tumor, or amyotrophic lateral sclerosis, and extradural spinal lesions, such as cervical disc disease or spondylosis, neurofibroma, or meningioma. Lesions of the brachial plexus involving the lower trunk or the medial cord (Pancoast tumor), entrapment of the ulnar nerve distally at the wrist (Guyon's canal), and polyneuropathy should also be ruled out.

Treatment

In early, minimally symptomatic cases, a conservative approach is recommended. The patient should wear an elbow pad for protection against direct pressure to the nerve and avoid excessive flexion of the elbow and strenuous exercise for some time, especially sports maneuvers that involve vigorous throwing, such as baseball. In persistent or highly symptomatic cases, surgical options should be considered. There is no other entrapment neuropathy for which the surgical options are more controversial than cubital tunnel syndrome. The available surgical methods are listed in Table 26.3. The simplest and most satisfactory procedure for uncomplicated cases is cubital tunnel release. (The steps of the procedure are shown in Figure 26.5.) In more involved cases complicated by elbow-joint abnormality, malunited fractures, or

Table 26.3 Surgical options for treating cubital tunnel syndrome

Simple decompression

Medial epicondylectomy

Subcutaneous anterior transposition

Intramuscular anterior transposition

Submuscular anterior transposition

other abnormalities, the nerve may be transposed anterior to the elbow joint, into the subcutaneous, intramuscular, or submuscular planes. Randomized prospective trials comparing these surgical options are not available at present, and the published results are tainted by considerable personal bias.

Meralgia paresthetica

Meralgia paresthetica[72–74] is a syndrome caused by the entrapment of the lateral femoral cutaneous nerve of the thigh in the inguinal region. The name refers to the burning sensation that affected individuals complain of in the anterolateral thigh (*meros*, thigh; *algos*, pain).

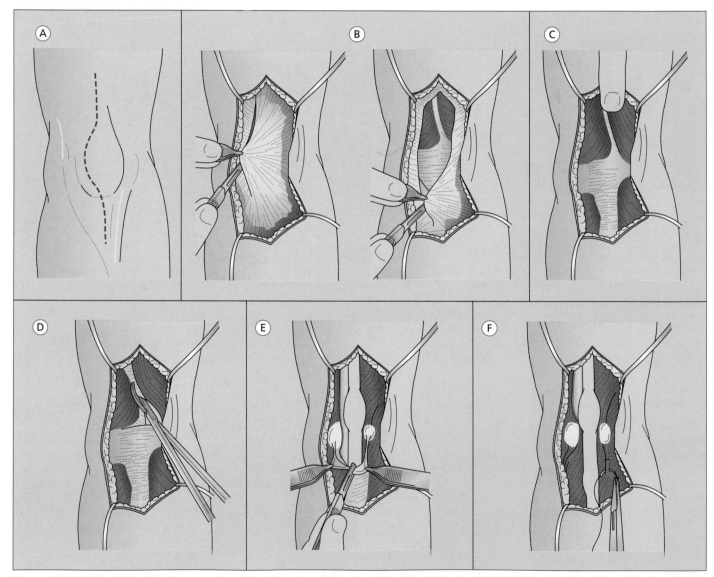

Figure 26.5 (A) Skin incision for decompression of the ulnar nerve. Note that the incision stops short of the basilic vein. **(B)** Incision of the deep fascia of the arm and forearm. **(C)** Digital palpation of the medial intermuscular septum and the ulnar nerve in the arm. **(D)** Section of the fascia over the ulnar nerve. **(E)** Section of the dense fascia spanning the two heads of the flexor carpi ulnaris; a bulbous enlargement of the ulnar nerve is noticeable. **(F)** The cut edges of the fascia are sewn over the flexor muscle on either side to prevent reformation of the cubital tunnel.

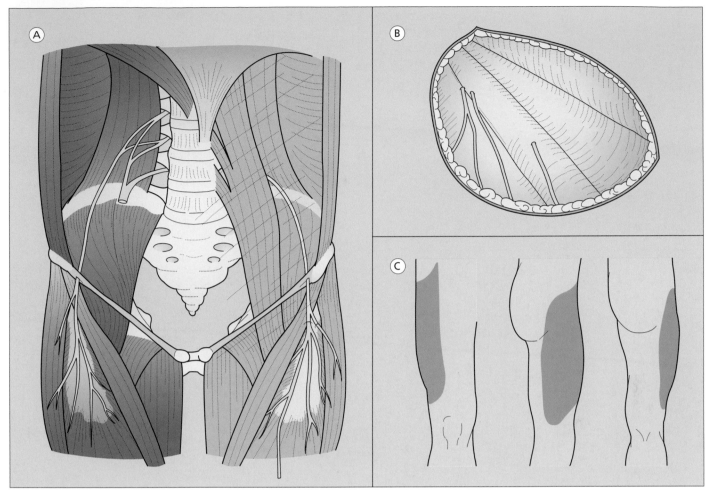

Figure 26.6 (A) Origin, course, and distribution of the lateral femoral cutaneous nerve of the thigh. On the right side of the specimen, the psoas major muscle and the fasciae have been removed. Not all branches of the lumbar plexus are shown. (B) Anatomy of the lateral femoral cutaneous nerve in the thigh. (C) Distribution of the lateral femoral cutaneous nerve in the thigh.

The lateral femoral cutaneous nerve of the thigh arises from the lumbar plexus, emerges at the lateral margin of psoas major muscle, descends obliquely downward and forward under the iliac fascia, pierces the inguinal ligament near the anterior superior iliac spine, courses under the fascia lata for about 5 cm, and then becomes subcutaneous by piercing the fascia lata (Figure 26.6A). It innervates the skin of the anterolateral aspect of the thigh and the gluteal region (Figure 26.6B, C).

Entrapment of the nerve occurs in the inguinal region at the point where it pierces the inguinal ligament. Obese individuals with the pendulous, flabby anterior abdominal wall are more prone to this disorder. Persons who are on their feet a lot, such as patrolmen, postal workers and traveling salesmen, are also more susceptible. Patients complain of a tingling, crawling, pricking, "pins and needles" sensation in the anterolateral thigh. Varying degrees of sensory loss may be present in the anterolateral thigh. Because the affected nerve is strictly a cutaneous nerve, there are no motor abnormalities or reflex changes. Indeed, if they are present an alternative diagnosis should be entertained.

Electrodiagnostic tests are generally not helpful in establishing the diagnosis of meralgia paresthetica. Rather, they are used to exclude other disorders that involve the lumbosacral plexus or the cauda equina. The best test for confirmation of the clinical

CLINICAL PEARLS

- Two factors predispose to entrapment neuropathy: repetitive motion and natural anatomical constraints around a peripheral nerve.

- The pathophysiological changes following nerve compression are dependent upon the degree, rate, and duration of compression.

- Carpal tunnel syndrome is the most common entrapment neuropathy.

- Diagnosis of entrapment neuropathy is established based on clinical history, objective findings, electro-myography, and study of nerve conduction velocity.

- If conservative measures fail, the offending compressing element should be surgically released.

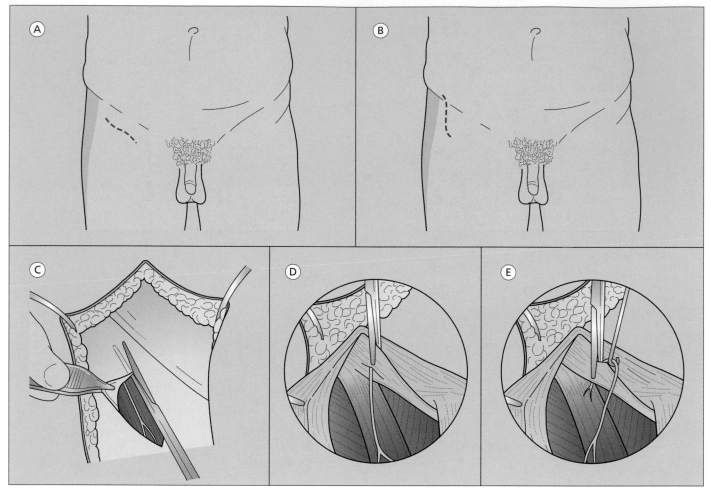

Figure 26.7 (A) Skin incision conventionally used to expose the lateral femoral cutaneous nerve. **(B)** Skin incision preferred by the author. **(C)** Section of the fascia lata at the anterior border of the sartorius. **(D)** Section of the superficial portion of the inguinal ligament. **(E)** Section of the fascial bands posterior to the nerve.

impression is a diagnostic nerve block, performed by injecting 5 mL of 0.5% lidocaine with epinephrine just medial to the anterior superior iliac spine. Complete relief of symptoms is generally predictive of a good operative result. The technique of section of the inguinal ligament and decompression is shown in Figure 26.7.

REFERENCES

1. Aguayo A, Nair CPV, Midgely R. Experimental progressive compression neuropathy in the rabbit. *Arch Neurol* 1971; 24: 358.
2. Bentley FH, Schlapp W. The effects of pressure on conduction in peripheral nerve. *J Physiol* 1943; 102: 72.
3. Dahlin LB, McLean WG. Effects of graded experimental compression on slow and fast axonal transport in rabbit vagus nerve. *J Neurol Sci* 1986; 72: 19–30.
4. Dahlin LB, Lundborg G. The neurone and its response to peripheral nerve compression. *J Hand Surg* 1990; 15B: 5–10.
5. Dahlin LB, Rydevik B, McLean WG, *et al.* Changes in fast axonal transport during experimental nerve compression at low pressures. *Exp Neurol* 1984; 84: 29–36.
6. Dahlin LB, Sjorstrand J, McLean WG. Graded inhibition of retrograde axonal transport by compression of rabbit vagus nerve. *J Neurol Sci* 1986; 76: 221–30.
7. Dahlin LB, Nordborg C, Lundborg G. Morphologic changes in nerve cell bodies induced by experimental graded nerve compression. *Exp Neurol* 1986; 95: 611–21.
8. Dahlin LB, Shyu BC, Danielsen N, *et al.* Effects of nerve compresson or ischemia on conduction properties of myelinated and non-myelinated nerve fibers: an experimental study in the rabbit peroneal nerve. *Acta Physiol Scand* 1989; 136: 97–105.
9. Denny-Brown D, Brenner C. Paralysis of nerve induced by direct pressure and by tourniquet. *Arch Neurol Psychiatr* 1944; 51: 1–26.
10. Duncan D. Alterations in the structure of nerves caused by restricting their growth with ligatures. *J Neuropathol Exp Neurol* 1948; 7: 261–73.
11. Fowler TJ, Ochoa J. Unmyelinated fibers in normal and compressed peripheral nerves of the baboon: a quantitative electron microscopic study. *Neuropathol Appl Neurobiol* 1975; 1: 247.
12. Fullerton PM, Gilliatt RW. Pressure neuropathy in the hindfoot of the guinea-pig. *J Neurol Neurosurg Psychiatr* 1967; 30: 18–25.
13. Fullerton PM, Gilliatt RW. Median and ulnar neuropathy in the guinea-pig. *J Neurol Neurosurg Psychiatr* 1967; 30: 393–402.

14. Lundborg G, Myers R, Powell H. Nerve compression injury and increase in endoneurial fluid pressure: a "miniature compartment syndrome." *J Neurosurg Psychiatr* 1983; 46: 1119.

15. Neary D, Eames RA. The pathology of ulnar nerve compression in man. *Neuropathol Appl Neurobiol* 1975; 1: 69–88.

16. Ochoa J. Nerve fiber pathology in acute and chronic compression. In: Omer GE Jr, Spinner M (eds). *Management of Peripheral Nerve Problems*. Philadelphia: WB Saunders Co.; 1980: 487–501.

17. Ochoa J, Marotte L. The nature of the nerve lesion caused by chronic entrapment in the guinea-pig. *J Neurol Sci* 1973; 19: 491.

18. Ochoa J, Fowler TJ, Gilliatt RW. Anatomical changes in peripheral nerves compressed by a pneumatic tourniquet. *J Anat* 1972; 113: 433.

19. Ogatta K, Naito M. Blood flow of peripheral nerve: effects of dissection, stretching and compression. *J Hand Surg* 1986; 11B: 10.

20. Rydevik B, Lundborg G. Permeability of intraneural microvessels and perineurium following acute, graded experimental nerve compression. *Scand J Plast Reconstr Surg* 1977; 11: 179.

21. Rydevik B, Nordborg C. Changes in nerve function and nerve fiber structure induced by acute, graded compression. *J Neurol Neurosurg Psychiatr* 1980; 43: 1070.

22. Upton ARM, McComas AJ. The double crush in nerve entrapment syndromes. *Lancet* 1973; 2: 359.

23. Barnes CG, Currey HLF. Carpal tunnel syndrome in rheumatoid arthritis: a clinical and electrodiagnostic survey. *Ann Rheum Dis* 1967; 26: 226–33.

24. Bauman TD, Gelbermann RH, Mubarak SJ, et al. The acute carpal tunnel syndrome. *Clin Orthop* 1981; 156: 151–6.

25. Bendler EM, Greenspun B, Yu J, et al. The bilaterality of carpal tunnel syndrome. *Arch Phys Med Rehabil* 1967; 58: 363–4.

26. Bradish CF. Carpal tunnel syndrome in patients on haemodialysis. *J Bone Joint Surg* 1985; 67B: 130–2.

27. Brain WR, Wright AD, Wilkinson M. Spontaneous compression of both median nerves in the carpal tunnel. *Lancet* 1947; 1: 277–82.

28. Carroll MP, Montero C. Rare anomalous muscle cause of carpal tunnel syndrome. *Orthop Rev* 1980; 9: 83–5.

29. Cseuz KA, Thomas JE, Lambert EH, et al. Longterm results of operation for carpal tunnel syndrome. *Mayo Clin Proc* 1966; 41: 232–41.

30. Dekel S, Papaioannou T, Rushworth G, et al. Idiopathic carpal tunnel syndrome caused by carpal stenosis. *Br Med J* 1980; 280: 1297–9.

31. Gelberman RH, Hergenroeder PT, Hargens AR, et al. The carpal tunnel syndrome. *J Bone Joint Surg* 1981; 63A: 380–3.

32. Goodman HV, Foster JB. Effect of local corticosteroid injection on median nerve conduction in carpal tunnel syndrome. *Ann Phys Med* 1962; 6: 287–94.

33. Gould JS, Wissinger HA. Carpal tunnel syndrome in pregnancy. *South Med J* 1978; 71: 144–5.

34. Green DP. Diagnostic and therapeutic value of carpal tunnel injection. *J Hand Surg* 1984; 9A: 850–4.

35. Halter SK, DeLisa JA, Stolov WC, et al. Carpal tunnel syndrome in chronic renal dialysis patients. *Muscle Nerve* 1980; 3: 438A.

36. Karpati G, Carpenter S, Eisen AA, et al. Multiple peripheral nerve entrapments: an unusual phenotypical variant of the Hunter syndrome (mucopolysaccharidosis II) in a family. *Arch Neurol* 1974; 31: 418–22.

37. Hartwell SW, Kurtay M. Carpal tunnel compression caused by hematoma associated with anticoagulant therapy. *Cleveland Clin* 1966; 33: 127–9.

38. Kremer M, Gilliatt RW, Golding JSR, et al. Acroparaesthesiae in the carpal-tunnel syndrome. *Lancet* 1953; 2: 590–5.

39. Phalen GS. Reflections on 21 years' experience with the carpal-tunnel syndrome. *JAMA* 1970; 212: 1365–7.

40. Phalen GS. The carpal-tunnel syndrome. *J Bone Joint Surg* 1966; 48A: 211–28.

41. Phalen GS, Kendrick JI. Compression neuropathy of the median nerve in the carpal tunnel. *JAMA* 1953; 164: 524–95.

42. Smith EM, Sonstegard DA, Anderson WH. Carpal tunnel syndrome: contribution of flexor tendons. *Arch Phys Med Rehabil* 1977; 58: 379–85.

43. Spinner M (ed.) *Management of Peripheral Nerve Problems*. Philadelphia: WB Saunders Co.; 1980: 487–501.

44. Spinner M, Spencer PS. Nerve compression lesions of the upper extremity. *Clin Orthop* 1974; 104: 46–67.

45. Tanzer RC. The carpal-tunnel syndrome: a clinical and anatomical study. *J Bone Joint Surg* 1959; 41A: 626–34.

46. Thomas JE, Lambert EH, Czeuz KA. Electrodiagnostic aspects of the carpal tunnel syndrome. *Arch Phys Med Rehabil* 1980; 16: 635–41.

47. Votik AJ, Mueller JC, Farlinger DE, Johnston RU. Carpal tunnel syndrome in pregnancy. *Can Med Assoc J* 1983; 128: 277–81.

48. Adelarr RS, Foster WC, McDowell C. The treatment of the cubital tunnel syndrome. *J Hand Surg* 1984; 9A: 90–5.

49. Apfelberg DB, Larson SJ. Dynamic anatomy of the ulnar nerve at the elbow. *Plast Reconstr Surg* 1973; 51: 76–81.

50. Broudy AS, Leffert RD, Smith RJ. Technical problems with ulnar nerves by Learmonth technique. *J Hand Surg* 1982; 7: 147–55.

51. Chan RC, Paine KWE, Varughese G. Ulnar neuropathy at the elbow: comparison of simple decompression and anterior transposition. *Neurosurgery* 1980; 7: 545–50.

52. Craven PR, Green DP. Cubital tunnel syndrome: treatment by medial epicondylectomy. *J Bone Joint Surg* 1980; 62A: 986–9.

53. Dahners LE, Wood FM. Aconeus epitrochlearis, a rare cause of cubital tunnel syndrome: a case report. *J Hand Surg* 1984; 9A: 579–80.

54. Eisen A. Early diagnosis of ulnar nerve palsy. *Neurology* 1974; 24: 256–62.

55. Eisen A, Danon J. The mild cubital tunnel syndrome: its natural history and indications for surgical intervention. *Neurology* 1974; 24: 608–13.

56. Feindel W, Stratford J. The role of the cubital tunnel in tardy ulnar palsy. *Can J Surg* 1958; 1: 287–300.

57. Harrison MJG, Nurick S. Results of anterior transposition of the ulnar nerve for ulnar neuritis. *Br Med J* 1970; 1: 27–9.

58. Jabre JF, Wilbourn AJ. The EMG findings in 100 consecutive ulnar neuropathies. *Acta Neurol Scand* 1979; 60(suppl.): 73–91.

59. Laha RK, Panchal PD. Surgical treatment of ulnar neuropathy. *Surg Neurol* 1979; 11: 393–8.

60. Leffert RD. Anterior submuscular transposition of the ulnar nerves by the Learmonth technique. *J Hand Surg* 1982; 7: 147–55.

61. Levy DM, Apfelberg DB. Results of anterior transposition for ulnar neuropathy at the elbow. *Am J Surg* 1972; 123: 304–8.

62. McGowan AJ. The results of transposition of the ulnar nerve for traumatic ulnar neuritis. *J Bone Joint Surg* 1950; 32B: 293–301.

63. Miller RG. The cubital tunnel syndrome: diagnosis and precise localization. *Ann Neurol* 1979; 6: 56–9.

64. Miller RG, Hummel EE. The cubital tunnel syndrome: treatment with simple decompression. *Ann Neurol* 1980; 7: 567–9.

65. Osborne G. Compression neuritis of the ulnar nerve at the elbow. *Hand* 1970; 2: 10–13.

66. Osborne GV. The surgical treatment of the tardy ulnar neuritis. *J Bone Joint Surg* 1957; 39B: 782.

67. Paine KWE. Tardy ulnar palsy. *Can J Surg* 1970; 13: 255–61.

68. Payan J. Cubital tunnel syndrome. *Br Med J* 1979; 2: 868.

69. Payan J. Electrophysiological localization of ulnar nerve lesions. *J Neurol Neurosurg Psychiatr* 1960; 32: 208–20.

70. Wadsworth TG, Williams JR. Cubital tunnel external compression syndrome. *Br Med J* 1973; 1: 662–6.

71. Wilson DH, Krout R. Surgery of ulnar neuropathy at the elbow: 16 cases treated by decompression without transposition. *J Neurosurg* 1973; 38: 780–5.

72. Ecker AD, Woltman HW. Meralgia paraesthetica. *JAMA* 1938; 110: 1650–2.

73. Stevens H. Meralgia paresthetica. *Arch Neurol Psychiatr* 1957; 77: 557–74.

74. Stookey B. Meralgia paresthetica. *JAMA* 1928; 90: 1705–7.

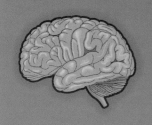

PAIN MANAGEMENT

27

Jeffrey A Brown

George Eliot wrote, "There is much pain that is quite noiseless, and vibrations that make human agonies are often a mere whisper in the ear of hurrying existence." Too often we concentrate on cure, never attending to the quiet, but more punishing, suffering that can debilitate or destroy a patient's daily life, livelihood and self-image. "Pain chokes us," wrote Ovid. Generations later physicians still seek to free us from this most private agony.

Physicians possess many tools to assist them in treating the suffering of their patients. This chapter outlines the basic neurosurgical approaches to the treatment of pain. To do this, the discussion reviews the physiology of pain transmission then examines the medical and surgical arsenal of pain management.

Pain and suffering present themselves in many forms. The experience of pain can be either *acute* or *chronic*. Chronic pain is defined as pain that persists for longer than 3 months. Chronic pain can be *nociceptive* or *neuropathic*. These distinctions will assist in determining a course of treatment. *Nociceptive pain* is commonly linked with an external stimulus. In contrast, *neuropathic pain* is usually caused by nerve damage rather than by stimuli to receptors (nociceptors). Unlike nociceptive pain, neuropathic pain is characterized by the absence of detectable ongoing tissue damage and is often present in combination with a sensory deficit. Neuropathic pain is characterized by *dysesthesias* (spontaneous unfamiliar, unpleasant sensations, often burning in quality), *paresthesias* (spontaneous paroxysmal, shooting or stabbing sensations) and associated with *allodynia* (when mild stimuli are perceived as painful). Distinguishing between these two types of pain will assist a physician in determining an appropriate treatment.

THE ANATOMY OF PAIN

To understand pain, a physician must first understand the process through which an individual feels pain. There are four steps between the cause and experience of pain. The first step, transduction, is the mechanism by which receptors are activated. During transduction, a mechanical, chemical, or thermal stimulus is converted to an electrochemical stimulus that, in turn, is converted to an electrochemical impulse by receptors (primary afferents). Free nerve endings typically function as pain receptors. Transmission is the process by which the electrochemical impulse travels from the originating sensory neuron to the spinal cord, brainstem, thalamus and cortex. During transmission, the central nervous system modifies the impulse (modulation). The final step, perception, is the subjective experience of pain. At any of these

steps, a physician can moderate pain through a variety of techniques to be discussed in this chapter.

If physicians understand the following principles of pain physiology and anatomy, then they will comprehend the principles and procedures that govern pain management. Anatomically and physiologically, axons are grouped into four populations by diameter or conduction velocity. The populations relevant to a discussion on pain are fiber group III (Aδ and B) and group IV (C fibers). Only Aδ and C fibers have a role in the sensation of pain. Aδ fibers are thinly myelinated, are 2–5 μm in diameter and conduct at 12–30 m/s. C fibers are unmyelinated, are 0.3–1.3 μm in diameter and conduct at 0.6–2.3 m/s. Most Aδ and C fibers are classified as nociceptors because their naked nerve endings act as pain receptors and because they respond maximally only when noxious stimuli are applied to their receptive fields. Aδ and C nociceptors increase their discharge as the stimulus intensity is increased into the range that produces tissue damage. This damage is expressed as classical erythema and edema associated with pain (*rubror, calor, dolor*).

Peripheral nervous system

The Aδ and C fibers are subclassified as Aδ mechanonociceptors, Aδ thermonociceptors, C-fiber chemonociceptors and polymodal nociceptors. All of these fibers are capable of sensitization. *Sensitization* occurs when repeated stimulation lowers the afferent fiber's threshold to application of a noxious stimulus. Aδ-fiber nociceptors evoke pricking pain, sharpness and aching pain. C-fiber activity is associated with a prolonged burning sensation. These anatomical differences and the perceptions that they evoke are important to know when considering treatment options (Figure 27.1).

Central nervous system

The central nervous system receives convergent input from the varied primary afferents. Two-thirds of dorsal root (sensory) axons are unmyelinated and become part of Lissauer's tract at the dorsolateral edge of the spinal gray matter. Aδ and C fibers enter the cord via the lateral division of the dorsal root entry zone. They enter the dorsolateral fasciculus (Lissauer's tract) and bifurcate into ascending and descending branches. Some collaterals terminate on interneurons in the spinal gray matter. The central target of nociceptive primary afferent fibers includes the dorsal horn Rexed laminae I, II, and V. The Rexed I lamina (postero-marginal nucleus) receives mostly input from Aδ fibers, which are

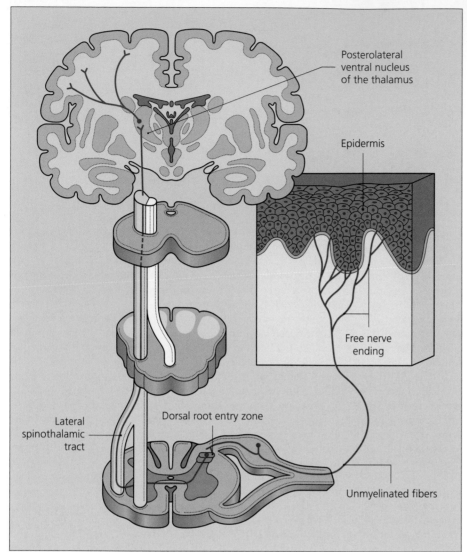

Posterolateral
ventral nucleus
of the thalamus

Epidermis

Free nerve
ending

Lateral
spinothalamic
tract

Dorsal root entry zone

Unmyelinated fibers

Figure 27.1 The nervous system pathway for nociception (pain) begins with the free nerve endings as receptors, which are present in the skin, mucous membranes, and periosteum. The nociceptive afferent fibers, represented by the unmyelinated C fibers and the thinly myelinated A-delta fibers with their cell bodies in the dorsal root ganglia, enter the dorsal root entry zone and synapse in the dorsal horn. Here, the first integration of pain occurs. The secondary nociceptive afferents decussate (cross) and then traverse the lateral spinothalamic tract to the rostral centers. Ultimately, pain is perceived at the cortical level.

related to pain and temperature. Projections from here go to other cord laminae, the brainstem reticular formation and the thalamus. Lamina II (substantia gelatinosa) contains both excitatory and inhibitory interneurons that project to other laminae of the dorsal horn. Lamina II has an outer II_O and an inner II_I layer. The input is primarily from C-fiber primary afferents, which then project to other laminae of the dorsal horn and supraspinal sites (for example, the thalamus). II_I also receives collaterals from non-nociceptor afferent fibers. Lamina V neurons also receive both nociceptive (mostly Aδ) and non-nociceptive inputs and project to medullary and mesencephalic reticular formation, thalamus and hypothalamus. Laminae III and IV (nucleus proprius) neurons receive non-nociceptive afferent inputs and project to deeper laminae of the cord, to the dorsal column nuclei, and other supraspinal relay centers (midbrain, thalamus and hypothalamus).

Fibers of the anterolateral system (ALS) participate in both direct and indirect spinothalamic pathways. Most Aδ fibers follow the direct (neospinothalamic) pathway that carries nondiscriminative tactile, innocuous thermal and nociceptive signals. Entering the dorsolateral fasciculus, the Aδ fibers bifurcate. The major branches ascend three to five spinal levels to terminate on the second-order neurons in lamina I of the dorsal horn. The second-

order fibers project to the thalamus. The great majority of the axons of the second-order fibers cross the midline of the cord obliquely via the ventral white commissure and ascend in the contralateral ALS. A few fibers ascend in the ipsilateral ALS. The third-order neurons of these crossed and uncrossed fibers are predominantly in the ventroposterolateral thalamic nucleus.

The polysynaptic indirect (paleospinothalamic) portion of the ALS whose major input is from C fibers, relays noxious and innocuous mechanical and thermal information to the brainstem reticular formation. Branches of these fibers ascend and descend by one or two levels in the dorsolateral fasciculus and synapse on interneurons in laminae II and III. The latter interneurons influence tract cells in laminae I to II, and V to VIII. Axons from these run obliquely across the ventral white commissure and join the contralateral ALS. These spinoreticular fibers terminate in the brainstem reticular formation, which then projects to the thalamus. Somatosensory information, including nociceptive input from dorsal horn cells, also ascends directly to the hypothalamus via the spinohypothalamic fibers of the ALS and indirectly via synaptic relays in the reticular formation and in the periaqueductal gray. Thus nociceptive information is carried to the limbic system, which relates emotional and autonomic responses to nociceptive stimuli. Neurons also project to the brainstem reticular nuclei and indirectly influence the thalamus. Reticulospinal fibers project to the intralaminar nuclei and posterior group of thalamic nuclei. From these posterior nuclei are fibers that project to the striatum and wide cortical areas that mediate the "alerting response to painful stimuli." Nuclei of the posterior thalamic group project to the secondary somatosensory cortex (SII) and retroinsular cortex and underlie the dull, poorly localized, but persistent painful sensation perceived after localized thalamic lesions (Figure 27.2).

ALS fibers are arranged somatotopically in the cord. Those from lower levels of the body are found dorsolaterally and those from rostral levels are added in an orderly ventromedial sequence. In the medulla, the ALS fibers are near the ventrolateral surface, being located ventral to the spinal trigeminal nucleus, dorsolateral to the inferior olive, and separated from the dorsal column–medial lemniscus system.

The spinothalamic tract terminates in six thalamic regions. The ventral posterior medial (facial sensation) and lateral (body sensation) nuclei, the posterior portion of the ventral median nucleus (insular projections for autonomic sensorimotor activity), the ventral lateral nucleus (motor cortex projections), the central lateral nucleus (projections to basal ganglia and motor cortex mediating somatomotor integration and orientation control), the parafascicular nucleus (projections to basal ganglia and motor cortex) and the ventral caudal portion of the medial dorsal nucleus. Thalamocortical axons carrying nondiscriminative tactile,

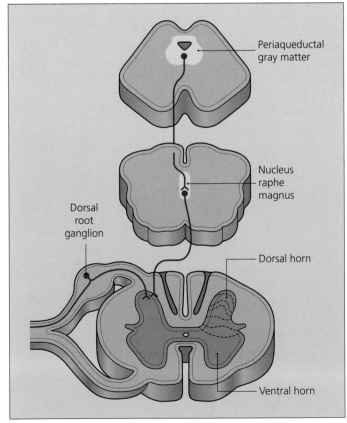

Figure 27.2 Neural pathways exist that inhibit pain at the dorsal horn level. These include brain stem pathways originating in the periaqueductal gray via the nucleus raphe magnus and peripheral nerve pathways involving the large A-alpha and A-beta fibers.

Labels in figure: Periaqueductal gray matter; Nucleus raphe magnus; Dorsal root ganglion; Dorsal horn; Ventral horn

nociceptive and thermal signals project via the posterior limb of the internal capsule to the somatosensory cortices. Fibers from the ventroposterolateral (VPL) nucleus project mainly to primary somatosensory (SI) cortex (areas 3,1,2) and from the posterior nucleus mostly to the SII cortex. Thalamocortical fibers from the lateral areas of VPL project to the posterior paracentral lobule (leg/foot) whereas progressively more medial parts of the VPL project to sequentially more lateral areas of the post central gyrus. Projections from the medial dorsal nucleus ascend to the anterior cingulate, orbitofrontal and prefrontal cortices. These projections are particularly important for the perception of pain. Activation of the anterior cingulate cortex may be related to the emotional/suffering aspect of chronic pain. In almost every positron emission tomography study of pain the anterior cingulate cortex is activated.

PRINCIPLES OF PAIN MANAGEMENT

Working from this anatomical knowledge, surgeons have developed a variety of treatment options. Strategies for pain management are divided into surgical and nonsurgical techniques. Medical treatment of pain can be systemic or regional. Surgical treatment is divided into two categories: ablative and augmentative. "Pain is as diverse as man, one suffers as one can," declared Victor Hugo. Ralph Waldo Emerson agreed, writing, "All pain is particular." In choosing an approach to pain management, the physician must keep these statements in mind, balancing the risks and benefits of a procedure for each individual.

Medical treatment

Pain management usually begins with medical treatment delivered systemically or regionally. Initial systemic treatment of nociceptive pain is usually accomplished by using oral nonsteroidal anti-inflammatory medications that act peripherally to inhibit the cyclo-oxygenase enzyme that induces synthesis of prostaglandins from arachidonic acid. They do not act on the central nervous system and are generally thus considered safer. These medications are effective in alleviating pain because prostaglandins cause hyperalgesia, an instance in which the same stimulus level will cause increased levels of pain.

Oral opioids, morphine derivates, are the next line of treatment. The level of pain dictates whether weak or strong opioids are used. Patients taking oral opioids must be carefully monitored. Opioids function by modulating pain pathways in the central nervous system. There are three opioid receptor types of which the μ-receptor agonists are the most effective analgesics. The μ opioids, such as morphine, modulate pain transmission at the midbrain periaqueductal gray and rostroventral medulla regions of the brainstem. The periaqueductal gray is connected with the rostral ventromedial medulla. The spinal terminals of the rostroventral medulla are most dense in laminae I, II and V of the dorsal horn and thus control nociceptive transmission from the spinal cord (Figure 27.2).

Neuropathic pain is treated medically with anticonvulsants, often in combination with antidepressants or other psychotropic drugs. The rationale for using antiepileptic drugs is that they suppress the pathological neural discharge that is presumed to be present in neuropathic pain. Carbamazepine and gabapentin, the most common drugs of this class, inactivate axonal sodium channels, thus reducing the generation of action potentials.

Antidepressants, especially tricyclics such as amitriptyline, are effective in treating coexisting depression and may have an independent effect on chronic pain by mediating central catecholamine release. Regional medical management involves the use of steroid solutions mixed with long-acting local anesthetic agents. These are injected into painful muscles or the epidural space.

Neurosurgical pain management

The neurosurgical approaches to chronic pain treatment are divided into surgery on the peripheral and central nervous systems. The approach may use decompression, ablation, drug infusion, or neuroaugmentation. The method selected must also consider whether the cause of the pain is malignant or benign. These approaches will be explained in sequence moving from the most peripheral to the more central procedures (Figure 27.3 and Table 27.1).

Neurectomy

Neurectomy (cutting a nerve) is performed in the case of injured sensory nerves. The end-bulb neuroma (sensitized sprouting of the cut nerve end) will recur as long as the dorsal root ganglion is in continuity with the fiber. The likelihood of pain recurrence can be limited by burying the nerve ending in adjacent soft tissue, which prevents repetitive mechanical trauma. The procedure is best performed on pure sensory nerves because of the loss of function associated with cutting a mixed sensorimotor nerve.

Decompression

Nerve decompression is the most frequently performed procedure in neurosurgery. In situations where an entrapped fragment of herniated disk or a thickened ligament is squeezing the nerve, removing the cause of the compression alleviates the noxious mechanical stimulation and thus relieves the pain. For example, pain derived from spinal nerve roots compressed by a laterally herniated disk or intraforaminal degenerative bone spur can be alleviated by surgical decompression at the site. Peripheral nerve decompression is most commonly performed for median nerve compression by a thickened transverse carpal ligament overlying the nerve. A neurosurgeon performing decompression must keep in mind that once pain has progressed from nociceptive to neuropathic, decompression alone may not fully resolve the pain, because the procedure does not repair nerve injury.

Dorsal ganglionectomy

Dorsal ganglionectomy is now recommended over dorsal rhizotomy for occipital neuralgia or chest wall pain. Dorsal rhizotomy (cutting an intraspinal dorsal nerve root) is an intraspinal, intradural operation that requires a laminectomy. Ganglionectomy is performed extradurally, requires less bone removal and may also section afferent fibers that go to the ventral root and sympathetic chain. In dorsal rhizotomy these fibers are spared injury and may be a source of persistent pain sensation. In a ganglionectomy, for

Table 27.1 Neurosurgical pain procedures		
Peripheral	**Central – spinal cord**	**Central – brain**
Peripheral neurectomy[4,5]	Cordotomy[11]	Mesencephalotomy[16]
Rhizotomy[6,7,8]	Midline myelotomy[12]	Brain stimulator[17,18]
Selective posterior rhizotomy[9]	Spinal stimulator[13]	Hypophysectomy[19]
Ganglionectomy[10]	Intraspinal narcotic analgesia[14,15]	
	Dorsal root entry zone (DREZ) lesion[21]	

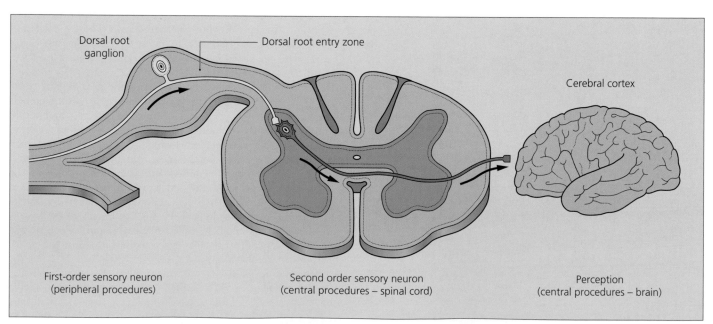

Figure 27.3 The sensory neural pathway beginning with the first-order neuron in the dorsal root ganglion, continuing with the second-order neuron in the dorsal root entry zone of the dorsal horn, and ultimately extending to the cortex where pain is perceived. Conceptually, palliative procedures for pain can be divided according to the level of the pathway approached.

example, a thoracic dorsal root ganglion is exposed by drilling the overlying lateral facet joint to expose the dural sheath containing both the dorsal and ventral roots. The neurosurgeon then amputates the distal margin of the ganglion and clips the proximal sensory root, preventing cerebrospinal fluid leakage. The operation is best performed at the thoracic level where the approach allows for minimal bone removal compared to the multiple laminectomies needed for intradural sections. Dorsal root ganglionectomy at C1–C2 is used to treat occipital neuralgia. At the thoracic level, it is used for post-thoracotomy pain. Unlike mid-cervical and lumbar level surgery, the ganglionectomy does not generally cause disabling loss of proprioception (Figure 27.4).

Dorsal root entry zone lesions (selective posterior intradural root section)

Here the small diameter sensory fibers that mediate pain and temperature are selectively sectioned in the lateral portion of the sensory rootlets as they enter Lissauer's tract in the dorsal horn of the spinal cord. A small incision is made into Lissauer's tract in the spinal cord (dorsal root entry zone) to injure the tract and outer laminar layers of the dorsal horn (Figure 27.5). This operation is used to treat limb pain where preservation of proprioception and tactile sensation is critical. It is also used for occipital neuralgia and brachial plexus avulsion injuries (Table 27.2). Because of the higher risk associated with intraspinal surgery, the operation is limited to the most severe and incapacitating pain conditions.

Sympathectomy

Sympathetic ganglion ablation or excision is often effective because of the involvement of the sympathetic autonomic system in mediating chronic pain, especially complex regional pain syndrome (neuropathic limb pain). Most often, sympathectomy is performed by excising the sympathetic ganglia at T1–T4 endoscopically (through the chest with the lung deflated). The diagnosis of sympathetically maintained pain must first be established for the operation to be successful. This is accomplished by a cervical, paravertebral trial injection of local anesthetic into the

Table 27.2 Dorsal root entry zone (DREZ) procedure

Brachial/lumbar plexus avulsion pain
Paraplegic/quadriplegic pain
Amputation phantom pain
Postherpetic neuralgia
Amputation stump pain
Postthoracotomy pain
Reflex sympathetic dystrophy pain

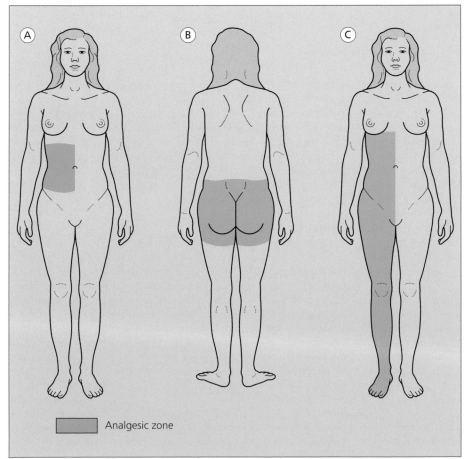

Analgesic zone

Figure 27.4 The effects of a variety of pain procedures on the sensory system can be described as: **(A)** *unilateral*, *segmental*, the result of a rhizotomy or ganglionectomy, creating a zone of analgesia useful for regional and lateralized pain in the thoracoabdominal area; **(B)** *bilateral*, *segmental*, the result of a midline myelotomy, providing a bilateral zone of analgesia particularly appropriate for lower pelvic pains; **(C)** *contralateral*, the result of an anterolateral cordotomy, creating a spinal level of analgesia that provides relief in diffuse, lateralized pains.

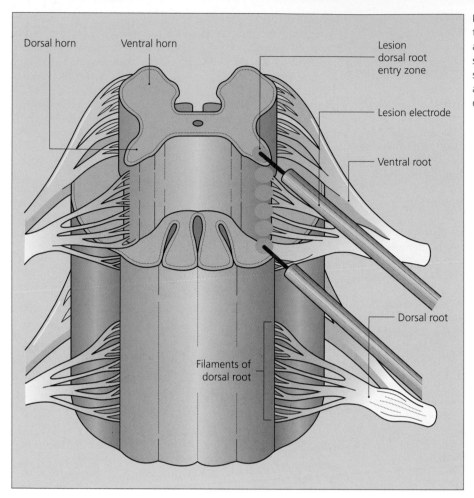

Dorsal horn   Ventral horn

Lesion
dorsal root
entry zone

Lesion electrode

Ventral root

Dorsal root

Filaments of
dorsal root

Figure 27.5 The DREZ procedure is designed to treat deafferentation pain by destroying the abnormally active dorsal horn neurons in the spinal cord at each segmental level of the pain. A small electrode is advanced into the spinal cord and radiofrequency lesions approximately 1 mm in diameter are created in a serial fashion.

stellate ganglon. If patients are not accurately diagnosed, a quarter of the patients will not benefit from the procedure.

Cordotomy

In percutaneous cordotomy, the spinothalamic and spinoreticular tracts are destroyed at the cervical level by making percutaneous radiofrequency thermal lesions. Lower body dermatomes are found in the dorsolateral spinothalamic tract and cervical dermatomes are anteroromedial, allowing for selective injury (Figure 27.4). Cordotomy is useful for pain caused by carcinomatous invasion of the brachial plexus in lung cancer. Because the pain tends to recur with time, cordotomy is not used in benign pain conditions. The risk of reducing respiratory drive when bilateral lesions are made additionally limits use to unilateral pain conditions.

To a great extent for both benign and malignant pain, ablative procedures, such as those listed above, have been replaced by the intrathecal infusion of opioids or by spinal neuromodulation (spinal cord stimulation). In general, ablative neurosurgical procedures are difficult to rationalize in noncancer patients because their effect is short term and the morbidity rate is higher than with drug infusion or neuromodulation.

Spinal opioid infusion

Spinal infusion of μ-opioid receptor agonists such as morphine at doses that have no effect on motor function will produce a potent increase in the nociceptive threshold. Intraspinal opioids are effective in nociceptive pain syndromes when the side-effects of oral or intravenous opioids are high, such as is seen with cancer patients. Infusion may also be effective for neuropathic pain, especially with the addition of nonopioids such as clonidine. In this procedure, an implanted, subcutaneous refillable pump infuses morphine at variably programmed rates into the spinal subarachnoid space. For benign conditions, such as persistent lower back pain after surgery, the gradual need for dose escalation limits the long-term effectiveness.

Spinal cord stimulation

Epidural spinal neuromodulation is effective for neuropathic limb pain. In this procedure either an electrode paddle is inserted into the extradural spinal space via a small laminotomy or a slender electrode wire is inserted percutaneously. After a trial for effectiveness the lead is connected to an external or fully implanted pulse generator. Spinal stimulation is used for failed back surgery syndrome with a predominant neuropathic component. It is also effective for cervical neuropathic pain (complex regional pain syndrome). Long-term neuropathic pain relief may be mediated by a suppressive effect on the hyperexcitability of the dorsal horn neurons with a wide dynamic range. Other indications for spinal cord stimulation include peripheral ischemic neuropathy and intractable angina. Effective long-term cervical stimulation using percutaneous leads for arm pain caused by complex regional pain syndrome is difficult to maintain. The leads often move from their original position because of the neck's flexibility.

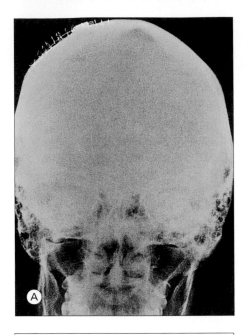
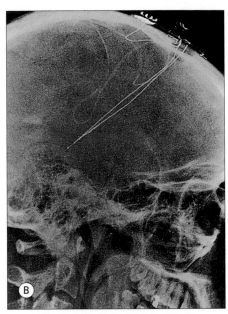

Figure 27.6 Anteroposterior (A) and lateral (B) skull radiographs show the placement of depth electrodes in the brain for stimulation-produced analgesia. The electrodes are placed either in the thalamus or the periaqueductal gray region.

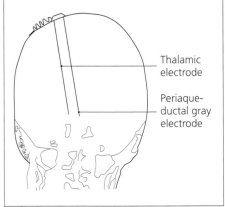
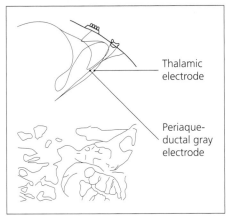

Deep brain stimulation

Deep brain stimulation is performed for both nociceptive and neuropathic pain. Electrodes are implanted into the periaqueductal gray and periventricular gray regions for nociceptive pain. For neuropathic facial pain electrodes are placed in the ventroposteromedial thalamic nucleus and for other unilateral regional body pain electrodes should be placed in the ventroposterolateral thalamic nucleus. Success rates decline with time and the best results have been in cancer patients and "failed back" patients. Thalamic pain and postherpectic neuralgia respond poorly (Figure 27.6).

Epidural motor cortex stimulation

Recently epidural motor cortex stimulation has been used for the treatment of formerly untreatable central pain caused by stroke, postherpetic neuralgia, phantom limb pain, and brachial plexus avulsion. The best results have been seen for neuropathic facial pain. In this operation, a craniotomy is performed to position an epidural electrode paddle over the motor cortex segment corresponding to the painful region using computer neuronavigation to identify the target site. Targeting is confirmed by cortical stimulation, which will elicit movement in the affected region of the body. Epidural motor cortex stimulation reduces pain by inhibiting thalamic hyperactivity resulting from deafferentation.

Motor cortex stimulation increases cingulate gyrus blood flow when it is effective in pain relief and may additionally reduce the suffering component of pain. The cingulate gyrus is involved in the emotional aspects of perception. Morbidity is low but patients must be able to undergo extradural cranial surgery. Results are best with neuropathic facial pain and worse when there is dense paresis associated with the affected painful region.

Whereas acute pain assists a physician in defining a physical source of illness, chronic pain may itself become the illness. Aeschylus wrote, "who apart from the gods is without pain for his whole lifetime?" What greater punishment is there for man than to be stricken with pain for the duration of a lifetime? The proper goal of neurosurgical pain management using the techniques briefly outlined above is the alleviation of suffering and the restoration of human well-being.

For a more extensive discussion of each of these topics, the references listed in the bibliography represent a selection of excellent textbooks and scientific papers.

ACKNOWLEDGMENT

I would like to acknowledge the assistance of Ben Pansky, MD.

CLINICAL PEARLS

- Neuropathic pain is characterized by an absence of detectable, ongoing tissue damage and is often seen with a sensory loss.

- Before acute pain is experienced there must be transduction, transmission, modulation then perception.

- Only Aδ and C fibers have a role in pain sensation.

- μ-Opioids, such as morphine, modulate pain transmission at the midbrain periaqueductal gray and rostroventral medullae. They work best in treating nociceptive not neuropathic pain.

- Spinal stimulation is most effective for neuropathic pain syndromes.

- Motor cortex stimulation is most effective in treating neuropathic facial pain.

BIBLIOGRAPHY

Burchiel KJ. *Surgical Management of Pain*. New York: Thieme; 2002.

Campbell JN, Meyer RA, LaMotte RH. Sensitization of myelinated nociceptive afferents that innervate monkey hand. *J Neurophysiol* 1979; 42: 1669–79.

Fields HL. *Pain*. New York: McGraw Hill; 1987.

Friedman AH, Nashold Jr BS. DREZ lesions for relief of pain related to spinal cord injury. *J Neurosurg* 1986; 65: 465–9.

Heinricher MM, Morgan MM, Fields HL. Direct and indirect actions of morphine on medullary neurons that modulate nociception. *Neuroscience* 1992; 48: 533–43.

Heinricher MM, Morgan MM, Tortorici V, Fields HL. Disinhibition of off-cells and antinociception produced by an opioid action within the rostral ventromedial medulla. *Neuroscience* 1994; 63: 279–88.

Kandel ER, Schwartz JH, Jessell TM. *Principles of Neural Science*, 4th edn. Elsevier Science Publishing Co., Inc.: New York; 2000.

LaMotte RH, Campbell JN. Comparison of responses of warm and nociceptive C-fiber afferents in monkey with human judgements of thermal pain. *J Neurophysiol* 1978; 41: 509–28.

Melzack R. The McGill Pain Questionnaire: major properties and scoring methods. *Pain* 1975; 1: 277–99.

Melzack R, Wall PD. *Textbook of Pain*. Edinburgh: Churchill Livingstone; 1999.

Mullan SF. Cordotomy and rhizotomy for pain. *Clin Neurosurg* 1983; 31: 344–50.

Nguyen JP, Lefaucheur JP, Decq P, *et al*. Chronic motor cortex stimulation in the treatment of central and neuropathic pain. Correlations between clinical, electrophysiological and anatomical data. *Pain* 1999; 82: 245–51.

North RB, Kidd DH, Zahurak M, James CS, Long DM. Spinal cord stimulation for chronic, intractable pain: experience over two decades. *Neurosurgery* 1993; 32: 384–94.

North RB, Kidd DH, Lee MS, Piantodosi S. A prospective, randomized study of spinal cord stimulation versus reoperation for failed back surgery syndrome: initial results. *Stereotact Funct Neurosurg* 1994; 62: 267–72.

North RB, Kidd DH, Wimberly RL, Edwin D. Prognostic value of psychological testing in patients undergoing spinal cord stimulation: a prospective study. *Neurosurgery* 1996; 39: 301–10.

Penn RD, Paice JA. Chronic intrathecal morphine for intractable pain. *J Neurosurg* 1987; 67: 182–6.

White JC, Sweet WH. *Pain: Its Mechanism and Neurosurgical Control*. Springfield, IL: Charles C. Thomas; 1955.

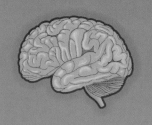

BRAIN AND SPINAL ABSCESS

28

Richard K Osenbach and Ash Pradhan

INTRODUCTION

Central nervous system (CNS) infections encompass a wide assortment of pathological processes that affect the brain, the spinal cord, their coverings, and adjacent anatomic compartments. Although many of the infectious processes that affect the CNS may threaten vital neurological functions and even life itself, the prognosis for patients with these illnesses has improved substantially over the past 20 years, in large measure as a result of technological advances in diagnostic and treatment modalities. The introduction and routine use of computed tomography (CT) and, more recently, magnetic resonance imaging (MRI) has revolutionized the diagnosis and management of both intracranial and intraspinal infections. Additionally, application of basic science research has further advanced the understanding of the pathogenic and pathophysiological mechanisms that underlie various infectious processes and has led to the development of adjuvant strategies for management. However, in spite of these advances, CNS infections continue to contribute to neurological morbidity and mortality. The purpose of this chapter is to review the contemporary diagnosis and management of pyogenic brain abscess and spinal epidural abscesses.

BRAIN ABSCESSES

Etiology of brain abscesses

Despite the improved treatment of underlying systemic infections and the development of more effective antibiotics, the overall incidence of bacterial brain abscess has remained relatively constant. Approximately 1500–2000 new cases of brain abscess are diagnosed annually. In some underdeveloped countries, brain abscess accounts for 8% or more of all intracranial space-occupying lesions, a sharp contrast to most industrialized nations where brain abscess constitutes only around 2% of all intracranial lesions.[1]

Although the age distribution of brain abscess varies somewhat depending on the underlying causes, it is primarily a disease of younger individuals. Most cases occur during the first four decades, the median age being around 30–40 years.[2] Cases related to an otitic source generally occur in persons younger than 20 or older than 40 years of age. The majority of abscesses related to an underlying sinus infection affect persons between 10 and 30 years of age. Overall, 25% of cases occur in children between 4 and 7 years of age, mostly as a result of cyanotic congenital heart disease or otitis media. Brain abscess is uncommon below the age of 2 years, and in this age group most often occurs as a compli-

cation of bacterial meningitis caused by selected Gram-negative organisms. There is a higher incidence of brain abscess in males for reasons that remain unclear.

Pathogenesis

Predisposing conditions

Microorganisms may reach the brain and cause focal suppuration by several different mechanisms: (1) direct spread from a contiguous site of infection, (2) hematogenous spread from a remote reservoir of infection, and (3) direct inoculation during a neurosurgical procedure or from penetrating craniocerebral trauma (Figure 28.1).[1–3] In addition, immunocompromised states such as acquired immune deficiency syndrome (AIDS),

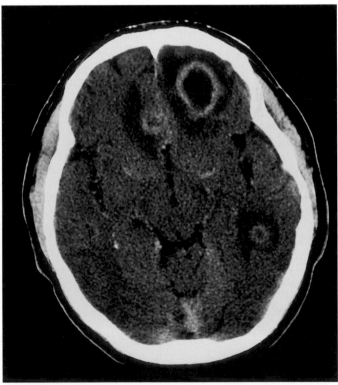

Figure 28.1 Contrasted CT scan shows multiple enhancing lesions consistent with brain abscesses. Note the relatively uniform enhancement of the capsule of the largest lesion in the left frontal region. Also note the white matter edema surrounding each of the lesions.

Table 28.1 Predisposing conditions for brain abscess

Predisposing condition	Most common pathogens
Contiguous site of infection	
Otitis media, mastoiditis	Streptococci (aerobic or anaerobic), Enterobacteriaceae, *Bacteroides* spp., *Provetella* spp.
Paranasal sinusitis	Streptococci, *Bacteroides* spp., Enterobacteriaceae, *Haemophilus* spp., *Staphylococcus aureus*
Metastatic sources of infection	
Pulmonary infection (lung abscess, empyema, bronchiectasis)	Streptococci, *Actinomyces* spp., *Nocardia* spp., *Bacteroides* spp., *Fusobacterium*, *Prevotella* spp.
Dental sepsis	Mixed *Fusobacterioum*, *Prevotella*, and *Bacteroides* spp., streptococci
Bacterial endocarditis	*Staphyloccus aureus*, streptococci
Congenital heart disease	Streptococci, *Haemophilus* spp.
Cutaneous/soft tissue infections	*Staphylococcus aureus*
Gastrointestinal (e.g. diverticulitis)	Anaerobes, Enterobacteriaceae
Genitourinary tract infection	Enterobacteriaceae
Penetrating head injury and post-craniotomy	*Staphylococcus aureus*, Streptococci, *Clostridium* spp., other anaerobes, Enterobacteriaceae
Immune compromised states/conditions	
HIV infection	*Toxoplasma gondii*, *Nocardia* spp., *Mycobacterium* spp., *Listeria monocytogenes*, *Cryptococcus neoformans*
Transplant recipients	*Aspergillus* spp., *Candida* spp., Mucorales, Enterobacteriaceae, *Nocardia* spp., *Toxoplasma gondii*
Neutropenic states	Aerobic Gram-negative bacilli, *Aspergillus* spp., Mucorales, *Candida* spp.

Modified from ref. 2.

malignancy, organ transplantation, and chronic corticosteroid therapy represent conditions that may place individuals at especially high risk for the development of brain abscess. A predisposing factor or condition can be identified in approximately 80% of patients with a brain abscess; the remaining 20% are cryptogenic (Table 28.1).[3]

Paranasal suppuration may spread to the brain in several ways. Bacteria may reach the brain through retrograde thrombophlebitis and spread via diploic or emissary veins, or by direct invasion following dehiscence of intervening bone (Figure 28.2). Brain abscesses that develop from contiguous sites of infection are usually solitary and in close proximity to the underlying infection. Abscesses related to frontal and/or ethmoidal sinusitis, and to a far lesser extent dental infection, usually occur in the frontal lobe while those due to sphenoid sinusitis more commonly occur in the temporal lobe or may result in pituitary abscess. Cerebral abscesses secondary to otogenic infections most often occur in the temporal lobe or the cerebellum.

A second mechanism of cerebral abscess formation is through hematogenous dissemination of bacteria from a remote site of infection. Unlike the lesions that are the result of contiguous infection, the incidence of metastatic abscesses is increasing.[4,5] These abscesses are not uncommonly multiple, deep-seated, and associated with a higher morbidity and mortality than those due to contiguous infection. Metastatic abscesses often occur at the corticomedullary junction, where blood flow is most sluggish. They are distributed proportionate to cerebral blood flow and therefore most commonly occur in the frontal and parietal lobes, although other sites such as the brainstem and cerebellum may also be involved. Another predisposing factor for the development of a metastatic abscess is the presence of cyanotic congenital heart disease, such as tetralogy of Fallot and transposition of the great vessels. In fact, brain abscess is one of the most common causes of

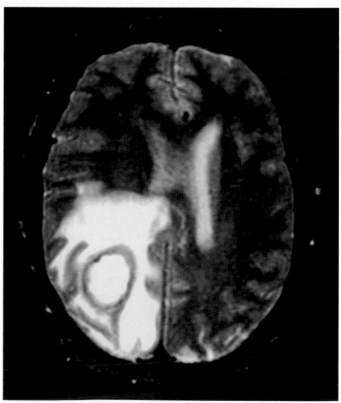

Figure 28.2 T2-weighted MRI demonstrates the typical findings of a mature brain abscess. There is a hyperintense core that corresponds to the necrotic center of the abscess. The capsule appears as a hypointense ring which is surrounded by a large zone of hyperintense signal that corresponds to edema.

morbidity in this population.[6] These congenital defects result in a right-to-left shunt of blood, thereby bypassing the normal filtering mechanism provided by the pulmonary capillary bed. In addition, these conditions result in hypoxemia, polycythemia, and increased blood viscosity. These in turn lead to areas of cerebral ischemia and microinfarction that provide the ideal milieu for the growth of microorganisms. Interestingly, endocarditis does not appear to be a major factor in the pathogenesis of brain abscess in this group.

Direct inoculation of microorganisms into the brain is another pathogenic mechanism in the development of brain abscess. Craniocerebral trauma is a well-established cause of post-traumatic brain abscess. An abscess may develop from retained bone fragments or foreign bodies or by secondary contamination of an initially "sterile" site from an overlying infection. A brain abscess is less likely to occur from retained bullet or missile fragments since the high temperature and friction generated by the projectile tend to sterilize the adjacent tissues. These abscesses, while rare, may actually present many years after the initial injury. Other causes and/or predisposing factors for the development of post-traumatic brain abscess include open depressed skull fracture, basilar skull fracture with associated cerebrospinal fluid (CSF) fistulas, animal bites, and, especially in children, injuries from lawn darts or pencil tips.[1] Many post-traumatic abscesses can probably be prevented by aggressive debridement of devitalized tissue, removal of accessible foreign material, and achievement of a water-tight dural closure.

Cerebral abscess may also occur following a neurosurgical procedure, most often the result of intraoperative contamination or secondary to an overlying bone flap infection. These complications usually require debridement, removal of the infected bone flap, and meticulous dural repair if cerebral abscess is to be prevented. Although infected CSF shunts are more likely to cause ventriculitis, they may occasionally result in a brain abscess.

Immunocompromised states currently represent an increasingly important predisposing factor for the development of brain abscess. There are numerous reasons for immune suppression, including AIDS, the use of immunosuppressive drugs in organ transplant recipients, chronic debilitating illnesses such as cancer or diabetes, and the use of chronic corticosteroids for various inflammatory and autoimmune conditions. In addition to abscesses caused by conventional bacteria, these patients frequently present with infections caused by opportunistic organisms, including atypical bacteria, fungi, and parasites. Brain abscess is responsible for up to 33% of infections in patients with cancer and nearly 45% of infections in heart and heart/lung transplant recipients.[7] Cerebral abscess represents the most common CNS infection in patients with leukemia; 4% of bone marrow transplant recipients develop brain abscess. Notwithstanding all the potential predisposing factors and sources of infection, there remains approximately 20% that are considered "cryptogenic" for which no underlying cause or factor can be identified.[1,3]

Clinical presentation
Contemporary clinical presentation of brain abscess differs negligibly from classical descriptions. The clinical course may range from indolent to fulminant. Most patients present with generalized signs of elevated intracranial pressure (ICP) and/or focal neurological findings that depend on the size, location, and multiplicity of the lesions, virulence of the organism, host response, and the severity of cerebral edema.[1-3,8] No particular constellation of symptoms or signs is pathognomonic for brain abscess. Although the symptoms of brain abscess are largely indistinguishable from those of any other space-occupying lesion, the tempo of progression tends to be more rapid, with 75% of patients having had symptoms for less than 2 weeks. However, immunocompromised patients may present more insidiously and a high index of suspicion is necessary to establish an early diagnosis in these patients.

Headache is prominent in 70–97% of patients; it is often constant, progressive, and refractory to therapy. Sudden worsening of headache associated with meningismus may herald rupture into the ventricular system, a complication associated with a high mortality.[2] Nausea and vomiting because of elevated ICP occur in 25–50% of patients. Slightly over 50% of patients have a low-grade fever, but fever exceeding 38.6 °C is relatively unusual and may indicate a concomitant systemic infection or meningitis. Two-thirds of patients have varying degrees of altered sensorium ranging from mild drowsiness and confusion to obtundation and coma. More than 60% of patients demonstrate focal neurological findings that are related to the size and location of the lesion. Supratentorial lesions may produce hemiparesis, aphasia, and visual field deficits while those located in the cerebellum are more likely to result in ataxia, dysmetria, and nystagmus. Brainstem lesions often present with facial weakness, dysphagia, and hemiparesis although the classic findings of a well-defined brainstem syndrome are usually lacking because the abscess is likely to extend longitudinally along fiber tracts rather than transversely.[2] Seizures occur in 30–50% of patients prior to any surgical intervention. Infants present with a combination of enlarging head circumference, bulging fontanelle, separation of the cranial sutures, vomiting, irritability, seizures, and poor feeding.[9]

Laboratory findings
Routine laboratory studies have proven to be of little value in the diagnosis of brain abscess. The peripheral white blood cell count is frequently normal or only mildly elevated (less than 15 000/cm^3) in up to 60–70% of patients.[8] In fact, white blood cell counts exceeding 20 000/cm^3 are usually indicative of concomitant meningitis or some other co-existing systemic infection. The erythrocyte sedimentation rate (ESR) is elevated in up to 90% of patients in whom it is measured. However, the ESR is a non-specific indicator of inflammation and provides no specific help in the diagnosis of brain abscess. Moreover, polycythemia lowers the ESR, and therefore the ESR is completely unreliable in patients with cyanotic congenital heart disease.

The results of CSF analysis are also non-specific. Opening pressure is usually elevated, indicative of raised ICP. There is generally a mild pleocytosis, with white cell counts < 100/cm^3 unless there is coexisting meningitis. CSF protein content is mildly elevated (usually < 100 mg%); hypoglycorrachia is generally absent except in the face of frank meningitis. Cultures are usually sterile, especially in patients who have been receiving antibiotics. Because lumbar puncture is potentially dangerous in the presence of an intracranial mass and given the fact that the CSF findings are non-specific at best, lumbar puncture is contraindicated in patients with suspected brain abscess.

Neuroimaging of brain abscesses
The development and widespread use of CT probably represents the single most important change in brain abscess management. Prior to the advent of CT, delay in diagnosis contributed signi-

ficantly to the high morbidity and mortality. In addition to being an excellent tool for examining the brain parenchyma, CT provides superior imaging of the contiguous bony anatomy of the calvarium, paranasal sinuses, mastoid, and middle ear. Indeed, CT has rendered diagnostic tests such as angiography, ventriculography, pneumoencephalography, and radionuclide brain scanning virtually obsolete. Consequently, these modalities will not be discussed further.

The imaging characteristics of brain abscess using CT are time-dependent and roughly correlate with the histopathological stages described by Britt and Enzmann (Table 28.2).[10,11]

During the early cerebritis stage, CT reveals an irregular area of low density with minimal if any enhancement. This area corresponds to an area of reactive cerebral edema surrounding the beginnings of the necrotic center. As the lesion progresses into the late cerebritis phase, the central area of hypodensity enlarges but still remains poorly demarcated. Early in this phase, there may be patchy contrast enhancement; later, if the lesion is sufficiently large, a typical pattern of ring-enhancement begins to become apparent. Immediately following contrast infusion, the ring may be thick and diffuse but with delayed scans contrast will diffuse into the central hypodense area. If the area of cerebritis is relatively small, a contrasted CT may show a nodular pattern of enhancement. The relative density of the lucent center is variable. A very low density or "black" center may indicate the presence of liquid pus. However, the center may have a density closer to normal brain parenchyma that may represent a combination of necrotic brain and pus. Notwithstanding, the density of the necrotic center during the stages of cerebritis does not appear to be of particular diagnostic value in predicting whether aspiration will yield pus.[11]

During early encapsulation, non-contrast CT demonstrates a faint ring of increased density compared with the surrounding brain and necrotic center. This correlates with the developing

Table 28.2 Correlation between abscess stage, histopathology, and neuroimaging studies

Abscess stage	Time course (days)	Histopathology	CT appearance	MRI appearance
Early cerebritis	0–3	Central zone of necrosis Local inflammatory response Marked peri-lesional edema Poor demarcation from adjacent brain Enlargement of necrotic center Initial formation of pus Surrounding zone of inflammatory cells and macrophages Maximal cerebral edema Reticulin network as precursor to capsule	Poorly marginated area of hypodensity Minimal if any enhancement with IV contrast	Edema may be more readily apparent
Late cerebritis	4–9		Hypodense area still may show poor margination Patchy enhancement during early part of phase Ring-enhancement begins later in phase Central hypodense areas fills in with contrast on delayed scans	Early patterns of ring enhancement more easily detectable Surrounding edema hypointense compared with normal brain Rim of lesion may be mildly hyperintense to white matter on T1WI
Early capsule formation	10–14	Continued formation of pus Development of collagen capsule Cerebral edema surrounding capsule	Non-contrast CT-faint ring of increased density Early in phase, center may fill in with contrast on delayed scans Enhancement of well-defined capsule Capsule usually thin, relatively uniform, and smoothly contoured on inner surface	
Late capsule formation	> 14	Five distinct histological zones: 1. necrotic center filled with pus 2. peripheral zone of inflammatory cells and fibroblasts 3. dense collagen capsule 4. neovascularity immediately external to capsule 5. peri-lesional edema and gliosis	Ring-enhancement of capsule which becomes thicker Daughter abscesses may be seen budding from 1. hyperintense liquefied core deep (medial) margin 2. hypointense capsule 3. hypointense capsule with surrounding hyperintense area of vasogenic edema and gliosis	Components on T2WI

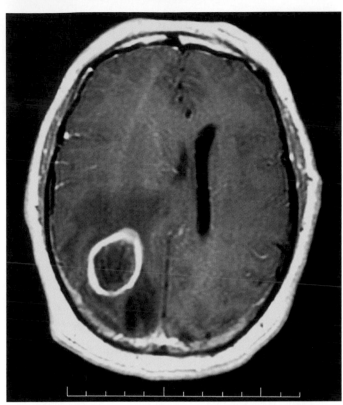

Figure 28.3 T1-weighted MRI with gadolinium (same patient as in Figure 28.2) demonstrates a well-encapsulated abscess. Note the relatively uniform thickness of the capsule as well as the smooth contour of the interior of the capsule. These features assist in differentiating a brain abscess from other enhancing lesions such as metastatic tumors.

capsule. Contrasted scans now show well-defined ring-enhancement of the developing capsule (Figure 28.3). Typically, the capsule is usually thin, relatively uniform in thickness, and smoothly contoured on the inner surface. Delayed scans after contrast infusion show reduction in the intensity of enhancement and minimal diffusion of contrast into the center. As the lesion progresses into the late capsule stage, the capsule can be clearly delineated on pre-contrast images. Following contrast administration, the ring-enhancing capsule appears denser and may become thicker. Peak enhancement occurs 5–10 minutes following infusion and then decays with time; delayed scans (30–60 minutes) during this stage show significant reduction in enhancement and there is virtually no diffusion of contrast into the center of the lesion. Administration of corticosteroids has been shown to influence the degree of enhancement. Enhancement may be significantly reduced during the cerebritis stage, shows an intermediate response during early encapsulation, but seems unaffected in the late capsule stage.[11]

Magnetic resonance imaging has now been extensively evaluated in the diagnosis of brain abscess and when available may be the imaging modality of choice. MRI in general is more sensitive than CT in detecting the very early changes of cerebritis, the extent of cerebral edema, the spread of inflammation into the subarachnoid space and/or ventricular system, and the earlier detection of small satellite lesions.[2,12] On T1-weighted images, a mature brain abscess is characterized by a central zone of marked signal hypointensity corresponding to the necrotic center

surrounded by a peripheral region of mild hypointensity. The intervening capsule appears as a discrete rim that is isodense to mildly hyperintense. An abscess typically has three components on T2W MRI; a hyperintense liquefied core, a hypointense capsule, and a surrounding area of hyperintense vasogenic edema or gliosis (Figure 28.4). Interestingly, the hypointense rim does not correspond exactly to the ring of enhancement seen after contrast administration, and is not thinned medially like the collagenous capsule.[12] Administration of gadolinium shows enhancement of the capsule and clearly differentiates the abscess core, enhancing rim, and surrounding brain.

Recently, diffusion weighted imaging (DWI) and magnetic resonance spectroscopy (MRS) have shown promise in differentiating abscess from a necrotic or cystic brain tumor. Abscess contents appear bright on DWI while cystic tumors appear dark. Using MRS, tumor spectra are characterized by an elevated choline peak, while abscess spectra are not. Abscesses also demonstrate elevated acetate and amino acid resonances, which are not seen in tumor spectra. For maximum accuracy, spectra should be obtained so that the wall of the lesion is dominant in the acquisition voxel. Given that DWI and MRS may be performed simultaneously with routine MRI, a combination of MR techniques may provide the diagnostic study of choice in the evaluation of suspected abscesses.[12]

Although the CT and MRI findings described above are characteristic of brain abscess, they are not pathognomonic. Indeed, the differential diagnosis of a ring-enhancing lesion includes a number of pathological entities including malignant glioma, metastatic tumors, infarction, resolving hematoma, and radiation necrosis. The characteristic features of the capsule described above help distinguish ring enhancement due to an abscess from that due to a neoplasm. Other findings, which favor a diagnosis of brain abscess, include multiloculation, multiplicity, and location at the corticomedullary junction. Additionally, leptomeningeal or ependymal enhancement favors the diagnosis of abscess.[8] In the absence of penetrating head trauma or prior craniotomy, the finding of gas within an intracranial lesion is highly suspicious of an abscess caused by a gas-forming organism. The emergence of a large population of immunocompromised patients has resulted in an increase in the incidence of abscesses caused by opportunistic infections. Fungi, parasites, and atypical bacteria cause a variety of pathological infections including brain abscess, meningitis, meningoencephalitis, and granuloma. Because of alterations in host defense mechanisms, parenchymal infection may not be well localized and may fail to become encapsulated.

In some cases, CT and/or MRI may be inconclusive, in which case radionuclide imaging with ^{111}In-labeled leukocytes may help clarify the diagnosis. Because a suppurative intracerebral process induces a significantly more intense inflammatory response than a tumor, this method should theoretically be able to distinguish abscess from neoplasm. In a series of 16 patients in whom the differential diagnosis included tumor versus abscess, ^{111}In white blood cell imaging was positive in four out of five (80%) patients proven to have a brain abscess and was negative in 10 of 11 (91%) patients who were found to have a tumor.[13] Overall, this modality has been reported to have a diagnostic accuracy between 88 and 96%, with sensitivity and specificity of 100% and 94%, respectively.[13,14] Leukocyte scanning is non-invasive, easily performed with virtually no side-effects, and provides useful information which might influence management. The main disadvantage is that optimal images are obtained 24 hours following injection of the cells, although positive images have been obtained as early as

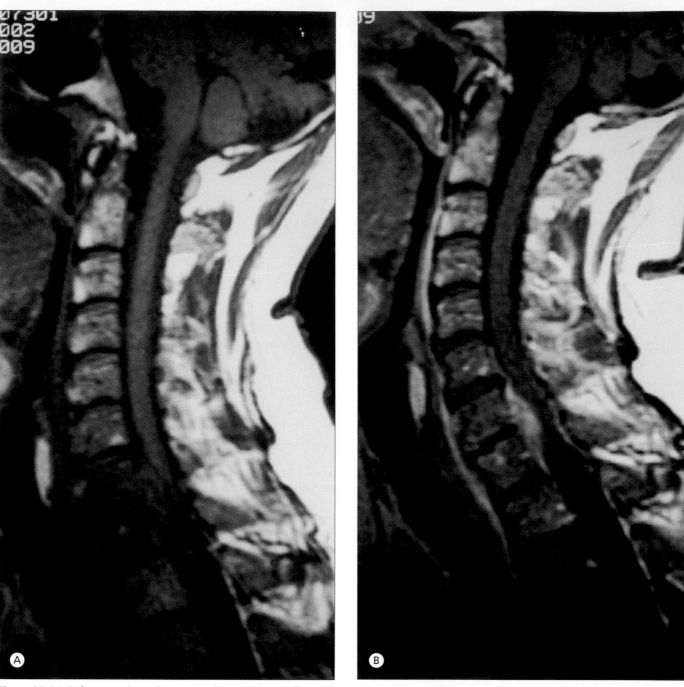

Figure 28.4 MRI from a patient who presented with neck pain, fever, and quadriparesis. The plain sagittal T1-weighted MRI **(A)** shows a confluent reduction in signal intensity in the C7 and T1 vertebral bodies as well as the intervening disk. There is a hypointense mass situated directly posterior to the vertebral bodies that is enhanced following administration of gadolinium **(B)**. Also note the anterior prevertebral soft tissue swelling. The abnormality is seen equally well on the T2-weighted images **(C)**. These findings are typical of osteomyelitis complicated by a contiguous epidural abscess.

Continued

6 hours following injection. Therefore, this modality is best suited to patients in good neurological condition who do not require emergent surgery. Although the sensitivity is extremely high, false-negative scans do occur. Modification of the inflammatory response and leukocyte function by prior antibiotic therapy may explain the rare false-negative results. Similarly, tumors that undergo extensive necrosis may incite an inflammatory response of sufficient magnitude to be detectable by labeled leukocytes. It should be kept in mind that metastatic tumors, particularly those of pulmonary origin, can be associated with concurrent bacterial infection. Therefore, it is generally recommended that histology and cultures be performed to verify the diagnosis. Despite these

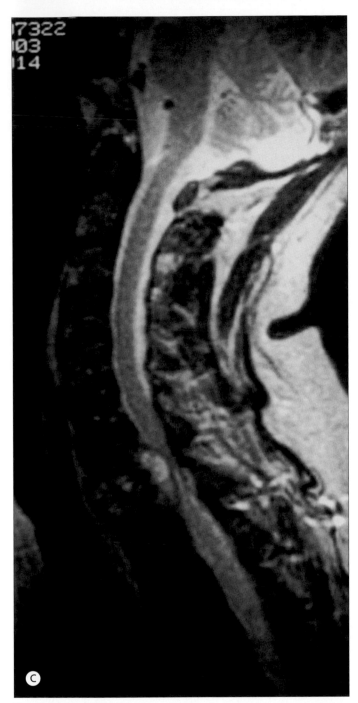

Figure 28.4, *cont'd.*

minor drawbacks, labeled leukocyte scintiscanning is a valuable adjunct that nicely complements the information provided by CT and/or MRI.

Other radionuclide scans such as [201]Th SPECT are useful for differentiating lymphoma from toxoplasmosis in AIDS patients. [201]Thallium is taken up by lymphoma but not by *Toxoplasma* abscesses. SPECT thallium may also help differentiate tumor from abscess in non-AIDS patients, although false-positive results have been reported.[12]

Management of brain abscesses

The management of brain abscess has changed over the past 20–30 years. Cerebral abscess was once considered strictly a surgical disease that demanded urgent surgical intervention. However, given the ability to establish the diagnosis earlier using CT and/or MRI, along with the development of newer more effective antibiotics, there has been a trend toward non-operative management in selected patients.[15–17] The fact is, there are no prospective randomized trials on the treatment of brain abscess and there is no consensus regarding ideal management. Consequently, the optimal management of brain abscess remains a subject of controversy. At present, the available treatment modalities include surgical excision, image-guided surgical aspiration, and empiric antibiotics.

Current treatment of brain abscess in most centers includes a combined surgical and medical approach. In many cases, brain abscesses result in relatively minimal destruction of brain tissue, producing their clinical effect through displacement of brain tissue and edema. Consequently, many of the neurological deficits may be reversible if appropriate treatment is initiated promptly. The goals of treatment of brain abscess include identification of the causative organism, establishment of antibiotic sensitivities, reduction of ICP and mass effect, and prevention of herniation and intraventricular rupture.

Principles of antibiotic therapy for brain abscesses

The introduction and widespread use of antibiotics in the 1940s has contributed in part to the reduction in mortality from brain abscess. Indeed, antibiotics continue to be an integral part of the treatment of brain abscess. A comprehensive discussion of antibiotics is well beyond the scope of this chapter; however, several principles should be kept in mind when prescribing antibiotics for brain abscess. Ideally, antibiotics should be prescribed based on culture and sensitivity testing of material obtained from the abscess. The efficacy of an antibiotic depends on a number of factors, including whether a particular antibiotic is bactericidal or bacteristatic for a particular organism, the route and duration of therapy, the host response to infection, and the concentration of the drug at the site of the abscess (Table 28.3).[2,18] Ample data exist on the penetration of antibiotics into CSF; however, CSF concentrations do not necessarily reflect the concentration within the abscess cavity. Antibiotics that achieve therapeutic concentrations within brain tissue include chloramphenicol, metronidazole, penicillin, methicillin, nafcillin, vancomycin, trimethoprim-sulfamethoxizole, and some of the third-generation cephalosporins.[2,18] However, despite antibiotic concentrations within an abscess in excess of the minimum inhibitory concentration, viable organisms may sometime be cultured from pus, especially in larger lesions.[8] This has been attributed to inhibition and ineffectiveness of antibiotics because of the acidic milieu within the abscess cavity. This would lend support to the argument that all large abscesses (> 2.5 cm) should be aspirated, not only potentially to reduce mass effect but also to provide an environment in which antibiotics can work optimally.

The empiric treatment of pyogenic brain abscess before culture results become available should take into account the underlying source of infection and the frequency with which certain organisms are isolated.[2] Abscesses of sinusitic origin are caused predominantly by carboxyphilic streptococci. These bacteria are extremely sensitive to penicillin and can be effectively treated with a third-generation cephalosporin, but are resistant to metronidazole. However, beta-lactamase-producing organisms

Table 28.3 Empiric antibiotic therapy for bacterial brain abscess

Underlying source of infection	Initial antibiotic regimen
Contiguous sources of infection	
Paranasal sinuses	Third-generation cephalosporin + metronidazole
Otogenic infection	Third-generation cephalosporin + metronidazole + PCN
Direct inoculation	
Postoperative	Vancomycin + third-generation cephalosporin
Post-traumatic	Vancomycin + third-generation cephalosporin + metronidazole
Metastatic infections	
Bacterial endocarditis	(1) Vancomycin + gentamicin or nafcillin
	(2) Nafcillin + ampicillin + gentamicin
Lung abscess, bronchietasis, empyema	PCN + metronidazole + trimethoprim-sulfamethoxazole
Dental and periodontal sepsis	PCN + metronidazole
Congenital heart disease	Third-generation cephalosporin
Source of infection unknown	Vancomyin + third-generation cephalosporin + metronidazole

Modified from ref. 2.

may also be present, and it is recommended that an agent active against obligate anaerobes, such as metronidazole, be included. A mixed flora of aerobic and anaerobic bacteria most often causes otogenic abscesses. Multiple broad-spectrum antibiotics should be administered initially, which will cover anaerobes as well as Gram-negative aerobes and streptococci. The combination of penicillin, metronidazole, and a third-generation cephalosporin such as cefotaxime fulfils this requirement. Metastatic abscesses are caused by a wide variety of bacteria, which depend on the source of the metastatic focus. In such cases, initial broad-spectrum therapy covering Gram-positive and Gram-negative bacteria as well as anaerobes is appropriate. In contrast, post-traumatic abscesses are most commonly the result of *Staphylococcus aureus* and are best treated with a semi-synthetic penicillinase-resistant penicillin or vancomycin. If *Pseudomonas aeruginosa* is considered a likely pathogen, ceftazadime should be given as the third-generation cephalosporin. In patients with an abscess of unclear etiology, an initial regimen consisting of vancomycin, a third-generation cephalosporin, and metronidazole should be selected. Therapy should be modified once culture results become available and unnecessary antibiotics should be discontinued to prevent the emergence of resistant strains.[2,19]

Nonoperative management

Successful non-operative management of brain abscesses was first reported in 1971.[16] Six patients, all of whom had co-existing infections (presumptively the source of the cerebral lesion) received 6 weeks of intravenous antibiotics which resulted in clinical cure. However, this report seems to indicate that all of the lesions may have been in the cerebritis stage. In 1985, 15 of 31 patients with apparently well-encapsulated abscesses were reportedly cured using antibiotics alone.[15] Four patients underwent stereotactic aspiration and 12 underwent surgical excisions. All patients had a comparable neurological status on admission. The outcome for the patients managed non-operatively was similar to that for patients who underwent aspiration or excision.[15] Based on these results, it was suggested that in many cases, brain abscesses could be successfully managed with antibiotics alone. Although these

results seem impressive, they should be viewed with caution since important differences in the treatment groups may have influenced the outcome. The patients managed medically had smaller abscesses (average 2.1 cm in diameter) compared with those managed by aspiration or excision (3.7 cm and 4.5 cm, respectively). In addition, nearly half the patients managed with antibiotics alone had deep-seated lesions that may not have been considered amenable to surgical management. In 1986, analysis of the five largest series concerning non-operative management of brain abscess totaling 67 patients revealed that the overall success rate of non-operative treatment was 74% in the collected series, with a mortality rate of 4%.[17] In 72% of the patients, antibiotics were selected based on organisms identified from blood, CSF, or other extracerebral body fluids (49%) or by aspiration of one of multiple abscesses (23%). Therefore, 28% of patients were treated without certainty of diagnosis. This is a critical point since there are any number of non-infectious processes that can mimic the radiographic appearance of brain abscess including primary and metastatic tumors, resolving hematoma, etc. Consequently, treatment without obtaining culture material from the lesion could lead to the erroneous treatment of a non-infectious lesion with antibiotics. Given the current availability and safety of stereotactic image-guided techniques, rarely should a lesion be treated with antibiotics before a culture or biopsy is obtained. An absolute contraindication to this approach would be patients with an uncontrollable bleeding diathesis in whom surgery cannot be performed safely. Another relative exception might be in a patient with a relatively small lesion (< 1.5 cm) who is neurologically intact, and in whom an *obvious* source of infection has been identified. In the cases of multiple abscesses, antibiotics are appropriate as the sole treatment for abscesses less than 2.5 cm as long as cultures obtained from one of the lesions have yielded a causative organism.[17]

Surgical treatment of brain abscess

Various procedures have been utilized in the operative management of brain abscess. Some of these, such as continuous drainage and marsupialization, are obsolete and will not be discussed.

Currently, the surgical management of brain abscess consists of image-guided stereotactic aspiration or craniotomy with complete excision. There continues to be some debate regarding which procedure represents optimal management. Each procedure has its distinct advantages and indications. Indeed, both methods have been and continue to be used successfully and each treatment has avid proponents. Aside from personal bias, the choice of one procedure over another may be influenced by the age of the patient, neurological condition, location and stage of the abscess, the type of abscess, and whether multiple lesions are present.

Excellent outcomes have been reported in patients managed by aspiration alone.[1,3–6,18,20,21] Stereotactic aspiration has a number of advantages. It can be accomplished rapidly and safely through a single bur hole under local anesthesia, making it particularly attractive in patients who are seriously ill. It allows precise localization and decompression of the abscess cavity using a minimally invasive technique. It is particularly valuable in treating deep-seated lesions, lesions in eloquent areas, and multiple abscesses. Indeed, with the stereotactic systems (frame-based and frameless) currently available, multiple lesions can frequently be aspirated through a single bur hole. During the earlier stages of cerebritis in which antibiotics alone may be curative, open procedures are more likely to cause significant neurological deficit whereas stereotactic aspiration/biopsy can safely retrieve tissue for culture. Additionally, removal of the purulent material creates a more favorable local environment in which antibiotics function effectively.

Although aspiration has certainly proven successful, excision via formal craniotomy has also been effective.[21,22] There are advantages and drawbacks to excision of an abscess. The primary disadvantage is that it is inappropriate for lesions in the cerebritis stages, a time during which aspiration can be performed with relative ease. Excision is also ill advised for deep abscesses and those abscesses located in eloquent regions in which excision might run the risk of disabling neurological dysfunction. Finally, multiple lesions are not amenable to excision. Notwithstanding, there are situations in which resection of an abscess is quite logical and in specific circumstances may be distinctly advantageous.[1] Many surgeons favor excision for cerebellar abscesses since failure of treatment for a lesion in this location can lead to rapid deterioration and death. Post-traumatic abscesses often contain retained foreign bodies, particularly bone fragments, that, if not removed, will probably result in recurrence. Excision, if feasible, is more likely to result in a cure in such cases. In cases where an abscess is associated with a CSF leak, operative excision of the abscess and repair of the CSF leak is mandatory. Excision has also been advocated for all abscesses containing gas within the abscess cavity.

Management of multiple brain abscesses

The incidence of multiple brain abscesses ranges from 10% to 50%. However, there is a paucity of literature on the appropriate management of multiple lesions. Various approaches have been suggested, including non-operative management with antibiotics alone, open excision combined with aspiration and antibiotics, and aspiration of a single lesion followed by antibiotics. Multiple repeated aspirations have been recommended when necessary.[1] Based on a review of 22 patients with multiple cerebral abscesses a number of recommendations and conclusions have evolved.[1] If multiple ring-enhancing lesions suspicious for brain abscess are discovered, emergent stereotactic aspiration should preferentially be performed for all lesions exceeding 2.5 cm in diameter. If all of the lesions are under 2.5 cm and are *not* producing mass effect,

then the largest suspected abscess should be aspirated for diagnostic cultures. In general, antibiotics should be withheld until culture material is obtained. Once culture material has been obtained, broad-spectrum antibiotic coverage should be initiated and then modified based on culture and sensitivity results. Antibiotic should be administered for at least 6–8 weeks. In immuno-compromised patients, the duration of therapy may sometimes exceed 1 year. Finally, postoperative imaging (CT or MRI) should be performed weekly or any time there is clinical evidence of deterioration. There should be little hesitation in considering repeated surgical aspiration if there is radiographic evidence of abscess enlargement after 2 weeks of therapy, failure of the abscess to diminish in size after 4 weeks of antibiotics, or in the face of clinical deterioration.[1]

Radiographic follow-up of brain abscesses

It is imperative that physicians involved in treating patients with brain abscess perform frequent clinical and radiographic evaluations. CT scans should be obtained at least weekly during the course of therapy, 1 week after antibiotics are discontinued, followed by a scan 1 month later and then at either monthly or bimonthly intervals until there has been radiographic resolution of the process. Although MRI can also be utilized, it has shown no advantage over CT. However, it is logical to use the same modality throughout the course of the disease in any given patient.

The time course of abscess resolution on CT is variable. In general, radiographic evidence of resolution lags well behind clinical improvement. In most cases, objective evidence of decrease in the size of the abscess first is noticeable 2–3 weeks following initiation of therapy. Complete resolution of the abscess cavity, mass effect, and contrast enhancement may not occur for 3–4 months and occasionally, residual contrast enhancement on CT may persist for up to 6–9 months[23] and even longer on MRI. In one series, it was noted that 20% of patients with persistent enhancement suffered recurrence. In all cases, this occurred within 6 weeks of discontinuation of therapy and discharge from the hospital. However, the majority of patients with residual enhancement do not experience recurrence. The precise cause of this prolonged enhancement is unknown, although it occurs in other conditions such as cerebral infarction. It may represent a non-specific response of the brain to various types of insults. Because the time required for radiographic resolution exceeds the duration of therapy in most cases, residual contrast enhancement should not in and of itself dictate the need for additional therapy. However, these patients bear close observation and follow-up. It should be noted that increase in contrast enhancement is commonly seen in patients who are withdrawn from steroids although, again, this does not necessarily indicate regrowth of the abscess.[23]

Corticosteroids

Corticosteroids continue to be utilized as an adjunct in the management of brain abscess although their use is controversial. Steroids have clearly been shown to reduce the cerebral edema and mass effect which accompany an abscess. However, despite the potential benefit in terms of reduction of mass effect, there may be detrimental side-effects. Overall, steroids tend to decrease both the rate and degree of capsule formation, a process critical to containing the abscess. This can potentially increase the amount of adjacent tissue destruction and negatively impact the outcome. Corticosteroids have also been shown to significantly reduce the degree of contrast enhancement on CT scans, particularly in the cerebritis stages. Therefore, in patients receiving steroids, reduction in contrast enhancement cannot be taken as *a priori* evidence of abscess resolution. In such cases, reduction in the diameter of the ring should be the criterion used to determine that an abscess is indeed regressing. Corticosteroids should be limited to patients who are debilitated by significant cerebral edema and mass effect or to patients in whom the mass effect poses an imminent danger to survival.[1,8] In such cases, steroids should be continued until the neurological condition stabilizes and then tapered rapidly as the clinical condition permits.

Prognosis and outcome of brain abscesses

Advances in diagnosis and treatment have resulted in a drastic reduction in mortality related to brain abscess. Mortality rates as high as 50% were commonplace in the older literature but are now the exception rather than the rule. The reduction in mortality has been attributed to a number of factors related to both diagnosis and management that have already been discussed. However, despite the significant reduction in mortality, brain abscess remains a serious illness that can result in death if misdiagnosed or managed improperly. Several factors influence mortality and outcome in this disease. With a trend toward non-surgical management there is sometimes an inappropriate delay in operative intervention that can result in death from herniation related to increased ICP or from rupture of the abscess into the ventricular system or subarachnoid space resulting in ependymitis or meningitis. Herniation can be avoided by identifying patients before they develop significant alteration in mentation. If these changes are discovered sufficiently early stereotactic drainage of the abscess cavity will immediately reduce the mass effect. Intraventricular rupture can be prevented by prompt drainage of deep-seated abscesses that are situated close to the ventricular system. Previously, intraventricular rupture was almost always fatal and although it remains a serious complication, it can frequently be managed with external ventricular drainage along with intraventricular antibiotics.

Even successfully treated brain abscesses can result in long-term neurological sequelae and disability. Long-term morbidity is most frequently related to seizures, cognitive dysfunction, and focal neurological deficits. Epilepsy is a common sequel of brain abscess; most series report an incidence of 30–50%. It has been suggested that the risk of developing late seizures is related to the location of the abscess although this has not been substantiated. Additionally, a trend toward reduction in seizures has been reported in patients treated with aspiration as opposed to excision.[8] Epilepsy that develops subsequent to a brain abscess can usually be controlled relatively easily with anticonvulsants. Those which are intractable to maximum medical therapy may sometimes be amenable to resection of the seizure focus. Given the high likelihood of developing seizures, all patients with supratentorial brain abscesses should probably be placed on prophylactic anticonvulsants. In the absence of seizures, the duration of therapy is unclear. However, a reasonable approach would be to continue anticonvulsants for at least 12 months following which they may be tapered providing the electroencephalogram shows no epileptogenic activity.

Recurrence of the abscess is seen in 5–10% of patients despite what is considered adequate therapy. Most recurrences become apparent within 6 weeks following therapy although recurrences have been reported many years following therapy. Reasons for recurrence include inadequate antibiotic therapy, incorrect choice of antibiotics, failure to aspirate large abscesses, presence of a retained foreign body or dural fistula, and failure to eradicate underlying sources of infection.

SPINAL EPIDURAL ABSCESS

Spinal epidural abscess (SEA) is a suppurative process, which may occur independently or in association with vertebral osteomyelitis. The first description of SEA was that of Morgagni in 1769[24] although it was not until well into this century that the condition was regularly recognized in living patients. Dandy was the first to comment on the regional distribution of SEA within the spinal axis.[25] He noted that the majority of cases of SEA were confined to the thoracic spine and that most occurred dorsally within the spinal canal. This observation has been confirmed in most published series on SEA.[26–29]

The most important anatomical factor is the regional variation in the size of the epidural space. In the cervical spine it is more of a potential space. The space becomes more apparent at the cervicothoracic junction and becomes wider in a rostral to caudal direction. Its maximum depth is between 0.5 and 0.75 cm between the fourth and eight thoracic segments. The space then tapers between approximately T11 and L2 caudal to which the epidural space attains its greatest depth.

These anatomical factors not only account for the rostral-caudal distribution of abscesses, but also for their preference for the dorsal epidural space. Posterior abscesses frequently result from hematogenous seeding of the epidural space from a distant site of infection. Because of the lack of resistance to rostral-caudal spread, abscesses located posteriorly may extend over several vertebral segments. In contrast, abscesses which occur ventrally are often associated with osteomyelitis and longitudinal extension over several segments is restricted by the adherence of the dura.[30,31] However, because of adherence of the dura, anterior abscesses are also more likely to penetrate the dura and lead to subdural empyema and/or spinal cord abscess.[30]

Risk factors and underlying disorders in spinal epidural abscess

A number of underlying illnesses and risk factors can be identified in patients with SEA. Hlavin *et al.* identified risk factors associated with altered immune status in over 50% of patients in their series.[29] These included diabetes mellitus, alcoholism, chronic renal failure, and underlying malignancy. The role of intravenous drug abuse as an underlying risk factor for infection has also been well documented. Although the number of patients with the human immunodeficiency virus has been rising, there does not seem to have been a concomitant rise in the incidence of SEA in this population.

Etiology and pathogenesis of spinal epidural abscess

Suppuration within the epidural space can arise in three ways: (1) by direct extension from a contiguous site of infection such as vertebral body osteomyelitis, (2) by hematogenous seeding from a distant source of infection, or (3) by direct contamination during procedures such as spinal surgery, administration of an epidural anesthetic, CT-guided needle biopsy, or lumbar puncture.[26,29,31]

A definitive etiology for a SEA is apparent in 50–80% of

patients.[28,29,32,33] The most frequent cause of SEA is hematogenous seeding of the epidural space from a metastatic source of infection, most commonly a skin or soft tissue focus.[28,29,34] Other common metastatic sources of infection include urinary or respiratory tract infections, intra-abdominal abscesses, subacute bacterial endocarditis, and septic arthritis. SEA not infrequently occurs as a complication of vertebral body osteomyelitis.[31–33,35,36]

Pathophysiology of epidural suppuration

The neurological deficit which results from SEA has been attributed to a variety of factors including mechanical compression of the cord, thrombosis of major arteries and veins supplying and draining the cord respectively, impairment of the intrinsic microcirculation of the cord, and infectious vasculitis.[30,32,33] The relative lack of correlative histopathological data make it difficult to define the exact pathophysiology in many cases.

SEA is a space-occupying lesion; therefore, mechanical compression would be the most obvious explanation for the neurological deficit, which occurs. Although mechanical compression is certainly a contributory factor, it alone does not adequately explain the often profound deficit associated with SEA.

To explain the precipitous onset of neurological deficit, some authors have hypothesized a vascular mechanism.[3,33,37,38] Browder and Meyers observed that the vessels of the pia and spinal cord were commonly congested and in some cases were thrombosed.[39] Baker and colleagues found inflammation and thrombosis of many small arteries and veins within the subarachnoid space.[32] They also noted inflammatory infiltrates in the pia directly involving the walls of blood vessels as well as organizing material within the lumen of the anterior spinal artery.

Clinical presentation and differential diagnosis

One of the most important aspects in the diagnosis of SEA is its variable presentation. Early findings may be subtle and overshadowed by other underlying problems that dominate the clinical picture making diagnosis more difficult. Therefore, one must have a high index of suspicion to make the diagnosis early and accurately and thereby prevent the development of neurological dysfunction. Heusner has described the classical clinical presentation of SEA as having four phases which evolve in sequence: (1) spinal pain; (2) radicular pain; (3) muscular weakness, sensory loss, sphincter dysfunction; and finally (4) complete paralysis.[33] The rapidity with which one stage progresses to another in a given patient will depend on the factors outlined above. With hematogenous seeding progression from spinal to radicular pain and neurological dysfunction is relatively rapid and systemic manifestations are often a prominent part of the clinical picture. On the other hand, cases secondary to vertebral osteomyelitis have a tendency to evolve more slowly and may take weeks or even months to become clinically apparent.[31,33,40]

Spinal pain is almost universally present with SEA and is most often associated with localized spinal tenderness to palpation or percussion.[28,29,40] Once spinal pain occurs, it often becomes progressively more severe and intractable. Over 90% of patients also develop radicular pain; this usually follows the onset of back pain by approximately 2 to 3 days but in some cases may precede the development of spinal pain.[40] Depending on the spinal level of involvement, root pain may mimic a variety of other conditions including classic sciatica due a herniated disc, acute abdominal processes, Herpes zoster as well as a variety of other conditions.[28]

Fever in excess of 38°C occurs at some point during the course of the illness in between two-thirds and three-quarters of patients irrespective of whether the presentation is acute or more chronic. In patients with a more chronic clinical course, constitutional symptoms such as weight loss and malaise are not unusual.[26,29] Headache and nuchal rigidity may also be present, reflecting either a parameningeal reaction or, rarely, frank meningitis.[29,33,40] In children, it must be cautioned that the characteristic features of SEA may not be prominent and the clinical picture may be dominated by nonspecific findings such as fever, malaise, irritability, headache, and vomiting.[41] Reluctance of the child to lie prone, irritability with movement, and rigidity of the spine may be the only clues to the diagnosis prior to the onset of neurological deficit.

Unfortunately, the diagnosis of SEA is all too frequently made after the onset of neurological dysfunction which occurs in as many as 90% of patients in some series.[29,32,42] Up to 75% of patients with SEA may have some degree of motor weakness, which may be unilateral, bilateral, or involve a single extremity. Sensory loss is usually incomplete and may occur in a radicular pattern or present as a discrete sensory level. However, complete loss of all sensory modalities with a discrete sensory level is associated with a very poor prognosis. The point at which neurological dysfunction begins is especially critical because once initiated, the time from onset of weakness to complete paralysis is often less than 24 hours and can occur in as little as 30 minutes.[29] This rapid progression emphasizes the need for rapid diagnosis and emergent surgical intervention. Indeed, the patient who presents with a chronic clinical course should not engender a feeling of complacency in the clinician as these patients can also deteriorate rapidly.

Although one must necessarily maintain a high index of suspicion for SEA, other more common conditions do occur which share the clinical features of epidural infection. Acute transverse myelitis should be part of the differential diagnosis in patients with back pain, fever, and progressive neurological deficit.[43] This disease is eight to 20 times more common than SEA. It usually differs from SEA in that back pain is somewhat less prominent and the progression to maximum neurological deficit is often more rapid than in SEA. The two can usually be differentiated on myelography, which is normal in cases of transverse myelitis but classically shows a subtotal to complete block in SEA. Most patients with transverse myelitis recover without specific treatment.

Metastatic neoplasms to the spine frequently invade the epidural space and may present a picture similar to a chronic epidural abscess. In particular, lymphoma may metastasize to the spine in up to 5% of cases; fever and systemic manifestations that are common with lymphoma may further complicate the clinical picture.

Bacteriology of spinal epidural abscess

The microbiological profile of SEA depends on a number of factors including the etiology of infection as well as the immunologic status of the host. Overall, *Staphylococcus aureus* is the organism most often isolated from patients harboring a SEA, accounting for 45–95% of cases.[26,28,29,32,33,37] *Staphylococcus aureus* is implicated in the majority of cases secondary to skin and soft tissue infections, cases related to intravenous drug use, and infections which occur as a sequel to spinal surgery.[26,29,42,44] It is also the most common organism isolated in cases occurring in young children.[41] Other Gram-positive cocci, such as *Staphylococcus epidermidis*, *Streptococcus pneumoniae*, and *Streptococcus viridans*, account for an additional 10% of cases.[28] In recent years, Gram-negative aerobes (*Escherichia coli*, *Pseudomonas aeruginosa*, *Klebsiella pneumoniae*, *Citrobacter* sp.) have accounted for a larger percentage of cases than in earlier series.[28] Anaerobic organisms have also been implicated in a small percentage of cases. Although not as prevalent as in earlier series, *Mycobacterium tuberculosis* continues to play an important role in this disease and in some large urban series accounts for nearly one-quarter of cases.[45] A number of less common organisms have also been implicated in SEA including atypical bacteria such as *Nocardia* and *Actinomyces israelii* and the gas-forming anaerobic organism *Clostridium perfringens*. Cases that are the result of infection with *Echinococcus*, *Cryptococcus*, *Brucella*, *Listeria*, *Blastomyces*, and *Aspergillus* have also been reported.[28,29,34]

Laboratory findings

Routine laboratory studies in patients with SEA are quite non-specific; in fact, no one laboratory study is pathognomonic of this condition. The majority of patients have a mild leukocytosis (10 000–13 000 mm^3) and an elevated sedimentation rate, usually in excess of 30 mm/hour. Blood cultures are positive in as many as 67% of patients.[29,46] If a lumbar puncture is performed, the CSF usually shows evidence of a parameningeal process manifested by pleocytosis, elevated protein, and normal glucose. However, the CSF can also be entirely normal or may reveal frank pus consistent with accompanying bacterial meningitis.[29]

Radiographic diagnosis

The cornerstone of diagnosis of SEA lies in contemporary neuroimaging studies, which, in the appropriate clinical setting, are confirmatory of SEA.[46] Plain radiographs of the spine may be normal or may demonstrate evidence of vertebral osteo-myelitis.[31,32] CT may better define the destructive bony changes and may be more sensitive in detecting subtle osseous changes not apparent on plain radiographs. Leys *et al.* reported the successful identification of five cases of SEA using plain CT alone; however, despite the optimistic report of these authors it is generally felt that CT is not particularly sensitive for demonstrating SEA.[45] Traditionally, the gold standard for the diagnosis of SEA has been myelography.[28,32] MRI has been shown to possess sensitivity equivalent to CT-myelography.[47] Additionally, MRI can readily exclude many entities included in the differential diagnosis, such as herniated disc, neoplasm, spinal hematoma, and transverse myelitis. MRI also provides greater anatomical detail in demon-strating the rostral-caudal extent of the lesion. In most cases, the T1- and T2-weighted images will display the abscess equally well.[47]

Treatment

Traditionally, SEA has been managed by surgery as soon as the diagnosis is made.[26,29,32,34,35] Surgery has been followed by aggressive antibiotic therapy of variable duration.[26,28,35] Surgical management of SEA has a number of advantages. Most important is the ability to decompress compromised neural tissues, thereby preventing further neurological deterioration. Devitalized tissue which acts as a nidus for infection can also be removed, which allows antibiotics to function more efficiently. Additionally, intraoperative cultures taken from the epidural space are the most

rewarding in terms of yielding the offending organism and in many cases may be the only source from which the organism can be cultured. This can be extremely important in terms of choosing the appropriate antibiotic regimen.

The type of surgical procedure chosen will depend on the site of neural compression. Under most circumstances, the procedure should be directed at the site of maximal compression. For abscesses located posteriorly, a laminectomy over the involved levels will generally provide adequate decompression. However, in patients with concomitant osteomyelitis and significant vertebral body destruction, extensive laminectomy must be used with caution as this may destabilize the spine.[31,48] When the abscess and compression are located ventrally, an anterior approach may be more suitable. Anterior cervical abscesses, which are usually associated with osteomyelitis, are ideally managed with a standard anterior cervical approach.[31,48] Anterior abscesses located in the thoracic and lumbar regions may be approached through a trans-pedicular approach, a posterolateral approach such as a costo-transversectomy, or through a transcavitary or lateral extracavitary approach.[49] In rare cases, a combined anterior and posterior approach may be necessary. Reconstruction of the spine should ideally be accomplished with autologous bone. The use of spinal instrumentation under these circumstances is controversial. Some authors have reported the successful use of instrumentation without sequelae as long as all obviously infected material has been removed.[31,48] It would seem that if there is a significant issue regarding spinal stability, that the use of instrumentation is certainly justified. Notwithstanding, there are still spine surgeons who believe that the presence of any degree of infection is a contraindication to the use of spinal implants.

Intravenous antibiotics specific for the offending organism should be initiated as soon as possible. If the organism has yet to be identified, then antibiotic coverage should be tailored according to the most likely organism based on the presumed etiology of infection. If there is no apparent etiology, institution of empiric therapy with an anti-staphylococcal agent along with broad-spectrum coverage for Gram-negative aerobes should be given. The duration of antibiotic therapy recommended in the literature has been variable. However, most authors advocate a 4–6-week course of intravenous antibiotics.[28,35,36] In the presence of vertebral osteomyelitis the duration of intravenous therapy should be extended to from 6 to 8 weeks.[31] Some authors[26] recommend additional oral therapy for up to several months although the efficacy and requirement for this is unclear.[50]

Although SEA has traditionally been considered a surgical disease, some authors have advocated conservative treatment of this condition, particularly in patients who are neurologically intact as well as selected patients in whom the surgical morbidity is unacceptable high.[45,51,52] This approach is predicated on early identification of the organism such that specific antibiotic therapy can be initiated. In selected patients who are neurologically intact, this may be a reasonable approach. However, these patients require vigilant monitoring as neurologic deterioration is not uncommon despite being on appropriate antibiotic therapy.[26,29,32] Any sign of neurological deficit should prompt one to abandon conservative therapy and proceed with surgical intervention.

Outcome

The ability to diagnose SEA in a timely fashion, coupled with improvements in antibiotics and surgical techniques have all resulted in a steady decline in mortality rates.[28,33] Despite these

CLINICAL PEARLS

- The diagnosis and management of pyogenic brain abscess has been revolutionized by contemporary neuroimaging techniques. When available, MRI represents the imaging modality of choice. The ability to perform diffusion weighting along with MR spectroscopy during the same examination adds to the diagnostic capabilities provided by MRI.

- Except for some exceptional cases noted previously, most patients with brain abscess should undergo surgery at least to obtain cultures that will assist in tailoring antibiotic therapy. Stereotactic aspiration is ideal in that it is minimally invasive, can be accomplished safely even in very ill patients, and allows for decompression of multiple lesions.

- Antibiotic therapy should be given for at least 6 weeks and should ideally be based on identification of the organism from the abscess itself. Close clinical and radiographic follow-up is critical to identify and treat recurrences. However, it is important to remember that radiographic improvement can be considerably slower than clinical improvement.

- Residual enhancement can persist for many months even following the successful treatment and resolution of a brain abscess.

- Spinal epidural abscess can no longer be considered rare or unusual. The incidence may be increasing. The diagnosis of spinal epidural abscess can sometimes be difficult and one needs to maintain a high index of suspicion in patients at risk. The diagnosis is most easily made with MRI, which is the imaging modality of choice In general, cervical and thoracic abscesses require surgical management. In many cases, an epidural abscess is associated with vertebral osteomyelitis. The issue of utilizing spinal instrumentation in the face of an active infection remains controversial. It would seem that in circumstances where surgical decompression will result in obvious spinal instability, that the advantages and benefits of spinal instrumentation may outweigh disadvantages and risks. Notwithstanding, the decision to use instrumentation under these circumstances should be made on a case-by-case basis.

advances the mortality rate has remained unacceptably high.[29,42] In addition, 20–32% of patients who survive will be left with significant neurological impairment resulting in long-term disability.[46]

The outcome of patients who survive depends primarily on the degree and duration of neurological impairment at the time of diagnosis. Not surprisingly, patients with severe neurological deficit have a much poorer prognosis than do patients who are neurologically intact.[26,28,29,34] Some authors have also pointed out that patients with a more chronic clinical course have a better prognosis than do patients who present with a rapid tempo.[32,33] Based on the literature, it cannot be sufficiently stressed that the single most important factor in reducing mortality and permanent neurological morbidity is early diagnosis and institution of treatment prior to the onset of any neurological deficit.

This chapter contains material from the first edition, and we are grateful to the authors of that chapter for their contribution.

REFERENCES

1. Gormley W, Rosenblum M. Cerebral abscess. In: Tindall G, Cooper P, Barrow D (eds). *The Practice of Neurosurgery*. Philadelphia: Lippincott Williams & Wilkins; 1996: 3343–54.

2. Tunkel A, Wispelwey B, Scheld W. Brain abscess. In: Mandell G, Bennett J, Dolin R (eds). *Principles and Practice of Infectious Diseases*. Philadelphia: Churchill Livingstone; 2000: 1016–27.

3. Kole M, Rosenblum M. Bacterial brain abscess. In: McCutcheon I, Hall W (eds). *Infections in Neurosurgery, American Association of Neurological Surgeons, Neurosurgical Topics Series*. Rolling Meadows, IL: American Association of Neurological Surgeons; 2001: 23–32.

4. Sharma B, Khosia V, Kak V, *et al*. Multiple pyogenic brain abscesses. *Acta Neurochirurg* 1995; 133: 36–43.

5. Sabiha P, Farida J, Cheah F. Microbiology of cerebral abscess: a four-year study in Malaysia. *J Tropical Med Hygiene* 1993; 96: 191–6.

6. Ciura A, Stocia F, Vasilescu G, *et al*. Neurosurgical management of brain abscesses in children. *Child's Nervous System* 1999; 15: 309–17.

7. Hall W. Neurosurgical infections in the compromised host. *Neurosurg Clin N Am* 1992; 3: 345–52.

8. Osenbach R, Loftus C. Diagnosis and management of brain abscess. *Neurosurg Clin N Am* 1992; 3: 403–20.

9. Graham DR, Band JD. Citrobacter diversus brain abscess and meningitis in neonates. *JAMA* 1981; 245: 1923–5.

10. Britt R, Enzmann D. Clinical stages of human brain abscess on serial CT scans after contrast infusion: computed tomographic, neuropathological, and clinical correlations. *J Neurosurg* 1982; 59: 972–89.

11. Britt R. Brain abscess. In: Wilkins RH, Rengachary SS (eds). *Neurosurgery*. New York: McGraw-Hill; 1985: 1928–56.

12. Cure J. Imaging of intracranial infection. In: Batjer H, Loftus CM (eds). *Textbook of Neurological Surgery*. Philadelphia: Lippincott Williams & Wilkins; 2003; 3108–30.

13. Rehncrona S, Brismar J, Holtas S. Diagnosis of brain abscess with indium-111-labelled leukocytes. *Neurosurgery* 1985; 16: 23–6.

14. Bellotti C, Aragno MG, Medina M, *et al*. Differential diagnosis of CT-hypodense cranial lesions with indium-111-oxine-labeled leukocytes. *J Neurosurg* 1986; 64: 750–3.

15. Rousseaux M, Lesoin F, Destee A, *et al*. Developments in the treatment and prognosis of multiple cerebral abscesses. *Neurosurgery* 1985; 16: 304–8.

16. Heinemann HS, Braude AI. Intracranial suppurative disease. *JAMA* 1971; 218: 1542–7.

17. Rosenblum ML, Mampalam TJ, Pons V. Controversies in the management of brain abscess. *Clin Neurosurg* 1987; 33: 603–32.

18. Takeshita M, Kagawa M, Izawa M, *et al*. Current treatment strategies and factors influencing outcome in patients with bacterial brain abscess. *Acta Neurochirurg* 1998; 140: 1263–70.

19. DeLouvois J, Gortavi P, Hurley R. The bacteriology and chemotherapy of brain abscess. *J Antimicrob Chemother* 1978; 4: 395–413.

20. Barlas O, Sencer A, Erkan K, *et al*. Stereotactic surgery in the management of brain abscess. *Surg Neurol* 1999; 52: 404–11.

21. Stephanov S. Surgical treatment of brain abscess. *Neurosurgery* 1988; 22: 724–30.

22. Taylor J. The case for excision of in the treatment of brain abscess. *Br J Neurosurg* 1987; 1: 173–8.

23. Whelan MA, Hilal SK. Computed tomography as a guide in the diagnosis and follow-up of brain abscesses. *Radiology* 1980; 135: 663–71.

24. Morgagni GB. *The Seats and Causes of Diseases, Investigated by Anatomy* [translated from the Latin by B Alexander, 1769]. New York Academy of Medicine Library, History of Medicine Series 13. New York: Hafner; 1960: vol. I, letter X, article 13, 220–22.

25. Dandy WE. Abscess and inflammatory tumors in the spinal epidural space (so-called pachymeningitis externa). *Arch Surg* 1936; 13: 477–94.

26. Curling OD, Gower DJ, McWhorter JM. Changing concepts in spinal epidural abscess: a report of 29 cases. *Neurosurgery* 1990; 27: 185–92.

27. Dacey RG, Winn HR, Jane JA, *et al*. Spinal subdural empyema: report of two cases. *Neurosurgery* 1978; 3: 400–3.

28. Danner RL, Hartman BJ. Update of spinal epidural abscess:35 cases and review of the literature. *Rev Infect Dis* 1987; 9: 265–74.

29. Hlavin ML, Kaminski HJ, Ross JS, *et al*. Spinal epidural abscess: a ten-year perspective. *Neurosurgery* 1990; 27: 177–84.

30. Hulme A, Dott NM. Spinal epidural abscess. *Br Med J* 1954; 1: 64–8.

31. Osenbach RK, Hitchon PW, Menezes AH. Diagnosis and management of pyogenic vertebral osteomyelitis in adults. *Surg Neurol* 1990; 33: 266–75.

32. Baker AS, Ojemann RG, Schwartz MN, *et al*. Spinal epidural abscess. *N Engl J Med* 1975; 293: 463–8.

33. Heusner AP. Nontuberculous spinal epidural infections. *N Engl J Med* 1948; 239: 845–54.

34. Ravicovitch MA, Spallone A. Spinal epidural abscess. Surgical and parasurgical management. *Eur Neurol* 1982; 21: 347–57.

35. Ericsson M, Algers G, Schliamser SE. Spinal epidural abscess in adults: review and report of iatrogenic cases. *Scand J Infect Dis* 1990; 22: 249–57.

36. Hitchon PW, Osenbach RK, Yuh TC, *et al*. Spinal infections. *Clin Neurosurg* 1992; 38: 373–90.

37. Russell NA, Vaughan R, Morley TP. Spinal epidural infection. *Can J Neurol Sci* 1979; 6: 325–8.

38. Feldenzer JA, McKeever PE, Schaberg DR, *et al*. The pathogenesis of spinal epidural abscess; microangiographic studies in an experimental model. *J Neurosurg* 1988; 69: 110–14.

39. Browder J, Meyers R. Pyogenic infections of the spinal epidural space. A consideration of the anatomic and physiologic pathology. *Surgery* 1947; 10: 296–308.

40. Verner EF, Musher DM. Spinal epidural abscess. Symposium on infections of the central nervous system. *Med Clin North Am* 1985; 69: 375–84.

41. Fischer EG, Greene CS, Winston KR. Spinal epidural abscess in children. *Neurosurgery* 1981; 9: 257–60.

42. Kaufman DM, Kaplan JG, Litman N. Infectious agents in spinal epidural abscesses. *Neurology* 1980; 30: 844–50.

43. Altrocchi PH. Acute spinal epidural abscess vs. acute transverse myelopathy. *Arch Neurol* 1963; 9: 17–25.

44. Koppel BS, Tuchman AJ, Mangiardi JR, *et al*. Epidural spinal infection in intravenous drug abusers. *Arch Neurol* 1988; 45: 1331–7.

45. Leys D, Lesoin F, Viaud C, *et al*. Decreased morbidity from acute bacterial spinal epidural abscesses using computed tomography and nonsurgical treatment in selected patients. *Ann Neurol* 1985; 17: 350–5.

46. Kraus WE, McCormick PC. Infections of the dural spaces. *Neurosurg Clin N Am* 1992; 3: 421–34.

47. Antuaco EJ, McConnell JR, Chadduck WM, *et al*. MR imaging of spinal epidural sepsis. *AJNR* 1987; 8: 879–83.

48. Eismont FJ, Bohlman HB, Prasanna SL, *et al*. Pyogenic and fungal vertebral osteomyelitis with paralysis. *J Bone Joint Surg* 1983; 65A: 19–29.

49. Vincent KA, Benson DR. Infectious diseases of the spine. Surgical treatment. In: Frymoyer JW (ed.). *The Adult Spine: Principles and Practice*. New York, NY: Raven Press; 1991: 787–809.

50. Sapico FL, Montgomerie JZ. Pyogenic vertebral osteomyelitis: report of nine cases and review of the literature. *Rev Infect Dis* 1979; 1: 754–76.

51. Mampalam TJ, Rosegay H, Andrews BT, *et al*. Nonoperative treatment of spinal epidural infections. *J Neurosurg* 1989; 71: 208–10.

52. Messer Hd, Lenchner GS, Brust JC, *et al*. Lumbar spinal abscess managed conservatively. Case report. *J Neurosurg* 1977; 46: 825–9.

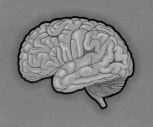

NEURO-ONCOLOGY: AN OVERVIEW

29

Michael Lim and Griffith R Harsh IV

Neuro-oncology is the study of tumors of the nervous system. A brain tumor can be defined at several levels (Figure 29.1).

1 Clinical: an intracranial neoplastic mass that because of size or location causes symptoms of mass effect or neurologic deficit.
2 Tissue: a group of cells and associated extracellular matrix whose growth exceeds and is uncoordinated with that of normal tissue;[1] as a result, tumors are often highly cellular and disrupt normal tissue architecture.
3 Cellular: individual cells altered in size, shape, nuclear to cytoplasmic ratio, nuclear appearance, and cytoplasmic organelles; as tumors become more malignant, features of cellular anaplasia become more pronounced and those of differentiation less apparent.
4 Biochemical: an altered assortment of regulatory and functional proteins that causes changes of cell structure and metabolism.
5 Immunologic: a set of epitopes that distinguishes neoplastic from normal cells.
6 Chromosomal: karyotypes that may appear normal or may have either aneuploid or polyploid abnormalities; integral changes in the number of chromosomes may be accompanied by amplification, deletion, and translocation of certain chromosomal segments.
7 Genetic: a constellation of alterations in DNA base sequence that changes either the expression of genes that normally regulate cell proliferation or the structure of the proteins these genes encode.

Primary intracranial tumors may arise from cells of the brain parenchyma or from its intracranial linings. Secondary intracranial tumors may arise in the skull or neighboring structures and extend through the skull or cranial foramina, or they may arise at distant sites and spread hematogenously to the brain or dura; both primary and metastatic tumors may be intra-axial, extra-axial, or both (Figure 29.2). Intra-axial tumors are located primarily within the brain parenchyma or ventricular system, whereas extra-axial tumors are located in the subarachnoid space or meninges. Unlike most systemic malignancies, primary brain tumors rarely metastasize to other regions of the body.

CLASSIFICATION OF BRAIN TUMORS

A classification scheme is valuable to the extent that it permits accurate predictions regarding the natural history of the disease and the response to therapy. Grouping together tumors with similar etiologies and neoplastic mechanisms is fundamental to

both preventive and therapeutic efforts. Ideally, a classification scheme should integrate clinical, tissue, cellular, biochemical, immunologic, chromosomal, and genetic criteria.

Classification by cell type

Traditional classifications of brain tumors are based on the premise that each type of tumor results from the abnormal growth of a specific cell type. This is the basis of the original classification of brain tumors by Bailey and Cushing[2] and is fundamental to the widely used World Health Organization (WHO) system (Table 29.1).[3] The nomenclature of these systems reflects this choice (e.g. astrocytomas are tumors of astrocytes). Categorization relies primarily on patterns of tissue and cellular histology identified by light microscopy.[3] Immunohistochemistry using monoclonal antibodies against structural proteins that serve as markers for specialized cell types has increased the specificity. Electron microscopy has also proven a valuable adjunct in cases where the basic cell type can be more accurately identified by the presence of specialized organelles (e.g. secretory granules in pituitary tumors).[4]

Difficulties with these classification systems arise when the tumor consists of more than one cell type or when the predominant cell type cannot easily be related to a normal adult cell type.[4] Cellular heterogeneity can occur to various degrees and may manifest a variety of mechanisms. The two cell types may be derived from different germ layers; this may occur as a result of differentiation within a germ cell tumor or after transformation of the stromal element of a glioma in the genesis of a gliosarcoma. The two cell types may be derived from a common precursor of the same germ layer (mixed malignant gliomas have both astrocytic and oligodendroglial elements). Multiple cell types may result from genotypic and consequent phenotypic evolution within the tumor (a glioblastoma may contain areas of lower degrees of malignancy).[4] Difficulties in relating the predominant cell type of a tumor to a normal cell type most commonly occur when the tumor consists of relatively primitive or undifferentiated cells (e.g. primitive neuroectodermal and embryonal cell tumors).

Grading the degree of malignancy

Tumors associated with a particular cell type can differ remarkably in their histologic and cytologic characteristics and in their clinical behavior. Clinically malignant central nervous system (CNS) tumors grow rapidly; they invade and destroy surrounding normal tissue but, unlike most systemic malignancies, they seldom metastasize. They often induce the formation of new blood vessels and produce areas of necrosis. Such changes are called tissue

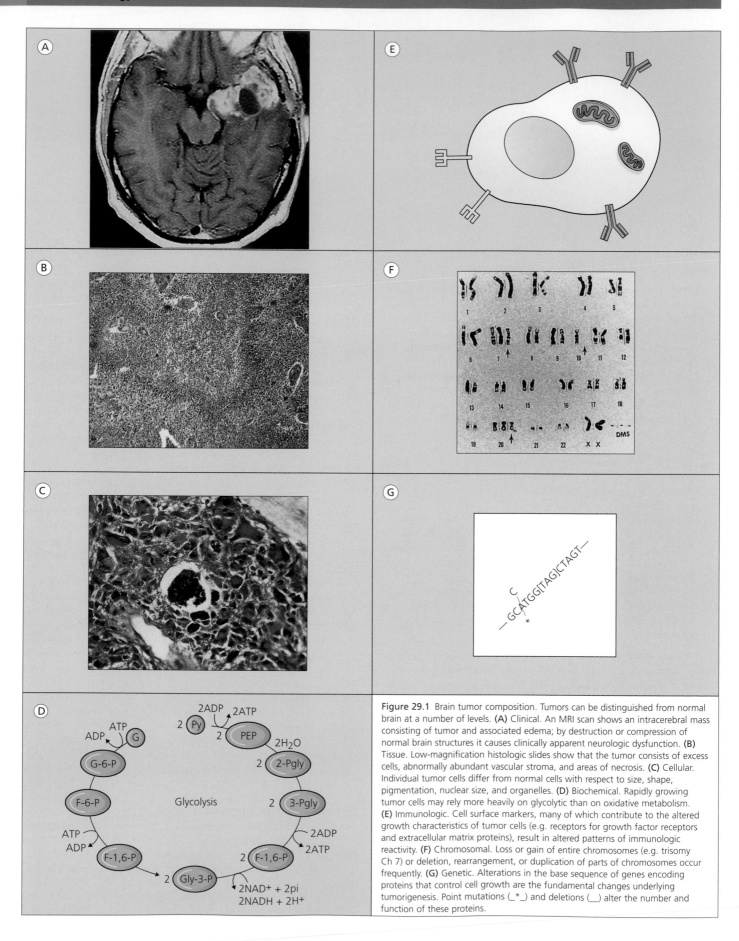

Figure 29.1 Brain tumor composition. Tumors can be distinguished from normal brain at a number of levels. **(A)** Clinical. An MRI scan shows an intracerebral mass consisting of tumor and associated edema; by destruction or compression of normal brain structures it causes clinically apparent neurologic dysfunction. **(B)** Tissue. Low-magnification histologic slides show that the tumor consists of excess cells, abnormally abundant vascular stroma, and areas of necrosis. **(C)** Cellular. Individual tumor cells differ from normal cells with respect to size, shape, pigmentation, nuclear size, and organelles. **(D)** Biochemical. Rapidly growing tumor cells may rely more heavily on glycolytic than on oxidative metabolism. **(E)** Immunologic. Cell surface markers, many of which contribute to the altered growth characteristics of tumor cells (e.g. receptors for growth factor receptors and extracellular matrix proteins), result in altered patterns of immunologic reactivity. **(F)** Chromosomal. Loss or gain of entire chromosomes (e.g. trisomy Ch 7) or deletion, rearrangement, or duplication of parts of chromosomes occur frequently. **(G)** Genetic. Alterations in the base sequence of genes encoding proteins that control cell growth are the fundamental changes underlying tumorigenesis. Point mutations (_*_) and deletions (_) alter the number and function of these proteins.

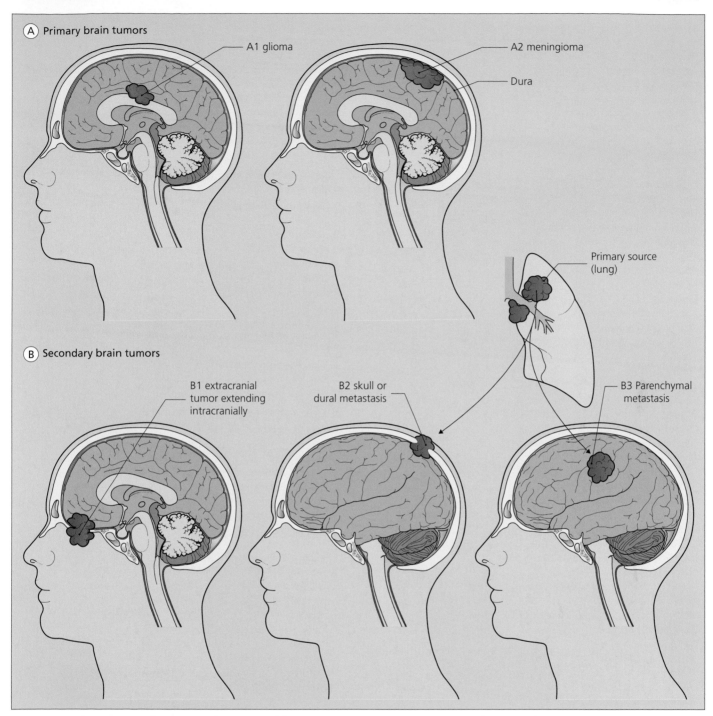

Figure 29.2 Primary or secondary, intra-axial or extra-axial brain tumors. Primary brain tumors, arising from cells of the brain parenchyma (e.g. gliomas, A1) or its meninges (e.g. meningiomas, A2), may be intra-axial or extra-axial, respectively. Secondary brain tumors that spread to the brain by local extension (e.g. esthesioneuroblastomas, B1, or skull metastasis) are extra-axial; those that spread hematogenously may be either extra-axial (e.g. dural-based metastasis, B2) or intra-axial (e.g. parenchymal metastasis, B3).

anaplasia. Cellular abnormalities, such as hypercellularity and an increased number of mitotic figures, also correlate with rapid growth. These and other cytologic features of rapid growth, including variability in cell size and shape, relative lack of cytoplasmic differentiation, and hyperchromatic, pleomorphic nuclei, are called cellular anaplasia.[4]

The correspondence between tissue and cellular anaplasia and malignant clinical behavior has led some classification systems to use the terms interchangeably. The strength of the correlation between histology and clinical behavior varies among tumor types. For ependymomas, the distinction between histologically benign and histologically malignant tumor has little prognostic value. For

Table 29.1 WHO histologic classification of tumors of the central nervous system

TUMORS OF NEUROEPITHELIAL TISSUE
Astrocytic tumors
Diffuse astrocytoma
  fibrillary astrocytoma
  protoplasmic astrocytoma
  gemistocytic astrocytoma
Anaplastic astrocytoma
Glioblastoma
  giant cell glioblastoma
  gliosarcoma
Pilocytic astrocytoma
Pleomorphic xanthoastrocytoma
Subependymal giant cell astrocytoma
Oligodendroglial tumors
Oligodendroglioma
Anaplastic oligodendroglioma
Mixed gliomas
Oligoastrocytoma
Anaplastic oligoastrocytoma
Ependymal tumors
Ependymoma
  cellular
  papillary
  clear cell
  tanycytic
Anaplastic ependymoma
Myxopapillary ependymoma
Subependymoma
Choroid plexus tumors
Choroid plexus papilloma
Choroid plexus carcinoma
Glial tumors of uncertain origin
Astroblastoma
Gliomatosis cerebri
Chordoid glioma of the third ventricle
Neuronal and mixed neuronal-glial tumors
Gangliocytoma
Dysplastic gangliocytoma of cerebellum
(Lhermitte–Duclos)
Desmoplastic infantile astrocytoma/ganglioglioma
Dysembryoplastic neuroepithelial tumor
Ganglioglioma
Anaplastic ganglioglioma
Central neurocytoma
Cerebellar liponeurocytoma
Paraganglioma of the filum terminale
Neuroblastic tumors
Olfactory neuroblastoma
(Esthesioneuroblastoma)
Olfactory neuroepithelioma
Neuroblastomas of the adrenal gland and sympathetic nervous system
Pineal parenchymal tumors
Pineocytoma
Pineoblastoma
Pineal parenchymal tumor of intermediate differentiation
Embryonal tumors
Medulloepithelioma
Ependymoblastoma

Medulloblastoma
  desmoplastic medulloblastoma
  large cell medulloblastoma
  melanotic medulloblastoma
Supratentorial primitive neuroectodermal tumor (PNET)
  neuroblastoma
  ganglioneuroblastoma
Atypical teratoid/rhabdoid tumor

TUMORS OF PERIPHERAL NERVES
Schwannoma
(Neurilemmoma, Neurinoma)
  cellular
  plexiform
  melanotic
Neurofibroma
  plexiform
Perineurioma
  intraneural
  soft tissue
Malignant peripheral nerve sheath tumor (MPNST)
  epithelioid
  MPNST with divergent mesenchymal and/or epithelial differentiation
  melanotic
  melanotic psammomatous

TUMORS OF THE MENINGES
Tumors of meningothelial cells
Meningioma
  meningothelial
  fibrous (fibroblastic)
  transitional (mixed)
  psammomatous
  angiomatous
  microcystic
  secretory
  lymphoplasmacyte-rich
  metaplastic
  clear cell
  chordoid
  atypical
  papillary
  rhabdoid
  anaplastic meningioma
Mesenchymal, non-meningothelial tumors
Lipoma
Angiolipoma
Hibernoma
Liposarcoma (intracranial)
Solitary fibrous tumor
Fibrosarcoma
Malignant fibrous histiocytoma
Leiomyoma
Leiomyosarcoma
Rhabdomyoma
Rhabdomyosarcoma
Chondroma
Chondrosarcoma
Osteoma

Continued

Table 29.1, cont'd.

Osteosarcoma	**GERM CELL TUMORS**
Hemangioma	Germinoma
Epithelioid hemangioendothelioma	Embryonal carcinoma
Hemangiopericytoma	Yolk sac tumor
Angiosarcoma	Choriocarcinoma
Kaposi sarcoma	Teratoma
Primary melanocytic lesions	mature
Diffuse melanocytosis	immature
Melanocytoma	teratoma with malignant transformation
Malignant melanoma	Mixed germ cell tumors
Meningeal melanomatosis	
Tumors of uncertain histogenesis	**TUMORS OF THE SELLAR REGION**
Hemangioblastoma	Craniopharyngioma
	adamantinomatous
LYMPHOMAS AND HEMOPOIETIC NEOPLASMS	papillary
Malignant lymphomas	Granular cell tumor
Plasmacytoma	
Granulocytic sarcoma	**METASTATIC TUMORS**
	UNCLASSIFIED TUMORS

meningiomas, the critical determinants for malignant behavior are the mitotic index and invasion of brain cortex. For astrocytomas, however, histologic features influence prognosis so strongly that multilevel grading schemes are used. The four-level grading system of Kernohan and colleagues,[5] Burger's modification of the three-level (astrocytoma, anaplastic astrocytoma, and glioblastoma multiforme) WHO system,[6] Davis's four-tiered scheme of anaplasia,[7] and Daumas-Duport's quantitative system[8] based on the presence of coagulative necrosis, endothelial proliferation, nuclear atypia, and mitotic figures have all shown predictive value for patient outcome.

Molecular neuropathology

The details of these multilevel grading schemes have proven controversial. The current trend in neuropathology is to use highly objective indices of tumor biology. The development of indices that register neoplastic changes at the molecular level heralds the arrival of molecular neuropathology.

Indices of proliferation

The first major advance in molecular neuropathology was in measurement of the rate of tumor cell proliferation. Counting of mitotic figures has been superseded by bromodeoxyuridine and Ki-67 labeling indices. The frequency of incorporation of the bromine analog of deoxyuridine (a marker for cells in the DNA synthesis phase of the cell cycle) in tumor cell DNA or of immunostaining for Ki-67 (a marker for cycling cells) provides an estimate of the portion of cells in a tumor that are actively dividing (Figure 29.3).[9,10] The mean bromodeoxyuridine labeling index is less than 1% in astrocytomas, 2.7% in anaplastic astrocytomas, and 7.3% in glioblastomas. It is higher in tumors with necrosis, vascular proliferation, high invasiveness, and absence of differentiation. These estimates of the growth fraction of brain tumors have predictive value for both tumor growth rate and clinical outcome that may exceed the predictive value of tumor histopathology.

Immunohistochemical markers

The second major advance in molecular neuropathology was the use of immunologic staining to characterize the assortment of structural and functional proteins produced in neoplastic cells. Immunohistochemical identification of marker proteins and glycolipids clarifies a tumor's cell type and degree of differentiation (Figure 29.4).[11] Expression of intermediate filaments, such as glial fibrillary acidic protein (GFAP) in glial tumors and neurofilaments in neuroepithelial tumors, has been studied extensively. GFAP is produced in normal astrocytes and in various tumors derived from astroglial cells: astrocytomas, some glioblastomas, mixed gliomas (oligodendroglioma–astrocytoma), and some ependymomas.[11] In many of these tumor types, the level of expression varies inversely with the degree of anaplasia. Neurofilaments are found in neurons and neural tumors, such as gangliocytomas, neuroblastomas, pineoblastomas, gangliogliomas, and some medulloblastomas.[11]

Panels of monoclonal antibodies against tumor-specific antigens on gliomas, melanomas, and neuroblastomas can be used to study the patterns of antigen expression in neuroepithelial tumors. The findings of such studies may prove valuable in selecting specific therapies. Tumor expression of other molecules commonly found in neuroglial cells, such as neuron-specific enolase, carbonic anhydrase isoenzymes, myelin basic protein, neuroendocrine proteins (e.g. neuropeptides, synaptophysin, and chromogranin), and a variety of glycolipids (e.g. 3′ iso-LM-1 ganglioside) can also be characterized, although their prognostic value has not yet been defined.[11]

Genetic markers

The third major advance in molecular neuropathology was in describing changes in the nucleic acids of tumor cells. Analysis of tumor DNA by flow cytometry is of little value in neuropathology. The degree of aneuploidy correlates poorly with clinical behavior; even highly malignant brain tumors can have a nearly diploid DNA content. Although karyotyping by itself adds little to a neuropathologic diagnosis, it can provide clues to genetic alterations of fundamental importance. Cytogenetic abnormalities, such as chromosome deletions, translocations, and amplifications (evident as homogeneously staining regions and double minute chromatin bodies), may signal the loss of tumor suppressor genes or the amplification of oncogenes. Because genetic changes underlie the

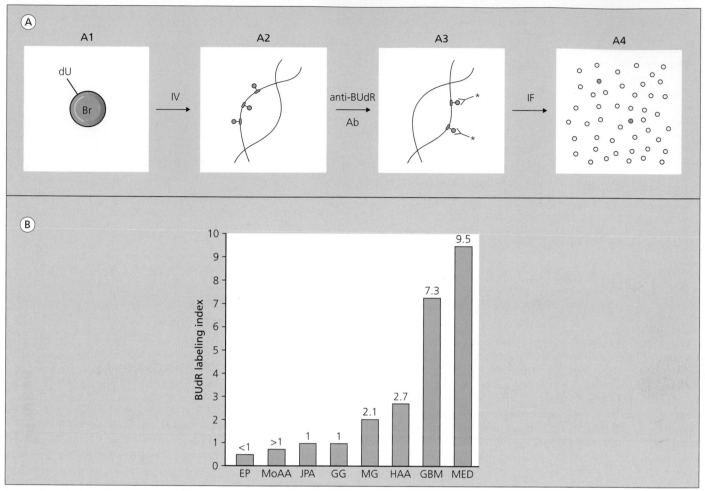

Figure 29.3 Indices of proliferation. **(A)** Immunofluorescent histochemical analysis of tumors exposed preoperatively to analogs of DNA bases can yield estimates of the rate of cell division. **(A1)** During the initial stages of surgery, BUdR is administered intravenously. **(A2)** Cells actively synthesizing DNA incorporate this thymidine analogue. **(A3)** Incubation of a histologic section of the tumor specimen with antibody specific for BUdR labels cells that have incorporated the marker in their DNA. **(A4)** The percentage of cells that are labeled provides an estimate of the proliferative fraction, i.e. the portion of the tumor cells that are actively dividing. **(B)** These estimates of proliferation rate correlate highly with tumor recurrence rate and clinical outcome.[9] EP, ependymoma; MoAA, moderately anaplastic astrocytoma; JPA, juvenile pilocytic astrocytoma; GG, ganglioglioma; MG, mixed glioma; HAA, highly anaplastic astrocytoma; GBM, glioblastoma multiforme; MED, medulloblastoma.

phenotypic progression of tumors to malignancy, these genetic markers should correlate well with the clinical behavior. Studies of the nature and consequences of primary and secondary genetic changes and the resulting alterations in the number, type, and immunologic structure of cell proteins should also suggest possibilities of therapeutic intervention.

EPIDEMIOLOGY

Epidemiologists attempt to identify patterns of disease in populations.[12] The frequency and distribution of brain tumors in a population and their change over time may provide clues to etiology.

Prevalence, incidence, and mortality rate

The prevalence of brain tumors at autopsy is 1–2%.[13] The annual incidence of newly diagnosed brain tumors in the United States is approximately 22 per 100 000 persons; one-half of these (22 000) are primary and the remainder are metastatic (Table 29.2).[14] The mortality rate for primary brain tumors in North America averages about 4 per 100 000 persons per year.[15] Less developed regions of the world report lower age-adjusted rates; this difference may reflect less accurate pre-mortem diagnosis or autopsy analysis.[16] The mortality rate from primary brain tumors varies with sex, race, and age. In the United States, it is higher for males than for females, is higher for whites than for blacks, and rises with age until 70 years and then declines.[15]

The incidence of primary parenchymal brain tumors of all histologic types varies with age: There is a small peak at 2 years, a decline for the rest of the first decade, and a slow increase from 2 per 100 000 per year at age 20 to 6 per 100 000 per year at age 40. During late adulthood the incidence doubles to a peak of 28 per 100 000 per year at age 75 before a final decline.[14] This pattern is essentially identical to that for malignant gliomas, reflecting the high proportion of primary brain parenchymal tumors that are of this pathologic type (Figure 29.5).

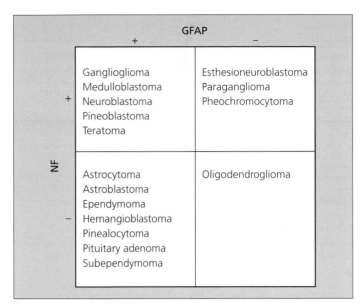

Figure 29.4 Markers of cellular differentiation. Immunohistochemical analysis with panels of monoclonal antibodies specific for glial or neuronal proteins helps classify tumors according to the predominant cell type.

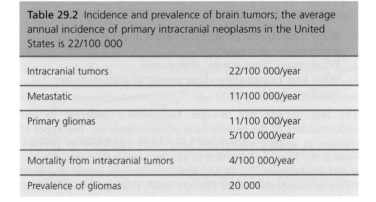

Table 29.2 Incidence and prevalence of brain tumors; the average annual incidence of primary intracranial neoplasms in the United States is 22/100 000

Intracranial tumors	22/100 000/year
Metastatic	11/100 000/year
Primary gliomas	11/100 000/year 5/100 000/year
Mortality from intracranial tumors	4/100 000/year
Prevalence of gliomas	20 000

Determinants of the incidence of specific tumor types

The incidence of different types of primary brain tumor varies with age.[17] In adults, metastatic lesions are the most common intracranial tumors and malignant gliomas and meningiomas are the most common primary brain tumors. In contrast, in children, medulloblastomas and less malignant astrocytomas are the most common tumor types (Figures 29.6, 29.7).[18] Sex and race are also influential. Unlike most types of gliomas, meningiomas and pituitary adenomas are more likely to occur in women than in men and are more frequent in African-Americans than in Caucasians.[19] Analysis of recent trends suggests a steady increase in the incidence of malignant brain tumors in various ethnic and sex groups, especially in persons over 70 years of age.[20,21]

Familial brain tumors

An increased incidence of brain tumors within a single family can usually be attributed to one of the phakomatoses (Table 29.3). These dominantly inherited predispositions to the development of

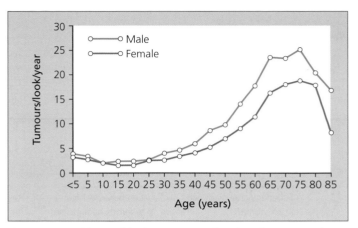

Figure 29.5 Incidence of brain tumors as a function of age. Recently, there has been a steady increase in the age-adjusted incidence of malignant central nervous system tumors.[21] This increased incidence is particularly prominent in the elderly with a slight male predominance.[20]

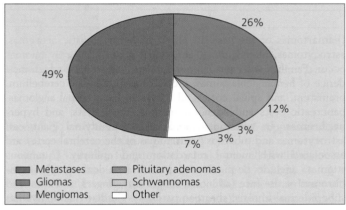

Figure 29.6 Brain tumors by histologic type.

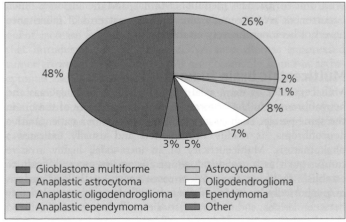

Figure 29.7 Gliomas by histologic type.

nervous system tumors include neurofibromatosis types 1 and 2 (NF-1 and NF-2), tuberous sclerosis, and von Hippel–Lindau disease.[22] Neurofibromatosis is the most common. In NF-1, nerve sheath tumors and optic, brainstem, and cerebellar gliomas are associated with café au lait spots, cutaneous neurofibromas, plexiform neurofibromas of peripheral nerves, and Lisch nodules

Angiogenesis

In the 1960s, experiments demonstrated that tumors are limited to a diameter of 2–3 mm unless new vessels form. New vessels are needed to provide oxygen and nutrients and to remove toxic metabolites.[119] The growth of new vessels, neovascularization or angiogenesis, is stimulated by angiogenic factors such as vascular epithelial growth factor (VEGF), TGF-α and TGF-β, and bFGF and opposed by inhibitory factors such as endostatin (collagen XVIII), angiostatin (plasminogen), fibronectin, platelet factor 4, interferon-α, EGF, and prolactin.[120–122]

Pharmaceuticals such as thalidomide and the fungus-derived AGM1470 also disrupt angiogenesis. Monoclonal antibodies against stimulatory angiogenic factors and their receptors have also been developed. Antibodies against the VEGF receptor and against the integrins have shown significant antiangiogenic activity only *in vitro*. Viral vectors expressing angiogenesis inhibitors have also shown promising antitumor effects *in vitro*, but the efficiency of viral delivery remains an obstacle.[120–123]

Immune suppression

Most of the central nervous system is immunologically privileged. Lymphocytic infiltration of a glioma is more limited than that of systemic tumors. In the 1960s, Medawar demonstrated the absence of an immune response to allogeneic cells placed intra-durally.[124] This diminished immune response has been variably attributed to the blood–brain barrier, the absence of brain lymph-atics, and suppression of antigen-presenting cells, which decreases both humoral and cell-mediated responses. CNS tumors also escape immune surveillance by lacking certain tumor antigens, loss of major histocompatibility complex (MHC) expression, and down-regulation of the antigen-processing mechanism. They also inactivate lymphocytes by secreting immunosuppressive factors such as TGF-2, prostaglandin E_2, and interleukin-10.[119,125–127] Recently, demonstration of the potent antigen-presenting capabilities of microglia and identification of MHCs at different stages of tumor growth have suggested the potential for enhancing an immune attack.[119]

Immunotherapy

Strategies for enhancing the immune response to CNS tumors are of four types:

1 cytokines;
2 antibodies;
3 adoptive immunotherapy; and
4 vaccines.

Cytokines, such as interleukin-2 (IL-2), IL-3, IL-4, tumor necrosis factor-α (TNF-α), granulocyte–macrophage colony-stimulating factor (GM-CSF), and interferon-γ, are lymphocyte-secreted peptide ligands that initiate an immune response.[119,124,129] Hypothetically, increase in local cytokine activity should augment the immune response to a tumor. Both immunogenic cytokines and vector cells transfected with the genes for these cytokines have been injected into tumors. *In vitro* work has demonstrated a spectrum of immune response, from recruitment of immune cells to cytolysis of tumor cells. In a Phase I/II study of recurrent gliomas, 51% of 65 patients intravenously injected with recombinant IFN-β had smaller or stable tumors.[130]

Antibodies have been used both to block critical components of tumor cell proliferation pathways and to deliver cytotoxic agents to tumor cells.[131] Identification of tumor-specific antigens, such as the truncated epidermal growth factor receptor (EGFRvIII), gp240, tenascin, and GFAP, prompted development of antibodies against these antigens alone or with delivery agents with cytotoxic agents.[131,132] A recent Phase II trial demonstrated extended median survival time when an ^{131}I-labeled anti-tenascin monoclonal antibody was injected into the surgical resection cavity of a malignant glioma.[133] A great deal of attention has also been focused on the EFGvIII monoclonal antibodies. EGFvIII is a mutant receptor, with an in-frame deletion of exons 2–7, found in more than 50% of glioblastomas multiforme. Two different receptor inhibitors have been developed. The first is a naked antibody that, in animal models, inhibits the receptor, reduces DNA transcription, and ultimately causes tumor cell death. Injection of murine brain tumors with antibodies to EGFvIII increased survival by an average of 286%. Intravenous delivery is restricted by the blood–brain barrier.[134] Use of antibodies coupled with toxins is also being investigated. Anti-EGFvIII antibodies coupled to the *Pseudomonas* endotoxin A increased the median duration of survival of rodents with gliomas by 430–657%.[135]

Adoptive immunotherapy involves injection of stimulated lymphokine-activated killer cells, tumor-infiltrating cells, or cyto-toxic T cells into patients with tumors. In one study, lymphokine-activated killer cells and IL-2 injected into the resection beds of gliomas improved patient survival (53-week median survival after lymphokine-activated killer cells + IL-2 versus 25.5 weeks with chemotherapy).[136] Although this approach is theoretically appealing, because harvesting and manipulating the cells to be injected is resource intensive, this strategy is impractical for widespread clinical use.

Vaccination strategies for gliomas have attempted to boost the immune response engendered by vaccinating a patient with irradiated autologous tumor cells by first transducing the tumor cells with cytokines, such as GM-CSF, a potent activator of T-helper 1 (Th1) and 2 (Th2) responses.[137] This approach was first investigated in prostate cancer and melanomas. In prostate cancer, Phase I and II trials found activated lymphocytes in tumor and a decline in prostate-specific antigen (PSA), suggesting that immune activation had been achieved.[138] Glioma cells transduced with either GM-CSF or IL-4 have been similarly tested. Rats harboring gliomas, when vaccinated peripherally with IL-4-transduced glioma cells, lived significantly longer than did control animals. In humans, a Phase I trial of vaccination with irradiated autologous glioma cells transduced with IL-4 is underway.[126] Other Phase I clinical trials are using autologous glioma cells admixed with fibroblasts expressing IL-4 or dendritic cells pulsed with tumor fragments.[126]

More recently, dendritic cells have been used for vaccination. These antigen-presenting cells are harvested from a patient's blood, exposed to cells, DNA, or proteins from the patient's tumor, expanded in cell culture, and re-injected into the patient's skin. Humoral and cytotoxic T-cell responses to EFGRvIII have also been demonstrated.[139] Dendritic cells pulsed with the EGFRvIII peptide elicit a specific cytotoxic T-cell response and prolonged survival in mice with gliomas. A Phase I trial using dendritic cells pulsed with EGFRvIII framents is underway.[134]

CONCLUSION

Three features – heterogeneity, invasiveness, and immuno-suppression – give malignant tumors a significant advantage in host–tumor interactions. Once a benign tumor accumulates suffi-

CLINICAL PEARLS

Etiology

● Alteration of tumor suppressor genes or oncogenes can produce tumors.

● Microarray techniques are revealing families of genes whose expression is changed.

● Tumorigenic genetic changes can be inherited or acquired.

Pathogenesis

● The annual incidence of brain tumors is 22 per 100 000 persons. The incidence of tumors varies with age. Approximately 50% of all brain tumors are primary, and the others are metastatic.

● Tumors are classified according to cell type, and the histology is predictive, in part, for prognosis of the patient. Molecular markers may improve tumor classification but that research is ongoing.

● Since actively dividing cells are more likely to sustain DNA injury; tumor progression occurs with acquisition of additional genetic defects as repeated cycles of division occur.

● It appears that invasivesness and angiogeneisis are found in more aggressive tumors.

● Attempts at immunotherapy for treatment of brain tumors are promising but preliminary.

cient genetic damage to progress to a more malignant phenotype, the all too frequent outcome is progressive tumor growth, clinical deterioration, and death. Additional research into the basic causes of tumor initiation and progression as well as the phenomena of genetic instability, phenotypic heterogeneity, invasiveness, and immunosuppression offers the best hope of altering this prognosis.

REFERENCES

1. Willis RA. *The Spread of Tumors in the Human Body*, 2nd edn. London: Butterworth; 1952.
2. Bailey P, Cushing H. *Classification of the Tumors of the Glioma Group on a Histogenetic Basis with a Correlated Study of Prognosis*. Philadelphia: JB Lippincott; 1926.
3. Zulch KJ. *International Histological Classification of Tumors, 21. Histological Typing of Tumors of the Central Nervous System*. Geneva: World Health Organization; 1979.
4. Garcia J. Classification of brain tumors. In: Salcman M (ed.). *Neurobiology of Brain Tumors: Concepts in Neurosurgery*. Baltimore: Williams & Wilkins; 1991: vol. 4; 19–32.
5. Kernohan JW, Mabon RF, Svien JH, *et al*. Symposium on a new and simplified concept of gliomas. *Proc Mayo Clin* 1949; 24: 71–5.

6. Burger PC. The grading of astrocytomas and oligodendrogliomas. In: Fields WS (ed.). *Primary Brain Tumors: A Review of Histologic Classification*. New York: Springer-Verlag; 1989: 171–80.
7. Davis RL. Grading of gliomas. In: Fields WS (ed.). *Primary Brain Tumors: A Review of Histologic Classification*. New York: Springer-Verlag; 1989: 150–8.
8. Daumas-Duport C. A new uniform grading system. In: Fields WS (ed.). *Primary Brain Tumors: A Review of Histologic Classification*. New York: Springer-Verlag; 1989: 159–70.
9. Hoshino T. Cell kinetics of brain tumors. In: Salcman M (ed.). *Neurobiology of Brain Tumors: Concepts in Neurosurgery*. Baltimore: Williams & Wilkins; 1991: vol. 4; 19–32.
10. Zuber P, Hamou M, de Tribolet N. Identification of proliferating cells in human gliomas using the monoclonal antibody Ki-67. *Neurosurgery* 1988; 22: 364–8.
11. Molenaar WM, Trojanowski JQ. Biological markers of glial and primitive tumors. In: Salcman M (ed.). *Neurobiology of Brain Tumors: Concepts in Neurosurgery*. Baltimore: Williams & Wilkins; 1991: vol. 4; 185–210.
12. Schoenberg BS. Epidemiology of primary intracranial neoplasms: disease distribution and risk factors. In: Salcman M (ed.). *Neurobiology of Brain Tumors: Concepts in Neurosurgery*. Baltimore: Williams and Wilkins; 1991: vol. 4; 3–18.
13. Green JR, Waggener JD, Kriesgsfield BA. Classification and incidence of neoplasms of the central nervous system. *Adv Neurol* 1976; 15: 51–5.
14. Walker AE, Robins M, Weinfield FD. Epidemiology of brain tumors: the national survey of intracranial neoplasms. *Neurology* 1985; 35: 219–26.
15. Chandra V, Bharucha NE, Schoenburg BS. Mortality data for the U.S. for death due to and related to twenty neurological diseases. *Neuroepidemiology* 1984; 3: 149–68.
16. Bahemuka M, Massey EW, Schoenberg BS. International mortality from primary nervous system neoplasms: distribution and trends. *Neuroepidemiology* 1983; 2: 196–205.
17. Helseth A, Mork SJ. Neoplasms of the central nervous system in Normal, III:epidemiological characteristics of intracranial gliomas according to histology. *APMIS* 1989; 97: 547–55.
18. Schoenberg BS, Christine BW, Whisnant JP. The descriptive epidemiology of primary intracranial neoplasms—the Connecticut experience. *Am J Epidemiol* 1976; 104: 499–510.
19. Heshmat MY, Kovi J, Simpson, *et al*. Neoplasms of the central nervous system: incidence and population selectivity in the Washington, DC, metropolitan area. *Cancer* 1979; 38: 2135–42.
20. Greig NH, Reis LG, Yancik R, Paroport SI. Increasing annual incidence of primary malignant brain tumors in the elderly. *J Natl Cancer Inst* 1990; 82: 1621–4.
21. National Institutes of Health. *Annual Cancer Statistic Review*, NIH publication 90-2789. Bethesda: National Cancer Institute; 1989.
22. Martuza RL. Neurofibromatosis as a model for tumor formation in the human nervous system. In: Salcman M (ed.). *Neurobiology of Brain Tumors: Concepts in Neurosurgery*. Baltimore: Williams & Wilkins; 1991: vol. 4; 53–62.
23. Shoenberg B, Christine B, Whisnant J. Nervous system neoplasms and primary malignancies of other sites: the unique association between meningiomas and breast cancer. *Neurology* 1975; 25: 705–12.
24. Seizinger BR, de la Monte S, Atkins L, *et al*. Molecular genetic approach to human meningioma: loss of genes of Ch 22. *Proc Natl Acad Sci USA* 1987; 84: 5419–23.
25. Knudson AG. Hereditary cancer, oncogenes, and antioncogenes. *Cancer Res* 1985; 45: 1437–43.

Presentation
- Headache in over 80%[70,74]
- Nausea and vomiting in 50–80%
- Others include cerebellar dysfunction and papilledema on examination
- Median duration of symptoms 4 months

Treatment
- Surgical resection
- Radiation therapy critical; dosing depends on tumor location, grade, and surgical outcome
- Repeat resection and/or chemotherapy are options at recurrence

Outcome
- Overall survival 35–60% at 5 years[1,70,73,74]
- One-third to two-thirds will recur, with increased incidence if anaplastic changes are present
- Most treatment failures are apparent within 2 years of therapy, and more than 90% of these are local recurrences

Comment
- Increased incidence of anaplastic changes in supratentorial lesions[70,71,74]
- No clear relationship between anaplastic changes and patient outcome[71,73,76]
- Rare to absent tumor progression to increased anaplasia on recurrence[71,74]

Figure 30.9, *cont'd.*

because of the heterogeneity of gliomas, sampling error is a concern: the tissue obtained from small needle biopsy may not be representative of the true nature of the tumor. The diagnostic accuracy of stereotactic biopsy ranges from 72 to 93% when compared with radical resection, while the risks of neurological complication are still significant (3.7%).[80]

Although a biopsy may provide an accurate pathologic diagnosis, surgical resection usually offers the best chance of improved survival. Debulking large tumors and those that cause mass effect can reduce intracranial pressure and lead to marked improvement in neurologically impaired patients. Superficial lesions are especially amenable to resection. Electrocorticography and other intraoperative mapping techniques, which are used to determine the potential extent of resection of tumors located near highly functional ("eloquent") cortex, require an open procedure. This may be an attempted resection or limited biopsy, depending on the mapping results. Highly vascular lesions cannot be approached safely by percutaneous stereotactic techniques and therefore a craniotomy should be performed for either biopsy or resection of such lesions. The various considerations for performing a biopsy versus a resection are illustrated in Figure 30.10.

The goal for surgery for most brain tumors is maximal resection of the tumor without producing new neurological deficits. This goal may be achieved by tailoring the operative approach and planning for each individual patient. Debulking large tumors can also markedly improve neurologic status, particularly for patients with large tumors in superficial locations. Studies have demonstrated that this improves survival.[50]

A traditional craniotomy under general anesthesia can be used for tumors in non-eloquent regions. However, for patients with lesions near eloquent regions, such as the motor or sensory areas, functional MRI and electrocorticography can be used preoperatively and intraoperatively (respectively) to identify functional regions of the brain and thus allow the surgeon to optimize the trajectory to maximize tumor resection while minimizing risk to eloquent brain (Figure 30.11). Endoscopy can also be useful for intraventricular lesions. Finally, highly vascular lesions should be approached through open procedures so that bleeding can be controlled.

While tissue diagnosis is optimal except for pediatric brainstem lesions,[37] observation is a viable option for low-grade astrocytomas and oligodendrogliomas once a definitive diagnosis is made, and should be considered. While there is increasing evidence that aggressive resection may be beneficial in most gliomas, this is probably only accurate in cases in which 95% or more of the enhancing tumor can be safely resected (as assessed by MRI).[50] There appears to be minimal benefit to subtotal resection compared to biopsy alone, particularly for tumor with minimal mass effect.[50,81] Recent studies also suggest that the benefit of early radiotherapy for patients with low-grade astrocytomas or oligodendrogliomas with minimal symptomatology is minimal.[38,39] Observation may also be a viable option if tissue diagnosis would not change the benefits. For example, a small non-enhancing, non-mass-producing lesion that is asymptomatic and has not demonstrated progression could be followed radiographically. A large tumor in an old, debilitated patient who would not be a candidate for treatment even if a definitive diagnosis were made should likewise not be subjected to surgery.

The mortality rate from craniotomy in most large series is 1–2%.[82,83] Surgical morbidity includes increased neurologic deficit from tumor resection or swelling (8.5–11%), hemorrhage at the operative site (4–5%), and wound infection (1–2%).[83,84] Medical complications, such as deep vein thrombosis, myocardial infarction and pneumonia, occur in 3–9% of patients.[47,84] Older, neurologically impaired patients with deep-seated, midline, or bilateral lesions are at relatively increased risk. Aggressive resection does not significantly increase the risks of surgery compared to subtotal debulking in most cases. Thus, since aggressive resection often improves symptoms and maximizes survival and quality of life, imaging complete resection should be the goal of surgery in most cases provided this can be done without significant risk of damage to eloquent brain.[50]

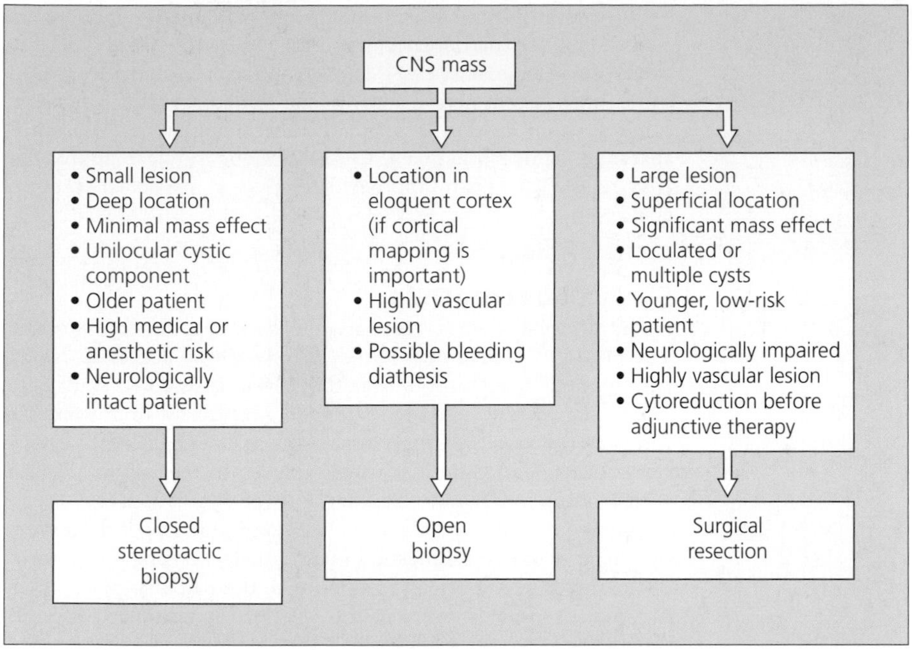
CNS mass
• Small lesion
• Deep location
• Minimal mass effect
• Unilocular cystic component
• Older patient
• High medical or anesthetic risk
• Neurologically intact patient
• Location in eloquent cortex (if cortical mapping is important)
• Highly vascular lesion
• Possible bleeding diathesis
• Large lesion
• Superficial location
• Significant mass effect
• Loculated or multiple cysts
• Younger, low-risk patient
• Neurologically impaired
• Highly vascular lesion
• Cytoreduction before adjunctive therapy
Closed stereotactic biopsy
Open biopsy
Surgical resection

Figure 30.10 Biopsy versus surgical resection in the treatment of the glioma patient. Open biopsy or resection may be advisable if mapping is required, if the lesion is vascular (increasing the risk of hemorrhage after biopsy), or if the patient has a bleeding diathesis. In most cases, resection offers the best chance for short-term improvement of neurologic deficits and improved long-term survival.

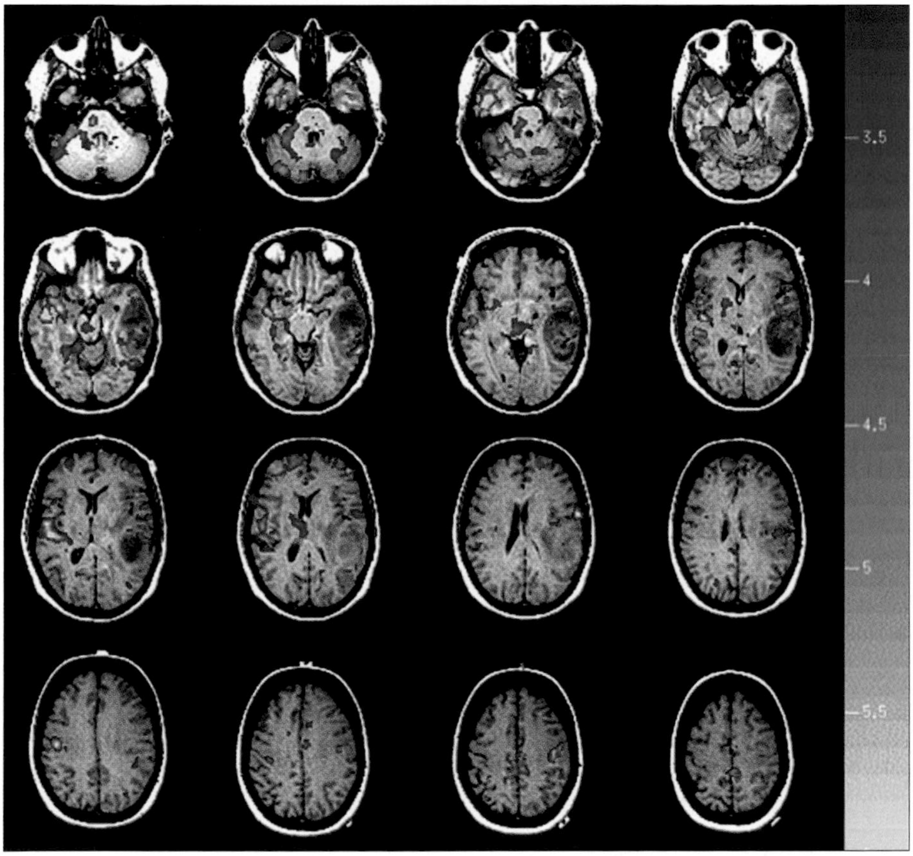
3.5
4
4.5
5
5.5

Figure 30.11 Functional MRI (fMRI). The patient is a 32-year-old ambidextrous female who presented with a 3-month history of headaches, expressive aphasia and memory loss. T1-weighted MRI with gadolinium demonstrated a large heterogeneous left temporo-parietal mass with surrounding edema and small regions of enhancement. Neurologic function markedly improved after administration of steroids and anticonvulsants. fMRI was performed to determine location of Wernicke's and Broca's areas. A silent counting task demonstrated activity in both temporal regions, with significant activity as illustrated by yellow and orange along the anterior–superior–lateral margin of the tumor, but no activity within the tumor itself. These findings were confirmed by reproducible speech arrest during stimulation of the corresponding region of the cortex with a threshold of 8 mA at 60 Hz. However, the lesion itself did not appear to have function. Accordingly, an imaging complete resection was performed. Postoperatively, the patient had mild expressive aphasia which returned to baseline by the fourth postoperative day. The tumor was a grade III oligoastrocytoma which was subsequently treated with PCV chemotherapy. The patient remains intact and tumor-free 3 years postoperatively.

Surgical techniques

The preparation for a particular case is determined by the goals (biopsy vs. resection), location of the mass (superficial vs. deep), risks (eloquent vs. non-eloquent brain), the experience of the surgeon, and the technical adjuncts available. The key to success is in adequate preparation and planning. After consideration of these factors, the surgeon considers the likely risks and the optimal way to minimize them. A general approach is illustrated in Table 30.5. Many points are self-explanatory and will not be specifically addressed here.

Perioperative and intraoperative steroids, anticonvulsants, antibiotics, and sequential compression stockings have become

Table 30.5 Preparation for brain tumor resection. (The order of presentation is roughly chronologic and is for a typical craniotomy. Not all steps are required for every operation.)

A. Preoperative
  1. Review presentation and studies
  2. Informed consent
B. Anesthesia
  Local sedation
  General anesthesia
C. Intraoperative preparation
  1. Radiographic studies selected
  2. Stereotactic equipment available
  3. Blood available
  4. Corticosteroids
  5. Anticonvulsants
  6. Antibiotics
  7. Minimize venous stagnation
  8. Urinary catheter
  9. Intravenous access
  10. Monitors (anesthesia and neurophysiologic)
  11. Intraoperative adjuncts available
    a. Microscope, ultrasound, X-ray equipment, iMRI
    b. Surgical tools
  12. Prepare operative field
  13. Plan incision
    a. Scalp flap
    b. Cranial opening
  14. Position patient
    a. Head fixation
    b. Avoid pressure points
  15. Draping
  16. Minimize exposure of personnel to blood
D. Surgical removal
  1. Approach
  2. Removal
  3. Avoid complications
E. Postoperative
  1. Immediate concerns
    a. General clinical status
    b. Bleeding in operative site
    c. Brain swelling
    d. Neurologic deficits
  2. Delayed concerns
    a. Hydrocephalus
    b. Infection
    c. Phlebitis and pulmonary emboli
    d. Wound healing
  3. Patient and family support

routine for craniotomies (see Chapter 6). Bipolar electrocautery, suction, microscopes and microneurosurgical instruments should always be available. An ultrasonic aspirator is frequently helpful for tumor debulking. Lasers offer few advantages for resection of gliomas, and are rarely used. With every maneuver of the surgeon, care is taken to protect adjacent normal brain and its vascular supply. Traction on the brain itself must be minimized. Traction should always be directed away from eloquent cortex and should be delivered gently using a self-retaining retractor system, which is released every 10–15 minutes.

Preoperative patient positioning and planning the incision and craniotomy are particularly important in neurosurgery because of the small cranial opening and operative field and the risks of retracting adjacent neural and vascular structures to gain access to tumors within, behind, or beneath functioning brain. Descriptive anatomic names are given to the various surgical approaches (Figure 30.12). Each approach requires a particular type of craniotomy.

Surgical approaches

For intracranial gliomas, there are four basic types of craniotomies. The pterional approach (Figure 30.13A) allows access to frontal and temporal lobe tumors near the sylvian fissure and skull base. The basic opening may be extended posteriorly or toward the vertex to expose the temporoparietal or lateral frontal regions, respectively. The patient is usually placed in the supine position with a bump under one shoulder and the head tilted 15° to 90° away from the involved side. The incision follows a gentle curve in the shape of a reverse question mark, usually starting just anterior to the tragus of the ear and posterior to the palpable pulse of the superficial temporal artery at the level of the zygomatic process, and ending behind the hairline between the mid-pupillary line and the midline superiorly. Care must be taken to preserve the frontotemporal branch of the facial nerve.[85]

The Sutar or bicoronal incision (Figure 30.13B) is used to approach the frontal region more anteriorly or medially than is suitable from a pterional craniotomy. This allows access to medial frontal lobe lesions and, via a subfrontal approach, to the chiasm or anterior hypothalamic region. The patient is usually supine with the head in the neutral position or at angles up to 30°. The skin incision may extend from one zygomatic process to the other if needed, approximately 1 cm posterior to the hairline. However, for unilateral craniotomy the incision is usually extended only to the contralateral superior temporal line. The forehead tissues are reflected forward in the supraperiosteal plane, and care is taken to preserve both the superficial temporal artery laterally and the supraorbital branch of the ophthalmic nerve as it exits the supraorbital foramen. The anterior third of the sinus may be sacrificed, but care should taken not to violate it inadvertently when the bone flap is elevated. If the frontal air sinus is entered during the craniotomy, it should be exenterated of mucosal lining and packed with fat or muscle to prevent communication between the sinus and the intradural space and subsequent infection.

The corpus callosum, interhemispheric fissure and intraventricular regions can be approached through a laterally based horseshoe-shaped incision extending at least 1 cm over the vertex medially (Figure 30.13C). If positioned anteriorly over the coronal suture, this opening also allows transcallosal access to the anterior third ventricle through the foramen of Monro. The horseshoe opening is suitable for gliomas near the midline of the frontal lobe, ependymomas near the lateral ventricles, and hypothalamic astrocytomas. The patient is supine, with the head in the neutral position and slightly flexed forward. Tumors of the parietal and occipital lobes can be approached through a more posterior opening. The patient can be positioned laterally for parietal tumors and prone or sitting for occipital tumors. Four burr holes, the medial pair directly over the sagittal sinus, are usually placed. Great care should be taken to protect the sinus during the opening.

The suboccipital craniectomy (Figure 30.13D) is used to expose infratentorial lesions, such as cerebellar pilocytic astrocytomas or ependymomas. It may be located either in the midline,

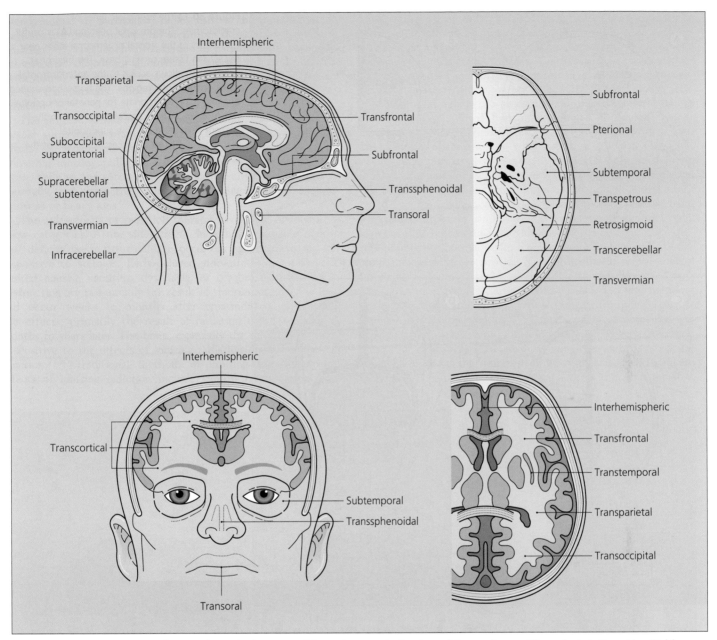

Figure 30.12 The various surgical approaches to brain tumors. Schematic anatomic drawings of the cranium and its contents in the midsagittal (upper left), axial skull base (upper right), coronal frontotemporal (lower left), and axial midcortical (lower right) planes.

as shown, or in a paramedian position. For a midline opening, the patient is usually placed in the prone, sitting, or "Concorde" position. If the sitting position is used, care is required to prevent an air embolism, and both the surgical and anesthetic teams must be prepared to act promptly in such an event. The surgical team floods the field with sterile saline, while the anesthesiology team lowers the head and evacuates an air embolus from the jugular vein. Preoperative preparation for this position includes placement of an intracardiac catheter to withdraw air and preoperative cardiac echocardiography to rule out cardiac septal defects that could allow right-to-left air passage. For more lateral openings, such as the retromastoid suboccipital craniectomy, the patient is placed in the lateral decubitus position with the head rotated away from the lesion toward the floor, and the vertex tilted downward.

The midline opening requires a linear incision from the inion to the second cervical spinous process. The incision is carried down to the bone of the occiput, and the semispinalis capitis and associated muscles are split and reflected laterally in a subperiosteal plane. In the region of the foramen magnum, the vertebral arteries must be carefully preserved as they loop over the lateral arches of the atlas toward the midline before they enter the dura. The craniectomy is limited rostrally by the transverse sinuses, laterally by the transverse-sigmoid junctions, and inferiorly by the margin of the foramen magnum. The surgeon must be careful to avoid injuring the intradural sinuses. The cisterna magna is opened just after opening the dura. For lesions in the lateral cerebellar hemispheres, a lateral approach using a linear or "lazy S" incision is often more suitable.

CHEMOTHERAPY

Chemotherapy combined with surgical resection and postoperative radiation therapy is moderately effective in the treatment of anaplastic astrocytomas and glioblastomas[89] and markedly effective in anaplastic oligodendrogliomas.[67–69] Anecdotal case reports suggest that chemotherapy may have some effectiveness against unresectable pilocytic astrocytomas in very young children[26] as well as in recurrent ependymomas[98] with anaplastic features and oligoastrocytomas.[99] Despite many investigational strategies and clinical trials, progress has been slow in terms of a real impact on patient survival and quality of life.

One of the first drugs used successfully to treat malignant astrocytomas was 1,3-bis(2-chloroethyl)-1-nitrosourea (BCNU).[89] Despite enormous effort to improve upon the early results, BCNU remains the standard against which other glioma treatment regimens are frequently judged. Another drug in this class is 1-(2-chloroethyl)-3-cyclohexyl-1-nitrosourea (CCNU), which has been used in many trials because it can be administered orally. More recently, other oral alkylating agents such as Procarbazine and Temodar have been studied either as conventional chemotherapy, or as neoadjuvant therapy in combination with radiotherapy.[99–101] There is also ongoing interest in Gleevec (STI-571), which was originally designed for the treatment of chronic myelocytic leukemia, but may also be active in glioma via the platelet-derived growth factor-α or c-*Kit* receptor.[102]

Multidrug regimens, intrathecal or intra-arterial injection with or without transient disruption of the blood–brain barrier, and even intratumoral delivery of drugs are also in testing. Intracavitary Gliadel, a biodegradable polymer that releases BCNU, had demonstrated efficacy in the treatment of recurrent glioma.[103] Clinical trials have been undertaken to increase the efficacy of chemotherapy by manipulating cell sensitivity or enhancing drug delivery to tumor cells using intra-arterial chemotherapy or convection-enhanced delivery, while decreasing toxicity to normal tissues. Inhibition of chemoresistance mechanisms used by tumors is another strategy which has been proven effective in pre-clinical studies,[104] and is now under investigation. A review of these efforts and future directions is presented in Chapter 47.

ALTERNATIVE THERAPEUTIC MODALITIES

The lack of improved survival from chemotherapy and radiation over more than two decades has strengthened interest in other therapeutic modalities. These include differentiating agents, biological response modifiers, gene therapy, antiangiogenesis factors and immunotherapy. Although these therapies are exciting because they exploit the molecular differences between glioma cells and normal glial cells, none has yet proven to be efficacious.

Biological response modifiers

Biological response modifiers are agents which can modify the phenotype of the tumor cells. The most common and most actively studied of these agents in gliomas are the interferons (IFN), interleukins (IL) and tumor necrosis factor-α (TNF-α).

Interferons are cytokines which modulate tumor cytotoxicity and immune modulation. Studies have demonstrated that human IFN-α and IFN-β inhibit tumor growth in rodent glioma models, and a large number of phase I and II clinical trials investigating these interferons have been reported over the past decade.[105–107] In general, IFN-β is more active than TNF-α.[106] Response rates have been encouraging in some studies.[106,107] IFN may be more effective if used in combination with other agents.[108]

Interleukins function by activating lymphocytes and leukocytes. IL-2 has demonstrated anti-glioma activity *in vitro*[109] and has been studied in combination with intracavitary immunotherapy with only modest efficacy.[110] IL-4 has also been studied, but only has efficacy in combination with other agents.[111]

Gene therapy

Gene therapy is a potentially attractive strategy for the treatment of brain tumors because of the lack of systemic toxicity and the ease of application during stereotactic procedures or craniotomy. Direct introduction of genes without any cellular or viral vector can be accomplished via aerosol, systemic delivery, or microcellular injection. Indirect gene delivery by transplantation of genetically engineered cells or inoculation of a recombinant defective virus is also feasible and constitutes a highly efficient means of transferring DNA to a target cell.

The best studied experimental paradigm for genetic treatment of gliomas has been the delivery of the herpes simplex virus thymidine kinase (*HSV-tk*) gene to the glioma using an adenovirus vector. Adenoviruses are highly stable, non-enveloped, double-stranded DNA-containing viruses with a low rate of genomic instability and, therefore, low risk of insertional mutagenesis. Adenoviruses transfer their DNA by binding to a specific cell surface receptor, entering the cytoplasm by endocytosis, and then forming a pore in the endosome to translocate genetic material to the nucleus. In principle, the *HSV-tk* construct should only be delivered to dividing cells. The thymidine kinase produced by these cells can phosphorylate nucleoside analogs such as ganciclovir to form nucleotide-like precursors that will block replication of DNA. Thus far, however, results have been disappointing.[112] Although the transduction process alone is not cytotoxic, cellular production of thymidine kinase confers susceptibility to those cells subsequently exposed to ganciclovir. The so-called "bystander effect" is the result of diffusion of phosphorylated nucleosides away from dying cells to adjacent non-transduced tumor cells resulting in their death.

Oncolytic viruses

There is increasing evidence that some viruses replicate selectively in neoplastic tissues inducing tumor lysis as a by-product of their growth. Unlike viral vectors used in gene therapy, oncolytic viruses do not deliver recombinant genes into tumors but lyse them directly as part of the viral growth cycle. Wilcox *et al.* have demonstrated that certain strains of reovirus can hijack the activated *Ras*-signaling pathways found in most human gliomas to lyse glioma cell lines and primary cultures *in vitro*, and *in vivo* in both subcutaneous and intracranial models.[113] However, neutralizing antibodies, complement and other factors in plasma impair viral activity[114] and this activity appears to be species specific.[115] ONYX-015 (dl1520) is another adenovirus construct designed to be differentially lethal to tumor cells with mutated or deleted *p53*, as in nearly 50% of gliomas, which is under active investigation. Thus, it remains to be seen whether this will translate into therapeutic efficacy in clinical trials.

Inhibitors of angiogenesis

Tumors must promote angiogenesis, the development of new blood vessels, to grow beyond 1–2 mm in diameter (about 10^6 cells). This is accomplished by altering the physiologic balance between positive and negative regulators of angiogenesis.[116] To the extent that tumors are dependent on this process, targeting these pathways has the potential to target tumors in a highly specific fashion.

Tumor neovascularization occurs through a number of mechanisms including overexpression and mobilization of angiogenic proteins from the extracellular matrix and recruitment of host cells such as macrophages, which in turn produce their own angiogenic proteins.[117] Key angiogenic proteins include vascular endothelial growth factor (VEGF), basic fibroblast growth factor (bFGF), platelet-derived growth factor (PDGF), and tenascin. Endogenous inhibitors of angiogenesis include angiostatin, endostatin and thrombospondin.[117] When the angiogenic process is triggered, a cascade of events occurs which includes activation of endothelial cells, proteolytic degradation of the extracellular matrix and basement membrane, proliferation and migration of endothelial cells, endothelial tube formation, and fusion and reassembly of the extracellular matrix. This complex process involves many enzymes, such as matrix metalloproteinases, serine proteases and cathepsins, which result in the release of stored growth factors and, in turn, promote further angiogenesis.[118]

Most experience with antiangiogenesis treatments in brain tumors has been with matrix metalloproteinase inhibitors (MMPIs). The MMPs are a family of over a dozen secreted and membrane-bound zinc endopeptidases. They require activation by other proteolytic enzymes to digest an extracellular matrix. MMPs are up-regulated in primary and metastatic brain tumors and correlate with malignant progression.[119] However, thus far there has been limited efficacy in clinical trials.

Immunotherapy

Immunotherapy is another area of active study for the treatment of gliomas. The high degree of specificity which characterizes the immune system, and the phenomenon of "immunologic memory" has led to the suggestion that immunotherapy may have the potential to eliminate infiltrating tumor without damaging the surrounding brain.[120] There are three general types of immunotherapy currently under investigation: passive, active and adoptive immunotherapy.[121]

Passive immunotherapy utilizes monoclonal antibodies to induce tumor death either directly, or by means of delivering radiotherapy or toxins. There is evolving evidence that both strategies may be effective[122,123] and this remains an area of active interest. Active immunotherapy utilizes vaccination with reproductive incompetent autologous or allogeneic tumor cells to induce a specific anti-tumor response. Most current efforts are based on dendritic cell vaccines and there is preliminary evidence of efficacy and increased lymphocytic infiltrate of the tumor.[124,125]

Adoptive immunotherapy employs *ex vivo* stimulation of the patient's own immune effector lymphocytes. Several studies have demonstrated the efficacy of this approach as well, with reported survival of more than three years.[126,127] Survival correlates with delayed-type hypersensitivity, a type of cell-mediated immune response.[127] Another approach to adoptive immunotherapy is the injection of activated LAK + IL-2 directly into the tumor via an Ommaya reservoir. Hayes *et al.* observed an objective radiographic response in four of 15 patients on this protocol.[128]

REOPERATION FOR RECURRENT GLIOMA

The only gliomas that can be cured by surgery alone are pilocytic astrocytomas and pleomorphic xanthoastrocytoma. Long-term survival is common in patients with low-grade astrocytomas, oligodendrogliomas, and occasionally ependymomas. Malignant astrocytomas are usually rapidly fatal despite multimodality therapy. When a recurrent lesion is detected, it is important to evaluate fully the diagnostic possibilities. Is the lesion at the site of the original tumor, a distant site, or both? Does the lesion represent true recurrence of the original histology? Other important possibilities, such as persistent residual tumor, malignant progression, or radiation necrosis, must also be considered.

Approximately 80% of gliomas occur locally, so a lesion at another location mandates consideration of other possible pathologies.[59] If it proves to be recurrent glioma, the consideration for surgery would be similar to that for newly diagnosed lesion. Recurrence at both local and distant locations is ominous and usually suggestive of rapid re-growth and invasion and is associated with a poor prognosis.[129] If there was no postoperative film demonstrating the extent of resection, one must consider the possibility that the lesion represents residual tumor from the earlier procedure, rather than true recurrence. Such lesions may be watched if there is no evidence of growth or progression of symptoms.

In the case of progressive lesions at the site of the original neoplasm, one must consider the possibility of recurrence of the original neoplasm vs. malignant progression or radiation necrosis. Nearly 50% of low-grade neoplasms are found to have progressed to higher grade at the time of recurrence.[130] Even GBMs occasionally recur as gliosarcomas. Radiation necrosis must also be considered, particularly for patients more than 6 months after high-dose radiation "boost" using conventional techniques, intensity-modulated radiotherapy (IMRT), stereotactic radiosurgery, or brachytherapy implants. Conventional MRI cannot usually distinguish between these possibilities, but MRI spectroscopy may be helpful, as is PET. In the case of symptomatic lesions with mass effect, the considerations for surgery are the same as for recurrent tumor. However, if the lesion is minimally symptomatic and consistent with radiation necrosis, biopsy is indicated to make the definitive diagnosis as these lesions may respond to medical management.[131]

In the case of confirmed tumor recurrence, one must consider factors related to the tumor itself as well as factors related to the patient in deciding whether reoperation is indicated. Tumor factors include: tumor biology (histology, grade, time to recurrence, growth rate and invasiveness), response to previous treatment, location and resectability. Factors related to the patient include age, neurologic status, medical condition, previous treatment, other treatment options and the goals of the patient and family. In general, reoperation is justified if it facilitates improved neurologic condition and quality of life or enhancement of response to adjuvant therapy. In some cases, it may also be indicated as part of experimental trials of new treatment regimens.

Several studies have demonstrated that aggressive resection of recurrent gliomas increases survival as well as quality of life. Reoperation for tumor recurrence significantly improved median survival by 88 and 36 weeks respectively for recurrent anaplastic astrocytoma or glioblastoma multiforme.[60,61] In one study, the proportion of additional survival time that was judged of high quality was substantially greater for anaplastic astrocytomas than for glioblastoma (90% vs. less than one-third).[61] Morbidity and mortality rates are no higher after reoperation than after the initial operation.[84,132]

The prognostic variables associated with a good outcome after reoperation for tumor recurrence are essentially the same as for the initial operation: young age, good functional status and apparent gross total resection. Age is a good predictor of total

CLINICAL PEARLS

- Making the correct diagnosis is crucial for deciding on appropriate goals and therapeutic intervention in patients with gliomas.

- A tissue diagnosis should always be sought except in the case of brainstem lesions or if the patient is a poor operative candidate.

- The role of surgery is to provide diagnosis, alleviate mass effect and increased intracranial pressure, and facilitate tolerance of future therapy.

- The goal of surgery should be to achieve an imaging complete resection whenever this can be done without compromising neurologic function.

- Non-invasive imaging should be employed pre-operatively to assess the location of eloquent brain with respect to the tumor and facilitate decisions regarding treatment strategy and goals whenever possible.

- Use of intraoperative computer-aided navigation and motor/language mapping can facilitate more aggressive resection while decreasing the risk to neurologic function.

- Many patients with local recurrence may benefit from reoperation which may improve neurologic status, quality of life, and response to treatment.

- Postoperative radiotherapy is indicated for most patients with Grade III–IV glioma except in the case of young children. The use of postoperative radiotherapy in lower grade gliomas remains controversial.

- Chemotherapy is highly dependent upon pathologic diagnosis. PCV chemotherapy is particularly effective in the treatment of anaplastic oligodendrogliomas.

- The failure of conventional radiation and chemotherapy to improve survival over two decades has led to increasing interest in alternative therapeutic modalities such as biological response modifiers, gene therapy, oncolytic viruses, angiogenesis inhibitors and immunotherapy. It is likely that these will play an increasingly important role in the treatment of gliomas in the future.

---

survival in patients undergoing reoperation, at least in part, because of the interval between operation and reoperation,[133] but it does not correlate with survival after reoperation.[60,61,133] The importance of preoperative functional status of the patient is demonstrated by the two and one half times greater length of survival of patients with Karnofsky performance scores of 70 or greater compared with those with lower scores.[60] In this same study, complete resection at reoperation resulted in survival after the second surgery more than twice that after partial resection. Thus, in selected patients with tumor recurrence or progression despite multimodality therapy, reoperation can be performed safely and with improved overall survival.

This chapter contains material from the first edition, and we are grateful to the authors of that chapter for their contribution.

REFERENCES

1. Kleihues P, Burger PC, Scheithauer BW. The new WHO classification of brain tumors. *Brain Pathol* 1993; 3: 255–68.
2. Berens ME, Rutka JT, Rosenblum ML. Brain tumor epidemiology, growth, and invasion. *Neurosurg Clin North Am* 1990; 1: 1–18.
3. Jellinger K. Pathology of human intracranial neoplasia. In: Jellinger K (ed.). *Therapy of Malignant Brain Tumors*. Berlin: Springer-Verlag; 1987: 23–7.
4. Ries LAG, Eisner MP, Kosary CL, *et al.* (eds). *SEER Cancer Statistics Review, 1973–1977*. National Cancer Institute, Bethesda, MD; 2000.
5. American Cancer Society. *Cancer Facts and Figures – 2000*. Atlanta, GA: American Cancer Society; 2000.
6. Legler JM, Ries LAG, Smith MA, *et al.* Brain and other central nervous system cancers: recent trends in incidence and mortalitiy. *JNCI* 1999; 91: 1382–90.
7. Wrensch M, Minn Y, Chew T, Bondy M, Berger MS. Epidemiology of primary brain tumors: current concepts and review of the literature. *Neuro-oncology* 2002; 4: 278–99.
8. Zulch KJ. *Brain Tumors: Their Biology and Pathology.* Berlin: Springer-Verlag; 1986.
9. Kernohan JW, Maborn RF, Svien HH, *et al.* A simplified classification of the gliomas. *Proc Staff Meeting Mayo Clin* 1949; 24: 71–5.
10. Ringertz N. Grading of gliomas. *Acta Pathol Microbiol Scand* 1950; 27: 51–64.
11. Burger PC, Vogel FS. *Surgical Pathology of the Nervous System and its Coverings*, 2nd edn. New York, NY: John Wiley and Sons; 1982: 226–66.
12. Zulch KJ. *Histological Typing of Tumors of the Central Nervous System.* Geneva: World Health Organization; 1979.
13. Daumas-Duport C, Scheithauer B, O'Fallon J, *et al.* Grading of astrocytomas: a simple and reproducible method. *Cancer* 1988; 62: 2152–65.
14. Bailey P, Cushing H. *A Classification of the Glioma Group on a Histogenetic Basis With a Correlated Study of Prognosis.* Philadelphia, PA: JB Lippincott; 1926.
15. Shaw EG, Scheithauer BW, O'Fallon JR, *et al.* Oligodendrogliomas: the Mayo Clinic experience. *J Neurosurg* 1992; 76: 428–34.
16. Daumas-Duport C, Tucker ML, Kolles H, *et al.* Oligodendrogliomas.

PartII: a new grading system based on morphological and imaging criteria. *J Neuro-oncol* 1997; 34: 61–78.

17. Coons SW, Johnson PC, Scheithauer BW, Yates AJ, Pearl DK. Improving diagnostic accuracy and interobserver concordance in the classification and grading of primary gliomas. *Cancer* 1997; 79: 1381–93.

18. Dean BL, Drayer BP, Bird CR, *et al.* Gliomas: classification with MR imaging. *Radiology* 1990; 174: 411–15.

19. Plate KH, Risau W. Angiogenesis in malignant gliomas. *Glia* 1995; 15: 339–47.

20. Moller-Hartmann W, Herminghaus S, Krings T, *et al.* Clinical application of proton magnetic resonance spectroscopy in the diagnosis of intracranial mass lesions. *Neuroradiology* 2002; 44: 371–81.

21. Taylor JS, Lanston JW, Reddick WE, *et al.* Clinical value of proton magnetic resonance spectroscopy for differentiating recurrent or residual brain tumor from delayed cerebral necrosis. *Int J Radiat Oncol Biol Phys* 1996; 36: 1251–61.

22. Rabinov JD, Lee PL, Barker FG, *et al.* In vivo 3-T MR spectroscopy in the distinction of recurrent glioma versus radiation effects: initial experience. *Radiology* 2002; 225: 871–9.

23. Glantz MJ, Hoffman JM, Coleman RE, *et al.* Identificaion of early recurrence of primary central nervous system tumors by [^{18}F]fluorodeoxyglucose positron emission tomography. *Ann Neurol* 1991; 29: 347–55.

24. Ribom D, Eriksson A, Hartman M, *et al.* Positron emission tomography ^{11}C-methionine and survival in patients with low grade gliomas. *Cancer* 2001; 92:1541–9.

25. Wallner KE, Gonzales MF, Edwards MFB, *et al.* Treatment results of juvinile pilocytic astrocytoma. *J Neurosurg* 1988; 69: 171–6.

26. Civitello LA, Packer RJ, Rourke LB, *et al.* Leptomeningeal dissemination of low grade gliomas in childhood. *Neurology* 1988; 38: 562–6.

27. Brown MT, Friedman HS, Oakes WJ. Chemotherapy of pilocytic astrocytomas. *Cancer* 1993; 71: 3165–72.

28. Danoff BF, Cowchock FS, Marquette C, *et al.* Assessment of long term effects of primary radiation therapy for brain tumors in children. *Cancer* 1982; 49: 1580–6.

29. Oxenhandler DC, Sayers MP. The dilemma of childhood optic gliomas. *J Neurosurg* 1978; 48: 34–41.

30. Naidich TP, Lin JP, Leeds NE, *et al.* Primary tumors and other masses of the cerebellum and fourth ventricle: differential diagnosis by computed tomography. *Neuroradiology* 1977; 14: 153–74.

31. Imes RK, Hoyt WF. Childhood chiasmal gliomas: update on the fate of patients in the 1969 San Francisco Study. *Br J Ophthalmol* 1986; 70: 179–82.

32. Palma L, Guidetti B. Cystic pilocytic astrocytomas of the cerebral hemispheres. *J Neurosurg* 1985; 62: 811–15.

33. Garcia DM, Fulling KH. Juvenile pilocytic astrocytoma of the cerebrum in adults: a distinctive neoplasm with favorable prognosis. *J Neurosurg* 1985; 63: 382–6.

34. Hadjipanayis CK, Kondziolka D, Gardner P, *et al.* Stereotactic radiosurgery for pilocytic astrocytomas when multimodal therapy is necessary. *J Neurosurg* 2002; 97: 56–64.

35. Philippon JH, Clemenceau SH, Fauchon FH, *et al.* Supratentorial low-grade astrocytomas in adults. *Neurosurgery* 1993; 32: 554–9.

36. Piepmeier J, Christopher S, Spencer D, *et al.* Variations in the natural history and survival of patients with supratentorial low-grade astrocytomas. *Neurosurgery* 1996; 38: 872–9.

37. Albright AI, Packer RJ, Zimmerman R, *et al.* Magnetic resonance scans should replace biopsies for the diagnosis of diffuse brain stem gliomas: a report from the Children's Cancer Group. *Neurosurgery* 1993; 33: 1026–30.

38. Karim AB, Afra D, Cornu P, *et al.* Randomized trial on the efficacy of radiotherapy for cerebral low grade glioma in the adult: European Organization for Research and Treatment of Cancer Study 22845 with the Medical Research Council study BRO4: an interim analysis. *Int J Radiat Oncol Biol Phys* 2002; 52: 316–24.

39. Shaw E, Arusell R, Scheithauer B, *et al.* Prospective randomized trial of low- versus high-dose radiation therapy in adults with supratentorial low-grade glioma: initial report of a North Central Cancer Treatment Group/Radiation Therapy Oncology Group/Eastern Cooperative Oncology Group study. *J Clin Oncol* 2002; 20: 2267–76.

40. Muller W, Afra D, Schroeder R. Supratentorial recurrences of gliomas: morphological studies in relation to time intervals with astrocytomas. *Acta Neurochir (Wien)* 1997; 37: 75–91.

41. Kleihaues P, Cavenee WK. Pathology and genetics of tumors of the nervous system. Lyon: IARC Press; 2000.

42. Tatter SB. Neurosurgical management of low- and intermediate-grade gliomas. *Sem Rad Oncol* 2001; 11: 113–23.

43. Kazner E, Wende S, Grumme T, *et al.* (eds). *Computed Tomography in Intracranial Tumors.* Berlin: Springer-Verlag; 1982.

44. Burger PC, Vogel S, Green SB, *et al.* Glioblastoma multiforme and anaplastic astrocytoma: pathologic criterion and prognostic implications. *Cancer* 1985; 56: 1106–11.

45. Levin VA, Silver P, Hannigan J, *et al.* Superiority of post-radiotherapy adjuvant chemotherapy with CCNU, procarbazine, and vincristine (PCV) over BCNU for anaplastic gliomas. NCOG 6G61 final report. *Int J Radiat Oncol Biol Phys* 1990; 18: 321–4.

46. Prados MD, Scott C, Curran WJ, *et al.* Procarbazine, lomustine, and vincristine (PCV) chemotherapy for anaplastic astrocytoma: a retrospective review of Radiation Therapy Oncology Group Protocols comparing survival with carmustine or PCV adjuvant chemotherapy. *J Clin Oncol* 1999; 17: 3389–95.

47. Mahaley MS, Mettlin C, Natarajan N, *et al.* National patterns of care for brain tumor patients. *J Neurosurg* 1989; 71: 826–36.

48. Newelt EA, Nazarro JM, Gumerlock MK. Is there a role for biopsy in the treatment of supratentorial high grade glioma? *Clin Neurosurg* 1990; 36: 384–407.

49. Wroe SJ, Foy PM, Shaw MDM, *et al.* Differences between neurological and neurosurgical approaches in the management of malignant brain tumors. *Br Med J* 1986; 293: 1015–18.

50. Lacroix M, Abi-Said D, Fourney DR, *et al.* A multivariate analysis of 416 patients with glioblastoma multiforme: prognosis, extent of resection, and survival. *J Neurosurg* 2001; 95: 190–8.

51. Ammirati M, Vick N, Liao Y, *et al.* Effect of the extent of surgical resection on survival and quality of life in patients with supratentorial glioblastomas and anaplastic astrocytomas. *Neurosurgery* 1987; 21: 201–6.

52. Burger PC, Green SB. Patient age, histologic features, and length of survival in patients with glioblastoma multiforme. *Cancer* 1987; 59: 1617–25.

53. Wood JR, Green SB, Shapiro WR. The prognostic importance of tumor size in malignant gliomas: a computed tomographic scan study by the Brain Tumor Cooperative Group. *J Clin Oncol* 1988; 6: 338–43.

54. Stenning SP, Freedman LS, Bleehen NM. Prognostic factors for high-grade malignant glioma: development of a prognostic index. *J Neuro-oncol* 1990; 9: 47–55.

55. Shipiro WR, Green SB, Burger PC, *et al.* Randomized trial of three chemotherapy regimens and two radiotherapy regimens in postoperative treatment of malignant glioma: Brain Tumor Cooperative Group Trial 8001. *J Neurosurg* 1989; 71: 1–9.

56. Stewart LA. Chemotherapy in adult high grade glioma: a systematic review and meta-analysis of individual patient data from 12 randomized trials. *Lancet* 2002; 359: 1011–18.

57. Davis F, Freels S, Grutch J, Barlas S, Brem S. Survival rates in patients with primary malignant brain tumor stratified by age and type: an analysis based on Surveillance Epidemiology and End Result (SEER) data, 1973–1991. *J Neurosurg* 1998; 88: 1–10.

58. Salcman M. Survival in glioblastoma: historical perspective. *Neurosurgery* 1980; 7: 435–9.

59. Wallner KE, Galicich JH, Krol G, et al. Patterns of failure following treatment for glioblastoma multiforme and anaplastic astrocytoma. *Int J Radiat Oncol Biol Phys* 1989; 16: 1405–9.

60. Ammirati M, Galicich JH, Arbit E, et al. Reoperation in the treatment of recurrent intracranial malignant gliomas. *Neurosurgery* 1987; 21: 607–14.

61. Harsh GR IV, Levin VA, Gutin PH, et al. Reoperation for recurrent glioblastoma and anaplastic astrocytoma. *Neurosurgery* 1987; 21: 615–21.

62. Fortin D, Cairncross G, Hammond RR. Oligodendroglioma: an appraisal of recent data pertaining to diagnosis and treatment. *Neurosurgery* 1999; 45: 1279–91.

63. Burger PC. What is an oligodendroglioma? *Brain Pathol* 2002; 12: 257–9.

64. Daumas-Duport C, Varlet P, Tucker ML, et al. Oligodendrogliomas, part I: patterns of growth, histological diagnosis, clinical and imaging correlations—a study of 153 cases. *J Neuro-oncol* 1997; 34: 37–59.

65. Chin HW, Hazel JJ, Kim Th, et al. Oligodendrogliomas, I: a clinical study of cerebral oligodendrogliomas. *Cancer* 1980; 45: 1458–66.

66. Van den Bent MJ, Kros JM, Heimans JJ, et al. Response rate and prognostic factors of recurrent oligodendroglioma treated with procarbazine, CCNU and vincristine chemotherapy. *Neurology* 1998; 51: 11140–5.

67. Cairncross G, Macdonald D, Ludwin S, et al. Chemotherapy for anaplastic oligodendroglioma. National Cancer Institute of Canada clinical trials group. *J Clin Oncol* 1994; 12: 2013–21.

68. Cairncross JG, Ueki K, Zlatescu MC, et al. Specific genetic predictors of chemotherapeutic response and survival in patients with anaplastic oligodendrogliomas. *J Natl Cancer Inst* 1998; 90: 1473–9.

69. Kristof RA, Neuloh G, Hans V, et al. Combined surgery, radiation, and PCV chemotherapy for astrocytomas compared to oligodendrogliomas and oligogastrocytomas. *J Neurooncol* 2002; 59: 231–7.

70. Barone BM, Elvidge AR. Ependymomas: a clinical survey. *J Neurosurg* 1970; 33: 428–38.

71. Fokes EC Jr, Earle KM. Ependymomas: clinical and pathologic aspects. *J Neurosurg* 1969; 30: 585–94.

72. Wallner KE, Wara WM, Sheline GE, et al. Intracranial ependymomas: results of treatment with partial or whole brain irradiation without spinal irradiation. *Int J Radiat Oncol Biol Phys* 1986; 12: 1937–41.

73. Salazar OM, Castro-Vita H, Van Houtte P, et al. improved survival in cases of intracranial ependymoma after radiation therapy. *J Neurosurg* 1983; 59: 652–9.

74. Shaw EG, Evans RG, Scheithauer BW, et al. Postoperative radiotherapy of intracranial ependymoma in pediatric and adult patients. *Int J Radiat Oncol Biol Phys* 1987; 13: 1457–62.

75. Ross GW, Rubinstein LJ. Lack of histopathological correlation of malignant ependymomas with postoperative survival. *J Neurosurg* 1989; 70: 31–6.

76. Korshunov A, Golanov A. Pleomorphic xanthroastrocytomas: immunohistochemistry, grading and clinico-pathologic correlations. An analysis of 34 cases from a single institute. *J Neuro-oncol* 2001; 52: 63–72.

77. Barker FG 2nd, Chang SM, Huhn SL, et al. Age and the risk of anaplasia in magnetic resonance-nonenhancing supratentorial cerebral tumors. *Cancer* 1997; 80: 936–41.

78. Konziolka D, Lunsford LD, Martinez AJ. Unreliability of contemporary neurodiagnostic imaging in evaluating suspected adult supratentorial (low-grade) astrocytoma. *J Neurosurg* 1993; 79: 533–6.

79. Young B, Oldfield EH, Markesberry WR, et al. Reoperation for glioblastoma. *J Neurosurg* 1981; 55: 917–21.

80. Jackson RJ, Fuller GN Abi-Said D, et al. Limitations of stereotactic biopsy in the initial management of gliomas. *Neuro-oncology* 2001; 3: 193–200.

81. Laws ER, Taylor WE, Clifton MB, et al. Neuro-surgical management of low-grade astrocytoma of the cerebral hemispheres. *J Neurosurg* 1984; 61: 665–73.

82. Ciric I, Vick NA, Mikhael MA, et al. Aggressive surgery for malignant supratentorial gliomas. *Clin Neurosurg* 1990; 36: 375–83.

83. Sawaya R, Hammoud M, Schoppa D et al. Neurosurgical outcomes in a modern series of 400 craniotomies for treatment of parenchymal tumors. *Neurosurgery* 1998; 42: 1044–56.

84. Fadul C, Wood J, Thaler H, et al. Morbidity and mortality of craniotomy for excision of supratentorial gliomas. *Neurology* 1988; 38: 1374–9.

85. Yasargil MG, Reichman MV, Kubak S. Preservation of the frontotemporal branch of the facial nerve using the interfascial temporalis flap for pterional craniotomy. Technical Note. *J Neurosurg* 1987; 67: 463–6.

86. Sloan AE, Perez R, Diaz, F. Stereotactic approaches for the treatment of metastatic brain tumors. In: Wilkins R, Rengachary S (eds). *Neurosurgery Operative Color Atlas*. Philadelphia: Williams & Wilkins; 2000.

87. Zamorano L, Jiang Z, Kadi AM. Computer-assisted neurosurgery system: Wayne State University hardware and software configuration. *Comput Med Imaging Graph* 1994; 18: 257–71.

88. Black PM, Alexander E 3rd, Martin C, et al. Craniotomy for tumor treatment in an intraoperative magnetic resonance imaging unit. *Neurosurgery* 1999; 45: 423–31.

89. Walker MD, Alexander E Jr, Hunt WE, et al. Evaluation of BCNU and/or radiotherapy in the treatment of anaplastic gliomas: a cooperative clinical trial. *J Neurosurg* 1978; 49: 333–43.

90. Woo SY, Maor MH. Improving radiotherapy for brain tumors. *Oncology* 1990; 4: 41–5.

91. Al-Mefty O, Kersh JE, Routh A, et al. The long-term side effects of radiation therapy for benign brain tumors in adults. *J Neurosurg* 1990; 73: 502–12.

92. Martins AN, Johnston JS, Henry JM, et al. Delayed radiation necrosis of the brain. *J Neurosurg* 1977; 47: 336–45.

93. Laperriere NJ, Leung PM, McKenzie S. Randomized study of brachytherapy in the initial management of patients with malignant astrocytoma. *Int J Radiat Oncol Biol Phys* 1998; 41: 1005–11.

94. Florell RC, Macdonald DR, Irish WD, et al. Selection bias, survival, and brachytherapy for glioma. *J Neurosurg* 1992; 76: 179–83.

95. Videtic GM, Gaspar LE, Zamorano L, et al. Use of RTOG recursive partitioning analysis to validate the benefit of iodine-125 implants in the primary treatment of malignant gliomas. *Int J Radiat Oncol Biol Phys* 1999; 45: 687–92.

96. Halligan JB, Stelzer KJ, Rostomily RC, et al. Operation and permanent low activity I-125 brachytherapy for recurrent high grade astrocytomas. *Int J Radiat Oncol Biol Phys* 1996; 35: 541–7.

97. Kondziolka D, Flickinger JC, Bissonette DJ, *et al*. Survival benefit of stereotactic radiosurgery for patients with malignant glial neoplasm. *Neurosurgery* 1997; 41: 776–83.

98. Levin VA, Lamborn K, Wara W, *et al*. Phase II study of 6-thioguanine, procarbazine, dibromodulcitol, lomustine, and vincristine chemotherapy with radiotherapy for treating malignant glioma in children. *Neuro-Oncology* 2000; 1: 22–8.

99. Buckner JC, Gesme D Jr., O'Fallon JR, *et al*. Phase II trial of procarbazine, lomustine and vincristine as initial therapy for patients with low-grade oligodendroglioma or oligoastrocytoma: efficacy and associations with chromosomal abnormalities. *J Clin Oncol* 2003; 21: 251–5.

100. Yung WK, Albright RE, Olson J, *et al*. A phase II study of temozolomide vs. procarbazine in patients with glioblastoma multiforme at first relapse. *Br J Cancer* 2000; 83: 588–93.

101. Brandes AA, Ermani M, Basso U, *et al*. Temozolamide in patients with glioblastoma at second relapse after first line nitrosourea-procarbazine failure: A phase II study. *Oncology* 2002; 63: 38–41.

102. Stanulla M, Welte K, Hadam MR, *et al*. Coexpression of stem cell factor and its receptor c-KIT in human malignant glioma cells lines. *Acta Neuropathol (Berlin)* 1995; 89: 158–65.

103. Brem H, Piantadosi S, Burger PC, *et al*. Placebo-controlled trial of safety and efficacy of intraoperative controlled delivery by biodegradable polymers of chemotherapy for recurrent gliomas. *Lancet* 1995; 345: 1008–12.

104. Rhines LD, Sampath P, Dolan ME, *et al*. O-6-benzylguanine potentiates the antitumor effect of locally delivered carmustine against an intracranial rat glioma. *Cancer Res* 2000; 60: 6307–10.

105. Yung WK, Prados M, Levin V, *et al*. Intravenous recombinant interferon beta in patients with recurrent malignant gliomas: a phase I/II study. *J Clin Oncol* 1991; 9: 1945–9.

106. Yung WKA, Steck PA, Kellcher P, *et al*. Growth inhibitory effect of recombinant alpha and beta interferon on human glioma cells. *J Neuro-oncol* 1987; 5: 323–30.

107. Hong YK, Chung DS, Joe YA, *et al*. Efficient inhibition of *in vivo* human malignant glioma growth and angiogenesis by interferon-beta treatment at early stage of tumor development. *Clin Cancer Res* 2000; 6: 3354–60.

108. Buckner JC, Brown LD, Kugler JW, *et al*. Phase II evaluation of recombinant interferon alpha and BCNU in recurrent glioma. *J Neurosurg* 1995; 82: 420.

109. Benveniste EN, Tozawa H, Gasson JC, *et al*. Response of human glioblastoma cells to recombinant interleukin-2. *J Neuroimmunol* 1988; 17: 301.

110. Merchant RE, Ellison MD, Young HF. Immunotherapy for malignant glioma using human recombinant interleukin-2 and activated autologous lymphocytes. A review of pre-clinical and clinical investigations. *J Neuro-oncol* 1990; 8: 173–88.

111. Iwasaki K, Rogers LR, Estes ML, *et al*. Modulation of proliferation and antigen expresson of a cloned human glioblastoma, by interleukin-4 alone and in combination with TNF-α and/or interferon activity. *Neurosurgery* 1993; 33: 489–93.

112. Varghese S, Rabkin SD. Oncolytic herspes simplex virus vectors for cancer vibrotherapy. *Cancer Gene Ther* 2002; 9: 967–78.

113. Wilcox ME, Yang W, Senger D, *et al*. Reovirus as an oncolytic agent against experimental human malignant gliomas. *J Natl Cancer Inst* 2001; 93: 903–12.

114. Ikeda K, Ichikawa T, Wakimoto H, *et al*. Oncolytic virus therapy of multiple tumors in the brain requires suppression of innate and elicited antiviral response. *Nat Med* 1999; 5: 881–9.

115. Wakimoto H, Ikeda K, Abe T, *et al*. The complement response against an oncolytic virus is species-specific in its activation pathways. *Mol Ther* 2002; 5: 275–82.

116. Hanahan D, Folkman J. Patterns and emerging mechanisms of the angiogenic switch during tumorigenesis. *Cell* 1996; 86: 353–64.

117. Folkman J. Clinical applications of research on angiogenesis. *N Eng J Med* 1995; 333: 1757–63.

118. Jekunen AP, Kairemo KJ. Inhibitors of malignant angiogenesis. *Cancer Treatment Rev* 1997; 23: 263–86.

119. VanMeter TE, Rooprai HK, Kibble MM, *et al*. The role of matrix metalloproteinase genes in glioma invasion: co-dependent and interactive proteolysis. *J Neuro-oncol* 2001; 53: 213–35.

120. Grolleau A, Sloan AE, Mule J. Dendritic cell vaccines for cancer therapy. In: Khleif S (ed.). *Tumor Immunology and Cancer Vaccines* (in press).

121. Parajulli P, Sloan AE. Dendritic cell immunotherapy for glioma. *Cancer Immunol Immunother* (in press).

122. Hall WA. Targeted toxin therapy for malignant astrocytoma. *Neurosurgery* 2000; 46: 544–51.

123. Cokgor I, Akabani G, Kuan CT, *et al*. Phase I trial results of iodine-131-labeled antitenascin monoclonal antibody 81C6 treatment of patients with newly diagnosed malignant gliomas. *J Clin Oncol* 2000; 18: 3862–72.

124. Liau LM, Black KL, Martin NA, *et al*. Treatment of a glioblastoma patient by vaccination with autologous dendritic cells pulsed with allogeneic major histocompatability complex class I-matched tumor peptides. *Neurosurg Focus* 2000; 8: 1–5.

125. Yu JS, Wheeler CJ, Zeltzer PM, *et al*. Vaccination of malignant glioma patients with peptide-pulsed dendritic cells elicits systemic cytotoxicity and intracranial T-cell infiltration. *Cancer Res* 2001; 61: 842–7.

126. Wood GW, Holladay FP, Turner T, *et al*. A pilot study of autologous cancer cell vaccination and cellular immunotherapy using anti-CD3 stimulated lymphocytes in patients with recurrent grade III/IV astrocytoma. *J Neuro-oncol* 2000; 48: 113–20.

127. Sloan AE, Sundrum H, Zamorano L, *et al*. Vaccination of patients with recurrent malignant astrocytoma with autologous whole cell vaccine and granulocyte macrophage colony stimulating factor (GM-CSF). *Neurosurgical Focus* 2000; 9: Article 9 1–8.

128. Hayes RL, Koslow M, Hiesiger EM, *et al*. Improved long term survival after intracavitary interleukin-2 and lymphokine-activated killer cells for adults with recurrent malignant glioma. *Cancer* 1995; 76: 840–52.

129. Harsh FR IV. Management of recurrent gliomas. In: Berger M, Wilson C (eds). *The Gliomas*. Philadelphia: WB Saunders; 1999: 549–659.

130. McCormick BM, Miller DC, Budzilovich GN, *et al*. Treatment and survival of low grade gliomas in adults, 1997–1988. *Neurosurgery* 1992; 31: 636–42.

131. Chuba PJ, Aronin P, Bhambhani K, *et al*. Hyperbaric oxygen therapy for radiation-induced brain injury in children. *Cancer* 1997; 80: 2005–12.

132. Chang S, Parney IF, McDermott M, *et al*. Perioperative complications and neurological outcome of first versus second craniotomy among patients enrolled in the Glioma Outcomes (GO) Project. *J Neurosurg* 2003; 98: 1175–81.

133. Salcman M, Kaplan RS, Ducker TB, *et al*. Effect of age and reoperation on survival in the combined multimodality treatment of malignant astrocytoma. *Neurosurgery* 1982; 10: 454–63.

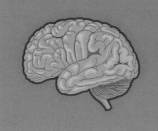

METASTATIC BRAIN TUMORS

31

Ian E McCutcheon

INTRODUCTION

Between 20 and 40% of patients with systemic cancer develop brain metastasis. Such tumors can be extra-axial in nature (e.g. involving the dura and subdural space, or the leptomeninges and subarachnoid space), but most commonly they occur within the brain parenchyma. This chapter focuses on these intra-axial tumors. Magnetic resonance imaging (MRI) confirms that the majority of such patients (two-thirds or more) have more than one metastatic deposit in the brain, a fact which influences current surgical practice. Classic solitary metastases are actually uncommon and therapeutic dilemmas abound in charting effective treatment for this challenging tumor subset. Available methods for treating brain metastasis include surgical excision, focused or diffuse irradiation, and chemotherapy.

The true incidence of brain metastasis is unknown. Computed tomography (CT) underestimates the burden of disease in any given patient, and is useful only as a screening study or in patients (e.g. those with pacemakers) who cannot undergo MRI, which is widely available and much more revealing than CT. Brain metastases are the most common intracranial neoplasm in adults. Certainly the recognized incidence of metastasis has risen over the past 30 years, partly as a result of the advent of MRI, and partly as a result of the longer survival from more effective systemic therapies. Because the biology, and nuances of surgical treatment, differ among the various histologies, it is a mistake to consider "brain metastasis" as a single disease. Although < 1–2% of ovarian and prostate cancers spread to the brain, at least half of melanomas do so. About 80% are located supratentorially and 20% in the posterior fossa. About two-thirds of these tumors are multiple (by MRI, fewer by CT). Metastatic brain tumors derived from cancer of the lung are the most common type, making up 40–60% of the total, followed by those derived from breast cancers (15–20%) and melanoma (10–20%) depending on whether the data come from a clinical or an autopsy series. Colorectal and renal cell carcinomas account for 5–10% each. These five sources are responsible for most cerebral metastases. Melanoma has the highest propensity to spread to the brain, but is less well represented than lung cancer in large series because of the much greater incidence of lung cancer in the general population. Intracerebral metastases occur in < 5% of children with systemic cancer, and arise typically from neuroblastoma, Wilm's tumor, or sarcoma (especially rhabdomyosarcoma).

CLINICAL FEATURES

Two-thirds of patients with brain metastasis complain of neurological decline, most often showing focal deficits like weakness or dysphasia or impairment of cognitive function. Indeed, neuropsychological testing reveals that many "asymptomatic" patients have disordered cognition which has gone unnoticed. Peritumoral edema and/or blockage of cerebrospinal fluid (CSF) pathways can raise the intracranial pressure, and edema and local ischemia or pressure effects can combine with local loss of brain substance to produce localized dysfunction. Seizures occur in 10–20% of patients and are more common with multiple metastases; vascular events include hemorrhage into the tumor or ischemic stroke from vascular compression. Overt intratumoral hemorrhage is seen in 5–15% of patients and even though it may occur with any neoplasm, two histologies are particularly prone to bleed: melanoma (40% of which bleed) and choriocarcinoma (of which almost 100% do so). On imaging, a large amount of edema around a *recent* hematoma (less than 6 hours old) suggests, but does not confirm, a tumor beneath the hematoma. Most metastases associated with an adjacent cyst derive from carcinomas of the breast or from adenocarcinoma of the lung, although a smattering of other histologies can also produce this phenomenon (Figure 31.1).

INVESTIGATIONS

Gadolinium-enhanced MRI is the most sensitive test available for detecting cerebral metastasis, even when compared with double-dose delayed post-contrast CT, which in turn is more sensitive than standard post-contrast CT. MRI is far superior in disclosing small or multiple lesions and should be used for surveillance unless contraindicated.

On non-enhanced T1-weighted MRI, most metastases are hypo- to isointense to gray matter and may be surrounded by a hypointense zone of edema. Such tumors tend to be hyperintense on T2-weighted images, on which cysts and edema are markedly hyperintense. Hemorrhagic tumor is suggested by the presence of a nonhemorrhagic area of enhancement with a "hemosiderin ring" that is hypointense on T2, as well as perilesional edema. Some small tumors may fail to enhance because of relative preservation of the blood–brain barrier. On MRI both melanotic melanoma (unlike *amelanotic* melanoma) and adenocarcinoma are relatively

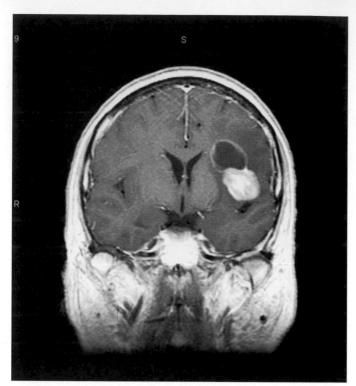

Figure 31.1 Cystic metastasis. This 45-year-old woman with carcinoma of the breast presented with expressive dysphasia. The tumor was just anterior to Broca's area and was resected by craniotomy; the lining of the cyst wall was also removed. For cystic metastases, which typically arise from carcinomas of the breast or lung, radiosurgery may be less effective than surgery as targeting only the tumor nodule may allow recurrence from tumor nests adherent to the cyst wall.

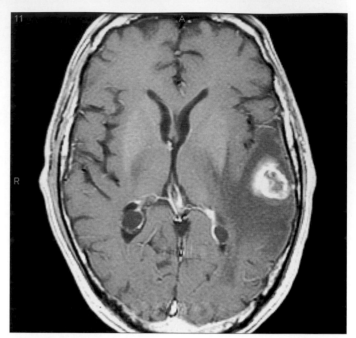

Figure 31.2 Radionecrosis after radiosurgery. This 70-year-old man had stereotactic irradiation to two foci of melanoma within the brain, one in the left cerebellum and one in the left temporal area. Seven months later, the cerebellar tumor had decreased in size but the left temporal enhancement had markedly increased. This was resected and proven as radionecrosis.

hyperintense on T1 and iso- to hypointense on T2, even in the absence of hemorrhage.

The classic location for brain metastasis is the gray–white matter junction. However, they can grow anywhere in the brain including the brainstem. Imaging remains inexact and tissue should be obtained for diagnosis in equivocal cases. Patchell *et al.* reported (in a series that relied on MRI) that 11% of patients presumed to harbor a single brain metastasis actually had other pathology.[1] Only 15% of patients with multiple brain lesions on CT or MRI, but no evidence for tumor outside the brain, have biopsy-proven metastasis. Other mimicking diagnoses include glioma, abscess, encephalitis, ischemic infarct, resolving hematoma, demyelinating disease, and postradiation necrosis (Figure 31.2). MRI can now show lesions as small as 1–2 mm in diameter. However, increased detection of minute subclinical lesions does not appear to improve outcome; patients may harbor additional microscopic disease beyond the ability of any scan to detect. Single photon emission CT, positron emission tomography, diffusion MRI, and magnetic resonance spectroscopy may each help to identify a lesion as a metastasis, but they are usually unnecessary.

UNKNOWN PRIMARY TUMORS

About one-third of patients with symptomatic brain metastasis have no known systemic cancer on presentation. Such patients should undergo a metastatic work-up that screens the most likely primary sites, namely the lung, breast, kidney, colon and skin. Most patients with unknown primary cancer have either bronchial (70%), gastrointestinal, or renal malignancies, or melanoma. Chest X-ray, mammography (in women), urinalysis and routine blood count and chemistry should be obtained, and the skin should be surveyed for lesions suspicious for melanoma. If the above tests are unrevealing then CT of the chest, abdomen, and pelvis should be performed. Bone scans have a low yield if CTs are negative but if the CT is positive, a bone scan may offer alternative sites for biopsy. In the absence of any accessible extracranial tumor, stereotactic biopsy or resection of the cerebral tumor should be undertaken to confirm the diagnosis prior to definitive treatment. However, even with exhaustive investigations the primary tumor remains undiagnosed in 15% of patients.

TREATMENT

The management of brain metastasis is complex and controversial. The current principal options for the treatment of cerebral metastasis include whole-brain radiotherapy, surgery and stereotactic radiosurgery.

Medical management

Steroids have been used since the 1950s to reduce the edema induced by brain metastases. The usual dose of dexamethasone (16 mg/day in divided doses after an initial dose of 10 mg) is a legacy of the arbitrarily chosen doses found to be beneficial during early studies of steroid efficacy. In truth, the dose required for an optimum response varies widely among patients, and ranges

Table 31.1 Summary of three randomized clinical trials comparing surgery plus subsequent radiotherapy with radiotherapy alone

	Patchell et al. (1990)[1]	Vecht et al. (1993)[2]	Mintz et al. (1996)[3]
n	48	63	84
Inclusion criteria	> 17 years old Single lesion KPS at least 70 Lesion accessible No LMD or very radiosensitive tumor	> 17 years old Single lesion Functional level at least 2 Life expectancy > 6 months No LMD, SCLC, or lymphoma	< 80 years old Single lesion KPS at least 50 Lesion accessible No LMD, SCLC, lymphoma, or nonmelanoma skin cancer
Disseminated cancer	18/48 (38%)	20/63 (32%)	38/84 (45%)
Imaging	MRI	CT	CT
Histological verification (in radiotherapy group)	Yes	No	Occasional
Radiotherapy regimen	36 Gy/12 fractions	40 Gy/20 fractions (b.i.d.)	30 Gy/10 fractions
Outcome	Survival longer with surgery 40 vs. 15 weeks	Survival longer with surgery 40 vs. 24 weeks	No significant difference in survival 24 weeks in each group

LMD, leptomeningeal dissemination of tumor; SCLC, small-cell carcinoma of lung; MRI, magnetic resonance imaging; CT, computed tomography; KPS, Karnofsky performance score.

from 3 mg to 96 mg/day. Once a therapeutic response has been achieved, its magnitude varies little by increasing the dose, but adverse effects are magnified. Steroids give clinical improvement within 12 hours in 70–80% of patients with brain metastasis, but the peak effect may be delayed for up to a week. Most patients can be tapered off perioperative steroids after surgery, with the taper usually taking 1–2 weeks.

Although seizures are usually treated with anticonvulsant drugs such as phenytoin, there is no evidence that prophylactic usage at the time of surgery lowers the incidence of seizures or improves outcome in patients with brain metastasis. If anticonvulsants are used, especially in conjunction with dexamethasone, levels should be monitored to avoid under-dosing.

Single brain metastasis

Without any treatment, patients with brain metastasis have a median survival of 6 weeks. The addition of steroids improves this to 3 months. External-beam radiotherapy given to the whole brain improves median survival to 4–6 months. Table 31.1 summarizes three randomized clinical trials that have compared surgery plus subsequent radiotherapy with radiotherapy alone.[1–3] The results obtained by the groups of Patchell and of Vecht are similar and confirm a significant benefit of surgery on overall survival and on quality of life. Obviously surgery within the brain does not impact systemic progression of cancer, which ultimately causes death in most patients. In the study of Vecht et al., the survival advantages of patients in the surgery group vanished with progressive systemic cancer. Only in those with controlled systemic disease is local cure likely to translate into a longer and/or more functional survival.

Three variables should be considered when selecting patients with a single metastasis for surgery: the patient's overall clinical status, the surgical accessibility of the tumor, and the tumor's radiosensitivity. The degree to which systemic (i.e. extracerebral) metastases are present and the patient's performance status (Karnofsky performance score; KPS) are the two most important prognostic variables. Only those with absent or controlled systemic disease and no leptomeningeal dissemination of tumor will derive significant benefit from removal of brain metastases. Although the distinction between the absence and presence of systemic cancer is straightforward, the definition of "controlled" or "limited" systemic disease is somewhat nebulous. Usually an expected survival of 4 months or more qualifies a patient for surgery, whereas advanced age, medical instability and a KPS < 70 argue against surgery. However, neurological dysfunction does not preclude surgery as correction may be sought through removal of a large tumor. If steroids give clinical improvement prior to surgery, postoperative benefit is more likely. Surgical accessibility depends on the skill of the surgeon to some degree, and is colored by the risk of neurological deficit that the patient is willing to accept. In deep tumor locations such as the basal ganglia, thalamus, brainstem, or white matter beneath eloquent cortex, the morbidity of surgical excision may overwhelm the benefits. Alternatives to surgery should be pursued in such patients or in those with highly radio- or chemosensitive tumors (Figure 31.3). Given that the results with post-contrast CT in the study of Vecht et al. are similar to those with MRI in the study by Patchell et al., it is logical that if a single tumor on CT is deemed "surgical" then the discovery of additional tumors on MRI should not automatically disqualify the patient from having surgery.

The best way to treat brain metastasis remains controversial. Although neurosurgical methods (resection and radiosurgery) address individual foci of disease, ultimately brain metastasis is often a multifocal or even diffuse process. Standard radiotherapy treats microscopic foci as well as radiographically evident tumors, but is less effective than radiosurgery for the latter because doses must be lowered to prevent toxicity to normal brain.

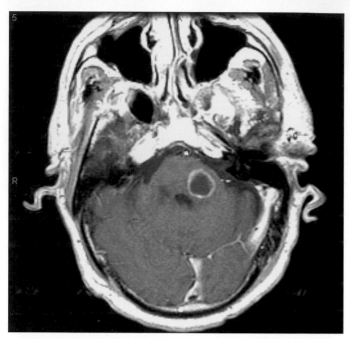

Figure 31.3 Deep tumor inaccessible to surgery but treatable by radiosurgery. This 64-year-old man with small cell carcinoma of the lung had active chest disease and was not given prophylactic brain irradiation. He presented with right hemiparesis and gait ataxia, and MRI showed a tumor occupying the left pons and brachium pontis. The lesion enhances peripherally and has a hypointense center. Its relatively spherical shape, deep location and size (diameter 15 mm) make it a good candidate for radiosurgery, to which it responded well.

Surgery vs. radiosurgery

To date no well-designed trials have been published which compare open resection with stereotactic irradiation. Retrospective analyses imply similar outcome but are unreliable because of selection bias. Advantages and disadvantages of radiosurgery are described in Table 31.2. At our institution the balance has shifted in favor of radiosurgery, which is now used to treat 60% of patients presenting to our neurosurgical clinic with a single metastasis and 30% of those with two sites of disease (Figure 31.4).

However, even when local control (or tumor kill) is achieved, patients with significant peritumoral edema may remain steroid-dependent for 3 months or even longer. Indeed, many tumors show temporary enlargement and intensification of enhancement during the first 1–2 months after radiosurgery; persistence of these changes, persistence of edema, development of radionecrosis exerting mass effect (Figure 31.2), or frank growth of tumor are all indications for definitive resection. Local control rates of 80–95% can be expected which are similar for various histologies, with median survivals of 8–13 months. As a result of the high dose used, "radioresistant" tumors such as melanoma, renal cell carcinoma, and soft tissue sarcomas respond to radiosurgery, as do the more "radiosensitive" tumors.

The overall odds of morbidity after radiosurgery are similar to those seen after surgery. In each, the local recurrence rate is about 15%. Hemorrhage, seizures and neurological decline as a result of such phenomena or of increased edema, can occur after either. Worsening of cerebral edema is unusual, however, after resecting a metastasis and the majority of post-surgical patients improve neurologically and can discontinue steroids within 1–2 weeks.

Table 31.2 Advantages and disadvantages of radiosurgery

Advantages
No incision
Treats surgically inaccessible lesions
More easily tolerated by physiologically compromised patients
Short hospital stay (usually 1 day)

Disadvantages
Poor targeting for tumors > 3 cm in diameter
Tumor persists on scans, so must be followed to prove success
No tissue diagnosis
Persistent edema or radionecrosis may require surgical removal of lesion
Cannot be used on targets within 5 mm of optic nerve or chiasm

Thirty-day postoperative mortality is 2–4% in major centers and morbidity overall is 10–15%.

We recommend surgery to patients with a single metastasis who present with marked mass effect and neurological decline. When systemic disease is controlled or eradicated, and the brain metastasis can probably be removed without inciting or increasing the neurological deficit, surgery is a reasonable option. Nonetheless, the optimal role of surgery relative to radiosurgery remains controversial. Very large tumors respond best to surgery (Figure 31.5). Radiosurgery is the preferred treatment for tumors < 3 cm in diameter in patients who are unfit for surgery because of age or medical condition, who have a tumor in a deep or otherwise inaccessible location (Figure 31.3), or who state an informed preference for this modality. Focal treatment is not warranted

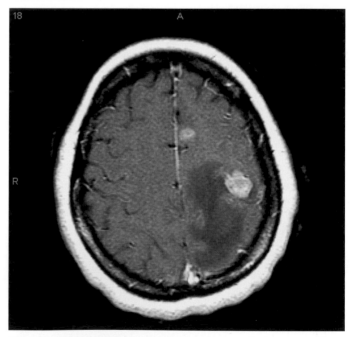

Figure 31.4 Small tumors in eloquent locations may be best treated by radiosurgery. This 40-year-old man with non-small cell carcinoma of lung presented with right arm weakness. MRI shows two metastases, one just anterior to the left motor strip with significant associated edema, and one adjacent to the falx in the frontal lobe. Although surgery is possible, radiosurgery was performed because of the small size of both tumors and the proximity of one to an eloquent area.

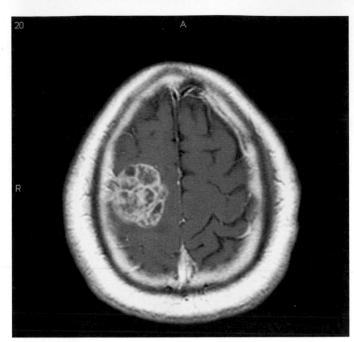

Figure 31.5 Tumor intimately associated with the motor strip. This 38-year-old woman with carcinoma of the breast developed left arm weakness and MRI revealed a tumor in the posterior right frontal lobe abutting the presumptive area of the motor strip. This patient underwent craniotomy rather than radiosurgery as the tumor measured 3.6 cm in maximum diameter; tumors > 3 cm cannot be as accurately targeted as those below that size.

in debilitated patients with advanced cancer who have a life expectancy of < 3–4 months as it offers no benefit over the palliation given by radiotherapy or steroids.

Radiotherapy after surgery

Whole-brain radiotherapy is often given after surgery to reduce local recurrence and eliminate any micrometastases that may (or may not) be present. The conventional dose of such radiotherapy is 30 Gy in 10 fractions; larger fraction sizes give an increased risk of neurotoxicity. However, this regimen does not eliminate the long-term cognitive effects of irradiating the entire brain. Given the longer survival produced by aggressive oncologic treatment of various cancers with a propensity for brain metastasis, this delayed toxicity has been seen more often in recent years, and is difficult or impossible to reverse.

Patchell *et al.* have described a randomized trial that assigned surgical patients to postoperative observation vs. whole-brain radiotherapy.[4] The study included 95 adult patients with a KPS > 70 and a single, completely resected metastasis. The radiotherapy consisted of 50.4 Gy in 28 fractions, a significantly longer course of treatment than is given in most centers. This regimen lowered both the local recurrence rate (from 46% to 10%) and the appearance of brain metastasis at new sites (from 37% to 14%). However, the differences in overall survival (48 vs. 43 weeks) and functionally independent survival (37 vs. 35 weeks) were not statistically significant, and the two groups were not compared for the delayed toxicity of the treatment.

Retrospective series evaluating radiotherapy following radiosurgery have also declared a lower rate of recurrence and perhaps

improved survival. Whole-brain radiotherapy for single lesions after surgical removal or after radiosurgery is thus a valid treatment option, as is withholding radiotherapy and monitoring closely for recurrence (at which point focal therapy may or may not be repeated, followed by radiotherapy or again by observation). The decision to give radiotherapy should be made based on the number of tumors in the brain and on their size and radiosensitivity. Radiotherapy is favored for patients with multiple tumors, small tumors (those > 2 cm in diameter respond poorly to radiotherapy), and radiosensitive tumors.

Multiple metastases

Traditionally multiple brain metastases have not been considered for surgery, and treatment has typically been confined to radiotherapy. Nevertheless, several retrospective series and case–control studies have advocated focal therapy in the form of multiple surgical resections via one or more craniotomies, or in the form of radiosurgery targeting up to four lesions in selected patients. In the case–control study by Bindal *et al.*, the survival of patients undergoing *complete* resection of up to three metastases through single or multiple concurrent craniotomies was significantly better than that of patients in whom one or more tumors was left unresected – and was similar to survival after removal of a single metastasis – without an increase in morbidity or mortality.[5] Surgery should be considered if there is a single dominant and surgically accessible tumor causing mass effect and neurological compromise (Figure 31.6), a need for histological diagnosis, or the possibility of removing a cluster of tumors through a single craniotomy.[6] In many larger centers (including this one) focal therapy followed by radiotherapy is offered for multiple metastases in patients with absent or controlled systemic cancer, KPS > 70, fewer than four brain metastases, and life expectancy > 3 months. Radioresistant tumors, such as renal cell carcinoma and melanoma, are also favored for focal therapy, as radiotherapy alone will provide poor control. In one typical scenario, any lesions > 3 cm in diameter are resected and the remainder, especially those that are surgically inaccessible, are treated with radiosurgery. For tumors < 3 cm in diameter all must be deemed resectable before surgery is undertaken, as resection of some but not all will not be beneficial. Generally, but not routinely, radiotherapy is given after focal therapy for multiple metastases (Figure 31.7).

Recurrence

Ten to twenty per cent of patients treated for a single brain metastasis will have a recurrence after focal therapy plus radiotherapy. The chance of recurrence is even higher in those with multiple tumors. The treatment choices facing the clinician in recurrent cases are similar to those at the time of initial presentation. When selecting the appropriate therapy, the time to recurrence should be noted: an interval of < 4 months predicts a poor outcome. In the many patients with recurrent brain metastasis who also harbor progressive extracranial disease, it may be best to offer supportive measures only. In the healthier subset of patients fulfilling the selection criteria already described for local therapy, radiosurgery or re-operation are the basic options, and radiotherapy may also be offered if it has not previously been given. Reoperation for recurrent metastasis gives a median survival of 9–11 months, with neurological improvement occurring in 62–75%.

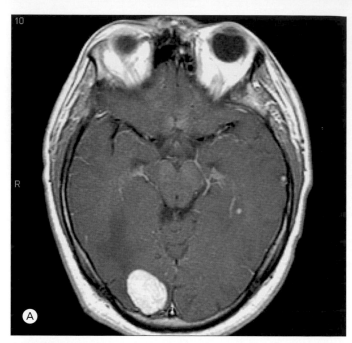
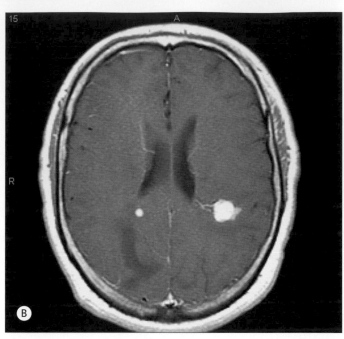

Figure 31.6 Multiple metastases with a dominant symptomatic lesion. This 24-year-old man with alveolar soft-part sarcoma presented with a worsening left visual field defect and gait ataxia. MRI showed a large tumor in the right occipital region with associated edema **(A)**, and also scattered smaller tumors in the left temporal area and within the deep parietal white matter of each hemisphere **(B)**. The large occipital lesion was removed and whole-brain irradiation was administered after surgery.

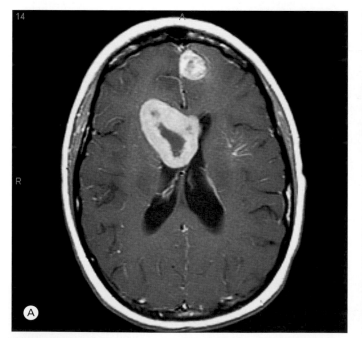
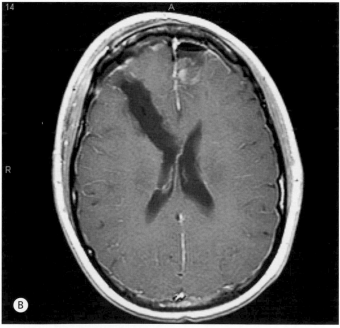

Figure 31.7 Multiple metastases from melanoma. This 20-year-old woman with melanoma by history presented with intractable headache. Several lumbar punctures revealed no malignant cells in cerebrospinal fluid. **(A)** MRI shows one large tumor in the frontal horn of the right lateral ventricle and a smaller tumor in the left frontal lobe. **(B)** Post-resection study showing complete resection of both tumors, accomplished at a single sitting through two simultaneous craniotomies. Whole-brain irradiation was then used to decrease the risk of recurrence.

Chemotherapy and brachytherapy

Chemotherapy has not been very successful in controlling cerebral metastasis. The notion of the blood–brain barrier as a pharmacological sanctuary for metastatic lesions has, however, been weakened by occasional responses by chemosensitive solid tumors like breast carcinoma, small cell carcinoma of the lung, and non-seminomatous germ cell tumors of the testis. Similar responses have been seen in a few patients with non-small cell lung cancer as well. Unlike brain metastasis from other histologies, those from small cell carcinomas and germ cell tumors are initially treated

CLINICAL PEARLS

- Post-contrast MRI shows the number of tumors best (better than CT), but still tends to underestimate the true extent of diseases because of the frequent presence of radiologically occult micrometastases.

- Minor tumor enlargement (10–20%) during the 3 months after radiosurgery may occur, as accurate delivery of the dose often causes the tumor to swell. Thus, such enlargement should be watched and must not prompt over-quick declaration of treatment failure leading to salvage operation.

- The ideal way to remove a brain metastasis is by *en bloc* technique, in which the surgeon enters the gliotic plane around the tumor while keeping the tumor capsule intact. Firm tumors (with low propen-

- sity to spill) with sharp borders may, however, be removed completely in a piecemeal fashion to eliminate the need to retract brain to visualize the deepest portion of the lesion.

- During removal of a melanoma metastasis, tumor fragments should not be allowed to spill as seeding may occur which permits early recurrence. Any associated hemorrhagic pocket should be evacuated first to prevent the blood from escaping and carrying tumor cells through the subdural space.

- To ensure completeness of tumor removal, the wall of any associated cyst should be excised along with the tumor mass itself.

with radiotherapy and chemotherapy, which allows the simultaneous treatment of extracranial disease. Chemotherapy is also an option in those patients with recurrent non-germ cell and non-small cell metastases who for a variety of reasons cannot be treated with surgery or radiosurgery. Because of their relatively greater ability to cross the blood–brain barrier, and their lower incidence of side-effects, oral regimens using newer drugs, such as temozolomide, are currently popular in this context. In most patients, however, chemotherapy gives little improvement in survival or quality of life and is usually a last resort after other therapies have failed.

Small cell carcinoma: a special case

Randomized prospective trials have shown that prophylactic whole-brain radiotherapy reduces the incidence of brain metastases in patients with small cell carcinoma of the lung, which is exquisitely sensitive to irradiation. Enthusiasm for routine prophylactic radiotherapy has been tempered by concern over possible detriment to neurological function in patients who survive for more than a year. As with any whole-brain radiotherapy, acute side-effects may include headaches, nausea, vomiting, and hair loss, and a syndrome of hypersomnia and increased fatigue may be noted 1–4 months later. Radiation necrosis can occur idiosyncratically beyond 6 months from radiation delivery. Neurological toxicity may be reduced by keeping dose fractions below 2 Gy and by forbidding concurrent chemotherapy. In this setting, the consensus is that prophylactic whole-brain radiotherapy confers a survival advantage of 5% at 3 years and a reduction in the incidence of brain metastasis by 25%, and it is considered standard treatment for patients with small cell carcinoma of the lung who are in complete remission after initial treatment. However, no data support this approach in patients who have not achieved complete remission.

CONCLUSIONS

The overall prognosis of patients with brain metastasis remains bleak. Median survival has only risen from 3–6 months with

radiotherapy and steroids, to 9–12 months with focal therapies. The 1-year and 2-year survivals for single brain metastasis are 40% and 20% respectively. Death is caused by progressive intracranial disease in about one-third of patients, with advancing systemic disease the more common culprit overall. Despite these discouraging statistics, the prognosis is not invariably dismal. Exceptionally long survivals (of 5–10 years or more) have been documented in our own series. Study after study has confirmed that the most important prognostic variables are the extent of systemic disease and the patient's functional status and age. These factors must guide treatment decisions as older patients with advanced disease and poor functional status not only receive less benefit from surgery but are more prone to complications. Both surgery and radiosurgery are reasonable choices for patients with good functional status and a limited number of metastases, and either may be followed by whole-brain radiotherapy at the physician's discretion. In the palliative care of patients with metastatic cancer, when treatments become toxic, inconvenient, and ineffective, quality of life and functional status assume even greater importance. The biggest gains for patients with brain metastasis in future will probably come through the development of targeted immunotherapy and biologically based therapy aimed at altering signal transduction or events at the genomic level.

This chapter contains material from the first edition, and I am grateful to the authors of that chapter for their contribution.

REFERENCES

1. Patchell RA, Tibbs PA, Walsh JW, *et al.* A randomized trial of surgery in the treatment of single metastases to the brain. *N Engl J Med* 1990; 322: 494–500.
2. Vecht CJ, Haaxma-Reiche H, Noordijk EM, *et al.* Treatment of single brain metastasis: radiotherapy alone or combined with neurosurgery? *Ann Neurol* 1993; 33: 583–90.
3. Mintz AH, Kestle J, Rathbone MP, *et al.* A randomized trial to assess the efficacy of surgery in addition to radiotherapy in patients with a single cerebral metastasis. *Cancer* 1996; 78: 1470–6.
4. Patchell RA, Tibbs PA, Regine WF, *et al.* Postoperative radiotherapy in

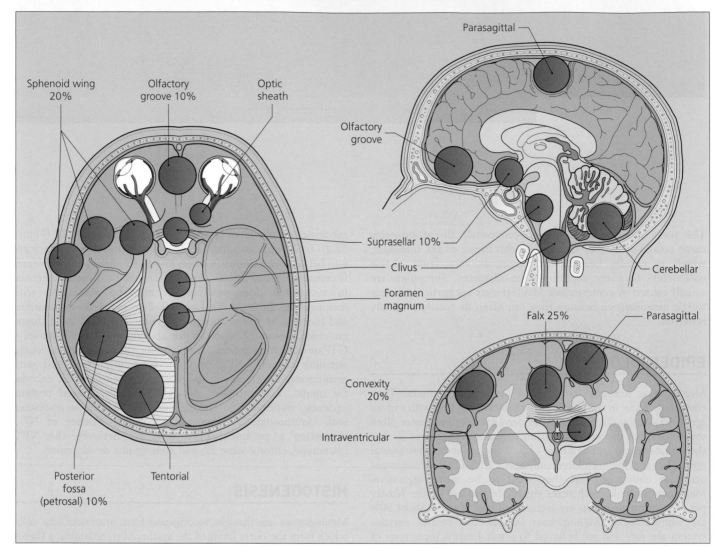

Figure 32.1 Three views of the skull and brain demonstrate the various locations of tumors and their relative occurrence at these sites.

small size of the tumor.[2] An *en plaque* meningioma, which has a flat pancake-like appearance under a thickened area of involved bone (Figure 32.6), occasionally occurs, usually in the area of the sphenoid ridge. Multiple meningiomas occur in 5–15% of patients, particularly in association with NF-2 (Figure 32.7).

Microscopic appearance

The histologic hallmark of meningiomas is whorls that form around a central hyaline material, which eventually calcify and form psammoma bodies (psammomatous type); interlacing bundles of elongated fibroblasts with narrow nuclei are found in the fibroblastic type (Figure 32.8). The World Health Organization recognizes nine subtypes of benign meningiomas[5] (Table 32.1), none of which predict tumor behavior. Several more recently described tumor subtypes – clear cell,[6] rhabdoid,[7] and chordoid[8] – join the papillary subtype as meningiomas that are more aggressive and more recurrence prone. Malignant tumors are defined by frequency of mitoses, invasion of the cortex, and metastasis.[5] The

angioblastic variety is histologically similar to the hemangiopericytoma with a high rate of recurrence.

BONY INVOLVEMENT, METASTASIS, AND ASSOCIATED LESIONS

Most meningiomas are adjacent to the skull, and they often involve it. Bone reacts to the neighboring tumors by *endostosis*, *exostosis*, or actual invasion (Figure 32.9). Surgical removal of the involved bone is necessary to eliminate recurrence. Bony changes that indicate the site and nature of the tumor are seen in about one-third of patients with meningiomas.

Meningiomas rarely spread locally to the temporal muscle or invade the surrounding cavities of the orbit, air sinuses, or middle ear, or pass through neural foramina into adjacent spaces (Figure 32.10). A malignant meningioma may occasionally metastasize to viscera, but this is more a pathologic oddity than the usual course. The most common site of metastasis is the lung.

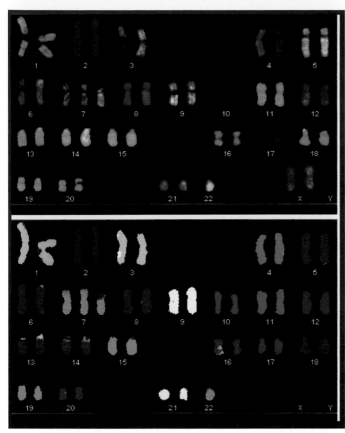

Figure 32.2 Chromosomal analysis demonstrating the loss of one of the two chromosomes 22.

Meningiomas may occur in association with other tumors, but this is coincidental; only the simultaneous occurrence of a meningioma and a breast carcinoma is significant. Patients with neurofibromatosis, however, are known concurrently to develop gliomas and vestibular schwannoma along with meningiomas (Figure 32.7). In patients without neurofibromatosis, the most common concurrent neoplasm is glioblastoma multiforme.[2]

DIAGNOSTIC STUDIES

Computed tomography (CT) is a definitive diagnostic method that shows the tumor as a homogeneously contrast-enhancing mass with well-defined borders (see Figure 32.11). Edema is well demonstrated on CT scans. Magnetic resonance imaging (MRI) has become the diagnostic study of choice, particularly with contrast enhancement, because it can reliably demonstrate the tumor and its relationship to neural and vascular structures. In multiple planes, these images show the extent of dural thickening, peritumoral edema, and associated hydrocephalus. MRI are particularly accurate in depicting encasement of major vessels (Figure 32.12).

Magnetic resonance angiography (MRA) and venography (MRV) are supplanting conventional angiography, because of their ability noninvasively to demonstrate vascular details that are critical for operative planning. MRA can demonstrate altered arterial anatomy, arterial constriction, and frequently the tumor's vascularity (Figure 32.13A). MRV can demonstrate the venous drainage pattern and venous sinus occlusion. Conventional angiography is recommended to evaluate meningiomas that appear

Figure 32.3 The architecture of the arachnoid villi, depicting arachnoid cap cells, the origin of meningiomas.

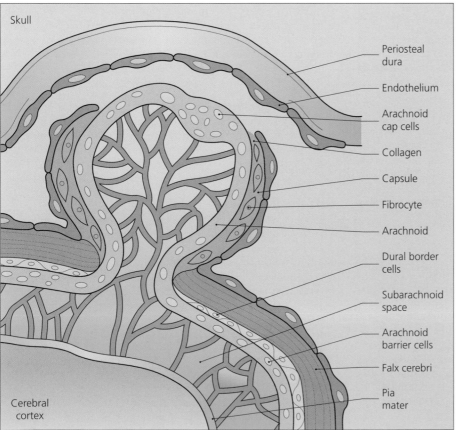

Skull

Periosteal dura

Endothelium

Arachnoid cap cells

Collagen

Capsule

Fibrocyte

Arachnoid

Dural border cells

Subarachnoid space

Arachnoid barrier cells

Falx cerebri

Pia mater

Cerebral cortex

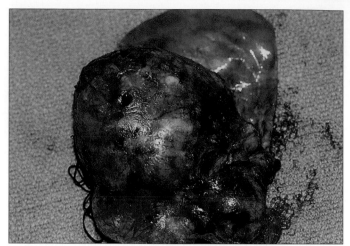

Figure 32.4 Surgical specimen of a meningioma demonstrating a well-demarcated multilobulated tumor on a dural base.

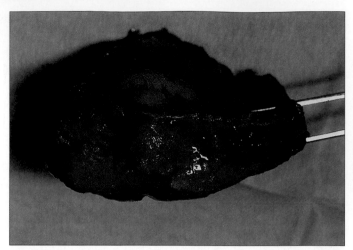

Figure 32.6 Operative photograph of *en plaque* meningioma with bony involvement.

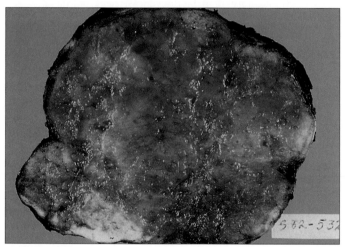

Figure 32.5 Cut surface of a meningioma demonstrating its firm character and pinkish color.

to be highly vascular on routine imaging or when preoperative tumor embolization is considered. Preoperative embolization can greatly facilitate surgical resection on conventional angiography; the vessels entering the tumor typically present a sunburst pattern (Figure 32.13B).

CLINICAL PRESENTATION

The clinical symptoms and signs of meningiomas are related to those of an intracranial mass lesion or seizure. The tumor has a predilection for certain regions and a tendency to produce hyperostosis of the skull, and some symptoms and signs are specific to the tumor's location. The clinical course of a meningioma characteristically spans a period of years. Depending on the location, the tumor may be giant before it becomes symptomatic, it may be discovered only after death because the patient was asymptomatic, or the patient may have a typical neurologic syndrome because adjacent neural structures are compressed (Figure 32.14).

Convexity

More than 70% of convexity meningiomas are frontal and anterior to the central sulcus. If located anteriorly, they may remain asymptomatic while growing to a large size. These tumors are usually concentrated around the coronal suture. Epilepsy and focal neurologic signs are common. These meningiomas have the best potential for total removal (Figure 32.15A,B).

Parasagittal

Parasagittal meningiomas arise in relation to the superior sagittal sinus, frequently in its middle third. They often cause focal epilepsy and later paralysis, particularly of the lower extremities. Hyperostosis often accompanies this tumor. The distinguishing feature of these meningiomas is that they involve the superior sagittal sinus and have an intimate relationship to the cortical veins draining into the sinus (Figure 32.16A,B).

Falx

Tumors arising from the falx also favor the anterior third and tend to be bilateral. Both falcine and sagittal meningiomas that involve the posterior part of the sagittal sinus or peritorcular area present a formidable surgical challenge and are likely to recur. The final outcome is guarded.

Olfactory groove

Olfactory groove meningiomas arise from the cribriform plate. They grow bilaterally and become large without causing significant neurologic deficits or evidence of increased intracranial pressure. Anosmia, which is rarely noticed, can be the only localizing sign. Changes in mental status are seldom striking until a tumor reaches an advanced stage. Once the tumor becomes large, it impinges on the optic nerves and chiasm, producing visual loss. These meningiomas may extend through the cribriform plate into the nasal cavity (Figure 32.17). The prognosis is excellent after surgical removal.

Tuberculum sellae

Tuberculum sellae meningiomas arise from the planum sphenoidale, tuberculum sellae, or the diaphragm sellae (Figure 32.18A,B).

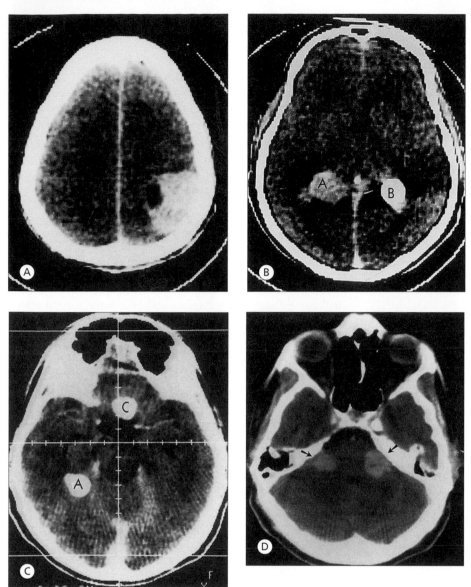

Figure 32.7 CT scan studies of multiple meningiomas in a patient with neurofibromatosis type II. (A) Left convexity meningioma. (B) A,B = bilateral intraventricular meningiomas. (C) C = tuberculum sella meningioma. (D) Bilateral acoustic neurofibromas (arrows).

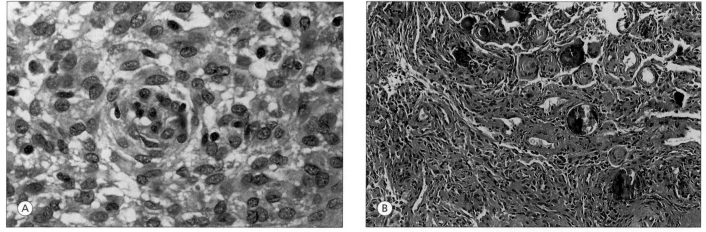

Figure 32.8 H & E stain of a typical meningioma showing characteristic whorl formations (A) and psammoma bodies (B).

Table 32.1 World Health Organization grading of meningiomas[5]

Meningioma	WHO grade
Meningothelial meningioma	I
Fibrous/fibroblastic meningioma	I
Transitional (mixed) meningioma	I
Psammomatous meningioma	I
Angiomatous meningioma	I
Microcystic meningioma	I
Secretory meningioma	I
Lymphoplasmacyte-rich meningioma	I
Metaplastic meningioma	I
Atypical meningioma	II
Clear cell meningioma	II
Chordoid meningioma	II
Rhabdoid meningioma	III
Papillary meningioma	III
Anaplastic (malignant) meningioma	III

They cause early and characteristic visual failure. Typically, loss of visual acuity and field is progressive and asymmetric, although it can be sudden. These tumors often cause hyperostosis over the planum sphenoidale.

Sphenoid ridge

Meningiomas of the sphenoid ridge are traditionally divided into three types: outer, middle, and inner. The outer sphenoid ridge usually harbors a large globoid tumor, accompanied by epilepsy, focal weakness, and, on the left side, aphasia. The rare *en plaque* variety is associated with hyperostosis, exophthalmos, and obvious swelling in the temporal region (Figure 32.19A,B). Tumors of the inner sphenoid ridge of the clinoidal type usually compress the optic nerve and present with early unilateral visual loss. They involve the cavernous sinus and may produce oculomotor palsies and facial hypesthesia. When the tumor becomes large, Foster–Kennedy syndrome (optic atrophy on one side and contralateral papilledema) is seen (Figure 32.20A,B). Meningiomas in the medial sphenoid ridge (Figure 32.21A,B) present a surgical challenge because they adhere to and encase the carotid artery (Figure 32.22).

Posterior fossa

Posterior fossa meningiomas constitute about 10% of all meningiomas. They frequently arise from the posterior surface of the petrous bone and are divided into four areas: petrosal, clival, foramen magnum, and the cerebellar convexities (Figure 32.1). When they arise from the tentorium, they can grow in both the

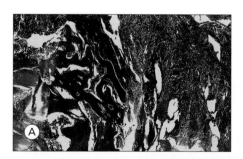

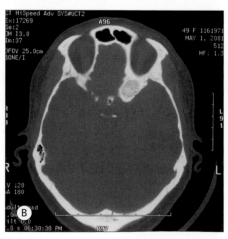

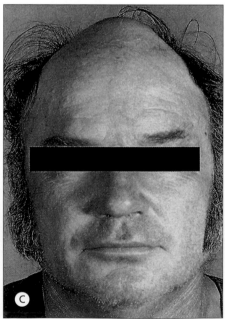

Figure 32.9 (A) H & E stain depicting invasion of the bone by a meningioma. (B) CT scan demonstrating hyperostotic bone in the sphenoid wing and orbital roof. (C) A patient with apparent bony growth secondary to invasion by a meningioma.

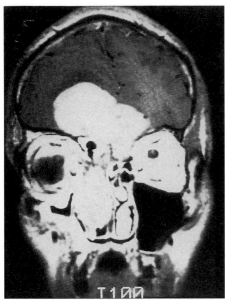

Figure 32.10 Local spread of a meningioma into adjacent skull base structures.

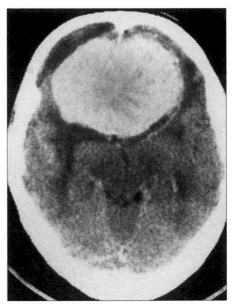

Figure 32.11 Contrast-enhanced CT scan of a typical benign meningioma.

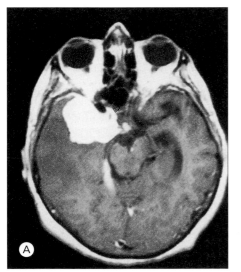 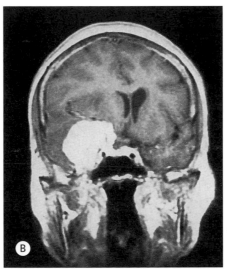 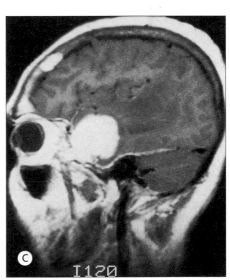

Figure 32.12 Gadolinium-enhanced MR image of a medial sphenoid wing meningioma in axial (**A**), coronal (**B**), and sagittal (**C**) planes.

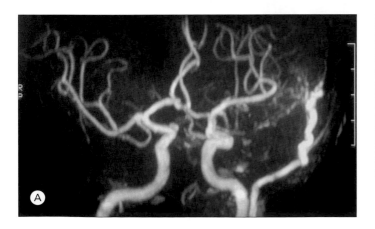

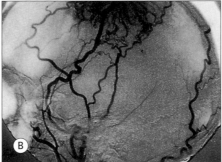

Figure 32.13 Magnetic resonance angiography can demonstrate arterial constriction or displacement as well as tumor vascularity, such as this dilated left middle meningeal artery (**A**). External carotid angiogram of a meningioma demonstrates a classical sunburst pattern (**B**).

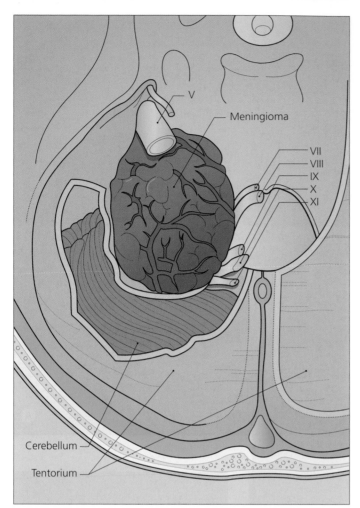

Figure 32.23 Tentorial meningioma growing above and below the tentorium and involving multiple cranial nerves.

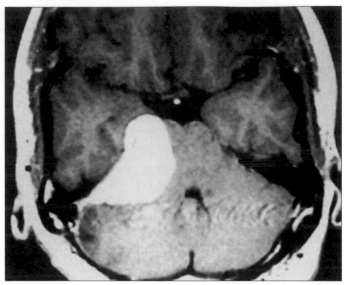

Figure 32.24 Contrast-enhanced MR image of a meningioma of the posterior fossa originating from the petrous portion of the temporal bone and filling the cerebellopontine angle.

size, however they have not been able to eradicate meningiomas.[13] Currently, medical management is a treatment option in unresectable meningiomas that have recurred or are progressive. More aggressive chemotherapeutic regimens have been reported for malignant meningiomas.[14]

RECURRENCE

Meningiomas are known to recur. Many factors relate to recurrence, the most important of which is the extent of the original removal. If the tumor has been totally removed, including

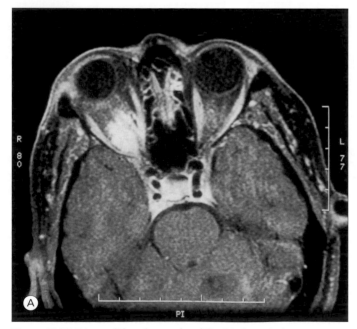

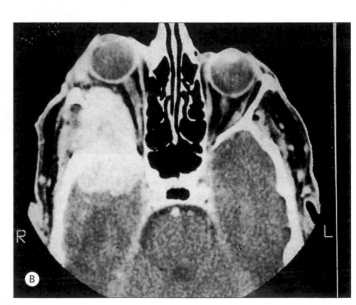

Figure 32.25 Primary (A) and secondary (B) orbital meningioma.

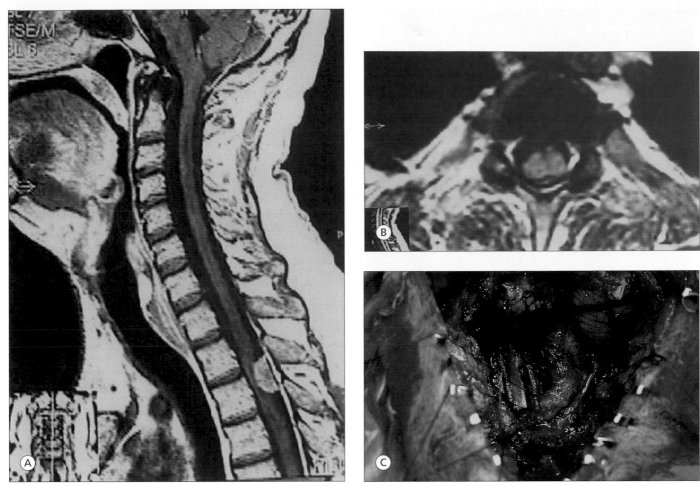

Figure 32.26 Sagittal (A) and axial (B) contrasted MR images of a spinal cord meningioma. Intraoperative photographs of spinal cord meningioma resection (C).

CLINICAL PEARLS

- Meningiomas are generally benign, circumscribed neoplasms arising from arachnoid cap cells with secondary attachment to the dura. They are distributed along the known locations of arachnoid granulations in the vicinity of major venous sinuses.

- Trauma, prior radiation, oncogenic viruses, hormones and defective genes are implicated in their causation.

- Several classic histologic types occur, the most common being the psammomatous type.

- Most meningiomas are benign; they generally do not recur if they are totally removed along with their dual attachment. Aggressive, frankly malignant, and metastasizing variants carry less favorable prognosis and higher risk of recurrence.

- Bone involvement is common.

- MRI, with and without contrast administration, is the single most useful test; CT, MRA, MRV and conventional angiograms may add further information in selected cases.

- The clinical syndrome is dictated by the location of the tumor.

- Total surgical excision when technically feasible is the treatment of choice. In unresectable, malignant, or recurrent tumors focused beam radiation therapy, fractionated external beam radiation therapy, hormonal manipulation and chemotherapy may slow the tumor growth and offer palliation.

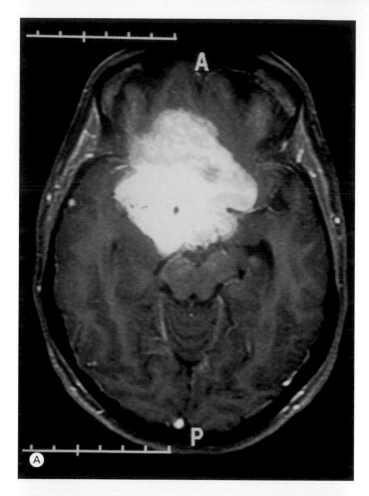

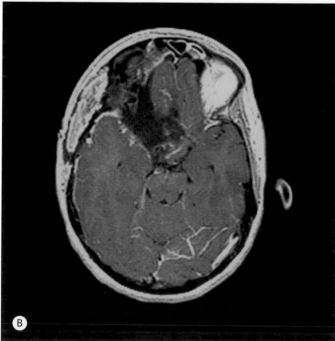

Figure 32.27 Original MR scan **(A)** and postoperative study **(B)** of a medial sphenoid meningioma

the margin of the dura and involved bone, recurrence is thought to be from a multicentric focus. Naturally, malignant and atypical tumors are associated with a higher incidence of recurrence, and radiation therapy is usually applied to these tumors. Symptomatic recurrence usually occurs within 5 years but can be detected within 2¹/₂ years with the newest methods of neurological imaging. Reasons for incomplete tumor removal include venous sinus invasion, investment of vital structures, and bone involvement.

REFERENCES

1. Cushing H, Eisenhardt L. *Meningiomas: Their Classification, Regional Behaviour, Life History, and Surgical End Results*. Springfield, IL: Charles C Thomas Publisher; 1938.
2. Al-Mefty O (ed.). *Meningiomas*. New York, NY: Raven Press; 1991.
3. Al-Mefty O, Kersh JE, Routh A, Smith RR. The long-term side effects of radiation therapy for benign brain tumors in adults. *J Neurosurg* 1990; 73: 502–12.
4. Kida S, Yamashima T, Kubota T, *et al*. A light and electron microscopic and immunohistochemical study of human arachnoid villi. *J Neurosurg* 1988; 69: 429–35.
5. Kleihues P, Cavenee WK (eds). *World Health Organisation Classification of Tumours: Pathology and Genetics of Tumours of the Nervous System*. Lyon: IARC Press; 2000.
6. Zorludemir S, Scheithauer BW, Hirose T, *et al*. Clear cell meningioma. A clinicopathologic study of a potentially aggressive variant of meningioma. *Am J Surg Pathol* 1995; 19: 493–505.
7. Perry A, Scheithauer BW, Stafford SL, *et al*. "Rhabdoid" meningioma: an aggressive variant. *Am J Surg Pathol* 1998; 2: 1482–90.
8. Couce ME, Aker FV, Scheithauer BW. Chordoid meningioma: a clinicopathologic study of 42 cases. *Am J Surg Pathol* 2000; 24: 899–905.
9. Kondziolka D, Levy EI, Niranjan A, *et al*. Long-term outcomes after meningiomas radiosurgery: physician and patient perspectives. *J Neurosurg* 1999; 91: 44–50.
10. Shafron DH, Friedman WA, Buatti JM, *et al*. LINAC radiosurgery for benign meningiomas. *Int J Rad Oncol Biol Phys* 1999; 43: 321–7.
11. Grunberg SM, Weiss MH, Spitz IM, *et al*. Treatment of unresectable meningiomas with the antiprogesterone agent mifepristone. *J Neurosurg* 1991; 74: 861–6.
12. Markwalder T-M, Seiler RW, Zava DT. Antiestrogenic therapy of meningiomas—A pilot study. *Surg Neurol* 1985; 24: 245–9.
13. Mason WP, Gentili F, Macdonald DR, *et al*. Stabilization of disease progression by hydroxyurea in patients with recurrent or unresectable meningioma. *J Neurosurg* 2002; 97: 341–6.
14. Chamberlain MC. Adjuvant combined modality therapy for malignant meningiomas. *J Neurosurg* 1996; 84: 733–6.

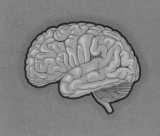

TUMORS OF THE PINEAL REGION

33

Christian Matula

Treatment of tumors in the pineal region remains one of the great intellectual and technical challenges to neurological surgeons. The mystique of the poorly understood function of the pineal gland, the beauty of its anatomy, and the elegance of the surgical approaches to this region, have fascinated generations of neurosurgeons. When coupled with the currently satisfactory clinical outcomes in the hands of experienced neurosurgeons, the allure of microsurgery or endoscopy of pineal region tumors is understandable.

Advances in microsurgical techniques, imaging, anesthesia, and critical-care medicine have led to a paradigm shift in the goals and approaches to treating pineal region tumors. In addition, minimally invasive techniques – such as neuroendoscopic techniques (classical neuroendoscopic operations or as endoscope-assisted or endoscope-guided procedures) – continue to evolve and have helped further revolutionize this subject.

HISTORY

The mystique of the pineal gland's function and the challenge of operating in this region make it worthwhile to provide a brief overview of the relevant historical facts The anatomists of ancient times knew about the pineal body and named it *Konareion* because of its cone-shaped appearance. It was first described by Herophilus of Alexandria (325–280 BC). Like all his contemporaries, he believed the ventricles to be the "seat of spirits" and thought that the pineal body acted like a sphincter, regulating the flow of thoughts between the third and the fourth ventricles. Galen (AD 129–201) was most likely the first to hypothesize that the pineal body served as a gland. During Galen's time, the structures of the pineal region were compared with the external genital organs of men. They named the pineal body, the "penis," the superior *colliculi* of the quadrigeminal plate "testes" and the inferior *colliculli of the quadrigeminal plate* "nates," simply based on their comparable appearance to these structures. Gibson in 1763, would later recapitulate these ideas in his *Epitome of Anatomy*.

Vesalius (1514–1564) described the pineal gland as being "similar to a cone from a pine tree." His description in 1543 was the basis for the current name "pineal gland." Descartes (1596–1650) during the 17th century suggested that the pineal gland be named *epiphysis cerebri* as he thought it was the "seat of the soul." He suggested that the pineal body acted like a valve, regulating the passage of spirits between the ventricles. He conceived the human body as a machine controlled by the pineal gland, which activated all the organs. His descriptions in 1677

suggested that consciousness and the power of imagination were located in the pineal gland.

Medical history therefore has three hypotheses about the function of the pineal gland:

1 a mechanical function, serving as a sphincter between the third and fourth ventricles;
2 a spiritual function, serving as a seat for the spirit and the soul; and
3 an organ with glandular function.

In general, tumors of the brainstem, as well as in the pineal region, were considered to be inoperable until the later part of the 20th century. There are only scattered reports on attempted or successful operations. In most cases, the patient died during the operation or shortly afterwards. One of the first clinical reports of a pineal region tumor in the 20th century was made by Cushing in 1904. He reported a bitemporal compression in a 28-year-old male with clinical evidence of a pineal region tumor. A few weeks later, the autopsy revealed the presence of a glioma of the quadrigeminal plate. The first direct surgical intervention was described by Horsley in 1905, and the first successful pineal region extirpation was described by Oppenheim and Krause in 1913. Since that time, a great number of neurosurgeons and investigators have written extensively on this topic, including McLean (1935), Dandy (1945), Pia (1954), Bailey (1964), Schmidek (1977), Pendl (1985), Schindler (1985), Slavin and Ausman (1991), and Tomita (2000) among others.

ANATOMY

The pineal region is defined as the area of the brain bordered dorsally by the splenium of the *corpus callosum* and the *tela choroidea*, ventrally by the quadrigeminal plate and midbrain tectum, rostrally by the posterior parts of the third ventricle, and caudally by the *cerebellar vermis* (Figure 33.1). The pineal gland itself, as an evagination of the diencephalic ependymal roof between the habenular commissure and the posterior commissure, lies between the *superior colliculi* and basal to the splenium of the *corpus callosum*. It has a thin stalk to the epithalamus and developmentally is considered to be a paired structure. The neural connections with adjacent centers are the topic of discussion but have yet to be clarified. The pineal body itself has an average length of 7.97 mm (range from 5.0 to 12.0 mm) and is 4.25 mm (2.5–7.0 mm) in height and width. It is oval in shape. The suprapineal recess projects posteriorly between the upper surface of the pineal gland and the lower layer of the *tela choroidea* in the roof.

Several authors have described different classification systems. The most current classification system for pure pineal parenchymal tumors is from the fascicle the *World Health Organization Classification of Tumors*, edited by Paul Kleihues and Webster K. Cavenee and published in 2000.

GERM CELL TUMORS

Germ cell tumors derive from pluripotential germ cells and span a wide range of differentiation and malignant characteristics. They constitute a unique class of rare tumors that affect mainly children and adolescents. Predominantly they occur in the midline when they arise in the central nervous system (CNS). Intracranial germ cell tumors, in general, account for 0.4–3.4% of intracranial neoplasms. Their average incidence is considered to be 0.1 per 100 000 persons per year. Pineal germ cell tumors occur primarily in males. Germ cell tumors in females are more common in the suprasellar region. Most germ cell tumors of the CNS occur in the first three decades (98%) with a peak in the second decade (65%) between 11 and 20 years. The histogenesis of germ cell tumors is a subject of controversy. For a long time, they have been assumed to represent the neoplastic offspring of primordial germ cells. During the last decade, however, a variety of speculative proposals have been published on this topic. As a reuslt of the etiology, certain observations suggest that gonadotropins play a role in the development or progression of CNS germ cell tumors. These include the predilection with Klinefelter syndrome, a condition characterized by chronically elevated serum levels of gonadotropins. Due to the variety of possible origins, the following entities are distinguished: germinoma, embryonal carcinoma, yolk sac tumor (endodermal sinus tumor), choriocarcinoma, mature teratoma, immature teratoma, teratoma with malignant transformation, and mixed germ cell tumors. An accurate histological identification and subclassification of CNS germ cell tumors is critical for current treatment planning and prognostication. In fact, only the germinoma and teratoma are likely to be encountered as pure tumor types.

Germinoma

Pure germinomas (Figures 33.3A–C, 33.4D,E) account for 65–72% of all intracranial germ cell tumors. These usually occur in the pineal region, although the second most common site is supra- and intrasellar. Germ cell tumors can be "synchronous," and can be found both in the the suprasellar region and in the pineal region approximately 10% of the time. In fact, the discovery of a synchronous lesion on MRI is indicative of a germ cell tumor. The germ cell tumors are usually poorly circumscribed, light gray in color, granular, solid neoplasms that destroy the pineal gland and infiltrate the ventricular system and subarachnoid space early in their course. Hemorrhage into the tumor and necrosis or cystic degeneration are not often found. This tumor is composed of uniform cells resembling primitive germ cells, with large, vesicular nuclei, prominent nucleoli, and a clear, glycogen-rich cytoplasm. Additional features include lymphoid or lymphoblasmacellular infiltrates and, less frequently, scattered syncytiotrophoblastic giant cells.

Teratoma

Teratomas (Figure 33.3D,E) derive from all germ layers and are composed of well-differentiated tissues in an organ-like pattern.

These tumors in the pineal region most often affect males. They are usually identified within the first two decades of life but occur more often in much younger children than other germ cell tumors (mostly in children younger than 9 years of age, about 20% occur between the ages of 16 and 18). By definition, the term "teratoma" can be used only in cases where tumor elements derive from two or three germ layers. These tumors are usually well-circumscribed, round or lobulated and multicystic, and compress the surrounding structures. The cystic component of the tumor may be watery, mucoid, or sebaceous. Sometimes bone, cartilage, hair, or teeth are present. Immature tumors are more frequently associated with a malignant course. Histologically, teratomas differentiate along ectodermal, endodermal, and mesodermal lines (e.g. they recapitulate somatic development from the three embryonic germ layers). Mature and immature variants as well as teratomas with malignant transformation must be distinguished from each other.

Mature teratoma

Mature teratomas are composed exclusively of fully differentiated, "adult-type" tissue elements that are sometimes arranged in patterns resembling normal tissue relationships. Mitotic activity is low or even absent.

Immature teratoma

This teratoma variant is composed of incompletely differentiated components resembling fetal tissue. Immature tumors are more frequently associated with a malignant course, but malignant potential may be explained by the presence of other germ cell tumor elements, such as choriocarcinoma or germinoma.

Teratoma with malignant transformation

This is the generic designation for occasional teratomatous neoplasm that contains as an additional malignant component a cancer of conventional somatic type. Detecting evidence of a malignant transformation within a germ cell tumor should state the specific histological form that this takes.

Yolk sac tumor (endodermal sinus tumor)

The histological appearance of endodermal sinus tumors classically features Schiller–Duval bodies, which resemble the yolk sac or endodermal sinus – an extra-embryonic endodermal derivative in lower animals. These bodies are composed of a blood vessel invaginating a space, with both being covered by a layer of cuboidal tumor cells with clear cytoplasm, small dark nuclei and prominent nucleoli set in a loose, variably cellular and often conspicuously myxoid matrix resembling extraembryonic mesoblasts. Eosinophilic hyaline globules, immunoreactive for alpha-fetoprotein, are a diagnostic feature. Endodermal sinus tumors are usually highly invasive.

Embryonal carcinoma

This type of germ cell tumor is the least frequently reported and is one that represents a primitive neoplasm consisting of pluripotential large cells that proliferate in cohesive nets and sheets. They form abortive papillae or line irregular, gland-like spaces. The tumor may exceptionally replicate the structure of the early embryo, forming "embryoid bodies" replete with germ discs and miniature amniotic cavities. A high mitotic rate and zones of coagulative necrosis complete the histological picture.

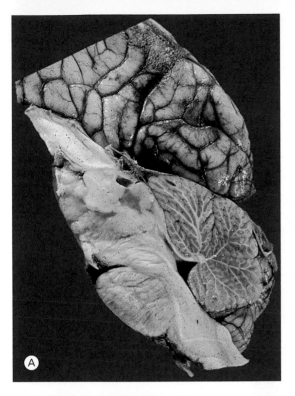

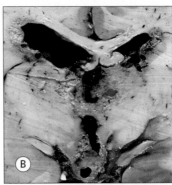

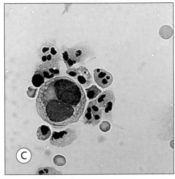

Figure 33.3 Midline sagittal section through the brain, with gross appearance of a germinoma. The tumor is infiltrating the brainstem at the level of the midbrain **(A)**. Frontal section through the brain, gross appearance of a germinoma growing into the ventricle **(B)**. Tumor cells of a germinoma in the postoperative cerebrospinal fluid representing a typical large cells with two prominent nucleoli (MGG, × 600) **(C)**. Histopathological features of a teratoma of the pineal region with fetal type glands and embryonic mesenchyme-like stroma (H&E, × 200) **(D)**. Immunohistochemistry out of **(D)** staining with synaptophysin representing the immature neuronal differentiated appearance (× 200) **(E)** (courtesy of O. Koperek, Neuropathological Institute, University of Vienna Medical School).

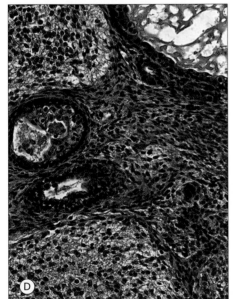

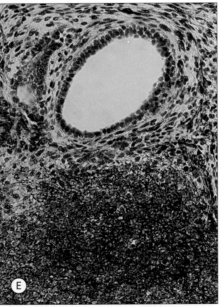

Choriocarcinoma

This type rarely arises extra-genitally and is characterized by extra-embryonic differentiation along trophoblastic lines. These tumors are characterized by two cell types: uniform cytotrophoblastic cells of medium size, with clear cytoplasm, vesicular nucleus, and distinct cell borders, and syncytio-trophoblastic cells, which are larger and multinucleated. The gross appearance of choriocarcinoma is a granular, reddish-brown mass, almost always with hemorrhage and necrosis As for all other tumors of germ cell origin, choriocarcinoma is usually accompanied by elements of other tumors of this group.

PINEAL PARENCHYMAL TUMORS

As described in the previous section of this article, these types of tumor constitute the second major group of pineal region tumors, accounting for 20–30% of all neoplasms in this location. They have to be considered to be the true neoplasm of the parenchyma of the pineal gland and are usually sharply delineated, with some formation of capsule and displacement of surrounding structures such as thalamus and midbrain. As a result of the variety of histological origins, the following entities are distinguished: pinealoblastoma, pinealocytoma, and pineal parenchymal tumor of intermediate differentiation.

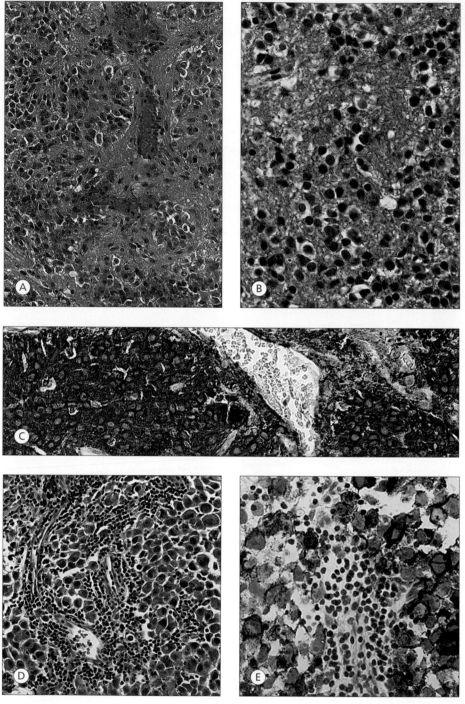

Figure 33.4 Histopathological features of a pinealocytoma with characteristic lobular pattern mimicking the structure of the normal pineal gland (H&E, 200×) **(A)**, isomorphic cells with small round nuclei and nucleus-free spaces filled with a fine meshwork of cell processes (neuropils) (H&E, 400×) **(B)**, and immunohistochemistry intensive diffuse staining with synaptophysin (× 200) **(C)**. Histopathological features of a germinoma with typical lymphocytic infiltrates along fibrovascular septae (H&E, × 200) **(D)** and immunohistochemistry staining of the cytoplasm and cytoplasmic membrane with placental alkaline phosphatase (PLAP) (× 400) **(E)** (courtesy of O. Koperek, Neuropathological Institute, University of Vienna Medical School).

Pinealoblastoma

This type of tumor (Figure 33.5A–D) is defined as a highly malignant, primitive embryonal tumor of the pineal gland itself and represents a true primitive neuroectodermal tumor (PNET). Although they are rare intracranial tumors, they constitute approximately 45% of all pineal parenchymal tumors. Usually they occur in the first two decades of life, more often in children, but principally can arise at any age. Some of these tumors may be present during the neonatal period. In larger series, pinealoblastomas are more common in males, with a male to female ratio of 2 : 1. The tumor usually replaces the tissue of the pineal gland. They are mostly soft, friable, and poorly demarcated and are pink,

white, or gray, smooth or granular when cut, sometimes cystic, and frequently hemorrhagic or necrotic. Calcifications are rare and infiltration of the surrounding structures, including the meninges, is common. Constituting the most primitive of pineal parenchymal tumors, pinealoblastomas are composed of patternless sheets of densely packed small cells with round to irregular nuclei and scant cytoplasm. Pinealocytomatous rosettes are lacking, but Homer–Wright and Flexner–Wintersteiner rosettes may be seen. Retinoblastomatous differentiation of pinealoblastomas sometimes occurs and supports the theory of the photoreceptive origin of pineal gland cells. Pinealoblastomas may accompany bilateral retinoblastomas, in which case together they are called trilateral

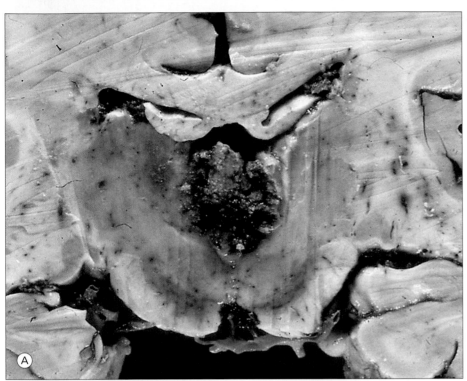

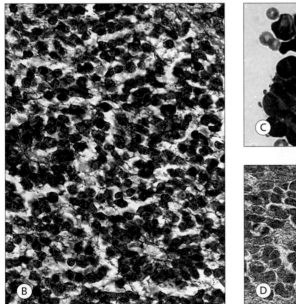

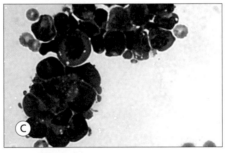

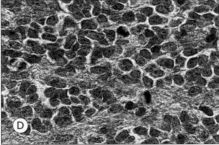

Figure 33.5 Frontal section of the brain, with gross appearance of a pinealoblastoma. The tumor is infiltrating the third ventricle **(A)**. Histopathological features of a pinealoblastoma with Flexner–Wintersteiner rosettes (H&E, × 400) **(B)**, typical tumor cells with mitotic activity in the cerebrospinal fluid (MGG, × 600) **(C)**, and high cellularity with numerous mitotic figures (H&E, × 400) **(D)** (courtesy of O. Koperek, Neuropathological Institute, University of Vienna Medical School).

retinoblastoma. Pinealoblastomas sometimes contain melanin pigment. Because of its infiltrating nature into surrounding structures, dissemination in the cerebrospinal fluid (CSF) is not so rare. Metastases to bone, lung, and lymph nodes have been reported.

Pinealocytoma

Pinealocytomas are defined as slow-growing pineal parenchymal neoplasms. They represent approximately 45% of all tumors with pineal parenchymal origin and occur throughout life, but most frequently in young adults (25–35 years). There is no sex predilec-

tion. Macroscopically, these tumors are well-circumscribed with a gray–tan, homogeneous or granular cut surface. Degenerative changes, such as hemorrhage and small cystic cavities, can be present. They may disseminate widely along the CSF pathways. The histological appearance is of a well-differentiated neoplasm composed of small, uniform, mature cells resembling pinealocytes. They grow in sheets, but also feature large pinealocytomatous rosettes composed of abundant, delicate tumor cell processes. Pinealocytomas may contain astrocytic or neuronal components or both (so-called ganglioma of the pineal). Such tumors are the most benign of the pineal parenchymal neoplasms.

Pineal parenchymal tumor of intermediate differentiation

This group of true pineal parenchymal tumors represents monomorphous types of lesions characterized by moderately high cellularity, mild nuclear atypia, occasional mitosis, and the absence of large pinealocytomatous rosettes. They occur in approximately 10% of all pineal parenchymal tumors and at all ages with a peak incidence in adulthood. The clinical behavior is variable.

TUMORS OF SUPPORTIVE AND ADJACENT STRUCTURES

There are several other tumors that can also be considered pineal parenchymal tumors, such as astrocytomas, ependymomas, or less frequently gliomas (glioblastomas or oligodendrogliomas). Glial cell tumors can also occur in the pineal gland, since astrocytes are normally present there, or may arise from the pluripotential pineal parenchymal cells. However, almost all glial tumors may arise from the glial tissue elements intimately surrounding the pineal gland. Real, true astrocytomas of the pineal gland itself are extremely rare. Tumors of other histological types may also occur as a substrate from the surrounding tissue, e.g. *choroidus plexus papillomas* or medulloepitheliomas. Tumors of mesenchymal origin that may occur include meningiomas, hemangiomas, and hemangiopericytomas or blastomas, which arise mostly from the falx and tentorium near their junction or from the *velum interpositum* at the roof of the third ventricle. Also reported are exceptionally rare cases of chemodectomas and craniopharyngiomas of the pineal region.

NON-NEOPLASTIC TUMOR-LIKE CONDITIONS

Sometimes of neurosurgical importance are non-neoplastic tumor-like malformations e.g. arachnoid cysts arising from the arachnoid cells of that region or "degenerative" cysts lined by fibrillary astrocytes (so-called pineal cysts). Cysticercosis and vascular lesions, such as arteriovenous malformations, cavernomas, and aneurysms of the vein of Galen, can also be included, but are very rare.

METASTASES TO THE PINEAL REGION

Although the absence of a blood-brain barrier in the pineal gland makes it a susceptible site for hematogenous metastases; however, despite this fact these tumors of the pineal region are surprisingly rare. The most common site of origin for metastases to the pineal region is the lung, followed by the breast and other organs, such as the stomach and kidney.

SIGNS AND SYMPTOMS

The presentation of patients with pineal region tumors relates to the anatomy being affected as well as to the specific tumor histology. However, the remarkable developments in neuroimaging are helping us to uncover more lesions in the pineal region in patients who have minimal symptoms and who might not normally be discovered until they became much more symptomatic. If the tumor is large enough to cause clinical symptoms, then these symptoms arise either because of local infiltration into surrounding neural structures or local compression to the adjacent structures. The most common symptom is Parinaud syndrome. It is present in 50–75% of all patients suffering from a pineal region tumor, characterized by its typical ocular movement disorder including paralysis of upward gaze, convergence or retraction nystagmus, and light-near dissociation. Direct pressure of the tumor on the tectum or dilatation of the proximal aqueduct causes the less common sylvian aqueduct syndrome, which includes paralysis of down gaze or horizontal gaze superimposed on Parinaud syndrome. Convergent nystagmus may be present when upward gaze is attempted. The anatomic substrate of these ocular functions is located below the posterior part of the third ventricle and anterior to the aqueduct. Lid retraction (Collier's sign) is quite rare; it is caused by compression of levator inhibitory fibers in the posterior commissure. Pupils are dilated and respond poorly to light, although they may respond to accommodation. Almost all patients with severe headaches have hydrocephalus by the time of presentation, causing the typical associated signs and symptoms, vomiting, lethargy and memory impairment. In infants, one typical sign is also an abnormally increasing head circumference and seizures. In the case of large tumors with invasive behavior, infiltration of the thalamic region or even the internal capsule can cause controlateral hemihypesthesia or paresthesia and sometimes can also be combined with typical thalamic pain syndromes. Depending on the extent of the invasion, extrapyramidal syndromes as well as different types of movement disorders can appear. Sudden occurrence of the sun-setting phenomenon, caused by hydrocephalus and Parinaud syndrome, together with decreased mental status, especially in infants, may be related to hemorrhage into the pineal tumor (pineal apoplexy). A commonly described endocrine disturbance in pineal region tumors is precocious puberty, which occurs in 10% of male patients with these lesions, and has been attributed to three hypothetical causes. One hypothesis connects the development of precocious puberty with ectopic secretion of beta human chorionic gonadotropin by choriocarcinoma or germinoma and thus explains the absence of precocious puberty in girls with pineal region tumors. Another hypothesis links precocious puberty with a mass effect in the region of the posterior diencephalon, which blocks its inhibitory effect on the median eminence of the hypothalamus, thereby augmenting secretion of gonadotropins. This hypothesis explains the association of precocious puberty with other symptoms of hypothalamic dysfunction (e.g. diabetes insipidus and polyphagia). According to a third hypothesis, the growth of a tumor in the pineal region causes a decrease in the secretion by the pineal gland of a substance (or substances) with antigonadotropic effect. If a pineal parenchymal tumor causes hypersecretion of such an agent, isolated hypogonadism may occur. In the case of drop metastases from the CSF, seeding radiculopathy or myelopathy can occur, sometimes from a nonspecific appearance. Signs and symptoms can occur in very rare cases as a result of hematogenous metastases to several structures outside the CNS.

DIAGNOSTIC STUDIES

Today, the two most important powerful diagnostic tools are laboratory tests including CSF cytology (tumor markers) and neuroradiological examinations using MRI and CT. Both are widely available and quite helpful for tumor detection.

Imaging

Diagnostic tools such as MRI have revolutionized the management of pineal region tumors (Figures 33.6A–C, 33.7A–C, 33.8A,B). The ability to obtain high-resolution images and multidimensional views makes it possible to show tumor location and extension clearly and accurately. Today, ventriculography or pneumencephalography have merely historical value. Skull radiography – formerly an important diagnostic study – has fallen into disuse because of its low sensitivity in detecting tumors. The normal pineal gland is seen on plain films as a calcified mass in 60% of the population over 20 years of age, and very rarely in children before the age of 6 years. Any calcified pineal gland that is larger than 1 cm in any dimension should be looked upon with suspicion. The appearance of a calcified pineal gland in early childhood is usually abnormal, but can, in fact, be physiologic in up to 5% of cases. CT superseded all other radiologic imaging methods for detection of pineal region tumors in the early 1980s. Currently, high-resolution CT with or without intravenous contrast administration is used to examine the pineal region, but is often more important for planning the appropriate approach than as a diagnostic tool. Carotid and vertebral arteriography are no longer used routinely. Superselective angiography has its undisputed value in detecting arterial or venous malformations such as aneurysms of the vein of Galen. Therefore, the current recommendation is to perform a high-resolution MRI examination and, when appropriate, in addition, CT scans with and without contrast. Table 33.2 gives an overview and comparison of the neuroradiological appearance of pineal region tumors in correlation to their pineal versus parapineal appearance, signal intensity (heterogeneous versus homogeneous), appearance of hemorrhage, calcification, brain edema or invasion, and contrast enhancement.

Tumor markers

Certain pineal region tumors manifest tumor markers that are identified in the serum and CSF. The identification is important not only for diagnostic purposes but also for monitoring response to treatment and relapse. The most important and useful markers

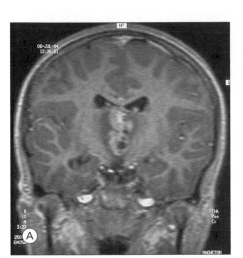 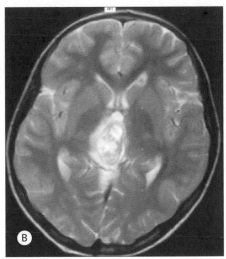 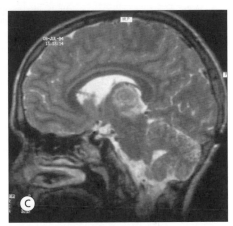

Figure 33.6 Coronal T1-weighted gadolinium enhanced MRI demonstrating an enhancing, demarcated mass lesion in the posterior part of the third ventricle representing a pinealoblastoma (A). Axial (B) and sagittal (C) T2-weighted MRI of the same patient.

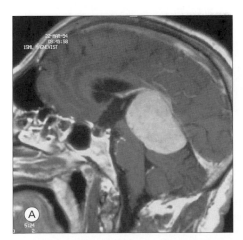 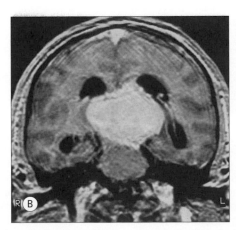 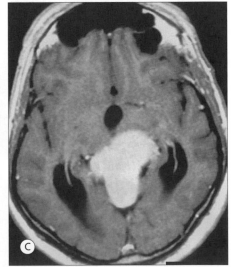

Figure 33.7 Infused MRI scans of a patient presenting a typical meningioma in the pineal region. Sagittal T1-weighted (A), coronal (B) and axial (C).

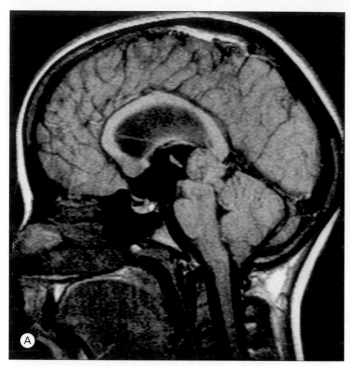
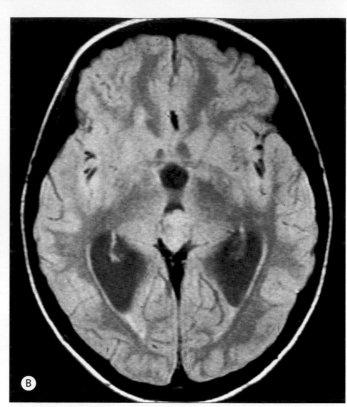

Figure 33.8 Infused T1-weighted MRI scans of a germinoma in sagittal direction **(A)** and axial direction **(B)** compressing the aqueduct, causing obstructive hydrocephalus.

Table 33.2 Pineal region tumors

	Germinoma	Teratoma	Pinealoblastoma	Pinealocytoma	Glioma	Meningioma
Age	Child	Child	Child	Adult	Child	Adult
Sex predilection	Male	Male	None	None	None	None
Pineal vs. parapineal	Pineal	Pineal	Pineal	Pineal	Parapineal (usually)	Parapineal (usually)
Signal intensity (heterogeneous vs. homogeneous)	Homogeneous (but often hemorrhagic)	Strikingly heterogeneous	Homogeneous (unless hemorrhagic)	Homogeneous	Homogeneous (usually)	Homogeneous
Hemorrhage	Common	Typical	Common	Common	Rare	Rare
Calcification	Rare	Typical	Common	Common	Uncommon	Common
Brain edema or invasion	Common	Variable	Common	Uncommon	Primarily midbrain neoplasm	Occasional
Tendency to metastasize	Yes	Variable	Yes	No	Variable	No
Enhancement	Dense	Variable	Dense	Dense	Variable	Dense
Prognosis (2-year survival rate, if available)	Excellent 83%	Variable 33%	Poor	Variable	Variable	Excellent

are the β-human chorionic gonadotropin and α-fetoprotein. α-Fetoprotein, a glycoprotein, is normally produced by the yolk sac and the fetal liver, and its production stops by the time of birth. An α-fetoprotein value of < 5 ng/mL in serum and CSF is considered to be normal. The greatest production of α-fetoprotein can be seen in cases of yolk sac tumors (endodermal sinus tumors). Embryonal carcinomas and immature teratomas produce α-fetoprotein to a lesser extent, < 1000 ng/mL. β-Human chorionic gonadotropin, also a glycoprotein, is normally produced by the syncytiotrophoblastic giant cells of placental trophoblastic tissue with a normal value in the serum and CSF of < 5 mIU/mL. Choriocarcinomas normally produce the highest amount,

Table 33.3 Tumor markers of pineal region tumors

	α-Fetoprotein (< 5 ng/mL)	Human chorionic gonadotropin (< 5 IU/mL)	Placental alkaline phosphatase	Melatonin
Germinoma	–	+ (< 770 IU/mL)	++	–
Teratoma	+ (< 1000 ng/mL)	–	–	–
Yolk sac tumor	+++	–	+/–	–
Embryonal carcinoma	++ (< 1000 ng/mL)	++ (< 770 IU/mL)	+	–
Choriocarcinoma	–	+++ (> 2000 IU/mL)	+/–	–
Pinealocytoma	–	–	–	+
Pinealoblastoma	–	–	–	++

> 2000 ng/mL. Mild elevations of < 770 ng/mL can be seen in cases of germinomas and embryonal carcinomas. The biological half-life is about 5 days for α-fetoprotein, but < 24 hours for β-human chorionic gonadotropin. In general, serum titers tend to show higher positivity than do CSF titers, because the tumor should be in direct contact with the CSF for positive markers. In recent studies, placental alkaline phosphatase was reported to be a specific marker for primary intracranial germinomas and is measured with an enzyme-linked immunosorbent assay in the serum as well as in the CSF. Melatonin as a tumor marker may be used in cases of tumors that destroy the pineal gland. The absence of melatonin in serum after surgery thereby indicates complete removal of the pineal gland. Elevation of the polyamines putrescine and spermidine in CSF has been reported in malignant brain tumors of childhood, especially PNETs.

Although the levels of markers in serum and CSF have been found to be extremely useful in assessing the efficacy of various treatment modalities and as indicators tumor recurrence; the tumor markers alone do not yield a definitive histological diagnosis. Table 33.3 gives a brief overview of the serum and CSF levels occurring in pineal region tumors. Both neuroimaging (MRI and possibly CT) and tumor marker evaluation improve diagnostic accuracy and should be routine measures for achieving an optimal diagnosis and planning the appropriate choice of treatment.

CHOICE OF TREATMENTS

Surgical treatment of pineal region tumors has been a topic of controversy and intellectual innovation for the past 100 years in neurological surgery. In the beginning of the 20th century, the lack of technical, anesthetic, and radiologic refinements led to uniformly poor surgical results and surgical mortality close to 90%. For decades, the treatment of these tumors was relegated to CSF diversion followed by radiotherapy. Even until the mid-1970s, the therapy of pineal region tumors consisted of ventricular shunting and radiation therapy, with 5-year survival rates as high as 60–80% with some histological types of tumor. Advanced techniques in microneurosurgery, neuroanesthesiology, neuroimaging, and intensive-care medicine have enabled modern neurosurgeons to operate on such lesions with more than acceptable outcomes. This has resulted in a much higher cure rate, decreased surgical mortality and morbidity, and increased longevity for those

individuals who have tumor recurrence after therapy. Today, control of hydrocephalus, which is associated with most of the tumors in this region, is no longer a problem and should be carried out routinely either through a shunting procedure or, more often, via endoscopic third ventriculostomy. Even in the case of non-resectable tumors, a safe and efficient histologic identification is advised and worth attempting by endoscopic stereotactic biopsy. This serves as the basis for further adjuvant radiotherapy and chemotherapy in these non-resectable lesions. There is a subset of tumors that lend themselves to resection despite their size and location. In these tumors a radical resection through a variety of approaches should be attempted by surgeons who are experienced with the technical refinements and surgical anatomy in this challenging region.

Stereotactic procedures

Stereotactic procedures, which have become increasingly more advanced and easy to use, may be used as a diagnostic tool for tumors that may not be amenable to resection. Most reports concerning this type of procedure indicate that the risks of intervention are minimal. However, caution is advised since the pineal region has numerous vessels, as described in the earlier section on anatomy. The vessels may be displaced from their normal position for several reasons (the pathology, brain swelling, etc). Also, some tumors, such as pinealoblastomas or choriocarcinomas, are highly vascular. However, the complication rate in stereotactic biopsy of these lesions is low: approximately 1.3% mortality and 7% morbidity, in skilled hands. The diagnostic is equivalently very high (94%), although sometimes stereotactic biopsy may fail to disclose the histological heterogeneity of some tumors, especially in the case of mixed malignant tumors.

Neuroendoscopy and hydrocephalus

Recent advances in neuroendoscopic techniques have enabled this technology to become a major component of the treatment strategies of pineal region tumors. In most of the cases, endoscopic biopsy can be performed with more than acceptable results, especially for tumors reaching into the posterior part of the third ventricle. There are case reports and series of pineal region tumors in which the hydrocephalus is treated by an endoscopic third ventriculostomy followed by a pineal region biopsy. The technique of endoscopic third ventriculostomy has proved to be highly effective and has obviated the need for placement of a permanent shunt. Alternatively, hydrocephalus may be controlled with either tumor mass reduction or a CSF diversion procedure such as a ventriculoperitoneal shunt. Patients presenting acutely with hydrocephalus may be treated using classical neuroendoscopic third ventriculostomy or, if not available, with external ventricular drainage. The ability of pineal cell tumors to metastasize through a diversionary CSF shunt is rare but has been reported. Certain germ cell tumors can reduce in size considerably within a short time following irradiation or chemotherapy, and hydrocephalus is resolved without any surgical procedure. However, these non-surgical procedures require at least several weeks and are not recommended in patients who present with acute hydrocephalus or local tumor compression syndromes. Steroid therapy should be used while awaiting the results of radiation, radiosurgery, and/or chemotherapy.

Surgical approaches and clinical examples

The efficacy of open microsurgery on pineal region tumors is undisputed in the 21st century. The main goal is complete tumor removal with minimal morbidity whenever possible. Even if that cannot be achieved for several reasons, histological verification, maximal cytoreduction, and, more often, restoration of CSF pathways may be achieved. For the benign pineal region tumor, surgery alone is often curative. Although about 80% of pediatric tumors are malignant, open surgery is recommended in most adult cases and selected pediatric cases in which resection is considered safe based on the appearance of the lesion by MRI. Radical resection is especially helpful in cases of the malignant non-germinoma germ cell tumors, as the extent of resection influences the prognosis of the patient. Because the pineal region is located in the geometric center of the intracranial cavity, operative approaches from every conceivable angle and direction have been developed (Figure 33.9). The five most common surgical approaches include:

1   the posterior transcallosal approach pioneered by Dandy;
2   the transventricular approach pioneered by Van Wagenen;
3   the occipital transtentorial approach pioneered by Foerster and Poppen;
4   the infratentorial-supracerebellar approach pioneered by Krause and popularized by Stein; and
5   the three-quarter-prone, operated side down, occipital transtentorial approach described by Ausman.

Other approaches include the frontal (anterior) transcallosal transventricular transvelum-interpositum approach by Sano, which is useful for large pineal tumors with anterior extension into the third ventricle, and represents a technical modifications of the first three approaches.

The posterior transcallosal approach

In 1921, Walter Dandy was one of the first to propose this approach to the pineal region. The primary anatomical structures exposed are the splenium of the *corpus callosum*, internal cerebral veins, basal vein of Rosenthal, vein of Galen, pineal body, posterior commissure, and the quadrigeminal plate. Patient position is similar to the position for the classical anterior transcallosal approach. However, a higher angle is required to provide the appropriate trajectory of about 40°. We prefer a semilunar skin incision over the midline. Craniotomy should include the lambdoid at the posterior margin of the bone flap (Figure 33.10). A semilunar

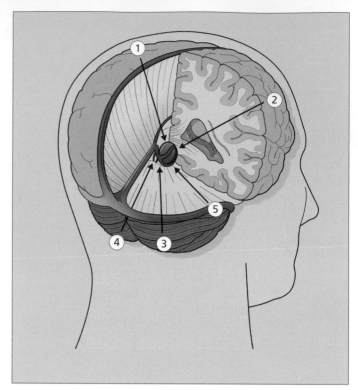

Figure 33.9 Schematic drawing of the various operative approaches to the pineal region from every direction (modified from Day *et al.*, *Color Atlas of Microneurosurgical Approaches*, Thieme, 1997).

dural flap is elevated to expose the cortical surface of the posterior parietal lobe. Entry point is the interhemispheric fissure (Figure 33.11). Bridging veins are rare posteriorly but should be preserved, whenever possible. Retraction of the mesial parietal lobe exposes the splenium of the *corpus callosum* and after splitting the splenium, the internal cerebral veins can be seen as they drain into the vein of Galen. The pineal gland is located inferior to the venous complex (Figure 33.12). The limitations of this approach include difficulty in visualization of inferiorly, the quadrigeminal plate, and laterally, the mesial occipital lobe, and the requirement to split the splenium of the *corpus callosum* and retract the mesial occipital lobe. Advantages of this approach are the superior access superior to the venous complex and the ability to visualize the veins so that they are not sacrificed. We recommend this approach for tumors spreading superior to the venous complex and expanding anteriorly into the third ventricle as well as those extending upward into the *corpus callosum* (Figure 33.13A–C). It is an approach that still has applications but has been supplanted by the other approaches, detailed above.

The occipital transtentorial approach

This approach was first proposed by Foerster in 1928 and described in detail by Poppen in 1966. Primary anatomical structures exposed are the splenium of the *corpus* callosum, internal cerebral veins, basal vein of Rosenthal, vein of Galen, the precentral cerebellar vermian vein, pineal body, posterior commissure, and the quadrigeminal plate. This approach comes from a more lateral direction and we prefer to have the patient in the recumbent, semi-sitting position with the chin tucked. Skin incision is an inverted L-shaped incision to expose the occipital

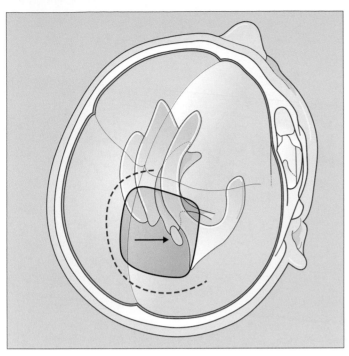

Figure 33.10 The posterior transcallosal approach. Direction of the approach, skin incision and postion of craniotomy (modified from Day *et al.*, *Color Atlas of Microneurosurgical Approaches*, Thieme, 1997).

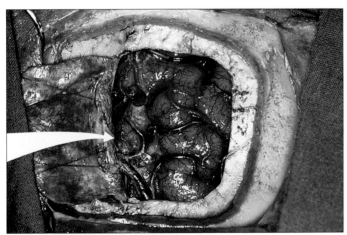

Figure 33.11 Dura opening and entrance into the interhemispheric fissure in an anatomic cadaver (modified from Day *et al.*, *Color Atlas of Microneurosurgical Approaches*, Thieme, 1997).

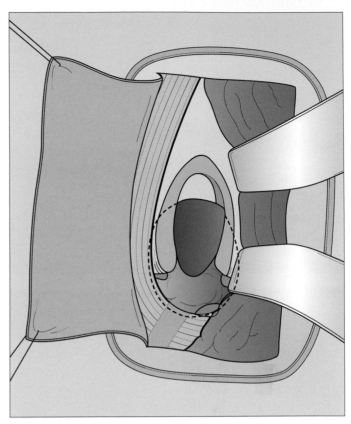

Figure 33.12 Approach to pineal region while performing the posterior transcallosal approach, demonstrating the relation from the pineal tumor to the venous system and surrounding structures (modified from Pendl, *Pineal and Midbrain Lesions*, Springer, 1985).

region. The inion should be clearly exposed and the bone flap is made with its superior margin approximately 1–2 cm below the lambdoid suture. The inferior margin is below the inion, thus placing the roecular within the inferior portion of the dural exposure (Figure 33.14). After opening the dura, the occipital lobe is retracted laterally to expose the posterior incisural edge and its junction with the falx cerebri. After the tentorium is incised, the lateral entry point has been reached and the venous complex can be explored (Figure 33.15). Sharp dissection of the arachnoid exposes the vein of Galen and the ipsilateral basal vein of Rosenthal. The pineal gland is most clearly visible inferior to the venous complex (Figure 33.16). Limitations of the approach

include poor visualization of the internal cerebral veins anteriorly, the quadrigeminal plate inferiorly, the falx cerebri and vein of Galen medially and the occipital lobe laterally. In addition, it is not uncommon to compress and injure the visual cortex through the extremes of retraction that are required to lift the occipital lobe. An advantage of this approach is the superb view – both above and below the tentorium. This approach is recommended for tumors growing through the tentorial hiatus with a supra- and infra-cerebellar extension, and especially in the case of meningiomas (Figure 33.17A–C). This approach is used in about 20% of the cases in our institution and makes this the second most common approach for dealing with tumors in the pineal region.

The infratentorial supracerebellar approach

The infratentorial supracerebellar approach was first described by Krause in 1913 and then modified and popularized by Stein in 1971. Performing this kind of approach in the sitting position means that gravity assists the cerebellum in falling down from the undersurface of the tentorium. Primary anatomical structures exposed are the cerebellum, the cerebellar veins, cerebellar vermian veins, the internal cerebellar veins, basal veins of Rosenthal, the vein of Galen, pineal body, posterior commissure, quadrigeminal plate, splenium of *corpus callosum*, and the posterior third ventricle. We prefer the patient to be placed in the sitting position with the head flexed anteriorly. The amount of flexion depends on the relationship of the tumor to the straight sinus. As an alternative position, we recommend the so-called modified "concord"

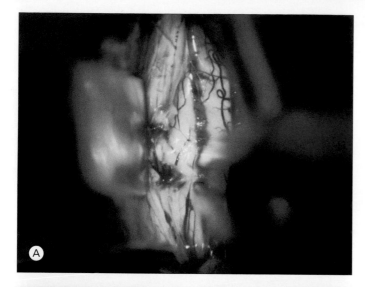

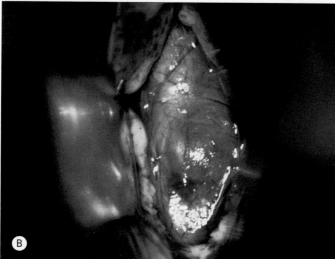

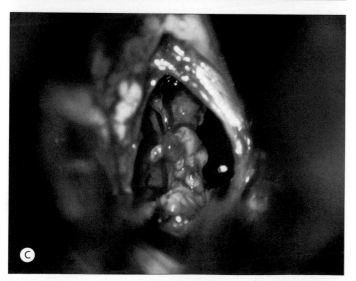

Figure 33.13 Intraoperative findings in case of a pinealoblastoma as presented in Figure 33.6A–C. Situation during splitting the splenium of the corpus callosum using a non-stick bipolar forceps (A). Appearance of the tumor located in the posterior part of the third ventricle before resection (B) and after complete tumor removal (C).

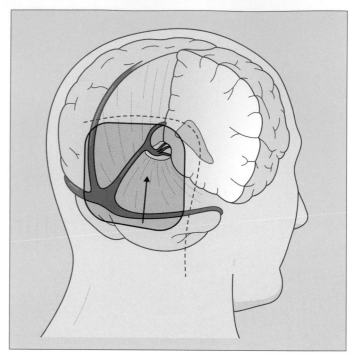

Figure 33.14 The occipital transtentorial approach: trajectory of the approach, skin incision and position of craniotomy (modified from Day *et al.*, *Color Atlas of Microneurosurgical Approaches*, Thieme, 1997).

position that allows the surgeon to sit comfortably behind the patient. One of the main advantages of the concord position is that it decreases the risk of air embolism. One of the disadvantages is that it is sometimes impossible when the tentorium is very steep. The skin incision is made in the midline, and we use either an S-shaped or a straight midline incision. The craniotomy is centered over the external occipital protuberance and includes the *torcular herophili* at the superior portion of dural exposure (Figure 33.18). This allows some upward retraction of the sinus complex, decreasing the degree of necessary downward retraction of the cerebellum. In most of the cases it is not necessary to open the foramen magnum. The preserved rim of bone inferiorly provides support for the cerebellum, decreasing traction on its superior connecting elements to the brain stem. Arachnoid dissection and division of the superomedial cerebellar bridging veins allow subsequent inferior retraction of the cerebellar hemispheres (Figure 33.19). In most of cases, a very thick arachnoid membrane is found spanning the interval between the cerebellar vermis and the central posterior incisura. After dissection of the arachnoid membrane the venous complex surrounding the pineal gland can be explored (Figure 33.20). Limitations of the approach are its restriction to the midline and limited extension to the lateral side. The most powerful advantage is the superior access inferior to the venous complex. We recommend this approach in most of the cases (more than 72%) in which the tumors are restricted to the midline and inferior to the venous complex. It also represents a perfect opportunity to use a rigid-angled endoscope as an adjuvant during surgery. This so-called endoscope-assisted or endoscope-guided procedure allows not only perfect illumination (which gives the anatomical structures more plasticity), but also enables the surgeon to have a "look around a corner" without even touching any anatomical structure. This helps the surgeon to detect any

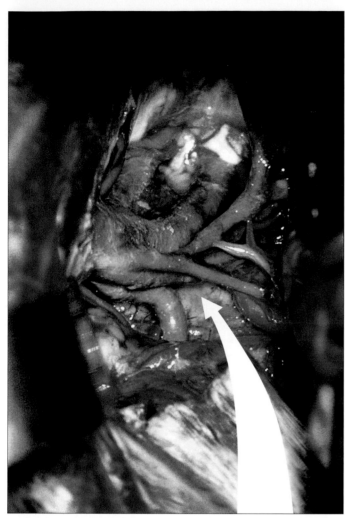

Figure 33.15 Dura opening and entrance after incision of the tentorium in an anatomic cadaver (modified from Day *et al.*, *Color Atlas of Microneurosurgical Approaches*, Thieme, 1997).

residual tumor hiding in the recesses of the pineal region, thus increasing the chance for a radical tumor resection (Figure 33.21).

The transventricular approach

The transventricular approach which was first described by Van Wagenen in 1931, is also useful in some select patients. This type of approach is indicated in very rare cases of large, eccentric lesions with ventricular dilatation. The entry point with this approach is usually via a cortical incision in the posterior portion of the superior temporal gyrus. Unfortunately, this exposes the patient to a high risk of visual impairment, seizure and dominant side language dysfunction. Therefore, this approach is limited to the non-dominant hemisphere.

In general, the main goal of pineal region microsurgery consist of having a complete tumor resection, combined with no additional neurological deficits. The routine use of transesophageal ultrasound in the sitting position to prevent air embolism, the widespread application of frameless stereotactic neuronavigational systems, and the increasingly common use of endoscopes have helped to refine and increase the safety associated with attempts at radical resection of pineal region tumors.

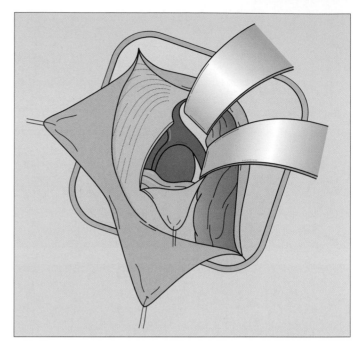

Figure 33.16 Pineal region after performing an occipital transtentorial approach presenting the relation of the pineal tumor to the venous system and surrounding structures (modified from Pendl, *Pineal and Midbrain Lesions*, Springer, 1985).

Other therapeutic modalities

Although in the majority of cases surgical removal is the treatment of choice, some tumors (like germinomas or non-germinoma germ cell tumors) may require further therapy. These tumors have shown a sensitivity to radiation therapy and chemotherapy, and thus these adjuvant therapies are now established as further therapeutic modalities.

Radiotherapy

Although more than 70% of tumors in the pineal region and the posterior third ventricle are highly radiosensitive, radiation therapy is still a subject of controversy. Select tumors respond to adequate courses of radiation therapy within 3–6 months. The current neurosurgical paradigm of the treatment of acute hydrocephalus followed by diagnostic biopsy or radical resection of tumor has obviated the need for preoperative empirical radiation therapy prior to diagnosis. However, it has been clinically proven that germinomas, like seminomas, are highly sensitive to radiation therapy. Therefore, in some institutions a pineal region tumor that has the classical appearance of a germinoma on MRI will receive a test dose of 5 Gy of radiation prior to any surgery. If the tumor shows shrinkage, then the diagnosis of germinoma is certain and radiation therapy will be continued without further surgery. There remain controversies regarding the optimal tumor dose, the volume to be irradiated, and the precise role of elective spinal irradiation and preradiation chemotherapy for germinomas. Radiotherapy is not a benign form of treatment, especially to the developing central nervous system, such as in the pediatric population. Serious consequences of such treatment include endocrine deficiencies, severe vasculitis, and significant intellectual impairment. All of these risks limit the dosage and modalities used in radiotherapy of pineal region tumors in young children. The application of preradiation chemotherapy and stereotactic

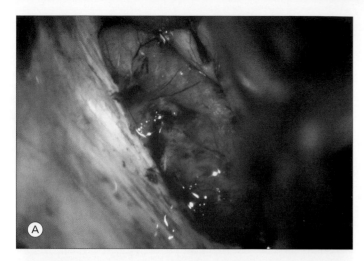

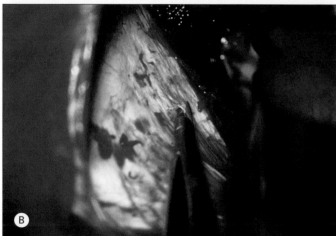

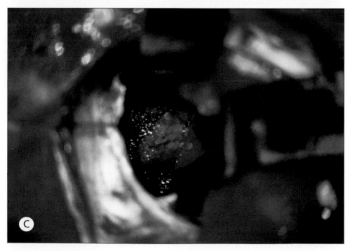

Figure 33.17 Intraoperative findings in case of a meningeoma as presented in Figure 33.7A–C. Photograph before the incision of the tentorium with the tumor in the background (A). Incision of the tentorium, as one of the key steps in performing the approach (B) and the situation after complete tumor removal, the surrounding tissue is covered with surgicel (C).

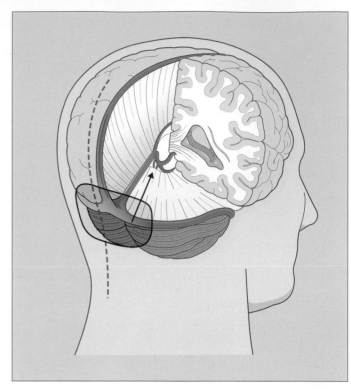

Figure 33.18 The infratentorial supracerebellar approach: trajectory of the approach, skin incision and position of craniotomy (modified from Day *et al.*, *Color Atlas of Microneurosurgical Approaches*, Thieme, 1997).

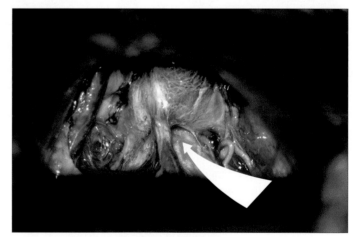

Figure 33.19 The infratentorial supracerebellar entry into the pineal region in an anatomic cadaver (modified from Day *et al.*, *Color Atlas of Microneurosurgical Approaches*, Thieme, 1997).

radiation techniques such as Linnac and gamma knife radiosurgery may provide some relief from the potential detrimental side-effects of radiation on the developing brain. Despite the well-established radiosensitivity of germinomas, about 10% of the patients may experience tumor recurrence.

Chemotherapy

Chemotherapy has gained considerable recognition for the treatment especially of malignant germ cell tumors. In 1977, de Tribolet and Barrelet reported the successful use of chemotherapy in a patient with a large pineal tumor. The chemotherapeutic

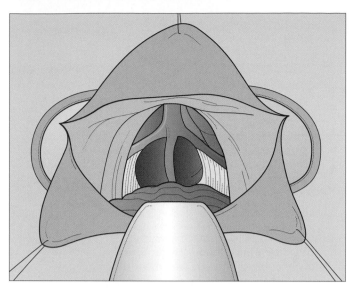

Figure 33.20 Pineal region while performing the infratentorial supracerebellar approach presenting the relation of the pineal tumor to the venous system and surrounding structures (modified from Pendl, *Pineal and Midbrain Lesions*, Springer, 1985).

regimen included daunorubicin, vincristine, and bleomycin. Later, the combination of cisplatin, bleomycin, and vincristine (PVB therapy) was employed to treat germ cell tumors in several series with limited success. In 1987, Takakura recommended the use

of ACNU (nimustine) and vincristine together with radiotherapy in cases of immature teratomas and PVB therapy after completing the entire course of radiotherapy to prevent recurrence. Responses to chemotherapy are apparent not only on MRI but also from tumor markers. Despite the known toxicity of chemotherapeutic agents, chemotherapy has an accepted role in the treatment of malignant pineal region tumors.

CONCLUSION

In the Western hemisphere, tumors of the pineal region constitute about 1% of all intracranial neoplasms and are more common in children (3–8% of all pediatric brain tumors). However, in Japan, pure germ cell tumors are more common for unknown reasons, and pineal region tumors constitute 4–7% of all intracranial neoplasms. The author's own data show a predominance of males (67%) to females (33%) in all cases. About 65% of all the cases involve patients who are younger than 20 years of age and about 35% who are aged between 21 and 70. Pathologically, primary tumors of the pineal region can be divided into: germ cell tumors (~60%), pineal parenchymal tumors (~30%), tumors of supportive and adjacent structures (~10%), non-neoplastic tumor-like conditions (less than 1%) and metastases (less than 0.1%). Symptoms of tumors in the pineal region are caused either by obstruction of CSF pathways or by local involvement (compression or invasion) of adjacent structures. Characteristic local signs include visual disturbances – the most common being Parinaud syndrome.

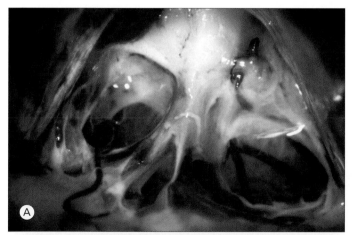

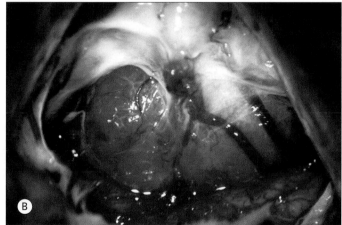

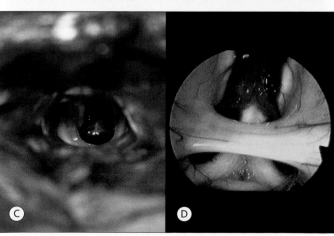

Figure 33.21 Intraoperative findings in case of a germinoma as presented in Figure 33.8A,B. Photograph during the opening of the arachnoid membranes in the pineal region with the tumor in the background (A). Appearance of the tumor before resection (B) and after complete tumor removal (C), and endoscope-assisted approach with the view into the third ventricle presenting the intermediate mass, the choroid plexus at the roof, both fornices and the anterior commissure (D).

CLINICAL PEARLS

- Pineal region tumors comprise about 1% of adult and 3–8% of all pediatric intracranial tumors.

- The histologic nature of pineal region tumors can be very variable and is moderately predictable based on the gender, age, neuroradiologic findings and tumor markers. Confirmation is required in cases where the histology is unclear. The author's recommendation is to perform surgery using individually tailored and appropriate approaches, such as open microsurgery, endoscopy or stereotactic biopsy, based on the tumor anatomy and surgeon's experience.

- In the majority of cases, the primary cause of symptoms in pineal region tumors, is the presence of hydrocephalus. The author recommends endoscopic third ventriculostomy including CSF studies such as cytology and tumor markers, as well as the possibility of a simultaneous endoscopic guided biopsy.

- Pineal region tumors can be removed with relatively low morbidity using either a posterior fossa approach (infratentorial/supracerebellar), supratentorial approaches (occipital transtentorial), or posterior transcallosal approach. Surgeons should be familiar with the anatomical structures in the pineal region, indications and limitations of each approach, as well as the risks and benefits of each approach.

- Other treatment modalities such as radiotherapy, chemotherapy, and radiosurgery should be incorporated into any treatment paradigm based on the extent of resection and histologic type of tumor.

The rate of incidental findings of pineal region tumors is currently increasing because of the high-resolution imaging modalities. The current diagnostic method of choice is MRI, and additional neuroradiological examinations such as MRI spectroscopy and positron emission tomography scans may eventually provide more information about the histological morphology. However, even today, imaging techniques cannot provide definitive information about the histological type of tumor. Biopsy (stereotactic or endoscopic), and surgical removal of the lesion represent the best way of establishing the histological diagnosis. Qualitative and quantitative assessment of tumor markers is non-specific in diagnostic evaluation, but useful for following the tumor after treatment and has become an important routine tool. It is well documented that the histology of any pineal tumor can be diverse. The treatment of tumors of the pineal region depends mostly on their histological type and may include a combination of surgery, radiation, and chemotherapy. In contrast to earlier times, microsurgery for radical resection of pineal region tumors is now increasingly safe (surgical mortality rate generally less than 5%) thanks to the evolution of technology and to intellectual discoveries in anesthesia, neurosurgery, imaging, and critical-care medicine.

ACKNOWLEDGMENTS

Grateful thanks are given to Mrs R.A. Klim for checking the language, to O. Koperek, Neuropathological Institute (H. Budka), University of Vienna, for arranging and preparing the histopathological figures, to F. Schindler from the neuroradiological department for helping with the radiological figures, to M. Tschabitscher, Anatomical Institute, University of Vienna, for preparing the neuroendoscopic figure, and last but not least to I. Dobsak, our medical illustrator, for her brilliant drawings on which the illustrations in this chapter are based.

This chapter contains material from the first edition, and I am grateful to the authors of that chapter for their contribution.

BIBLIOGRAPHY

Abay EO II, Laws ER Jr, Grado GL, *et al*. Pineal tumors in children and adolescents: treatment by CSF shunting and radiotherapy. *J Neurosurg*. 1981; 55: 889–95.

Allen JC, Nisselbaum J, Epstein F, Rosen G, Schwartz MK. Alphafetoprotein and human chorionic gonadotropin determination in cerebrospinal fluid: an aid to the diagnosis and management of intracranial germ-cell tumors. *J Neurosurg* 1979; 51: 368–74.

Arita N, Ushio Y, Hayakawa T, *et al*. Tumor markers: their role and limit for management of pineal tumor. In: Samii M (ed.). *Surgery in and Around the Brain Stem and the Third Ventricle*. Berlin: Springer-Verlag; 1986: 318–25.

Atlas SW (ed.). *Magnetic Resonance Imaging of the Brain and Spine*. New York: Raven Press; 1991.

Ausman JI, Malik GM, Pearce J, Rogers JS. A new operative approach to the pineal region. In: Samii M (ed.). *Surgery in and Around the Brain Stem and the Third Ventricle*. Berlin: Springer-Verlag; 1986: 326–8.

Bruce JN, Stein BM. Infratentorial approach to pineal tumors. In: Wilson CB (ed.). *Neurosurgical Procedures: Personal Approaches to Classic Operations*. Baltimore, MD: Williams & Wilkins; 1992: 63–76.

Bruce JN, Stein BM. Surgical management of pineal region tumors. *Acta Neurochir (Wien)* 1995; 134: 130–5.

Budka H, Schmidbauer M. Pathology of tumors of the pineal region (Pathologie der Tumoren der Pinealisregion). In: Bamberg M, Sack H (eds). *Therapy of Primary Brain Tumors (Therapie primärer Hirntumoren)*. Munich: W. Zuckerschwerdt Vlg.; 1988: 334–42.

Cho BK, Wang KC, Nam DH, *et al*. Pineal tumors: experience with 48 cases over 10 years. *Childs Nerv Syst* 1998; 14: 53–8.

Citow JS, Wollmann RL, Macdonald RL (eds). *Neuropathology and Neuroradiology. A Review*. Stuttgart: Thieme; 2001.

Clark WK. Occipital transtentorial approach. In: Apuzzo MLJ (ed.). *Surgery of the Third Ventricle*. Baltimore, MD: Williams & Wilkins; 1987: 591–610.

Colombo F, Benedetti A, Pozza F, *et al*. External stereotaxic irradiation on a linear accelerator. *Neurosurgery* 1985; 16: 154–60.

Connolly ES, McKhann II GM, Huang J, Choudhri TF. *Fundamentals of Operative Techniques in Neurosurgery*. Stuttgart: Thieme; 2002.

Dandy WE. An operation for the removal of pineal tumors. *Surg Gynecol Obstet* 1921; 33: 113–19.

Day JD, Koos WT, Matula C, Lang J (eds). *Color Atlas of Microneurosurgical Approaches. Cranial Base and Intracranial Midline*. Stuttgart: Thieme; 1997.

Edwards MSB, Levin V. Chemotherapy of tumors of the third ventricular region. In: Apuzzo MLJ (ed.). *Surgery of the Third Ventricle*. Baltimore, MD: Williams & Wilkins; 1987: 838–42.

Fukui M, Natori Y, Matsushima T, Nishio S, Ikezaki K. Operative approaches to the pineal region tumors. *Childs Nerv Syst* 1998; 14: 49–52.

Fukushima T. Endoscopic biopsy of intraventricular tumors with the use of a ventriculofiberscope. *Neurosurgery* 1978; 2: 110–13.

Gangemi M, Maiuri F, Colella G, Buonamassa S. Endoscopic surgery for pineal region tumors. *Minim Invasive Neurosurg* 2001; 44: 70–3.

Ganti SR, Hilal SK, Stein BM, Silver AJ, Mawad M, Sane P. CT of pineal region tumors. *AJNR* 1986; 7: 97–104.

Greenberg MS (ed). *Handbook of Neurosurgery*. Stuttgart: Thieme; 2002.

Grimoldi N, Tomei G, Stankov B, *et al*. Neuroendocrine, immunohisto-chemical, and ultrastructural study of pineal region tumors. *J Pineal Res* 1998; 25: 147–58.

Haimovich IC, Sharer L, Hyman RA, Beresford HR. Metastasis of intracranial germinoma through a ventriculoperitoneal shunt. *Cancer* 1981; 48: 1033–6.

Herrmann HD, Winkler D, Westphal M. Treatment of tumours of the pineal region and posterior part of the third ventricle. *Acta Neurochir (Wien)* 1992; 116: 137–46.

Hirato J, Nakazato Y. Pathology of pineal region tumors. *J Neuro-oncol* 2001; 54: 239–49.

Jakacki RI. Pineal and nonpineal supratentorial primitive neuroectodermal tumors. *Child's Nerv Syst* 1999; 15: 586–91.

Jooma R, Kendall BE. Diagnosis and treatment of pineal tumors. *J Neurosurg* 1983; 58: 654–65.

Kang JK, Jeun SS, Hong YK, Park CK, Son BC, Lee IW, Kim MC. Experience with pineal region tumors. *Child's Nerv Syst* 1998; 14: 63–8.

Kleihus P, Cavenee WK (eds). *Pathology & Genetics. Tumours of the Nervous System. World Health Organization Classification of Tumours*. Lyon: IARC Press; 2000.

Koos WT, Pendl G. Lesions of the cerebral midline. *Acta Neurochir (Wien)* 1985; Suppl. 35.

Koos WT, Spetzler RF, Lang J (eds). *Color Atlas of Microneurosurgery*, Vol. 1. Stuttgart: Thieme; 1993.

Korogi Y, Takahashi M, Ushio Y. MRI of pineal region tumors. *J Neuro-oncol* 2001; 54: 251–61.

Kurisaka M, Arisawa M, Mori T, *et al*. Combination chemotherapy (cisplatin, vinblastin) and low-dose irradiation in the treatment of pineal parenchymal cell tumors. *Child's Nerv Syst* 1998; 14: 564–9.

Lapras C, Patet JD. Controversies, techniques, and strategies for pineal tumor surgery. In: Apuzzo MLJ (ed.). *Surgery of the Third Ventricle*. Baltimore, MD: Williams & Wilkins; 1987: 649–62.

Neuwelt EA (ed.). *Diagnosis and Treatment of Pineal Region Tumors*. Baltimore, MD: Williams & Wilkins; 1984.

Nomura K. Epidemiology of germ cell tumors in Asia of pineal region tumor. *J Neuro-oncol* 2001; 54: 211–17.

Oi S, Shibata M, Tominaga J, *et al*. Efficacy of neuroendoscopic procedures in minimally invasive preferential management of pineal region tumors: a prospective study. *J Neurosurg* 2000; 93: 245–53.

Oi S, Kamio M, Joki T, Abe T. Neuroendoscopic anatomy and surgery in pineal region tumors: role of neuroendoscopic procedure in the "minimally-invasive preferential" management. *J Neuro-oncol* 2001; 54: 277–86.

Pendl G (ed.). *Pineal and Midbrain Lesions*. Berlin: Springer; 1985.

Pernkopf E. *Topographische Anatomie des Menschen*. München: Urban und Schwarzenberg; 1960.

Phillips PC, Kremzner LT, De Vivo DC. Cerebrospinal fluid polyamines: biochemical markers of malignant childhood brain tumors. *Ann Neurol* 1986; 19: 360–4.

Regis J, Bouillot P, Rouby-Volot F, Figarella-Branger D, Dufour H, Peragut J. Pineal region tumors and the role of stereotactic biopsy: review of the mortality, morbidity, and diagnostic rates in 370 cases. *Neurosurgery* 1996; 39: 907–12; discussion 912–14.

Raco A, Raimondi AJ, D'Alonzo A, Esposito V, Valentino V. Radiosurgery in the management of pediatric brain tumors. *Child's Nerv Syst* 2000; 16: 287–95.

Regis J, Bouillot P, Rouby-Volot F, *et al*. Microsurgery of the third ventricle, 2: operative approaches. *Neurosurgery* 1981; 8: 357–73.

Rieger A, Rainov NG, Brucke M, Marx T, Holz C. Endoscopic third ventriculostomy is the treatment of choice for obstructive hydrocephalus due to pediatric pineal tumors. *Minim Invasive Neurosurg* 2000; 43: 83–6.

Robertson PL, DaRosso RC, Allen JC. Improved prognosis of intracranial non-germinoma germ cell tumors with multimodality therapy. *J Neuro-oncol* 1997; 32: 71–80.

Robinson S, Cohen AR. The role of neuroendoscopy in the treatment of pineal region tumors. *Surg Neurol* 1997; 48: 360–5; discussion 365–7.

Sano K. Pineal region tumors: problems in pathology and treatment. *Clin Neurosurg* 1983; 30: 59–91.

Sano K. Treatment of tumors in the pineal and posterior third ventricular region. In: Samii M (ed.). *Surgery in and Around the Brain Stem and the Third Ventricle*. Berlin: Springer-Verlag; 1986: 309–17.

Satoh H, Uozumi T, Kiya K, *et al*. MRI of pineal region tumours: relationship between tumours and adjacent structures. *Neuroradiology* 1995; 37: 624–30.

Sawaya R, Hawley DK, Tobler WD, Tew JM Jr, Chambers AA. Pineal and third ventricle tumors. In: Youmans JR (ed.). *Neurological Surgery*, 3rd edn. Philadelphia: WB Saunders Co; 1990: 3171–203.

Scheithauer BW. Neuropathology of pineal region tumors. *Clin Neurosurg* 1985; 32: 351–83.

Schindler E (ed.). *Tumors of the Pineal Region (Die Tumoren der Pinealisregion)*. Berlin: Springer; 1985.

Schmidek HH (ed.). *Pineal Tumors*. New York, NY: Masson Publishing USA; 1977.

Schmidek HH, Waters A. Pineal masses: clinical features and management. In: Wilkins RH, Rengachary SS (eds). *Neurosurgery*. New York, NY: McGraw-Hill; 1985: 688–93.

Shinoda J, Yamada H, Sakai N, Ando T, Hirata T, Miwa Y. Placental alkaline phosphatase as a tumor marker for primary intracranial germinoma. *J Neurosurg* 1988; 68: 710–20.

Stein BM, Fetell MR. Therapeutic modalities for pineal region tumors. *Clin Neurosurg* 1985; 32: 445–55.

Takakura K. Intracranial germ cell tumors. *Clin Neurosurg* 1985; 32: 429–44.

Takakura K, Matsutani M. Therapeutic modality selection in management of germ cell tumors. In: Apuzzo MLJ (ed.). *Surgery of the Third Ventricle*. Baltimore, MD: Williams & Wilkins; 1987: 843–6.

Tien RD, Barkovich AJ, Edwards MSB. MR imaging of pineal tumors. *AJNR* 1990; 11: 557–65.

Timmermann B, Kortmann RD, Kuhl J, *et al*. Role of radiotherapy in the treatment of supratentorial primitive neuroectodermal tumors in childhood: results of the prospective German brain tumor trials HIT 88/89 and 91. *J Clin Oncol* 2002; 20: 842–9.

Tomita T. Pineal region tumors. In: Albright AL, Pollack IF, Adelson PD (eds). *Principles and Practice of Pediatric Neurosurgery*, Stuttgart: Thieme; 2001.

Tribolet N, Barrelet L. Successful chemotherapy for pinealoma. *Lancet* 1977; 2: 1228–9.

Van Wagenen WP. A surgical approach for the removal of certain pineal tumors: report of a case. *Surg Gynecol Obstet* 1931; 53: 216–20.

Vorkapic P, Waldhauser F, Bruckner R, Biegelmayer C, Schmidbauer M, Pendl G. Serum melatonin level: a new diagnostic tool in pineal region tumors. *Neurosurgery* 1987; 21: 817–24.

Wara W, Gutin PH. Radiotherapy of pineal and suprasellar tumors. In: Apuzzo MLJ (ed.). *Surgery of the Third Ventricle*. Baltimore, MD: Williams & Wilkins; 1987: 831–7.

Williams DL, Warwick R, Dyson M, Bannister LH (eds). *Gray's Anatomy*, 37th edn. Edinburgh: Churchill Livingstone; 1989.

Yamamoto I, Rhoton AL Jr, Peace DA. Microsurgery of the third ventricle, 1: microsurgical anatomy. *Neurosurgery* 1981; 8: 334–56.

Yamamoto I. Pineal region tumor: surgical anatomy and approach. *J Neuro-oncol* 2001; 54: 263–75.

Zimmerman RA. Pineal region masses: radiology. In: Wilkins RH, Rengachary SS (eds). *Neurosurgery*. New York, NY: McGraw-Hill; 1985: 680–7.

Zülch KJ. Reflections on the surgery of the pineal gland (a glimpse into the past). *Neurosurg Rev* 1981; 4: 159–62.

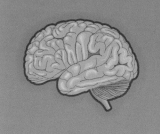

CEREBELLOPONTINE ANGLE TUMORS

34

Marcelo D Vilela, Gavin Wayne Britz, and Robert C Rostomily

INTRODUCTION

The cerebellopontine angle (CPA) is the region where the petrosal surface of the cerebellum wraps around the pons and upper medulla, with the middle cerebellar peduncle being its floor.[1] The CPA is a common location for tumor occurrence (8–10% of all intracranial tumors) with vestibular schwannoma, meningioma, and epidermoid cyst accounting for 95% of these.[2–13] This chapter provides an overview of tumors involving the CPA, including the relevant surgical anatomy, patient evaluation, surgical approaches, and the clinical and surgical features of the most common CPA tumors.

SURGICAL ANATOMY OF THE CEREBELLOPONTINE ANGLE

The cerebellopontine "angle" is formed by the superior and inferior limbs of the cerebellopontine fissure with the apex oriented laterally. The anatomy of the CPA can be conceptualized by breaking down the various neurovascular elements into three complexes (Figure 34.1).

The upper neurovascular complex consists of the trigeminal nerve contained within the superior cerebellopontine cistern, the superior cerebellar artery, and the petrosal vein. The trigeminal nerve courses toward the petrous apex anterior to the superior petrosal vein. The vein is identified by its typical inverted Y configuration at its entrance into the superior petrosal sinus at the tentorial–petrosal dural junction deep and anteriorly (Figure 34.2). The superior cerebellar artery usually runs along the superior aspect of the fifth nerve.

The second or middle neurovascular complex includes the facial and vestibulocochlear nerves, which arise from the lateral part of the pontomedullary sulcus, and the anterior inferior cerebellar artery (Figures 34.1, 34.2). The VIIth and VIIIth nerves course in the cerebellopontine cistern and enter the internal auditory canal (IAC) located in the petrous portion of the temporal bone. At the brainstem, the facial nerve is medial and inferior to the vestibulocochlear nerves (Figures 34.1, 34.2). The nerves rotate in the basal cisterns such that once inside the IAC, the facial and cochlear nerves are anteriorly situated and the vestibular nerves are posteriorly located (Figure 34.3). The superiorly located facial and superior vestibular nerves are separated from the inferiorly located cochlear and inferior vestibular nerves by a ridge of bone at the fundus, called the transverse crest, while the facial and superior vestibular nerves are separated by an island of bone, called "Bill's Bar" or the "vertical crest."

The anterior inferior cerebellar artery courses in association with nerves VII and VIII in the subarachnoid space and has three branches relevant to CPA surgery: the internal auditory artery (labyrinthine artery), the recurrent perforating artery and the subarcuate artery (Figure 34.4). The internal auditory artery travels into the IAC and provides blood supply to the inner ear and nerves in the IAC and must be spared to preserve hearing. The recurrent artery goes towards the canal and then makes a loop before going back to supply the VII–VIII nerve complex and the brainstem near the root entry zones for these nerves. The subarcuate artery enters the petrous bone at the subarcuate fossa, located near the IAC.

The lower complex consists of the IXth, Xth, and XIth nerves and the posterior inferior cerebellar artery (Figures 34.1, 34.5). The IXth, Xth, and XIth nerves arise posterior to the rostral pole of the olive just a few millimeters inferior to nerves VII and VIII. They run through the cerebellomedullary cistern and enter the jugular foramen, having an intimate relationship to the posterior inferior cerebellar artery and vertebral artery. A tuft of choroid plexus protruding from the foramen of Luschka is commonly visualized and sits on the glossopharyngeal and vagus nerves. The flocculus is situated superior to this tuft of choroid plexus and is posterior to the facial and vestibulocochlear nerves. The posterior inferior cerebellar artery courses in variable relationship to nerves IX, X, XI, and XII and occasionally loops superiorly, close to the VII–VIII nerve complex, before supplying the lateral medulla and the posterior inferior cerebellum.

The abducens and hypoglossal nerves, although not in the CPA *per se*, can also be encountered during surgery for large tumors in this region. The finer details of the surgically relevant anatomy are beyond the scope of this chapter but have been carefully documented elsewhere[1] and should be studied carefully prior to undertaking surgical resection of CPA tumors.

PATIENT EVALUATION AND SURGICAL CONSIDERATIONS

The preoperative evaluation of the patient with a CPA tumor is tailored to the precise location, size, and anticipated surgical approach. Careful neurologic evaluation for cranial nerve dysfunction is essential to determine potential perioperative risks and to counsel patients regarding potential postoperative deficits. Preoperative audiogram is generally indicated to help determine surgical approach and the potential for intraoperative monitoring of evoked auditory potentials. In selected cases, angiography is useful for surgical planning by defining arterial and venous

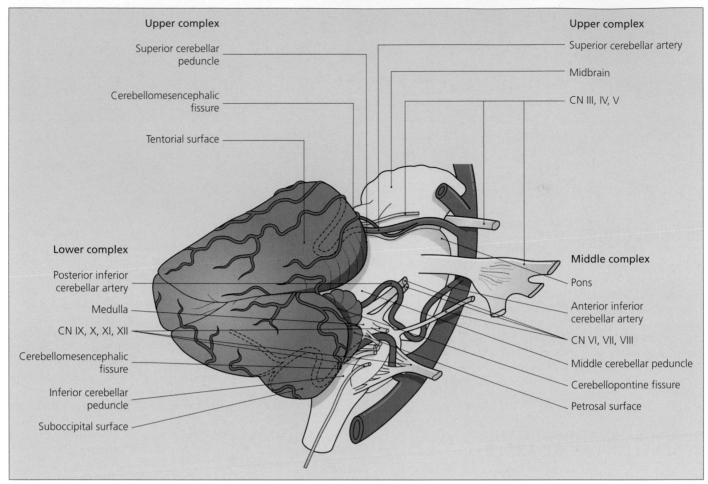

Figure 34.1 Schematic diagram demonstrating the CPA formed by the superior and inferior limbs of the cerebellopontine fissure with the apex oriented laterally. Also demonstrated are the three neurovascular complexes, the upper, middle and lower complex and the elements that form each of these complexes. Adapted from Rhoton.[65]

anatomy and also for embolization of highly vascular lesions when early access to the tumor blood supply is difficult.

General anesthesia is used without paralytics when cranial nerve electromyographic (EMG) monitoring is planned intraoperatively. Electrodes can be placed to monitor motor branch of cranial nerve V, and cranial nerves VII, X, XI, XII. Auditory pathways can be monitored with brainstem auditory-evoked potentials (BAEPs) recorded on the scalp or directly from the cochlear nerve with a small electrode that gives more immediate feedback and anatomic localization of the cochlear nerve. For large lesions the addition of somatosensory-evoked potential (SSEP) monitoring provides a broader sampling of signal transmission through the brainstem than BAEPs.

Although a large number of surgical approaches can provide access to the CPA, the vast majority of CPA tumors can be managed with the retrosigmoid sub-occipital approach. Options for positioning include supine, sitting, lateral, or three-quarter prone or park-bench. The sitting position can be particularly useful for large patients, and has the advantages of excellent exposure in the caudal to rostral direction for identification of the lower cranial nerves and brainstem origin of the VII–VIII nerve complex, and minimizes obscuration of the surgical field from blood and spinal fluid. However, because of the increased risk of air embolus and

even spinal cord injury as a result of ischemia or direct compression with neck flexion, patients in the sitting position require monitoring for air embolus and spinal cord injury in cases at risk for ischemia or mechanical compression. The non-sitting positions largely avoid these complications. The best position ultimately depends on many factors including the surgeon's preference and experience, the size and location of the lesion, the patient's medical condition and risk factors, anticipated surgical time, and limitation of surgical access imposed by the patient's body habitus.

Proper patient positioning provides optimal surgical exposure and comfortable surgical ergonomics while preventing complications from direct pressure, vascular occlusion, or neural compression. For non-sitting cases the head is most commonly positioned parallel to the floor. Axial rotation towards or away from this plane determines the angle of view out the IAC versus that back towards the brainstem, while lateral flexion of the head relative to the floor will influence the "steepness" of the tentorium and should be considered when positioning large CPA tumors that extend to the tentorium (Figure 34.6). The skin incision can be vertical, C-shaped or inverted U-shaped and should be tailored to provide adequate exposure for the extent of the lesion at the petrous bone and brainstem. After exposure of the sub-occipital

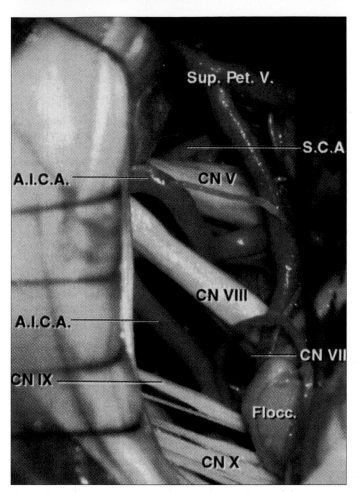

Figure 34.2 The upper neurovascular complex consisting of the trigeminal nerve (CN V – cranial nerve V) contained within the superior cerebellopontine cistern, the superior cerebellar artery (SCA) and the superior petrosal vein (Sup. Pet. V). The trigeminal nerve courses toward the petrous apex anterior to the superior petrosal vein which is identified by its typical inverted Y configuration at its entrance into the superior petrosal sinus at the tentorial–petrosal dural junction. The superior cerebellar artery usually runs along the superior aspect of the fifth nerve. The middle neurovascular complex consists of the facial (CN VII) and vestibulocochlear nerves (CN VIII), which arise from the lateral part of the pontomedullary sulcus, and the anterior inferior cerebellar artery (AICA). The VIIth and VIIIth nerves course in the cerebellopontine cistern and enter the internal auditory canal. Also seen are the glossopharyngeal nerve (CN IX), vagal nerve (CN X) and the flocculus (Flocc.) of the cerebellum. From Rhoton.[1]

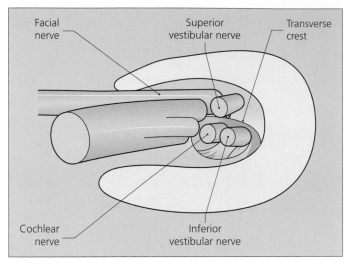

Figure 34.3 A schematic diagram of the right internal acoustic meatus demonstrating the facial nerve and nerve VIII dividing into its three parts, the superior vestibular nerve above the transverse crest and the cochlear and inferior vestibular nerve below the crest. Adapted from Rhoton.[1]

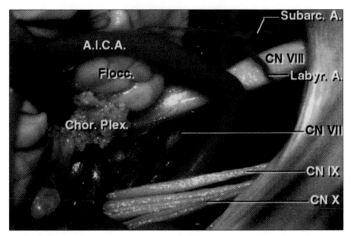

Figure 34.4 Intraoperative view demonstrating the relationship of the anterior inferior cerebellar artery and its two major branches in the CPA, the internal auditory artery (Labyr. A.), and the subarcuate artery (Subarc. A.). The internal auditory artery travels into the IAC and provides a blood supply to the inner ear and nerves in the IAC. Also demonstrated are the vestibularcochlear nerve (CN VIII), facial nerve (CN VII), and the glossopharyngeal nerve (CN IX), vagal nerve (CN X) and the flocculus (Flocc.). From Rhoton.[66]

bone either by dividing muscle layers or performing an anatomic muscle plane dissection a craniotomy or a craniectomy is performed. The extent of bony removal is variable but helpful landmarks include visualization of the angle of the transverse and sigmoid sinus and the medial borders of the sigmoid sinus to the jugular bulb (Figure 34.7). Externally, the junction of the transverse and sigmoid sinus is approximated by the position of the asterion. A linear dural opening along a portion of the transverse and the entire length of the sigmoid sinus is used and the dura is left in place on the cerebellum for protection. Relaxation of the cerebellum is critical to provide adequate surgical exposure and prevent complications from excessive retraction. This can be achieved by opening the cisterna magna, medullary cistern, or with lumbar drainage.

SPECIFIC CEREBELLOPONTINE ANGLE TUMORS

Vestibular schwannoma

Vestibular schwannomas are the most common tumor (80–90%) in the CPA and arise from Schwann cells at the junction of central nervous system glia and peripheral nervous system Schwann cells

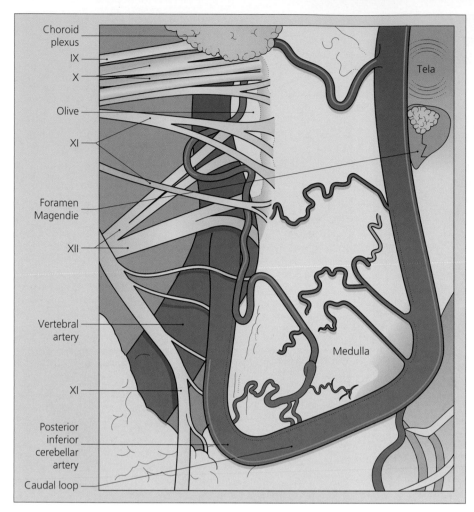

Choroid plexus
IX
X
Olive
XI
Foramen Magendie
XII
Vertebral artery
XI
Posterior inferior cerebellar artery
Caudal loop
Tela
Medulla

Figure 34.5 Schematic of the lower neurovascular complex consisting of cranial nerves IX, X, XI and the posterior inferior cerebellar artery coming off the vertebral artery (VA). The IXth, Xth, XIth nerves can be demonstrated to arise just posterior to the rostral pole of the olive, just a few millimeters inferior to the VII–VIIIth nerves. A tuft of choroid plexus protruding from the foramen of Luschka is commonly visualized and sits on the glossopharyngeal and vagus nerves. Also seen are the foramen Magendie, and the hypoglossal nerve (CN XII). Adapted from Rhoton.[1]

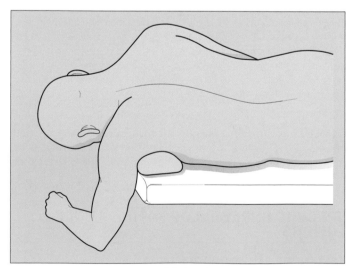

Figure 34.6 Schematic of the modified park-bench operative position during a retrosigmoid craniotomy/craniectomy to expose the CPA. Adapted from Day et al.[67]

(Redlech–Obersteiner zone) of the vestibular nerve at the entrance of the IAC.[14] There is a slight female preponderance to the incidence of vestibular schwannomas and the mean age at diagnosis is in the fifth or sixth decade.[15–18] An estimated 2000 to 3000 new cases of unilateral vestibular schwannomas are diagnosed in the USA each year, which reflects an average incidence of 1 per 100 000 per year.[19] They are slow growing tumors and usually enlarge 1–3 mm/year but may do so by more than 5 mm/year.[17,20–22] A reasonable percentage (9–21%) may remain quiescent for several years and even involute with time (6–15%).[17,20,21,23,24] There appears to be some correlation between changes in tumor volume and deterioration of hearing function.[24] The most common presenting symptoms are hearing loss (75–95% of cases), tinnitus (15–75%), dizziness (40–57%), and disequilibrium.[15–17,21,23,25] Mild facial hypoesthesia, tic-like pain, hypoesthesia in the external auditory canal, ataxia, facial paresis, facial twitching, hemifacial spasm, positive Romberg's test, dysmetria, or headaches are encountered in 5–20% of cases.[15,16] Sudden deafness occurs in around 10% of cases and of those there is a 19% risk of being permanently deaf in that ear.[15,16]

Macroscopically, the tumor is generally firm, encapsulated, rounded and smooth, often gray, yellow, or slightly red, and with

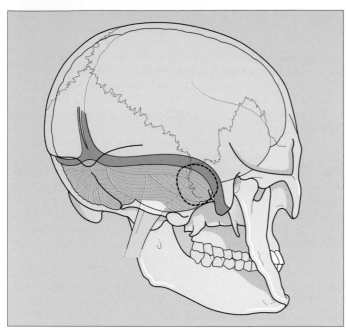

Figure 34.7 Schematic of the limited retrosigmoid craniotomy/craniectomy performed posteriorly and inferiorly to the junction of the transverse and sigmoid sinus. Adapted from Day et al.[67]

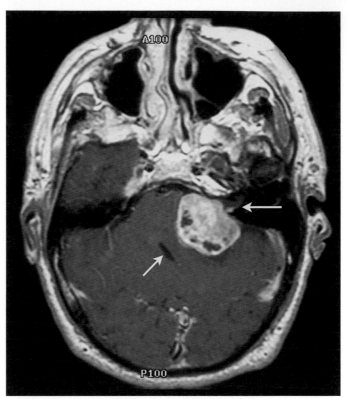

Figure 34.8 Axial T1-weighted MRI with gadolinium, demonstrating a mass lesion in the right CPA, with compression of the brainstem and displacement of the fourth ventricle (large white arrow). Also demonstrated are a slight "extension" into the right IAC and some enhancement of the VII–VIIIth nerve complex (smaller white arrow), all consistent with the diagnosis of a vestibular schwannoma.

some degree of vascularization on the surface. Some tumors contain foci of hemorrhage and cystic formations. Microscopically, there are spindle-shaped cells, with elongated nuclei and fibrillary cytoplasm. Two different microscopic patterns predominate: Antoni A, which is a compact pattern, and Antoni B, which is looser in appearance. Pleomorphism and bizarre nuclei are frequent. Rare mitotic figures are encountered and necrosis is common. Malignant transformation is very rare. Hemosiderin deposits and cystic formations correlate with heterogeneous tumors on magnetic resonance imaging (MRI).[26]

Audiograms usually show more prominent hearing loss for high-frequency tones. When the pure tone average (PTA) is more than 50 dB and speech discrimination score (SDS) is less than 50% (the so-called "50–50 rule"), hearing is considered non-serviceable. The American Association for Otolaryngology-Head and Neck Surgery established guidelines in 1995 for the classification of hearing function as follows:[24,27]

- Class A: PTA < 30 db and SDS > 70%.
- Class B: PTA > 30 db and < 50 db and SDS > 50%.
- Class C: PTA > 50 db and SDS > 50%.
- Class D: SDS < 50%.

Imaging

On CT imaging, vestibular schwannomas are round, lobular, isointense, intensely enhancing tumors centered in the CPA, with an intracanalicular component and some degree of erosion of the IAC. MRI shows an isodense lesion on T1-weighted images that enhances strongly and homogeneously with gadolinium. T2 weighted images show a hyperintense lesion, sometimes heterogeneous with cystic formations or prior evidence of hemorrhage (Figures 34.8, 34.9). Some radiological features, such as high signal in the inner ear in MRI–CISS (constructive interference in steady state) sequences, length and widening of the IAC, extension of the tumor anterior and caudal to the IAC and cystic

formations, have been correlated to be predictive of facial and cochlear preservation during microsurgical removal.[28,29] Tumor size assessed on imaging is an important factor in managing patients with vestibular schwannoma. Tumor size directly correlates with surgical and radiation treatment morbidity for hearing and facial nerve function.[30,31] The larger the tumor, the greater the chance that the vestibular and facial nerves will be compromised by surgery. In addition, tumors > 3 cm in diameter are not considered candidates for single-fraction radiation. One commonly used classification stratifies tumors as purely intracanalicular or by largest diameter in the subarachnoid space as small (≤ 10 mm), medium (11–20 mm), large (21–40 mm) and giant (> 40 mm).

Treatment options

Various surgeons have adopted the "wait and image" policy based on the fact that tumors are slow growing or even quiescent for a long time and a large proportion of patients are elderly and can have a good quality of life despite some symptoms.[23,24,32–34] This management has been advocated for small tumors, whether hearing has been compromised or not, and for medium-sized tumors when patients have already lost the ability to hear and there is no significant brainstem compression or other symptoms.[23,24,32–34] However, other surgeons adopt a more aggressive treatment philosophy given that treatment complications are directly related to tumor size, functional outcome is related to pre-treatment function, and changes in individual tumor growth rates are unpredictable. Additionally, a great percentage of

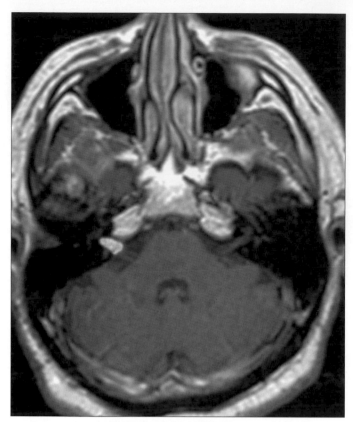

Figure 34.9 High-resolution axial T1-weighted MRI with gadolinium, demonstrating a mass lesion in the right internal auditory canal consistent with the diagnosis of an intracanicular schwannoma.

patients show a deterioration in their hearing during observation and commonly lose their eligibility for hearing preservation surgery on subsequent follow-up.[20] Tumors in a patient with only one functional hearing ear should be treated when there is hearing deterioration, tumor growth, and/or compression of the brainstem.[23]

MICROSURGERY Surgery has an aim of total tumor removal and cure, together with preservation of facial and cochlear function (when preoperative hearing is serviceable). Surgery is indicated for symptomatic medium-sized tumors and for large tumors with compression of the brainstem. For small tumors, some authors state that if the tumor is small and the patient has serviceable hearing, surgery should be offered since there is a chance of total tumor removal and hearing preservation, with a high chance of preservation of normal facial nerve function. This philosophy is also based on reports that patients with serviceable hearing may lose hearing function during observation, even if there is no tumor growth.[20,29,33] Results seem to depend on the experience of the surgical team.[35] Recurrences may occur several years after surgery in subtotal resection but the rate is variable.[36,37]

There are three surgical approaches that can be used to resect vestibular schwannomas.

The *middle fossa approach* is used for small intracanalicular tumors, especially those located laterally in the IAC when hearing preservation is an option.[18,27,38–40] Some surgeons use this approach even for medium–large tumors.[18,39] It consists of a subtemporal craniotomy designed to access the IAC antero-superiorly. The course of the IAC in the temporal bone can be projected by a line that bisects the angle formed by the greater superficial petrosal nerve and arcuate eminence.

The *translabyrinthine approach* involves a retroauricular incision, a mastoidectomy and drilling of the semicircular canals with exposure of the IAC and can be used for tumors when hearing preservation is not an issue.[25]

The *retrosigmoid transmeatal approach* is the most common approach used by neurosurgeons to resect vestibular schwannomas. It has been advocated for small and large tumors, whether hearing preservation is an issue or not.[27,37–39,41–43] It consists of a retrosigmoid craniotomy about 3–4 cm in diameter, exposing the edges of the transverse and sigmoid sinus. The dura is opened and the cerebellum is retracted, exposing the tumor. The tumor is progressively debulked, preserving the arachnoid plane in order to protect neurovascular structures. The IAC in the petrous bone is then opened using a high-speed drill. The tumor is dissected off the nerves in a medial to lateral fashion so as not to pull on the cochlear nerve fibers. The location of the facial nerve is usually in the antero-superior surface of the tumor and the cochlear nerve is located at the antero-inferior surface.[41,44] The nerves rarely travel through or are enfolded by the tumor.[41] Cerebrospinal fluid (CSF) leaks can be avoided in almost all cases by careful waxing of the mastoid air cells and air cells exposed around the IAC as well as packing the IAC with a piece of muscle and fibrin glue and securing it by suturing the dura back over the IAC. CSF leaks are reported to occur in up to 15% of the patients but they can usually be managed successfully simply with lumbar drainage.[31]

Microsurgical series report rates of facial nerve preservation with respect to size that demonstrate excellent results in 96% of small tumors (< 2 cm), 74% of medium tumors (2.0–3.9 cm), and 38% of large tumors (≥ 4 cm). Functional hearing preservation, can be achieved in 48% of small tumors and 25% of medium tumors and in very few to none of the large tumors.[31]

RADIATION THERAPY Radiosurgery employing both gamma-knife and linac-based radiation delivery systems, has evolved in the last two decades and has been used more frequently in the treatment of vestibular schwannomas. Its safety and efficacy have been supported by a growing body of literature. However, considerable controversy exists in centers around the world as to whether or not radiosurgery should be used as the primary modality in the treatment of vestibular schwannoma. Much of the decision of whether to use microsurgery or radiosurgery depends on the experience and personal preference of the treatment team, as well as the informed consent of the patient. In contrast to microsurgery, the goal in radiosurgery is to arrest tumor growth rather than eradicate the tumor while preserving neurological function. Tumor shrinkage, when it occurs, is believed to be the result of radiation-induced vessel damage with resultant diminished blood supply to the tumor but a direct effect on the tumor cells has also been shown.[45] Radiosurgery as a primary modality of treatment is usually indicated for patients that are poor surgical candidates because of medical conditions or advanced age, patients that refuse an open surgical procedure, patients operated on previously in which there is a remnant of tumor that is growing, and for tumors in the only hearing ear or when hearing is still serviceable but would unlikely be preserved with microsurgical removal.[45–47]

After radiosurgical treatment, the tumor may enlarge but after 6–12 months, regression in size is usually observed.[45] Tumor control rates have been reported in the range of 87–91% at

3–5 years with good hearing preservation rates and results comparable to microsurgery.[45,47–49] Complications reported include facial nerve paresis (15%), hearing deterioration (21%), worsening tinnitus (15%), and trigeminal sensory dysfunction (11%).[45,47,49]

Neurofibromatosis type 2

Neurofibromatosis type 2 (NF-2) is an autosomal dominant disorder involving deletion or mutation of the NF-2 gene on the long arm of chromosome 22 with an incidence of about 100 new cases per year in the USA.[50] This gene encodes the tumor suppressor protein, *merlin/schwannomin*, which impairs cell adhesion, motility, and spreading properties.[50] The hallmark of the disease is the appearance of bilateral vestibular schwannomas.

The best management of CPA vestibular schwannomas in the patient with NF-2 is controversial. Ultimately the treatment goal is to preserve cranial nerve function as long as possible while controlling tumor growth. Treatment options include radiosurgery,[45] early surgical intervention with partial[14] or total[40] tumor resection, or simply bone removal with decompression of the IAC.[40] Patients with large tumors and brainstem compression should be offered surgical debulking/excision of the lesion.

Meningiomas

CPA meningiomas comprise 3–15% of all CPA tumors and arise from the arachnoid villae adjacent to the sinuses or cranial nerve foramina.[6–8,51] The CPA is the commonest location for meningiomas in the posterior fossa, which by definition arise lateral to the trigeminal nerve.[13] The prevalence of meningioma predominates in women over men with a ratio of 4:1 to 5:1.[7,8] Anatomically, meningiomas can be classified based on their location anterior/posterior or inferior/superior to the IAC, or purely intracanalicular.[6,7,13,52,53] Notably, although meningiomas located anterior to the meatus present at a significantly smaller size than those growing posterior to the IAC, premeatal tumors have been demonstrated to carry a significantly higher risk of pre- and postoperative auditory and facial nerve dysfunction, presumably because of their location ventral to the neurovascular complex.[53]

Meningiomas usually grow as globular masses that displace, stretch, and compress neurovascular structures. Less commonly they grow in an en-plaque-like[51] configuration or encase neural and/or vascular elements, making total resection difficult if arachnoid planes that envelop the nerves are not recognized.[8] Hearing loss (70% of cases), vestibular symptoms and tinnitus (40–60%), and headaches (40%) are the most common presenting complaints.[6–8] Facial numbness/weakness, tic-like facial pain, hemifacial spasm, vertigo, visual disturbances, ataxia, and lower cranial nerves deficits are encountered in fewer cases.[6,8,10]

On imaging studies, meningiomas are large, oval or flat, broad-based, sessile, arising from the petrous surface of the temporal bone and are usually larger than 3 cm at the time of diagnosis (Figure 34.10).[8,10] When they invade the IAC, it is not usually eroded.[6] CT scans show an isointense, rounded mass, with strong enhancement. Calcifications and hyperostosis may be seen.[6,10,51] On MRI scans, they are hypointense or isointense on T1, hyperintense or hypointense on T2, show intense homogeneous enhancement and usually have a dural tail.[6,7,10,51] Angiograms typically show a tumor blush and embolization can be used to diminish the blood supply, which usually comes from the ascending pharyngeal,

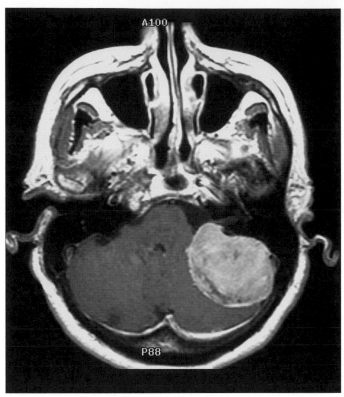

Figure 34.10 Axial T1-weighted MRI with gadolinium, demonstrating a mass lesion in the right CPA which is somewhat oval and appears to be arising from the petrous surface of the temporal bone.

meningohypophyseal, or meningeal branches of the occipital or middle meningeal artery.

The ideal treatment for meningiomas is total resection of the tumor and involved dura and bone. Gross total removal in some series varies between 80% and 95% of cases, but near-total or subtotal resection may be comtemplated in order to preserve neurological function.[6–8] The chance of hearing preservation is higher in meningiomas than vestibular schwannomas.[6] Even when patients have poor hearing preoperatively, cochlear nerve preservation should be attempted since there are reports of complete restoration of serviceable hearing function after a preoperative state of deafness.[6,8] Therefore, surgical approaches that destroy the labyrinth should be avoided. The suboccipital retrosigmoid is currently the preferred approach.[8]

Patients usually improve early with regard to trigeminal and vestibular function. Cochlear nerve function can improve but takes longer and facial nerve function improves in a period of a few months.[8] The overall results are good, but complications can be expected in some patients.[7] Recurrences can occur in cases of incomplete resection and the rate is much higher than in vestibular schwannomas.[6–8] Options after subtotal resection include observation, radiosurgery, or a repeat operation for confirmed tumor growth and good results can still be expected.[6,8]

Radiosurgery

Radiosurgery has been shown to control the growth of skull-base meningiomas, including those in the CPA, effectively and with acceptable morbidity.[54,55] It has been used either as a primary treatment or after subtotal resection.[54] Usually the tumor has to be less than 3 cm in diameter. Major mass effect is usually a contraindication and open surgery and debulking have to be considered. The control rate and survival have been considerably higher for benign meningiomas in comparison to atypical or malignant meningiomas and this implies that the biology of the tumor has a direct impact on outcome.[55] Malignant meningiomas have a poor prognosis despite an aggressive approach with surgery and radiotherapy.[55]

Epidermoid cysts

Epidermoid cysts represent 4.6–6.3% of the lesions in the CPA, the most common intracranial location for this tumor.[2,5] They are congenital, non-neoplastic, slowly growing lesions that are believed to arise from displaced or sequestered epithelial remnants during the 3rd to 5th weeks of gestation, when closure of the neural tube is taking place.[2] Its enlargement occurs by desquamation of cells into a cystic cavity, enveloping neurovascular structures rather than displacing or compressing them.[5] They are usually cauliflower-shaped, have a pearly appearance and a thin wall formed by a basal cell layer and stratified squamous epithelium.[2,5] The inner core is avascular and rich in cholesterol crystals, being either waxy or oily. Cyst rupture may occur and induce a granulomatous meningeal reaction, clinically manifesting as aseptic meningitis.[2,5] Malignant degeneration to squamous cell carcinoma is extremely rare.

Patients with epidermoids of the CPA usually present during their fourth decade of life.[4,5] Hearing loss, gait disturbance, tinnitus, dizziness, tic douloureux, headache, diplopia, facial paresis, and facial numbness are the most common symptoms.[2,4,5] The VIIIth and Vth nerves are affected in 50–70% of cases.[4]

Head CT scans may show a hypo-, hyper-, or isodense lesion in relation to the brain. The cyst wall may show some enhancement after injection of intravenous contrast but this is rare.[4,5,56] Erosion of the petrous apex may be observed in some cases.[4] On T1 images the lesion is hypointense to brain and slightly hyperintense to CSF (Figure 34.11A–C). Hyperintense T1 lesions are usually the result of high lipid content. On T2 images, they are hyperintense to brain tissue and slightly hyperintense to CSF.[2,5] MR diffusion images are useful in that epidermoids are hyper-

intense to CSF and brain and are distinguished from the low-signal arachnoid cysts and encephalomalacia.[57] Additionally, epidermoids are very irregular and indent into cisterns and brain tissue whereas arachnoid cysts have walls with a smooth appearance.[5]

Most tumors extend either into the foramen magnum, supratentorially, into the pineal region, the middle fossa, or to the other side.[2,4,5]

Surgical treatment

The surgical approach used most commonly is the suboccipital retrosigmoid.[4,5,56] The subtemporal approach can be used for tumors with large middle fossa extensions in a combined or staged procedure.[4,56] One should perform an initial debulking by aspiration of the cyst contents and then proceed with extracapsular dissection remembering that the neurovascular elements are coursing through the tumor and can be very adherent to the capsule. Total removal is possible but may result in serious neurological deficits and/or death due to cranial nerve palsies or brainstem injury.[4,5,56]

UNCOMMON CEREBELLOPONTINE ANGLE LESIONS

A number of other less common but unique lesions can occur in the CPA. The CPA is the second most common location for intracranial *arachnoid cysts*.[51,58] Symptoms are usually headaches, vomiting, cerebellar disturbances or cranial nerve involvement. They can be distinguished from CPA epidermoids by their lack of bright signal on diffusion-weighted MRI. Treatment options include fenestration of the cyst or cystoperitoneal shunting.[10,58] *Choroid plexus papillomas* in the CPA are almost exclusively found in adults and present with headaches, cerebellar dysfunction, cranial nerve involvement, and hydrocephalus. Total removal is not always possible because of their adherence to neurovascular structures.[9,10] *Trigeminal neuromas* enlarge Meckel's cave and those that extend into the posterior fossa have a dumbbell appearance. Facial sensory symptoms usually predominate over

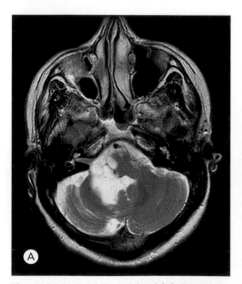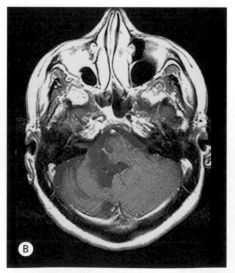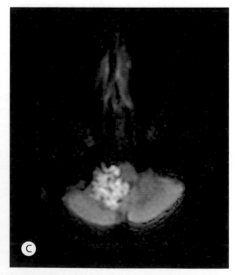

Figure 34.11 Axial T2-weighted **(A)**, T1-weighted with gadolinium **(B)** and diffusion-weighted MRI **(C)** through the posterior fossa that demonstrates a mass lesion in the right CPA. The findings are consistent with an epidermoid with signal characteristics of the tumors showing increased signal on T2, decreased signal on T1 with no enhancement, and increased signal noted on diffusion.

symptoms of VIIIth nerve involvement.[51] *Facial nerve neuromas* comprise 1% of CPA tumors. They manifest clinically by involvement of the VIIIth cranial nerve followed by the VIIth nerve. Imaging is similar to vestibular schwanomma but some tumors may show Fallopian canal enlargement.[51] *Metastatic lesions* arise most commonly from lung, breast, kidney, prostate and melanoma. The progression of symptoms is rapid. Treatment is usually surgery plus radiotherapy.[10,11,51,59] *Cholesterol granulomas* usually arise at the petrous apex and cause bone erosion. Treatment is surgical evacuation of the cyst contents. *Paragangliomas* usually erode the jugular foramen and have a salt-and-pepper appearance. They are very vascular tumors. MRI shows multiple flow voids inside the tumor and angiography shows a marked tumor blush in the region of the jugular bulb.[51] *Cavernous angiomas* are very rare. Facial weakness is usually present despite the small size of the tumor. Calcifications are common and high signal on T2 is classical.[51,59] *Lipomas* are also very rare. Very characteristic is the high signal on T1-weighted MRI scans. They also enlarge the IAC and can be very adherent to the cochlear nerve.[51,59] Other rare lesions described include osteomas, lymphomas, primitive neurecto-dermal tumor, gliomas, ependymomas, hamartomas, and lymphangiomas.[3,11,12,52,60,61]

COMPLICATIONS OF CEREBELLOPONTINE ANGLE TUMOR SURGERY

The most common complication is new or worsening cranial nerve deficit and the trigeminal, facial, and cochlear nerves are especially affected.[6–8,37,62,63] The combination of corneal hypoesthesia and facial paresis is dangerous and one should be vigilant so as to prevent corneal ulceration. Sometimes partial tarsorrhaphy or gold-weight implantation is necessary.

CSF leaks can be paradoxical or direct and usually resolve with a period of lumbar drainage or compressive dressings. Surgical intervention may be required for those that persist after conservative treatment and some cases require packing of the mastoid cells.[6,8,15,36] Meningitis is also a possible complication, especially when there is a CSF leak.[15] Treatment should use the appropriate antibiotics, directed by CSF cultures. Air embolism is a risk, especially when patients are operated on in the sitting position but can occur in the supine or park-bench position if the head is above the level of the heart.[15] Hydrocephalus can occur postoperatively and in most cases can be managed with a few lumbar taps and removal of high volumes of CSF. External ventricular drainage for a few days may be necessary postoperatively in some cases and uncommonly will need conversion to a permanent shunt.[7,8,64]

Temporal lobe contusion is possible when the middle fossa approach is used.[6] Injury to the vein of Labbé can cause significant edema with mass effect or temporal lobe hemorrhage. Brainstem injury can occur during the dissection of large tumors.[14,37] Stroke secondary to manipulation or inadvertent injury of vessels is uncommon when arachnoidal planes are well preserved. Postoperative hematomas, although rare, can be intradural or extradural. Large clots may require surgical evacuation.[6,8,15,37] Mortality in large series is around 1% and the major causes are brainstem injury or hematoma.[15,37]

CLINICAL PEARLS

- The surgically relevant anatomy of the CPA is composed of three compartments that include specific neurovascular structures; the upper component contains the Vth cranial nerve, superior cerebellar artery and petrosal veins within the trigeminal cistern; the middle complex contains the VIIth and VIIIth cranial nerves, anterior inferior cerebellar artery and its branches and the lower complex contains the IXth and XIIth cranial nerves and posterior inferior cerebellar artery. A thorough understanding of the anatomic landmarks that define the relationships of these structures to one another is necessary to manage CPA tumors successfully.

- A large variety of tumors with unique biological and surgical characteristics arise within the CPA. While imaging and angiographic characteristics can generally distinguish between the most common lesions, the surgeon must consider and be prepared to deal with all possible lesions at the time of surgery.

- The majority of tumors confined to the CPA can be managed through a retrosigmoid approach in either a sitting or lateral/three-quarter prone position. More extensive lesions extending beyond the CPA may require more complex combined skull-base approaches.

- Identifying the arachnoid plane between tumor and normal structures will allow ease of dissection and improved outcome.

- Treatment options for CPA tumors vary considerably depending on tumor type. While some lesions are amenable to observation, surgery, radiation, or surgery with adjuvant radiation (i.e. vestibular schwannoma, meningioma), other lesions, such as epidermoid cysts, are restricted to observation or surgical management alone.

- The vast majority of CPA tumors are benign and individualized treatment strategies must take into account the best option for long-term tumor control as well as the long-term consequences of treatment-related morbidity.

SUMMARY

The cerebellopontine angle is a region of the posterior fossa where the lateral cerebellum wraps around the brainstem. Several lesions can grow in that region and cause impairment of hearing, facial nerve, and trigeminal nerve function. The most common tumors are vestibular schwannomas, meningiomas, and epidermoid cysts. Treatment is usually surgery with the aim of tumor removal and improvement of neurological function. Radiosurgery has been a good alternative to surgery with good tumor growth control rates and minimal morbibity/mortality.

This chapter contains material from the first edition, and we are grateful to the author of that chapter for his contribution.

REFERENCES

1. Rhoton, AL, Jr. The cerebellopontine angle and posterior fossa cranial nerves by the retrosigmoid approach. *Neurosurgery* 2000; 47: S93–S129.

2. Cobbs CS, Pittls LH, Wilson CB. Epidermoid and dermoid cysts of the posterior fossa. *Clin Neurosurg* 1997; 44: 511–28.

3. Davis TC, Thedinger BA, Greene GM. Osteomas of the internal auditory canal: a report of two cases. *Am J Otol* 2000; 21: 852–6.

4. Mohanty A, Venkatrama, SK, Rao BR, et al. Experience with cerebellopontine angle epidermoids. *Neurosurgery* 1997; 40: 24–9; discussion 29–30.

5. Samii M, Tatagiba M, Piquer J, Carvalho GA. Surgical treatment of epidermoid cysts of the cerebellopontine angle. *J Neurosurg* 1996; 84: 14–19.

6. Voss NF, Vrionis FD, Heilman CB, Robertson JH. Meningiomas of the cerebellopontine angle. *Surg Neurol* 2000; 53: 439–46; discussion 446–7.

7. Thomas NW, King TT. Meningiomas of the cerebellopontine angle. A report of 41 cases. *Br J Neurosurg* 1996; 10: 59–68.

8. Matthies C, Carvalho G, Tatagiba M, et al. Meningiomas of the cerebellopontine angle. *Acta Neurochir Suppl (Wien)* 1996; 65: 86–91.

9. Talacchi A, De Micheli E, Lombardo C, et al. Choroid plexus papilloma of the cerebellopontinbe angle: a twelve patient series. *Surg Neurol* 1999; 51: 621–9.

10. Brunori A, Scarano P, Chiappetta F. Non-acoustic neuroma tumor (NANT) of the cerebellopontine angle: a 15 year experience. *J Neurosurg Sci* 1997; 41: 159–68.

11. Kohan D, Downey LL, Lim J, Cohen NL, Elowitz E. Uncommon lesions presenting as tumors of the internal auditory canal and cerebellopontine angle. *Am J Otol* 1997; 18: 386–92.

12. Kalamarides M, Dewolf E, Couvelard A, et al. Extraaxial primitive neuroectodermal mimicking a vestibular schwannoma: diagnostic and therapeutic difficulties. *J Neurosurg* 2001; 94: 612–16.

13. Martinez Devesa PM, Wareing MJ, Moffat DA. Meningioma in the internal auditory canal. *J Laryngol Otol* 2001; 115: 48–9.

14. Wigand ME, Haid T, Goertzen W, Wolf S. Preservation of hearing in bilateral acoustic neurinomas by deliberate partial resection. *Acta Otolaryngol* 1992; 112: 237–41.

15. Jannetta PJ. Vestibular neurilemmomas. *Clin Neurosurg* 1997; 44: 529–48.

16. Matthies C, Samii M. Management of 1000 vestibular schwannomas (acoustic neuromas): clinical presentation. *Neurosurgery* 1997; 40: 1–9; discussion 9–10.

17. Rosenberg SI. Natural history of acoustic neuromas. *Laryngoscope* 2000: 110: 497–508.

18. Gjuric M, Wigand ME, Wolf SR. Enlarged middle fossa vestibular schwannoma surgery: experience with 735 cases. *Otol Neurotol* 2001; 22: 223–30; discussion 230–1.

19. Tos M, Charabi S, Thomsen J. Incidence of vestibular schwannomas. *Laryngoscope* 1999; 109: 736–40.

20. Charabi S, Tos M, Thomsen J, Charabi B, Mantoni M. Vestibular schwannoma growth: the continuing controversy. *Laryngoscope* 2000; 110: 1720–5.

21. Mirz F, Jorgensen B, Fiirgaard B, Lundorf E, Pedersen CB. Investigations into the natural history of vestibular schwannomas. *Clin Otolaryngol* 1999; 24: 13–8.

22. Nutik SL, Babb MJ. Determinants of tumor size and growth in vestibular schwannomas. *J Neurosurg* 2001; 94: 922–6.

23. Shin YJ, Fraysse B, Cognard C, et al. Effectiveness of conservative treatment of acoustic neuromas. *Am J Otol* 2000; 21: 857–62.

24. Massick DD, Welling DB, Dodson EE, et al. Tumor growth and audiometric change in vestibular schwannomas managed conservatively. *Laryngoscope* 2000; 110: 1843–9.

25. Lanman TH, Brackmann DE, Hitselberger WE, Subin B. Report of 190 consecutive cases of large acoustic neuromas (vestibular schwannomas) removed via the translabyrinthine approach. *J Neurosurg* 1999; 90: 617–23.

26. Gomez-Brouchet A, Delisle MB, Cognard C, et al. Vestibular schwannomas: correlation between magnetic resonance imaging and histopathologic appearance. *Otol Neurotol* 2001; 22: 79–86.

27. Holsinger FC, Coker NJ, Jenkins HA. Hearing preservation in conservation surgery for vestibular schwannoma. *Am J Otol* 2000; 21: 695–700.

28. Matthies C, Samii M, Krebs S. Management of vestibular schwannomas (acoustic neuromas): radiological features in 202 cases – their value for diagnosis and their predictive importance. *Neurosurgery* 1997; 40: 469–81; discussion 481–2.

29. Somers T, Casselman J, de Ceulaer G, Govaerts P, Offeciers E. Prognostic value of magnetic resonance imaging findings in hearing preservation surgery for vestibular schwannoma. *Otol Neurotol* 2001; 22: 87–94.

30. Pollock BE, Lunsford, LD, Kondziolka D, et al. Outcome analysis of acoustic neuroma management: a comparison of microsurgery and stereotactic radiosurgery. *Neurosurgery* 1995; 36: 215–24; discussion 224–9.

31. Gormley WB, Sekhar LN, Wright DC, Kamerer D, Schessel D. Acoustic neuromas: results of current surgical management. *Neurosurgery* 1997; 41: 50–8; discussion 58–60.

32. Thomsen J, Charabi S, Tos M, Mantoni M, Charabi B. Intracanalicular vestibular schwannoma – therapeutic options. *Acta Otolaryngol Suppl* 2000; 543: 38–40.

33. Charabi S, Thomsen J, Tos M, et al. Management of intrameatal vestibular schwannoma. *Acta Otolaryngol* 1999; 119: 796–800.

34. Walsh RM, Bath AP, Bance ML, Keller A, Rutka JA. Consequences to hearing during the conservative management of vestibular schwannomas. *Laryngoscope* 2000; 110: 250–5.

35. Welling DB, Slater PW, Thomas RD, McGregor JM, Goodman JE. The learning curve in vestibular schwannoma surgery. *Am J Otol* 1999; 20: 644–8.

36. Cerullo L, Grutsch J, Osterdock R. Recurrence of vestibular (acoustic) schwannomas in surgical patients where preservation of the facial and cochlear nerve is the priority. *Br J Neurosurg* 1998; 12: 547–52.

37. Samii M, Matthies C. Management of 1000 vestibular schwannomas (acoustic neuromas): surgical management and results with an

emphasis on complications and how to avoid them. *Neurosurgery* 1997; 40: 11–21; discussion 21–3.

38. Staecker H, Nadol JB, Jr, Ojeman R, Ronner S, McKenna MJ. Hearing preservation in acoustic neuroma surgery:middle fossa versus retrosigmoid approach. *Am J Otol* 2000; 21: 399–404.

39. Kumon Y, Sakaki S, Kohno K, et al. Selection of surgical approaches for small acoustic neurinomas. *Surg Neurol* 2000; 53: 52–9; discussion 59–60.

40. Brackmann DE, Fayad JN, Slattery WH, III, et al. Early proactive management of vestibular schwannomas in neurofibromatosis type 2. *Neurosurgery* 2001; 49: 274–80; discussion 280–3.

41. Sampath P, Rini D, Long DM. Microanatomical variations in the cerebellopontine angle associated with vestibular schwannomas (acoustic neuromas): a retrospective study of 1006 cases. *J Neurosurg* 2000; 92: 70–8.

42. Mazzoni A, Calabrese V, Danesi G. A modified retrosigmoid approach for direct exposure of the fundus of the internal auditory canal for hearing preservation in acoustic neuroma surgery. *Am J Otol* 2000; 21: 98–109.

43. Fahlbusch R, Neu M, Strauss C. Preservation of hearing in large acoustic neurinomas following removal via suboccipito-lateral approach. *Acta Neurochir (Wien)* 1998; 140: 771–7; discussion 778.

44. Rhoton AL, Jr, Tedeschi H. Microsurgical anatomy of acoustic neuroma. *Otolaryngol Clin North Am* 1992; 25: 257–94.

45. Bertalanffy A, Dietrich W, Aichholzer M, Brix R, Ertl A, Heimberger K, Kitz K, et al. Gamma knife radiosurgery of acoustic neurinomas. *Acta Neurochir (Wien)* 2001; 143: 689–95.

46. Kida Y, Kobayashi T, Tanaka T, Mori Y. Radiosurgery for bilateral neurinomas associated with neurofibromatosis type 2. *Surg Neurol* 2000; 53: 383–89; discussion 389–90.

47. Foote KD, Friedman WA, Buati JM, et al. Analysis of risk factors associated with radiosurgery for vestibular schwannoma. *J Neurosurg* 2001; 95: 440–9.

48. Kaylie DM, Horgan MJ, Delashaw JB, McMenomey SO. A meta-analysis comparing outcomes of microsurgery and gamma knife radiosurgery. *Laryngoscope* 2000; 110: 1850–6.

49. Flickinger JC, Kondziolka D, Niranjan A, Lunsford LD. Results of acoustic neuroma radiosurgery: an analysis of 5 years experience using current methods. *J Neurosurg* 2001; 94: 1–6.

50. Evans DG, Sainio M, Baser ME. Neurofibromatosis type 2. *J Med Genet* 2000; 37: 897–904.

51. Moffat DA, Saunders JE, McElveen JT, Jr, McFerran DJ, Hardy DG. Unusual cerebello-pontine angle tumors. *J Laryngol Otol* 1993; 107: 1087–98.

52. Kawamura S, Yamada M, Nonoyama Y, Yasui N, Yoshida Y, Ishikawa K, et al. Intrameatal tumors presenting as a hearing disturbance: case reports of meningioma and lymphoma. *Acta Neurochir (Wien)* 1998; 140: 675–9.

53. Schaller B, Merlo A, Gratzl O, Probst R. Premeatal and retromeatal cerebellopontine angle meningioma. *Acta Neurochir (Wien)* 1999; 141: 465–71.

54. Black PM, Villavicencio AT, Rhouddou C, Loeffler JS. Aggressive surgery and focal radiation in the management of meningiomas of the skull base: preservation of function with maintenance of local control. *Acta Neurochir (Wien)* 2001; 143: 555–62.

55. Stafford SL, Pollock BE, Foote RL, et al. Meningioma radiosurgery: tumor control, outcomes, and complications among 190 consecutive patients. *Neurosurgery* 2001; 49: 1029–37; discussion 1037–8.

56. Lunardi P, Missori P, Innocenzi G, Gagliardi FM, Fortuna A. Long-term results of surgical treatment of cerebello-pontine angle epidermoids. *Acta Neurochir (Wien)* 1990; 103: 105–8.

57. Moritani T, Shrier DA, Numaguchi Y, et al. Diffusion-weighted echo-planar MR imaging:clinical applications and pitfalls. a pictorial essay. *Clin Imaging* 2000; 24: 181–92.

58. Jallo GI, Woo HH, Meshki C, Epstein FJ, Wisoff JH. Arachnoid cysts of the cerebellopontine angle:diagnosis and surgery. *Neurosurgery* 1997; 40: 31–7; discussion 37–8.

59. Krainik A, Cyna-Gorse F, Bouccara D, et al. MRI of unusual lesions in the internal canal. *Neuroradiology* 2001; 43: 52–7.

60. Ajal M, Roche J, Turner J, Fagan P. Unusual lesions of the internal auditory canal. *J Laryngol Otol* 1998; 112: 650–3.

61. Simmons MA, Luff DA, Banerjee SS, Ramsden RT. Primitive neuroectodermal tumor (PNET) of the cerebellopontine angle presenting in adult life. *J Laryngol Otol* 2001; 115: 848–52.

62. Ohata K, Nunta-aree S, Morino M, et al. Aetiology of delayed facial palsy after vestibular schwannoma surgery: clinical data and hypothesis. *Acta Neurochir (Wien)* 1998; 140: 913–17.

63. Grant GA, Rostomily RR, Kim DK, et al. Delayed facial palsy after resection of vestibular schwannoma. *J Neurosurg* 2002; 97: 93–6.

64. Pirouzmand F, Tator CH, Rutka J. Management of hydrocephalus associated with vestibular schwannoma and other cerebellopontine angle tumors. *Neurosurgery* 2001; 48: 1246–53; discussion 1253–4.

65. Rhoton AL, Jr. Microsurgical anatomy of posterior fossa cranial nerves. In: Barrow DL (ed.). *Surgery of the Cranial nerves of the Posterior Fossa, Neurosurgical Topics.* Rolling Meadows, IL: American Association of Neurological Surgeons; 1993: 1–103.

66. Rhoton AL, Jr. The cerebellar arteries. *Neurosurgery* 2000; 47: S29.

67. Day JD, Koos WT, Matula C, Lang J (eds). *Color Atlas of Microneurosurgical Approaches.* New York: Thieme Medical Publishers; 1997: 198.

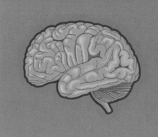

POSTERIOR FOSSA TUMORS

35

Marion L Walker and Joseph Petronio

Considerable progress has been made in the management of tumors of the posterior fossa. While some lesions, such as the cerebellar astrocytoma, were surgically curable even in the early days of neurosurgery, advances in diagnostic imaging, microsurgical techniques, neuroanesthesia, and critical-care medicine have reduced the operative mortality and morbidity associated with the removal of posterior fossa tumors. Advances in radiation and chemotherapy and an improved understanding of the cellular and molecular biology of brain tumors have resulted in significant improvements in the long-term prognosis for patients with even the most malignant tumors. For example, while the cerebellar medulloblastoma was universally fatal in Cushing's first reported series of 61 patients,[1] current 5-year survival rates exceed 60% for all patients and 70% for certain "good-risk" individuals.[2,3]

This chapter focuses primarily on intrinsic tumors arising in the posterior fossa. Anatomically, tumors in this location can arise in the cerebellar hemispheres, the cerebellar vermis, the fourth ventricle, or the brainstem. This discussion excludes extra-axial tumors such as posterior fossa meningiomas and nerve sheath tumors.

INCIDENCE AND EPIDEMIOLOGY

Tumors of the posterior fossa occur more commonly in children than adults. Between 54% and 70% of all childhood tumors arise in the posterior fossa, compared with 15–20% in adults.[4–11]

Although most histopathologic varieties of posterior fossa tumors have been reported at any age, certain types, including primitive neuroectodermal tumors (PNET), medulloblastomas, ependymomas, and astrocytomas of the cerebellum and brainstem, more commonly affect infants and children.[9] Certain types of glial tumors, including mixed gliomas, are common in children. They are more frequently located in the cerebellum (67%) than the cerebrum and are usually histologically benign. The most common combination is that of neoplastic astrocytes and oligodendroglia.[9] As a rule, astrocytic tumors of adults more commonly display the histologic features of malignancy than those of children. Certain tumors, including metastatic lesions, hemangioblastoma, and lymphoma, more commonly affect adults than children.

SIGNS AND SYMPTOMS

The clinical presentation of a posterior fossa tumor depends on the anatomical site of origin, rate and pattern of growth, and the age of the patient. Obstruction of cerebrospinal fluid (CSF) circulation at the cerebral aqueduct, fourth ventricle, or the foramina of Magendie or Luschka produces hydrocephalus. Patients present with headache, vomiting, papilledema, meningismus, dizziness, and strabismus.[12,13] Very young children and infants may not express their symptoms, leaving signs such as irritability, frequent vomiting, failure to thrive, and increasing head circumference.

Tradition has accorded "classic" syndromes to determine anatomic localization for cerebellar lesions. In practice, however, clinical presentation rarely allows for a completely accurate anatomical localization. The *vermian syndrome* consists primarily of truncal ataxia, while the *hemicerebellar syndrome* presents with appendicular ataxia, dysmetria, dysdiadochokinesia, and nystagmus. In children, these signs and symptoms may prove very subtle.

Brainstem tumors usually present with focal signs of cranial nerve and long-tract dysfunction. Truncal ataxia is more commonly associated with pontine and medullary tumors,[14] while hemiparesis is more commonly associated with cerebral peduncle lesions.[15] Tumors of the tectal plate frequently present with hydrocephalus and only occasionally with symptoms referable to opthalmoplegia.[16]

Headache is the most common symptom of patients with a cerebellar mass, a condition reported in nearly 100% of patients in some series.[17] The headache associated with most cerebellar tumors is generalized or frontal in location.[12,13,18] It may eventually localize to the occipital region. Associated neck pain and stiffness, or a head tilt suggest tonsillar herniation into the foramen magnum.[13] The headache of a posterior fossa tumor is insidious and intermittent initially and is often most severe in the morning or after a nap.[12] Hypoventilation during sleep results in a relative increase in arterial vasodilatation, which in turn increases intracranial pressure. This, in combination with an increase in intracranial pressure associated with recumbency, probably explains the more severe headache on awakening. In infants, headache may only manifest itself as irritability, particularly on waking, and a reluctance to be handled. In general, headache is an uncommon complaint in early childhood, and its persistence or recurrence should suggest increased intracranial pressure in this age group. Headache is uncommonly associated with brainstem tumors unless hydrocephalus is present.

Vomiting associated with posterior fossa tumors may represent a generalized response to increased intracranial pressure or direct involvement of the area postrema of the fourth ventricle or the vagal nuclei. In association with hydrocephalus and increased intracranial pressure, vomiting is frequently limited to awakening. So called "projectile vomiting" occurs rarely and its absence should not provide comfort to the physician in the face of other signs of increased intracranial pressure. Vomiting and its associated hyperventilation may relieve the headache. Emphasized more than 30 years ago by Matson,[12] *persistent* vomiting is unfortunately still commonly misinterpreted, even in pediatric patients, as a symptom of a gastrointestinal ailment or emotional disturbance. Most gastrointestinal ailments are self-limiting, while the vomiting associated with posterior fossa tumors is usually persistent and associated with headaches.

A patient with a posterior fossa tumor who presents with protracted vomiting as the primary symptom usually harbors an ependymoma. Medulloblastomas and cerebellar astrocytomas more commonly present with headache as the initial symptom, with vomiting occurring later in the course. "If the vomiting occurs before the headache, the tumor is most likely to be an ependymoma. If the headache precedes the vomiting, then the tumor is more likely to be a medulloblastoma or astrocytoma." This axiom, known as "Robin's Rule," named after pediatric neurosurgeon, Dr Robin Humphreys, is rarely broken.

Commonly associated with cerebellar tumors, *ataxia* depends on the location of the lesion. The midline vermian tumors such as medulloblastoma, ependymomas, and vermian astrocytomas generate a truncal ataxia with relative sparing of the extremities. In children, this presents as a tendency to fall, a lurching wide-based gait, and an abnormal Romberg maneuver.[12] The hemispheric tumors, such as metastases, hemangioblastomas, and cerebellar astrocytomas, often generate the hemicerebellar syndrome of unilateral ataxia or dysmetria of the extremities.

Eye findings are common and include nystagmus, strabismus, and papilledema. While considered a "classic" sign of cerebellar lesions, nystagmus is usually absent until late in the clinical course. Nevertheless, it offers localizing value. Lateral nystagmus suggests involvement of the cerebellar hemisphere, while vertical nystagmus suggests a lesion of the anterior vermis, periaqueductal region, or craniocervical junction.[12] Strabismus and its associated diplopia result primarily from sixth nerve palsies secondary to hydrocephalus.[12,13] Third and fourth nerve palsies may also occur. Intrinsic tumors of the brainstem may directly involve the nuclei or tracts of the third, fourth, and sixth cranial nerves, producing ocular palsies and diplopia.

NEURODIAGNOSTIC EVALUATION

Magnetic resonance imaging (MRI) has generally superseded computed tomography (CT) for nearly all types of posterior fossa tumors.[4,19,20] It offers the obvious advantage of superior anatomic resolution, multiplanar imaging, and lack of radiation exposure. However, while neither MRI nor CT can distinguish one tumor type from another with certainty, certain trends exist which, when combined with the clinical information, can narrow the differential diagnosis. As the strength of MRI magnets increases and the understanding of the physics behind MRI expands, magnetic resonance spectroscopy (MRS) has great potential to narrow or eliminate the confusion over preoperative diagnosis.[21]

Medulloblastoma

The medulloblastoma, often classified as a PNET, presents as an intraventricular midline or paramedian mass on MRI. It is usually of a homogenous signal intensity isointense to brain on T1 images and enhances prominently (Figure 35.1). It can appear heterogeneous with areas of cystic degeneration and central necrosis,

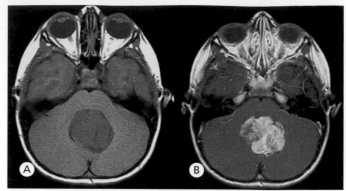

Figure 35.1 Axial precontrast **(A)** and postcontrast **(B)** T1 MRI appearance of a cerebellar medulloblastoma (PNET).

which may indicate a poorer prognosis.[4] Other atypical features, found in up to 10% of cases, include calcification, failure to enhance, and an eccentric location. The CT appearance of a medulloblastoma typically reveals a lesion hyperdense to normal brain, as opposed to the usual appearance of an astrocytoma, which is usually iso- or hypodense.

Since up to 43% of patients have myelographic evidence of asymptomatic subarachnoid metastasis at the time of diagnosis,[22–24] and metastatic lesions are present in over 50% of patients at autopsy,[25] patients suspected of having a medulloblastoma merit an MRI of the spine with contrast. Enhanced MRI has become the standard initial screen for leptomeningeal metastases, particularly "sugar coating" of the spinal cord and nerve roots, because it is more sensitive than CT-myelography[26] (Figure 35.2). It is important to obtain the spinal MRI prior to surgery to avoid confusion in the postoperative period when there is blood in the spinal canal.

Ependymoma

Since ependymomas commonly present on gross inspection as multicystic, hemorrhagic, and calcified, MRI often demonstrates these features.[4,27] Commonly located within the fourth ventricle, they often present with evidence of hydrocephalus on imaging studies. Since calcification occurs more commonly in ependymoma (nearly 45%) than in any other posterior fossa tumor,[28] MRI or CT evidence of calcification strongly supports this diagnosis, but it does not exclude other tumors. Extension of the tumor through the foramen of Luschka into the cerebellopontine angle is essentially pathognomonic of ependymoma. The classic designation "plastic ependymoma" refers to tumors that extend through the foramina of Magendie and Luschka to compress the craniocervical junction and lateral brainstem[29] (Figure 35.3). Nearly all ependymomas enhance, though they often appear more heterogeneous than the uniformly enhancing medulloblastoma.[28] Since subarachnoid seeding may occur, these patients should also undergo imaging of their spine.

Cerebellar astrocytoma

The cerebellar astrocytoma typically appears on MRI as an intra-axial mass, either midline or hemispheric, often accompanied by a prominent cystic component and an enhancing mural nodule (Figure 35.4). The mass usually displaces or effaces the fourth ventricle. Evidence of hydrocephalus, with ventriculomegaly and

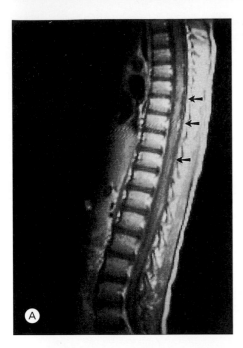
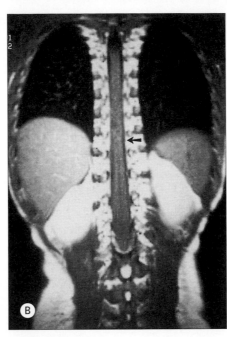

Figure 35.2 Sagittal (A) and coronal (B) postcontrast T1 sagittal MRI demonstrating subarachnoid metastases (arrows) of a cerebellar medulloblastoma.

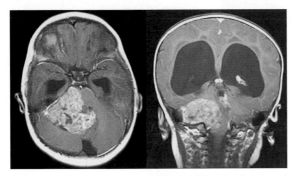

Figure 35.3 Fourth ventricular ependymoma with extension into the cerebellopontine angle and subarachnoid spaces, i.e. the so-called plastic ependymoma, shown with T1 MRI imaging following gadolinium administration in the axial and coronal planes.

occasionally periventricular low signal intensity on T1 and high signal intensity on T2 images, is common at the time of diagnosis. The solid portion of the cystic cerebellar astrocytoma is commonly hyperintense to brain on T2 images, while the cystic portion can be slightly hyperintense to CSF on T1 images secondary to increased protein content.[4] The mural nodule or solid portion of the cyst often enhances with paramagnetic contrast agents, while the cyst wall may or may not enhance. While signal heterogeneity and calcification occur less prominently than in the ependymoma, both may occur in the cerebellar astrocytoma.

Choroid plexus papilloma

This tumor typically presents on MRI as an intraventricular mass with a lobulated margin and hypointense signal to gray matter on T1 images. Calcification and hypervascularity may appear as linear and patchy regions of hypointensity. The tumor usually enhances prominently (Figure 35.5), and heterogeneity in the pattern of enhancement suggests calcifications, cysts, or old hemorrhage. T2 images may reveal regions of hyperintensity from calcifications

and old hemorrhage. The tumor may extend from the fourth ventricle through the foramina into the basal cisterns. Most choroid plexus tumors in children are found in the lateral ventricles, while the posterior fossa is a more common location in adults. Hydrocephalus is usually present, sometimes without evidence of obstruction of the CSF pathways.[4]

Hemangioblastoma

The typical features of a posterior fossa hemangioblastoma on MRI include a cystic mass with a pial-based mural nodule that enhances prominently, associated with abnormally prominent vessels within or adjacent to the tumor (Figure 35.6). These findings in the setting of an intra-axial mass in an adult are virtually pathognomonic for hemangioblastoma.[4] A history of von Hippel–Lindau disease adds to the certainty of the diagnosis. The pial-base for the mural nodule helps to distinguish it from the mural nodule of the cystic cerebellar astrocytoma. The MRI signal intensity of the cyst fluid varies with its composition from isointense to hyperintense to CSF on all images.[20] Typically only slightly hyperintense in comparison to cortex on T1 images, the mural nodule enhances brightly. Large tumor-associated vessels appear readily on spin-echo MRI images as regions of signal void.[20] Variations in the MRI appearance include the presence of hemorrhage into the cyst and solid rather than cystic masses. This can occur in approximately 30–40% of hemangioblastomas but primarily in the supratentorial lesions.[30] Other variations include multiple lesions and medullary or cervical tumors with an associated syrinx.[20]

Dermoid tumors

Dermoid cysts typically appear on MRI as hypointense on T1 and T2 images and are difficult to separate from CSF. They are best seen on diffusion or flair images.[4,31] They most commonly arise in the posterior fossa in the midline. Rupture of the fatty contents of the cyst into the subarachnoid space or ventricles may be visible radiographically.[4]

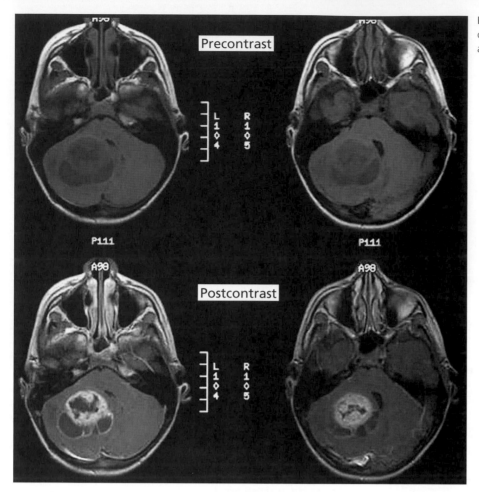

Precontrast

Postcontrast

Figure 35.4 Axial T1 MRI appearance of a cystic cerebellar astrocytoma prior to and following the administration of paramagnetic contrast material.

OPERATIVE STRATEGY AND APPROACH

Initial management

Initial management of a patient with a posterior fossa tumor often involves correction of the secondary effects of the tumor and increased intracranial pressure, including headache, nausea, vomiting, and occasionally dehydration. Children with posterior fossa tumors are frequently very ill on presentation, with severe headache and vomiting as a result of obstructive hydrocephalus. Since brainstem compression is often present, rapid and catastrophic deterioration is always a danger. Shunting prior to craniotomy has largely fallen out of favor since a majority of posterior fossa tumors can be excised sufficiently to re-establish the CSF pathways.[32–34] Shunting exposes the patient to the potential perils of shunt dependency and its attendant risks. Some neurosurgeons now perform a third ventriculostomy at the beginning of the surgical procedure as a means of controlling hydrocephalus.[35]

While some neurosurgeons have advocated initial management of the hydrocephalus with external ventricular drainage, most advocate preoperative treatment with glucocorticoids followed by tumor removal.[13,36] Patients with posterior fossa tumors receive glucocorticoids, usually dexamethasone, with surgery scheduled within the next few days. If the patient deteriorates neurologically or presents having experienced a rapid deterioration, the tumor is resected on an emergent basis.

Operative management

Virtually all posterior fossa tumors can be resected with the patient in a prone or modified prone position. This position almost eliminates the risk of air emboli and greatly reduces fatigue to the surgeon's arms in comparison with the sitting position. The patient's head is immobilized in three-point head fixation if over 2 years of age or in a padded horseshoe headrest if below 2 years of age. A moderate amount of cervical flexion allows access to the superior vermis and aqueduct.

For patients with significant hydrocephalus or obstruction of the fourth ventricle, an occipital burr hole may be placed at the beginning of surgery, establishing external ventricular drainage for postoperative management. In planning the surgery, the surgeon must consider the location of the tumor and the relevant anatomy. For a comprehensive review of the microsurgical anatomy and surgical approaches to the posterior fossa, surgeons may consult Rhoton's excellent supplement to *Neurosurgery*.[37]

Tumors of the vermis, fourth ventricle, and paramedian cerebellar hemisphere

These tumors may be approached through a midline incision extending from the inion to the upper cervical spine. The paracervical and suboccipital musculature is then elevated with electrocautery in the suboccipital plane. In children, we have advocated a free craniotomy flap extending from the transverse sinus to the area just above the foramen magnum. The foramen

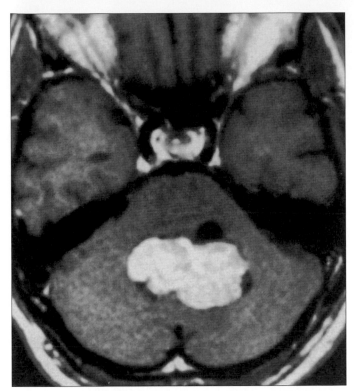

Figure 35.5 Axial T1 MRI appearance of choroid plexus papilloma of the fourth ventricle following administration of intravenous gadolinium.

will welcome if reoperation proves necessary, particularly after radiation therapy. Craniectomy has been associated with a statistically significant increased incidence of postoperative CSF leak, pseudomeningocele, and wound reclosures.[38] Replacement of the bone flap may limit the stress on the dural suture line.

The dura is best opened in a Y-shaped fashion, extending below the cerebellar tonsils. However, especially in children, the occipital and circular sinuses may be quite prominent and the surgeon must be prepared for potentially significant bleeding. In children under the age of 2 there are often large venous lakes between the leaves of the dura. Opening through this type of dura often requires the surgeon to clip the edges of the dura, cut between the clips, clip again, and cut, progressing slowly to an adequate dural opening. The clips are then removed after the edges of the dura are oversewn. Care should be taken to keep the dura moist and on a stretch to facilitate a watertight closure at the conclusion of the case. If this proves difficult, particularly if the edges retract with cautery, the pericranium provides an excellent source for a graft.

For midline tumors, the cerebellar vermis is opened in the midline using a combination of bipolar electrocautery and gentle suction. Self-retaining retractors facilitate exposure. Surgeons should be aware of *akinetic mutism*, a syndrome encountered primarily in pediatric patients. The syndrome generally results after resection of a cerebellar mass, has a delayed onset after relatively normal speech for 1–2 days after surgery, consists of transient mutism that lasts from 1 day to 6 months, and is often followed by severe dysarthria that recovers slowly over months. It is frequently associated with other neurological signs such as long tract signs and behavioral abnormalities.[39–41] While the exact mechanism remains unknown, Pollack and colleagues suggest that paravermal manipulation may result in damage to the dentate and interpositus nuclei. Their concept is based on the work of Fraioli and Guidetti who report mutism after bilateral stereotactic lesions in these regions.[39,40]

While a surgeon may use a variety of techniques to remove the tumor, he or she should adhere to certain general principles. The surgical goal for nearly all tumors is complete resection[13,42] provided the floor of the fourth ventricle and brainstem are not

magnum is removed with the combination of a high-speed drill and sharp rongeurs. The arch of C1 may be removed separately. Patients have traditionally received craniectomies. However, in the era of high-speed drills and microplates, craniotomy is feasible. Adults have a more prominent internal midline keel that must be carefully separated from the underlying dura. One advantage to replacement of the bone flap, aside from better protection, is that it preserves an anatomical plane that a surgeon

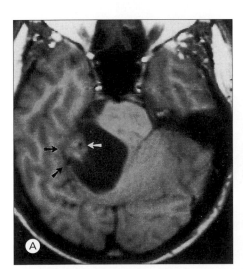
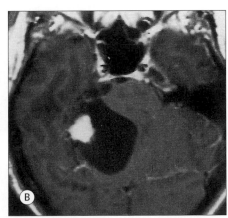
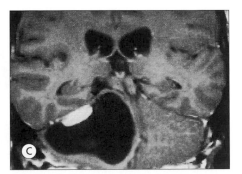

Figure 35.6 T1 MRI appearance of a cystic cerebellar hemangioblastoma in the axial plane before **(A)** and after **(B)** contrast administration and in the coronal plane **(C)**, demonstrating pial-based, contrast-enhancing mural nodule. Note the signal voids (arrows) corresponding to flow through feeding vessels.

infiltrated. In most cases, decompression of the brainstem and reduction of tumor bulk is the initial objective. Mass effect associated with cystic or hemorrhagic lesions is quickly and effectively reduced by early aspiration. Removal of CSF via the ventriculostomy is another effective method to reduce mass effect after the dura is open.

Large solid tumors with a capsule or pseudocapsule are safely debulked from within using either gentle suction, the ultrasonic surgical aspirator, or, less commonly, lasers, allowing the capsule to limit resection and protect adjacent vital structures. It is often safer for the surgeon to remove a large tumor in a piecemeal fashion than to apply needless traction on the brainstem or lower cranial nerves. After tumor debulking, the capsule or pseudo-capsule can be removed in an extratumoral plane under magnification. Use of cottonoid patties protects the surrounding structures and preserves the plane of dissection. Attachments of tumor to the brainstem, cerebellar peduncles, or lower cranial nerves can be removed last. All radiographically enhancing tissue, including the cyst wall if it enhances, should be removed if possible.[36,43] Unusually fibrous or tough tumors may be effectively removed with the ultrasonic aspirator.

Meticulous attention to proper wound closure is necessary in the posterior fossa, especially in the presence of hydrocephalus. The surgeon should close the dura in a watertight fashion to reduce the likelihood of cerebellar hernias, pseudomeningoceles, and CSF fistulas. A variety of substances may be used for grafting including pericranium, fascia lata, and bovine pericardium. Fibrin glue may be used to facilitate attachment of the graft and to repair small defects.

Tumors of the cerebellar hemispheres

These tumors are more effectively approached through a para-median or retromastoid incision. Care should be taken to avoid injury to the vertebral artery as it transverses from the C1 vertebral canal to the foramen magnum. If the surgeon requires access to the cerebellopontine angle, the craniotomy or craniectomy can be extended laterally to the transverse sinus or beyond: the trans-sigmoid approach. Opened mastoid air cells should be sealed with bone wax while larger exposures may require mastoidectomy and obliteration. Intraoperative ultrasound can be used to locate sub-cortical tumors and plan the corticectomy. The corticectomy is then made in the horizontal plane parallel to the cerebellar folia. Bipolar electrocautery and gentle suction are used for the incision. Self-retaining retractors help maintain exposure. Some cases may benefit from stereotactic techniques.

Intrinsic tumors of the cervicomedullary junction

These tumors can be approached through a midline incision with the patient in a prone position. Exposure of the cerebellum, lower brainstem, and upper cervical spinal cord should be carried out under magnification. The midline incision begins just below the obex and extends to the upper cervical region as necessary. It is important to avoid incising through the obex unless the tumor is truly exophytic at that level. The dorsally exophytic tumors allow easy access to the brainstem. Tumors that are not exophytic usually lie immediately beneath the surface. Approach to these tumors through a midline incision minimizes deficits. The laser is ideal for this opening, allowing a precise and sharp incision with little damage to surrounding neural tissue. Once identified, the tumor is removed through internal debulking with the ultrasonic aspirator and/or laser. The distinct tumor texture and coloration compared with the normal white color of the brainstem allows for

creation of a plane of dissection and, often, a gross total resection (Figure 35.7). Occasionally the tumor tissue is not distinct from the surrounding normal brain. We have found this to be true most often in cases with an associated diagnosis of neurofibromatosis. When this occurs, biopsy is the only appropriate therapeutic choice. Attempts at gross total removal should be limited to those tumors that are visually distinct when compared with surrounding normal tissue. Fortunately, this is the usual case.

TUMORS OF THE CEREBELLUM AND FOURTH VENTRICLE

Tumors of the cerebellum and fourth ventricle comprise a diverse group of neoplasms that can arise congenitally though senescence. Generally, these represent pediatric tumors; however, they do not spare adults. Nevertheless, considerable differences with respect to anatomic location, histology, and prognosis exist between the tumors that commonly affect children and those that affect adults.

Medulloblastoma

Cerebellar medulloblastomas, currently considered a form of PNET, represent the prototypical posterior fossa brain tumor, presenting with morning headache and vomiting.[44] Pediatric medulloblastomas arise in the inferior medullary velum, grow to fill the fourth ventricle, may infiltrate surrounding structures including the floor of the fourth ventricle, and metastasize along CSF pathways as well as systemically.[2,44] Bailey and Cushing first reported the tumor in 1925 and gave it the name "medullo-blastoma cerebelli," based on their theory that it arises from a "pluripotential medulloblast."[45] This presumptive progenitor cell has never been located.

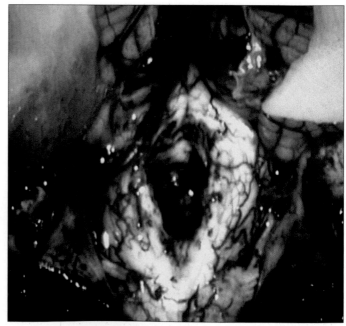

Figure 35.7 A view of the dorsal medulla post resection of an intrinsic low-grade astrocytoma. The distinctive coloration of the tumor allowed a gross total resection.

Epidemiology

The medulloblastoma competes with the cerebellar astrocytoma as the most common pediatric posterior fossa brain tumor, representing between 20 and 25% of all brain tumors and 30% of all posterior fossa tumors in children.[44,46] The majority of medulloblastomas occur in children, with 50% arising within the first decade and 80% within the first 15 years of life. The peak incidence is between 5 and 9 years of age.[47,48] A second peak exists in young adults between the ages of 20 and 24 years.[47]

Studies have found a male predominance, with ratios between 1.4 : 1 and 4.8 : 1.[44,48–52] Medulloblastoma develops sporadically, and no environmental factors have been reported to increase the incidence;[44] rare familial cases have been reported. Hung and colleagues reported the tumor in two non-twin siblings and reviewed six reports in the literature for a total of fourteen cases.[53] Evans and associates reported four children with evidence of a genetic syndrome in a series of 174 children with medulloblastoma.[54] Furthermore, an increased incidence exists in Turcot syndrome,[51,55] while between 3 and 5% of patients with Gorlin's or nevoid basal cell carcinoma syndrome develop medulloblastoma, often before the age of 5 years.[56,57] Medulloblastoma has been reported in a family with Li–Fraumeni syndrome.[58,59] Finally, an association between medulloblastoma and the blue rubber bleb nevus syndrome has been reported.[58,60]

These hereditary syndromes have raised fascinating insights into the possible mechanisms of tumor genesis, which have been comprehensively reviewed by Taylor and colleagues.[61] Patients with Gorlin syndrome have an autosomal dominant disorder involving a mutation of the human homolog of the *Drosophila melanogaster Patched* gene (*PTCH*) which is a transmembrane receptor for *Sonic Hedgehog* (*Shh*).[61–63] The *Shh* signal pathway is critical in central nervous system development.[64,65]. *PTCH* is localized on 9q, which is a region where some medulloblastomas lose heterozygosity, particularly the desmoplastic variety. A minority of sporadic medulloblastomas have mutations of *PTCH*. Between 10 and 20% of mice with a loss of one gene (*PTCH*) develop a tumor similar to human medulloblastoma.[61] The theory is that *PTCH* behaves as a tumor suppressor gene to *Shh*, which behaves as an oncogene.[61] Purkinje cells secrete *Shh*, which acts as a strong mitogen for granule cell precursors in the external granule layer, and blockage of *Shh* dramatically decreases their proliferation.[61,66]

Pathology

The precise cell of origin for the medulloblastoma remains unknown. Since the 1930s, it has been noted that the fetal external granular layer persists during the first year and may be found in scattered foci in the posterior medullary velum during the first 18 months of life.[44] In 1973, Hart and Earle first described the PNET, and in 1983 Rorke proposed classification of the medulloblastoma as a PNET.[67,68] PNETs include ependymoblastoma, pineoblastoma, cerebral neuroblastoma, retinoblastoma, medulloepithelioma, and pigmented medulloblastoma, also known as the melanotic vermian PNET of infancy. These tumors cannot be distinguished on the basis of light microscopic, immunocytochemical, or ultrastructural analysis.[68] Rorke proposed that PNETs arise from a pool of undifferentiated cells in the subependymal region of the fetal brain.[68] Her theory can explain the ability of PNETs to differentiate along multiple lines including the neuronal, spongioblastic, glial, and ependymal. However, Rubinstein considered the inclusion of these tumors under the general classification of PNET an indiscriminate application of a simplistic concept that fails to recognize actual differences between the tumors such as the distinctive differentiating capacity of the medulloblastoma compared with the pineoblastoma and retinoblastoma.[69]

Immunohistochemical techniques have demonstrated that medulloblastomas may be divided into the following subgroups:

1 undifferentiated neuroepithelial cells;
2 undifferentiated cells with some neuronal differentiation;
3 undifferentiated cells with some glial differentiation; and
4 a combination of the three with melanin containing cells or muscle.[70]

Cells that cannot be distinguished by light microscopy may stain positively for specific intermediate filament proteins, and many cells may express more than one.[70]

The most reported chromosome abnormality in medulloblastoma involves chromosome 17.[44] An isochromosome of 17q has been reported in 36–66% of cases;[44] however, this may result from tumor progression.[71,72] Roughly 50% of cases have an absence of 17p,[73,74] which appears significant since the tumor suppressor gene *p53* is located in this region.[44] The Li–Fraumeni syndrome involves a mutation in *p53*;[58,59] however, the gene is normal in most tumors[74] with only about 10% of medulloblastomas not associated with the Li–Fraumeni syndrome demonstrating a *p53* mutation.[75,76]

Macroscopically, the medulloblastoma is soft and friable. Areas of necrosis and focal hemorrhage are sometimes present but rare,[2,44] and calcification is uncommon. While the tumor may confine itself to the vermis and fourth ventricle, it will infiltrate the brainstem or adjacent cerebellar hemisphere in approximately 30% of cases. Isolated involvement of one cerebellar hemisphere is much less common,[77] and usually consists of the desmoplastic variant found in young adults. This desmoplastic variant is firmer, better demarcated, and may involve the meninges.[25,78] Park and colleagues demonstrated only 1 of 21 (5%) desmoplastic medulloblastomas occurring in the 10–16-year age group.[77] The distribution tended towards younger children, with 11 of 21 (52%) occurring in the 0–4-year age group. However, 18 of 21 desmoplastic medulloblastomas occurred in the midline rather than the cerebellar hemisphere.

Dissemination through the subarachnoid space is common. Between 11 and 43% of patients have myelographic evidence of asymptomatic subarachnoid metastasis at the time of diagnosis,[22–24] and metastatic lesions are present in over 50% of patients at autopsy.[25] Extraneural metastases occur in 5% of patients and primarily involve the bone marrow, along with the peritoneum, lungs and pleura, liver, and multiple organs.[77–81]

Microscopically, the medulloblastoma appears as a highly cellular tumor composed of round to oval cells with scant cytoplasm and hyperchromatic nuclei, giving it the appearance of a "blue tumor" on staining with hematoxylin & eosin (Figure 35.8). Homer–Wright rosettes, which suggest neuronal differentiation, as well as pseudorosettes are commonly present.

Treatment

The surgical goal is aggressive but sensible resection. The surgeon should attempt to remove all grossly visible tumor. Invasion of the floor of the fourth ventricle will limit the extent of resection. The temptation to remove tumor invading the floor should be avoided unless a clean anatomic plane of separation exists. Medulloblastoma invades the floor in between 15% and 36% of cases.[15,77] Albright recommends ending the resection flush with the floor

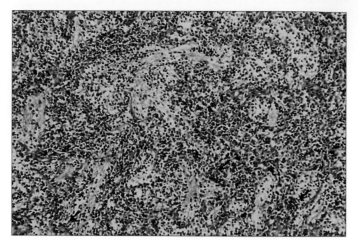

Figure 35.8 Photomicrographs of a cerebellar medulloblastoma stained with hematoxylin & eosin. Note Homer–Wright rosettes (arrows). (H&E; × 100.)

because leaving microscopic residual for irradiation does not worsen the prognosis.[44]

Patients may be separated into a "good-risk" and a "bad-risk" group based on the age at diagnosis, extent of surgical resection, and the presence of leptomeningeal dissemination or metastatic disease.[2] Children have a significantly worse prognosis if they are under 2 years of age at the time of diagnosis, have less than 80% resection, have subarachnoid metastasis, have brainstem invasion, or have persistently positive CSF cytology more than 2 weeks following surgery.[2] Chang and associates proposed a staging system based on residual tumor size,[82] brainstem invasion, and metastases.[44] More recent studies indicate that tumor size is unimportant, while multicenter trials have confirmed that age at the time of diagnosis and presence of metastases correlate with outcome.[44,77,83,84]

Postoperative adjuvant therapy is universally indicated in patients with medulloblastomas. All of our patients over 3 years of age with newly diagnosed medulloblastomas receive adjuvant radiotherapy. Five-year survival rates of 70% or greater are considered routine for the "good-risk" patients. "Poor-risk" patients receive adjuvant chemotherapy in addition to radiotherapy.

Ependymoma, anaplastic ependymoma, and ependymoblastoma

Ependymomas derive from and have the appearance of differentiated ependymal cells. While considered favorable tumors in the past, it has been stressed that ependymomas may recur relentlessly and force the surgeon to decide between a radical resection that risks serious neurologic complications or a more limited resection that spares the patient deficits but promises inevitable recurrence.[85]

Epidemiology

Ependymomas tend to occur in younger patients, with nearly 50% presenting in children less than 3 years of age.[12,86–89] They represent roughly 10% and 30% of brain tumors in children under 14 and 3 years of age respectively[85,90,91] and are the third most common pediatric brain tumor after medulloblastoma and astrocytoma.[91] There exists a slight sex predilection for boys, with a ratio ranging between 1 : 1 and 1.4 : 1.[91,92] Roughly two-thirds

of pediatric ependymomas originate in the posterior fossa;[85] thus, the presenting signs and symptoms are similar to those for other posterior fossa masses. The most common presenting symptoms are nausea, vomiting, and headache.[91,92] The most common presenting signs in children are ataxia, papilledema, nystagmus, cranial nerve palsies, weight loss, and increasing head circumference in children less than 2 years of age.[92,93] Since this tumor may occur in very young children, the presenting symptoms and signs may prove nonspecific such as developmental delay, irritability, and weight loss.[92] As noted previously, the patient who presents with a long history of vomiting prior to the onset of headache usually harbors an ependymoma.

No environmental factor that contributes to the development of ependymomas has been identified.[85] Since 2–5% of patients with neurofibromatosis type two (NF-2) develop ependymomas, research has focused on chromosome 22.[46,85] Several reports of losses on chromosome 22[94–98] suggest the loss of a tumor suppressor gene.[85] Smyth and colleagues provide an excellent review of studies of chromosomal abnormalities.[99]

For many years it has been known that inoculation of newborn hamsters with simian virus 40 (SV 40) induces ependymomas.[99–101] Several studies using the polymerase chain reaction to detect the presence of simian virus 40 reported its presence in high percentages.[99,100,102,103] This remains an active area of investigation.

Pathology

Most ependymomas fall under the histological classification of ependymoma or anaplastic ependymoma.[87] Numerous alternative schemes of classification have been proposed[104–106] without much bearing on prognosis, time to recurrence, and response to therapy.[72,107] The World Health Organization II (WHO-II) classification has become generally accepted.[99,108] The WHO-II Grade I represents the myxopapillary ependymoma of the cauda equina. The WHO-II Grade II represents the classical ependymoma. These display the three following classic histologic features:

1 perivascular pseudorosettes;
2 true ependymal rosettes; and
3 blepharoplasts.

In the absence of the diagnostic true ependymal rosettes and pseudorosettes, many ependymomas resemble astrocytomas and may contain gemistocytic cells indistinguishable from gemistocytes in anaplastic astrocytomas and glioblastomas.[107]

The WHO-II Grade III ependymoma is the anaplastic or malignant ependymoma. Anaplastic ependymomas display malignant histological features: cytoplasmic and nuclear pleomorphism, nuclear hyperchomatism, mitoses, necrosis, and cytoarchitectural disorganization. Patients with what is now regarded as a grade III or anaplastic ependymoma have a significantly worse prognosis than those with less malignant phenotypes.[92,105,109,110]

Ependymoblastomas are PNETs with ependymal differentiation.[99] Symth and colleagues feel that the term "ependymoblastoma" has fallen by the wayside and more properly represents the WHO-II Grade IV which microscopically consist of densely packed, small, undifferentiated cells arranged in rosettes with concentric rings around the lumina.[99,111] Nevertheless, small foci with classical pseudorosettes or true rosettes characteristic of ependymomas may be found in some PNETs.[107] Differentiation between an ependymoma and a PNET is difficult in tumors mostly composed of rosettes and pseudorosettes, with relatively small and subtle areas of diffuse architecture containing primitive cells.[107]

Most ependymomas react to antibodies to glial fibrillary acidic protein (GFAP), particularly in the perivascular pseudorosettes.[112] More anaplastic tumors appear to react better to epithelial markers, such as epithelial membrane antigen, than to GFAP.[112–114]

Treatment

The surgical approach for ependymomas is identical to that for all other vermian and midline posterior fossa tumors. Ependymomas may prove quite vascular. However, the blood supply derives from small branches off the posterior inferior cerebellar artery, which renders the risks of preoperative embolization significant.[85] The ependymoma can usually be identified in the vallecula; the vermis is split early to provide access to the fourth ventricle. While most originate in the midline, roughly 25% of ependymomas arise in the cerebellopontine angle and the lateral cerebellum.[112,115,116] Reports on postoperative cerebellar mutism suggest surgeons should try to avoid splitting the inferior vermis greater than 1 cm.[99,117–120]

The tumor generally does not adhere to the walls of the ventricle except at the site of origin, which usually allows for a gross total or near gross total excision. Nevertheless, the surgeon must take care to remove the entire tumor in the lateral recess of the ventricle and to follow any extension out of the foramina of Luschka. The tumor frequently molds to the available spaces without adhering to them, earning the description "plastic ependymoma."[29] Lifting the cerebellar tonsil on the involved side and taking the small arachnoidal adhesions can facilitate exposure of the lateral recess and cerebellopontine angle. This often gives a wide exposure to this area. The tumor often arises in the subependymal region of the lateral wall of the ventricle and displaces the ventricle laterally.[85] It also has a tendency to arise from the obex, which risks sleep apnea, swallowing dysfunction, and chronic aspiration.[85] Furthermore, the tumor may encase the posterior inferior cerebellar artery and cranial nerves,[85] and even if the nerves appear intact at the conclusion of surgery the patient may have prolonged difficulty with swallowing.[116] Unfortunately, the tumor can invade the parenchyma locally. Nazar and colleagues reported that 10 out of 14 children with ependymoma who presented with focal cerebellar, brainstem, or cranial nerve signs had tumor invasion at the time of surgery.[91]

It has become clear in recent years that the most important and consistent prognostic factor for posterior fossa ependymoma is the extent of surgical resection.[40,91,99,121–125] Since total resection is possible in only about 50% of patients,[6,112,126] most require adjuvant therapy. Postoperative radiation therapy improves survival in many retrospective studies.[87,89,121,122,125,127–129] The benefits versus the risks of craniospinal axis irradiation have become clearer in recent years. Since posterior fossa ependymomas tend to recur locally, spinal radiation is generally withheld unless evidence exists for metastasis.[112,125,129–132] Subarachnoid seeding appears more frequent with anaplastic ependymomas.[128,133] Craniospinal axis radiation is usually reserved for patients over 3 years of age with anaplastic ependymomas or with subarachnoid seeding on enhanced MRI.[112] For non-disseminated ependymomas clinicians can limit the radiotherapy volume to the tumor bed.[134] Depending on the residual size, clinicians may consider stereotactic radiosurgery.[135]

The severe detrimental effects of radiation on young children and the lack of complete tumor control drive the investigation into chemotherapeutic agents. Unfortunately, the results of clinical trials involving ependymoma have been discouraging.[112,136] A randomized study on the effects of lomustine and vincristine with postoperative radiation therapy compared with radiotherapy alone showed no improvement in outcome. Other retrospective studies demonstrate a 20% response rate, with cisplatin being the most effective single agent.[112,126] A French multicenter trial could only demonstrate a radiologically documented response in less than 50% and achieved overall 40% and 23% survival rates after 2 and 4 years respectively.[137] High-dose chemotherapy with stem-cell rescue has failed to provide radiological evidence of disease regression or longer survival in multiple trials.[99,137–139]

Cerebellar astrocytoma

While the "classic" astrocytoma of the cerebellum is the cystic pilocytic or "juvenile" astrocytoma encountered primarily in pediatric patients, higher-grade astrocytomas, including glioblastoma multiforme, may arise in the cerebellum.

Pilocytic astrocytoma

EPIDEMIOLOGY The term juvenile pilocytic astrocytoma originally conveyed a contrast with the "piloid" astrocytomas encountered in adults,[107] which Rubinstein considered high grade neoplasms.[25] This distinction has largely passed, leaving pilocytic astrocytomas to refer to tumors with the distinctive features of juvenile pilocytic astrocytoma and the adult "piloid" to refer to a variant of high-grade fibrillary astrocytomas.[107]

The pilocytic astrocytoma comprises between 12 and 28% of all pediatric brain tumors and nearly one-third of all posterior fossa tumors in children.[13,34,140–143] Although almost exclusively a tumor of children and young adults, cases have been reported in older patients.[34,144] In Cushing's original series the average age of presentation was 13 years. However, most of these children suffered symptoms for two or more years prior to presentation and many were blind from chronic papilledema by the time of presentation.[18] In his 76 cases, two-thirds never experienced a recurrence after resection.[18] More modern series report ages of presentation ranging from 8 months to 29 years, with median ages ranging from 6 to 8 years.[143,145–150] In all of the modern series, between 70 and 80% of pilocytic astrocytomas of the cerebellum develop before the age of 10 years. A recent review of pilocytic cerebellar astrocytomas presenting at the time of recurrence showed patients ranging from 3 to 52 years of age, with a median age of 14 years.[151]

Pilocytic astrocytomas present like other tumors of the posterior fossa, demonstrating signs and symptoms referable to increased intracranial pressure and direct effect. Headache and vomiting represent the two most frequent symptoms, occurring in 72–97% and 58–84% of patients respectively.[143,145,146,152–155] Headache follows the pattern of increased intracranial pressure: worse on awakening, developing frontally, relieved by emesis, and often related to developing hydrocephalus.[143] Similarly, vomiting relates more to increased intracranial pressure and hydrocephalus than to local irritation of the area postrema seen in ependymomas.[143]

Given the frequency of hydrocephalus-related headache and vomiting, papilledema is one of the most frequent signs, occurring in between 69 and 90% of patients.[143,145,146,153,155] Ataxia and other signs reflective of cerebellar impairment are exhibited in 56–95% of patients.[143,145,146,153,155] Rarely, a cerebellar pilocytic astrocytoma may present with a spontaneous hemorrhage.[156]

PATHOLOGY The pilocytic astrocytoma classically arises laterally in a cerebellar hemisphere forming a cyst with a well-defined mural nodule and yellow–brown cyst fluid. Involvement of the vermis has been shown to occur in over 40% of cases.[33,34,144]

However, only 2% of the vermian tumors are truly cystic. The majority of vermian astrocytomas are solid and higher-grade astrocytomas.[145,155]

Rubinstein defined juvenile pilocytic astrocytomas based on the presence of piloid fibrocytic astrocytes.[25,150] While the pilocytic astrocyte refers to elongated "hair-like" bipolar astrocytes,[157] the majority of astrocytes that comprise such pediatric tumors are typical fibrillary astrocytes with round to oval nuclei, some cytoplasmic pleomorphism, and Rosenthal fibers. The tumor appears histologically as alternating areas of dense and loose cellular areas resembling a honeycomb (Figure 35.9). The Rosenthal fibers, intracellular densely eosinophilic rod-like structures composed largely of the heatshock protein α-B crystalin, are found particularly in cells located in the compact zones.[107]

Little definitive information is known concerning the pathogenesis of pilocytic astrocytomas. A recognized risk in children with neurofibromatosis type-1 (NF-1) exists[158] and a history of NF-1 and cerebellar astrocytoma should prompt investigation for other tumors such as optic pathway astrocytomas.[107] Kluwe and colleagues report that 11 of 12 NF-1 patients with pilocytic astrocytomas had a loss of the NF-1 allele, while only 1 in 24 patients with sporadic pilocytic astrocytomas exhibited allelic loss in the NF-1 region. Thus supporting a different mechanism of tumor genesis from sporadic pilocytic astrocytomas.[159]

TREATMENT Complete resection is the goal of surgical therapy for pilocytic astrocytomas. Considerable controversy remains concerning whether or not to resect the walls of the cyst. The presence or absence of contrast enhancement of the cyst wall does not accurately reflect actual presence of tumor.[148] Any macroscopically abnormal cyst wall should be removed. An important issue is whether or not resection of the cyst wall impacts on recurrence. Extent of resection appears to be the most important prognostic factor.[148] Cystic pilocytic tumors carry an excellent prognosis with 2-, 5-, and 10-year survivals reported to be 94%, 87%, and 73% respectively.[145]

Solid pilocytic astrocytomas of the vermis have a propensity to involve cerebellar peduncles and the brainstem. Involvement of the brainstem heralds a worse prognosis.[145] Tumors involving the

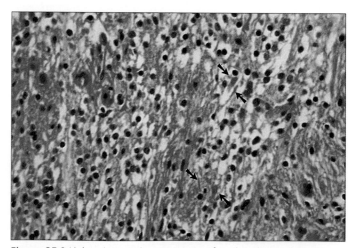

Figure 35.9 Light microscopic appearance of a pilocytic astrocytoma, consisting of alternating areas of densely and loosely packed cells, imparting a "honeycomb" appearance. Note the presence of Rosenthal fibers (arrows). (H&E; × 250.)

brainstem are usually not pilocytic and up to 40% are reported as high-grade fibrillary astrocytomas.

RECURRENCE AND ADJUVANT THERAPY Since the most significant factor for recurrence and prognosis is the extent of resection, adjuvant therapy is not indicated for pilocytic astrocytoma unless the lesion proves to be a higher-grade astrocytoma on recurrence or the surgeon cannot achieve complete resection. However, pilocytic astrocytomas may recur after a complete resection. A case report exists of the recurrence of a cerebellar pilocytic astrocytoma 45 years after a complete resection in a 54-year-old man.[160] Repeat surgery with the goal directed towards complete resection remains the treatment of choice. A gross total resection at the second surgery can usually be achieved. The difficulty arises when complete resection or re-resection does not prove safe or practicable. Given the apparent benign behavior of the tumor, an argument can be made for close observation, reserving adjuvant therapy for patients who experience disease progression.[150,151,161,162]

In evaluating the efficacy of adjuvant therapy, investigators frequently group pilocytic astrocytomas with the pathologically distinct low-grade fibrillary astrocytoma.[163] Nevertheless, chemotherapy has been used successfully in patients with recurrent and progressive pilocytic astrocytomas.[163] Radiation therapy has some promise, particularly based on recent studies of stereotactic or focused therapy.[151,164] However, stereotactic radiosurgery is not without risk. Fulminant radiation necrosis has been noted after stereotactic radiosurgery for a recurrent pilocytic astrocytoma of the cerebellum.[165] Radiation therapy may also present a risk of transformation into a more aggressive tumor.[150,166,167]

Anaplastic astrocytoma

EPIDEMIOLOGY While rarer than the typical pilocytic astrocytoma of the cerebellum, higher-grade astrocytomas, including glioblastomas, arise in the cerebellum. As noted previously, the higher-grade solid astrocytomas far more frequently involve the midline,[155] and may represent the "transitional" astrocytoma reported by Pencalet and colleagues.[148] Viano and co-workers report that 12% of their cerebellar astrocytomas proved malignant.[155] Spontaneous malignant astrocytomas of the cerebellum behave similarly to, if not worse than, their more notorious supratentorial counterparts.[168–171] Malignant cerebellar astrocytomas may also develop from progression of a cerebellar pilocytic astrocytoma.[13,147,172–178]

PATHOLOGY Anaplastic astrocytomas meet the criteria of WHO grade III. Low-grade fibrillary astrocytomas demonstrate mild to moderate nuclear pleomorphism, little to no mitosis, and neither vascular hyperplasia nor necrosis. While some argue that the existence of one mitotic figure pushes the tumor into the category of anaplastic astrocytoma,[179] Miller cautions that one or two mitotic figures do not truly alter the grade of the tumors and will demonstrate increased cellularity, pleomorphism, and mitotic activity.[107] While vascular hyperplasia pushes the tumor into the WHO grade IV glioblastoma multiforme, Miller allows some degree of vascular hyperplasia in the anaplastic astrocytoma, and argues that the classification neglects the far more prognostically significant presence of necrosis to separate the anaplastic astrocytoma from the glioblastoma.[107]

Some pilocytic astrocytomas that develop anaplastic changes have been shown on review of the original pathological slides to show increased perivascular cellularity.[147] This may suggest that pilocytic astrocytomas with a risk for progression may demonstrate elements of a low-grade astrocytoma on presentation.

TREATMENT As with the pilocytic astrocytoma, the primary goal of therapy for the anaplastic astrocytoma is complete surgical removal. However, the greater tendency of the anaplastic astrocytoma to involve central structures such as the cerebellar peduncle and the brainstem limits the resection. Based on the clinical behavior of the tumor, most patients received adjuvant therapy.

Glioblastoma multiforme

Though even rarer than the anaplastic astrocytoma, glioblastoma does develop in the cerebellum and, unfortunately, shares the behavior and prognosis of its supratentorial namesake.

EPIDEMIOLOGY Currently, glioblastoma of the cerebellum is rare enough to generate case reports on its presentation and behavior. Dorhman and Dunsmore presented a review of 33 patients with primary cerebellar glioblastoma, which remains one of the largest series.[180] Several reviews from several large neurosurgical series have shown only sporadic cases of cerebellar glioblastoma.[155,169,170,181]

The primary glioblastoma of the cerebellum appears in a wide range of ages, from congenital to middle age.[169,181–185] Consistent with its aggressive nature, the glioblastoma presents clinically in a relatively short time, symptoms usually present for only 4–6 weeks.[169,181,186] Kulkarni and colleagues reported a patient who had a normal CT scan 2 months prior to the diagnosis of a 42 mm midline cerebellar glioblastoma.[181] Headache, nausea, and vomiting are the most frequently reported symptoms, while ataxia and other cerebellar signs are the most frequently reported signs.[169,181,183,186]

PATHOLOGY Cerebellar glioblastoma has the same histopathological criteria as the supratentorial glioblastoma. Along with the features of anaplastic astrocytoma, glioblastomas demonstrate necrosis and often pseudopallisading.[107] Almost all of the tumors display hypercellularity, pleomorphism, mitoses, pseudopallisades, necrosis, and endothelial proliferation.[181]

TREATMENT Cerebellar glioblastomas show the unfortunate prognosis of their supratentorial counterparts. Despite resection and adjuvant therapy, patients ultimately succumb within 12–13 months after the onset of symptoms.[180,183] There have been occasional reports of longer survival.[170] It appears reasonable to attempt a complete a resection and offer adjuvant therapy. Radiotherapy appears to offer prolongation of survival.[181,187] Chemotherapy remains unproven, but it remains the only adjuvant therapy available for very young children.

Astrocytomas of the fourth ventricle

Astrocytomas may arise from the floor, walls, or roof of the fourth ventricle and project into it, often invading other local structures.[15] It can become a matter of debate as to whether or not a tumor arises from the vermis and infiltrates the floor of the fourth ventricle or vice versa.[15] Thus, these tumors include those described earlier by Hoffman and associates[188] in which the lesion arises within the pons just beneath the surface of the fourth

ventricle without deep extension, instead growing exophytically into the fourth ventricle. While one may argue that these merely represent variants of cerebellar or brainstem astrocytoma, by both location and behavior, these tumors merit attention.[15,188]

Epidemiology

Tomita and co-workers report that 21 of 75 children with benign cerebellar astrocytoma seen over a 10-year period had tumors of the fourth ventricle.[15] Ages ranged from 3 months to 16 years, with a mean age at diagnosis of 6 years. Given that these tumors in one way or another involve the fourth ventricle, symptoms and signs referable to increased intracranial pressure secondary to hydrocephalus are the most frequent: headache, vomiting, papilledema, gait disturbance, and truncal ataxia.

Pathology

In all of these cases, the fourth ventricle contains solid tumor. Cysts may be present within or outside the solid portion. Many patients have subependymal invasion of the floor. Less commonly, the tumors involve a cerebellar peduncle but not the brainstem.

Histopathological examination reveals the relatively benign nature of these tumors. Eighteen out of the 21 patients in the Tomita series were pilocytic.[15] Pilocytic astrocytomas represent the majority of tumors that invade the floor of the fourth ventricle.[15,189]

Treatment

Surgical resection remains the primary goal. An attempt at complete resection should be attempted. Any portion invasive of the floor of the fourth ventricle is left behind. Surgeons should not pursue tumor that infiltrates the brainstem since residual benign astrocytoma may fail to grow even without adjuvant therapy. Tomita and colleagues recommend reserving adjuvant therapy for unresectable recurrences.[15] Radiotherapy is not indicated unless significant tumor remains or the tumor progresses.

Cerebellar pleomorphic xanthroastrocytoma

The pleomorphic xanthroastrocytoma represents an interesting but rare tumor considered to be part of the spectrum of desmoplastic neuroepithelial tumors which include the desmoplastic astrocytoma of infancy and the desmoplastic infantile ganglioglioma.[190,191] While almost exclusively tumors of the cerebral hemispheres, case reports have appeared describing pleomorphic xanthroastrocytoma arising in the cerebellum.[192–194]

EPIDEMIOLOGY These tumors were first described in 1989 by VandenBerg and colleagues;[195] they presented 11 supratentorial cases of desmoplastic infantile ganglioglioma occurring in children under 18 months of age, the majority under 4 months of age. These tumors presented as large masses with intense desmoplasia, divergent astrocytic and ganglionic differentiation, and a favorable prognosis. Subsequent reports demonstrated that desmoplastic infantile ganglioglioma, pleomorphic xanthroastrocytoma, and desmoplastic astrocytoma of infancy all shared the common characteristics of giant size on presentation, intense desmoplasia, near identical histology, associated cysts, and attachment to the overlying dura.[190,191] The few cases reported demonstrate a wide range of ages for the cerebellar pleomorphic xanthroastrocytoma. Lim and colleagues present a 3-month-old diagnosed after a 1-month history of upward gaze difficulty,[193] while others describe patients in their sixth decade.[192,194]

PATHOLOGY As noted, the pleomorphic xanthroastrocytoma shares elements wth other tumors under the rubric of desmoplastic neuroepithelial tumor. These tumors are desmoplastic with pleomorphic astrocytes admixed with neoplastic ganglion cells, involve the overlying leptomeninges, and demonstrate rare mitotic activity.[192]

TREATMENT It proves difficult to recommend established guidelines with only a few case reports in the literature. However, the tumor appears to have the favorable prognosis of the supratentorial desmoplastic neuroepithelial tumors. Gross total resection should be attempted when safe and practicable. Residual tumor may undergo another resection should it progress. Experience in infants with desmoplastic infantile ganglioglioma reveals little evidence of benefit from radiotherapy and only some for chemotherapy.[190,196] The supratentorial desmoplastic neuroepithelial tumors attach or envelop a major artery and venous sinus in 50% and 60% of cases, respectively.[190] Similar findings may occur in the posterior fossa variety.

BRAINSTEM GLIOMAS

> It is unfortunate that one of the more common locations of gliomas in childhood is within the brainstem. Despite the specific histology, they must all be classified as malignant tumors, since their location renders them inoperable.
>
> (Donald Matson, 1969)

The term *brainstem glioma* has for many years signified an inoperable and inexorably fatal tumor. Matson's regretful observation[12] bears respect since these tumors may represent 15% of all intracranial tumors and between 25% and 35% of pediatric posterior fossa tumors.[188] However, experience over the past 15–20 years has shown that location of the tumor within the brainstem greatly influences the histology and prognosis, whether or not the tumor is amenable to surgery.[14,197–200] Epstein and McCleary,[14] Hoffman and colleagues,[188] Tomita and colleagues[199] and Walker and Storrs[200] have all suggested a scheme for classification of tumors within the brainstem. Most of the non-pontine gliomas are focal pilocytic astrocytomas amenable to therapy. While the overwhelming majority of these tumors are astrocytomas, other tumor types such as ganglioglioma, may arise in the brainstem parenchyma.[197,198,201]

Tumors of the cervicomedullary junction

Epidemiology

The proportion of brainstem gliomas confined to the cervicomedullary junction varies widely in the literature. Epstein and McCleary report eight cervicomedullary junction tumors out of 34 brainstem tumors[14] while Epstein and Farmer reported 44 out of 88 brainstem gliomas.[198] Weiner and colleagues present 39 cervicomedullary junction tumors treated over a 10-year period.[202] The age at presentation ranged from 6 to 12 years.[201]

As expected, the signs and symptoms of cervicomedullary junction tumors reflect their location and growth patterns. Lower cranial nerve palsies, pyramidal tract signs, ataxia, spinal cord dysfunction, and nystagmus are the usual findings.[14,201–203] Lower cranial nerve dysfunction manifests itself as a difficulty

with swallowing, nasal speech, nausea, vomiting, apnea, irregular nocturnal breathing patterns, and failure to thrive in infants.[202]

Pathology

The cervicomedullary junction astrocytomas tend to be low grade.[14,198,202,203] These tumors tend to grow in a predictable fashion, with the rostral portion expanding posteriorly at the level of the obex.[198] This is consistent with the observations of Scherer that surrounding anatomical structures, such as the fiber tracts and pial structures, influence the growth of lower grade gliomas, with higher grade tumors having the ability to infiltrate through them.[204] The anatomical barriers, which include the pyramid decussation, internal arcuate fibers, medial lemniscus, and efferents from the inferior olivary complex, direct the growth of low-grade tumors towards the obex and the dorsal medulla.[198]

Treatment

The location and behavior of cervicomedullary tumors offers the potential for surgical resection. While slow-growing tumors tend to displace adjacent structures, they do invade at the margin. A cleavage plane does not exist, and the apparent interface between the tumor and brainstem proves extremely vulnerable.[205] A significant advantage on outcome with gross total resection has not been demonstrated. While high-grade tumors frequently recur despite gross total resection, many low-grade lesions may not recur despite incomplete resection although long-term follow-up is required to verify this observation.[202]

Tumors of the medulla oblongata

Epidemiology

While somewhat rare, tumors of the medulla occur almost exclusively in children. As expected, children present with signs and symptoms referable to the location and size of their tumors. Ataxia, quadraparesis, incontinence, and vomiting are the typical signs and symptoms. Many children curiously present with small stature and are often referred to an endocrinologist for failure to thrive[200, 202] (Figure 35.10).

Pathology

Like their cervicomedullary counterparts, tumors that originate within the medulla are usually histologically benign.[14,188,197,200] While Epstein noted a few cases of malignancy in his series,[197] most were low-grade astrocytomas. Histopathologically, these lesions may appear identical to the pilocytic astrocytomas of the cerebellum.

Treatment

Since many of these tumors are histologically benign, surgery offers potential benefits. However, the surgeon should expect temporary postoperative difficulties with increased ataxia and swallowing in patients following surgery. Ataxia may remain permanently, but with only slight impairment. We feel that part of the success of this surgery is based on not violating the obex during tumor removal.

Histologically benign lesions do not require nor benefit from adjuvant radiation therapy or chemotherapy. Currently, no series in the literature supports routine postoperative adjuvant therapy. A prolonged recurrence-free interval can be expected in most of these patients. Even with recurrence, the patients often enjoy a

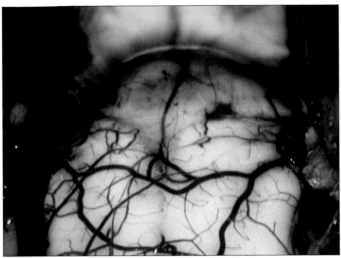

Figure 35.10 Gross appearance of a tumor of the medulla extending through the region of the obex. The surgical approach is through a midline incision in the medulla, avoiding direct incision through the obex itself.

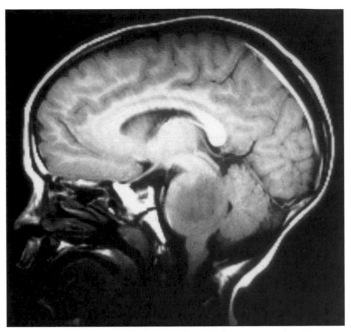

Figure 35.11 Characteristic T1 non-enhanced MRI appearance of a diffuse pontine glioma. Note expanded brainstem with areas of hypointense signal.

significant period of disease-free existence. Should the tumor recur, the surgeon should give serious consideration to reoperation and then, depending on the results, adjuvant therapy.

Pontine glioma

Epidemiology

The term *brainstem glioma* traditionally evokes the image of a large infiltrative tumor of the pons with a disastrous prognosis. Unfortunately the pontine glioma justifies this image. Almost all patients with diffuse pontine tumors who have undergone a stereotactic biopsy have had at least an anaplastic astrocytoma.[200,206] Some have obvious glioblastomas. Few patients survive more than 12–15 months.[14,201]

Pathology

Patients who present with the rapid onset and progression of signs and symptoms with a diffusely enlarged pons revealed by MRI usually harbor a malignant astrocytoma. Although another disease process, such as encephalitis, may exist, the usual pontine glioma exhibits a very classic presentation and typical findings on MRI (Figure 35.11). This typical MRI appearance has changed opinions on diagnostic biopsies. Little evidence exists that the procedure yields information that changes therapy.[207] Diffuse brainstem tumors in children are clinically and histologically malignant gliomas. Demyelinating disease can be excluded because demyelination is multifocal, nonenhancing, and does not enlarge the brainstem. No case of encephalitis confined to the brainstem has been reported.

Treatment

Attempts at radical surgical removal remain futile. Most patients are treated with radiation therapy. While this offers initial relief of the symptoms associated with the rapid progression of their disease, all patients eventually suffer recurrence. Radiation therapy may allow survival for 12–15 months. There appears to be little long-term benefit from adjuvant chemotherapy.[208] Until advances in adjuvant therapy become realized, the diffuse pontine glioma will remain an injustice inflicted all too frequently on young children.

Tumors of the mesencephalon

Mesencephalic tumors are usually low-grade astrocytomas and typically occur in either the cerebral peduncle or tectal plate.

Tumors of the cerebral peduncle

Astrocytomas of the cerebral peduncle are often amenable to surgical excision. Frequently, these lesions have an associated large cyst (Figure 35.12). Evacuation of the cyst and removal of the surrounding tumor tissue offers relief of symptoms and potentially many years of stability before recurrence. Some have advocated stereotactic aspiration of the cyst as the only surgical therapy.[209] However, an attempt at complete resection is justified in a patient with progressive symptoms from a mostly solid lesion.

We utilize an orbitozygomatic exposure or a subtemporal transtentorial approach. If the lesion is in the anterior portion of the cerebral peduncle, the orbitozygomatic approach gives excellent exposure. With the subtemporal approach the tentorial notch can be split and affords an excellent exposure of the lateral cerebral peduncle. These lesions typically extend to the peduncular surface, which provides an access that limits involvement of normal neural tissue. These tumors can extend rostrally towards the thalamus and caudally into the pons, beyond the visual limits of the surgical approach. In our experience, many of these tumors will continue to deliver themselves into the operative field, allowing for gross total resection. Removal of the mass promises relief of symptoms for many years without further adjuvant therapy. Decompression and removal of distinct tumor tissue that disengages easily is the goal of surgery. Many patients have a postoperative contralateral hemiparesis, which is frequently less than their preoperative deficit.

CLINICAL PEARLS

- Posterior fossa tumors are a diverse group of tumors, more common in children than adults. The most common posterior fossa tumors in children are astrocytoma and medulloblastoma (PNET). Most posterior fossa tumors are amenable to surgical resection.

- Patients with posterior fossa tumors often present with headache and vomiting. Depending on where the tumor is located (midline or lateral in the cerebellar hemisphere) the patient may possess neurologic symptoms associated with midline cerebellar dysfunction, such as truncal ataxia, or unilateral cerebellar hemispheric dysfunction, such as appendicular ataxia, weakness, nystagmus, and dysmetria.

- Posterior fossa tumors are often associated with hydrocephalus as a result of obstruction of the aqueduct of Sylvius or the fourth ventricular outflow. Treatment of the posterior fossa mass often, but not always, obviates the need for permanent CSF diversion. Alternative approaches to the treatment of clinically symptomatic hydrocephalus include external ventricular drainage at the time of tumor resection or endoscopic third ventriculostomy.

- Robin's Rule: If vomiting precedes the headache, the tumor is most likely to be an ependymoma. If the headache precedes the vomiting, then the tumor is more likely to be a medulloblastoma or astrocytoma.

- The typical features of a posterior fossa hemangioblastoma on MRI include a cystic mass with a pial-based mural nodule that enhances prominently associated with abnormally prominent vessels within or adjacent to the tumor. These findings in the setting of an intra-axial cerebellar mass in an adult are virtually pathognomonic for hemangioblastoma. The cystic nodule associated with a cerebellar astrocytoma is not pial based.

- Dermoid tumors can be easily confused with arachnoid cysts. Diffusion weighted MRI is the best way to differentiate them.

- When resecting a tumor in the fourth ventricle, the surgeon should find the floor of the fourth ventricle near the region of the obex, then resect rostally to find normal anatomy in the region of the aqueduct and upper fourth ventricle. The rule of thumb is to work from normal fourth ventricle and cerebellar/brainstem anatomy to abnormal to avoid damage to the floor of the fourth ventricle. Resection should continue until normal ventricular floor is seen; tumor invading the floor should not be pursued into the brainstem.

3. Packer R, Sutton L, Goldwein J, et al. Improved survival with the use of adjuvant chemotherapy in the treatment of medulloblastoma. *J Neurosurg* 1991; 74: 433–40.

4. Atlas S, Lavi E, Fischer P. Intraaxial brain tumors. In: Atlas S (ed.). *Magnetic Resonance Imaging of the Brain and Spine*, 3rd edn. Philadelphia: Lippincott Williams & Wilkins; 2002: 565–693.

5. Cushing H. The intracranial tumors of preadolescence. *Am J Dis Child* 1927; 33: 551–84.

6. Duffner P, Cohen M, Freeman A. Pediatric brain tumors: an overview. *Cancer* 1985; 35: 287–301.

7. Gold J, Smith K. Childhood brain tumors: a 15-year survey of treatment in a university pediatric hospital. *South Med J* 1975; 68: 1337–40.

8. Keith H, Craig W, Kernohan J. Brain tumors in children. *Pediatrics* 1949; 3: 839–43.

9. Rorke L, Schut L. Introductory survey of pediatric brain tumors. In: McLaurin R, Schut L, Venes J, et al. (eds). *Pediatric Neurosurgery: Surgery of the Developing Nervous System*. Philadelphia: WB Saunders Co.; 1989: 335–7.

10. Schiffer D. Morbid anatomy of the tumors of the posterior fossa in childhood. *Mod Probl Paediatr* 1977; 18: 131–46.

11. Walker M. Diagnosis and treatment of brain tumors. *Pediatr Clin N Am* 1976; 23: 131–46.

12. Matson D. *Neurosurgery of Infancy and Childhood*. Springfield: Charles C Thomas; 1969.

13. Sutton L, Schut L. Cerebellar astrocytomas. In: McLaurin R, Schut L, Venes J, et al. (eds). *Pediatric Neurosurgery: Surgery of the Developing Nervous System*, 2nd edn. Philadelphia: WB Saunders Co; 1989: 338–46.

14. Epstein F, McCleary EL. Intrinsic brain-stem tumors of childhood: surgical indications. *J Neurosurg* 1986; 64: 11–15.

15. Tomita T, Chou P, Reyes-Mugica M. IV ventricle astrocytomas in childhood: Clinicopathological features in 21 cases. *Child's Nerv Syst* 1998; 14: 537–46.

16. Vandertop WP, Hoffman HJ, Drake JM, et al. Focal midbrain tumors in children. *Neurosurgery* 1992; 31: 186–94.

17. Geissinger J, Bucy P. Diagnosis and treatment of brain tumors. *Arch Neurol* 1971; 24: 125–35.

18. Cushing H. Experiences with the cerebellar astrocytomas. *Surg Gynecol Obstet* 1931; 52: 129–204.

19. Kucharczyk W, Brant-Zawadzki M, Sobel D, et al. Central nervous system tumors in children: detection by magnetic resonance imaging. *Radiology* 1985; 155: 131–6.

20. Lee B, Kneeland J, Deck M, et al. Posterior fossa lesions: magnetic resonance imaging. *Radiology* 1984; 153: 137–43.

21. Burtscher I, Holtas S. Proton magnetic resonance spectroscopy in brain tumors: clinical applications. *Neuroradiology* 2001; 43: 345–52.

22. Deutsch M, Reigel D. The value of myelography in the management of childhood medulloblastoma. *Cancer* 1980; 45: 2194–7.

23. Dorwart R, Wara W, Norman D, *et al*. Complete myelographic evaluation of spinal metastases from medulloblastoma. *Radiology* 1981; 139: 403–8.

24. O'Reilly G, Hayward R, Harkness W. Myelography in the assessment of children with medulloblastoma. *Br J Neurosurg* 1993; 7: 183–8.

25. Rubinstein L (ed.). *Tumors of the Central Nervous System*. Washington: Armed Forces Institute of Pathology; 1972; fascicle 6.

26. Kramer E, Rafrto S, Packer R, *et al*. Comparison of myelography with CT follow-up versus gadolinium MRI for subarachnoid metastatic disease in children. *Neurology* 1991; 41: 46–50.

27. Spoto G, Press G, Hesslink J, *et al*. Intracranial ependymoma and subependymoma: MR manifestations. *AJNR* 1990; 11: 83–91.

28. Fitz C, Rao K. Primary tumors in children. In: Lee S, Rao K (eds). *Cranial Computed Tomography and MRI*. New York: McGraw-Hill; 1987: 365–412.

29. Courville C, Broussalian S. Plastic ependymoma of the lateral recesses: report of eight verified cases. *J Neurosurg* 1962; 18: 792–9.

30. Silbergeld J, Cohen W, Maravilla K, *et al*. Supratentorial and spinal cord hemangioblastomas: gadolinium enhanced MR appearance with pathologic correlation. *J Comput Assist Tomogr* 1989; 13: 1048–51.

31. Peter JC, Sinclair-Smith C, de Villiers JC. Midline dermal sinuses and cysts and their relationship to the central nervous system. *Eur J Pediatr Surg* 1991; 1: 73–9.

32. Stein B, Tenner M, Fraser R. Hydrocephalus following removal of cerebellar astrocytomas in children. *J Neurosurg* 1972; 36: 763–8.

33. Page L. Astrocytomas involving the cerebellar midline. In: Marlin A (ed.). *Concepts in Pediatric Neurosurgery*, Vol. 7. Basel: Karger; 1987: 93–104.

34. Gol A, McKissock W. The cerebellar astrocytomas: a report on 98 verified cases. *J Neurosurg* 1959; 16: 287–96.

35. Sainte-Rose C, Cinalli G, Roux FE, *et al*. Management of hydrocephalus in pediatric patients with posterior fossa tumors: the role of endoscopic third ventriculostomy. *J Neurosurg* 2001; 95: 791–7.

36. Lapras C, Palet J, Lapras C, *et al*. Cerebellar astrocytomas in childhood. *Child's Nerv Syst* 1986; 2: 55–9.

37. Rhoton A. The posterior cranial fossa: microsurgical anatomy and surgical approaches. *Neurosurgery* 2000; 47 Supplement.

38. Gnanalingham K, Lafuente J, Thompson D, *et al*. Surgical procedures for posterior fossa tumors in children: does craniotomy lead to fewer complications than craniectomy? *Neurosurgery* 2002; 97: 821–6.

39. Catsman-Berrevoets C, Van Dongen H, Mulder P, *et al*. Tumour type and size are high risk factors for the syndrome of "cerebellar" mutism and subsequent dysarthria. *Neurol Neurosurg Psychiatr* 1999; 67: 755–7.

40. Pollack I, Gerszten P, Martinez A, *et al*. Intracranial ependymomas of childhood: Long-term outcome and prognostic factors. *Neurosurgery* 1995; 37: 665–7.

41. Proctor M, Scott R. Special considerations for children in neurosurgery. In: Kaye A, Black P (eds). *Operative Neurosurgery*. London: Harcourt Publishers Limited; 2000: 33–44.

42. Matson D. Surgery of the posterior fossa in childhood. *Clin Neurosurg* 1968; 15: 247–64.

43. Zimmerman R, Bilaniuk L, Bruno L, *et al*. Computed tomography of cerebellar astrocytoma. *Am J Roentgenol* 1978; 130: 929–33.

44. Albright L (ed.). *Medulloblastomas*. New York: Thieme Medical Publishers, Inc.; 1999.

45. Bailey P, Cushing H. Medulloblastoma cerebelli, a common type of mid-cerebellar glioma of childhood. *Arch Neurol Psychiatr* 1925; 42: 1–15.

46. Russell D, Rubinstein L (eds). *Pathology of Tumors of the Nervous System*. Baltimore: Williams & Wilkins; 1994.

47. Russell D, Rubinstein L (eds). *Pathology of Tumors of the Nervous System*. Baltimore: Williams & Wilkins; 1989.

48. Roberts R, Lynch C, Jones M, *et al*. Medulloblastoma: a population-based study of 532 cases. *J Neuropathol Exp Neurol* 1991; 50: 134–44.

49. Chatty E, Earler K. Medulloblastoma. A report of 201 cases with emphasis on the relationship of histological variants to survival. *Cancer* 1991; 28: 911.

50. Hershatter B, Halpern E, Cox E. Medulloblastoma: the Duke University Medical Center experience. *Int J Radiat Oncol Biol Phys* 1986; 12: 1771.

51. Finley J. Natural history and epidemiology of medulloblastoma. In: Zeltzer P, Pochedly C (eds). *Medulloblastomas in Children. New Concepts in Tumor Biology, Diagnosis, and Treatment*. New York: Praeger; 1986: 22–36.

52. Lannering B, Marky I, Norborg C. Brain tumors in childhood and adolescence in west Sweden 1970–1984. Epidemiology and survival. *Cancer* 1990; 66: 604–9.

53. Hung K, Wu C, Huang J, How S. Familial medulloblastoma in siblings: report in one family and review of the literature. *Surg Neurol* 1990; 33: 341–6.

54. Evans G, Burnell L, Campbell R, *et al*. Congenital abnormalities and genetic syndromes in 173 cases of medulloblastoma. *Med Pediatr Oncol* 1993; 21: 443–434.

55. Anseline P. Turcot's syndrome. *Austr NZ J Surg* 1992; 62: 587–90.

56. Evans D, Farndon P, Burnell L, *et al*. The incidence of Gorlin syndrome in 173 consecutive cases of medulloblastoma. *Br J Cancer* 1991; 64: 959–61.

57. LaCombe D, Chateil J, Fontan D, Battin J. Medulloblastoma in the nevoid basal-cell carcinoma syndrome: case reports and review of the literature. *Genet Couns* 1990; 1: 273–7.

58. Burger M, Lorenzo M, Geyer R (eds). *Medulloblastoma and Primitive Neuroectodermal Tumors*. Edinburgh: Churchill Livingstone; 1995.

59. Santibanez-Koref M, Birch J, *et al*. p53 germline mutations in Li-Fraumeni syndrome. *Lancet* 1991; 338: 1490–1.

60. Rice J, Fischer D. Blue rubber bleb nevus syndrome. *Arch Dermatol* 1962; 86: 503–11.

61. Taylor M, Mainprize T, Rutka J. Molecular insight into medulloblastoma and central nervous system primitive neuroectoderm tumor biology from hereditary syndromes: a review. *Neurosurgery* 2000; 47: 888–901.

62. Hahn H, Wicking C, Zaphiropoulous P, *et al*. Mutations of the human homolog of Drosophila patched in the nevoid basal cell carcinoma syndrome. *Cell* 1996; 85: 841–51.

63. Johnson R, Rothman A, Xie J, *et al*. Human homolog of patched, a candidate gene for the basal cell nevus syndrome. *Science* 1996; 272: 1668–71.

64. Ingham P. The patched gene in development and cancer. *Curr Opin Genet Dev* 1998; 8: 88–94.

65. Ingham P. Transducing Hedgehog: the story so far. *EMBO J* 1998; 17: 3505–11.

66. Wechsler-Reya R, Scott M. Control of neuronal precursor proliferation in the cerebellum by Sonic Hedgehog. *Neuron* 1999; 50: 103–14.

67. Hart M, Earle K. Primitive neuroectodermal tumors of the brain in children. *Cancer* 1973; 32: 890–7.

68. Rorke L. The cerebellar medulloblastoma and its relationship to primitive neuroectodermal tumors. *J Neuropathol Exp Neurol* 1983; 42: 1–15.

69. Rubinstein L. Embryonal central neuroepithelial tumors and their differentiating potential. A cytogenetic view of a complex neuro-oncological problem. *J Neurosurg* 1985; 62: 795–805.

70. Sutton L, Packer R. Medulloblastomas. In: Cheek W, Marlin A, McLone D, *et al.* (eds). *Pediatric Neurosurgery: Surgery of the Developing Nervous System*, 3rd edn. Philadelphia: WB Saunders Co; 1994: 362–73.

71. Biegel J, Rorke L, Packer R, *et al.* Isochromosome 17q in primitive neuroectodermal tumors of the central nervous system. *Genes Chromosomes Cancer* 1988; 1: 139–47.

72. Bigner S, Mark J, Friedman H, *et al.* Structural chromosomal abnormalities in human medulloblastoma. *Cancer Genet Cytogenet* 1988; 30: 91–101.

73. Badiali M, Iolascon A, Loda M, *et al.* p53 gene mutations in medulloblastoma. Immunohistochemistry, gel shift analysis, and sequencing. *Diagn Mol Pathol* 1993; 2: 23–8.

74. Raffel C, Thomas GA, Tishler DM, Lassoff S, Allen JC. Absence of p53 mutations in childhood central nervous system primitive neuroectodermal tumors. *Neurosurgery* 1993; 33: 305–6.

75. Cogen P. Prognostic significance of molecular genetic markers in childhood brain tumors. *Pediatr Neurosurg* 1991; 17: 245–50.

76. Ohgaki H, Eibl R, Wiester O, *et al.* p53 mutations in non astrocytic human brain tumors. *Cancer Res* 1991; 51: 6202–5.

77. Park T, Hoffman J, Hendricks E, *et al.* Medulloblastoma: clinical presentation and management. *J Neurosurg* 1983; 58: 543–52.

78. Hughes P. Cerebellar medulloblastoma in adults. *J Neurosurg* 1984; 60: 994–7.

79. Allen J. Childhood brain tumors: current status of clinical trials in newly diagnosed and recurrent disease. *Pediatr Clin N Am* 1985; 32: 633–51.

80. Jamjoon Z, Jamjoon A, Sulaiman A, *et al.* Systemic metastasis of medulloblastomas through ventriculoperitoneal shunt: report of a case and critical analysis of the literature. *Surg Neurol* 1993; 40: 403–10.

81. Kleinman G, Hochberg F, Richardson E. Systemic metastases from medulloblastoma. Report of two cases and review of the literature. *Cancer* 1981; 48: 2296–309.

82. Chang C, Housepian E, Herbert C. An operative staging system and a megavoltage radiotherapeutic technique for cerebellar medulloblastoma. *Radiology* 1969; 93: 1351–9.

83. Albright L, Wisoff J, Zeltzer P, *et al.* Effects of medulloblastoma resections on outcome in children: a report from the Children's Cancer Group. *Neurosurgery* 1996; 38: 934–9.

84. Maleci A, Cervoni L, Delfini R. Medulloblastoma in children and in adults: a comparative study. *Acta Neurochir* 1992; 119: 62–7.

85. Sutton L, Goldwein J, Schwartz D. Ependymomas. In: Albright L, Pollack I, Adelson D (eds). *Principles and Practice of Pediatric Neurosurgery*. New York: Thieme Medical Publishers; 1999: 609–28.

86. Coulon R, Till K. Intracranial ependymomas in children. *Child's Brain* 1977; 3: 154–68.

87. Dorhman G, Farwell J, Flannery J. Ependymomas and ependymoblastomas in children. *J Neurosurg* 1976; 45: 273–83.

88. Koss W, Miller M. *Intracranial Tumors of Infants and Children*. St Louis: CV Mosby Co; 1971.

89. Salazar O, Castro-Vita H, Van Houtte P, *et al.* Improved survival in cases of intracranial ependymoma after radiation therapy. *J Neurosurg* 1983; 59: 652–9.

90. Choux M (ed.) *Ependymomas of the Posterior Fossa in Children*. Springfield, IL: Charles C. Thomas; 1983.

91. Nazar G, Hoffman H, Becker L, *et al.* Infratentorial ependymomas in childhood: prognostic factors and treatment. *J Neurosurg* 1990; 72: 408–17.

92. Hendrick E, Raffel C. Tumors of the fourth ventricle: ependymomas, choroid plexus papillomas, and dermoid cysts. In: McLaurin R, Schut L, Venes J, *et al.* (eds). *Pediatric Neurosurgery: Surgery of the Developing Nervous System*, 2nd edn. Philadelphia: WB Saunders Co; 1989: 366–72.

93. Duncan J, Hoffman H (eds). *Intracranial Ependymomas*. Edinburgh: Churchill Livingston; 1995.

94. Rubio MP, Correa KM, Ueki K, *et al.* The putative glioma tumor suppressor gene on chromosome 19q maps between APOC2 and HRC. *Cancer Res* 1994; 54: 4760–3.

95. Sawyer JR, Sammartino G, Husain M, Boop FA, Chadduck WM. Chromosome aberrations in four ependymomas. *Cancer Genet Cytogenet* 1994; 74: 132–8.

96. Slavc I, MacCollin MM, Dunn M, *et al.* Exon scanning for mutations of the NF2 gene in pediatric ependymomas, rhabdoid tumors and meningiomas. *Int J Cancer* 1995; 64: 243–7.

97. Vagner-Capodano AM, Gentet JC, Gambarelli D, *et al.* Cytogenetic studies in 45 pediatric brain tumors. *Pediatr Hematol Oncol* 1992; 9: 223–35.

98. Weremowicz S, Kupsky WJ, Morton CC, Fletcher JA. Cytogenetic evidence for a chromosome 22 tumor suppressor gene in ependymoma. *Cancer Genet Cytogenet* 1992; 61: 193–6.

99. Smyth M, Biljana N, Russo C, Berger M. Intracranial ependymomas of childhood: current management strategies. *Pediatr Neurosurg* 2000; 33: 138–50.

100. Bergsagel D, Finegold M, Butel J, *et al.* DNA sequences similar to those of simian virus 40 in ependymomas and choroid plexus tumors of childhood. *N Engl J Med* 1992; 326: 988–93.

101. Kirschstein R, Gerger P. Ependymomas produced after intracerebral inoculation of SV 40 into newborn hamsters. *Nature* 1962; 195: 299.

102. Lednicky J, Garcea R, Bergsagel D, Butel J. Natural simian virus 40 strains are present in human choroid plexus and ependymoma tumors. *Virology* 1995; 212: 710–17.

103. Martini F, Iaccheri L, Lazzarin L, *et al.* SV 40 early region and large T antigen in human brain tumors, peripheral blood cells, and sperm fluids from healthy individuals. *Cancer* 1996; 56: 4820–5.

104. Kernohan J, Fletcher-Kernohan E. Ependymomas: a study of 109 cases. *Res Publ Assoc Res Nerv Ment Dis* 1937; 16: 182.

105. Kernohan J, Sayre G (eds). *Tumors of the Central Nervous System*. Washington: Armed Forces Institute of Pathology; 1952.

106. Ringertz N, Reymond A. Ependymomas and choroid plexus papillomas. *J Neuropathol Exp Neurol* 1949; 8: 355–80.

107. Miller D. Surgical neuropathology. In: Keating R, Goodrich J, Packer R (eds). *Tumors of the Pediatric Central Nervous System*. New York: Thieme Medical Publishers Inc; 2001: 44–102.

108. Kleiheus P, Cavenee W. *Pathology and Genetics of Tumors of the Nervous System. World Health Organization International Histological Classification of Tumours*. Berlin: Springer-Verlag; 1993.

109. Renaudin J, DiTullio M, Brown W. Seeding of intracranial ependymomas in children. *Child's Brain* 1979; 5: 408–12.

110. Rubinstein L. The definition of ependymoblastoma. *Arch Pathol* 1970; 90: 35–45.

111. Becker L (ed.). *Ependymoma*. Lyon: International Agency for Research on Cancer; 1997.

112. Weitman D, Cogen P. Infratentorial ependymoma. In: Keating R, Goodrich J, Packer R (eds). *Tumors of the Pediatric Central Nervous System*. New York: Thieme Medical Publishers, Inc.; 2001: 232–8.

113. Figarella-Branger D, Gambarelli D, Dollo C, *et al.* Infratentorial ependymomas of childhood: correlation between histological features, immunohistological phenotype, silver nucleolar organizer

region staining values and postoperative survival in 16 cases. *Acta Neuropathol* 1991; 82L: 208–16.

114. Kaneko Y, Takeshita I, Matsushima T, *et al*. Immunohistochemical study of ependymal neoplasms: histological subtypes and glial and epithelial characteristics. *Virchows Arch A Pathol Anat Histopathol* 1990; 417: 97–103.

115. Ikezaki K, Matsushima T, Inoue T, *et al*. Correlation of microanatomical localization with postoperative survival in posterior fossa ependymomas. *Neurosurgery* 1993; 32: 38–44.

116. Nagib M, O'Fallon M. Posterior fossa lateral ependymoma in childhood. *Pediatr Neurosurg* 1996; 24: 299–305.

117. Dailey AT, McKhann GM, 2nd, Berger MS. The pathophysiology of oral pharyngeal apraxia and mutism following posterior fossa tumor resection in children. *J Neurosurg* 1995; 83: 467–75.

118. Erashin Y. Is splitting of the vermis responsible for cerebellar mutism? (Letter). 1998.

119. Kellogg J, Piatt J. Resection of fourth ventricle tumors without splitting the vermis: the cerebellomedullary fissure approach. *Pediatr Neurosurg* 1997; 27: 28–33.

120. Rekate H, Grubb R, Aram D, *et al*. Muteness of cerebellar origin. *Arch Neurol* 1985; 42: 697–8.

121. Perilongo G, Massimino M, Sotti G, *et al*. Analyses of prognostic factors in a retrospective review of 92 children with ependymoma: Italian pediatric neuro-oncology group. *Med Pediatr Oncol* 1997; 29: 79–85.

122. Rousseau P, Habrand J, Sarrazin D, *et al*. Treatment of intracranial ependymomas of children: review of a 15-year experience. *Int J Radiat Oncol Biol Phys* 1994; 28: 381–6.

123. Paulino A, Wen B, Bautti J, *et al*. Intracranial ependymomas: an analysis of prognostic factors and patterns of failure. *Am J Clin Oncol* 2002; 25: 117–22.

124. Sutton L, J G, Perilongo G, *et al*. Prognostic factors in childhood ependymomas. *Pediatr Neurosurg* 1990–91; 16: 57–65.

125. van Veelen-Vincent ML, Pierre-Kahn A, Kalifa C, *et al*. Ependymoma in childhood: prognostic factors, extent of surgery, and adjuvant therapy. *J Neurosurg* 2002; 97: 827–35.

126. Bouffet E, Perilongo G, Canete A, Massimino M. Intracranial ependymomas in children: a critical review of prognostic factors and a plea for cooperation. *Med Pediatr Oncol* 1998; 30: 319–29.

127. Bloom H. Intracranial tumors: response and resistance to therapeutic endeavors, 1970–1980. *Int J Radiat Oncol Biol Phys* 1982; 8: 1083–113.

128. Sheline G. Radiation therapy of tumors of the central nervous system in childhood. *Cancer* 1975; 35: 957–64.

129. Shaw E, Evans E, Scheithauer B, *et al*. Postoperative radiotherapy of intracranial ependymoma in pediatric and adult patients. *Int J Radiat Oncol Biol Phys* 1987; 13: 1457–62.

130. Carrie C, Mottolese C, Bouffet E, *et al*. Non-metastatic childhood ependymomas. *Radiother Oncol* 1995; 36: 101–6.

131. Goldwein J, Corn B, Finlay J, *et al*. Is craniospinal irradiation required to cure children in malignant (anaplastic) intracranial ependymomas? *Cancer* 1991; 67: 2766–71.

132. Merchant T, Haida T, Wang M, *et al*. Anaplastic ependymoma: treatment of pediatric patients with or without craniospinal radiation therapy. *J Neurosurg* 1997; 86: 943–9.

133. Oi S, Raimondi A. Ependymomas in children. In: McLaurin R, Schut L, Venes J, *et al*. (eds). *Pediatric Neurosurgery: Surgery of the Developing Nervous System*, 1st edn. New York: Grune & Stratton; 1982: 419–28.

134. Paulino A. The local field in infratentorial ependymoma: does the entire posterior fossa need to be treated? *Int J Radiat Oncol Biol Phys* 2001; 49: 757–61.

135. Raco A, Raimondi A, D'Alonzo A, Esposito V, Valentino V. Radiosurgery in the management of pediatric brain tumors. *Child's Nerv Syst* 2000; 16: 287–95.

136. Evans A, Anderson J, Lefkowitz-Boudreaux I, Finlay J. Adjuvant chemotherapy of childhood posterior fossa ependymoma: craniospinal irradiation with or without adjuvant CCNU, vincristine, and prednisone: a Children's Cancer Group study. *Med Pediatr Oncol* 1996; 27: 8–14.

137. Grill J, le Deley M, Gambarelli D, *et al*. Postoperative chemotherapy without irradiation for ependymoma in children under 5 years of age: a multicenter trial of the French Society of Pediatric Oncology. *J Clin Oncol* 2001; 19: 1288–96.

138. Kalifa C, Valteau D, Pizer B, *et al*. High-dose chemotherapy in childhood brain tumours. *Child's Nerv Syst* 1999; 15: 498–505.

139. Mason W, Goldman S, Yates A, *et al*. Survival following intensive chemotherapy with bone marrow reconstitution for children with recurrent intracranial ependymoma. *J Neurooncol* 1998; 37: 135–43.

140. Dorhman G, Farwell J, Flannery J. Astrocytomas in childhood: a population-based study. *Surg Neurol* 1985; 23: 64–8.

141. Gjerris F, Klinken L. Long-term prognosis in children with benign cerebellar astrocytoma. *J Neurosurg* 1978; 71: 661–4.

142. Rutka J, Hoffman H, Duncan J. Astrocytomas of the posterior fossa. In: Cohen A (ed.). *Surgical Disorders of the Fourth Ventricle*. Boston: Blackwell Science; 1996: 189–208.

143. Steinbok P, Mutat A. Cerebellar astrocytomas. In: Albright L, Pollack I, Adelson D (eds). *Principles and Practice of Pediatric Neurosurgery*. New York: Thieme Medical Publishers Inc; 1999: 641–62.

144. Obrador S, Blazquez M. Benign cystic tumors of the cerebellum. *Acta Neurochir* 1975; 32: 55–68.

145. Desai K, Nadkarni T, Muzumdar D, Goel A. Prognostic factors for cerebellar astrocytomas in children: a study of 102 cases. *Pediatr Neurosurg* 2001; 35: 311–17.

146. Garcia D, Latifi H, Simpson, JR, Picker, S. Astrocytomas of the cerebellum in children. *J Neurosurg* 1989; 49: 179–84.

147. Krieger MD, Gonzalez-Gomez I, Levy ML, McComb JG. Recurrence patterns and anaplastic change in a long-term study of pilocytic astrocytomas. *Pediatr Neurosurg* 1997; 27: 1–11.

148. Pencalet P, Maixner W, Wainte-Rose C, *et al*. Benign cerebellar astrocytomas in children. *J Neurosurg* 1999; 90: 265–73.

149. Schneider J, Raffel C, McComb J. Benign cerebellar astrocytomas of childhood. *Neurosurgery* 1992; 30: 58–63.

150. Wallner K, Gonzales M, Edwards M, *et al*. Treatment results of juvenile pilocytic astrocytoma. *J Neurosurg* 1988; 69: 171–6.

151. Hadjipanayis C, Kondziolka D, Gardner P, *et al*. Stereotactic radiosurgery for pilocytic astrocytomas when multimodal therapy is necessary. *J Neurosurg* 2002; 97: 56–64.

152. Abdollahzedeh M, Hoffman H, Blazer S, *et al*. Benign cerebellar astrocytoma in childhood: experience at the Hospital for Sick Children. *Child's Nerv Syst* 1994; 10: 380–3.

153. Davis C, Joglekar V. Cerebellar astrocytomas in children and young adults. *Neurol Neurosurg Psychiatr* 1981; 44: 820–8.

154. Sgouros S, Fineron P, Hockley A. Cerebellar astrocytoma of childhood: long-term follow-up. *Child's Nerv Syst* 1995; 11: 89–96.

155. Viano J, Herrera E, Suarez J. Cerebellar astrocytomas: a 24-year experience. *Child's Nerv Syst* 2001; 17: 607–10.

156. Mesiwala A, Avellino A, Roberts T, Ellenbogen R. Spontaneous cerebellar hemorrhage due to a juvenile pilocytic astrocytoma. *Pediatr Neurosurg* 2001; 34: 235–8.

157. Russell D, Rubinstein L (eds). *Pathology of Tumors of the Nervous System*. Baltimore: Williams & Wilkins; 1977.

158. Medlock M. Infratentorial astrocytoma. In: Keating R, Goodrich J, Packer R (eds). *Tumors of the Pediatric Central Nervous System*. New York: Thieme Medical Publishers Inc; 2001: 199–205.

159. Kluwe L, Hagel C, Tatagiba M, *et al*. Loss of NF1 alleles distinguish sporadic from NF1-associated pilocytic astrocytomas. *J Neuropathol Exp Neurol* 2001; 60: 917–20.

160. Boch A, Cacciola F, Mokhtari K, *et al*. Benign recurrence of a cerebellar pilocytic astrocytoma 45 years after gross total resection. *Acta Neurochir (Wien)* 2001; 142: 341–6.

161. Palma L, Russo A, Mercuri S. Cystic pilocytic astrocytomas in infancy and childhood: long-term results. *Child's Brain* 1983; 10: 79–91.

162. Palma L, Guidetti B. Cystic pilocytic astrocytomas of the cerebral hemispheres. Surgical experience with 51 cases and long-term results. *J Neurosurg* 1985; 62: 811–15.

163. Bowers D, Krause T, Aronson L, *et al*. Second surgery for recurrent pilocytic astrocytoma in children. *Pediatr Neurosurg* 2001; 34: 229–34.

164. Samoza S, Kondziolka D, Lansford D, Fleckinger J, Bissonette D, Albright A. Early outcome after stereotatic radiosurgery for growing pilocytic astrocytomas in childhood. *Pediatr Neurosurg* 1996; 25: 109–15.

165. Tandon N, Vollmer D, New P, *et al*. Fulminant radiation-induced necrosis after stereotactic radiation therapy to the posterior fossa. case report and review of the literature. *J Neurosurg* 2001; 95: 507–12.

166. Panchawagh J, Muzumdar D, Goel A. Cerebellar astrocytoma in an adult with extensive leptomeningeal spread. *Br J Neurosurg* 2000; 14: 364–6.

167. Schwartz A, Ghatak N. Malignant transformation of benign cerebellar astrocytoma. *Cancer* 1990; 65: 333–6.

168. Bristot R, Santoro A, Raco A, *et al*. Malignant cerebellar astrocytomas: clinico-pathological remarks on 10 cases. *J Neurosurg Sci* 1999; 43: 271–6.

169. Bristot R, Raco A, Vangelista T, Delfini R. Malignant cerebellar astrocytomas in childhood: experience with four cases. *Child's Nerv Syst* 2001;14:532–6.

170. Rizk T, Remond J, Alhayek G, *et al*. Malignant astrocytoma of the cerebellum. Apropos of 10 cases. Review of the literature. *Neurochirurgie* 1994; 40: 121–6.

171. Shinoda J, Yamada H, Sakai N, *et al*. Malignant cerebellar astrocytic tumours in children. *Acta Neurochir* 1989; 98: 1–8.

172. Alpers C, Davis R, Wilson C. Persistence and late malignant transformation of childhood cerebellar astrocytoma: case report. *J Neurosurg* 1982; 57: 548–51.

173. Bernell W, Kepes J, Seitz E. Late malignant recurrence of childhood cerebellar astrocytoma: report of two cases. *J Neurosurg* 1972; 37: 470–4.

174. Budka H. Partially resected and irradiated cerebellar astrocytoma of childhood: malignant evolution after 28 years. *Acta Neurochir* 1975; 32: 139–46.

175. Casadei G, Arrigoni G, D'Angelo V, Bizzozero L. Later malignant recurrence of childhood cerebellar astrocytoma. *Clin Neuropathol* 1990; 9: 295–8.

176. Kleinman G, Schoene W, Walshe T, Richardson E. Malignant transformation in benign cerebellar astrocytoma: case report. *J Neurosurg* 1978; 49: 111–18.

177. Scott R, Ballantine H. Cerebellar astrocytoma: malignant recurrence after prolonged post-operative survival: case report. *J Neurosurg* 1973; 39: 777–9.

178. Ushio Y, Arita N, Yoshimine T, *et al*. Malignant recurrence of childhood cerebellar astrocytoma: case report. *Neurosurgery* 1987; 21: 251–5.

179. McCormack B, Miller D, Budzilovich G, *et al*. Treatment and survival of low-grade astrocytoma in adults – 1977–1988. *Neurosurgery* 1992; 31: 636–42.

180. Dorhman G, Dunsmore R. Glioblastoma multiforme of the cerebellum. *Surg Neurol* 1975; 3: 219–23.

181. Kulkarni A, Becker L, Jay V, *et al*. Primary cerebellar glioblastomas multiforme in children: report of four cases. *J Neurosurg* 1999; 90: 546–50.

182. Chamberlain M, Silver P, Levin V. Poorly differentiated gliomas of the cerebellum. A study of 18 patients. *Cancer* 1990; 65: 337–40.

183. Kuroiwa T, Numaguchi Y, Rothman M, *et al*. Posterior fossa glioblastoma multiforme: MR findings. *AJNR* 1995; 16: 583–9.

184. Nishioka H, Saito F, Haraoka J, Miwa T. Glioblastoma of the cerebellum: report of an autopsy case associated with intratumoral hemorrhage and CSF seedings. *No Shinkei Geka* 1991; 19: 547–52.

185. Ota T, Yamada S, Samejima N, *et al*. A case of cerebellar glioblastoma with massive cerebellar hemorrhage. *No Shinkei Geka* 2001; 29: 1201–5.

186. Dorhman G, Farwell J, Flannery J. Glioblastoma multiforme in children. *J Neurosurg* 1976; 44: 442–8.

187. Kopelson G. Cerebellar glioblastoma. *Cancer* 1982; 50: 308–11.

188. Hoffman HJ, Becker L, Craven MA. A clinically and pathologically distinct group of benign brain stem gliomas. *Neurosurgery* 1980; 7: 243–8.

189. Hoffman HJ. Dorsally exophytic brain stem tumors and midbrain tumors. *Pediatr Neurosurg* 1996; 24: 256–62.

190. Mallucci C, Lellouch-Tubiana A, Salazar C, *et al*. The management of desmoplastic neuroepithelial tumours in childhood. *Child's Nerv Syst* 2000; 16: 8–14.

191. Paulus W, Schlote W, Perentes E, Jacobi G, Warmuth-Metz M, Roggendorf W. Desmoplastic supratentorial neuroepithelial tumours of infancy. *Histopathology* 1992; 21: 43–9.

192. Evans AJ, Fayaz I, Cusimano MD, Laperriere N, Bilbao JM. Combined pleomorphic xanthoastrocytoma-ganglioglioma of the cerebellum. *Arch Pathol Lab Med* 2000; 124: 1707–9.

193. Lim SC, Jang SJ, Kim YS. Cerebellar pleomorphic xanthoastrocytoma in an infant. *Pathol Int* 1999; 49: 811–15.

194. Rosemberg S, Rotta JM, Yassuda A, Velasco O, Leite CC. Pleomorphic xanthoastrocytoma of the cerebellum. *Clin Neuropathol* 2000; 19: 238–42.

195. VandenBerg SR, May EE, Rubinstein LJ, *et al*. Desmoplastic supratentorial neuroepithelial tumors of infancy with divergent differentiation potential ("desmoplastic infantile gangliogliomas"). Report on 11 cases of a distinctive embryonal tumor with favorable prognosis. *J Neurosurg* 1987; 66: 58–71.

196. Duffner PK, Burger PC, Cohen ME, *et al*. Desmoplastic infantile gangliogliomas: an approach to therapy. *Neurosurgery* 1994; 34: 583–9.

197. Epstein FJ. Prognosis in pediatric brain-stem gliomas. *J Neurosurg* 1987; 67: 323–4.

198. Epstein FJ, Farmer JP. Brain-stem glioma growth patterns. *J Neurosurg* 1993; 78: 408–12.

199. Tomita T, McLone DG, Naidich TP. Brain stem gliomas in childhood. Rational approach and treatment. *J Neuro-oncol* 1984; 2: 117–22.

200. Walker M, Storrs B. Surgical therapy for intrinsic brain stem gliomas. *Concepts Pediatr Neurosurg* 1985; 5: 178–86.

201. Farmer JP, Montes JL, Freeman CR, Meagher-Villemure K, Bond MC, O'Gorman AM. Brainstem gliomas. A 10-year institutional review. *Pediatr Neurosurg* 2001; 34: 206–14.

202. Weiner HL, Freed D, Woo HH, Rezai AR, Kim R, Epstein FJ. Intra-axial tumors of the cervicomedullary junction: surgical results and long-term outcome. *Pediatr Neurosurg* 1997; 27: 12–18.

203. Behnke J, Christen H, Bruck W, Markakis E. Intra-axial endophytic tumors in the pons and/or medulla oblongata: I. Symptoms, neuroradiological findings, and histopathology in 30 children. *Child's Nerv Syst* 1997; 13: 122–34.

204. Scherer H. Structural development in gliomas. *Am J Cancer* 1938; 34: 333–51.

205. Ragheb J, Epstein F, Goh K. Brain-Stem gliomas. In: Kaye A, Black P (eds). *Operative Neurosurgery*. London: Harcourt Publishers Ltd; 2000: 437–45.

206. Albright L. Biopsy of brainstem masses. *J Neurosurg* 1996; 84: 304–6.

207. Albright AL, Packer RJ, Zimmerman R, Rorke LB, Boyett J, Hammond GD. Magnetic resonance scans should replace biopsies for the diagnosis of diffuse brain stem gliomas: a report from the Children's Cancer Group. *Neurosurgery* 1993; 33: 1026–9.

208. Levin VA, Edwards MS, Wara WM, Allen J, Ortega J, Vestnys P. 5-Fluorouracil and 1-(2-chloroethyl)-3-cyclohexyl-1-nitrosourea (CCNU) followed by hydroxyurea, misonidazole, and irradiation for brain stem gliomas: a pilot study of the Brain Tumor Research Center and the Children's Cancer Group. *Neurosurgery* 1984; 14: 679–81.

209. Hood TW, McKeever PE. Stereotactic management of cystic gliomas of the brain stem. *Neurosurgery* 1989; 24: 373–8.

210. Oka K, Kin Y, Go Y, *et al*. Neuroendoscopic approach to tectal tumors: a consecutive series. *J Neurosurg* 1999; 91: 964–70.

211. Bowers DC, Georgiades C, Aronson LJ, *et al*. Tectal gliomas: natural history of an indolent lesion in pediatric patients. *Pediatr Neurosurg* 2000; 32: 24–9.

212. Russell D, Rubinstein L. *Pathology of Tumors of the Nervous System*. London: Edward Arnold; 1959.

213. Ellenbogen R, Scott R. Choroid plexus tumors. In: Kaye A, Laws E (eds). *Brain Tumors: An Encyclopedic Approach*, 2nd edn. London: Churchill Livingston; 2001: 551–62.

214. Harwood-Nash D, Fitz C. *Neuroradiology in Infants and Children*. St Louis, MO: CV Mosby Co.; 1976.

215. Raimondi AJ, Gutierrez FA. Diagnosis and surgical treatment of choroid plexus papillomas. *Child's Brain* 1975; 1: 81–115.

216. Milhorat TH, Davis DA, Hammock MK. Choroid plexus papilloma. II. Ultrastructure and ultracytochemical localization of Na-K-ATPase. *Child's Brain* 1976; 2: 290–303.

217. Ellenbogen RG, Winston KR, Kupsky WJ. Tumors of the choroid plexus in children. *Neurosurgery* 1989; 25: 327–35.

218. Ellenbogen R, Donovan D. Choroid plexus tumors. In: Keating R, Goodrich J, Packer R (eds). *Tumors of the Pediatric Central Nervous System*. New York, NY: Thieme Medical Publishers, Inc.; 2001: 339–50.

219. Matson D, Crofton F. Papilloma of the choroid plexus in childhood. *J Neurosurg* 1960; 17: 1002–27.

220. McGirr SJ, Ebersold MJ, Scheithauer BW, Quast LM, Shaw EG. Choroid plexus papillomas: long-term follow-up results in a surgically treated series. *J Neurosurg* 1988; 69: 843–9.

221. Eisenberg H, McComb J, Lorenzo A. Cerebrospinal fluid overproduction and hydrocephalus associated with choroid plexus papilloma. *J Neurosurg* 1974; 40: 381–5.

222. Ghatak NR, McWhorter JM. Ultrastructural evidence for CSF production by a choroid plexus papilloma. *J Neurosurg* 1976; 45: 409–15.

223. Rekate H, Erwood S, Brodkey J, *et al*. Etiology of ventriculomegaly in choroid plexus papilloma. *Pediatr Neurosci* 1985; 12: 196–201.

224. Hawkins JC, 3rd. Treatment of choroid plexus papillomas in children: a brief analysis of twenty years' experience. *Neurosurgery* 1980; 6: 380–4.

225. Morello G, Migliavacca F. Primary choroid papillomas in the cerebellopontine angle. *Neurol Neurosurg Psychiatr* 1964; 27: 445–50.

226. van Swieten JC, Thomeer RT, Vielvoye GJ, Bots GT. Choroid plexus papilloma in the posterior fossa. *Surg Neurol* 1987; 28: 129–34.

227. Nassar S, Mount L. Papillomas of the choroid plexus. *J Neurosurg* 1968; 29: 73–7.

228. Ausman J, Shrontz C, Chason J, *et al*. Aggressive choroid plexus papilloma. *Surg Neurol* 1984; 22: 472–6.

229. Paulus W, Janisch W. Clinicopathological correlations in epithelial choroid plexus neoplasms: a study of 52 cases. *Acta Neuropathol (Berlin)* 1990; 80: 635–41.

230. Newbould M, Kelsey A, Arango J, *et al*. The choroid plexus carcinomas of childhood: histopathology, immunocytochemistry and clinicopathological correlations. *Histopathology* 1995; 26: 137–43.

231. Fujii K, Lenkey C, Rhoton AL Jr. Microsurgical anatomy of the choroidal arteries. Fourth ventricle and cerebellopontine angles. *J Neurosurg* 1980; 52: 504–24.

232. Zhang W. Choroid plexus papilloma of the cerebellopontine angle, with special reference to vertebral angiographic study. *Surg Neurol* 1982; 18: 367–71.

233. Leblanc R, Bekhor S, Melanson D, Carpenter S. Diffuse craniospinal seeding from a benign fourth ventricle choroid plexus papilloma. Case report. *J Neurosurg* 1998; 88: 757–60.

234. Russell D, Rubinstein L. *Pathology of Tumors of the Nervous System*, 2nd edn. Baltimore: Williams & Wilkins; 1963.

235. Araki K, Aori T, Takahashi JA, *et al*. [A case report of choroid plexus carcinoma]. *No Shinkei Geka* 1997; 25: 853–7.

236. St Clair S, Humphreys R, Pillay P, *et al*. Current management of choroid plexus carcinoma in children. *Pediatr Neurosurg* 1991; 17: 225–33.

237. Cobb C, Youmans J. Sacromas and neoplasms of blood vessels. In: Youmans J (ed.). *Neurological Surgery*, 3rd edn. Philadelphia: WB Saunders Co.; 1990: 3152–70.

238. Horten B, Urich H, Rubinstein L, *et al*. The angioblastic meningioma: a reappraisal of the nosological problems: light-, electron-microscopic, tissue, and organ culture observations. *J Neurosurg Sci* 1977; 31: 387–410.

239. Singounas EG. Haemangioblastomas of the central nervous system. *Acta Neurochir (Wien)* 1978; 44: 107–13.

240. Jeffreys R. Clinical and surgical aspects of posterior fossa haemangioblastomata. *J Neurol Neurosurg Psychiatr* 1975; 38: 105–11.

241. Mondkar VP, McKissock W, Russell RW. Cerebellar haemangioblastomas. *Br J Surg* 1967; 54: 45–9.

242. Obrador S, Martin-Rodriguez JG. Biological factors involved in the clinical features and surgical management of cerebellar hemangioblastomas. *Surg Neurol* 1977; 7: 79–85.

243. McDonnell DE, Pollock P. Cerebral cystic hemangioblastoma. *Surg Neurol* 1978; 10: 195–9.

244. Conway JE, Chou D, Clatterbuck RE, Brem H, Long DM, Rigamonti D. Hemangioblastomas of the central nervous system in von Hippel–Lindau syndrome and sporadic disease. *Neurosurgery* 2001; 48: 55–62.

245. Rengachary S, JP B. Hemangioblastoma. In: Wilkins R, Rengachary S (eds). *Neurosurgery*, 2nd edn. New York: McGraw-Hill; 1996: 1205–19.

246. Neumann HP, Bender BU. Genotype–phenotype correlations in von Hippel–Lindau disease. *J Intern Med* 1998; 243: 541–5.

247. Maher ER, Kaelin WG, Jr. von Hippel–Lindau disease. *Medicine*

(Baltimore) 1997; 76: 381–91.

248. Taylor M, Thapar K, Rutka J. Neurogenetics and the molecular biology of human brain tumors. In: Kaye A, Laws E (eds). *Brain Tumors: An Encyclopedic Approach*, 2nd edn. London: Churchill-Livingston; 2001: 71–103.

249. Weitman D, Cogen P. The phakomatoses. In: Albright L, Pollack I, Adelson D (eds). *Principles and Practice of Pediatric Neurosurgery*. New York: Thieme Medical Publishers, Inc.; 1999: 741–63.

250. Hubschmann OR, Vijayanathan T, Countee RW. Von Hippel–Lindau disease with multiple manifestations: diagnosis and management. *Neurosurgery* 1981; 8: 92–5.

251. Maher ER, Yates JR, Harries R, *et al*. Clinical features and natural history of von Hippel–Lindau disease. *Q J Med* 1990; 77: 1151–63.

252. Richard S, Beigelman C, Gerber S, *et al*. Does hemangioblastoma exist outside von Hippel–Lindau disease? *Neurochirurgie* 1994; 40: 145–54.

253. Melmon K, Rosen S. Lindau's disease: review of the literature and study of a large kindred. *Am J Med* 1964; 36: 595–617.

254. Tachibana O, Yamashima T, Yamashita J, Takinami K. Immunohistochemical study of basic fibroblast growth factor and erythropoietin in cerebellar hemangioblastomas. *Noshuyo Byori* 1994; 11: 169–72.

255. Olivecrona H. The cerebellar angioreticulomas. *J Neurosurg* 1952; 9: 317–30.

256. Rawe S, Van Gilder J, Rothman S. Radiographic diagnostic evaluation and surgical treatment of multiple cerebellar, brain stem, and spinal cord hemangioblastomas. *Surg Neurol* 1978; 9: 337–41.

257. Ludwin S, Rubinstein L, Russell D. Papillary meningioma. A malignant variant of meningioma. *Cancer* 1975; 36: 1363–73.

258. Knudson A, Strong L. Mutation and cancer: neuroblastoma and pheochromocytoma. *Am J Hum Genet* 1972; 24: 514–32.

259. Latif F, Tory K, Gnarra J, *et al*. Identification of the von Hippel–Lindau disease tumor suppressor gene. *Science* 1993; 260: 1317–20.

260. Lee JY, Dong SM, Park WS, *et al*. Loss of heterozygosity and somatic mutations of the VHL tumor suppressor gene in sporadic cerebellar hemangioblastomas. *Cancer Res* 1998; 58: 504–8.

261. Seizinger B, Rouleu G, Ozelius L, *et al*. Von Hippel–Lindau disease maps to the region of chromosome 3 associated with renal cell carcinoma. *Nature* 1988; 322: 268–9.

262. Gijtenbeek JM, Jacobs B, Sprenger SH, *et al*. Analysis of von Hippel–Lindau mutations with comparative genomic hybridization in sporadic and hereditary hemangioblastomas: possible genetic heterogeneity. *J Neurosurg* 2002; 97: 977–82.

263. Maxwell P, Wiesener M, Chang G, *et al*. The tumour suppressor protein VHL targets hypoxia-inducible factors for oxygen-dependent proteolysis. *Nature* 1999; 399: 271–5.

264. Wizigmann-Voos S, Breijer G, Risau W, *et al*. Up-regulation of vascular endothelial growth factor and its receptors in von Hippel–Lindau associated and sporadic hemangioblastomas. *Cancer Res* 1995; 55: 1358–64.

265. Wykoff CC, Pugh CW, Maxwell PH, Harris AL, Ratcliffe PJ. Identification of novel hypoxia dependent and independent target genes of the von Hippel–Lindau (VHL) tumour suppressor by mRNA differential expression profiling. *Oncogene* 2000; 19: 6297–305.

266. Glasker S, Bender BU, Apel TW, *et al*. Reconsideration of biallelic inactivation of the VHL tumour suppressor gene in hemangioblastomas of the central nervous system. *J Neurol Neurosurg Psychiatr* 2001; 70: 644–8.

267. Kanno H, Kondo K, Ito S, *et al*. Somatic mutations of the von Hippel–Lindau tumor suppressor gene in sporadic central nervous system hemangioblastomas. *Cancer Res* 1994; 54: 4845–7.

268. Oberstrass J, Reifenberger G, Reifenberger J, Wechsler W, Collins VP. Mutation of the Von Hippel–Lindau tumour suppressor gene in capillary haemangioblastomas of the central nervous system. *J Pathol* 1996; 179: 151–6.

269. Tse JY, Wong JH, Lo KW, Poon WS, Huang DP, Ng HK. Molecular genetic analysis of the von Hippel–Lindau disease tumor suppressor gene in familial and sporadic cerebellar hemangioblastomas. *Am J Clin Pathol* 1997; 107: 459–66.

270. Sung DI, Chang CH, Harisiadis L. Cerebellar hemangioblastomas. *Cancer* 1982; 49: 553–5.

271. Smalley S, Schomberg P, Earle J, *et al*. Radiotherapeutic considerations in the treatment of hemangioblastomas of the central nervous system. *Int J Radiat Oncol Biol Phys* 1990; 18: 1165–71.

272. Page KA, Wayson K, Steinberg GK, Adler JR, Jr. Stereotaxic radiosurgical ablation: an alternative treatment for recurrent and multifocal hemangioblastomas. A report of four cases. *Surg Neurol* 1993; 40: 424–8.

273. Martinez-Lage JF, Ramos J, Puche A, Poza M. Extradural dermoid tumours of the posterior fossa. *Arch Dis Child* 1997; 77: 427–30.

274. Lekias J, Stokes B. Dermoid lesions of the central nervous system in childhood. *Aust N Z J Surg* 1970; 39: 335–40.

275. Groen RJ, van Ouwerkerk WJ. Cerebellar dermoid tumor and occipital meningocele in a monozygotic twin: clues to the embryogenesis of craniospinal dysraphism. *Child's Nerv Syst* 1995; 11: 414–17.

276. Kavar B, Kaye A. Dermoid, epidermoid, and neuroenteric cysts. In: Kaye A, Laws E (eds). *Brain Tumors: An Encyclopedic Approach*, 2nd edn. London: Churchill Livingston; 2001: 965–81.

277. Amirjamshidi A, Ghodsi M, Edraki K. Teeth in the cerebellopontine angle: an unusual dermoid tumour. *Br J Neurosurg* 1995; 9: 679–82.

278. Corkill G, McCulloch GA, Tonge RE. Cranial dermal sinus: value of plain skull X-ray examination and early diagnosis. *Med J Aust* 1974; 1: 885–7.

279. Galicich J, Aribit E. Metastatic brain tumor. In: Youmans J (ed.). *Neurological Surgery*, 3rd edn. Philadelphia: WB Saunders Co.; 1990: 3204–22.

280. Silverberg E. Cancer statistics. 1986. *CA Cancer J Clin* 1986; 36: 9–25.

281. Delattre JY, Krol G, Thaler HT, Posner JB. Distribution of brain metastases. *Arch Neurol* 1988; 45: 741–4.

282. Haar F, Patterson RH, Jr. Surgical for metastatic intracranial neoplasm. *Cancer* 1972; 30: 1241–5.

283. Posner JB, Chernik NL. Intracranial metastases from systemic cancer. *Adv Neurol* 1978; 19: 579–92.

284. Sawaya R, Bindal R, Lang F, Abi-Said D. Metastatic brain tumors. In: Kaye A, Laws E (eds). *Brain Tumors: An Encyclopedic Approach*, 2nd edn. London: Churchill Livingston; 2001: 999–1026.

285. Takakura K, Sano K, Hojo S, *et al*. *Metastatic Tumors of the Central Nervous System*. Tokyo: Igaku-Shoin; 1982.

286. Chason J, Walker F, Landers J. Metastatic carcinoma in the central nervous system and dorsal root ganglia. *Cancer* 1963; 16: 781–7.

287. Landis SH, Murray T, Bolden S, Wingo PA. Cancer statistics, 1998. *CA Cancer J Clin* 1998; 48: 6–29.

288. Tsukada Y, Fouad A, Pickren J, *et al*. Central nervous system metastasis from breast carcinoma. Autopsy study. *Cancer* 1983; 52: 2349–54.

289. Timothy J, Kerawala C, Brazil L, Bartlett J, Doshi B. Medullary cell carcinoma of the thyroid: metastases to the central nervous system. *Eur J Surg Oncol* 1995; 21: 329–30.

290. Pacak K, Sweeney DC, Wartofsky L, *et al*. Solitary cerebellar metastasis from papillary thyroid carcinoma: a case report. *Thyroid* 1998; 8: 327–35.

291. Cha ST, Jarrahy R, Mathiesen RA, Suh R, Shahinian HK. Cerebellopontine angle metastasis from papillary carcinoma of the thyroid: case report and literature review. *Surg Neurol* 2000; 54: 320–6.

292. Perri F, Bisceglia M, Giannatempo GM, Andriulli A. Cerebellar metastasis as a unique presenting feature of gastric cancer. *J Clin Gastroenterol* 2001; 33: 80–1.

293. Papatsoris AG, Mpadra FA, Karamouzis MV. Prostate cancer presenting as a solitary cerebellar metastasis. A case report and review of the literature. *Tumori* 2002; 88: 61–4.

294. Lewanski CR, Botwood N, Glaser MG. Bilateral cerebellopontine metastases in a patient with an unknown primary. *Clin Oncol (R Coll Radiol)* 1999; 11: 272–3.

295. Chang TC, Jain S, Ng KK, Hsueh S, Tsai CS, Chen HL, *et al.* Cerebellar metastasis from papillary serous adenocarcinoma of the ovary mimicking Meniere's disease. A case report. *J Reprod Med* 2001; 46: 267–9.

296. Cairncross JG, Kim JH, Posner JB. Radiation therapy for brain metastases. *Ann Neurol* 1980; 7: 529–41.

297. Vannucci RC, Baten M. Cerebral metastatic disease in childhood. *Neurology* 1974; 24: 981–5.

298. Gercovich FG, Luna MA, Gottlieb JA. Increased incidence of cerebral metastases in sarcoma patients with prolonged survival from chemotherapy. Report of cases of leiomysarcoma and chondrosarcoma. *Cancer* 1975; 36: 1843–51.

299. Graus F, Walker RW, Allen JC. Brain metastases in children. *J Pediatr* 1983; 103: 558–61.

300. Jaffe N. Metastases in malignant childhood tumors – the role of "adjuvant" therapy and the utility of multidisciplinary treatment. *Semin Oncol* 1977; 4: 177–86.

301. Bannayan G, Huvos A, D'Angio G. Effect of irradiation on the maturation of Wilms' tumor. *Cancer* 1971; 27: 812–18.

302. Klapproth H. Wilms' tumor: a report of 45 cases and an analysis of 1351 cases reported in the world literature from 1940 to 1958. *J Urol* 1959; 81: 633–48.

303. Mohammad AM, Meyer J, Hakami N. Long-term survival following brain metastasis of Wilms' tumor. *J Pediatr* 1977; 90: 660.

304. Gandolfi A, Orsoni JG. Occult nephroblastoma (Wilms' tumor) presenting with symptoms of central nervous system involvement. *Acta Neurol (Napoli)* 1979; 1: 424–8.

305. O'Brien M, Prats A. Metastatic tumors. In: McLaurin R, Schut L, Venes J, *et al.* (eds.) *Pediatric Neurosurgery: Surgery of the Developing Nervous System*, 3rd edn. Philadelphia: WB Saunders Co.; 1989: 417–20.

306. Alpert JN, Mones R. Neurologic manifestations of neuroblastoma. *J Mt Sinai Hosp N Y* 1969; 36: 37–47.

307. Danzinger J, Wallace S, Handel S, *et al.* Metastatic osteogenic sarcoma to the brain. *Cancer* 1979; 43: 707–10.

308. Mandybur TI. Intracranial hemorrhage caused by metastatic tumors. *Neurology* 1977; 27: 650–5.

309. Takamiya Y, Toya S, Otani M, *et al.* Wilms' tumor with intracranial metastases presenting with intracranial metastases presenting with intracranial hemorrhage. *Child's Nerv Syst* 1985; 1: 291–4.

310. Arbit E, Wronski M, Burt M, Galicich JH. The treatment of patients with recurrent brain metastases. A retrospective analysis of 109 patients with nonsmall cell lung cancer. *Cancer* 1995; 76: 765–73.

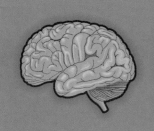
The pituitary gland regulates the function of the thyroid gland, the adrenal glands, the ovaries and the testes. It controls lactation, uterine contractions during labor and linear growth and it regulates the osmolality and volume of the intravascular fluid by providing resorption of water in the kidney (Table 36.1). Symptoms and signs of disorders that affect the pituitary reflect the normal function and anatomy of the pituitary gland.

The pituitary gland rests in the sella turcica, a saddle-shaped concavity of the sphenoid bone. The optic nerves, chiasm and tracts lie just above the diaphragma sella, through which passes the pituitary stalk (Figure 36.1). The cavernous venous sinuses, the medial walls of which form the lateral walls of the sella, contain the IIIrd, IVth and VIth cranial nerves that provide eye movement, the ophthalmic and maxillary division of the trigeminal nerves, and the internal carotid arteries.

The pituitary gland is comprised of anterior and posterior lobes. The gland secretes eight peptide hormones, two from the posterior lobe and six from the anterior lobe (see Table 36.1). Disorders that alter pituitary function produce symptoms by (1) excess or deficient secretion of the pituitary hormones, (2)

extrinsic compression on the pituitary and adjacent structures by mass lesions, or (3) interruption of the blood supply to the pituitary.

Assessment of pituitary function requires clinical evaluation for hormonal deficiency or excess and laboratory testing of the various pituitary–target organ axes. Endocrine evaluation confirms endocrinopathy, defines it, and helps establish the etiology. In addition, endocrine evaluation of patients with tumors in the sellar region is used to document pre- and postoperative hypothalamic–pituitary deficiencies and to assess the effects of treatment, such as surgery and radiation therapy.

ANTERIOR PITUITARY HORMONES

In the anterior lobe five distinct types of cells produce and release six different hormones: corticotrophs, adrenocorticotropic hormone (ACTH); somatotrophs, growth hormone (GH); lactotrophs, prolactin (PRL); thyrotrophs, thyroid-stimulating hormone (TSH); and gonadotrophs, follicle-stimulating hormone

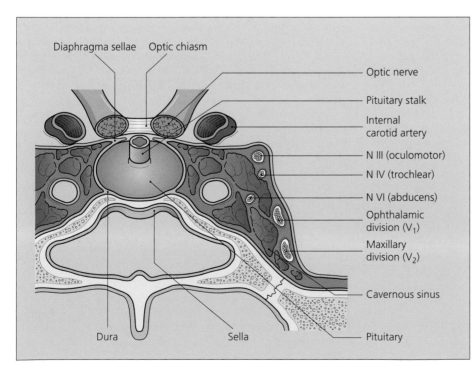

Diaphragma sellae   Optic chiasm

Optic nerve

Pituitary stalk

Internal carotid artery

N III (oculomotor)

N IV (trochlear)

N VI (abducens)

Ophthalmic division (V_1)

Maxillary division (V_2)

Cavernous sinus

Dura   Sella   Pituitary

Figure 36.1 Anatomic relationships of the pituitary gland. A coronal section through the sella turcica shows the pituitary gland in relation to surrounding structures: the cavernous sinuses, carotid arteries, and cranial nerves II, III, IV, V (V_1, V_2) and VI.

Table 36.1 Summary of pituitary functions

| Hypothalamus | Pituitary | | End-organ | | |
	Pituitary cell	Pituitary hormone	Organ	Hormone	Primary functions
Anterior lobe					
Releasing factors					
Corticotropin releasing hormone (CRH)	Corticotroph	Adrenocorticotropin (corticotropin, ACTH)	Adrenals	Cortisol	General metabolism; required for physiologic adaptation to stress
Thyrotropin releasing hormone	Thyrotroph	Thyroid-stimulating hormone (TSH)	Thyroid	Thyroid hormones (T_3, T_4)	General metabolism; influences pace of metabolism
Gonadotropin releasing hormone (GnRH)	Gonadotroph	Follicle-stimulating hormone (FSH)	Ovaries	Estradiol, progesterone	Required for normal female sexual development and fertility
		Luteinizing hormone (LH)	Testes	Testosterone	Required for normal male sexual development and fertility
Growth hormone releasing hormone (GHRH)	Somatotroph	Growth hormone (somatotropin, GH)	Liver and other tissues	Somatomedin (insulin-like growth factor-I, IGF-I)	Growth, glucose regulation
Inhibiting factors					
Dopamine (PIF)	Lactotroph	Prolactin (PRL)	Breast, gonads	Prolactin	Lactation
Somatostatin	Somatotroph	Growth hormone (GH)	Liver and other tissues	Somatomedin (insulin-like growth factor-I, GF-I)	Growth, glucose regulation
Posterior lobe					
Antidiuretic hormone (vasopressin, ADH)	ADH produced in hypothalamus stored in posterior pituitary		Kidney	Antidiuretic hormone (ADH)	Resorption of water in the kidney
Oxytocin	Oxytocin produced in hypothalamus; stored in posterior pituitary		Uterus	Oxytocin	Uterine contractions during labor

(FSH) and luteinizing hormone (LH). The secretion of these hormones is regulated by the hypothalamus and by negative (inhibitory) feedback regulation by the hormonal product of the target organ (Figures 36.2 and 36.3). The posterior lobe of the pituitary, the neurohypophysis, secretes antidiuretic hormone (ADH) and oxytocin, which are produced by hypothalamic neurons and released directly from nerve terminals in the posterior pituitary. For ACTH, TSH, LH and FSH, the corresponding hypothalamic regulating factors, corticotropin-releasing hormone (CRH), thyrotropin-releasing hormone (TRH), and gonadotropin-releasing hormone (GnRH), appear to be exclusively stimulatory. In contrast, GH secretion receives both positive and negative hypothalamic influence, via GH-releasing hormone (GHRH) and somatostatin, respectively, and prolactin release is primarily under tonic inhibition by dopamine, also known as prolactin-inhibiting factor, from the hypothalamus. Several of these hypothalamic factors affect more than one type of anterior pituitary cell and influence the secretion of more than one anterior pituitary hormone. For instance, TRH, which stimulates TSH production, also stimulates prolactin release.

Prolactin

Physiology

PRL is secreted by the lactotrophs; these cells are unique in that they have the capacity to proliferate during adulthood. PRL interacts with receptors in the gonads and acts on the breast to initiate and maintain lactation. Hypothalamic restraint of PRL secretion occurs by the release of dopamine (prolactin-inhibiting factor, PIF) into the portal circulation from nerve processes that originate in the arcuate nucleus of the hypothalamus (Figure 36.4). PRL-releasing factors include TRH, vasoactive intestinal peptide (VIP), GnRH and peptide histidine methionine (PHM). Although pharmacologic doses of TRH result in a rapid release of prolactin the physiologic role of TRH in prolactin secretion is unclear.

During pregnancy, estrogen stimulates lactotroph hyperplasia and hyperprolactinemia but blocks the action of PRL on the breast, inhibiting lactation until after delivery. Within 4–6 months after delivery, basal PRL levels are normal.

PRL is secreted episodically, with 13 or 14 peaks per day and an interpulse interval of about 90 minutes. Small postprandial rises occur secondary to central stimulation by the amino acids from meals.

Hyperprolactinemia

Stimulation of prolactin release and increased serum prolactin levels have many causes (Table 36.2). Sleep, TRH, VIP, opiates and estrogen stimulate the release of PRL. Hyperprolactinemia can be caused by: (1) excess autonomous production (PRL-secreting pituitary adenomas) (Figure 36.5A); (2) diminished hypothalamic production of dopamine or interruption of dopamine delivery to the pituitary [hypothalamic disorders, such as tumors and sarcoidosis; drugs, such as reserpine and methyldopa, which block

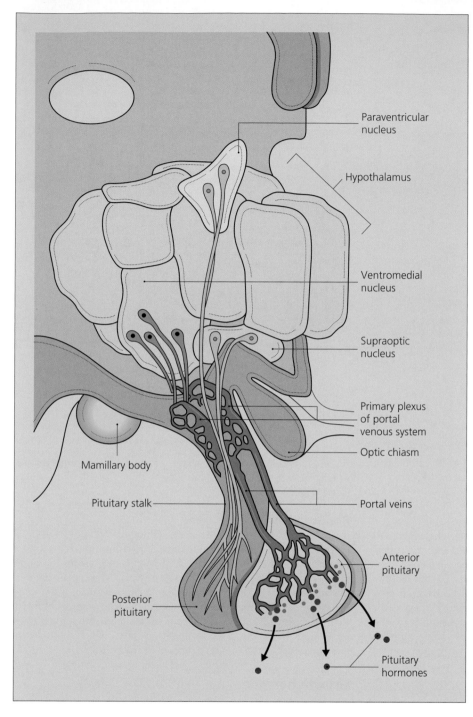

Figure 36.2 Hypothalamic control of the pituitary. Anterior pituitary: the neural processes of the hypothalamic nuclei (green) terminate on fenestrated vessels of the portal venous system in the median eminence. The portal veins (blue) carry releasing and inhibiting factors to the anterior lobe of the pituitary, where they regulate the release of anterior pituitary hormones (red). Posterior pituitary: the neural processes of the hypothalamic neurons of the supraoptic and paraventricular nuclei (yellow) carry the posterior pituitary hormones, antidiuretic hormone, and oxytocin, which are released directly from nerve terminals in the posterior pituitary.

Paraventricular nucleus

Hypothalamus

Ventromedial nucleus

Supraoptic nucleus

Primary plexus of portal venous system

Optic chiasm

Mamillary body

Pituitary stalk

Portal veins

Anterior pituitary

Posterior pituitary

Pituitary hormones

dopamine production; interruption of the portal venous system in the pituitary stalk by a sellar mass (pituitary tumor, aneurysm); following pituitary irradiation, or in the empty sella syndrome] (Figure 36.5B); (3) inhibition of dopamine activity on the lactotrophs (drugs that block interaction of dopamine with its receptor; e.g. the phenothiazines; and (4) stimulation of PRL secretion by estrogens, TRH, or opiates. Physiologic stimulation of PRL secretion and sporadic hyperprolactinemia occur with exercise and other forms of stress and with postpartum suckling.

Hyperprolactinemia causes hypogonadism and galactorrhea. The symptoms of hyperprolactinemia in women are amenorrhea and galactorrhea, diminished libido, and infertility. Gonadal deficiency with diminished estrogen secretion leads to osteoporosis in susceptible women. In males, hyperprolactinemia results in diminished libido, impotence, and infertility with decreased sperm counts.

EVALUATION AND LABORATORY TESTING Laboratory testing in patients with suspected hyperprolactinemia consists of repeated measurements of basal, resting serum PRL levels by radioimmunoassay. Normal PRL levels are gender-specific, random values may be above the normal limit and peak levels occur during the late

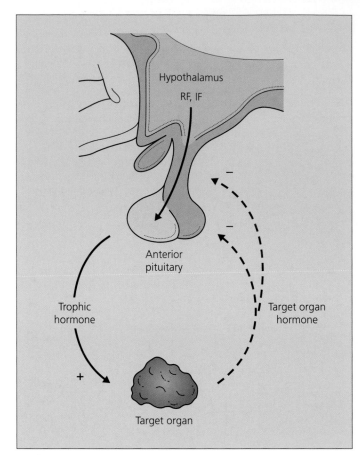

Figure 36.3 Feedback regulation of the anterior pituitary. The production and secretion of anterior pituitary hormones is inhibited by the hormonal products of the target organs (negative feedback).

Table 36.2 Causes of hyperprolactinemia

I **Neurogenic**
  1 Suckling or nipple stimulation
  2 Stress (transient)

II **Hypothalamic and interruption of portal circulation**
  1 Granulomatous diseases of hypothalamus; sarcoid, histiocytosis
  2 Neoplasms: craniopharyngiomas, hypothalamic astrocytomas
  3 Stalk section: surgical or traumatic
  4 Empty sella
  5 Nonlactotropic cell pituitary tumors (which affect portal venous blood flow)
  6 Radiation treatment to sella

III **Pituitary**
  1 Prolactinomas

IV **Other endocrine factors**
  1 Pregnancy
  2 Estrogen administration, contraceptive pills
  3 Hypothyroidism

V **Drugs that inhibit dopamine secretion and action**
  1 Psychotropic (phenothiazines, butyrophenones, thioxanethenes, reserpine)
  2 Opiates (morphine)
  3 Antiemetics (metoclopramide)
  4 Anithypertensives (methyldopa, reserpine)
  5 Histamine-receptor blockers (cimetidine)

hours of sleep. PRL levels rise in response to psychological and physical stress, nipple stimulation, intercourse and estrogens. Therefore, minimally elevated PRL levels must be confirmed from several samples or by the measurement of PRL in a pooled sample. Serum PRL levels in normal subjects range between 5 and 20 ng/mL (Figure 36.6). A PRL level greater than 200 ng/mL is nearly always the result of a prolactinoma. Prolactinomas are the most common type of secreting pituitary tumors and comprise about 30% of all pituitary tumors. In patients with amenorrhea, pregnancy has to be excluded, as it is associated with PRL levels of 100–250 ng/mL by the third trimester (see Figure 36.6). An intermediate degree of serum PRL elevation, 20–250 ng/mL, can result from several other conditions. The conditions that inhibit hypothalamic suppression of the lactotrophs by dopamine, such as distortion of the pituitary stalk, rarely cause serum PRL greater than 100 ng/mL, but elevations as high as 250 ng/mL occasionally occur. Medications can cause PRL levels greater than 100 ng/mL. Because there are numerous causes of hyperprolactinemia, the history and physical findings, blood chemistries, thyroid function tests and a pregnancy test should be reviewed to exclude nonhypothalamic–pituitary causes.

Stimulation of PRL secretion during the TRH-stimulation test is not sufficiently reliable for diagnosing the presence of a prolactinoma, but can provide information that supports this diagnosis. In normal subjects intravenous administration of TRH (200–500 µg) stimulates a three- to fivefold rise in serum prolac-

tin levels within an hour, whereas patients with a prolactinoma usually have a blunted response (less than a twofold increase) (Figure 36.7).

Prolactin deficiency

Deficiency of prolactin can cause failure of lactation, which is often one of the early indications of peripartum pituitary necrosis (Sheehan syndrome). Lymphocytic hypophysitis, an autoimmune pituitary disorder usually associated with hyperprolactinemia during the active phase and usually occuring during or immediately after pregnancy, also produces hypopituitarism. A blunted PRL response (less than a twofold increase in serum PRL over basal values) in the TRH-stimulation test, which heralds an inadequate lactotroph reserve, occurs in hypopituitarism.

Growth hormone

Physiology

GH is anabolic, lipolytic, and diabetogenic. Growth *in utero* and during the first year of life is independent of GH, the role of GH in growth being maximal at puberty. GH is required for normal linear growth and is secreted in pulses by the somatotrophs. Two hypothalamic peptides control the release of GH: (1) GHRH, which stimulates GH release; and (2) somatostatin, which inhibits GH secretion (Figure 36.8A). GH controls growth by stimulating the production and release of somatomedin-C (also known as insulin-like growth factor I; IGF-I) that is synthesized in the liver and other tissues. Changes in the serum concentration of somatomedin-C closely parallel GH deficiency or excess. Somatomedin-C exerts a negative feedback on GH release at the hypothalamus, where it stimulates somatostatin release, and at the

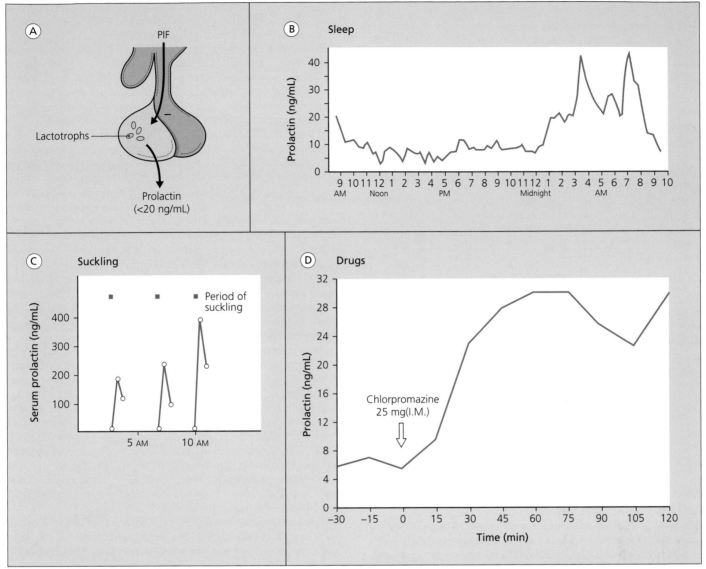

Figure 36.4 Normal control of prolactin secretion. **(A)** Lactotrophs of the anterior pituitary are primarily under inhibitory control of prolactin-inhibiting factor (PIF; probably dopamine). **(B)** Serum prolactin levels follow a diurnal pattern with increased levels several hours after the onset of sleep (data from Sassin JF, Frantz AG, Weitzman ED, Kapen S. Human prolactin: 24-hour pattern with increased release during sleep. *Science* 1972; 177:1205–07). Elevation in prolactin levels can be caused by a variety of stimuli, including suckling **(C)** (data from Hwang P, Guyda H, Friesen H. A radioimmunoassay for human prolactin. *Proc Natl Acad Sci USA* 1971; 68:1902–6) or medications such as chlorpromazine **(D)** (data from Sachar EJ. Hormonal changes in stress and mental illness. In: Krieger DT, Hughes JC (eds). *Neuroendocrinology*. Sunderland, MA: Sinauer Associates; 1980: 177–83).

pituitary, where it inhibits GH secretion and suppresses GHRH-induced GH release. Hypothalamic control also mediates various neurogenic, metabolic and hormonal influences on GH secretion. For instance, sleep, stress, arginine and exercise stimulate GH release, whereas hyperglycemia and obesity inhibit GH secretion (Figure 36.8B–D). Glucocorticoids inhibit somatic growth and suppress GHRH-induced GH release, a finding commonly seen in Cushing syndrome. Hypoglycemia reduces hypothalamic somatostatin release and is a potent trigger for GH secretion; this is the basis of a diagnostic test of GH reserve. Conversely, hyperglycemia blocks GH release. Elevation of free fatty acids suppresses GH release, and the converse is true. GH is anabolic and increases tissue uptake of amino acids. Therefore, elevation of amino acids increases GH discharge, which is the basis for the arginine infusion test for GH release.

In normal subjects serum GH is undetectable for most of the day. GH secretion is pulsatile, with between two and seven peaks per 24 hours. Although it is secreted in bursts associated with meals, much of the 24-hour secretion of GH occurs during the early stages of sleep. Since GH has a half-life in serum of only 20–30 minutes and is secreted in brief pulses, during the waking hours serum levels of GH fluctuate greatly (see Figure 36.8B). In contrast, the serum half-life of somatomedin-C is prolonged (3–18 hours) and serum levels of somatomedin-C are relatively stable. Thus, the serum level of somatomedin-C provides a more reliable indication of the exposure of the body to GH than does random determination of serum GH.

Excess growth hormone

Excess GH secretion, which results in excess growth of the

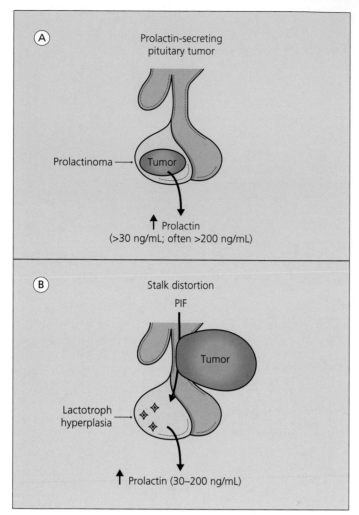

Figure 36.5 (A) Abnormal prolactin regulation. Prolactin-secreting adenomas (prolactinomas) can cause marked elevation of serum prolactin levels. **(B)** Distortion of the pituitary stalk by pathologic processes, such as tumors arising in the suprasellar region, can cause mild to moderate hyperprolactinemia.

soft tissues, bony changes and various biochemical effects linked to excess GH and somatomedin-C, produces the syndromes of acromegaly in adults (Figure 36.9) and gigantism in children (who are affected before epiphyseal closure). Evidence of acromegaly includes enlargement of the paranasal sinuses with frontal bossing and deepening of the voice; coarse facial features with prognathism and separation of the teeth with malocclusion; enlargement of the hands and feet requiring a change in shoe, glove and ring size; increased skin sweating, oiliness and areas of cutaneous pigmentation (acanthosis nigricans); hypertrichosis; and organomegaly. Tongue enlargement produces obstructive sleep apnea. Accumulation of excess soft tissue in the hands results in a wet, doughy handshake and in the feet it produces increased heel-pad thickness, which can be detected radiographically. Many patients have headaches. The insulin resistance associated with excess GH causes glucose intolerance and diabetes mellitus. Additional common accompaniments of acromegaly are proximal myopathy with weakness, osteoarthritis, carpal tunnel syndrome with nocturnal paresthesias and pain in the hands, and hypertension and cardiomegaly. The metabolic derangements lead to

accelerated atherosclerosis and a shortened life expectancy as a result of cardiovascular, cerebrovascular and respiratory causes.

Excess GH with acromegaly or gigantism almost always results from a GH-secreting pituitary adenoma. Because the average patient with acromegaly has had symptoms for 8–10 years before the diagnosis is made, most pituitary tumors are large. Many compress the optic system and produce loss of visual acuity or bitemporal hemianopsia by the time the tumor is recognized.

EVALUATION AND LABORATORY TESTING In a patient with suspected acromegaly or gigantism, endocrine evaluation includes measurement of basal GH and somatomedin-C levels and testing to assess suppression of GH secretion by hyperglycemia. Since exercise and stress stimulate GH secretion, serum GH levels are ideally obtained in the early morning, before the patient arises from bed, or 2 hours after a meal, when GH levels would normally be suppressed. GH is elevated to > 10 ng/mL in over 90% of patients with acromegaly. However, most patients have wide fluctuations in the serum levels of GH (Figure 36.10A) and some patients have levels between 5 and 10 ng/mL, or even, rarely, less than 5 ng/mL (Figure 36.10B). Thus, GH levels in patients with GH-secreting pituitary tumors may occasionally be within the range found in normal subjects. In patients with active acromegaly, the normal pulsatile GH secretory pattern is replaced by a consistent elevation of GH throughout the day. To confirm the diagnosis of acromegaly, a glucose suppression test is performed (Figure 36.10D), in an abnormal GH–glucose suppression test GH fails to suppress to < 2 μg/L (2 ng/mL) with glucose loading.

Somatomedin-C, with rare exceptions, is elevated in all acromegalics, including patients in whom basal or random serum GH levels are within the range considered normal (Figure 36.10C). Unlike GH, somatomedin-C is not affected by stress or physical exercise. Circulating somatomedin-C is bound to carrier proteins that regulate its function. Normal values of somatomedin-C are gender-specific, ranging from 0.34 to 2.0 U/mL in men and 0.45 to 2.2 U/mL in women. Its half-life is 2–4 hours.

Additional endocrine testing may be required to confirm the diagnosis of GH excess. TRH usually causes at least a 50% rise of GH in untreated acromegaly, whereas normal subjects generally have little change in serum GH in response to TRH injection (Figure 36.10E). This test is also used to identify patients who, despite normalized GH levels after pituitary surgery, have residual GH-secreting adenoma and are at risk for tumor recurrence.

Recently, measurement of plasma GHRH has become available. Acromegaly as a result of extra-central nervous system causes, ectopic acromegaly (e.g. islet tumor of the pancreas, bronchial carcinoid) results in a measurable level of GHRH in the circulation, whereas in other forms of acromegaly GHRH is barely detectable.

Insulin-like growth-factor binding proteins (IGFBPs) are relatively new in the diagnosis of acromegaly. IGF circulates in the blood bound to IGFBPs. Of the four IGFBPs identified, IGFBP-1 and IGFBP-3 are most relevant to acromegaly. IGFBP-1 is inversely related to GH levels, while IGFBP-3 correlates directly with GH levels.

Since patients with acromegaly often have large tumors, evaluation of patients who prove to have excess GH secretion also includes magnetic resonance imaging (MRI) or the sella, formal visual field assessment, and endocrine testing for hypopituitarism.

Acromegaly can also be caused, rarely, by an ectopic GHRH-secreting tumor. In acromegalic patients who do not have a discrete pituitary tumor on MRI, and in patients in whom tissue

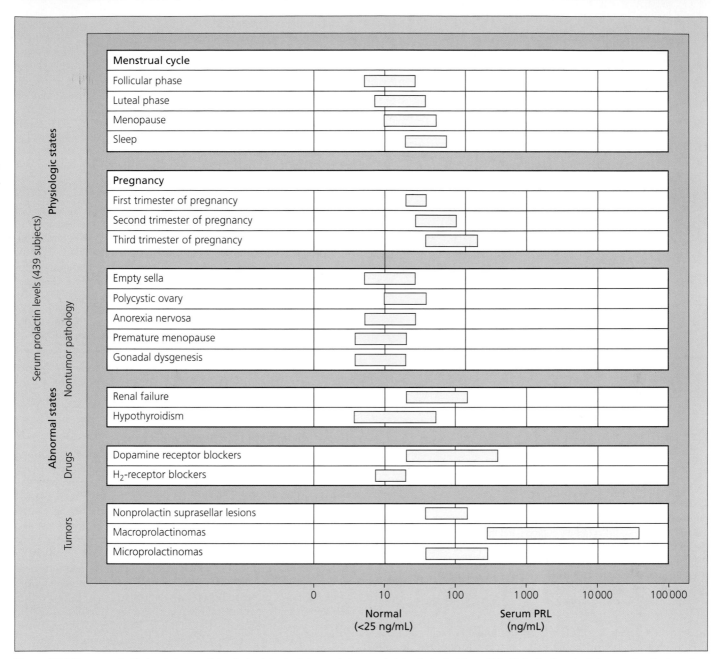

Figure 36.6 Serum prolactin levels in a variety of physiologic states and abnormal states (adapted from Tolis G. Prolactin: physiology and pathology. In: Krieger DT, Hughes JC (eds). *Neuroendocrinology*. Sunderland, MA: Sinauer Associates; 1980; 321–30).

from surgery indicates somatotroph hyperplasia, serum GHRH should be measured.

Growth hormone deficiency

Although adult GH deficiency is clinically silent, GH deficiency in children produces dwarfism. Random GH levels are rarely helpful in assessing GH deficiency. Serum somatomedin-C levels are useful (see Figure 36.10C) if they are interpreted with consideration of the age-related differences of normal values. Therefore the diagnosis of GH deficiency is dependent on the demonstration of a subnormal rise in serum GH in response to one or more dynamic stimulation tests. Options include the insulin tolerance test, glucagon test, arginine stimulation and combinations of arginine

and GHRH or GH secretagogs. Of these possibilities, the best validated is the insulin tolerance test which has been demonstrated to distinguish reliably between the GH responses of patients with structural pituitary disease and those of age-matched controls across the adult age range. A variety of serum GH cut-off points has been used to define GH deficiency. However, an international consensus (convened by the Growth Hormone Research Society) has defined severe GH deficiency in adults as a peak response to insulin-induced hypoglycemia of < 9 mU/L (< 3 ng/mL).

Additional tests include stimulation of GH secretion with exercise (brisk exercise for 20 minutes with GH levels at 0, 20 and 40 minutes) or with clonidine (dose adjusted for body concentrations (Figure 36.11C), and in response to emotional, biochemical and physical stressors.

The hypothalamic–pituitary–adrenal axis is regulated by the balance between the stimuli for secretion of CRH, ACTH and cortisol and the inhibition (negative feedback) of cortisol on production and secretion of CRH and ACTH, and by suppression of CRH-induced ACTH secretion (see Figure 36.11A).

ACTH and cortisol secretion are pulsatile. ACTH levels decline over the morning and reach a nadir in the evening. ACTH secretion is also regulated by circadian rhythms and therefore is affected by light and by major time-zone shifts. Stresses such as trauma, major surgery, hypoglycemia and fever increase ACTH and cortisol secretion. The bioactive half-life of ACTH is 4–8 minutes, whereas its immunoreactive half-life is variable.

Glucocorticoids increase gluconeogenesis, and inhibit glucose uptake and utilization by peripheral tissues. Lipolysis is enhanced, and body fat redistribution occurs with alteration in body habitus. Glucocorticoids decrease peripheral lymphocytes and monocytes and suppress the inflammatory response but increase the level of circulating granulocytes. Glucocorticoids increase osteoclast formation but inhibit osteoblasts and decrease new bone formation. Their catabolic effect on muscle protein results in the myopathy of hypercortisolism. Linear growth in children is suppressed. Fibroblast proliferation and function is inhibited, as is the synthesis of some extracellular matrix components, the net clinical effect is impaired wound healing. Glucocorticoids have behavioral effects, for example alteration of mood, sleep, and cognition.

Hypercortisolism (Cushing syndrome)

Prolonged excess exposure to cortisol produces Cushing syndrome (Figure 36.12). Several different processes can cause Cushing syndrome (Table 36.3, Figure 36.13), therefore establishing the specific cause can occasionally be difficult. Late evening plasma levels (normally 5–25 ng/mL) are elevated, early morning plasma cortisol levels may be normal, but the circadian rhythm is lost and mean plasma cortisol is elevated. The chronic hypercortisolemia suppresses hypothalamic CRH and inhibits ACTH secretion by the normal corticotrophs, which atrophy. Plasma free cortisol is filtered into saliva and urine, and these levels are more sensitive indicators of increased cortisol secretion than urinary 17-hydroxysteroids because they increase more rapidly after the plasma cortisol exceeds the binding capacity of transcortin. Cortisol urinary excretion products, 24-hour urinary free cortisol levels are elevated (normal 20–90 μg; Cushing syndrome > 150 μg) as are some of its metabolites, 17-hydroxysteroids (normally under 12 mg/day), and some of its precursors, 17-ketosteroids and dihydroepiandrosterone sulfate.

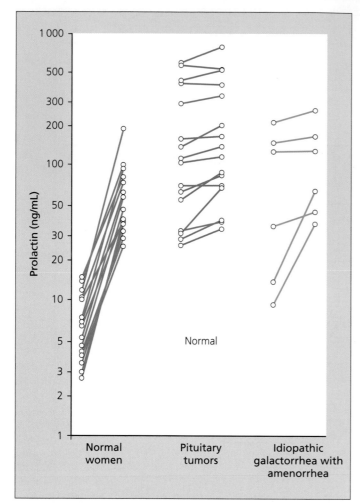

Figure 36.7 Serum prolactin before and after administration of TRH, 500 mg intravenously, in normal subjects and in patients with galactorrhea, due to either a prolactinoma or idiopathic galactorrhea with amenorrhea (data from Kleinberg DL, Noel GL, Frantz AG. Galactorrhea: a study of 235 cases, including 48 with pituitary tumors. *N Engl J Med* 1977; 296: 589–600).

weight, GH levels at 0, 60 and 90 minutes), which stimulates GH levels to ≥ 7 ng/mL in normal subjects but does not do so in those with GH deficiency.

Pituitary–adrenal axis

Physiology

Cortisol is necessary for the maintenance of life and for the homeostatic biochemical and physiological responses to stress. The hypothalamic–pituitary–adrenal axis regulates cortisol secretion (Figure 36.11A). The adrenal glands secrete cortisol in response to ACTH. The corticotrophs synthesize and store ACTH as a portion of a larger prohormone, pro-opiomelanocortin (Figure 36.11B). As ACTH is cleaved from pro-opiomelanocortin and secreted, β-lipoprotein, also a component of pro-opiomelanocortin, is secreted simultaneously.

CRH stimulates pituitary ACTH production and secretion. Hypothalamic secretion of CRH occurs in response to signals from the brain to produce the circadian rhythm of plasma cortisol

Table 36.3 Etiology of Cushing syndrome

ACTH-dependent	85%	ACTH-independent	15%
Cushing's disease	80–85%	Adrenal adenoma	7%
Ectopic ACTH-secreting tumor	15–20%	Adrenocortical carcinoma	7%
Ectopic CRH-secreting tumor	Rare	Primary adrenal nodular hyperplasia	Rare
Diffuse corticotroph hyperplasia	Rare		

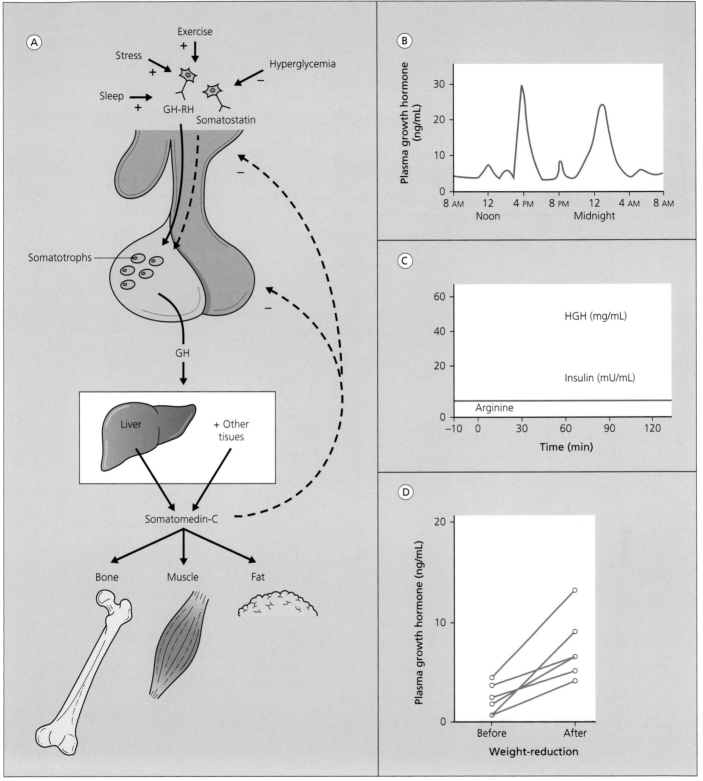

Figure 36.8 Regulation of growth hormone secretion. **(A)** Hypothalamic–pituitary axis. Somatotrophs of the anterior pituitary are stimulated to release GH by GHRH and are inhibited by somatostatin. Stress, exercise, sleep rhythms and hyperglycemia modify GH secretion. Somatomedin-C exerts negative feedback on GH release at the pituitary and hypothalamus. **(B)** Plasma GH levels fluctuate during a 24-hour period with peaks related to stress, exercise and sleep. **(C)** Arginine infusion stimulates GH secretion. **(D)** Obesity suppresses GH secretion. Peak plasma GH levels during arginine infusion are shown for patients before and after weight reduction (data from El-Khodary AZ, Ball MF, Stein B, *et al*. Effect of weight loss on the growth hormone response to arginine infusion in obesity. *J Clin Endocrinol Metab* 1971; 32: 42–51).

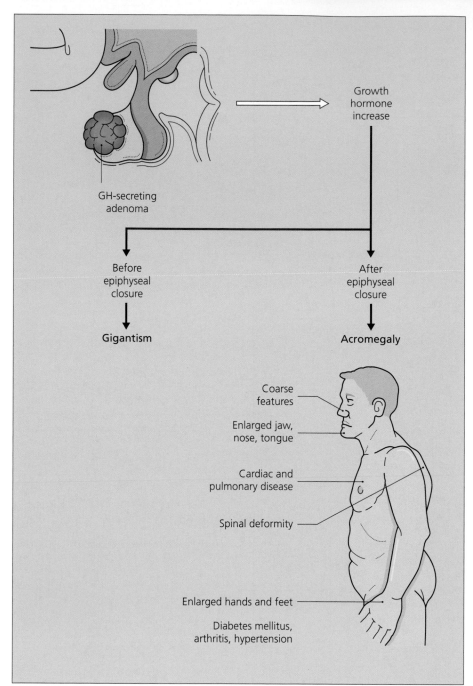

Figure 36.9 Clinical manifestations of acromegaly.

Evaluation and laboratory testing The first step in the differential diagnosis is to establish that the patient has abnormal, excess secretion of cortisol (Table 36.4). This is accomplished by tests that (1) directly or indirectly measure cortisol production over 24 hours, by 24-hour urine collection for free cortisol and 17-hydroxyglucocorticoid excretion (Figure 36.14A,B), and (2) assess whether normal sensitivity of the hypothalamic–pituitary–adrenal axis to negative feedback by glucocorticoids is present (Figure 36.14C), using one of the low-dose glucocorticoid tests (the overnight test or the low-dose portion of the 6-day dexamethasone suppression test). Furthermore, since in Cushing syndrome the diurnal rhythm of the plasma cortisol levels is disturbed, plasma cortisol levels between 06.00 and 08.00 h and 23.00 and 01.00 h reveal the loss of the normal circadian rhythm in patients with Cushing syndrome.

If the results of the tests described above indicate that the patient has Cushing syndrome, the final portion of the diagnostic assessment – establishing the specific cause of Cushing syndrome – is performed. For the differential diagnosis of Cushing syndrome the causes are classified as ACTH-dependent processes, which cause Cushing syndrome by excess secretion of ACTH (ACTH-secreting pituitary tumors, ectopic ACTH-secreting tumors, diffuse corticotroph hyperplasia, and ectopic CRH secretion), or ACTH-independent processes, which cause Cushing syndrome by a primary process of excess cortisol secretion (cortisol-secreting adrenal disease) (see Table 36.4). Since the hypothalamic and

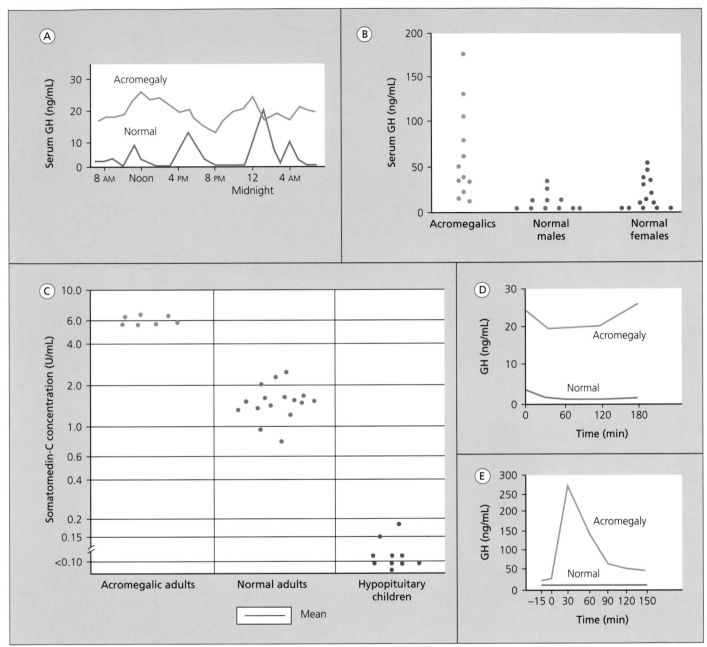

Figure 36.10 Evaluation of patients suspected of having excess GH secretion. **(A)** GH levels fluctuate widely in acromegalics and normal subjects over 24 hours (data from Carlson HE. The diagnosis of acromegaly. In: Robbins RJ, Melmed S (eds). *Acromegaly: A Century of Scientific and Clinical Progress*. New York: Plenum Press; 1987: 197–208). **(B)** Acromegalics may have low GH levels that overlap with those of normal subjects (data from Carlson HE. The diagnosis of acromegaly. In: Robbins RJ, Melmed S (eds). *Acromegaly: A Century of Scientific and Clinical Progress*. New York: Plenum Press; 1987: 197–208). **(C)** Thus, somatomedin-C levels more reliably distinguish acromegalics from normal subjects (data from Van Wyk JJ, Underwood LE. Growth hormone, somatomedins and growth failure. In: Krieger DT, Hughes JC (eds). *Neuroendocrinology*. Sunderland, MA: Sinauer Associates; 1980: 299–309). **(D)** GH levels are suppressed after an oral glucose load in normal subjects but not in acromegalics, who, paradoxically, may have a rise in GH level (data from Raiti S, Tolman RA (eds). *Human Growth Hormone*. New York: Plenum Medical Book Co; 1986). **(E)** TRH stimulates a rise in GH levels in acromegalics but not normal subjects (data from Raiti S, Tolman RA (eds). *Human Growth Hormone*. New York: Plenum Medical Book Co; 1986).

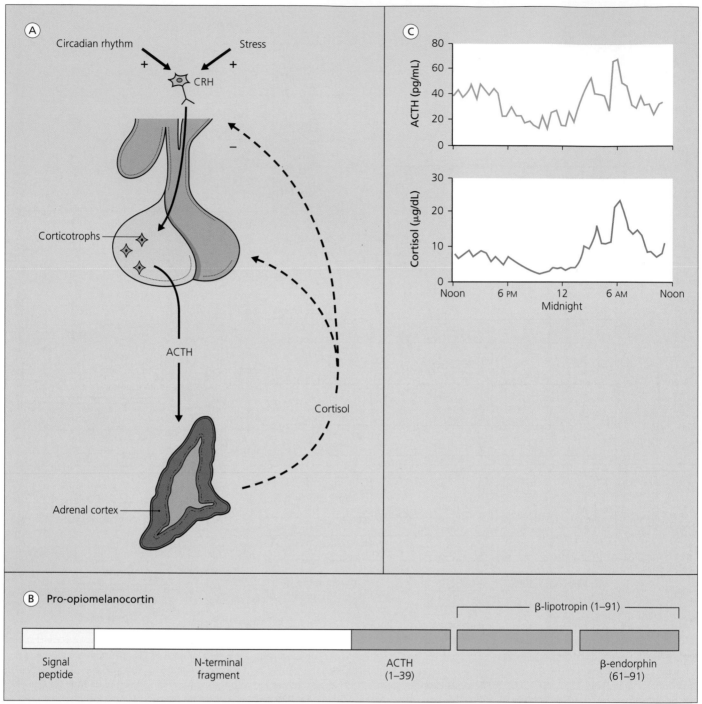

Figure 36.11 Regulation of cortisol secretion. **(A)** Regulation of the hypothalamic–pituitary–adrenal axis. CRH is released by the hypothalamus to stimulate the corticotrophs of the anterior pituitary to secrete adrenocorticotropic hormone (ACTH), which stimulates cortisol secretion from the adrenal cortex. Cortisol exerts negative feedback at the pituitary and hypothalamus. **(B)** Schematic representation of pro-opiomelanocortin, the prohormone from which ACTH is cleaved. **(C)** The circadian rhythm of serum ACTH and cortisol levels (data from Tanaka K, Nicholson WE, Orth DN. Diurnal rhythm and disappearance half-time of endogenous plasma immunoreactive B-MSH (LPH) and ACTH in man. *J Clin Endocrinol Metab* 1978; 46: 883–90).

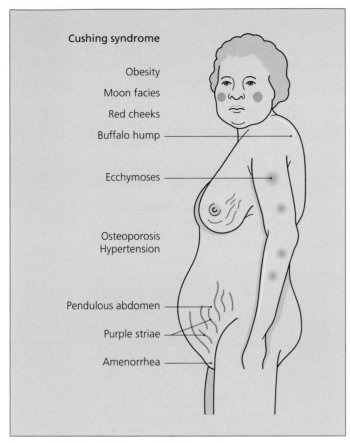

Cushing syndrome

Obesity

Moon facies

Red cheeks

Buffalo hump

Ecchymoses

Osteoporosis
Hypertension

Pendulous abdomen

Purple striae

Amenorrhea

Figure 36.12 Clinical features of Cushing syndrome.

Table 36.4 Clinical approach to patients suspected of having Cushing syndrome

I Establish presence of Cushing syndrome
A Establish hypercortisolism
  24-hour urinary free cortisol
  or
  24-hour urinary 17-hydroxysteroid per gram of urinary creatinine
B Establish resistance to dexamethasone suppression
  Overnight low-dose (1 mg) dexamethasone suppression test

II Differential diagnosis of Cushing syndrome
A Distinguish between ACTH-independent and ACTH-dependent types of Cushing syndrome
  1 Plasma ACTH
B ACTH-independent Cushing syndrome (adrenal disease)
  1 Adrenal CT or MRI
C ACTH-dependent Cushing syndrome
  1 CRH stimulation test
  2 High-dose dexamethasone suppression test
    a Overnight high-dose (8 mg)
    or
    b 6-day low-dose, high-dose test (Liddle)
  3 Bilateral petrosal vein sampling for ACTH (with and without CRH)
D Confirm diagnosis
  1 If tests indicate Cushing's disease: pituitary MRI
  2 If tests indicate ectopic ACTH secretion: MRI of chest and abdomen

---

pituitary portions of the adrenal axis are normal with primary adrenal disease, hypercortisolism suppresses pituitary ACTH secretion and plasma ACTH levels are either undetectable or very low (Figure 36.15; see Fig. 36.13). In contrast, since the ACTH-dependent forms of Cushing syndrome act via excess ACTH secretion, with the ACTH-dependent etiologies the plasma ACTH levels are inappropriately elevated for the level of cortisol secretion (see Figures 36.13 and 36.15). Thus, the ACTH-independent and ACTH-dependent forms are distinguished by the level of plasma ACTH in the presence of hypercortisolism. If cortisol is ACTH-dependent, then the ACTH assay shows increased or high–normal levels (normal < 10 pg/mL, 2 pmol/L) as in Cushing's disease, a high plasma ACTH is also seen in ectopic ACTH-producing tumors. A simultaneous plasma cortisol measurement is necessary to evaluate properly the plasma ACTH.

In almost 100% of patients with adrenal tumors, the most common form of ACTH-independent Cushing syndrome, adrenal imaging with MRI or computed tomography (CT) scanning identifies the adrenal tumor as the source of the excess cortisol secretion. Thus, the combined results of the plasma ACTH levels and adrenal imaging are used either to diagnose a primary adrenal disorder or to eliminate primary adrenal disease as the etiology.

Differential diagnosis of ACTH-dependent Cushing syndrome

Because of the very small size of most ACTH-secreting pituitary tumors and ectopic ACTH-secreting tumors, the differential diagnosis in patients with ACTH-dependent Cushing syndrome is often not obvious. The differential diagnosis of patients with ACTH-dependent Cushing syndrome is based on endocrinologic and anatomic principles. (1) ACTH-secreting pituitary adenomas are well-differentiated tumors that originate from pituitary corticotrophs. They are more likely to retain the negative-feedback response to glucocorticoids (dexamethasone suppression) and to respond to CRH stimulation than the ectopic ACTH-secreting tumors, which arise from tissues that do not normally secrete ACTH, respond to negative feedback by glucocorticoids, or contain receptors for CRH. (2) The source of excess ACTH secretion must be localized [inferior petrosal sinus sampling (IPSS) and radiographic imaging]. Thus, the high-dose, 8-mg overnight dexamethasone suppression test (Figure 36.16A) or the high-dose portion of the 6-day dexamethasone suppression test, the Liddle test (Figure 36.16B), the CRH stimulation test (Figure 36.16C), bilateral catheterization and simultaneous sampling of the inferior petrosal sinuses for ACTH concentrations (Figure 36.16D,E), and high-resolution imaging of the pituitary with MRI before and after contrast enhancement with gadolinium are used today to determine the differential diagnosis of Cushing syndrome.

The low-dose dexamethasone suppression test differentiates patients with Cushing syndrome of any cause from those without hypercortisolism. In the overnight, or standard 2-day, low-dose dexamethasone suppression test, an oral dose of 0.5 mg (low-dose) of dexamethasone in normal individuals will suppress the ACTH–adrenal axis; therefore, serum cortisol levels are less than 140 nmol (5 µg/dL), urinary 17-hydroxysteroids are less than 6.9 µmol (2.5 mg)/24 h, and urinary free cortisol is less than 55 nmol (20 µg)/24 h. Patients with Cushing syndrome do not show suppression. In the 2-mg (high-dose) dexamethasone suppression test, most patients with Cushing's disease should suppress their parameters by more than 50% of baseline. An ectopic source of ACTH or an adrenal tumor will not be significantly suppressed by either the high or low doses.

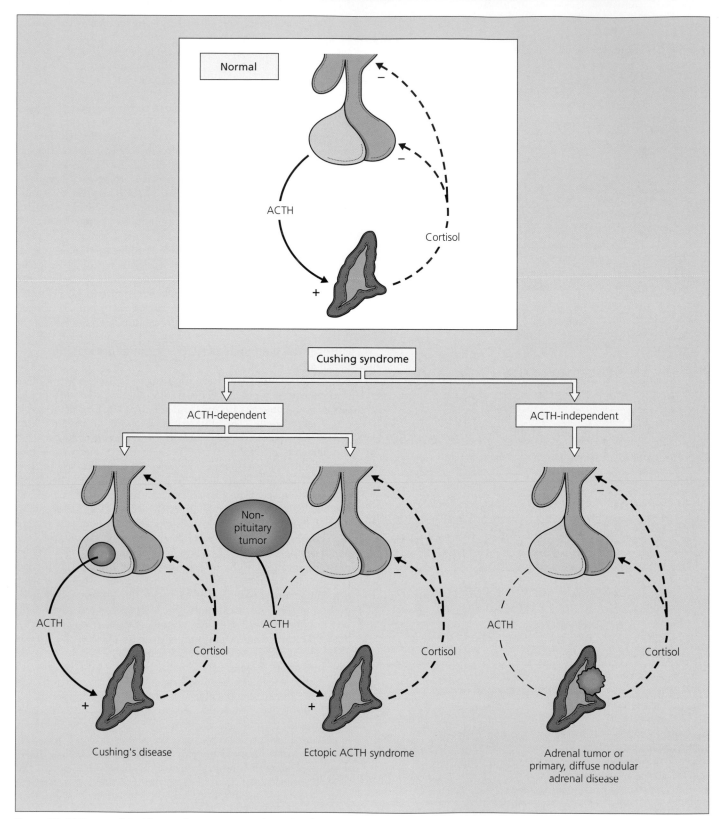

Figure 36.13 Causes of Cushing syndrome. In ACTH-dependent hypercortisolism, cortisol secretion is excessive in response to ACTH secretion by either a corticotroph pituitary adenoma or a nonpituitary (ectopic) tumor. In ACTH-independent hypercortisolism, there is autonomous overproduction of cortisol because of an adrenal gland abnormality.

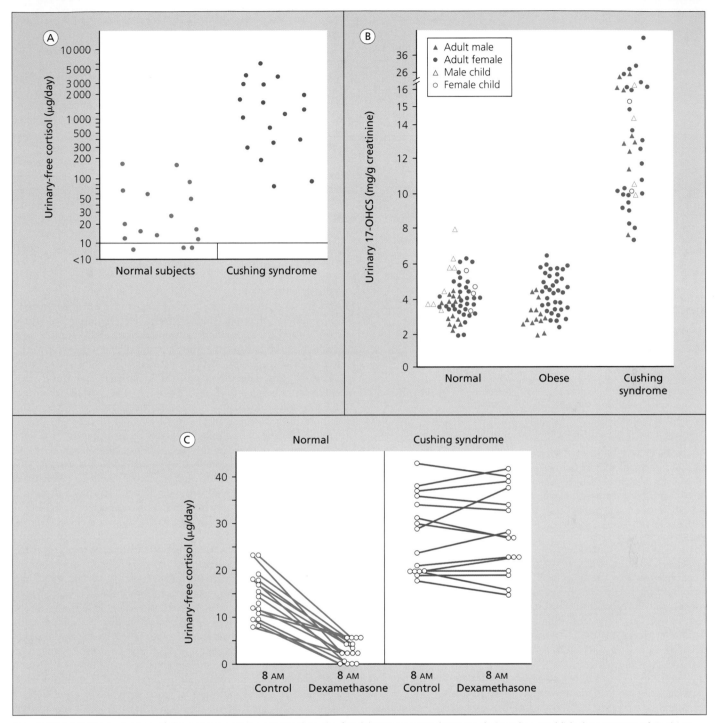

Figure 36.14 In the evaluation of the patient with hypercortisolism the first laboratory procedures are designed to establish the presence of Cushing syndrome. Cortisol production is measured by 24-hour urinary free cortisol excretion **(A)** (data from Loriaux DL, Cutler GB Jr. Disease of the adrenal glands. In: Kohler PO (ed.). *Clinical Endocrinology*. New York: John Wiley & Sons; 1986) and 24-hour urinary 17-hydroxysteroid excretion **(B)** (data from Streeten DHP, Stevenson CT, Dalakos TG, *et al*. The diagnosis of hypercortisolism: biochemical criteria differentiating patients from lean and obese normal subjects and from females on oral contraceptives. *J Clin Endocrinol Metab* 1969; 29: 1191–211), and by dexamethasone suppression testing. **(C)** In the overnight low-dose dexamethasone suppression test, plasma cortisol levels are measured at 08.00 h on two successive days before and after 1 mg of dexamethasone is taken orally at 23.00 h on the first day. The lack of suppression in patients with Cushing syndrome contrasts with the response of normal subjects (adapted from Melby JC. Assessment of adrenocortical function. *N Engl J Med* 1971; 285: 735–9).

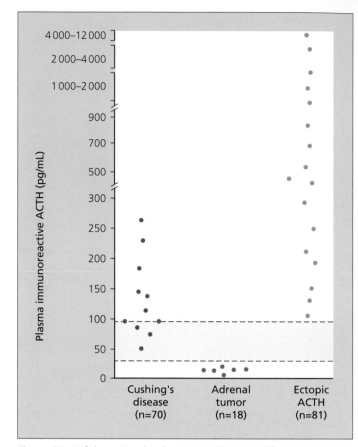

Figure 36.15 If the patient has hypercortisolism, the differential diagnosis of the etiology of Cushing syndrome must be established. Initially, this is accomplished by distinguishing ACTH-dependent and ACTH-independent causes by measuring plasma ACTH levels and by evaluating the adrenal glands for an adrenal tumor with CT or MRI (data from Besser GM, Edwards CRW. Cushing's syndrome. *Clin Endocrinol Metab* 1972; 1: 451–90).

The CRH, or arginine vasopressin, test may differentiate Cushing's disease from ectopic ACTH secretion. CRH and arginine vasopressin are physiologic secretagogs and most micro-adenomas will respond. In Cushing's disease, there is a significant rise in ACTH following administration of CRH, whereas in patients with ectopic ACTH secretion and adrenal tumors, ACTH fails to respond to CRH. CRH can also be administered during petrosal sinus sampling.

The IPSS test was developed to establish a pituitary origin for Cushing's disease in patients with negative results on MRI or CT scans and to lateralize the tumor within the gland by establishing a differential in ACTH levels between the left and right sinuses draining the pituitary gland. Because of the episodic pattern of ACTH release, samples may not be drawn at the precise moment of a spontaneous secretory episode; therefore, the yield from the study can be enhanced by peripheral intravenous injection of CRH to stimulate a secretory episode. CRH also releases PRL, which can be a useful adjunctive measurement.

Most patients receive a combination of these tests. In addition to being important tests for the differential diagnosis of Cushing syndrome, in patients with Cushing's disease the IPSS test and MRI often provide information that localizes a small ACTH-secreting tumor within the pituitary gland. The latter information is helpful during pituitary surgery, since these tumors are often so

small that they are difficult to localize during exploratory transsphenoidal procedures.

It is critical to establish the presence of Cushing syndrome before proceeding with the differential diagnostic portion of the evaluation described above. Since in subjects without Cushing syndrome ACTH secretion from the pituitary is suppressed by dexamethasone and responds to CRH and the concentration of ACTH is greater in IPSS than in peripheral blood, the results of these endocrine tests will suggest, erroneously, Cushing's disease, potentially resulting in pituitary surgery in a normal subject.

In patients with Cushing's disease who are treated by bilateral adrenalectomy, the loss of the suppressive effects of the excess cortisol on tumor ACTH secretion and growth results in very high levels of plasma ACTH, levels frequently sufficient to increase both skin pigmentation and the progression of the ACTH-secreting pituitary tumor, which occasionally becomes invasive or even metastatic. This clinical condition is known as Nelson syndrome.

Hypocortisolism

Adrenocortical insufficiency causes weakness, anorexia, nausea and vomiting, abdominal pain, weight loss, hypotension, hypo-natremia, and the incapacity to respond to stressful stimuli. It is classified on the basis of whether it results from a disorder of the adrenal gland (primary adrenocortical insufficiency – Addison's disease) or from a disturbance of the hypothalamic–pituitary axis (secondary adrenocortical insufficiency). The adrenal disorders tend to produce more severe and life-threatening symptoms and are more likely to result in disturbance in salt metabolism (hypo-natremia, hyperkalemia and hypovolemia as a result of absent aldosterone secretion). In the past, tuberculous infection of the adrenals was the most common cause of Addison's disease, but today primary adrenal insufficiency is more likely to result from autoimmune disorders that produce adrenal atrophy (idiopathic adrenal atrophy), other types of granulomatous infection, adrenal hemorrhage associated with severe stress, or after surgical removal of both adrenals.

Although secondary adrenocortical insufficiency occurs with hypothalamic–pituitary disorders that produce panhypopitui-tarism, ACTH secretion is the most resistant to loss of all the pituitary hormones. Thus, selective pituitary ACTH insufficiency is uncommon. The exception is the selective ACTH deficiency that occurs with prolonged hypercortisolism associated with glucocorticoid administration or with the excess endogenous production of glucocorticoids in Cushing syndrome. Prolonged hypercortisolism, whether endogenous or exogenous, suppresses hypothalamic CRH secretion and pituitary ACTH secretion such that after the excess exposure to glucocorticoids is eliminated it requires 6–24 months for the hypothalamic–pituitary–adrenal axis to resume normal function and for recovery of the normal response to CRH and ACTH. In these circumstances hypo-cortisolism is only evident after withdrawal of prolonged glucocorticoid therapy or after successful treatment of Cushing syndrome.

EVALUATION AND LABORATORY TESTING In severe adrenal insufficiency, cortisol secretion (assessed by morning plasma cortisol levels and 24-hour urine collections for free cortisol and 17-hydroxysteroids) is low. However, basal cortisol secretion may be in the low–normal range in even moderately severe hypo-adrenalism. Thus, dynamic testing is usually required to detect and confirm adrenal insufficiency.

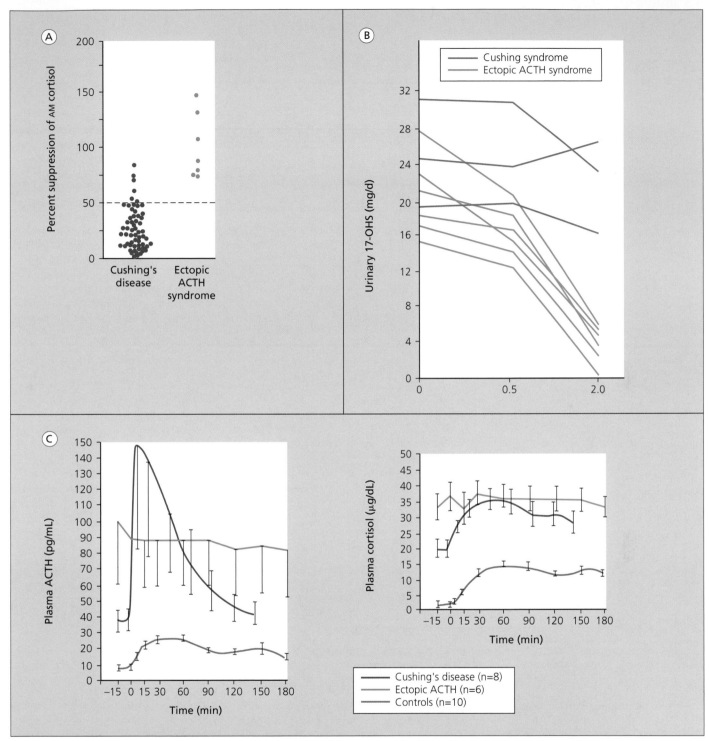

Figure 36.16 With ACTH-dependent Cushing syndrome, the differential diagnosis of Cushing's disease (ACTH-secreting pituitary adenoma) versus ectopic ACTH syndrome is made with one or more of the following tests: high-dose dexamethasone suppression test, either the overnight suppression test **(A)** (data from Tyrrell JB, Findling JW, Aron DC, Fitzgerald PA, Forsham PH. An overnight high-dose dexamethasone suppression test for rapid differential diagnosis of Cushing syndromes. *Ann Intern Med* 1986; 104: 180–6), or the Liddle test **(B)**; **(C)** the CRH stimulation test (data from Chrousos GP, *et al.* The corticotropin-releasing factor stimulation test: an aid in the evaluation of patients with Cushing syndrome. *N Engl J Med* 1984; 310: 622–6). *Continued*

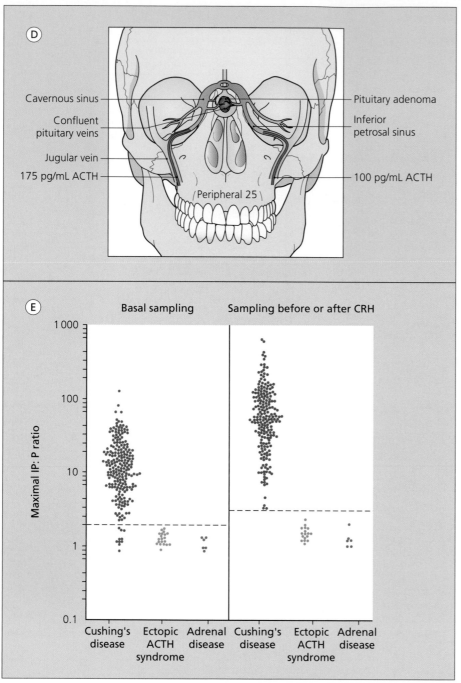

Figure 36.16, *cont'd*. With ACTH-dependent Cushing syndrome, the differential diagnosis of Cushing's disease (ACTH-secreting pituitary adenoma) versus ectopic ACTH syndrome is made with one or more of the following tests: **(D)** anatomy and catheter placement in bilateral simultaneous blood sampling of the inferior petrosal sinuses (data from Oldfield EH, Chrousos GP, Schulte HM, *et al.* Preoperative lateralization of ACTH-secreting micro-adenomas by bilateral and simultaneous inferior petrosal sinus sampling. *N Engl J Med* 1985; 312: 100–3); **(E)** bilateral inferior petrosal vein sampling in the differential diagnosis of Cushing syndrome; maximum ratio of ACTH concentration from one of the inferior petrosal sinuses to the simultaneous peripheral venous ACTH concentration in patients with Cushing syndrome in basal samples (left) and in basal and CRH-stimulated samples (right) (data from Oldfield EH, Doppman JL, Nieman LK, *et al.* Bilateral petrosal sinus sampling with and without corticotropin-releasing hormone for the differential diagnosis of Cushing syndrome. *N Engl J Med* 1991; 325: 897–905).

Since the adrenal cortex atrophies without normal ACTH stimulation, the response to ACTH stimulation in primary or secondary adrenal insufficiency is suppressed. In the short ACTH stimulation test 0.25 mg (25 units) of cosyntropin, a synthetic short form of ACTH (α^{1-24}-ACTH), which retains the biological activity of ACTH, is injected intravenously or intramuscularly and plasma cortisol is measured just before and at 30 and 60 minutes after injection. An increment of ≥ 7 µg/dL over basal levels or a peak value ≥ 20 µg/dL is expected in normal subjects. In contrast, patients with longstanding ACTH deficiency or suppression have a definite, but blunted, response, and patients with primary adrenal insufficiency generally have no response. When the diagnosis of adrenal insufficiency is confirmed, basal plasma ACTH measurements and the CRH stimulation test are used to establish the location and etiology of the disorder (Figure 36.17). In primary adrenal insufficiency, because diminished cortisol production provides reduced negative feedback of the pituitary corticotrophs, basal plasma ACTH levels are high (Figure 36.17A) and the ACTH response to CRH is exaggerated (Figure 36.17B). On the other hand, with pituitary disease, or after prolonged excess glucocorticoid exposure, basal plasma ACTH levels are low and do not respond, or respond minimally, to CRH infusion.

Glycoprotein hormones

The glycoprotein pituitary hormones, TSH, FSH and LH are comprised of two glycopeptide chains, an α-chain common to all and a unique β-chain (Figure 36.18). The α- and β-chains are synthesized separately, and join to form the functional dimer. There is normally slight excess production of the α-chain, which is secreted alone, and which can be detected in the serum by radioimmunoassay.

Pituitary–thyroid axis

Physiology

Production and secretion of the thyroid hormones, thyroxine (T_4) and tri-iodothyronine (T_3), are regulated via hypothalamic secretion of TRH into the portal venous system. In response to TRH the thyrotropes release TSH, which acts on the thyroid gland to release T_4 and T_3. Both T_3 and T_4 inhibit TRH secretion by the hypothalamus and TSH release by the pituitary (Figure 36.19). Somatostatin, glucocorticoids and dopamine also suppress TRH release and suppress the TSH response to TRH.

Hyperthyroidism

Hyperthyroidism causes tremulousness, anxiety, heat intolerance, diarrhea and changes in mental status. The majority of hyperthyroid patients have either a circulating "thyroid-stimulating" antibody, a thyroid adenoma, or thyroiditis. These disturbances elevate the serum levels of free T_4, which results in low plasma TSH measurements in screening tests for thyroid function (Figure 36.20A). Because of the negative feedback of the excess thyroid hormones on the pituitary thyrotrophs, hyperthyroidism also suppresses the TSH response to TRH stimulation (Figure 36.20B), which helps to confirm hyperthyroidism in a minimally symptomatic patient.

Hypersecretion of TSH by a pituitary adenoma is a rare cause of hyperthyroidism (less than 1% of patients) (Figure 36.21A). In TSH-secreting tumors the production of α- and β-subunits is sufficiently imbalanced that excess α-subunit is secreted, which produces a ratio of plasma α-subunit (mol/L) to plasma TSH (mol/L) greater than 1.0 (Figure 36.21B). In a patient with hyperthyroidism, or a patient with a pituitary tumor who has had thyroid treatment for hyperthyroidism, an elevated TSH level combined with a ratio of the molar concentration of α-subunit to TSH greater than 1.0 indicates the presence of a TSH-secreting pituitary adenoma and calls for further evaluation of the pituitary. Many TSH-secreting pituitary tumors also secrete GH or PRL. Table 36.5 summarizes the expected findings on thyroid screening tests.

Since hyperthyroidsim is common and TSH-secreting tumors are very rare, many patients with TSH-secreting pituitary tumors are initially misdiagnosed and receive ablative therapy of the thyroid gland. Thus, they may not have hyperthyroidism when the pituitary tumor is recognized (see Figure 36.21). In these patients the high plasma TSH levels do not fully suppress when the patient is given thyroid hormone and the TSH response to TRH is blunted. Because of the delay in diagnosis, TSH-secreting pituitary adenomas are often large, invasive tumors by the time they are recognized. In patients who receive thyroid ablation as treatment for hyperthyroidism, the evolution to a large and invasive tumor seems to be analogous to the circumstance that occurs in Nelson syndrome with the ACTH-secreting tumors after adrenalectomy.

Hypothyroidism

The signs and symptoms of hypothyroidism include fatigue, dry skin, cold intolerance, alopecia and, in severe cases, progression to myxedema coma. The majority of patients with hypothyroidism have primary hypothyroidism as a result of failed thyroid gland function. This most often results from autoimmune Hashimoto's thyroiditis or from thyroid destruction after ^{131}I therapy or surgery for hyperthyroidism. In these conditions of primary hypothyroidism, the absence of the feedback inhibition of the thyroid hormones on the pituitary and hypothalamus typically results in increased TRH secretion and elevated TSH levels (Figure 36.22A). In untreated patients the increased TRH secretion stimulates thyrotroph hyperplasia and, in some instances, pituitary enlargement. Since the TRH also stimulates PRL secretion, these patients may be misdiagnosed as having a PRL-secreting or a TSH-secreting tumor and may, mistakenly, receive pituitary surgery.

Table 36.5 Thyroid screening tests

	Free T_4	TSH
Hypothyroidism		
Primary	↓	↑
Secondary (pituitary)	↓	↓
Hyperthyroidism		
Primary	↑	↓
Secondary (pituitary)	↑	↑

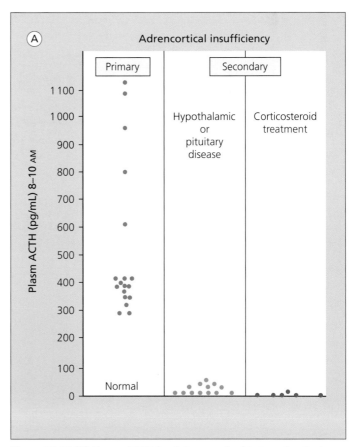

Figure 36.17 (A) Plasma ACTH levels in normal subjects and patients with primary and secondary adrenal cortical insufficiency (data from Rees LH, Holdaway IM, Phenekos C, *et al.* ACTH secretion and clinical investigations. In: *Some Aspects of Hypothalamic Regulation of Endocrine Functions: Symposium, Vienna, June 3–6, 1973.* Stuttgart: F Schattaur Verlag; 1974: 451–63). *Continued*

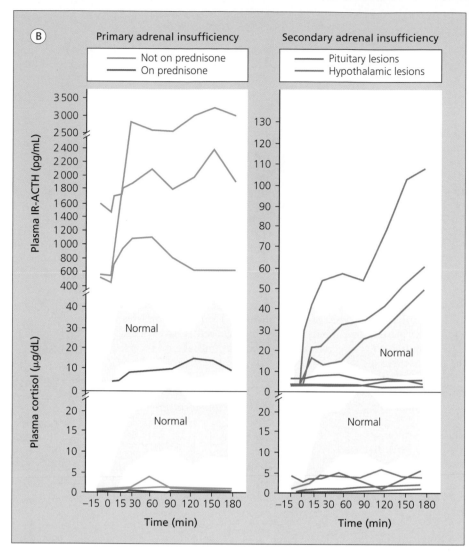

Figure 36.17, *cont'd.* (B) CRH stimulation test in adrenal insufficiency. Plasma ACTH (top) and cortisol (bottom) responses to oCRH (1 µg/kg UV) in patients with primary (left) and secondary (right) adrenal insufficiency (data from Schulte HM, Chrousos GP, Avgerinos PC, Oldfield EH, Gold PW, Cutler GB Jr, Loriaux DL. The corticotropin-releasing factor stimulation test: an aid in the evaluation of patients with adrenal insufficiency. *J Clin Endocrinol Metab* 1984; 58: 1064–7).

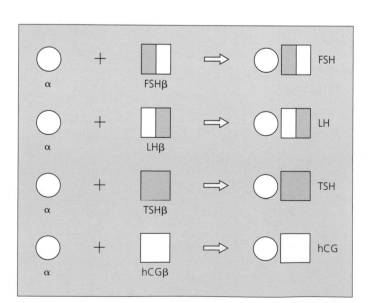

Figure 36.18 Glycoprotein hormones. Follicle-stimulating hormone (FSH), luteinizing hormone (LH), thyroid-stimulating hormone (TSH), and human chorionic gonadotropic hormone (hCG) have a common α-subunit but a unique β-subunit, which confers binding specificity. The α- and β-subunits are linked by hydrogen binding.

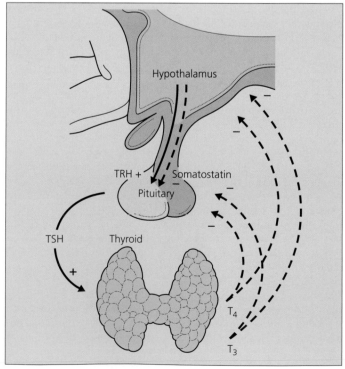

Figure 36.19 Hypothalamic–pituitary–thyroid axis.

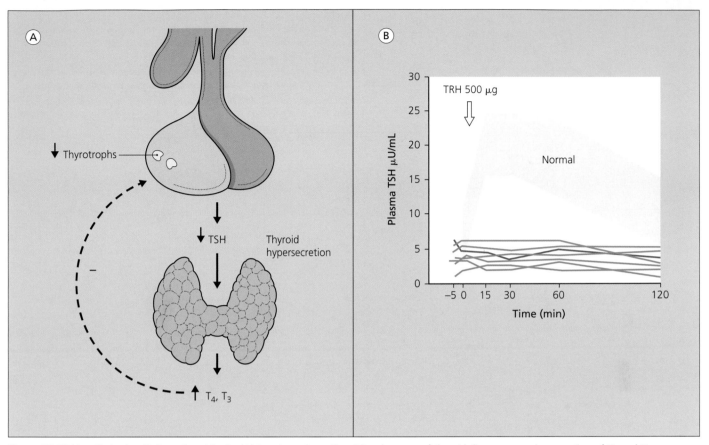

Figure 36.20 Hypothalamic–pituitary–thyroid axis. **(A)** In primary hyperthyroidism because of thyroid disease, excessive secretion of T_4 and T_3 occurs and provides feedback inhibition of the pituitary thyrotrophs (decreased TSH secretion). **(B)** The graph depicts the flat response to TRH in patients with hyperthyroidism compared with the range of responses in normal subjects (data from Gaul C, Wilber JF, Tello C, Rios E. Administration of thyrotropin release hormone (TRH) as a clinical test for pituitary thyrotropin reserve. *Rev Invest Clin* 1972; 24: 35).

TSH deficiency, which causes secondary hypothyroidism, results from pituitary or hypothalamic disease. Often it accompanies multihormonal pituitary deficiency from large pituitary adenoma or a suprasellar tumor (Figure 36.22B).

EVALUATION AND LABORATORY TESTING In primary or secondary hypothyroidism, the serum level of free thyroxine (free T_4) is low (see Table 36.5). Free T_4 can be measured by direct radioimmunoassay of serum dialysate or it can be estimated by the free thyroxine index (FTI = total $T_4 \times T_3$ resin uptake). Although it is usually reliable, the FTI can be misleading in euthyroid "sick" patients in whom prolonged illness causes a low FTI despite clinical euthyroidism and normal serum levels of free T_4. When serum free T_4 is low, measurement of plasma TSH is used to distinguish primary (TSH elevated) from secondary (TSH low) hypothyroidism (Figure 36.22C). However, various non-thyroidal illnesses (e.g. liver failure, sepsis) can also alter TSH levels. A TRH stimulation test further differentiates primary and secondary hypothyroidism, and in secondary hypothyroidism may distinguish between pituitary and hypothalamic disorders (Figure 36.22D). TRH (200–500 μg) is given intravenously over 30 minutes and serum TSH levels are obtained at −5, 0, 15, 30 and 60 minutes. In primary hypothyroidism basal TSH levels are elevated and respond briskly and excessively to TRH. In normal subjects serum TSH peaks at 15 minutes and increases ≥ to 6 μU/mL over the basal values, and in subjects with primary hypothyroidism TRH stimulates a rise in plasma TSH levels. Patients with pituitary lesions that destroy the thyrotrophs have no TSH response to TRH, whereas patients with hypothalamic disorders and surviving thyrotrophs have a delayed TSH response which peaks at 60 minutes.

Gonadotropins

Physiology

FSH and LH are produced and released by the gonadotrophs of the adenohypophysis to regulate ovarian and testicular function (Figure 36.23). Normally the α-subunit is produced in slight excess. The plasma levels of FSH, which has a half-life of 3–4 hours, are more stable than those of LH, which has a half-life of 50 minutes.

FSH stimulates the growth of the granulosa cells of the ovarian follicle and controls estrogen secretion by them. During the midportion of the menstrual cycle, the increasing concentration of estradiol stimulates a surge of LH secretion, which in turn triggers ovulation. After ovulation, LH supports the formation of the corpus luteum. Exposure of the ovary to FSH is required for expression of the receptors for LH.

In men, LH is responsible for the production of testosterone by the Leydig cell. The combined effects of FSH and testosterone on the seminiferous tubule stimulate sperm production.

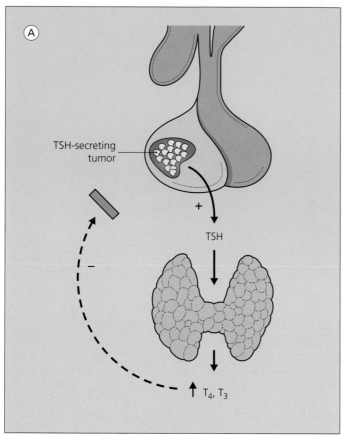

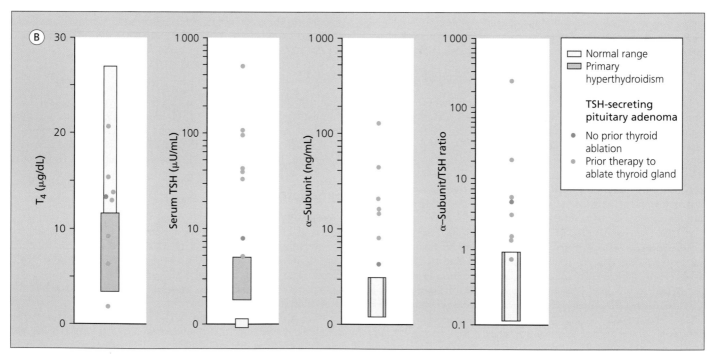

Figure 36.21 (A) In secondary hyperthyroidism, a TSH-secreting thyrotroph adenoma of the pituitary secretes excessive amounts of TSH, which stimulates increased T_4 and T_3 output from the thyroid. **(B)** In contrast to patients with primary hyperthyroidism, who have low serum levels of TSH, α-subunit levels in the normal range, and an α-subunit/TSH molar ratio less than 1.0, patients with TSH-secreting tumors have high serum TSH levels, high α-subunit levels, and an α-subunit/TSH molar ratio greater than 1.0 (data from McCutcheon IE, Weintraub BD, Oldfield EH. Surgical treatment of thyrotropin-secreting pituitary adenomas. *J Neurosurg* 1990; 73: 674–83).

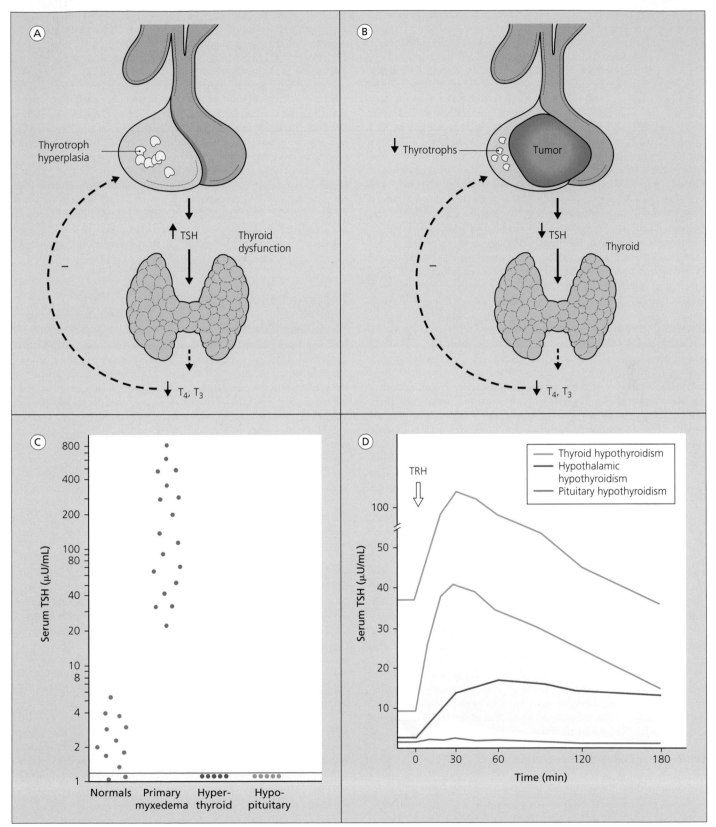

Figure 36.22 **(A)** In primary hypothyroidism, disease of the thyroid gland results in insufficient secretion of T_4 and T_3 and reduced feedback inhibition, pituitary thyrotroph hyperplasia, and increased TSH secretion. **(B)** In secondary hypothyroidism, any type of tumor in the sellar region can compress and destroy the pituitary thyrotrophs or distort the pituitary stalk and disrupt delivery of TRH to the pituitary, reducing TSH secretion and leading to decreased T_4 and T_3 output from the thyroid. **(C)** Serum TSH levels as determined by radioimmunoassay. The shaded area represents levels below the minimum detectable level (data from Hershman JM, Pittman JA. Utility of the radioimmunoassay of serum thyrotropin in man. *Ann Intern Med* 1971; 74: 481–90). **(D)** Typical changes of serum TSH with TRH-stimulation test. Patients with pituitary (secondary) hypothyroidism have a flat TSH response to TRH in contrast to the excess levels and the rise in serum TSH in patients with thyroidal (primary) hypothyroidism. Patients with hypothalamic hypothyroidism have a delayed and intermediate response (data from Utiger RD. Tests of the hypothalamic–pituitary–thyroid axis. In: Werner SC (ed.). *The Thyroid*, 4th edn. Hagerstown: Harper & Row; 1978).

FSH and LH secretion is stimulated in a pulsatile fashion in response to pulses of secretion of GnRH from the hypothalamus. GnRH is also known as LH-releasing hormone (LHRH) because it is a potent stimulator of LH secretion. Levels of FSH and LH are regulated by the balance of GnRH stimulation, negative feedback regulation exerted by inhibin, a peptide secreted by the ovaries and the testes, and the effect of the sex steroids on the pituitary and the hypothalamus (see Figure 36.23). Appropriate levels of FSH and LH are needed for normal sexual development and reproductive function in men and women. Although GnRH can stimulate gonadotropin secretion from the pituitary for the first few months of life, the pituitary then becomes unresponsive to GnRH until puberty, when pulsatile secretion of FSH and LH occurs in response to pulses of GnRH. After the gonadal failure associated with menopause the negative feedback provided by the hormonal products of the gonads is eliminated and serum levels of FSH and LH increase. Because of the pulsatile nature of serum GnRH, LH and FSH, and their fluctuation during the menstrual cycle, isolated and random FSH and LH levels are of little diagnostic use, but must be correlated with the results of simultaneous levels of estradiol or testosterone and the results of dynamic testing.

Excess gonadotropin secretion

Although FSH-secreting and LH-secreting pituitary adenomas are rarely recognized clinically, about 5% of pituitary adenomas have immunohistochemical staining for the gonadotropins or their subunits. Nearly all of these tumors are clinically "nonfunctional" pituitary macroadenomas that cause symptoms because of their mass effect on sellar or parasellar structures, as there is no characteristic hypersecretory endocrinopathy, as occurs with the other types of tumors described above. About 20% of these tumors hypersecrete the α-subunit, the level of which can be determined by radioimmunoassay. It is not yet known if measurements of FSH, LH, or α-subunit will accurately indicate response to therapy or tumor recurrence.

Precocious puberty is often associated with hypothalamic hamartomas, which, by interrupting the normal suppression of pituitary gonadotropin function by higher neural centers in children, lead to pulsatile secretion of GnRH and, in turn, to secretion of FSH and LH, estrogen and testosterone and thus to premature sexual development. Sustained, nonpulsatile exposure to GnRH desensitizes the gonadotrophs to GnRH and inhibits the release of FSH and LH. Knowledge of this phenomenon and the development of a long-acting analog of GnRH is now used to suppress pituitary gonadotropin secretion and reverse sexual development in children with idiopathic precocious puberty and precocious puberty associated with hypothalamic hamartomas. Ectopic production of gonadotropin, usually of human chorionic gonadotropin (which has LH-like activity), by germinomas of the nonseminiferous type, lung carcinomas, and other types of tumors can also cause precocious puberty.

Deficient gonadotropin secretion

Hypogonadism is suspected in women who develop loss of libido and amenorrhea associated with uterine and vaginal atrophy. In men, low testosterone results in loss of libido, impotence, decreased body hair (including reduced beard growth) and testicular softening. In patients suspected of having hypogonadism, endocrine evaluation includes measurement of plasma FSH, LH and the sex steroids, estradiol in women and testosterone in men. Primary hypogonadism as a result of end-organ failure (e.g. premature ovarian failure) is associated with low levels of sex steroids

and high levels of FSH and LH (Figure 36.24A). If FSH and LH are inappropriately low and are associated with a decreased level of sex steroids, the patient has hypogonadotropic hypogonadism (Figure 36.24B). This may be primary and result from congenital causes, as in Kallman syndrome, in which GnRH deficiency is associated with anosmia and defective development of the midline structures of the brain. More commonly, hypogonadotropic hypogonadism is a secondary, acquired defect of GnRH production associated with hypothalamic dysfunction, as in anorexia nervosa or bulimia, or as a result of destruction of the pituitary gonadotrophs or interruption of function of the pituitary stalk from a sellar mass, or from surgery or radiation therapy used to treat a sellar or parasellar tumor. GnRH stimulation testing can be used to determine the presence of adequate gonadotroph reserves (Figure 36.25). If a detectable elevation of FSH and LH levels occurs after GnRH administration (the response to GnRH often requires "priming" of the gonadotrophs by repeated injections of GnRH), functional gonadotropic cells are still present.

Posterior pituitary hormones

ADH (or vasopressin) and oxytocin are stored and secreted in the posterior lobe of the pituitary (Figure 36.26). Although these hormones are normally stored in secretory granules in the nerve terminals of the neurohypophysis and released from the posterior lobe into the systemic circulation in response to various stimuli, if the pituitary is selectively damaged and the median eminence and hypothalamus are intact, they can be secreted from the median eminence.

ADH conserves water. Derangements in ADH secretion can result in severe, potentially lethal, disturbances in plasma osmolality and volume.

Oxytocin stimulates uterine contractions at parturition and acts to expel milk from the secretory tissue of the breast to the nipple during suckling. The major biologic action of oxytocin is to facilitate nursing by stimulating the contraction of myoepithelial cells in the lactating mammary gland. Oxytocin is not routinely assayed in the assessment of pituitary function.

Antidiuretic hormone (ADH)

The most important action of ADH is to conserve body water by reducing the rate of urine output. This antidiuretic effect is achieved by promoting the reabsorption of solute-free water in the distal or collecting tubules of the kidney. The hormone has little or no pressor effect in healthy humans. Despite large daily variations in sodium intake and water loss, plasma osmolality and its principal determinant – plasma sodium concentration – are maintained within a narrow range.

Although multiple hypothalamic inputs influence ADH secretion, the primary stimuli for ADH release are an increase in plasma osmolality (Figure 36.27) or a decrease in plasma volume. As little as a 2% increase in plasma osmolality caused by an impermeable solute, such as NaCl, causes shrinkage of hypothalamic osmoreceptor cells and stimulates ADH release. Thirst is also stimulated. The osmoregulatory mechanism functions like a discontinuous or set-point receptor, the sensitivity and "set" of the osmoregulator is highly variable. The osmoregulatory mechanism is differentially sensitive to plasma solutes. Sodium cations and their associated anions, which normally contribute more than 95% of the osmotic pressure of plasma, are the most potent solutes in stimulating ADH release. Sugars, such as sucrose and mannitol,

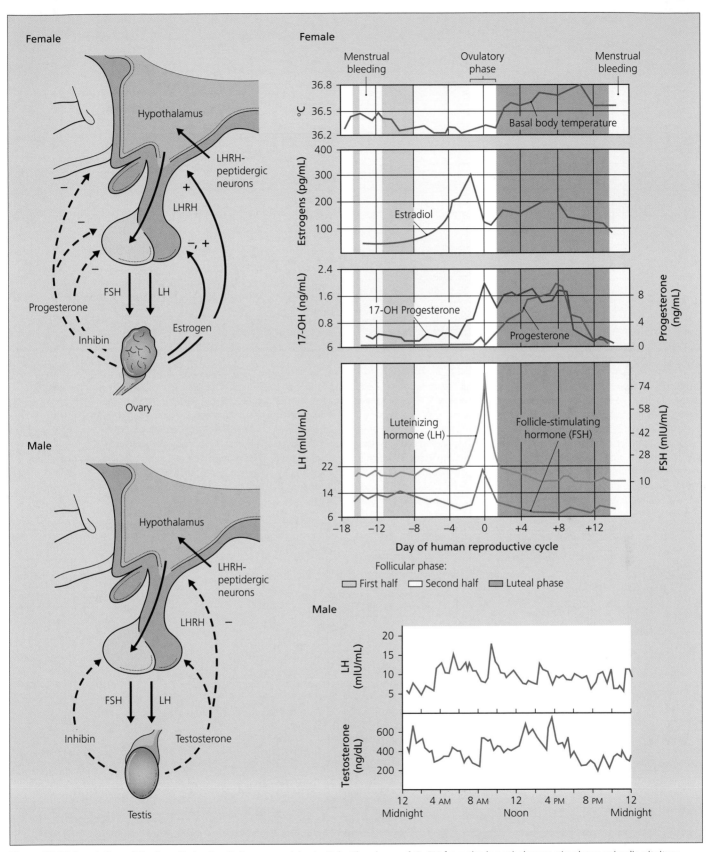

Figure 36.23 Regulation of the hypothalamic–pituitary–gonadal axis. Pulsatile release of GnRH from the hypothalamus stimulates episodic pituitary release of FSH and LH. Negative feedback regulation is exerted by the sex steroids and the peptide inhibin (data from Yen SSC. Neuroendocrine regulation of the menstrual cycle. In: Krieger DT, Hughes JC (eds). *Neuroendocrinology*. Sunderland, MA: Sinauer Associates; 1980: 259–72; Griffin JE, Wilson JD. The testis. In: Bondy PK, Rosenberg LE (eds). *Metabolic Control and Disease*, 8th edn. Philadelphia: WB Saunders Co.; 1980: 1535).

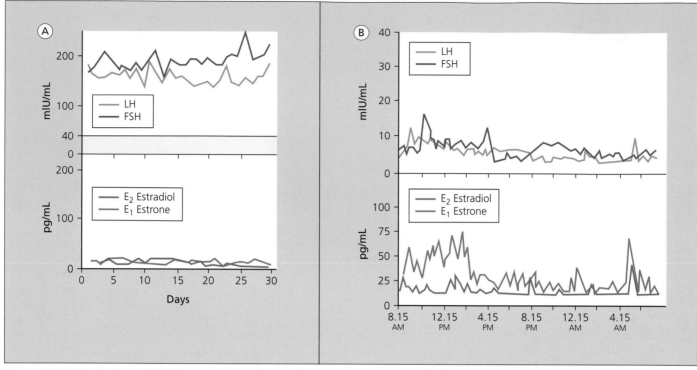

Figure 36.24 Typical pattern of FSH, LH, and corresponding ovarian estrogen and androgen levels in daily samples from a woman with premature ovarian failure. **(A)** Primary hypogonadism. Ovarian failure is associated with low levels of sex steroids and high levels of FSH and LH. The yellow-shaded area represents concentrations up to 40 mIU/mL; FSH levels above this are considered to represent ovarian failure (data from Rebar RW, Erickson GF, Yen SSC. Idiopathic premature ovarian failure: clinical and endocrine characteristics. *Fertil Steril* 1982; 37: 35–41). **(B)** Hypogonadotropic hypogonadism. Typical pattern of FSH, LH, and corresponding ovarian estrogen and androgen levels in samples obtained at 15-min intervals over a 24-h period in a woman with hypogonadotropic hypogonadism, in which inadequate secretion of FSH and LH results in decreased levels of the sex steroids. This can result from destruction of pituitary gonadotrophs, distortion of the pituitary stalk, and interruption of delivery of GnRH, or hypothalamic dysfunction with insufficient GnRH release (data from Yen SSC. Chronic anovulation due to CNS–hypothalamic–pituitary dysfunction. In: Yen SSC, Jaffe RB (eds). *Reproductive Endocrinology*. Philadelphia: WB Saunders; 1978: 341–72).

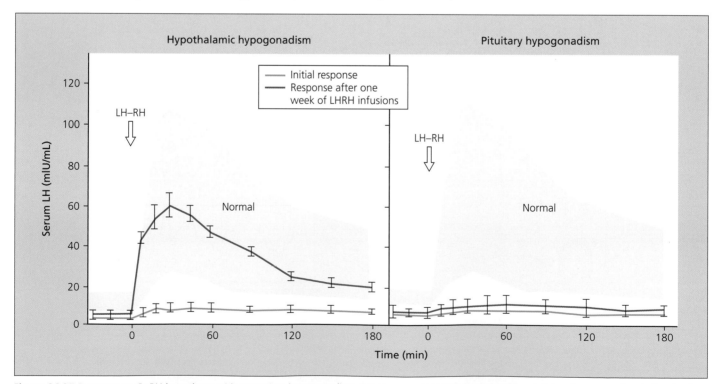

Figure 36.25 Response to GnRH in patients with secondary hypogonadism. Mean serum LH levels in men with secondary hypogonadism before and after a 250 μg intravenous bolus of GnRH before and after priming with daily infusions (500 μg over 4 h) of GnRH for 1 week. Patients with pituitary hypogonadism lack gonadotropin secretion (data from Snyder PJ, Rudenstein RS, Gardner DF, *et al*. Repetitive infusion of gonadotropin-releasing hormone distinguishes hypothalamic from pituitary hypogonadism. *J Clin Endocrinol Metab* 1979; 48: 864–8).

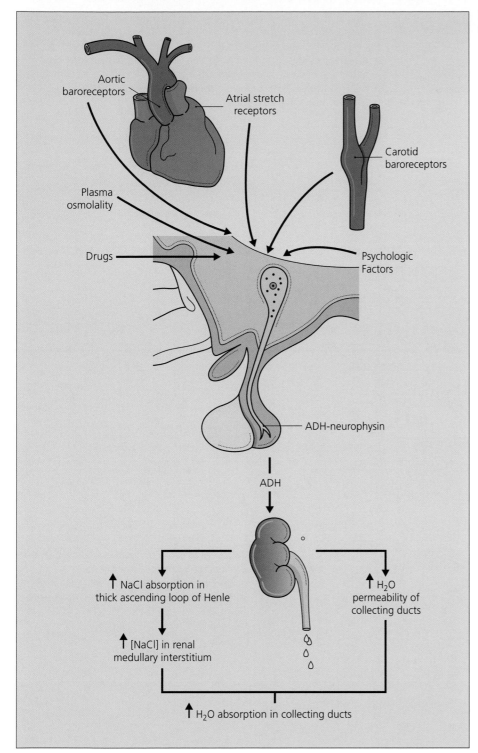

Figure 36.26 Control of antidiuretic hormone (ADH, vasopressin) secretion.

appear to be nearly as potent. The other major physiologic stimulus to ADH release is decreased intravascular volume. Small decreases stimulate ADH secretion by activation of stretch receptors in the left atrium, whereas decreases in circulating volume of approximately 10% stimulate ADH release by baroreceptors in the carotid arteries and the aortic arch. Higher neural centers also influence ADH release. Both β-adrenergic and cholinergic agonists stimulate the release of ADH, while α-adrenergic agonists and atropine inhibit its release. Thus, psychological factors, pain and stress increase ADH release. Nausea is an extremely potent stimulus for ADH secretion in humans. Its effect on ADH is instantaneous and extremely potent. Other stimuli for ADH release include hypoglycemia, angiotensin, many hormones and drugs (nicotine, morphine and the barbiturates stimulate, while alcohol, phenytoin and narcotic antagonists inhibit ADH secretion).

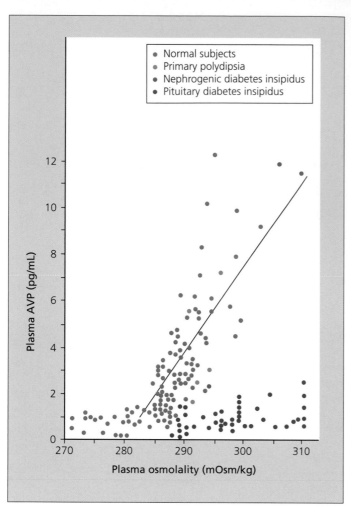

Figure 36.27 There is a close relationship between plasma osmolality and plasma arginine vasopressin (AVP) in normal subjects, patients with nephrogenic diabetes insipidus and primary polydipsia, but not with pituitary diabetes insipidus (data from Robertson GL. Diseases of the posterior pituitary in endocrinology and metabolism. In: Felig P, Baxter JD, Broadus AE, Frohman LA (eds). *Endocrinology and Metabolism.* New York: McGraw-Hill; 1981: 251–80).

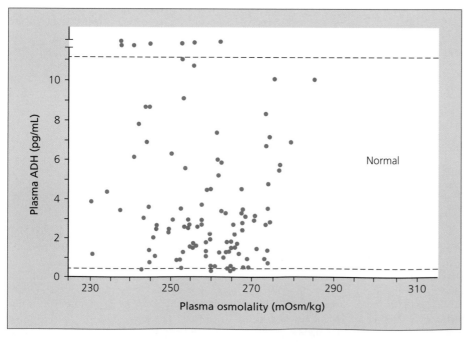

Figure 36.28 Levels of plasma vasopressin (ADH) as a function of plasma osmolality are inappropriately high in patients with the syndrome of inappropriate ADH secretion (SIADH) (adapted from Martin JB, Reichlin S. *Clinical Neuroendocrinology*, 2nd edn. Philadelphia: FA Davis Co.; 1987).

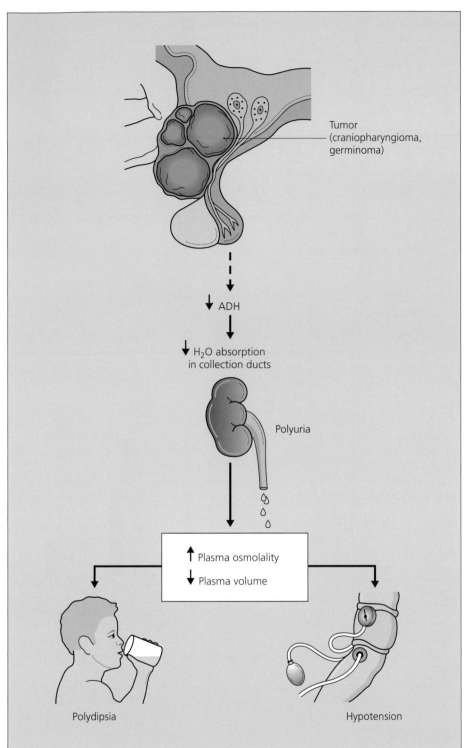

Figure 36.29 Deficient ADH secretion. Destruction of hypothalamic neurons by hypothalamic masses or injury, including surgery, produces pituitary diabetes insipidus.

Excess ADH (syndrome of inappropriate ADH secretion, SIADH)

SIADH results from excess ADH secretion, either from the hypothalamus or from an ectopic source. Excess ADH secretion stimulates excess retention of free water associated with the inability to excrete dilute urine and results in hyponatremia and hypotonicity of the plasma. Continued nonsuppressible ADH release in association with elevated urine osmolality above plasma osmolality is considered inappropriate in patients with low plasma osmolality and hyponatremia. The many causes of SIADH include ectopic production of ADH by tumors (especially oat-cell carcinoma) or by lung tissue during inflammatory diseases (tuberculosis), excessive neuro-hypophyseal release of ADH caused by a variety of intracranial disorders (head trauma, subarachnoid hemorrhage, meningitis, etc.), or by drugs that stimulate ADH release (e.g. chlorpropamide, carbamazepine, tricyclic antidepressants).

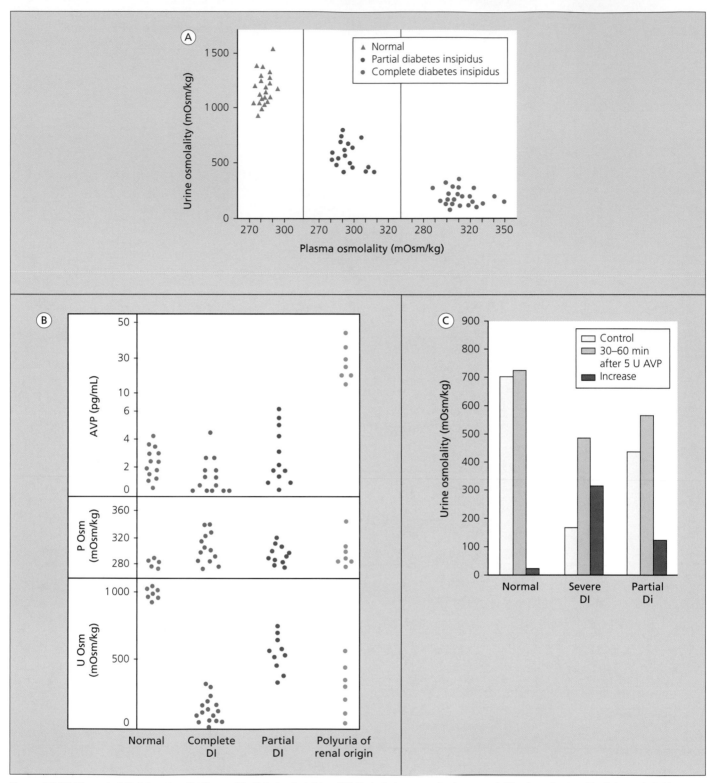

Figure 36.30 Characteristic laboratory findings with diabetes insipidus. **(A)** Typical plasma and urine osmolalities in patients with diabetes insipidus compared to normal subjects. **(B)** Characteristic plasma and urine osmolality and plasma AVP level after water deprivation in patients with diabetes insipidus, normal subjects, and patients with polyuria of renal origin. **(C)** The differences in the increase in urine osmolality after 5 units of subcutaneous vasopressin in patients with central (hypothalamic–pituitary) diabetes insipidus compared with normal subjects after water deprivation. Urine osmolality rises less than 5% in normal subjects but more than 9% in patients with central diabetes insipidus (data from Verbalis J, Robinson A, Moses S. Postoperative and posttraumatic diabetes insipidus. *Front Horm Res* 1985; 13: 247–65).

SIADH can also occur after transsphenoidal surgery or pituitary apoplexy.

The clinical features of SIADH include weight gain, weakness, lethargy and mental confusion. As the serum sodium drops below 120 mEq/L seizures and coma ultimately occur.

EVALUATION AND LABORATORY TESTING The laboratory features of SIADH include hyponatremia, hypotonicity of plasma, urine osmolality that is hypertonic to plasma, and urinary sodium concentration $\geq$ 20 mEq/L (except in patients who are chronically depleted of sodium). The diagnosis of SIADH is made when these features are present and adrenal, thyroid, renal, or hepatic dysfunction and prior diuretic use have been excluded. Measurement of plasma ADH reveals inappropriately elevated levels despite low plasma osmolality (Figure 36.28) and confirms, but is not essential for, the diagnosis.

Deficient ADH (diabetes insipidus)

Deficient ADH secretion in response to physiological stimuli, pituitary diabetes insipidus, impairs renal conservation of water. Causes of diabetes insipidus include sellar and parasellar tumors (especially craniopharyngiomas, large nonfunctional pituitary adenomas, germinomas and metastatic tumors), infiltrative processes (hypothalamic sarcoidosis and histiocytosis X), pituitary or hypothalamic surgery, head trauma, ruptured intracranial aneurysms, and idiopathic causes. The typical clinical features include polyuria, excessive thirst and polydipsia, and nocturia (Figure 36.29). Urine volumes can vary from a few liters a day to more than 15 liters per day. If access to water is restricted or interrupted, dehydration can rapidly become severe and result in altered mental status, fever, hypotension and death.

EVALUATION AND LABORATORY TESTING The laboratory findings of diabetes insipidus include persistent urine osmolality of < 300 mOsm/kg H_2O associated with a urine specific gravity $\leq$ 1.005 and plasma osmolality greater than the normal 287 mOsm/kg H_2O (Figure 36.30A; see Figure 36.27). To confirm the diagnosis, patients are tested to document that there is inadequate release of ADH to an osmotic stimulus. The simplest, safest, and most widely used test to raise plasma osmolality is the water deprivation test (Figure 36.30B,C).

In the water deprivation test all oral intake is stopped after obtaining baseline body weight, urine and plasma osmolality, and vital signs. Water deprivation begins the night before the test in patients with mild polyuria, and early on the day of the test in patients with severe polyuria. The test should be performed only while the patient is under constant supervision. For patients with diabetes insipidus this test may be hazardous. Hourly measurements of urine osmolality and weight are obtained. Dehydration continues until either two sequential urine osmolalities vary by less than 30 mOsm/kg H_2O or loss of greater than 3% of body weight occurs or orthostatic hypotension and postural tachycardia appear. Subjects then receive 5 units of aqueous ADH subcutaneously and a final urine osmolality is measured 1 hour later. In normal subjects endogenous ADH secretion concentrates the urine and preserves normal plasma osmolality. Thus, urine osmolality normally exceeds 500 mOsm/kg H_2O and plateaus, and plasma osmolality remains below 300 mOsm/kg H_2O before ADH injection, and urine osmolality rises less than 5% after injection. In patients with central (pituitary or hypothalamic) diabetes insipidus, urine osmolality usually plateaus at 300–500 mOsm/kg H_2O, plasma osmolality may exceed 300 mOsm/kg H_2O, and

urine osmolality rises greater than 9% after ADH injection. This test not only establishes whether or not diabetes insipidus is present, it also distinguishes central diabetes insipidus from other causes of polyuria. In patients with polyuria from renal disease or nephrogenic diabetes insipidus (renal tubular insensitivity to ADH), the rise in urine osmolality with dehydration is limited and does not increase after ADH administration. In patients with primary polydipsia (compulsive water drinking), water deprivation has to be prolonged for urine osmolality to plateau and urine osmolality does not increase after the dose of ADH.

Plasma ADH measurements by radioimmunoassay can also be used during or as an adjunctive test to the water deprivation test (see Figure 36.28), but because of the simplicity and reliability of the measurements of plasma and urine osmolality, ADH determinations are rarely required. Furthermore, radioimmunoassay is difficult to perform and is not routinely available.

CLINICAL PEARLS

- A PRL level greater than 200 ng/mL is nearly always due to a prolactinoma, and a value greater than 300 ng/mL is diagnostic of one.

- The serum level of somatomedin-C (IGF-I) provides a more reliable indication of the exposure of the body to GH than does random determination of serum GH.

- GH is the most sensitive of the pituitary hormones to be lost in adults and children with pituitary and hypothalamic disorders.

- The ACTH-independent and ACTH-dependent forms of hypercortisolism are distinguished by the level of plasma ACTH in the presence of hypercortisolism.

- Hypersecretion of TSH by a pituitary adenoma is a rare cause of hyperthyroidism. Since hyperthyroidism is common and TSH-secreting tumors are very rare, many patient with TSH-secreting pituitary tumors are intially misdiagnosed and receive ablative therapy of the thyroid gland. Thus, they may not have hyperthyroidism when the pituitary tumor is recognized.

BIBLIOGRAPHY

General

Becker KL (ed.). *Principles and Practice of Endocrinology and Metabolism*, 2nd edn. Philadelphia: Lippincott-Raven; 1995: 112–13

Bennett JC, Smith LH, Wyngaarden JB (eds). *Cecil Textbook of Medicine*, 19th edn. Philadelphia: WB Saunders Co.; 1992.

Cooper PR (ed.). *Contemporary Diagnosis and Management of Pituitary Adenomas*. Park Ridge: American Association of Neurological Surgeons; 1991.

Gilman AG. Guanine nucleotide-binding regulatory proteins and dual control of adenylate cyclase. *J Clin Invest* 1984; 73: 1–4.

Kannan CR. *The Pituitary Gland*. New York, NY: Plenum Publishing Corp.; 1987.

Klibanski A, Zervas NT. Diagnosis and management of hormone-secreting pituitary adenomas. *N Engl J Med* 1991; 324: 822–31.

Lechan RM. Neuroendocrinology of pituitary hormone regulation. *Endocrinol Metab Clin North Am* 1987; 16: 475.

Martin JB, Reichlin S. *Clinical Neuroendocrinology*, 2nd edn. Philadelphia: FA Davis Co.; 1987.

Reeves WB, Andreoli TE. The posterior pituitary and water metabolism. In: Foster DW, Wilson JD (eds). *Williams Textbook of Endocrinology*, 8th edn. Philadelphia: WB Saunders Co.; 1992: 311–56.

Reichlin S. *Neuroendocrinology*. In: Foster DW, Wilson JD (eds). *Williams Textbook of Endocrinology*, 8th edn. Philadelphia: WB Saunders Co.; 1992: 135–220.

Thorner MO, Vance ML, Horvath E, Kovacs K. The anterior pituitary. In: Foster DW, Wilson JD (eds). *Williams Textbook of Endocrinology*, 8th edn. Philadelphia: WB Saunders Co.; 1992: 221–310.

Vance ML. Hypopituitarism. *N Engl J Med* 1994; 330: 1651–62 [Erratum: *N Engl J Med* 1994; 331: 487].

Prolactin
Boyd AE III, Reichlin S, Turksoy RN. Galactorrhea–amenorrhea syndrome: diagnosis and therapy. *Ann Intern Med* 1977; 87: 165–75.

Frantz AG. Prolactin. *N Engl J Med* 1978; 298: 201.

Hwang P, Guyda H, Friesen H. A radioimmunoassay for human prolactin. *Proc Natl Acad Sci USA* 1971; 68: 1902–6.

Koppelamn MCS, Jaffe MJ, Reith KG, *et al*. Hyperprolactinemia, amenorrhea, and galactorrhea. *Ann Intern Med* 1984; 100: 115.

Sachar EJ. Hormonal changes in stress and mental illness. In: Krieger DT, Hughes JC (eds). *Neuroendocrinology*. Sunderland, MA: Sinauer Associates; 1980: 177–83.

Sassin JF, Frantz AG, Weitzman ED, Kapen S. Human prolactin: 24-hour pattern with increased release during sleep. *Science* 1972; 177: 1205–7.

Schlechte J, Dolan K, Sherman B, *et al*. The natural history of untreated hyperprolactinemia: a prospective analysis. *J Clin Endocrinol Metab* 1989; 68: 412.

Tolis G. Prolactin: physiology and pathology. In: Krieger DT, Hughes JC (eds). *Neuroendocrinology*. Sunderland, MA: Sinauer Associates; 1980: 321–30.

Growth hormone
Barkan AL, Beitins IZ, Kelch RP. Plasma insulin-like growth factor-I/somatomedin-C in acromegaly: correlation with the degree of growth hormone hypersecretion. *J Clin Endocrinol Metab* 1988; 67: 69–73.

Carlson HE. The diagnosis of acromegaly. In: Robbins RJ, Melmed S (eds). *Acromegaly: A Century of Scientific and Clinical Progress*. New York: Plenum Press; 1987; 197–208.

Clemmons DR, Van Wyk JJ, Ridgeway EC, *et al*. Evaluation of acromegaly by radioimmunoassay of somatomedin C. *N Engl J Med* 1979; 301: 1138–42.

El-Khodary AZ, Ball MF, Stein B, *et al*. Effect of weight loss on the growth hormone response to arginine infusion in obesity. *J Clin Endocrinol Metab* 1971; 32: 42–51.

Melmed S. Acromegaly. *N Engl J Med* 1990; 322: 966–77.

Melmed S, Braunstein GD, Horvath E, *et al*. Pathophysiology of acromegaly. *Endocr Rev* 1983; 4: 271–90.

Raiti S, Tolman RA (eds). *Human Growth Hormone*. New York: Plenum Medical Book Co.; 1986.

Van Wyk JJ, Underwood LE. Growth hormone, somatomedins and growth failure. In: Krieger DT, Hughes JC (eds). *Neuroendocrinology*. Sunderland, MA: Sinauer Associates; 1980: 299–309.

Pituitary–adrenal axis
Besser GM, Edwards CRW. Cushing's syndrome. *Clin Endocrinol Metab* 1972; 1: 451–90.

Chrousos GP, Schulte HM, Oldfield EH, Gold PW, Cutler GB Jr, Loriaux DL. The corticotropin-releasing factor stimulation test: an aid in the evaluation of patients with Cushing's syndrome. *N Engl J Med* 1984; 310: 622–6.

Doppman JL, Oldfield EH, Cruddy AG *et al*. Petrosal sampling for Cushing's syndrome: Anatomical and technical considerations. *Radiology* 1984; 150: 99.

Kaye TB, Crapo L. The Cushing syndrome: an update on diagnostic tests. *Ann Intern Med* 1990; 112: 434–44.

Krieger DT. Physiopathology of Cushing's disease. *Endocr Rev* 1983; 4: 22–43.

Liddle GW. Tests of pituitary-adrenal suppressibility in the diagnosis of Cushing's syndrome. *J Clin Endocrinol Metab* 1960; 20: 1539–60.

Loriaux DL, Cutler GB Jr. Disease of the adrenal glands. In: Kohler PO (ed.). *Clinical Endocrinology*. New York: John Wiley & Sons; 1986.

Melby JC. Assessment of adrenocortical function. *N Engl J Med* 1971; 285: 735–9.

Nieman LK, Loriaux DL. Corticotropin-releasing hormone: clinical applications. *Annu Rev Med* 1989; 40: 331–9.

Oldfield EH, Chrousos GP, Schulte HM, *et al*. Preoperative lateralization of ACTH-secreting micro-adenomas by bilateral and simultaneous inferior petrosal sinus sampling. *N Engl J Med* 1985; 312: 100–3.

Oldfield EH, Doppman JL, Nieman LK, *et al*. Bilateral petrosal sinus sampling with and without corticotropin-releasing hormone for the differential diagnosis of Cushing's syndrome. *N Engl J Med* 1991; 325: 897–905.

Rees LH, Holdaway IM, Phenekos C, *et al*. ACTH secretion and clinical investigations. In: *Some Aspects of Hypothalamic Regulation of Endocrine Functions: Symposium, Vienna, June 3–6, 1973*. Stuttgart: F Schattaur Verlag; 1974: 451–63.

Schulte HM, Chrousos GP, Avgerinos PC, *et al*. The corticotropin-releasing factor stimulation test: an aid in the evaluation of patients with adrenal insufficiency. *J Clin Endocrinol Metab* 1984; 58: 1064–7.

Streeten DHP, Stevenson CT, Dalakos TG, *et al*. The diagnosis of hypercortisolism: biochemical criteria differentiating patients from lean and obese normal subjects and from females on oral contraceptives. *J Clin Endocrinol Metab* 1969; 29: 1191–211.

Tanaka K, Nicholson WE, Orth DN. Diurnal rhythm and disappearance half-time of endogenous plasma immunoreactive B-MSH (LPH) and ACTH in man. *J Clin Endocrinol Metab* 1978; 46: 883–90.

Tyrrell JB, Findling JW, Aron DC, Fitzgerald PA, Forsham PH. An overnight high-dose dexamethasone suppression test for rapid differential diagnosis of Cushing's syndromes. *Ann Intern Med* 1986; 104: 180–6.

Glycoprotein hormones

Bousfield GR, Perry, WM, Ward DN. Gonadotropins: chemistry and biosynthesis. In: Knobil E, Neill JD (eds). *The Physiology of Reproduction*. New York, Raven Press 1994; 1749.

Demura R, Kubo O, Demura H, *et al*. FSH and LH secreting pituitary adenoma. *J Clin Endocrinol Metab* 1977; 45: 653–7.

Gaul C, Wilber JF, Tello C, Rios E. Administration of thyrotropin release hormone (TRH) as a clinical test for pituitary thyrotropin reserve. *Rev Invest Clin* 1972; 24: 35–55.

Gesundheit N, Petrick PA, Nissim M, *et al*. Thyrotropin-secreting pituitary adenomas: clinical and biochemical heterogeneity. *Ann Intern Med* 1989; 111: 827–35.

Gharib H, Carpenter PC, Scheithauer BW, *et al*. The spectrum of inappropriate pituitary thyrotropin secretion associated with hyperthyroidism. *Mayo Clin Proc* 1982; 57: 556–63.

Griffin JE, Wilson JD. The testis. In: Bondy PK, Rosenberg LE (eds). *Metabolic Control and Disease*, 8th edn. Philadelphia: WB Saunders Co.; 1980: 1535.

Hershman JM, Pittman JA. Utility of the radioimmunoassay of serum thyrotropin in man. *Ann Intern Med* 1971; 74: 481–90.

Ishibashi M, Yamaji T, Takaku F, *et al*. Secretion of glycoprotein hormone alpha-subunit by pituitary tumors. *J Clin Endocrinol Metab* 1987; 64: 1187–93.

Jackson IMD. Thyrotropin-releasing hormone. *N Engl J Med* 1982; 306: 145–55.

Klibanski A. Nonsecreting pituitary tumors. *Endocrinol Metab Clin North Am* 1987; 16: 793–804.

Kourides IA, Weintraub BD, Rosen SW, Ridgeway EC, Kliman B, Maloof F. Secretion of alpha subunit of glycoprotein hormones by pituitary adenomas. *J Clin Endocrinol Metab* 1976; 43: 97–106.

McCutcheon IE, Weintraub BD, Oldfield EH. Surgical treatment of thyrotropin-secreting pituitary adenomas. *J Neurosurg* 1990; 73: 674–83.

Morley JE. Neuroendocrine control of thyrotropin secretion. *Endocr Rev* 1981; 2: 396.

Pierce JG, Parsons TF. Glycoprotein hormones: structure and function. *Annu Rev Biochem* 1981; 50: 465–95.

Rebar RW, Erickson GF, Yen SSC. Idiopathic premature ovarian failure: clinical and endocrine characteristics. *Fertil Steril* 1982; 37: 35–41.

Snyder PJ. Gonadotroph cell adenomas of the pituitary. *Endocr Rev* 1985; 6: 552–63.

Snyder PJ, Rudenstein RS, Gardner DF, *et al*. Repetitive infusion of gonadotropin-releasing hormone distinguishes hypothalamic from pituitary hypogonadism. *J Clin Endocrinol Metab* 1979; 48: 864–8.

Utiger RD. Tests of the hypothalamic–pituitary–thyroid axis. In: Werner SC (ed.). *The Thyroid*, 4th edn. Hagerstown: Harper & Row; 1978: 1000–47.

Weintraub BD, Gershengorn MC, Kourides IA, *et al*. Inappropriate secretion of thyroid-stimulating hormone. *Ann Intern Med* 1981; 95: 339–51.

Yen SSC. Chronic anovulation due to CNS–hypothalamic–pituitary dysfunction. In: Yen SSC, Jaffe RB (eds). *Reproductive Endocrinology*. Philadelphia: WB Saunders Co.; 1978: 341–72.

Yen SSC. Neuroendocrine regulation of the menstrual cycle. In: Krieger DT, Hughes JC (eds). *Neuroendocrinology*. Sunderland, MA: Sinauer Associates; 1980: 259–72.

Posterior pituitary

Andreoli TE. The polyuric syndromes. In: Andreoli TE, Hoffman JF, Fanestil DD (eds). *Physiology of Membrane Disorders*. New York: Plenum Medical Book Co.; 1978: 1063–91.

Brownstein MJ, Russell JT, Gainer H. Synthesis, transport and release of posterior pituitary hormones. *Science* 1980; 207: 373–8.

Kovacs L, Robertson GL. Syndrome of inappropriate diuresis. *Neuroendocrinology* 1992; 63: 859–75.

Miller M, Dalakos T, Moses AM, Fellerman H, Streeten DHP. Recognition of partial defects in antidiuretic hormone secretion. *Ann Intern Med* 1970; 73: 721–9.

Robertson GL. Diseases of the posterior pituitary in endocrinology and metabolism. In: Felig P, Baxter JD, Broadus AE, Frohman LA (eds). *Endocrinology and Metabolism*. New York: McGraw-Hill; 1981: 251–80.

Robertson GL. Thirst and vasopressin function in normal and disordered states of water balance. *J Lab Clin Med* 1983; 101: 351–71.

Sklar AH, Schrier RW. Central nervous system mediators of vasopressin release. *Physiol Rev* 1983; 63: 1243–80.

Verbalis J, Robinson A, Moses S. Postoperative and posttraumatic diabetes insipidus. *Front Horm Res* 1985; 13: 247–65.

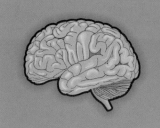

NONFUNCTIONING PITUITARY ADENOMAS

37

Nelson M Oyesiku

CLINICAL PRESENTATION

Nonfunctioning pituitary adenomas account for approximately 30% of pituitary tumors.[1] The term nonfunctioning reflects the fact that these tumors do not cause clinical hormone hypersecretion.[1-4] The nonfunctioning tumors are uniquely heterogeneous (Table 37.1). They typically are quite large, and cause hypopituitarism or blindness from regional compression.[5] The tumors are usually solid (Figure 37.1), although they may be both solid and cystic (Figure 37.2).

Despite the lack of clinical hormone hypersecretion, immunocytochemical staining for hormones reveals evidence for hormone expression in up to 79% of these tumors. The remainder are negative for hormone expression.[1,4] Cell culture studies also demonstrate that some nonfunctioning tumors secrete hormone *in vitro*.[6] Unlike the functional pituitary tumors, there is no available effective medical therapy for the nonfunctioning tumors.

Nonfunctioning tumors are usually seen in the fourth and fifth decades of life and there is no sexual bias. The tumors may be classified into two main groups: null cell adenomas and silent adenomas. Null cell adenomas may be divided into non-oncocytic and oncocytic adenomas. Oncocytomas contain large numbers of mitochondria, show focal immunostaining for anterior hormones, and produce hormones *in vitro*. Silent adenomas consist of three morphological subtypes of well-differentiated tumors. The cell of origin is unknown. Silent corticotrope adenoma subtype 1 is morphologically indistinguishable from the corticotrope adenomas associated with Cushing's disease.[4] This type is more common in

women and many are associated with symptoms of recent hemorrhage. Silent corticotrope adenoma subtype 2 occurs mostly in men (4 : 1 sex bias). Silent adenoma subtype 3 morphologically resembles glycoprotein-hormone-secreting tumors.

Enlargement of a tumor into the suprasellar area results in optic chiasmal compression, which may cause visual field deficits. Because the inferior nasal fibers located in the inferior aspect of the optic chiasm subserve the superior temporal field, the first visual field deficits are frequently bitemporal superior quadrant defects (Figure 37.3). Occasionally the tumors extend into the cavernous sinus (Figure 37.4). Extraocular muscle palsies are rare even if there is cavernous sinus extension, presumably because these tumors grow slowly.

Enlargement of a nonfunctioning adenoma causes progressive loss of pituitary function over months or years.[7] Gonadotropin function is usually lost first; followed by loss of growth hormone function, then loss of thyroid function, and finally loss of adrenocorticotropic hormone (ACTH) function. Loss of antidiuretic hormone function is almost never a presenting symptom.

Although progressive bitemporal visual field loss and progressive hypopituitarism are the typical presenting clinical manifestations, occasionally large pituitary adenomas become

Table 37.1 Classification of non-functional (NF) adenomas by cell of origin

Cell type	Hormone expression	NF tumors
Null cell	None	17%
Oncocytoma	None	6%
Silent corticotrope	ACTH	8%
Silent somatotrope	GH	3%
Gonadotropes	Intact LH/FSH or subunits	40–79%

GH, growth hormone; LH, luteinizing hormone; FSH, follicle-stimulating hormone.

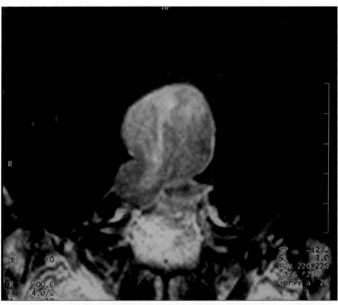

Figure 37.1 Coronal contrast MRI showing a large solid sellar–suprasellar nonfunctioning pituitary adenoma.

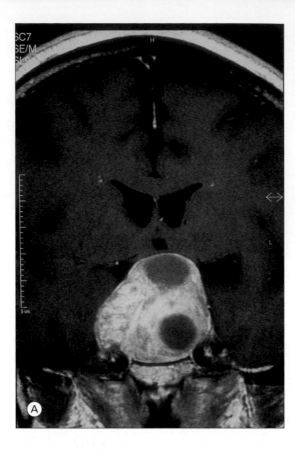

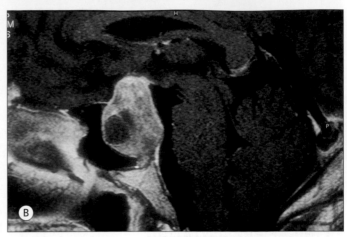

Figure 37.2 Coronal **(A)** and sagittal **(B)** MRI showing a large sellar-suprasellar nonfunctioning pituitary adenoma that has a solid and a cystic portion.

Figure 37.3 Visual field examination on a patient with a pituitary tumor causing inferior chiasmal compression. The largest defects are in the superior temporal fields.

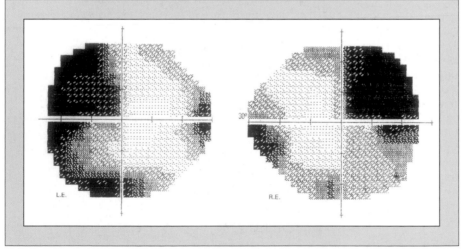

apparent suddenly, secondary to hemorrhage or infarction (apoplexy).[8] When there is a large hemorrhage into the pituitary tumor, the patient may have a sudden headache, a decreased level of consciousness, vision loss, and acute hormonal insufficiency (Figure 37.5).

EVALUATION

Since the tumors are usually large, the sella turcica also enlarges. The floor of the sella (lamina dura) frequently thins, and if the enlarged adenoma is asymmetrical, the lateral radiograph may show a double floor. The sella becomes more rounded. Also, the dorsum sellae may be thinned and pushed back, and the anterior clinoids may be undercut (Figure 37.6).

Magnetic resonance imaging (MRI) and computed tomography (CT) show the exact anatomical configuration of the adenoma.[9,10] MRI is preferable to CT because it better demonstrates the carotid arteries and chiasm and has better anatomical definition. However, CT may be better than MRI for demonstrating the bony anatomy of the sphenoid sinus (Figure 37.7).

Visual acuity and visual field examinations are necessary preoperatively and postoperatively to document visual deficit and monitor improvement or worsening (Figures 37.3, 37.8E–F).

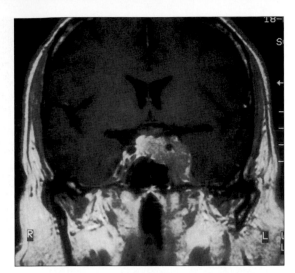

Figure 37.4 MRI of the sella and cavernous sinuses of a patient with a large pituitary adenoma – cavernous sinus extension of tumor on the left.

Endocrine function testing is needed to determine loss of hormonal function – basal levels by themselves may not reveal hypofunction. Stimulation testing is frequently performed in a clinical research unit.

DIFFERENTIAL DIAGNOSIS

The differential diagnosis of a nonfunctioning pituitary adenoma is quite extensive. Tuberculum sellae meningiomas may mimic pituitary adenoma, but MRI usually does not show significant enlargement of the sella. A large internal carotid artery aneurysm may also fill the sella turcica but an aneurysm can be diagnosed as a flow void seen on an MRI. Although craniopharyngiomas are generally suprasellar tumors, they may present as intrasellar tumors (Figure 37.9). Patients with metastasis to the sella frequently have associated extraocular muscle palsies or diabetes insipidus (Figure 37.10), findings almost never seen in pituitary adenomas. Rathke's pouch cleft cysts occasionally present as large sellar and suprasellar cystic masses (Figure 37.11). Tuberculoma, giant cell hypophysitis

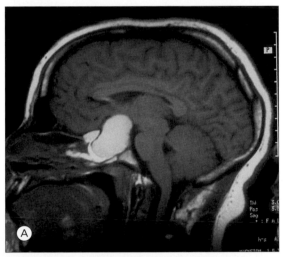

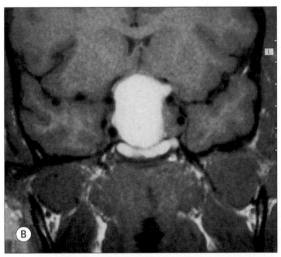

Figure 37.5 Sagittal (A) and coronal (B) unenhanced MRI of a patient with pituitary apoplexy.

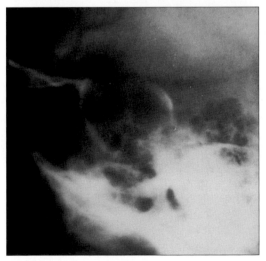

Figure 37.6 Lateral skull radiograph in a patient with a large pituitary tumor. The sella is rounded and enlarged with thinning of the floor and dorsum.

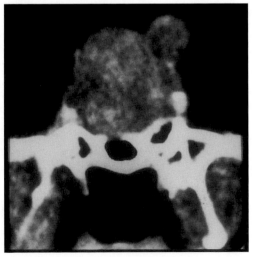

Figure 37.7 Coronal enhanced CT scan of a patient with a large sellar–suprasellar nonfunctioning pituitary adenoma.

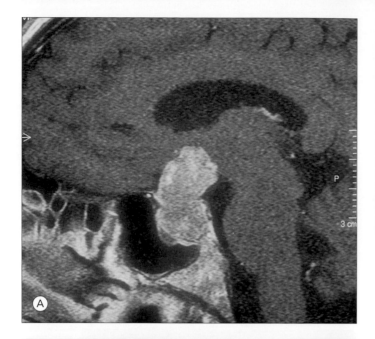

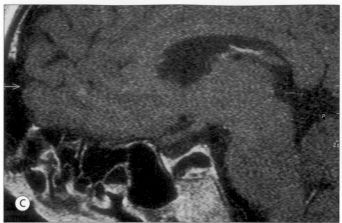

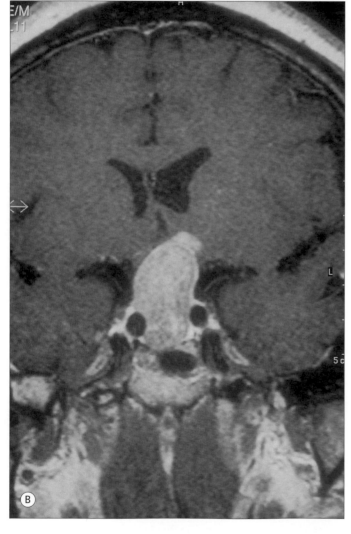

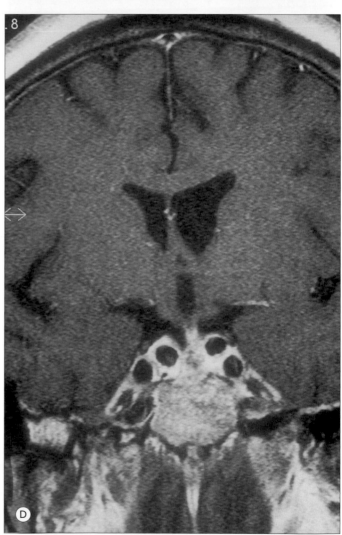

Figure 37.8 Surgical outcome: preoperative sagittal **(A)** and coronal **(B)** enhanced MRI of nonfunctioning pituitary adenoma. Postoperative sagittal **(C)** and coronal **(D)** enhanced MRI of nonfunctioning pituitary adenoma showing gross total tumor resection.

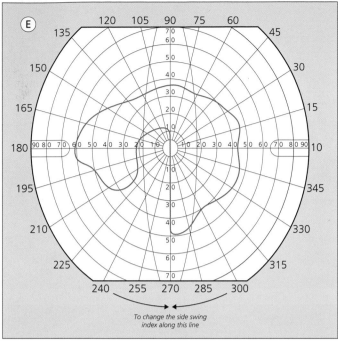
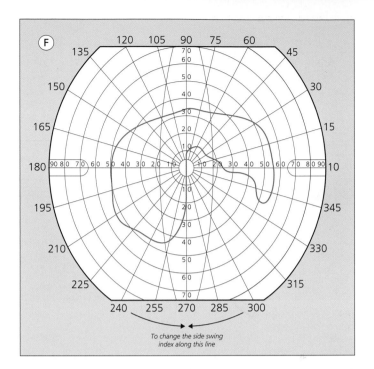
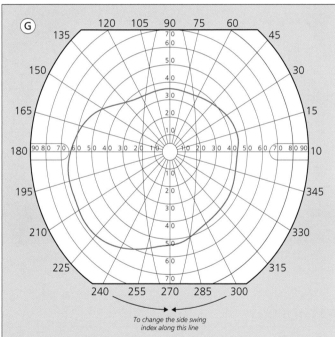
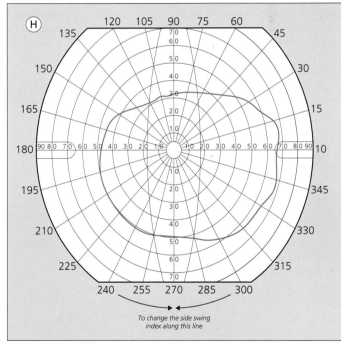

Figure 37.8, *cont'd* Surgical outcome: preoperative visual fields of left **(E)** and right eye **(F)**; and postoperative visual fields visual of left eye **(G)** and right eye **(H)**.

(Figure 37.12), and sarcoidosis may mimic nonfunctioning adenoma, but they are seen infrequently.

TREATMENT

The usual treatment of a nonfunctioning pituitary adenoma in a medically stable patient is microscopic or endoscopic transsphenoidal removal of the tumor.[4,5,7,11] In most cases this is an elective procedure. The typical indications are visual loss or hypopituitarism. If the patient has loss of thyroid or ACTH function preoperatively, surgery is usually delayed so that the patient can begin thyroid or hydrocortisone replacement therapy.[7] If vision loss is rapid or the adenoma is associated with hemorrhage or abscess, a more urgent surgical approach is needed.[8] Sellar and suprasellar tumors can be removed from the transsphenoidal approach by either a sublabial, transseptal, or direct endonasal approach using the endoscope or microscope. Some surgeons

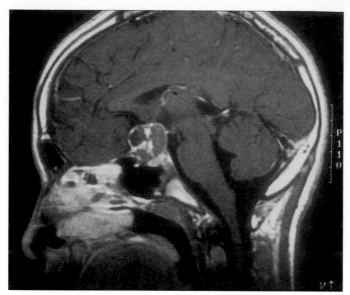

Figure 37.9 Sagittal contrast-enhanced MRI of intrasellar craniopharyngiomas.

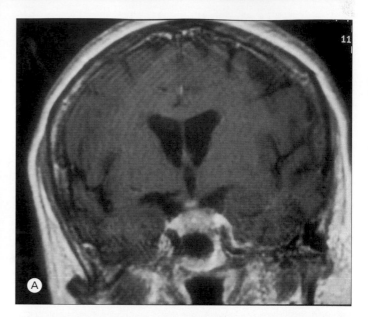

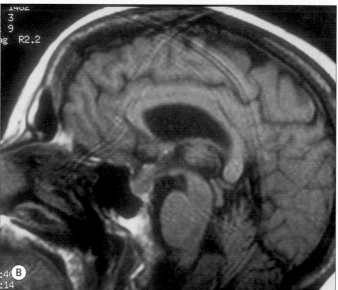

Figure 37.10 Enhanced MRI scan of a patient presenting with a metastasis (adenocarcinoma) to the sella. Coronal (**A**) and sagittal (**B**).

insert a lumbar drain and instill saline to help bring down the suprasellar extension. C-arm guidance or MRI image-guidance may be used with the transsphenoidal approach to orient the surgeon intraoperatively. The surgeon needs a thorough understanding of sphenoid sinus and parasellar anatomy (Figure 37.13).

Relative contraindications to transsphenoidal surgery include a dumbbell tumor (Figure 37.14A), which has an extremely narrow waist at the junction of the sellar and suprasellar portions; a tumor with a large subfrontal or parasellar extension (Figure 37.14B,C); a tumor with massive suprasellar extension; and, sometimes, an extremely fibrous tumor. Occasionally, craniotomy will be needed in patients who are contraindicated for transsphenoidal surgery.

Significant complications from transsphenoidal surgery are not common. The incidence of rhinorrhea is about 5%. Approximately 20% of patients develop diabetes insipidus; however, permanent diabetes insipidus is uncommon. Approximately 10% of patients have partial worsening of their hormone function. The chances of visual loss, stroke, and death are less than 1%.

Radiation therapy can be used in patients with nonfunctioning pituitary adenomas.[12–14] If the patient is elderly or medically unstable, radiation therapy may be the only viable treatment. The patient who postoperatively has a significant amount of residual tumor or who shows regrowth may be a candidate for fractionated radiation therapy, generally 4000–5000 cGy over 25 treatments. Stereotactic radiosurgery is preferable to conventional external radiotherapy when the tumor configuration relative to the chiasm and optic nerves is favorable.

Radiation therapy controls tumor growth in 80–98% of patients with nonfunctioning tumors.[12–14] Hypopituitarism is the most common side-effect of pituitary irradiation with an incidence of 13–56%. Long-term overall risk for brain necrosis in a total of 1388 analyzed patients was estimated to be 0.2%. Other side-effects are rare, they include deterioration of vision in 1.7%, vascular changes in 6.3%, neuropsychological problems in 0.7% and secondary malignancies in 0.8%.[13]

Despite the frequent dural invasion of these tumors, many patients do well for long periods of time without radiation therapy.

PATHOLOGY

Pathologic staining with hematoxylin & eosin stain usually shows the adenoma arranged in a papillary fashion (Figure 37.15). A touch preparation done at surgery shows a monolayer of adenomatous cells (Figure 37.16). In many nonfunctioning pituitary adenomas, the immunohistochemical staining is negative. Immunohistochemical staining is performed to detect if the tumor is producing any of the anterior pituitary hormones (Figure 37.17).

More recently, cDNA microarray analysis has revealed that the folate receptor (FR-α) is significantly over-expressed in clinically non-functional adenomas. FR-α is a high-affinity folate transporter that is over-expressed by other tumors and may provide a growth advantage to cells that express it.[15] Analysis of FR-α expression by Western blotting confirmed that FR-α protein is specifically over-expressed in non-functional tumors. It is known from studies

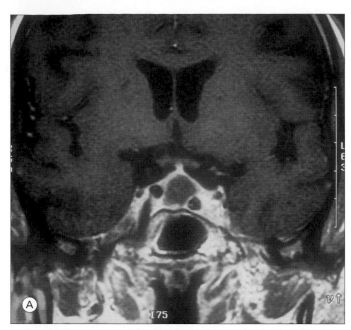
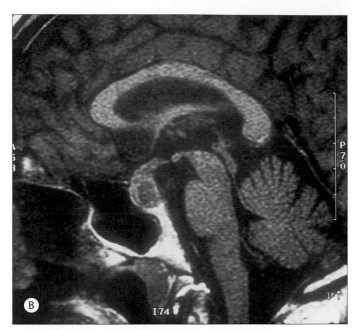

Figure 37.11 Enhanced MRI scan of a patient with a large sellar Rathke's pouch cleft cyst. Coronal **(A)** and sagittal **(B)**.

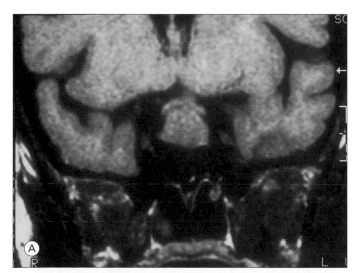
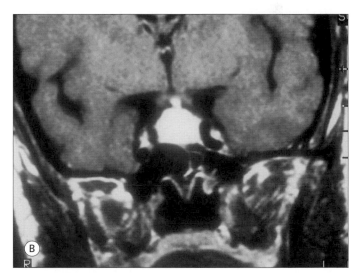

Figure 37.12 Coronal **(A)** unenhanced and **(B)** enhanced MRI of lymphocytic hypophysitis.

Figure 37.13 Operative set-up for a transsphenoidal operation.

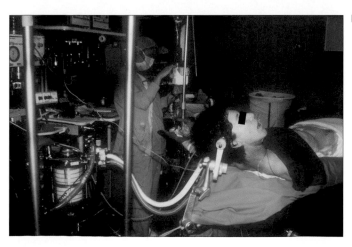

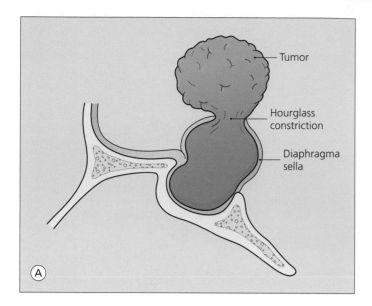

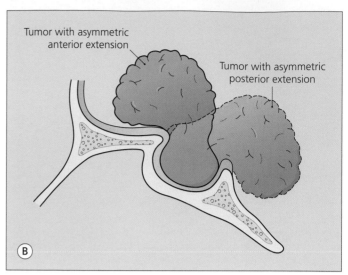

Figures 37.14 Line illustrations of extension and tumor configurations of pituitary tumor. **(A)** A dumbbell tumor, which has an extremely narrow waist at the junction of the sellar and suprasellar portions; a tumor with a large subfrontal or parasellar extension **(B,C).**

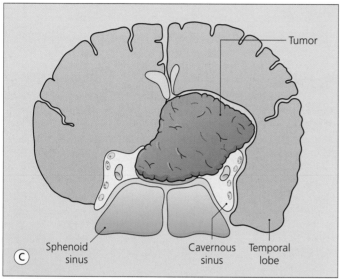

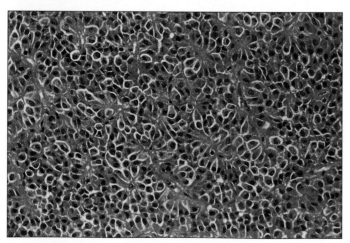

Figure 37.15 A nonfunctional pituitary adenoma arranged mostly in a papillary fashion. (H & E; × 250)

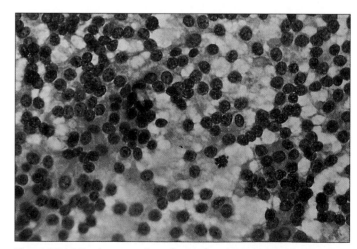

Figure 37.16 Touch preparation of a nonfunctioning pituitary adenoma showing a monolayer of adenomatous cells. Some nuclear atypism and prominent nucleoli are noted. The cytoplasm is barely visible. (H&E; × 250.)

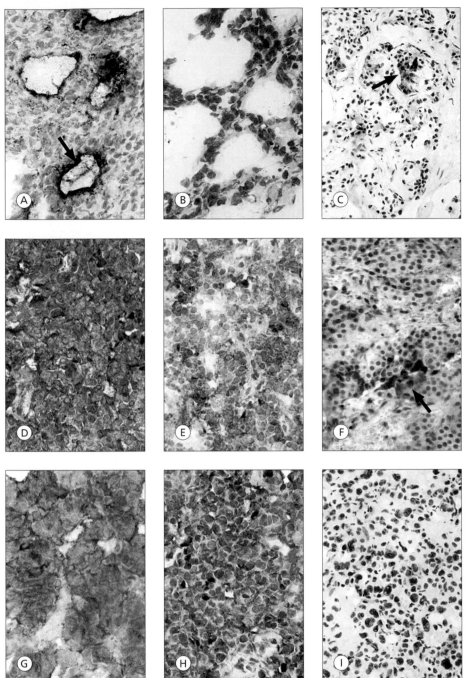

Figure 37.17 Immunohistochemistry (IHC) demonstrating cytoplasmic folate receptor (FR-α) in anterior pituitary gland, nonfunctioning pituitary adenomas, and functional pituitary adenoma. Ovarian adenocarcinoma served as a positive control for FRα receptor IHC. Strong immunoreactivity for FR-α was present on the luminal membrane of ovarian adenocarcinoma glands and to a lesser extent within the cytoplasm (**A**) (arrow). Ovarian adenocarcinoma did not show any immunoreactivity when the primary antibody directed against FR-α was replaced with phosphate-buffered saline (**B**) (negative control). Normal (non-neoplastic) anterior pituitary gland showed focal weak staining for FR-α in glandular cells but none in stromal cells (**C**) (arrow). Nonfunctioning adenomas that did not show any evidence of hormone production by IHC were all immunoreactive for FR-α, with the intensity of staining varying from strong (**D**) to moderate (**E**). Immunoreactivity for FR-α was limited to the cytoplasm of adenoma cells and was not present in stromal cells or blood vessels. Nonfunctioning adenomas that showed only focal, weak immunoreactivity for hormones [IHC for luteinizing hormone shown by arrow in (**F**)] also showed strong cytoplasmic expression FR-α (**G**). Pituitary adenomas, such as a prolactinoma showing cytoplasmic immunoreactivity for prolactin by IHC (**H**), did not show appreciable cytoplasmic FR-α (**I**).

using ³H-labeled folic acid that FR-α is capable of binding folates, indicating that the over-expressed receptor was properly folded and may mediate vitamin uptake. Comparison of binding levels for protein and ³H-labeled folic acid in subtypes of non-functional adenomas suggests that the immunhistochemically negative adenomas produced more properly folded FR-α than adenomas that stained positively for anterior pituitary hormones. Finally, immunohistochemistry demonstrated that FR-α was specifically expressed in nonfunctioning adenoma cells. These results demonstrate that over-expression of FR-α mRNA by nonfunctioning pituitary adenomas results in production of properly folded FR-α

protein, may mediate vitamin transport, and could potentially facilitate the growth of these tumors (Figure 37.17).[16]

SURGICAL OUTCOME

Following operative decompression of nonfunctioning adenomas, vision improves in approximately 80% of patients. Generally, endocrine function is the same pre- and postoperatively, although transsphenoidal surgery usually stops progressive loss of hormonal function. Unfortunately, approximately one-third of patients with nonfunctioning adenomas already exhibit panhypopituitarism before their surgical treatment.[7]

Postoperative evaluation with MRI and CT has several limitations. It is difficult to evaluate the sella immediately after surgery because of postoperative bleeding and intrasellar changes. It is probably best to delay the initial postoperative anatomical study for at least 4–6 weeks. In most cases, no suprasellar mass is seen following operative decompression. Persistent mass effect seen in the early postoperative period will generally resolve. The gradual resolution of the mass effect can be documented with serial MRI studies.[17] If vision is improved following transsphenoidal surgery, it may be best simply to follow the patient, even if he or she has persistent suprasellar mass effect.

FOLLOW-UP

Most patients with nonfunctioning pituitary adenomas should have annual CT scan or MRI, visual field, and endocrine evaluations whether or not they have had surgical or radiation treatment. If these tumors are not treated, they grow slowly over months or years. There is a significant recurrence rate following transsphenoidal surgery (approximately 20%). The recurrence rate following both surgical decompression and radiation therapy is approximately 10%. A significant number of patients who undergo postoperative radiation therapy can develop further hormonal loss. Replacement hormonal therapy should be monitored by an endocrinologist. Patients must be aware that hydrocortisone replacement doses may need to be increased during illness or stressful periods.

CONCLUSION

Nonfunctioning pituitary adenomas are found in a significant proportion of patients with pituitary tumors. The tumors are usually large before they are discovered. Bitemporal visual field loss or loss of pituitary function are the most common presenting clinical manifestations. Transsphenoidal removal of the adenoma with appropriate replacement therapy is the most common treatment for this disorder. Radiation therapy may be used in selected patients.

Unlike the functional pituitary tumors, there is no available effective medical therapy for the nonfunctioning tumors and only a better understanding of the molecular biology of these tumors will provide a medical treatment option. The goal of transsphenoidal surgery is to remove the adenomas as completely as possible while leaving any remaining normal gland. However, invasion of the cavernous sinus and frequent invasion of the surrounding dura may limit the ability to remove a large adenoma totally.

This chapter contains material from the previous edition, and I am grateful to the author of that chapter for his contribution.

REFERENCES

1. Asa SL, Kovacs K. Clinically non-functioning human pituitary adenomas. *Can J Neurol Sci* 1992; 19: 228–35.
2. Asa SL, Ezzat S. The cytogenesis and pathogenesis of pituitary adenomas. *Endocr Rev* 1998; 19: 798–827.
3. Black PM, Hsu DW, Klibanski A, *et al.* Hormone production in clinically nonfunctioning pituitary adenomas. *J Neurosurg* 1987; 66: 244–50.

CLINICAL PEARLS

- Nonfunctioning pituitary adenomas comprise a significant portion of patients with pituitary tumors.

- They typically are quite large, and cause hypopituitarism or blindness from regional compression.

- The term nonfunctioning reflects the fact that these tumors do not cause clinical hormone hypersecretion.

- The usual treatment of a nonfunctioning pituitary adenoma in a medically stable patient is microscopic or endoscopic transsphenoidal removal of the tumor.

- Unlike the functional pituitary tumors, there is no available effective medical therapy for the nonfunctioning tumors.

4. Katznelson L, Alexander JM, Klibanski A. Clinical review 45: clinically nonfunctioning pituitary adenomas. *J Clin Endocrinol Metab* 1993; 76: 1089–94.
5. Greenman Y, Melmed S. Diagnosis and management of nonfunctioning pituitary tumors. *Annu Rev Med* 1996; 47: 95–106.
6. Yamada S, Asa SL, Kovacs K, Muller P, Smyth HS. Analysis of hormone secretion by clinically nonfunctioning human pituitary adenomas using the reverse hemolytic plaque assay. *J Clin Endocrinol Metab* 1989; 68: 73–80.
7. Nelson PB, Goodman M, Flickenger JC. Endocrine function in patients with large pituitary tumors treated with operative decompression and radiation therapy. *Neurosurgery* 1989; 24: 398–400.
8. Biousse V, Newman NJ, Oyesiku NM. Precipitating factors in pituitary apoplexy. *J Neurol Neurosurg Psychiatr* 2001; 71: 542–5.
9. Mikhael M, Ciric I. MR imaging of pituitary tumors before and after surgical and/or medical treatment. *J Computer Assisted Tomogr* 1988; 12: 441–5.
10. Dolinskas C, Simeone F. Transsphenoidal hypophysectomy: postsurgical CT findings. *Am J Neuroradiol* 1985; 6: 45–50.
11. Ebersold MJ, Quast LM, Laws ER, Scheithauer B, Randall RV. Long-term results in transsphenoidal removal of nonfunctioning pituitary adenomas. *J Neurosurg* 1986; 64: 713–19.
12. Marcou Y, Plowman PN. Stereotactic radiosurgery for pituitary adenomas. *Trends Endocrinol Metab* 2000; 11: 132–7.
13. Becker G, Kocher M, Kortmann RD, *et al.* Radiation therapy in the multimodal treatment approach of pituitary adenoma. *Strahlenther Onkol* 2002; 178: 173–86.
14. Milker-Zabel S, Debus J, Thilmann C, Schlegel W, Wannenmacher M. Fractionated stereotactically guided radiotherapy and radiosurgery in the treatment of functional and nonfunctional adenomas of the pituitary gland. *Int J Radiat Oncol Biol Phys* 2001; 50: 1279–86.
15. Evans CO, Young AN, Brown MR, *et al.* Novel patterns of gene expression in pituitary adenomas identified by complementary deoxyribonucleic acid microarrays and quantitative reverse transcription-polymerase chain reaction. *J Clin Endocrinol Metab* 2001; 86: 3097–107.
16. Evans CO, Reddy P, Brat DJ, *et al.* Differential expression of folate receptor in pituitary adenomas. *Cancer Res* 2003; 63: 4218–24.
17. Rajaraman V, Schulder M. Postoperative MRI appearance after transsphenoidal pituitary tumor resection. *Surg Neurol* 1999; 52: 592–8.

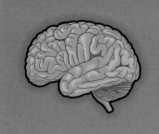

The anterior pituitary gland is responsible for the secretion and regulation of a variety of peptide hormones and stimulating factors. Pituitary adenomas are benign monoclonal tumors that arise from the cells comprising the anterior pituitary gland. They account for approximately 15% of all intracranial tumors. Tumors originating in the anterior pituitary gland may, therefore, produce excess quantities of a particular peptide hormone. When this occurs the resulting adenoma is classified as a functioning or secretory adenoma. Tumors without hormonal activity are logically classified as nonfunctioning or nonsecretory adenomas (see Chapter 37). In this chapter we will review the different types of functioning pituitary adenomas. A brief review of the hypothalamic–pituitary–end organ axis will be helpful in understanding the diagnosis and treatment of patients with functioning pituitary tumors.

The anterior pituitary gland is under predominantly stimulatory control by the hypothalamus. Function of the normal pituitary gland depends on the integrity of the hypothalamus, the portal circulation, and the pituitary stalk. The pituitary hormones adrenocorticotropic hormone (ACTH), growth hormone (GH), prolactin, thyroid-stimulating hormone (TSH), luteinizing hormone (LH), and follicle-stimulating hormone (FSH) are controlled by the hypothalamic hormones corticotropin-releasing hormone (CRH), growth-hormone-releasing factor (GRF), dopamine [also known as prolactin inhibitory factor (PIF)], thyroid-releasing hormone (TRH), and gonadotropin-releasing hormone (GnRH) respectively. This is efficiently accomplished via a portal vascular system connecting the hypothalamus with the anterior pituitary gland. The fact that prolactin is under inhibitory control by the hypothalamus becomes advantageous in the medical treatment of prolactin-secreting tumors. These hypothalamic releasing factors are then under negative feedback control from the end-organ products, i.e. adrenal gland products, thyroid hormone, etc., thereby completing the axis loop.[1] The predominant net hypothalamic regulatory influence is stimulatory for all pituitary hormones except prolactin, which is under dominant inhibitory control.[2] Any interruption or compression of the network of portal vessels as a result of pressure or invasion by any parasellar mass can alter the delivery of these hypothalamic factors to the anterior pituitary and cause impairment in its function.

Anterior pituitary gland adenomas are identified pathologically both by their *in vivo* endocrine activity and by their *in vitro* immunohistochemical staining characteristics. The advent of immunohistochemical staining for the various peptide hormones has revealed the fact that many adenomas once thought to be nonsecretory actually secrete endocrinologically inactive peptides.[3]

The alpha subunit, which has no known systemic effects, is one of the commonly found peptides.

Adenomas may be further subdivided into micro- or macroadenomas based upon size (Figure 38.1).[4] Tumors less than 1 cm in diameter are considered microadenomas and are predictably located solely within the sella turcica. They characteristically do not invade neighboring structures such as the sphenoid and cavernous sinuses. Macroadenomas, by definition greater than 1 cm, typically enlarge the sella turcica and frequently invade neighboring structures. Microadenomas usually are discovered because of an endocrinopathy, whereas macroadenomas present with compressive effects of the tumor, i.e. bitemporal hemianopsia, as well as endocrinopathy. The endocrinopathy may be one of either oversecretion or undersecretion.

The evaluation of a patient with a suspected functioning pituitary tumor will be discussed in relation to each tumor type; however, because of the protean and often subtle manifestations of these endocrinopathies, a detailed history and physical examination are mandatory in guiding the rest of the work-up. Subtle changes in hair growth, skin texture or color, and body mass may be the only heralds of early endocrine dysfunction.

The radiographic evaluation of patients with pituitary adenomas has been dramatically changed with the advances of magnetic resonance imaging (MRI) technology. MRI with and without gadolinium enhancement is now considered the study of choice in evaluating patients with suspected pituitary abnormalities (Figures 38.2–38.4).[5–8] The normal pituitary gland will enhance within 5 minutes of contrast administration, leaving the adenoma hypointense compared with the surrounding pituitary tissue. If the study is performed more than 5 minutes after contrast administration, the tumor will appear enhanced while the normal gland will appear unenhanced. It is therefore imperative that the neuroradiologist indicates the timing of the study in relation to contrast enhancement. Findings on high-resolution MRI studies are highly sensitive, with a 60–70% sensitivity on unenhanced studies, increasing by 10% on postcontrast studies. Computed axial tomography (CT) is helpful in evaluating bony changes in the sella and surrounding structures but is much less sensitive than MRI in detecting small adenomas (Figure 38.5).[9–12] Patients with endocrinologically silent tumors may infrequently require angiography to exclude a carotid artery aneurysm, although MRI has made this very rare.

Patients with macroadenomas must undergo detailed visual-field testing that may reveal previously unnoticed abnormalities. This will also serve as a baseline for comparison to subsequent visual-field testing. With all this in mind, it is appropriate to focus

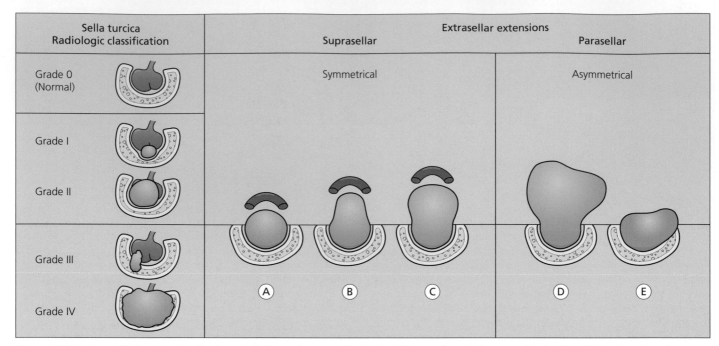

Figure 38.1 Radiographic/imaging classification of pituitary adenomas. Grades I and II are enclosed adenomas. Grades III and IV are invasive adenomas. Extensions A, B, C are directly suprasellar, while D is asymmetric intracranial and E is asymmetric into the cavernous sinus. (Adapted from ref. 4.)

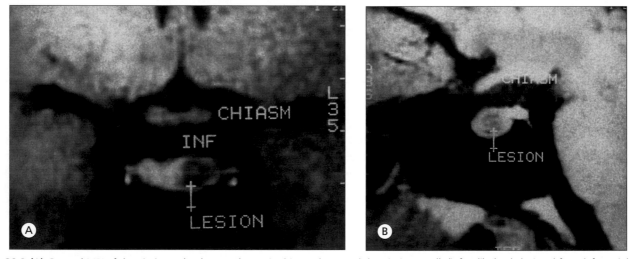

Figure 38.2 (A) Coronal MRI of the pituitary gland. Note the optic chiasm above and the pituitary stalk (infundibulum) deviated from left to right (grade I). **(B)** Sagittal MRI of the pituitary gland with a central lesion.

on the management of patients with various secretory pituitary adenomas.

PROLACTIN-SECRETING ADENOMAS

Prolactin-secreting pituitary adenomas are the most common form of pituitary tumor and represent the most common cause of hyperprolactinemia. Prolactin is classified as a somatomammotropic hormone along with GH and chorionic somatomammotropin.[13] It is a peptide chain, 198 amino acids long, necessary for the normal lactation in postpartum women. Prolactin levels begin to rise shortly after conception and reach levels of 150–200 ng/mL at

term, however it is not until the postpartum decline in estrogen is complete that lactation may occur. Stimulation of tactile receptors on the nipple and areola of the breast leads to prolactin secretion that in the postpartum estrogen-primed breast results in lactation. TRH and vasoactive intestinal peptide both appear to have minor prolactin-releasing activity, although their significance is presently unclear. Although the above stimuli lead to increases in prolactin secretion, the overwhelming control of prolactin release is inhibitory in nature, via dopamine. Dopamine, also known as prolactin-inhibiting factor (PIF), is released by the hypothalamus and leads to a decrease in prolactin secretion. As mentioned earlier, this inhibitory control becomes vitally important in the medical management of prolactinomas.[14,15] Normal prolactin levels are less

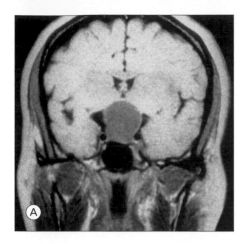

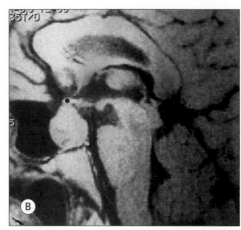

Figure 38.3 (A) Coronal MRI of the sella. Note the large adenoma with suprasellar extension. The optic chiasm is compressed and is not visible (grade IIc). **(B)** Sagittal MRI of the sella. Adenoma is seen reaching the lower surface of the optic chiasm (asterisk) (grade IIa).

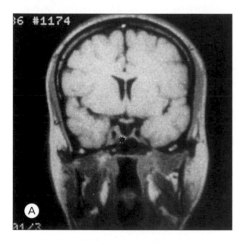

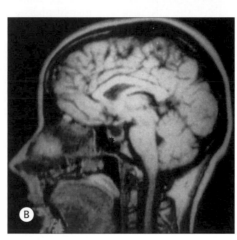

Figure 38.4 (A) Coronal MRI of sella postoperatively. Note the residual gland at the bottom of the sella (asterisk). The stalk is seen midline. **(B)** Sagittal MRI of the sella postoperatively. The residual gland is seen at the bottom of the sella (asterisk).

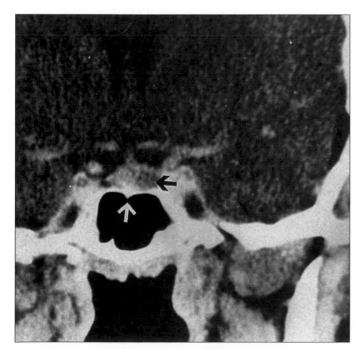

Figure 38.5 Coronal enhanced CT scan of sella. Note the adenoma (dark arrow) in the left side of the pituitary gland. The white arrow points to a bony septation within the sphenoid sinus.

than 15 ng/mL in men and less than 20 ng/mL in nonpregnant women. Causes of hyperprolactinemia other than a pituitary adenoma include pregnancy, stress, hypoglycemia, renal failure, hypothyroidism, and phenothiazine-like medications. These, as well as several other etiologies, must be considered prior to a detailed investigation of a patient's pituitary gland.[16]

Signs and symptoms

Prolactin-secreting tumors represent 40% of all pituitary adenomas and are typically more symptomatic in women. Hyperprolactinemia in women leads to amenorrhea, galactorrhea, and osteoporosis, while in men it may result in diminished sexual drive and impotence or it may be asymptomatic. Because of this difference, men are not usually diagnosed until the tumor has reached a size sufficient to cause compressive effects on neighboring structures.[17]

Diagnosis

Random measurements of the serum prolactin level are reliable to establish the diagnosis of hyperprolactinemia (Table 38.1). In the absence of the other above-mentioned disorders investigation of the pituitary gland is necessary. This should begin with a gadolinium-enhanced MRI, which will often disclose a pituitary macroadenoma. Hyperprolactinemia in the presence of a macroadenoma does not mean *a priori* that the tumor is a prolactinoma.

Table 38.1 Diagnosis of pituitary function

1 Thyroid function tests, e.g. thyroxine, triiodothyronine resin uptake, TSH
2 Baseline a.m. plasma cortisol and response to ACTH
3 LH, FSH, and testosterone in men; no tests if menstruating female
4 Prolactin – no stimulation test
5 Growth hormone, IGF-1

Table 38.2 Differential diagnosis of hyperprolactinemia

Nonpathologic causes
Pregnancy
Early periods of nursing
Stress

Primary pituitary causes
True prolactinomas
Stalk compression secondary to nonprolactin-secreting adenomas
Traumatic stalk section
Empty sella syndrome

Systemic disorders
Hypothyroidism
Renal failure
Liver disease
Chest wall surgery/trauma

Pharmacologic causes
Dopamine antagonists, e.g. phenothiazine-like drugs
Monoamine oxidase inhibitors
Monoamine oxidase depleters
Opiate derivatives
Oral contraceptives

The degree of prolactin elevation is directly related to the level of tumor function. Serum prolactin levels greater than 250 ng/mL correlate very well with the presence of a prolactinoma; however, milder elevations may be the result of stalk compression leading to interference with the inhibitory effects of dopamine (Table 38.2).

Treatment

Dopamine agonists such as bromocriptine and cabergoline have radically changed the treatment of symptomatic prolactinomas (Figure 38.6).[18–32] Except for the specific situations discussed below, dopamine agonist therapy has virtually replaced transsphenoidal resection as the therapy of choice for this group of tumors. Bromocriptine is a dopamine agonist that directly stimulates the dopamine receptors located on lactotrophs (prolactin-secreting cells). Dosages of 2.5–7.5 mg/day are usually sufficient to treat most patients. Cabergoline dosage is usually 2.5 mg/week. The response to dopamine agonists is remarkable. Prolactin levels will begin to decrease in a matter of hours following the first dose and tumor size will often diminish within a few days. Patients with visual-field deficits may begin to improve after a few days of treatment. Other than pregnancy or rapidly deteriorating visual function, there are virtually no contraindications to an initial trial of bromocriptine therapy. Follow-up, with periodic serum prolactin measurements and imaging studies of the sella, is necessary to ensure that therapy is effective. In approximately 66% of patients, tumor size will be reduced by as much as 75%, with the best response seen in patients with large tumors (Figures 38.7, 38.8).[21] Endocrine function often returns to normal, with establishment of cyclic menses in women and return of libido in men. Many previously infertile women have, in fact, been able to conceive while on bromocriptine therapy.

Since bromocriptine and cabergoline are not tumoricidal, it is said that tumor re-expansion will occur as soon as therapy is stopped.[33] There is, however, a small subset of patients in which neither discontinuation of therapy nor microdosage leads to a return of symptoms or hyperprolactinemia.[20,34] Because it is impossible to predict which patients will have such a dramatic response, it is prudent to stop therapy every few years and determine whether there is continued need for treatment.[35]

While dopamine agonists appear to be a true panacea, they are not without problems and side-effects. Most commonly, patients complain of nausea and vomiting and the need for potential lifelong therapy. Although there are as yet no definite teratogenic effects from bromocriptine or cabergoline, pregnancy is a relative contraindication to dopamine agonist therapy. Women harboring tumors larger than 12 mm who wish to conceive are often referred for tumor resection prior to pregnancy to avoid pregnancy-induced enlargement of the tumor and neurologic symptoms. In women with tumors smaller than 12 mm, the risk of neurologic dysfunction during pregnancy is less than 1%.[36]

Bromocriptine has greatly limited the indications for transsphenoidal resection of prolactinomas. Surgery is usually reserved for patients who are either completely intolerant or show zero to minimal response to medical therapy, patients with severe or worsening visual-field deficits, and patients with deficits that do not improve after 2 months of medical therapy (Figure 38.6).[37] Young women with microadenomas are excellent surgical and medical candidates and may opt for surgery where there is a high likelihood of cure, rather than a prolonged period of time on medication. Giant prolactinomas often do extremely well with just dopamine agonists as they may be exquisitely responsive. The main indication for early surgery is intratumoral hematoma, whereas our main indications for late surgery are cerebrospinal fluid leakage caused by medical treatment, or an increasing prolactin level and tumor growth despite medical therapy.[37]

Radiation therapy has a very limited role in the treatment of prolactinomas. Primary radiation therapy is reserved for elderly or debilitated patients who have large tumors that threaten vital neurovascular structures and who are not adequately helped by medical therapy. Secondary radiation therapy as an adjunct to transsphenoidal surgery is indicated in patients with residual tumor who are unresponsive to or intolerant of bromocriptine.

Pretreatment with bromocriptine to "shrink" the tumor has been suggested to increase the surgical cure rate.[38,39] Thus far, there has been no appreciable benefit. If surgery is contemplated, it is best performed within a year of bromocriptine therapy. Long-term bromocriptine use has been associated with tumor fibrosis, making surgical resection more difficult.[40,41]

Do all patients with prolactinomas require treatment of some sort? There is a subset of patients with so-called asymptomatic microprolactinomas whose treatment remains controversial. Both tumor size and serum prolactin levels may remain unchanged or even decrease over many years in some women with microprolactinomas who receive no treatment.[42,43] Aside from regular surveillance it would not appear that any treatment is indicated. Many favor treatment to normalize prolactin and thereby decrease the future risks of osteoporosis.[44,45]

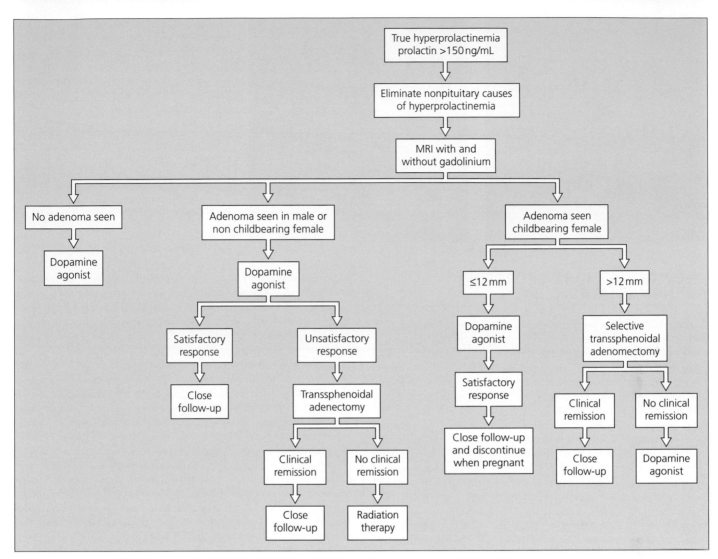

Figure 38.6 Management of prolactinomas.

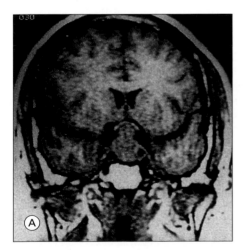

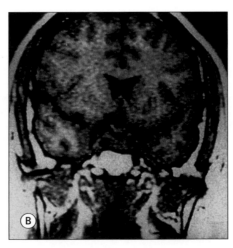

Figure 38.7 (A) Prebromocriptine coronal MRI demonstrating a large prolactin-secreting pituitary adenoma. The chiasm (white arc above tumor) is distorted. **(B)** Coronal MRI of same patient after 4 months of bromocriptine therapy. Note the dramatic decrease in the size of the tumor. The chiasm is no longer compressed.

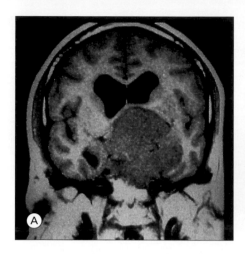 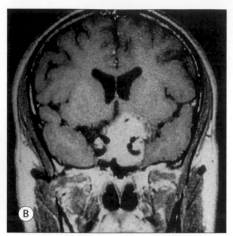

Figure 38.8 (A) Prebromocriptine MRI demonstrating enormous prolactin-secreting pituitary adenoma with hydrocephalus. **(B)** The same patient 2 years later, treated only with bromocriptine. The tumor is dramatically smaller and the hydrocephalus is resolved.

GROWTH-HORMONE-SECRETING ADENOMAS (ACROMEGALY)

Acromegaly or gigantism results from the hypersecretion of GH, and although it was described before the turn of the century, Cushing is credited with relating it to the overproduction of GH from a pituitary source.[46] The term acromegaly is derived from the Greek *akron* (extremity) and *megale* (great) but describes only one aspect of the clinical features. GH is a polypeptide hormone, 191 amino acids long, normally produced and released by the somatotropic cells found in the anterior pituitary in response to hypothalamic GRF.[47] Somatostatin is a 14-amino-acid cyclic peptide-releasing factor that inhibits GH release.[48] Three or four bursts of GH secretion occur per day, punctuating a basal state of minimal activity.[49] Sleep, physical exertion or stress, hyper- and hypoglycemia, and a variety of pharmacologic agents may also precipitate GH release. Circulating GH results in the secretion from the liver of a family of peptides called somatomedins. Somatomedin-C [insulin-like growth factor 1 (IGF-1)] is the most familiar somatomedin measured in clinical practice. These secondary hormones, in turn, produce a variety of anabolic effects throughout the body and mediate the effects of GH at the end-organ level. Unlike GH, the somatomedins do not exhibit significant diurnal variation in serum levels and therefore may be a better means of evaluating patients.[50] To summarize, GH is released in response to GRF from the hypothalamus, leading to increased levels and activity of IGF-1, which, in turn, negatively feeds back to limit the production of GH. In addition, GH secretion is tightly regulated by somatostatin.

Hypersecretion of GH may result from a number of conditions. The most common, and the focus of this section, is a pituitary adenoma. However, GH may also be produced by ectopic adenomas derived from remnants of the embryonic pituitary diverticulum or from tumors of the breast, lung, or ovary.[51] Acromegaly may rarely be caused by excessive production of GRF by a hypothalamic tumor or from peripheral sources such as carcinoid tumors of the abdomen.[52]

Signs and symptoms

Acromegaly affects males and females equally, most often in the fifth decade.[53] The effects of chronically elevated growth hormone are gradual and will result either in gigantism in a child whose epiphyseal plates have not yet closed or in classic acromegalic features in an adult. Typically there is an insidious coarsening of the facial features and an increase in the soft tissues. A significant number of patients present because of the local compressive effects of an expanding pituitary mass, rather than because of somatic disturbances. The somatic changes may be so insidious as to go unnoticed until old snapshots are used for comparison. Classically patients first note an increase in shoe size or inability to wear rings that were previously a good fit. Later in the disease process patients may develop visceromegaly, arthralgias, nerve entrapment syndromes, hyperhidrosis, prognathism, and acrochordon (skin tags). The development of skin tags is interesting and deserves some comment because of its relationship to potentially malignant colonic polyps. It has been noted in several studies that as many as 46% of patients with acromegaly will have colonic polyps, of which more than 50% are adenomatous.[54] Some studies have also shown that the incidence of true colon carcinoma in acromegalics may be higher than in the general population. Because of this relationship it has been recommended that acromegalic patients older than 50 years, patients with more than a 10-year history of acromegaly, or patients with more than three skin tags should have careful screening for colonic disease.[55]

Diagnosis

The laboratory diagnosis of acromegaly is hampered by the normally wide daily variations in serum GH levels. In fact, the daily bursts of secretion are maintained even in the presence of oversecretion of GH from an adenoma. Unlike the other secretory adenomas, static measurements of serum GH are, therefore, unreliable in establishing the diagnosis of acromegaly. Normal basal GH levels are generally below 1 ng/mL, with several secretory bursts seen throughout the day.[56] In acromegaly the basal level is often elevated to levels above 5 ng/mL, although some patients may have normal basal levels with elevations only during the daily secretory bursts (Table 38.3).

Fortunately, IGF-1 levels are even throughout the day, and are consistently elevated in acromegaly. Static measurements of IGF-1 are an effective and reliable method for confirming the diagnosis of acromegaly.[57,58] Alternatively, a glucose tolerance test can be performed. Normally, GH is suppressed to levels below 1 ng/mL after an oral glucose load (100 g). Failure of this normal suppression is consistent with hypersecretion of GH. In addition, infusions of either GRF or TRH will lead to increased GH in affected individuals but not in normal subjects.

Table 38.3 Diagnosis of acromegaly
Usual studies
Plasma GH
Response to oral glucose (OGTT)
MRI
Other studies
Somatomedin-C (IGF-1)
Response to TRH
GRF

Once a patient is confirmed as having a hypersecretory state, the goal is to discover the source. The overwhelming majority of patients will have an anterior pituitary adenoma and, therefore, the radiographic work-up should begin with a contrast-enhanced MRI. Only in the few cases where no pituitary mass is demonstrated should a search be made for ectopic sources of growth hormone.

Treatment

The effects of untreated acromegaly are eventually fatal. Patients will develop cardiac failure, diabetes, disfigurement, and possibly blindness, leading to a markedly shortened life expectancy.[59] The goal of treatment, therefore, is the safe and rapid reduction of GH levels, elimination of any mass effect, and preservation of normal hormonal balance. The type of treatment must be judged on its ability to normalize GH levels and thereby to eliminate the development of the various metabolic derangements associated with hypersecretory states. The criteria for successful treatment of acromegaly are quite controversial. The accepted postoperative levels of GH that are indicative of a cure have declined in recent years. The current standard for cure is clinical remission associated with a postoperative GH level of less than 1 ng/mL following oral glucose tolerance test with a normal IGF-1 level.[60] GH levels may return to normal in hours or days, but it has been our experience that IGF-1 levels may take weeks or months to normalize. Postoperative adjuvant therapy should be reserved for patients who do not meet these criteria (Figure 38.9).

Transsphenoidal resection remains the primary treatment modality for acromegaly (Figure 38.10). Successful resection results in a rapid reduction in GH levels and can be achieved with very low morbidity and mortality, even in older patients.[4,61–64] In addition, the preservation of pituitary function has been reported to be as high as 95%, avoiding the need for lifelong hormone replacement. For larger tumors not amenable to curative resection, surgery still plays a significant role in reducing tumor load prior to any adjuvant therapy.

While transsphenoidal resection of pituitary adenomas is a safe and well-tolerated procedure, there are still many patients who

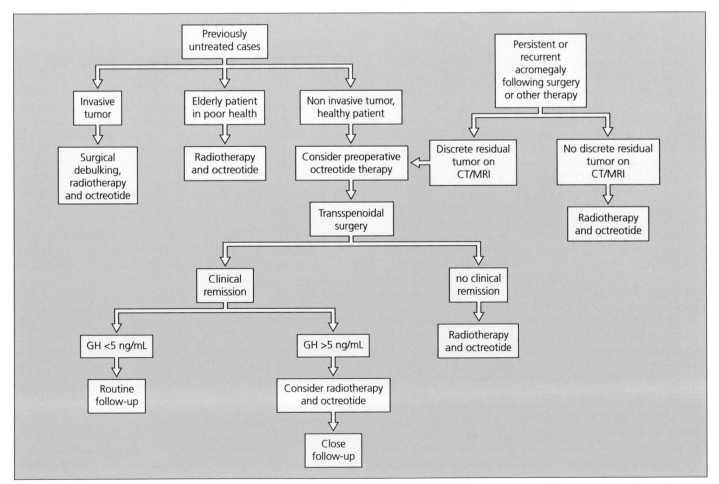

Figure 38.9 Management of acromegaly.

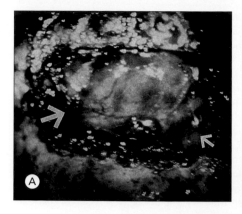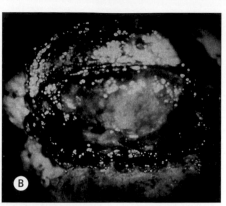

Figure 38.10 (A) Transsphenoidal exposure of the pituitary gland (large arrow). Microadenoma is seen in right lower corner (smaller arrow). **(B)** Same exposure with the adenoma removed. The normal gland remains.

simply are not surgical candidates. In those cases medical treatment and radiotherapy have great therapeutic importance. The medical treatment of acromegalics has undergone considerable change in the past 10–15 years. Medical therapy, which included estrogens, chlorpromazine, and antiserotonergic agents, had met with only limited success. Bromocriptine therapy, then used for its dopaminergic effects, was able to reduce GH levels to 5–10 ng/mL in more than 20% of patients.[65,66] Most patients did achieve some relief of their somatic symptomatology, with reduced soft-tissue swelling and decreased perspiration, even though GH levels were still elevated. The dosages necessary to achieve these effects are much higher than the dosages needed to control a prolactinoma and the consequent incidence of side-effects and drug intolerance is much higher. The same has been true of cabergoline.[67]

Since somatostatin naturally suppresses GH production, the ideal would be to give somatostatin. A somatostatin analog named octreotide has a longer half-life and has been shown to be very effective.[68–79] It initially had to be administered three times each day as a subcutaneous injection or as a continuous subcutaneous infusion. The most common side-effects reported include diarrhea and cholelithiasis, and the incidence of these side-effects increases the longer the drug is administered. Some studies have shown dramatic reductions in GH levels and moderate tumor shrinkage. The perioperative period may be significantly improved by using octreotide for 3–4 months preoperatively.[75] The reversal of soft-tissue changes about the tongue and throat may lessen the risks of anesthesia. With the newer long-acting somatostatin analogs, there has been more reason to utilize this as adjunctive therapy for those tumors not cured by surgery, and even as primary therapy for some.[76] It has become imperative to normalize the GH and IGF-1 utilizing the strictest criteria as it has been shown that cardiac performance is dramatically improved, with a return to normal cardiac function.[78] All patients not achieving cure with surgery are considered candidates for adjunctive therapy with either somatostatin analogs, radiation, or a combination of the two. With long-acting release (LAR) there is a 70% chance of controlling GH to < 2.5 ng/mL with a 61% likelihood of a normal IGF-1 level. In this same series there was a 50% incidence of 50% decrease in tumor size.[77]

The only other treatment option for patients is radiation therapy. Not only is this treatment fraught with difficulties such as hypopituitarism in up to 80% and radiation necrosis, but it has not been shown to be uniformly effective.[80–84] Many patients will have persistently elevated GH levels for years following radiation therapy and may never reach normal levels, resulting in delayed or incomplete remission. However, there clearly is efficacy in utilizing radiation when surgery has not been curative and the tumor has not been responsive to adjunctive LAR therapy. Conventional radiotherapy, utilizing a total dose of 40–54 Gy in 1.8–2 Gy per fraction has led to normalization in 65–70% of patients after 6–15 years.[80,81] Stereotactic radiosurgery has had more recent application to target residual tumor within the cavernous sinus and greater than 4 mm distant from the optic nerves and chiasm.[85,86] Thus far it does show promise for tumor control with less morbidity to the surrounding structures including the normal pituitary gland, but longer follow-up studies are needed before final recommendations are established. At the present time, we utilized stereotactic radiosurgery for this type of residual disease.

GLYCOPROTEIN-SECRETING ADENOMAS (TSH, FSH, LH)

The glycoprotein hormones produced in the mammalian pituitary gland are TSH, LH, and FSH. Although these hormones are clearly related structurally, their roles are markedly different. TSH, as its name implies, regulates the metabolic rate via thyroid hormones, while the gonadotropic hormones LH and FSH are responsible for sexual maturation and play pivotal roles in reproduction. Structurally, all three are composed of a common alpha subunit bonded to a beta subunit that is unique to each hormone.

A number of laboratory advances have changed our understanding of glycoprotein-secreting adenomas. Two in particular were the development of specific immunohistochemical techniques for looking at tumor specimens and the improved techniques of measuring hormone and subunit levels *in vivo*. It had always been taught that glycoprotein-secreting adenomas represent a very small percentage of all pituitary tumors (approximately 1%). These improved techniques have revealed that many so-called "nonfunctioning" adenomas have evidence of glycoprotein production by immunohistochemical staining and serum radio-immunoassay techniques.[3]

Signs and symptoms

Except for TSH-secreting tumors, which may present as hyperthyroidism, the glycoprotein-secreting adenomas do not produce any specific clinical syndrome referable to the hypersecretory state. Consequently, these adenomas are not discovered until they produce compressive effects upon juxtaposed structures such as the optic chiasm or pituitary stalk. This unfortunately means that many of these adenomas will grow to a size and extent that precludes any type of curative resection.

Hyperthyroidism caused by a TSH adenoma differs markedly from Graves' disease, for which it is very often mistaken.[87] The typical features of Graves' disease, including ophthalmopathy, pretibial edema, female preponderance, and serum thyroid-stimulating immunoglobulin, are lacking in hyperthyroidism of pituitary origin. While these differences are not usually enough to make a clear distinction, it should raise some questions as to the accuracy of the diagnosis of Graves' disease. Of note is a rare inherited disorder (autosomal dominant) designated as "selective pituitary resistance to thyroid hormone," in which the normal negative feedback effect of thyroid hormone upon TSH secretion is defective. This leads to TSH hypersecretion and continued production of active thyroid hormone, resulting in clinical hyperthyroidism. The TSH levels increase with TRH stimulation, and this disorder is often associated with deaf-mutism, stippled epiphyses, and goiter, distinguishing it from a pituitary adenoma.

Diagnosis

As mentioned above, these tumors do not typically present with symptoms of hormone hypersecretion. As a result the determination that a pituitary tumor is secreting one of the glycoproteins is usually made after the tumor itself is discovered. Each of the hormones is composed of an alpha subunit and a beta subunit. Although the alpha subunit is the same for all three hormones, the beta subunit is specific to each type. We are currently only able to measure serum intact hormone levels (alpha + beta), or alpha subunit levels alone. The measurement of beta subunit levels is possible, but is only available in some research laboratories. We have learned that not all patients will have an elevated intact hormone level and some may in fact have low intact hormone levels with evidence of hormone production seen on pathologic examination.[88] Fortunately, alpha subunit levels are elevated fairly consistently in these tumors, decrease after successful treatment, and rise with tumor recurrence, although 22% of truly nonfunctional adenomas will have an associated alpha subunit elevation.[89,90] Even with this small false-positive rate, alpha subunit measurements serve as reliable guides to tumor therapy and recurrence.

As with all other pituitary adenomas, MRI with gadolinium has nearly replaced all other imaging modalities for evaluation of tumor anatomy. Specific to glycoprotein-secreting adenomas is the tendency to be larger and involve adjacent structures more often. Aside from this, there is no way to distinguish these adenomas from any other pituitary adenoma based on radiographic studies alone.

Treatment

The treatment of patients with glycoprotein-secreting adenomas is often unrewarding. Because of the delay in clinical presentation these tumors usually have suprasellar extension and involvement of the cavernous sinuses, lowering the chances for a surgical cure. Transsphenoidal resection is necessary for tissue diagnosis as well as decompression of the optic chiasm. Most patients have adequate symptomatic relief postoperatively; however, surgery is very often combined with radiotherapy or adjuvant medical therapy. Since the response of the tumor to radiation has not been impressive, the indications for it remain controversial.[89] Trials with

a somatostatin analog and bromocriptine in the treatment of these tumors have met with some success, but not as much as in the treatment of acromegaly and prolactinomas, respectively.[90,91] At our institution, these patients are managed with transsphenoidal adenomectomy followed by radiation therapy if residual tumor is seen on postoperative scans. If the postoperative studies suggest a "cure," MRIs are repeated every 6 months initially, followed by yearly intervals.

ACTH-SECRETING ADENOMAS (CUSHING'S DISEASE)

By definition, Cushing syndrome is a condition of hypercortisolemia from any source, while the term Cushing's disease refers exclusively to an ACTH-producing pituitary adenoma. More than any other secretory tumor of the pituitary gland, the basophilic ACTH-producing adenoma responsible for Cushing's disease continues to provide the clinician with diagnostic and therapeutic challenges. Other pituitary tumors that synthesize excessive amounts of hormones often present with annoying or disfiguring symptoms or mass effect related to large adenoma size (e.g. tumors making prolactin or GH), MRI or CT are usually positive, and treatment options, while not always effective, are at least straightforward.

Hypercortisolemia, on the other hand, can cause a myriad of problems of significant clinical importance.[92] Patients tend to feel poorly, have diffuse muscle weakness and pain, emotional lability, and profound fatigue. The presence of cortisol-induced or accelerated atherosclerosis, hypertension, diabetes mellitus, osteoporosis, obesity, susceptibility to infection, and perhaps peptic ulcer disease and thrombosis provide compelling impetus to identify and resolve the problem.

Until recently, in most surgical series examining the diagnostic usefulness of standard radiologic imaging in Cushing's disease, scans have often been either negative or nonspecifically (misleadingly) positive.[8,93–104] Because of the high frequency of incidental pituitary tumors (reported by Burrow and colleagues to be found in 27% of nonselected patients studied at autopsy), which may be causally unrelated to a patient's Cushing's disease, and because most ACTH-producing tumors tend to be small, radiographic findings must be interpreted cautiously. In our experience, even with modern MRI, including rapid sequence studies, 45% of patients with Cushing's disease have normal MRI studies. Rapid sequence imaging has not proven as effective as we had anticipated.

Most cases of hypercortisolemia seen in the adult population are caused by microadenomas of the anterior pituitary gland.[106] Other sources, including ectopic overproduction of ACTH[107,108] and/or CRH,[109,110] benign or malignant adrenal tumors synthesizing cortisol autonomously, iatrogenic or other exogenous hypercortisolemias, and alcoholic or depressive "pseudo-Cushing's" states,[111] are less common. The distinction between Cushing's disease and other causes of Cushing syndrome often poses a challenging (and frustrating) diagnostic dilemma. We will not discuss nonpituitary sources of hypercortisolemia in this chapter, except in relation to their distinction from Cushing's disease.

The histopathologic findings from pituitary tissue removed during surgery for Cushing's disease can be variable, and this is discussed in more detail below. The presence of neural tissue within an adenoma and either a distinct adenoma or diffuse or nodular hyperplasia may support the concept that pituitary

Cushing's disease is actually a heterogeneous disorder.[112] The implications for clinical management are important. Primary pituitary Cushing's (with a single adenoma) might be curable by selective adenomectomy. Hyperplasia (perhaps resulting from central overstimulation of the pituitary) might best be treated by complete hypophysectomy or drugs aimed at modulating that stimulation.[113]

Signs and symptoms

There appears to be a female preponderance, with an average age of approximately 40 years. All patients present with clinical evidence of hypercortisolemia of varying degrees. Typically patients will have truncal obesity, hypertension, easy bruisability, abdominal striae, and plethoric or moon facies (Figure 38.11). This impressive endocrinologic display means that patients generally present early in terms of tumor growth, making detection and identification of a source quite frustrating.

Diagnosis

Prior to a detailed discussion of the various tests available to establish the diagnosis of Cushing's disease, it is important to understand the normal hypothalamic–pituitary–adrenal axis. Briefly, CRH is released from the hypothalamus and stimulates ACTH secretion from the adenohypophysis. ACTH increases the production and secretion of cortisol from the adrenal cortex. Aldosterone secretion is controlled by the renin–angiotensin

system and is therefore essentially unaffected by ACTH. There is a normal diurnal pattern to cortisol release, with the highest levels seen in the morning and the lowest seen in the evening. In addition, cortisol levels normally increase any time the body is subjected to stress, either physical or metabolic. Cortisol then negatively feeds back to reduce ACTH secretion. Since ACTH is difficult to measure clinically, circulating levels of cortisol or its urinary metabolites are used to diagnose states of adrenal excess.

While Cushing syndrome is usually easy to recognize clinically, it is not always so easy to define etiologically. The various diagnostic testing protocols have been extensively reviewed and appear to be always increasing.[106,111–122] Measurements of plasma and urinary cortisol and cortisol derivatives, basally and in response to dexamethasone or metyrapone, as well as determination of plasma ACTH, may suggest either a primary adrenal, pituitary, or ectopic neoplastic source of disease (Table 38.4). If these data are equivocal, CRH measurements[109,110,123] and CRH stimulation testing with measurement of ACTH and/or cortisol[114,116,117,121] peripherally or in the bilateral venous effluent from the petrosal sinuses,[115,118,120,122] are now frequently employed to provide additional biochemical evidence for the diagnosis of Cushing's disease (Table 38.4).

Once it has been determined that a patient has a pituitary source of ACTH hypersecretion (Cushing's disease) it can be extremely difficult to identify the pituitary lesion. Since most ACTH-producing adenomas are small, their radiographic detection is difficult at best. Improvements in MRI with gadolinium enhancement have identified many microadenomas that would otherwise be radiographically invisible. Because many cases have no evidence of tumor on the MRI, the technique of petrosal sinus sampling has been developed to confirm the diagnosis and guide the surgical resection. The rationale behind this technique, which has been described in detail elsewhere, is quite straightforward (Figure 38.12).[120] Patients with Cushing's disease should have high (or inappropriately high) levels of ACTH production coming directly from the pituitary gland,[115] and the levels should lateralize[120,122] to the side containing the adenoma. Comparison of pituitary to peripheral ACTH levels should demonstrate a gradient. Those with ectopic ACTH secretion whose pituitary glands are suppressed should have neither an elevated pituitary-to-peripheral gradient nor a difference between sides. Patients without a discrete pituitary tumor (i.e. with hyperplasia of the corticotrophs) may have an increased central level of ACTH that is equal in blood from both sides of the gland. Some have advocated petrosal sinus sampling in all patients with ACTH-dependent disease, either to supplement or to supplant the conventional methods for establishing the etiology of the hypercortisolism.[118,123] Published series indicate that the usefulness and reliability of this technique may be variable.

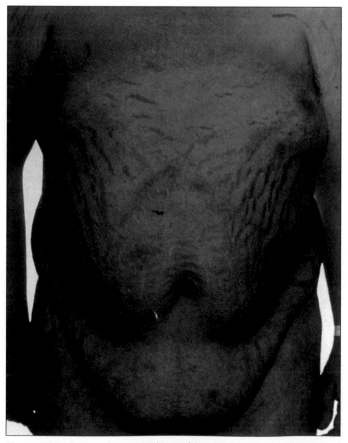

Figure 38.11 Patient demonstrating cushingoid changes.

Table 38.4 Diagnosis of Cushing's disease
Usual studies
Plasma and urinary free cortisol – baseline and response to dexamethasone
Plasma ACTH
MRI
Other studies
CRH stimulation test
Petrosal sinus ACTH sampling with CRH stimulation

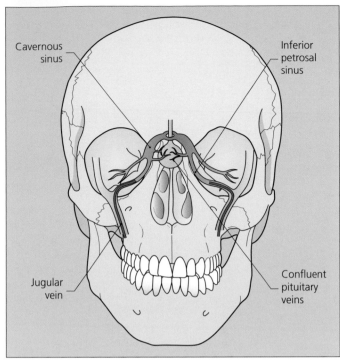

Figure 38.12 Catheter placement for simultaneous blood sampling of the inferior petrosal sinuses. The confluent pituitary veins empty laterally into the cavernous sinuses, which drain into the inferior petrosal sinuses. (Adapted from ref. 120.)

In Mampalam's series,[97] 39 of 116 subjects (34%) had selective venous sampling of ACTH. An inferior petrosal sinus to peripheral gradient was seen in 36. Of these 36, 31 (86%) were found to have adenomas. In three patients without a significant gradient, two had adenomas. Nine per cent had false localization as to the side of the adenoma. In Ludecke's series,[119] six of 19 (31%) had incorrect lateralization of the adenoma by inferior petrosal sinus sampling. Ludecke recommended intraoperative measurement of ACTH in the peripituitary blood as a means of lateralizing the adenoma.

In practice, it is clear that ACTH secretion is pulsatile, and that random sampling may not demonstrate either a gradient or laterality in patients with Cushing's disease. When ACTH levels are measured after the intravenous injection of CRH even a basally quiescent gland will respond with a localizing increase in ACTH secretion if the patient has pituitary-dependent Cushing's disease.[118,119]

In our institution, we use the technique in the following situations:

1 Patients with definite Cushing syndrome, but doubt exists as to the source of ACTH overproduction, and radiographic studies are not helpful.
2 Patients with laboratory data clearly pointing to the pituitary gland but with normal radiographic studies. A petrosal-sinus-directed hemihypophysectomy is performed if an adenoma is not seen at surgery.
3 Young patients, especially women, for whom preservation of fertility is an important consideration and whose radiologic studies are not grossly abnormal. Even when the laboratory studies clearly indicate pituitary-dependent disease, we

routinely study these patients to lateralize the tumor. If nothing is found at the time of surgery, hemihypophysectomy on the side with the higher CRH-stimulated ACTH levels would then be performed.
4 Patients who have not been cured following transsphenoidal surgery. In these patients the question to be answered is whether the diagnosis of Cushing's disease, which had obviously been thought sound enough to justify the initial surgery, was truly correct. Lack of a gradient would suggest ectopic production.

In the most skilled hands, this sampling of venous effluent from the petrosal sinuses appears to be reliable and safe. Because of our experience with false lateralization and inability to cannulate both sides simultaneously (problems that become less frequent as we do more procedures), we consider the information gained from the study along with, not in place of, the more conventionally acquired data.

Treatment

The treatment of Cushing's disease has been advanced significantly by the development and refinement of transsphenoidal pituitary microsurgery (Figure 38.13). The dramatic results of selective adenomectomy include immediate reversal of hypercortisolism and eventual return of normal pituitary corticotroph function.

Most cases of Cushing's disease are caused by isolated adenomas of the anterior gland. In less than 2% of patients with pituitary ACTH excess there occurs basophilic hyperplasia involving the entire gland. The treatment of choice for Cushing's disease is transsphenoidal exploration of the pituitary gland, with either selective adenomectomy or partial or hemihypophysectomy.[94–99,124,125] For those with very large or invasive tumors, most would suggest surgery for diagnosis and debulking, followed by conventional radiation therapy, medications, and, rarely, adrenalectomy. The large majority of these tumors (89%)[99] are microadenomas (< 1 cm in diameter) and can be difficult to localize on imaging. In 25–45% of cases, MRI does not demonstrate an identifiable neurosurgical target despite biochemical confirmation of pituitary-driven Cushing syndrome.[100] In these cases, surgical exploration reveals a seemingly identifiable adenoma in 94% of cases, which is verified histologically in 82% of cases. Intraoperative ultrasound can aid in tumor localization with 73% sensitivity and 84% positive predictive value in patients with no demonstrable tumor on MRI.[100] Frozen section and immunohistochemical analyses are often confounded by the paucity of pathologic tissue. Intraoperative cytologic examination may provide improved sensitivity for adenomatous cells as compared with traditional immunohistochemistry.[101]

In cases where preoperative imaging is nondiagnostic and no lesion is identifiable at the time of surgery, preoperative bilateral inferior petrosal sinus sampling may help to identify which side of the sellar region is pathologic. In experienced hands, inferior petrosal sinus sampling preceded by CRH stimulation can correctly lateralize a tumor in 83% of cases (compared with 74% with MRI) where there is an ACTH gradient of more than 1.4 between the two sides.[126] Depending on the severity of the patient's symptomatology and the patient's expressed desires, the operating surgeon may opt for hemihypophysectomy or complete hypophysectomy with the knowledge that such measures may result in lifelong hypopituitarism requiring hormone replacement.

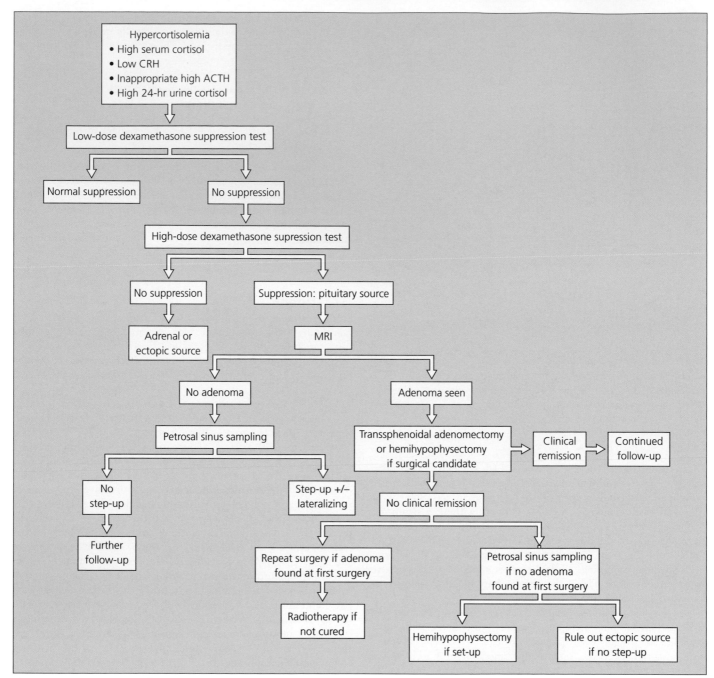

Figure 38.13 Management of Cushing's disease.

Hemihypophysectomy in these cases is usually guided by the results of preoperative inferior petrosal sinus sampling, whereas complete hypophysectomy is usually reserved for patients in whom resolution of the hypercortisolemic state is an absolute necessity.

Probably because there are different etiologic and pathologic subtypes within the category of Cushing's disease (as discussed under the preceding section), the cure rate for this illness in all series remains under 90%. Repeat surgeries and nonselective partial or total hypophysectomies often must be done to attain those cures. Thus, some controversy exists as to what the initial surgical intervention should be. Some suggest visual exploration of

the gland, with removal of abnormal tissue for frozen section; if an adenoma is seen, its selective excision would be the only intervention. If permanent disease remission is not achieved, only then would more extensive surgery be suggested.[97] Others feel that petrosal-sinus-directed or blind partial hemihypophysectomy is a more reasonable initial approach. Because incidental (non-functioning) adenomas or small inhomogeneities in the gland are common, the surgeon may be guided toward an abnormal part of the gland that is not responsible for the Cushingoid state. Since frozen section is not always reliable, some recommend removal of more than just the grossly abnormal tissue identified intraoperatively. That same type of argument, as well as the controversy over whether a higher source of stimulation (e.g. CRH[127]) is responsible for Cushing's disease, has caused others to suggest total hypophysectomy as the surest way of achieving permanent disease remission.

Macroadenomas are easier to identify on preoperative imaging and to localize intraoperatively. However, they portend a worse prognosis and higher surgical failure rate than microadenomas. In a series of 137 patients with microadenomas at Massachusetts General Hospital, 123 (90%) were cured with transsphenoidal surgery with or without adjuvant therapy. This contrasts with a 65% surgical cure rate in 11 of 17 patients from the same series who harbored macroadenomas.[99] The 5-year cure rates in this series for patients with microadenomas versus macroadenomas were 96% and 91%, respectively, whereas the 10-year cure rates were 93% and 55%.[99]

Outcomes do not correlate with the presence of a lesion on preoperative imaging or histology-documented tumor. In a recent study of Cushing's disease patients with normal preoperative MRI scans, a tumor could be identified at the time of surgery in 94% of cases and verified histologically in 78%. Long-term remission was obtained in 89% of patients for a mean follow-up period of 21 months. Despite the short follow-up period, these results surpass those of larger complete series of patients with Cushing's disease, underscoring the better prognosis of patients harboring microadenomas versus macroadenomas.

Similarly, in a series of 161 patients undergoing operation for Cushing's disease at the University of Virginia, surgical specimens in 29 (18%) failed to demonstrate adenomatous cells despite an identifiable lesion on preoperative MRI in 21 (72%) and identification of seemingly abnormal tissue in 26 (90%).[127] Both abnormal-appearing tissue and a discrete lesion on MRI did not correlate statistically with outcome. Nonetheless, 19 patients (66%) demonstrated disease remission with one recurrence at a mean follow-up period of 38 months. These results are similar to those from the UCSF group that demonstrated a remission rate of 69% in patients with no histological confirmation of tumor despite resection of a suspected adenoma or hypophysectomy.[97] This remission rate did not differ significantly from that of the remaining 171 patients with histologically confirmed tumor (88% remission). These studies emphasize the lack of prognostic importance attributable to histological confirmation of tumor in the hands of an experienced surgeon after a meticulous preoperative endocrine workup has been completed.

Recurrence rates have been reported from 3.7% to 9.3%.[94,96–98] However, relapse rates of 7 to 11% have been reported from 12 to 158 months following surgery (average 68–76 months).[99,103] Thus, long-term remission rates following surgery range from 67 to 77% of cases (follow-up 72–88 months).[103,128] A recent study involving an extensive biochemical examination of patients in long-term remission (8 years) has demonstrated that virtually full normalization of pulsatile, 24-hour, regulated ACTH, cortisol, GH, and prolactin secretion can be attained following successful surgery.[129] Furthermore, recent survival analysis of a large surgical series of Cushing's patients demonstrates mortality rates similar to that of age- and sex-matched population controls.[99]

Because of the relatively high rate of relapse, attention has recently focused on the determination of immediate postoperative factors that predict long-term remission. Serum ACTH and cortisol levels may remain unchanged or even elevate presumably due to the stress of surgery and anesthesia, however, levels that remain elevated beyond the first postoperative day indicate surgical failure except for a few rare cases in which "late remission" has been documented in the literature.[104] Currently, we measure morning cortisol and ACTH in postoperative patients for 2 days following surgery before instituting replacement therapy. Undetectable or very low values suggest that cure has been achieved.

Cortisol levels that are low or undetectable predict long-term remission in more than 95% of cases. Simmons and colleagues recently reported that a comparison of serum cortisol levels measured preoperatively at midnight and approximately 30 hours after operation offer the most sensitive indication of long-term remission. Using these two measurements, a lower postoperative level offers 95% sensitivity and a 95% positive predictive value for remission up to 2 years following surgery. They stress that the administration of exogenous steroids in the immediate postoperative period is unnecessary except in a small percentage of patients who demonstrate laboratory-documented hypocortisolemia accompanied by symptoms of steroid withdrawal. In fact, routine administration of postoperative steroids only delays accurate biochemical assessment in the remaining majority of patients.[104]

Although potentially a dramatic decrease from preoperative values, 1-week postoperative serum cortisol levels within the normal range are not predictive of remission. Another indication of viable tumor cells in the immediate postoperative period is a measurable response of serum ACTH level to CRH stimulation. In a series of 82 patients, a normal or exaggerated response predicted recurrence in 18% and 43% of patients, respectively, whereas an absent response predicted long-term remission at 2 years follow-up.[129]

Repeat surgery

Patients who are not cured by selective resection fall into several groups:[2]

1. those with invasive adenomas;
2. those with microadenomas not identified;
3. those with corticotrope hyperplasia without a discrete adenoma;
4. those with ectopic secretion of ACTH or CRH; and
5. those with defined tumors, but inadvertent incomplete removal.

Patients who demonstrate elevated postoperative ACTH and cortisol levels are candidates for attempted surgical re-exploration. In addition, some authors advocate repeat surgery in the immediate postoperative period when cortisol levels are within the normal range because of the chance of recurrence as discussed above.[130] They argue that in early re-exploration the lack of scar formation and the surgeon's acquaintance with the surgical target facilitate access and resection. In all cases of repeat surgery, the biochemical and radiologic work-up must be re-scrutinized and possibly repeated to verify a pituitary origin of disease. Mandatory tests in this setting include MRI, static and dynamic biochemical testing, as well as inferior petrosal sinus sampling for ACTH with or without CRH stimulation, if it has not been previously performed. In this setting, the likelihood of intraoperatively identifying a lesion is > 50%. A small percentage of patients may in fact harbor an ectopic source of abnormal ACTH-secreting cells, such as within the cavernous sinus, which would not be amenable to repeat surgery.[131] However, Oldfield and colleagues have presented data on recurrent or non-cured Cushing's patients where the majority had cavernous sinus dura and actual sinus invasion, which they approached surgically with resection of the dura and removal of the intracavernous tumor, We are not enthusiastic about entering the cavernous sinus as it clearly changes the morbidity of the surgery to potentially unacceptable levels. Withstanding such cases, if no discrete adenoma is found at the time of repeat exploration, the surgeon may opt for hemi-hypophysectomy or complete hypophysectomy as described above. Remission rates following repeat surgery for residual or recurrent disease ranges from 30 to 53%.[99,103,132] Hypopituitarism as well as complications including infection (33%) and cerebro-spinal fluid leaks (20%) are more common following repeat surgery, most likely because of the tendency to perform more aggressive procedures.[130,132] Friedman and colleagues[133] studied the efficacy of repeat surgery for recurrent or persistent Cushing's disease. They operated upon 31 patients who had previously undergone a transsphenoidal operation and two patients who were previously irradiated. In 24 (73%) of the 33 patients, remission of hypercortisolism was achieved by surgery. The incidence of remission of hypercortisolism was greatest if an adenoma was identified at surgery and the patient received selective adenomec-tomy (19, or 95%, of 20 patients), if there was evidence at surgery or on the preoperative CT scan of incomplete initial exposure, or if the patient had only radiation. In contrast, only five of 12 (42%) who received subtotal or total hypophysectomy had remission following repeat surgery. Thirteen per cent of their patients in remission subsequently had recurrent hypercortisolism. Those with lateral invasive extension will not be cured by any surgical procedure and, therefore, hypophysectomy is not a consideration.

While transsphenoidal resection remains the primary procedure of choice, as illustrated above, it does not carry a 100% success rate. There are other treatment modalities available for use as adjuvants for those cases in which initial or repeat surgical therapy has failed.

Stereotactic radiation has been used alone or in combination with surgery for the treatment of Cushing's disease;[134,135] reports on its efficacy (cure rates) vary from 50% to 100%. In recent studies radiation after failed surgery, administered by linear accelerator or gamma knife, has provided long-term remissions in 83% (42-month follow-up)[136] and 63% (12-month follow-up)[137] respectively. Average time from radiation to clinical remission was 12–18 months.[136,137] These results are significantly better than those obtained with pituitary irradiation as stand-alone treat-ment.[137] Hypopituitarism is a common side-effect of pituitary irradiation if the gland is irradiated. We currently prefer stereo-tactic radiosurgery for residual or recurrent tumor in the cavernous sinus if there is at least a 5-mm distance from the optic nerves and chiasm to the irradiated area. Because of the length of time needed to effect a cure and because of the high incidence of hypopituitarism, we currently suggest that radiation therapy be used only when pituitary surgery has failed.

In addition to radiotherapy, there are a number of medical therapies available. One immediate drawback to medical therapy for Cushing's disease is that all currently available medications block ACTH or cortisol production; in doing so, however, they treat symptoms rather than abolish the tumor, and often ameliorate them incompletely and at a high price in terms of unpleasant and potentially dangerous side-effects.

Ketoconazole, a potent antifungal agent, inhibits adrenal steroidogenesis by blocking the 11β-hydroxylase (and other enzymes involved in both cortisol and testosterone production as well). It is generally well tolerated, although sedation is not uncommon. While it may be possible to titrate the dose carefully to achieve eucortisolemia, this may be difficult. Often, the aim is to achieve complete adrenal suppression, at which time supple-mental steroid treatment is begun.[138,139] Because several steps in steroid production are halted, effects on cholesterol, vitamin D, mineralocorticoid, and estrogen and androgen production need to be evaluated more closely before ketoconazole's use on a long-term basis should be recommended. We often use this drug if there is to be a delay between diagnosis and treatment, or if precise etiologic diagnosis is in doubt (depression versus mild Cushing's disease) and some interim treatment is desirable.

CONCLUSION

As illustrated above, patients with functioning pituitary adenomas pose very different management problems and decisions than do patients with nonfunctioning adenomas. The issue of medical versus surgical treatment is ever-present in the management of this group of patients. One must weigh all the factors such as age,

CLINICAL PEARLS

- Even with highly sophisticated radiologic imaging techniques, it is still difficult preoperatively to demonstrate a pituitary tumor causing Cushing's disease. Indeed, gland asymmetry or inhomogeneity is common in patients without Cushing's disease. Such findings may not correlate with intraoperative tumor localization and, thus, abnormal scans need to be interpreted cautiously.

- Tumors causing Cushing's disease tend to be small. Thus, even at the time of exploration, it is possible to locate the tumor in only 79% of the cases.

- Using standard biochemical parameters, errors in the diagnosis of Cushing's disease are made in 1% of cases. In our series, CRH stimulation testing has been helpful in resolving some diagnostic ambiguity.

- Petrosal venous sampling may confirm a questionable diagnosis of Cushing's disease by showing a clear step-up between peripheral and petrosal blood levels of ACTH. The use of CRH stimulation during this test adds to the accuracy. Lateralization of the tumor may be suggested by a side-to-side gradient so that surgery will be more successful.

- Transsphenoidal surgery is the overwhelming choice of therapy unless surgery is clearly contraindicated for other reasons. Selective adenomectomy directed by definitive radiologic abnormality is preferred. Petrosal sinus sampling laterality may direct a curative hemihypophysectomy. If an adenoma is not found in an adult and hemihypophysectomy is not curative, then hypophysectomy is considered. In a child with Cushing's disease, if an adenoma is not found and laterality is not demonstrated, then radiation, adrenalectomy, or medical treatment is preferred before hypophysectomy. Radiosurgery may be the preferred second step in adults if the pituitary etiology is secure.

medical condition, and tumor size before choosing any course of action. The most important thing to remember in the management of these patients is that they require meticulous follow-up for evidence of tumor regrowth regardless of the treatment plan chosen.

REFERENCES

1. Reichlin S. Anatomical and physiological basis of hypothalamic-pituitary regulation. In: Post KD, Jackson IMD, Reichlin S (eds). *The Pituitary Adenoma*. New York, NY: Plenum Medical Book Co.; 1980: 3–28.

2. Cunnah D, Besser M. Management of prolactinomas. *Clin Endocrinol (Oxf)* 1991; 34: 231–5.

3. Klibanski A. Nonsecreting pituitary tumors. *Endocrinol Metab Clin North Am* 1987; 16: 793–804.

4. Hardy J, Somma M. Acromegaly: surgical treatment by transsphenoidal microsurgical removal of the pituitary adenoma. In: Tindall GT, Collins WF (eds). *Clinical Management of Pituitary Disorders*. New York, NY: Raven Press; 1979: 209–17.

5. Litt AW, Kricheff II. Magnetic resonance imaging of pituitary tumors. In: Cooper PR (ed.). *Contemporary Diagnosis and Management of Pituitary Adenomas*. Illinois: American Association of Neurologic Surgeons; 1991: 1–19.

6. Macpherson P, Hadley DM, Teasdale E, *et al*. Pituitary microadenomas: does gadolinium enhance their demonstration? *Neuroradiology* 1989; 31: 293–8.

7. Kulkarni MV, Lee KF, McArdle CB, *et al*. 1.5T MR imaging of pituitary microadenomas: technical considerations and CT correlation. *AJNR* 1988; 9: 5–11.

8. Doppman JL, Frank JA, Dwyer AJ, *et al*. Gadolinium DTPA enhanced MR imaging of ACTH-secreting microadenomas of the pituitary gland. *J Comput Assist Tomogr* 1988; 12: 728–35.

9. Marcovitz S, Wee R, Chan J, *et al*. The diagnostic accuracy of preoperative CT scanning in the evaluation of pituitary ACTH-secreting adenomas. *AJR* 1987; 149: 803–6.

10. Marcovitz S, Wee R, Chan J, *et al*. Diagnostic accuracy of preoperative scanning of pituitary prolactinomas. *AJNR* 1988; 9: 13–17.

11. Marcovitz S, Wee R, Chan J, *et al*. Diagnostic accuracy of preoperative CT scanning of pituitary somatotroph adenomas. *AJNR* 1988; 9: 19–22.

12. Davis PC, Hoffman JC Jr, Tindall GT, *et al*. Prolactin-secreting pituitary microadenomas: inaccuracy of high-resolution CT imaging. *AJR* 1985; 144: 1541–6.

13. Frantz AG. Prolactin. *N Engl J Med* 1978; 298: 201–7.

14. Jaquet P, Guibout M, Lucioni J, *et al*. Hypothalamopituitary regulation of prolactin in hypersecreting prolactinoma. In: Robyn C, Harter M (eds). *Progress in Prolactin, Physiology and Pathology*. New York, NY: Elsevier-North Holland Biochemical Press; 1978: 371–82.

15. Boyd AE III, Reichlin S. Neural control of prolactin secretion in man. *Psychoneuroendocrinology* 1978; 3: 113–30.

16. Kleinberg DL, Noel GL, Frantz AG. Galactorrhea: a study of 235 cases including 48 with pituitary tumors. *N Engl J Med* 1977; 296: 589–600.

17. Goodman RH, Molitch MD, Post KD, Jackson, IMD. Prolactin secreting adenomas in the male. In: Post KD, Jackson IMD, Reichlin S (eds). *The Pituitary Adenoma*. New York, NY: Plenum Press; 1980: 91–108.

18. Thorner MO, McNeilly AS, Hagan C, Besser GM. Long-term treatment of galactorrhea and hypogonadism with bromocriptine. *Br Med J* 1974; 2: 419–22.

19. Vance ML, Evans WS, Thorner MO. Bromocriptine. *Ann Intern Med* 1984; 100: 78–91.

20. Zarate A, Canales ES, Cano C, Pilonieta CJ. Follow-up of patients with prolactinomas after discontinuation of long-term therapy with bromocriptine. *Acta Endocrinol (Copenh)* 1983; 104: 139–42.

21. Molitch ME, Elton RL, Blackwell RE, *et al*. Bromocriptine as primary therapy for prolactin-secreting macroadenomas: results of a prospective multicenter study. *J Clin Endocrinol Metab* 1985; 60: 698–705.

22. Thorner MO, Martin WH, Rogol AD, *et al*. Rapid regression of pituitary prolactinomas during bromocriptine treatment. *J Clin Endocrinol Metab* 1980; 51: 438–45.

23. Tindall GT, Kovacs K, Horvath E, *et al*. Human prolactin-producing adenomas and bromocriptine: a histological, immunocytochemical, ultrastructural, and morphometric study. *J Clin Endocrinol Metab* 1982; 55: 1178–83.

24. Barrow DL, Tindall GT, Kovacs K, *et al*. Clinical and pathological effects of bromocriptine on prolactin-secreting and other pituitary tumors. *J Neurosurg* 1984; 60: 1–7.

25. Barrow DL, Mizuno J, Tindall GT. Management of prolactinomas associated with very high serum prolactin levels. *J Neurosurg* 1988; 68: 554–8.

26. Molitch ME, Reichlin S. Hyperprolactinemic disorders. *Dis Mon June* 1982; 28: 1–58.

27. Reichlin S. The prolactinoma problem. *N Engl J Med* 1979; 300: 313–15.

28. Thorner MO, Schran HF, Evans WS, *et al*. A broad spectrum of prolactin suppression by bromocriptine in hyperprolactinemic women: a study of serum prolactin and bromocriptine levels after acute and chronic administration of bromocriptine. *J Clin Endocrinol Metab* 1980; 50: 1026–33.

29. Thorner MO, Edwards CRW, Charlesworth M, *et al*. Pregnancy in patients presenting with hyperprolactinemia. *Br Med J* 1979; 2: 771–4.

30. Tindall GT, Barrow DL, Tindall SC. Current management of pituitary tumors, II. *Contemp Neurosurg* 1988; 10: 1–6.

31. Vance ML, Cragun JR, Reimnitz C, *et al*. CV 205–502 treatment of hyperprolactinemia. *J Clin Endocrinol Metab* 1989; 68: 336–9.

32. Wang C, Lam KSL, Ma JTC, *et al*. Long-term treatment of hyperprolactinaemia with bromocriptine: effect of drug withdrawal. *Clin Endocrinol (Oxf)* 1987; 27: 363–71.

33. Thorner MO, Perryman RL, Rogol AD, *et al*. Rapid changes of prolactinoma volume after withdrawal and reinstitution of bromocriptine. *J Clin Endocrinol Metab* 1981; 53: 480–3.

34. Liuzzi A, Dallabonzana D, Oppizzi G, *et al*. Low doses of dopamine agonists in the long-term treatment of macroprolactinomas. *N Engl J Med* 1985; 313: 656–9.

35. Kleinberg DL, Boyd AE III, Wardlaw S, *et al*. Pergolide for the treatment of pituitary tumors secreting prolactin or growth hormone. *N Engl J Med* 1983; 309: 704–9.

36. Molitch ME. Pregnancy and the hyperprolactinemic woman. *N Engl J Med* 1985; 312: 1364–70.

37. Shrivastava RK, Arginteanu MS, King WA, Post KD. Giant prolactinomas: clinical management and long-term follow up. *J Neurosurg* 2002; 97: 299–306.

38. Fahlbusch R, Buchfelder M, Schrell U. Short-term preoperative treatment of macroprolactinomas by dopamine agonists. *J Neurosurg* 1987; 67: 807–15.

39. Hubbard JL, Scheithauer BW, Abboud CF, Laws ER Jr. Prolactin-secreting ademonas: the preoperative response to bromocriptine

120. Oldfield EH, Chrousos GP, Schulte HM, *et al*. Preoperative lateralization of ACTH-secreting pituitary microadenomas by bilateral and simultaneous inferior petrosal venous sinus sampling. *N Engl J Med* 1985; 312: 98–103.

121. Schrell U, Fahlbusch R, Buchfelder M, *et al*. Corticotropin-releasing hormone stimulation test before and after transsphenoidal selective microadenomectomy in 30 patients with Cushing's disease. *J Clin Endocrinol Metab* 1987; 64: 1150–9.

122. Zovickian J, Oldfield EH, Doppman JL, *et al*. Usefulness of inferior petrosal sinus venous endocrine markers in Cushing's disease. *J Neurosurg* 1988; 68: 205–10.

123. Findling JW, Tyrell JB. Occult ectopic secretion of corticotropin. *Am J Med* 1986; 146: 929–33.

124. Boggan JE, Tyrell JB, Wilson CB. Transsphenoidal microsurgical management of Cushing's disease: a report of 100 cases. *J Neurosurg* 1983; 59: 195–200.

125. Tindall GT, Herring CJ, Clark RV, *et al*. Cushing's disease: results of transsphenoidal microsurgery with emphasis on surgical failures. *J Neurosurg* 1990; 72: 363–9.

126. Kaltsas GA, Giannulis MG, Newell-Price JD, *et al*. A critical analysis of the value of simultaneous inferior petrosal sinus sampling in Cushing's disease and the occult ectopic adrenocorticotropin syndrome. *J Clin Endocrinol Metab* 1999; 84: 487–92.

127. Sheehan JM, Vance ML, Sheehan JP, Ellegala DB, Laws ER, Jr. Radiosurgery for Cushing's disease after failed transsphenoidal surgery. *J Neurosurg* 2000; 93: 738–42.

128. Sonino N, Zielezny M, Fava GA, Fallo F, Boscaro M. Risk factors and long-term outcome in pituitary-dependent Cushing's disease. *J Clin Endocrinol Metab* 1996; 81: 2647–52.

129. Bochicchio D, Losa M, Buchfelder M. Factors influencing the immediate and late outcome of Cushing's disease treated by transsphenoidal surgery: a retrospective study by the European Cushing's Disease Survey Group. *J Clin Endocrinol Metab* 1995; 80: 3114–20.

130. Trainer PJ, Lawrie HS, Verhelst J, *et al*. Transsphenoidal resection in Cushing's disease: undetectable serum cortisol as the definition of successful treatment. *Clin Endocrinol (Oxf)* 1993; 38: 73–8.

131. Ohnishi T, Arita N, Yoshimine T, Mori S. Intracavernous sinus ectopic adrenocorticotropin-secreting tumours causing therapeutic failure in transsphenoidal surgery for Cushing's disease. *Acta Neurochir* 2000; 142: 855–64.

132. Ram Z, Nieman LK, Cutler GB, Jr, Chrousos GP, Doppman JL, Oldfield EH. Early repeat surgery for persistent Cushing's disease. *J Neurosurg* 1994; 80: 37–45.

133. Friedman RB, Oldfield EH, Nieman LK, *et al*. Repeat transsphenoidal surgery for Cushing's disease. *J Neurosurg* 1989; 71: 520–7.

134. Degerblad M, Rahn T, Bergstrand G, Thoren M. Long-term results of stereotactic radiosurgery to the pituitary gland in Cushing's disease. *Acta Endocrinol (Copenh)* 1986; 112: 310–14.

135. Sandler LM, Richards NT, Carr DH, *et al*. Long term follow-up of patients with Cushing's disease treated by interstitial irradiation. *J Clin Endocrinol Metab* 1987; 65: 441–7.

136. Estrada J, Boronat M, Mielgo M, *et al*. The long-term outcome of pituitary irradiation after unsuccessful transsphenoidal surgery in Cushing' disease. *N Engl J Med* 1997; 336: 172–7.

137. Sheehan JM, Lopes MB, Sheehan JP, Ellegala D, Webb KM, Laws, ER, Jr. Results of transsphenoidal surgery for Cushing's disease in patients with no histologically confirmed tumor. *Neurosurgery* 2000; 47: 33–6; discussion 37–9.

138. Loli P, Berselli ME, Tagliaferri M. Use of ketoconazole in the treatment of Cushing's syndrome. *J Clin Endocrinol Metab* 1986; 63: 1365–71.

139. Sonino N. The use of ketoconazole as an inhibitor of steroid production. *N Engl J Med* 1987; 317: 812–18.

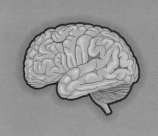

CRANIOPHARYNGIOMAS

39

Dachling Pang

Craniopharyngiomas are unique lesions in that they are histologically benign, but because of the technical difficulties and potential hazards involved in their radical excision, a surgical cure is seldom achieved except in expert hands. Their intimate adherence to the infundibular stalk and hypothalamus predisposes to a number of endocrinologic and neurobehavioral problems rarely seen in other brain tumors. They are slow-growing, but a mere fleck of residual tumor virtually guarantees a recurrence. With all these surgical idiosyncracies, microsurgery is still the mainstay of management, although recent advances in radiotherapy offer a number of nonsurgical options that could arguably be the treatments of choice in special circumstances. The treatment algorithm recommended in this chapter must therefore be regarded merely as the personal viewpoint of the author, not as the undisputed answer to this complex lesion. Neurosurgeons and oncologists must continue to modify their protocols along with advances in the frontiers of treatment for this tumor.

INCIDENCE

Craniopharyngiomas are relatively rare tumors, constituting between 2.5% and 4% of all intracranial tumors.[1,2] They are much more common among children, forming 9% of Matson's series of childhood brain tumors[3] and making up 54% of neoplasms in the sellar–chiasmal region in children. There is a bimodal age distribution, with the first peak at 5–10 years[4,5] and a second peak between 55 and 65 years,[6] but the tumor may become symptomatic at any age. Recent large series show equal sex distribution.[7,8]

EMBRYOLOGIC ORIGIN

For several decades, craniopharyngiomas were thought to arise exclusively from epithelial rests along the embryologic migration path of the anterior pituitary lobe. At the end of the third gestational week, the stomodeal ectoderm invaginates toward the diencephalon and eventually meets the downwardly projecting infundibular bud. As the sphenoid bone forms ventral to the diencephalon, the stomodeal cleft is pinched off from the pharyngeal epithelium to become a pouch (of Rathke), whose wall eventually thickens to form the various parts of the anterior pituitary lobe (Figure 39.1). Ectoblastic cell rests have been found along this migration path (called the hypophysiopharyngeal duct), from the partes tuberalis and distalis of the gland to the posterior pharyngeal mucosa (Figure 39.2). The frequent occurrence of craniopharyngiomas around the infundibular stalk, their occasional occurrence within the sphenoid bone and pharynx, and the striking histologic resemblance between some craniopharyngiomas and tumors of known ectoblastic origin, such as adamantinomas, led Erdheim[9] and others[10–12] to implicate these embryonic ectoblastic remnants as the sole source of all craniopharyngiomas.

During the 1950s, the embryonic origin of craniopharyngiomas was challenged when it was discovered that the pituitary squamous cell rests are rarely seen in children under 10 years but are found with increasing frequency in each succeeding decade of life, even though the peak incidence of craniopharyngiomas is between the ages of 5 and 10 years.[13] It was then postulated that the squamous cell rests from which craniopharyngiomas originate are products of metaplasia of the mature cells of the anterior pituitary gland, and not embryonic remnants.[10,13]

There is evidence to suggest that craniopharyngiomas may indeed have dual origins. The so-called childhood type, which occurs in all ages and contains palisading columnar cells that resemble the ameloblasts of fetal tooth buds (adamantinomatous type, see below), may be of embryonic origin.[14,15] The adult type, which occurs mostly in adults and consists mainly of mature stratified squamous cells (papillary type, see below), may be of metaplastic origin.

Recent gene studies support this theory of dual origins. Sekine and colleagues found a *β-catenin* gene mutation in 100% of adamantinomatous craniopharyngiomas studied but in none of the papillary tumors.[16] Since β-catenin acts as a transcriptional activator of the Wnt signaling pathway, mutation of the *β-Catenin* gene results in stabilization of β-catenin and up-regulation of specific transcription activities that are presumably important in the tumorigenesis of adamantinomatous craniopharyngiomas but not in the tumorigenesis of the papillary types.

There is also molecular evidence to suggest that the adamantinomatous craniopharyngiomas are in fact a heterogeneous group made up of diverse genomic subtypes.[17] Lefranc and associates found that biologically aggressive adamantinomatous craniopharyngiomas that were characterized by rapid recurrence after resection, compared to those with a more benign course, had consistently low expressions of galectin-3 and macrophage migration-inhibiting factor.[18] Galectin-3 and migration-inhibiting factor play a significant role in the various intracellular signaling pathways that control apoptosis. Their low levels suggest that this subtype of adamantinomatous tumor may originate from a defect in the apoptosis-mediated elimination of embryological remnants of epithelial tissue.

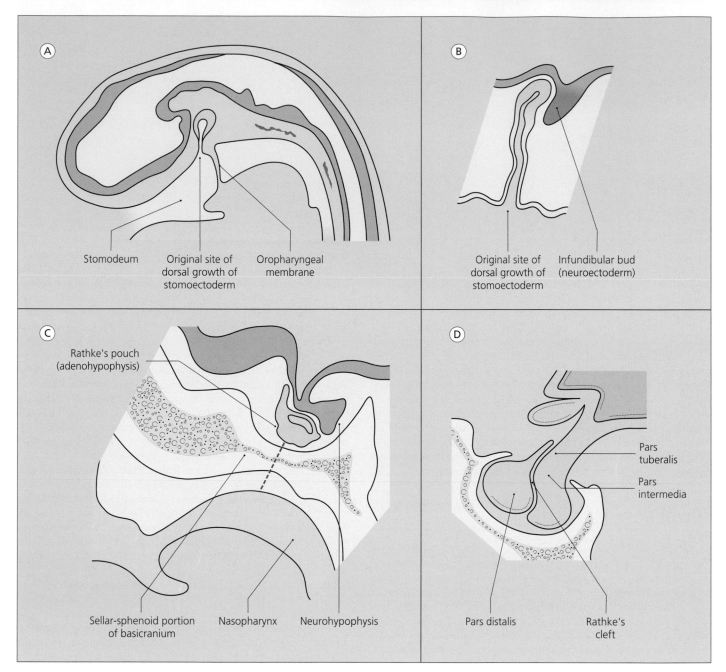

Figure 39.1 Embryogenesis of the pituitary gland. **(A)** Formation of Rathke's pouch from the stomodeal epithelium. **(B)** Fusion of stomodeal ectoderm, with downgrowing infundibular bud, from neuroectoderm. **(C)** Interposition of mesoderm of basicranium to form the sella–sphenoid complex ventral to the pituitary gland, after Rathke's pouch has been pinched off from the stomodeum. Dotted line denotes the tract of the upgrowth, the hypophysiopharyngeal duct. **(D)** Final development of the adenohypophysis from thickening of Rathke's pouch wall.

SURGICAL ANATOMY AND PATHOLOGY

Most craniopharyngiomas originate near the infundibular stalk and distort or completely obliterate the suprasellar cistern, depending on their size and direction of growth. Approximately one-third of cases are retrochiasmatic (Figure 39.3) – the tumor displaces the pituitary forward and the chiasm upward and forward towards the tuberculum so that both optic nerves appear shortened and acquire the false appearance of being prefixed (pseudoprefixity). Another one-third of cases are subchiasmatic – the tumor displaces the stalk backwards and the chiasm directly upward so that the optic nerves are stretched. Both of these types are solid tumors and therefore have the solid consistency required to indent and elevate the floor of the third ventricle all the way to the level of the foramen of Monro. The hypothalamic structures accommodate gradually by displacing to the sides, but generally maintain

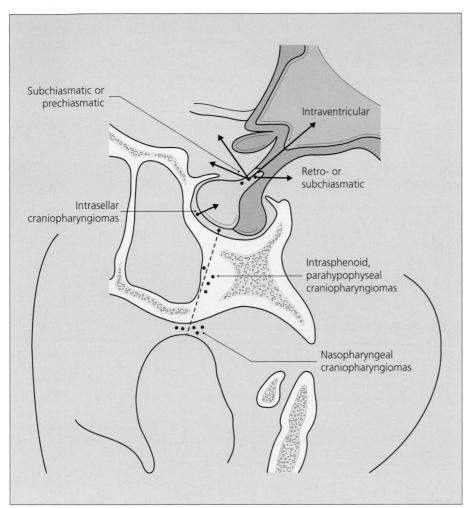

Figure 39.2 Possible sites of embryonic ectoblastic remnants and their relationship to subsequent locations of craniopharyngiomas. Dots indicate sites of ectoblastic remnants. Arrows indicate direction of growth and final location of tumors.

Subchiasmatic or prechiasmatic

Intraventricular

Retro- or subchiasmatic

Intrasellar craniopharyngiomas

Intrasphenoid, parahypophyseal craniopharyngiomas

Nasopharyngeal craniopharyngiomas

most of their normal functions, judging from the rarity of severe hypothalamic insufficiency in children with craniopharyngiomas. The third ventricular floor, no matter how attenuated, keeps the tumor dome outside the third ventricle even though the passage of cerebrospinal fluid (CSF) is often obstructed and the superior pole of the tumor appears on neuroimaging studies to be within the third ventricle (Figure 39.4). True intraventricular craniopharyngiomas have been reported[19–21] and probably arise from dislocated tuberal ectoblastic cells, but they are exceedingly rare. For most craniopharyngiomas, the transventricular approach from above risks injuring the hypothalamus and is not recommended.

About 20% of craniopharyngiomas are prechiasmatic. These tumors are frequently cystic and, by burrowing under and expanding within the frontal lobes, may reach enormous sizes (Figures 39.5 and 39.6). The soft cystic component of the tumor may also extend, like fingers, to the sylvian fissure laterally and over the dorsum sellae into the prepontine cistern posteriorly, becoming extensively multilobulated. This explains the occurrence of psychomotor seizures and cranial neuropathies in large rambling cystic tumors. Intrasellar craniopharyngiomas are the least common (10–15%),[22,23] but because they expand within the sella and cause pituitary insufficiencies early, they are often diagnosed when still relatively small (Figure 39.7) and thus may be removed by the transsphenoidal route.

Craniopharyngiomas may be predominantly solid, predominantly cystic, or cystic with a large solid component that may in turn contain small cysts. The solid part is usually smooth, rubbery, firm, and pinkish gray, resembling fish flesh. The cyst wall may be diaphanous or a thick shell of solid tumor. The fluid is typically dark green with suspended birefringent cholesterol crystals.

Microscopically, the cyst lining is composed of simple stratified squamous epithelium supported by a collagenous basement membrane. Two histologic types have been described in the solid parts. The more common *childhood* or *adamantinomatous* type is found in both children and adults.[14,15] It consists of epithelial trabeculae supported by a loose connective tissue stroma. These trabeculae are lined by palisading columnar cells radially arranged around a central cord of round or polygonal cells with transparent cytoplasm and intercellular bridges (prickle cells). In other areas there are masses of dead cells that show whorled or laminated arrangements reminiscent of keratinization. It is this combination of palisading columnar cells and central transparent cells that suggests a link with fetal tooth buds and other oral mucosal appendages (Figure 39.8). The less common *adult* or *papillary* type is found predominantly in adults[14,15] and consists of sheets of stratified squamous epithelium embedded in a matrix of vascular connective tissue. There are no laminellae or keratinization, and calcification is much less common (Figure 39.9).

Either the solid part or the cyst wall, or both, may be calcified. Calcification marks the site of regressive changes in the epithelium and is therefore particularly prevalent within the laminated whorls

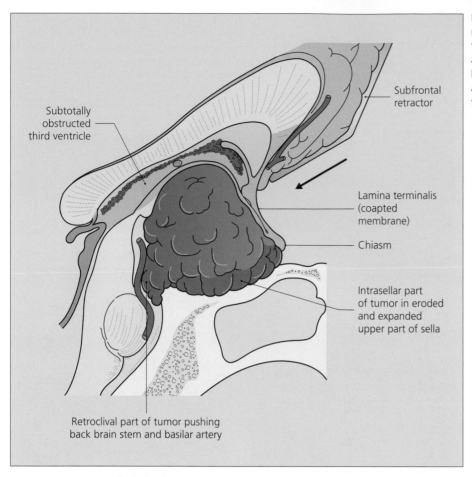

Figure 39.3 Schematic view of a large retrochiasmatic craniopharyngioma pushing the third ventricular floor upwards and coapting the attenuated midline basal hypothalamus with the lamina terminalis into a single membrane. The arrow indicates the direction of the translamina terminalis approach.

Subtotally obstructed third ventricle

Subfrontal retractor

Lamina terminalis (coapted membrane)

Chiasm

Intrasellar part of tumor in eroded and expanded upper part of sella

Retroclival part of tumor pushing back brain stem and basilar artery

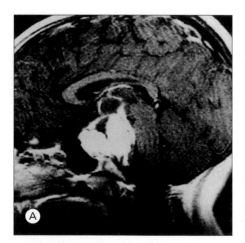

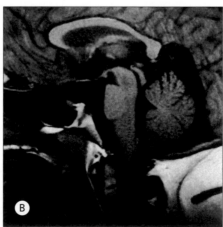

Figure 39.4 Postcontrast sagittal MRI of a large solid craniopharyngioma. **(A)** Note severe elevation of hypothalamus and third ventricular floor up to the level of foramen of Monro and distortion of the mamillary bodies. **(B)** After total resection of the tumor, the third ventricle resumes its normal location and its intact floor is again seen well. Note that the previously compressed mamillary body is now seen well.

of dead cells in the childhood type but not in the adult type. This explains why calcium is seen on computed tomography (CT) in almost all childhood craniopharyngiomas but in only slightly over 50% of adult craniopharyngiomas.[4] Small calcium foci may become confluent to form large stones, and actual bone formation has been reported.[14] It is important not to mistake a large stone as a sign of "burnt-out" tumor. Thin layers of *live* tumor cells are sandwiched between lamellae of calcium within the stone, which grows by further concretions being laid down after more live cells undergo regressive changes. In fact, reappearance of calcium or enlargement of a stone invariably means recurrence of an actively growing tumor.

The anterior, inferior, and lateral walls of the tumor capsule are normally separated from surrounding structures by a single layer of arachnoid. In contrast, the posterior wall is separated from the basilar artery and brainstem by the double-layered membrane of Liliequist. However, the dome of the tumor is almost always adherent to the infundibulum and basal hypothalamus as a result of an intense glial reaction in this region of the brain where most craniopharyngiomas arise. This tenacious glial sheath frequently

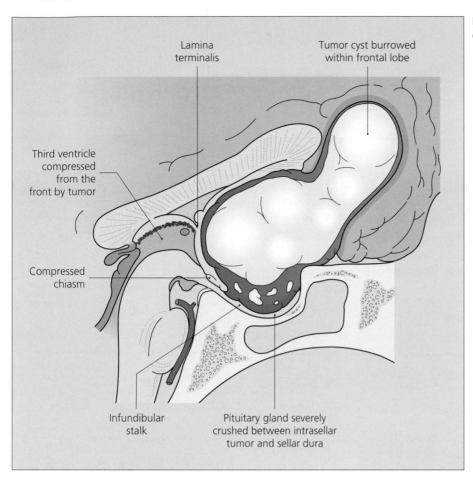

Lamina terminalis

Tumor cyst burrowed within frontal lobe

Third ventricle compressed from the front by tumor

Compressed chiasm

Infundibular stalk

Pituitary gland severely crushed between intrasellar tumor and sellar dura

Figure 39.5 Prechiasmatic, predominantly cystic craniopharyngioma.

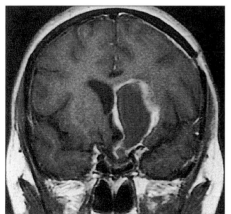

Figure 39.6 Postcontrast coronal MRI of a large, predominantly cystic craniopharyngioma that has expanded upwards and burrowed within the left frontal lobe.

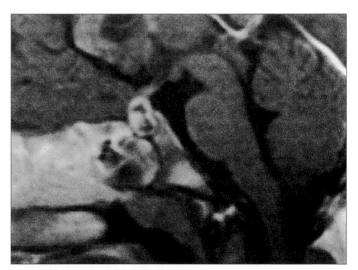

Figure 39.7 Postcontrast sagittal MRI of a mostly intrasellar craniopharyngioma. About two-thirds of the tumor is intrasellar, and only one-third is above the diaphragm.

contains pseudopods of tumor extending beyond the capsule. Occasionally, the inferior pole of the tumor expands within the sella and the capsule fuses tightly with the sellar dura and the medial walls of the cavernous sinus.

Having a common embryologic origin, craniopharyngiomas share the same blood supply as the anterior diencephalon (Figure 39.10).[11,24,25] The anterior portion of the tumor thus receives arterial feeders from the anterior communicating artery and the A1 segment of the anterior cerebral arteries, and its lateral portion receives branches from the posterior communicating artery. If the tumor involves the sella, it will also pick up arterial supply

from the capsular and meningohypophyseal arteries. However, the tumor almost never receives a blood supply from the posterior cerebral or basilar artery, no matter how far posteriorly it extends,[11,26] since these vessels do not normally irrigate the anterior diencephalon. This fact is crucial to the safe removal of the retrosellar portion of the tumor.

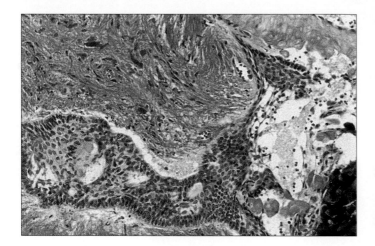

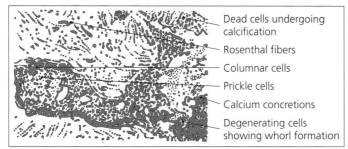

Dead cells undergoing calcification
Rosenthal fibers
Columnar cells
Prickle cells
Calcium concretions
Degenerating cells showing whorl formation

Figure 39.8 Histology of the so-called juvenile-type or adamantinomatous craniopharyngioma, showing a pseudopod of tumor lined with palisading columnar cells surrounding central cells with transparent cytoplasm ("prickle cells"). Note intense gliosis of the brain around the tumor, with abundant Rosenthal fibers. (H & E; ×100.)

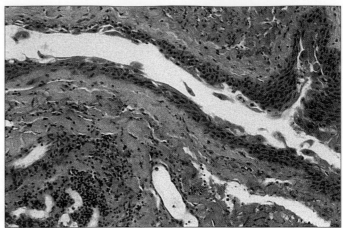

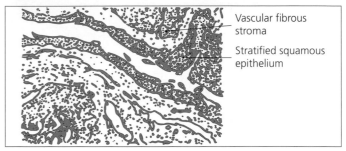

Vascular fibrous stroma
Stratified squamous epithelium

Figure 39.9 Histology of the so-called adult-type craniopharyngioma, showing stratified squamous epithelium overlying vascular fibrous stroma. Note absence of calcium and whorls (laminellae). (H & E; ×100.)

CLINICAL FEATURES

The clinical presentation of craniopharyngiomas differs between children and adults (Figure 39.11). Even though the optic chiasm and nerves are affected first by enlargement of the tumor, only 20–30% of children present with visual symptoms. This is because children tolerate progressive visual failure amazingly well, and they seldom complain until one eye is totally blind and the other can barely count fingers.[4,6,11,26] Subtle clues of progressive visual loss in young children include inexplicable deterioration in school performance, frequent stumbling, and an insistence on sitting very close to the television.

Other symptoms of an expanding intracranial mass such as headaches, personality changes, or even disturbance in orientation are likely to be overlooked in a young child. Diagnosis is therefore often delayed until the mass is enormous or hydrocephalus is already present due to third ventricular obstruction. Thus, 75–80% of children with craniopharyngiomas present with severe headache and vomiting without focal neurologic deficits.[4,6,11]

The two most frequent presenting endocrinopathies in children are short stature and delayed puberty (hypogonadism) in adolescents.[1,6] Diabetes insipidus[6,7] is less common and is usually only partial. Hypothyroidism and hypocortisolemia are unusual, although a blunter corticotropin response to provocative testing is common. Galactorrhea and hyperprolactinemia have been associated with craniopharyngiomas[24,27] and are thought to result from suppression of hypothalamic prolactin-inhibiting factor as a result of infundibular stalk compression.

The most common hypothalamic syndrome encountered in children is central hyperphagia and obesity, which is sometimes disproportionate to the food intake and may be partly the result of metabolic derangement. An unusual disturbance of fat metabolism causing emaciation in spite of adequate food intake has been described by Northfield.[28] Precocious puberty has also been reported in four cases of craniopharyngiomas,[6,29–31] presumably because of compression of the arcuate nucleus luteinizing-hormone-releasing hormone (LHRH) pacemaker. Flagrant disturbances of sleep and of thirst or temperature regulation are rarely seen in these children.

Neurobehavioral abnormalities occur in 20% of children with craniopharyngiomas.[1,4,6] In recent years, the author has repeatedly recognized signs of abulia minor in these children, such as psychomotor retardation, flattening of affect, and loss of enthusiasm toward the environment. Severely affected children also show significant recent memory deficits; the abulia and amnesia contribute most to the poor school performance. The amnesic syndrome has been attributed to compression of the hypothalamic component of the limbic memory circuit, such as the mamillary bodies. The abulia probably results from injury to the dopaminergic mesolimbic pathway, either within the medial forebrain bundle or at the medial septal region. This pathway is thought to be responsible for exploratory behaviors in animals and motivation in humans.[32–34] Thus, the typical child with a craniopharyngioma is short and obese with poor eyesight and learning difficulties.

Unlike children, most adults are very sensitive to visual disturbance, and 80% of adults in Banna's series[35] presented with assorted patterns of field deficits, scotomas, and decreasing visual acuity. In contrast, less than one-third of adults have signs of increased intracranial pressure (ICP). Nevertheless, neurobehav-

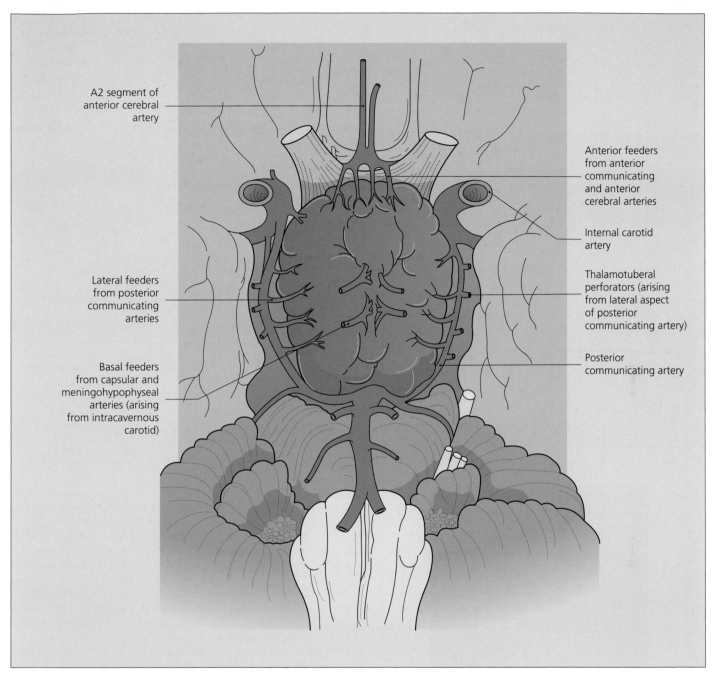

A2 segment of anterior cerebral artery

Anterior feeders from anterior communicating and anterior cerebral arteries

Internal carotid artery

Lateral feeders from posterior communicating arteries

Thalamotuberal perforators (arising from lateral aspect of posterior communicating artery)

Basal feeders from capsular and meningohypophyseal arteries (arising from intracavernous carotid)

Posterior communicating artery

Figure 39.10 Blood supply of a craniopharyngioma.

ioral syndromes unrelated to raised ICP are also much more common in adults than children.[1,4,11] Bartlett estimated that 31.5% of patients older than 45 years had dementia,[36] and an even higher percentage had intermittent confusion and hypersomnia. A Korsakoff-like amnesia was found in 30% of adults,[37–39] and occasionally severe depression and apathy will complicate the intellectual deterioration.[36] The most common endocrinopathy in adults is gonadal failure (37%),[11] presenting as secondary amenorrhea in women and loss of libido in men.[11]

RADIOGRAPHIC DIAGNOSIS

Even though plain skull radiographs are seldom obtained for headache or visual symptoms today, craniopharyngioma is one of few intracranial tumors that can be accurately diagnosed with a skull film. Two-thirds of adults and 95% of children with this tumor have an abnormal skull X-ray. The usual findings are erosion of the anterior clinoids and dorsum sellae, expansion of the upper sella, and suprasellar calcification (Figure 39.12). Intrasellar extension of a craniopharyngioma may produce a "ballooned" sella that mimics a pituitary adenoma, but the intrasellar calcium should exclude most adenomas.

Both CT and magnetic resonance imaging (MRI) are important for craniopharyngiomas, for different reasons. CT is less ambiguous than MRI in distinguishing the solid from the cystic parts of the tumor. The MR signal intensity of the cyst fluid varies widely depending on protein, lipid, and methemoglobin contents, and may be confused with that of the solid part. The cyst fluid

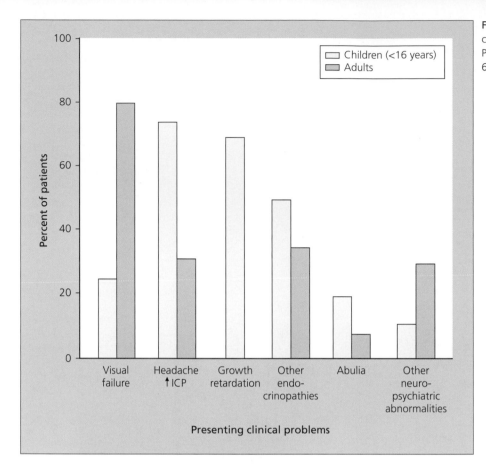

Figure 39.11 Presenting clinical problems of children and adults with craniopharyngiomas. Pooled data from references 11, 12, 17, 23, 36, 60, 62, 63, 65, and author's unpublished series.

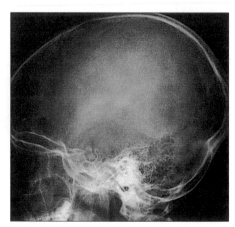

Figure 39.12 Lateral skull radiograph showing calcification within the sella and suprasellar regions in a child with a predominantly intrasellar craniopharyngioma.

is always hypodense on CT and thus is easily distinguished from the solid or calcified tumor (Figure 39.13). CT is therefore vital in classifying the tumor according to the solid/cyst ratio. A predominantly solid tumor is one that is at least 70% solid (Figure 39.14), and a predominantly cystic tumor is less than 30% solid. This classification is important in choosing the optimal therapy.

Another important function of CT is to define the bony anatomy of the sphenoid sinus, tuberculum sellae, and sella in preparation for the frontobasal transsphenoidal approach to a low

extension of the tumor (see below). The contiguous 3–5-mm coronal CT cuts using bone algorithms through the anterior skull base far surpass the old standard plain tomography. In addition, CT is much better than MRI in picking out small calcified parts of the tumor, particularly when these are close to the skull base.

On the other hand, MRI is better than CT in delineating the interface and relationship between tumor and brain in multiplane displays. The sagittal image, for instance, shows the distortion of the third ventricle and hypothalamic structures to great advantage and will frequently suggest whether a translamina terminalis approach to the dome of the tumor is necessary or feasible. Coronal images show the relationship of the lower pole of the tumor to the sella, sphenoid sinus, and cavernous sinus, and help determine whether the combined frontobasal transsphenoidal approach is necessary. Thus the MRI details enable the surgeon to select the surgical approach most likely to achieve total resection. Improving systems for MR and CT angiography now completely replace conventional angiography in defining the relationship of the tumor to the circle of Willis, except when an aneurysm of the cavernous carotid is strongly suspected.

MODALITIES AND OPTIONS FOR TREATMENT

Primary tumor, predominantly solid

Four treatment options are available for predominantly solid tumors diagnosed for the first time. The initial choice of therapy

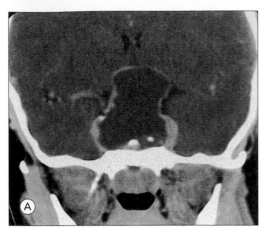

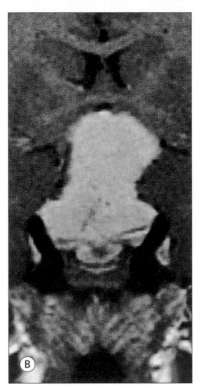

Figure 39.13 Predominantly cystic craniopharyngioma. **(A)** Postcontrast coronal CT shows clear distinction betwen cyst, cyst wall, basal solid part, and calcified part. **(B)** Postcontrast coronal T1-weighted MRI shows high-intensity cyst fluid and no distinction between solid, cyst, or calcium.

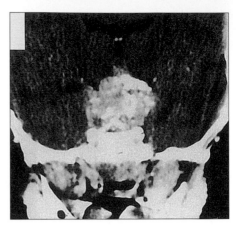

Figure 39.14 Postcontrast coronal CT of a predominantly solid craniopharyngioma.

is guided by several factors: (1) the experience of the surgeon, (2) the availability of stereotactic radiosurgery, (3) the age and medical condition of the patient, (4) the size and extent of the tumor on neuroimaging studies, and (5) the surgical anatomy, the degree of adherence, and the texture of the tumor capsule at surgery. A recommended treatment algorithm is summarized in Figure 39.15.

Total resection

Total resection of craniopharyngiomas is feasible with low mortality and morbidity in skilled and experienced hands. Even though total resection is the starting objective for most craniopharyngiomas, the aggressiveness of tumor removal must be tempered by the degree of difficulty encountered at surgery. Resectability depends on the tumor size (tumors larger than 4 cm are less likely to be totally resected), the degree of tumor adherence to the chiasm and great vessels, and the extent of rambling of the capsule within the basal cisterns and deep brain structures. Thus, the ratio of the number of cases in which total resection was accomplished (confirmed by postoperative neuroimaging) to the number in which total resection was attempted varies between 30% and 90%.[4,8,40–44] The realistic expectation for total resection is probably around 80–90%. MRI with and without contrast should be performed within 24 hours after surgery to eliminate "false cure," i.e. to rule out residual tumor fragments in "blind spots" such as the underside of the chiasm, deep inside the sella, and behind the dorsum sellae in the prepontine cistern. Unexpected residual tumor should be reoperated on within 7–10 days, before the formation of troublesome adhesions in the surgical field.

The overall operative mortality is probably around 1–2%, and the best reported serious postoperative morbidity is well below 10%.[7,8,40,41,44]

In spite of meticulous technique and diligent screening for false cures, a number of tumors will nonetheless recur after what has been deemed "complete" resection. Recurrences are usually detected within 5 years of the surgery,[4,41] but late recurrences after 20 years have been reported.[7] A long-term review by Katz[45] of Matson's original series[46] reported recurrences in 25% of patients 4–19 years after "total" resection, and most other series recorded recurrence rates of 15–25%, with a mean of 20%.[7,8,40,41,43] Recent updating of results including the author's personal series (author's unpublished results) shows a 10-year recurrence rate of less than 15%. In any case, the 10-year survival rate of patients who have undergone total resection is well over 85%[47] (Figure 39.16). Thus, the overall results of total resection for solid craniopharyngiomas are excellent, and it is the treatment of choice in children and young adults.[47] Obviously, the associated morbidity and, to an extent, the recurrence rate are dependent on the experience of the surgeon. Total resection should therefore be attempted only in centres where a large number of these tumors are managed.

That having been said, there is recent evidence to suggest that the biological behavior of craniopharyngiomas, long thought to be indolent, may be as important as surgical technique in determining recurrence. The proliferative activity of craniopharyngiomas has been studied using MIB-1 immunostaining for the Ki-67 antigen, which is expressed during all phases of the cell cycle except G0.[48] MIB-1 immunoreactivity is mainly confined to the peripheral palisaded epithelium. In a mixed age population, Raghavan and colleagues found that the mean MIB-1 labeling index of adult craniopharyngiomas was 8.9% ± 9.8, versus 6.3% ± 3.7 for childhood tumors, suggesting an inherently more aggressive class of lesions in adults.[48] Furthermore, Nishi and co-workers found that the mean MIB-1 labeling index for craniopharyngiomas that showed no recurrence (3.4% ± 2.3) was significantly lower than

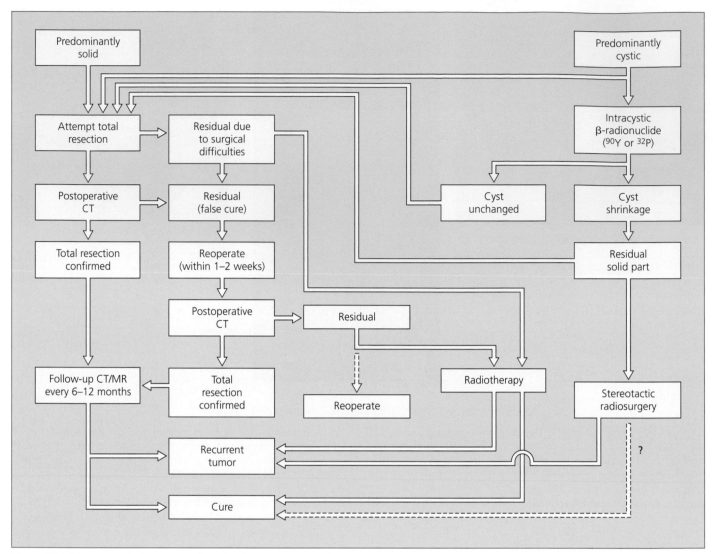

Figure 39.15 Recommended treatment algorithm for primary craniopharyngiomas in young and relatively healthy patients. Planned partial resection and postoperative radiation therapy is recommended for elderly and medically infirm patients.

the mean index for tumors that showed rapid recurrence (13.2% ± 7.7).[49] An MIB-1 labeling index higher than 7% was a statistically helpful predictor for regrowth in an otherwise seemingly homogeneous cohort of craniopharyngiomas patients. Perhaps the most cogent argument for the role of tumor biology in influencing regrowth rate was the discovery that the MIB-1 labeling index in the regrown specimen was unmistakably greater than that of the original specimen in all recurrence cases,[48] suggesting that clonal selection may have produced a more aggressive cell line. In this regard, rapidly recurring tumors have also been shown to express lower levels of retinoic acid receptor β, galectin-3, and migration-inhibiting factor than nonrecurring tumors, all three factors being intimately involved in apoptosis pathways.

Subtotal resection with postoperative radiation

When only subtotal resection is achieved, the recurrence rate is unacceptably high if postoperative radiation therapy is not given. The combined recurrence rate from several large series for subtotal resection without radiation therapy is about 75%,[4,8,41,50–54]

with a 10-year survival rate of only 25%. Postoperative radiation therapy significantly improves outcome and increases 10-year survival to between 75% and 80%.[12,40,53] External beam radiotherapy is usually delivered by a three- or four-field technique over a field size of 6 × 7 cm, with a total dose of 50–60 Gy fractionated over 6–7 weeks, with the daily dose not exceeding 2 Gy.

Postoperative radiation therapy is an excellent adjunct after an attempt at total resection has proven unfeasible. Because of the good 10-year survival rate of subtotal resection and radiation therapy, and the sometimes unusually taxing nature of radical excision, some surgeons are adopting a planned incomplete resection combined with radiation therapy. Others have advocated limited surgery and conventional radiotherapy in children because they reported a better neurologic, cognitive and endocrine outcome compared to radical surgery in their institution,[55] but this bias against an "upfront" attempt for curative surgery is not shared by centres experienced in craniopharyngioma surgery (author's unpublished series).[44]

Conventional radiation therapy is not without hazard, especially in children. Visual failure, hypopituitarism, organic brain

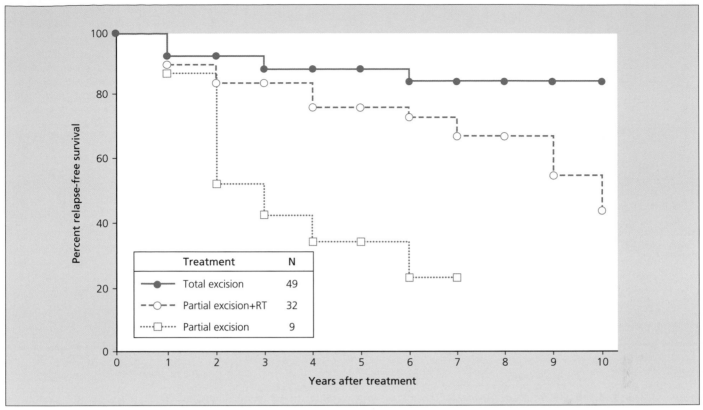

Figure 39.16 Actual relapse-free survival rates in patients with craniopharyngioma, comparing total excision (combined data from reference 66 and the author's unpublished series), subtotal or partial resection plus radiation (data from reference 17); and partial resection without radiation (data from reference 66). RT = radiation therapy.

syndromes, dementia, and sensorimotor deficits have all been reported.[27,42,56–58] Frontal lobe dysfunction translating into severe learning disabilities is especially troublesome in children,[59] and radiation therapy has also been etiologically implicated in malignant mesenchymal tumors arising *de novo* in the radiated field.[60–62] Furthermore, recent long-term follow-up studies[1,63] are beginning to reveal that subtotal resection with radiation therapy delays, but does not prevent, the eventual recurrence of the tumor. This treatment option is therefore not recommended as first choice for children and healthy young adults with potentially long life spans, but it is a wise alternative if total resection is found to be too risky at surgery, as when a piece of tumor is obstinately adherent to a great vessel. It is also a reasonable option for older patients with large tumors.

Biopsy and radiation

Most workers now believe that simple tumor biopsy and post-operative radiation therapy are inferior to either total resection or subtotal resection and radiation therapy. Shapiro and colleagues[40] reported 5- and 10-year survival rates for biopsy and radiation therapy of only 62% and 50%, respectively. Sung and colleagues[64] and Manaka and colleagues[53] reported comparable figures. Thus, this option is only endorsed for the old, the infirm, or those patients refusing more radical approaches. Because the biologic effects of radiation therapy may take 6–9 months to occur, patients suffering from imminent optic compression or high ICP as a result of the mass effect of the tumor will not benefit from this treatment method. If a cyst contributes significantly to the mass effect, an in-dwelling catheter connected to a subcutaneous

reservoir may be implanted in the cyst to permit periodic percutaneous aspiration of fluid during the waiting period.

Stereotactic radiosurgery

In several treatment centers in Europe and the United States, stereotactic radiosurgery using the gamma irradiation unit[65–68] and the linear accelerator has been used for the primary control of small solid craniopharyngiomas and solid recurrences following cyst aspiration. Radiosurgery is based on the principle that the biologic effects produced by a single radiation dose are greater than those produced by the same dose fractionated. Thus, if the single dose is delivered to sharply circumscribed and precisely targeted areas of tissue, tumor necrosis may be induced with comparatively low morbidity to the surrounding brain.[69] The gamma unit delivers 201 radially directed narrow beams of cobalt-60 gamma radiation towards a target region within a spherical sector (Figure 39.17). The system of apertures for each individual beam and the spatial arrangements of the ^{60}Co sources are designed to give oval-shaped isodose fields with very steep dose gradients in the border zones of the lesions to minimize radiation damage to the adjacent optic pathways and hypothalamus. To adapt the irradiated volume to the shape of the target, a number of adjacent target points in a predetermined spatial pattern can be used.[65] For solid craniopharyngiomas, approximately 50 Gy are directed at the main parts of the tumor.[70] For an in-depth discussion of stereotactic radiosurgery see Chapter 46.

To date, relatively few patients who have undergone this treatment are available for long-term analysis. In spite of exuberant interest and improved technology in this modality of treatment,

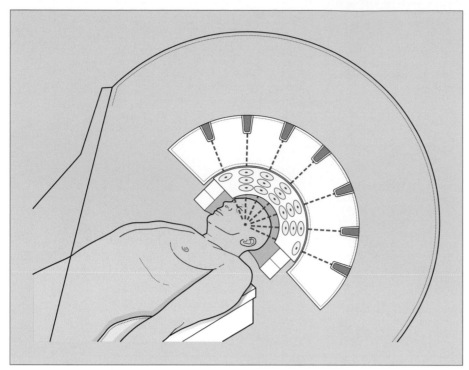

Figure 39.17 Schematic diagram of stereotactic radiosurgery using the gamma irradiation unit illustrating the principle of cross-firing with multiple beams stereotactically aimed at the target. The number of beams is under-represented to preserve clarity. (Adapted with permission from Coffey RJ, Lunsford LD. Stereotactic radiosurgery using the 201 cobalt-60 source gamma knife. *Neurosurg Clin North Am* 1990; 1: 955–90.[125])

there is a distinct dearth of carefully designed studies with reasonable cohort size and adequate follow-up for craniopharyngioma patients. Plowman and associates reported on only six patients and their endorsement of radiosurgery for "low-lying lesions" was unjustified, having only a 1–2-year observation.[71] Mokry's cohort size was larger, but the follow-up was only 6 years, and the patients also received concomitant intracystic bleomycin so that the "pure" efficacy of radiosurgery was difficulty to assess.[72] The 31 patients reported by Chung and co-workers had relatively uniform marginal dosage (9.5–16 Gy) and no radionuclide or chemical treatment; the tumor control rate was 87% with acceptable clinical outcome, but the median follow-up was only 3 years, and even within the 55 months of follow-up, there was 15% tumor progression rate.[73] Backlund's original series from Sweden had incomplete analysis of post-treatment clinical status, but showed high preliminary tumor control rate and low mortality.[74–76] However, a subsequent study on these same patients with follow-up as long as 34.3 years (mean follow-up 18.2 years) revealed that 82% of 11 tumors in children and 50% of 10 tumors in adults ultimately showed tumor progression.[77] Most of these patients received 3–25 Gy prescription dose and approximately 6 Gy at the margin. This meticulous meta-analysis emphasizes the desperate need for a much larger series with comprehensive reporting of late complications and survival quality to ascertain the long-term value and late adverse effects of stereotactic radiosurgery for this slow-growing tumor. At the moment, it is a tempting nonsurgical alternative for small solid craniopharyngiomas as well as for tumor remnants found to be too hazardous to excise.

Primary tumor, predominantly cystic

Approximately 30% of craniopharyngiomas are predominantly cystic.[40,53] If the wall of the cyst is relatively thick and the tumor is not extensively multilobulated within the substance of the frontal or temporal lobes, radical excision should probably be attempted. Puncturing the cyst will collapse the wall towards the central operative field. As long as the cyst wall is tough enough to be pulled on, the collapsed "bag" can be extracted piecemeal. However, if the cyst wall is too thin or fragile to be used as a "handle" during tumor dissection and is likely to fragment into little pieces behind collapsing cisterns, or if the cystic part is too intimately enwrapped within brain tissue, total resection will be difficult to achieve and may even result in unacceptable surgical trauma to the brain.

An alternative treatment is the instillation of beta-emitting radionuclide into the cyst cavity so that a high radiation dose can be delivered to the inner cyst wall to cause cell necrosis and arrest fluid production. A small probe is used to puncture the cyst under stereotactic guidance. The cyst volume can be estimated either by MRI volumetric analysis or by a radionuclide dilution method, in which a known quantity of a radioactive colloid such as technetium-99m-sulphur is injected into the cyst and the cyst fluid–radiocolloid mixture is withdrawn for scintillation counting.[67] The radiation dose planned for the cyst wall is from 200 to 400 Gy, depending on the wall thickness. The amount of beta activity injected is determined using the measured cyst volume and a volume–dosimetry function approximated from a spherical cyst model.[75] Pure beta-emitting isotopes, such as yttrium-90 and phosphorus-32, are used because beta rays have short tissue penetration and can exert a tumoricidal effect at the cyst wall without injuring the structures immediately outside the wall, such as optic and hypothalamic tissues. ^{90}Y has a half-life of 2.67 days and a half-value tissue depth of 1.1 mm. As more than 95% of the radiation dose is delivered within the first five half-lives, decompression of the cyst can be carried out without mitigating treatment efficacy 2 weeks after the radionuclide injection, if required.[56,75] ^{32}P has a longer half-life, of 14.2 days, but a shorter half-value tissue depth of 0.8 mm. It is a less desirable agent if cyst evacuation is necessary within a few days (as

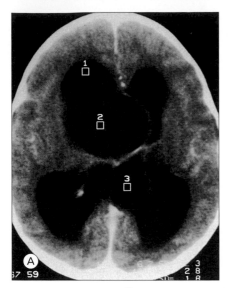 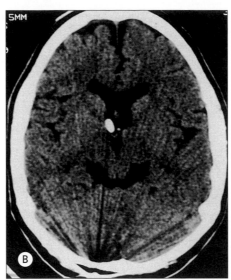 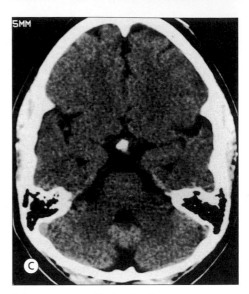

Figure 39.18 Intracystic ^{32}P treatment in a child with a large predominantly cystic craniopharyngioma. **(A)** Pretreatment CT showing large tumor cyst and hydrocephalus. **(B)** CT 12 months after treatment showing disappearance of the cyst and resolution of hydrocephalus with ventriculoperitoneal shunting. **(C)** Posttreatment residual of the calcified solid basal portion of the tumor in suprasellar cistern.

with impending visual failure), but is preferable to ^{90}Y if the cyst wall is very thin (Figure 39.18).[75]

Preliminary results reported by Backlund[76] and Kobayashi and colleagues[51] are encouraging. Backlund reported 14 cyst injections using ^{90}Y, with an average follow-up of 3 years. Contamination of CSF and blood was minimal. The procedures were tolerated well and most patients were ambulatory on the first postoperative day. All patients obtained immediate symptomatic relief, and the cyst shrinkage rate was around 90%. The complication rate was low but not zero. Partial blindness, partial hypopituitarism, third nerve palsy, and mild psychiatric disturbances have been documented.[76–78] Experience with ^{32}P shows similar promise. Pollock and colleagues injected ^{32}P into predominantly cystic craniopharyngiomas in 30 patients.[79] After a mean follow-up of 46 months, 88% of cysts showed regression, with improvement of visual function in 63%, preservation of pretreatment endocrine functions in 67%, and maintenance of overall pretreatment functional level in 70% of patients. Mortality was 10%, mainly as a result of tumor progression in nonresponders. The results of Voges and associates with either ^{90}Y or ^{32}P were similar and the follow-up periods were longer.[78] Thus, intracavitary radionuclide is a viable alternative to radical resection for large, rambling cystic craniopharyngiomas if a larger study with at least 10 years follow-up continues to support its effectiveness in arresting tumor growth and if postoperative morbidity remains less than with total excision.

However, there are also pitfalls to this treatment modality. Most thin-walled cystic craniopharyngiomas have thickened portions of the wall not affected by the intracavitary beta radiation. These thickened parts will continue to grow as solid tumors. Second-stage stereotactic radiosurgery for the solid parts has been given to 46 patients by Yu and co-workers with 85–90% tumor control rate, but the follow-up is less than 3 years.[80] A follow-up period of at least 8–10 years is needed to reach meaningful conclusions. Currently, the author is evaluating the efficacy of a two-stage treatment protocol for large, rambling cystic tumors, first using intracavitary irradiation to collapse the cyst toward the solid basal

part, and then removing the remaining cyst–solid composite by elective microsurgery. Four patients have been treated this way with excellent results.

Recurrent craniopharyngioma

Several options may be considered in the case of recurrent tumors: a second attempt at total excision, subtotal resection and postoperative radiation therapy, or radiation alone. It has been said that a second attempt at radical excision carries a higher morbidity and a lower probability of a cure.[7,41] That may well be true for some recurrent tumors, but more recent reports of reoperations,[4] as well as my own experience (author's unpublished results), show that total excision can be accomplished in many cases with low morbidity. Reoperation is still my first choice of treatment for recurrent tumors, especially if the patient is a child and in good medical condition. Reoperation is especially recommended for those who have already received conventional radiation, or if the solid component of a cystic tumor regrows after intracavitary radionuclide treatment. In unradiated cases, the recurrent tumor is not much more adherent to the brain than during the initial operation, but it may be densely fused with the dural wall of the sella and the cavernous sinus. In postradiation cases, tumor fragments are usually more adherent to vessel walls and hypothalamus, and good sense must be exercised to dictate how aggressive the dissection should be.

If a total excision is again thought to have been achieved, the patient is followed by the same protocol as for the primary operation. If only a subtotal excision is accomplished, conventional radiation or stereotactic radiosurgery should be given to control the residual disease. If a patient returns with recurrence after multiple attempts at radical resection, radiosurgery should also be considered to prolong symptom-free survival.[81]

If the recurrent tumor is purely cystic, and the surgeon is unsure whether the thin adherent wall of the cyst would be amenable to re-resection, intracavitary ^{90}Y may be useful as a salvage procedure compatible with relatively long progression-free survival.[82] It can be used alone in cases refractory to multiple operations, or as an adjunct to simultaneous radiosurgery for adjacent solid recurrences. In situations where focal radiation is undesirable due to proximity of the visual apparatus, intracavitary bleomycin has been used with some success.[83–85]

Finally, progressive craniopharyngiomas that had failed all conventional therapies have been treated with interferon-α2a with variable responses in 50% of patients.[86] This and other systemic chemotherapies[87] are experimental and require much more experience before they become practical.

SURGICAL MANAGEMENT

Preoperative evaluation and management

A complete endocrinologic evaluation is routinely performed before therapy. This should include challenging tests for subtle hormonal deficiencies such as arginine infusion, insulin-induced hypoglycemia, and thyrotropin-releasing hormone and LHRH administration. An 8-hour partial water deprivation test should be performed to stress the pitressin axis if the patient has symptoms of diabetes insipidus. These results are important both for the academic records and for establishing a baseline endocrine profile against which the effects of therapy and future impairments can be gauged. These results do not assist immediate management if radical resection is planned, since the patient is then expected at least to have panhypopituitarism for some time after surgery and full hormone replacement is routine, but preoperative adreno-corticotropic hormone (ACTH) and thyroid status comprise important information that will guide selective intraoperative replacement if the therapy chosen is not expected to destroy pituitary functions abruptly, such as stereotactic radiation or intracystic radionuclide injection.

Adequate thyroid replacement takes several days to 2 weeks with oral L-thyroxine and should be started immediately if the patient is found to be hypothyroid. Intravenous L-thyroxine may be given if the patient's condition demands immediate surgical intervention, but it must be infused extremely carefully in elderly patients lest it produce arrhythmias and acute myocardial ischemia. If the patient is euthyroid before surgery, L-thyroxine can be prescribed at leisure 1–2 weeks after surgery or as dictated by the postoperative serum free L-thyroxine level.

Pre- and intraoperative replacement of corticosteroids is mandatory and should be carried out rapidly. All but the smallest craniopharyngiomas with proven normal ACTH axes should be given preoperative stress steroid doses. The first crisis of physiologic stress requiring stress levels of circulating corticosteroids is during induction of general anesthesia. Patients should therefore be given stress doses before the morning of surgery equivalent to three times the physiologic daily corticosteroid production (the mean physiologic cortisone requirement is 13 mg/m^2/day for normal individuals over 4 months of age[88]). For adults, this can be given by infusing intravenous Solu-Cortef beginning the night before, but for children it is simpler to avoid the intravenous line and give a single intramuscular injection of the daily stress dose of cortisone acetate both the night before and on the morning of surgery, followed by Solu-Cortef drip during the operation.

Detailed neuro-ophthalmologic evaluation is obtained to follow the patient's postoperative or postradiation visual status. Intraoperative visual evoked response monitoring using either contact lenses with a built-in flash unit or wick electrodes directly applied to the optic nerves is being evaluated with limited success.

The former method carries a real risk of corneal abrasion for long procedures, and the latter is all too often in the way of the dissection.

Because of the recent interest in neurobehavioral syndromes following treatment of craniopharyngiomas,[59,89] the author has been obtaining detailed preoperative neuropsychologic testing. This has included the standard Wechsler Intelligence Scale for Adults and Children (WISC), the Wechsler Memory Scale and its modified form for children, verbal and nonverbal selection memory tests, complex figure duplication, and a variety of subtests to measure frontal lobe functions.[59] The lower age limit for this test is around 6 years, and there is no optimal test for younger children. These tests are extremely important for monitoring the child's intellectual as well as psychosocial progress after initial treatment.

Finally, for children with this tumor, the magnitude of the therapeutic problem, the long-term prognosis, and most importantly, the neurobehavioral sequelae following treatment should be discussed openly and extensively with the family before surgery. Parents must understand that their participation is vital in the postoperative management of endocrinopathies, hyperphagia, obesity, memory deficits, body-image distortion, and psychosocial maladjustment, to name a few. A conscientious social worker experienced in this field and with psychotherapeutic training would be a valuable member of the treatment team.

Management of hydrocephalus

Over 60% of children with craniopharyngiomas have obstructive hydrocephalus at diagnosis. If the symptoms of high ICP are not disabling, it is preferable to obtain all preoperative testing without preoperative shunting, and then to put in an external ventricular drain (EVD) at the time of tumor resection. The hydrocephalus usually resolves after total or subtotal resection. After surgery, the EVD chamber is set at physiologic level (10 cm above the external auditory meatus) for 3–4 days and then gradually elevated to test the patient's CSF absorptive capacity. If the patient remains asymptomatic and the CT does not show ventriculomegaly, the EVD is removed. Only rarely will the EVD "chamber test" indicate the need for permanent shunting.

If the patient presents with severe symptoms of raised ICP as a result of hydrocephalus, a temporary EVD is still preferable to preresection shunting. A temporary EVD allows time for the necessary preoperative testing but does not carry the risk of shunt infection, which is not negligible, considering the long exposure time of the CSF during the radical excision operation.

Surgical approaches

Subfrontal approach

This is my preferred approach because it affords total excision of most craniopharyngiomas except for those eccentric large tumors that require staged procedures from diverse angles. Unilateral frontal lobe retraction is usually adequate for exposure, and it avoids the potentially disastrous problem of bifrontal damage. The right side is used by the right-handed surgeon unless there is significant lateral extension of the tumor into the left sylvian fissure. A bicoronal scalp flap is fashioned. An osteoplastic right frontal craniotomy is made so that the medial margin crosses the midline by 1.5 cm to gain control of the superior sagittal sinus. The anterior margin of the bone flap is flush with the orbital roof. The posterior margin of the bone flap may also be extended

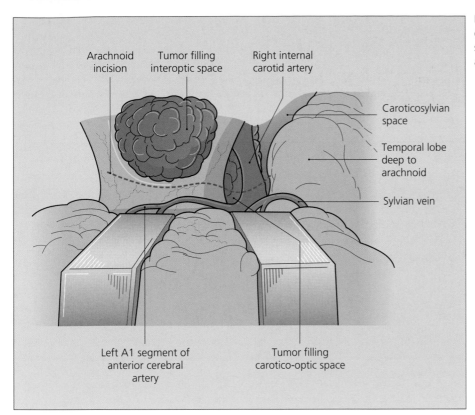

Figure 39.19 Exposure of optic nerves and chiasm, right internal carotid artery, and all three surgical spaces. Dotted line represents line of arachnoid incision.

Labels in figure:
Arachnoid incision
Tumor filling interoptic space
Right internal carotid artery
Caroticosylvian space
Temporal lobe deep to arachnoid
Sylvian vein
Left A1 segment of anterior cerebral artery
Tumor filling carotico-optic space

posteriorly to the sphenoid ridge if the pterional approach is to be adopted for certain parts of the exposure.

With large tumors and high-riding domes, where high frontal lobe retraction is anticipated, the orbital–zygomatic bar can be removed to gain an additional 5° to 10° of ventral–basal vision. A small burr hole is made in the medial orbital roof. A Gigli saw is passed through the burr hole and a low cut is made across the glabella medially, and then laterally along the anterior orbital roof all the way through the fronto-zygomatic pillar at the level of the fronto-zygomatic suture.

The anteriormost portion of the superior sagittal sinus is doubly ligated and transected. The anterior falx is completely detached from the crista galli. For large tumors, it is usually necessary to divide the right olfactory tract. Gradually deepening the subfrontal retraction will bring the right optic nerve, chiasm, and right carotid artery into view, at which time the carotid and prechiasmal cisterns are opened along a line stretching from the right temporal lobe to the left carotid cistern (Figure 39.19). Time is well spent in patiently aspirating CSF at this point so that after the "tethering" arachnoid has been cut to release the deep frontal lobules from the chiasm and carotid arteries, further retraction of the frontal lobe can be performed with minimal force to reveal the entire anterior surface of the chiasm and anterior cerebral arteries.

The anterior lower aspect of the tumor is now visible behind dense arachnoid adhesions between the optic nerves and between the optic nerve and carotid artery. It is at once obvious that the surgical exercise involves extracting a large but (fortunately) usually soft bulk through a series of relatively small holes. These small holes are the important "surgical spaces," namely, interoptic (between the optic nerves), carotico-optic (between optic nerve and carotid), and caroticosylvian (between carotid and the lateral sylvian fissure) (see Figure 39.19). The tactic thus consists of

debulking and collapsing the center of the bulk, pulling in and freeing the capsule from surrounding structures, and finally grabbing and pulling out the morsellated capsule through these spaces. It is advisable to follow a drilled sequence of maneuvers, because each preceding step makes the next one easier and safer. The recommended sequence is as follows: (1) interoptic debulking, (2) separation of capsule from optic structures, (3) right lateral dissection, (4) left lateral dissection, (5) detaching upper pole of tumor from hypothalamus, (6) basilar tip dissection, and finally, (7) dorsum sellae–intrasellar dissection.

Tumor reduction begins with aspiration of cyst fluid in the interoptic space followed by generous excision of tumor capsule for biopsy. With further debulking, the chiasm falls away from the tuberculum and its "pseudoprefixity" is lost, thereby widening the interoptic space further. As the capsule pulls away from the underside of the chiasm and optic nerves, the arachnoid plane between lesion and brain is carefully exploited to peel tumor from the optic structures. The arterial feeders to this part of the capsule from the anterior cerebral and anterior communicating arteries are taken without affecting the vascular supply to the optic chiasm and nerves.

With the arterial feeders from the anterior cerebral arteries already interrupted, the only remaining blood supply comes from the posterior communicating arteries from the sides and the meningohypophyseal arteries from below. The main objectives of the lateral dissection are therefore to eliminate the lateral blood supply and detach the capsule from the medial temporal lobe and carotid artery. Right lateral dissection is best done through the carotico-optic space. The lateral capsule is manipulated medially towards the collapsed central cavity to put the lateral feeders on stretch, which are then cauterized and cut, while the important thalamotuberal perforators from the lateral aspect of the posterior

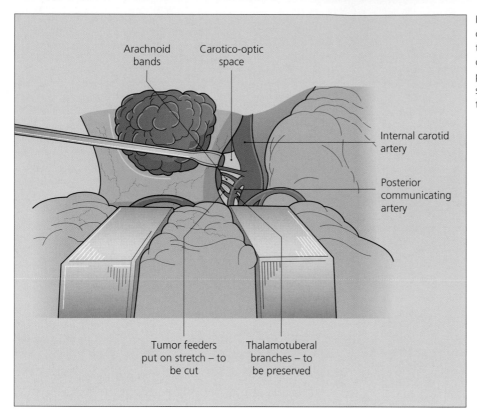

Figure 39.20 Right lateral dissection within carotico-optic space. The right lateral surface of the tumor capsule is pulled away from the internal carotid and posterior communicating arteries, putting the lateral feeders on stretch. The superiorly coursing thalamotuberal perforators to the hypothalamus and basal ganglia are preserved.

Labels in figure:
Arachnoid bands
Carotico-optic space
Internal carotid artery
Posterior communicating artery
Tumor feeders put on stretch – to be cut
Thalamotuberal branches – to be preserved

communicating artery that normally supply the basal ganglia are preserved (Figure 39.20). In tumors with extreme lateral extension, the caroticosylvian space may have to be used, but the arachnoid plane here is usually very well preserved. Because of the convenient microscope angle for the right-handed surgeon, the left lateral dissection can be performed through the now much larger interoptic space by rotating the operating table to the left.

Removal of the two lateral portions of the capsule should create enough room in the suprasellar cistern to allow the upper pole of the tumor to be firmly pulled downwards away from the hypothalamus and into view through the interoptic space. The capsule can be peeled off the underside of the chiasm and anterior floor of the third ventricle along a well-defined arachnoid plane, but near the infundibular stalk the capsule is always seemingly fused with the hypothalamus. This unique part of the tumor is more tenacious than brain tissue and can literally be torn away from the hypothalamus by firmly grasping and pulling it downwards using the alternating right and left tumor microforceps (Figure 39.21). This technique is likened to pulling a large rag out of a deep bag with both hands alternating. The split usually occurs within the gliotic plane surrounding the capsule, and the firm pulling motion ensures that the tumor pseudopods are avulsed intact from the gliotic brain rather than amputated and retained if the usual sweeping dissection technique is used. The distorted pituitary stalk is recognized by its striated long portal vessels.[4,7,90] It can occasionally be preserved, but in large lesions the stalk is hopelessly encased in tumor and must be divided.

The posterior pole of the tumor can now be rolled forward into the interoptic space. Because of the absence of feeders from the posterior circulation, and the double-layered membrane of Liliequist insulating brainstem and basilar artery from the tumor, even large and low-lying retrosellar extensions can be safely pulled

forward so that the ample arachnoid adhesions can be cut under direct vision.

The remaining inferior pole is now examined. If the coronal MRI does not show tumor expanding the sella, the lower capsule is usually not fused with the diaphragma or the sellar dura. The remaining tumor can simply be lifted upwards and the meningo-hypophyseal branches can be cauterized and cut or tamponaded (Figure 39.22).

Translamina terminalis approach

In patients with prefixed chiasm, the interoptic space is too small for the extensive maneuvers needed to extract a large craniopharyngioma. The lamina terminalis can then be traversed to gain access to the tumor dome (Figure 39.23). Normally the lamina terminalis is a narrow structure that delimits the anterior third ventricle, but with large suprasellar tumors the tuberal portion of the basal hypothalamus, from the mamillary bodies to the chiasm, is stretched very thin and may actually be coapted with the lamina terminalis to form a single membrane (see Figure 39.3). Both the infundibular and supraoptic recesses are obliterated, so that traversing this coapted membrane instantly gives access to the tumor without actually entering the third ventricle. In most large solid tumors, the lamina terminalis is widely expanded behind the chiasm, and the yellowish, gritty tumor can often be seen through the diaphanous coapted membrane in between the splayed-out optic tracts (Figure 39.24). Opening this membrane carefully behind the crossing macular fibers of the chiasm (to avoid severe loss of acuity) will afford an excellent view of the tumor dome (Figure 39.25). It appears likely that the basal hypothalamic nuclei are displaced laterally by the slow expansion of the tumor, since using the translamina terminalis route does not usually produce hypothalamic deficiency.

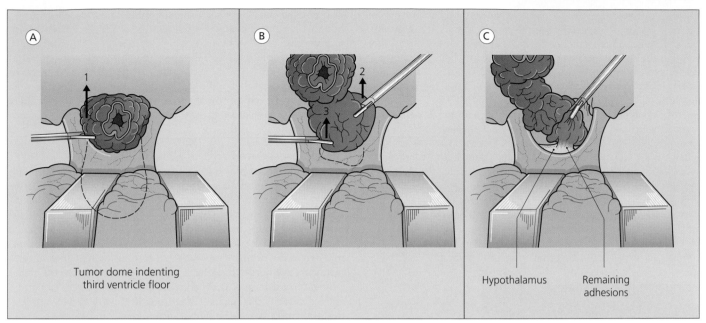

Figure 39.21 Detaching the upper pole of the tumor from the hypothalamus. **(A)** After considerable reduction of tumor volume through interoptic debulking, the base of the upper tumor piece (indenting third ventricular floor) is firmly grasped by the left microforceps and pulled down towards the suprasellar cistern (grasp 1). **(B)** When more tumor appears in the interoptic space, it is, in turn, grasped by the right microforceps, which continues the downward pull (grasp 2), alternating with the left hand (grasp 3). **(C)** The upper pole is pulled down, and the previously severely elevated basal hypothalamus is now visible through the interoptic space.

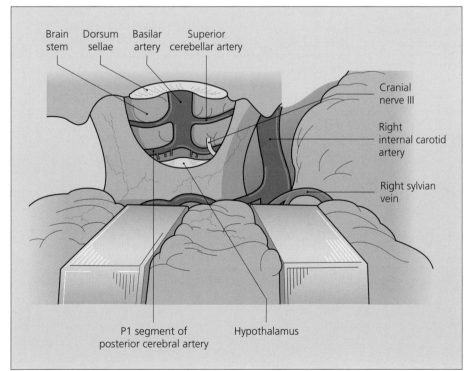

Figure 39.22 View after total resection of tumor.

Subfrontal–transsphenoidal approach

There are situations where the inferior tumor capsule is densely fused with the sellar dura, walls of the cavernous sinus, and even the lining of the sphenoid sinus. It would then not be possible to lift the inferior portion of the tumor upward into the suprasellar cistern from above through the standard subfrontal approach.

The lower pole of the tumor must first be dissected free from the sellar and/or sphenoid lining under direct vision. This calls for a combined subfrontal–transsphenoidal approach.

Four radiographic signs are associated with this situation, which should alert the surgeon to pre-plan for the combined approach, such as preparing the thigh for fascia lata graft harvesting. These signs are (1) wide expansion and "excavation" of the sella by tumor, especially with dramatic lateral extensions into the cavernous sinuses (Figure 39.26); (2) frank invasion of tumor through the sella floor into the sphenoid sinus (Figure 39.27); (3) calcium flecks within the cavernous sinus (Figure 39:28), and (4) "fluffy–flaky" erosion of the sellar or sphenoid floor and the dorsum sellae (Figure 39.29).

Intraoperatively, basal adhesion of the tumor is recognized when upward pulling of the inferior capsule through the intraoptic space encounters obvious resistance. Direct access to the intrasellar tumor can be gained by drilling through the tuberculum sellae into the sphenoid sinus, sweeping aside the sphenoid mucosa, and then finally breaking open the anterior sellar wall (Figure 39.30). A thin shell of pituitary gland is often sandwiched between the tumor capsule and the dura. If the pituitary stalk has already been cut, as with most of these tumors with large sellar extensions, there is no point in saving the gland. The sella is thus completely exenterated together with the tumor (Figure 39.31).

The circular and cavernous sinuses sometimes bleed profusely, but this type of venous bleeding can be readily controlled with tamponade.

After complete tumor resection, the confluent sella sphenoid cavity is packed with fat, and a piece of fascia lata is sutured to the edge of the tuberculum dural defect and laid over the sella (Figures 39.32 and 39.33). If the sphenoid mucosa is accidentally perforated, a lumbar drain may be needed to prevent postoperative CSF leak.

Staged procedures

Extension of the tumor far away from the primary suprasellar site occasionally requires a second procedure, usually 2–3 weeks after the removal of the central core of the tumor. Lateral rambling of tumor cyst far into the Sylvian fissure or in the posterior choroid fissure necessitates using the subtemporal or pterional approach (Figure 39.34). By itself the subtemporal route is not recommended as the primary approach, because of the high incidence of postoperative nerve III, IV, and VI palsies, and because the translamina terminalis and modified transsphenoidal options cannot be exercised from this angle. Sometimes the cyst extends into the posterior fossa below the line of vision from the subfrontal angle, e.g. behind the dorsum sellae and the clivus and even down into the upper cervical canal (Figure 39.35). A separate retrosigmoid exposure will be required to peal the cyst wall off the branches of the basilar tree and the cranial nerves.

Because most craniopharyngiomas do not actually penetrate the floor of the third ventricle no matter how high the hypothalamus has been lifted up by the tumor mass, using a primary transventricular approach from above has been associated with significant hypothalamic damage and poor results.[21,91] This approach is only used as a first procedure for the truly rare intraventricular craniopharyngiomas. It is also recommended as a second procedure if after the subfrontal operation a portion of the

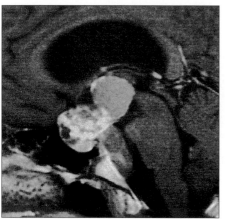

Figure 39.23
Postcontrast sagittal MRI of a partially solid craniopharyngioma with a large solid upper dome and a large retroclival part. Interoptic space is not adequate for removal of the upper part, nor does it afford the angle for the removal of the retroclival part.

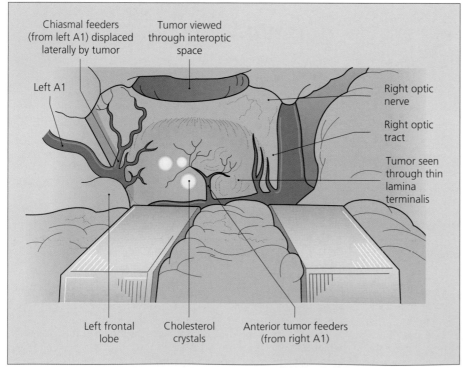

Chiasmal feeders (from left A1) displaced laterally by tumor

Tumor viewed through interoptic space

Left A1

Right optic nerve

Right optic tract

Tumor seen through thin lamina terminalis

Left frontal lobe

Cholesterol crystals

Anterior tumor feeders (from right A1)

Figure 39.24 Large craniopharyngioma and prefixed chiasm. Only the most posterior segments of the optic nerves are seen. The small interoptic space is too small for tumor extraction. Tumor is seen bulging through the thin (coapted) lamina terminalis, splaying open the optic tracts. The chiasmal feeders from the anterior cerebral arteries are also displaced laterally by the tumor, and thus can be selectively preserved while the more medial feeders to the tumor are taken.

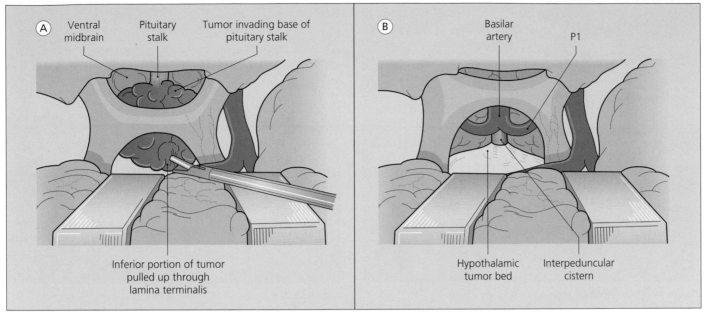

Figure 39.25 (A) Translamina terminalis resection of large craniopharyngioma. After debulking the main retrochiasmal portion of the tumor, the inferior pole is pulled up from the sella through the large opening in the lamina terminalis. **(B)** After total resection of tumor, the tip of the basilar artery and the posterior cerebral arteries (P1), the midbrain, and the now "hanging" hypothalamic floor are seen through the lamina opening.

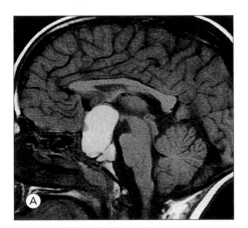
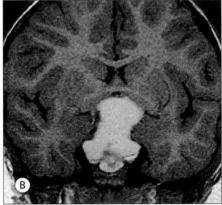

Figure 39.26 Precontrast MRI of a child with a partially cystic craniopharyngioma. **(A)** Sagittal image shows wide expansion of the sella and encroachment of the sphenoid sinus. Note level of the tumor dome almost at the level of the foramen of Monro and mamillary bodies just behind the tumor dome. **(B)** Coronal image shows wide lateral displacement of the cavernous sinuses, wide expansion of the sella, and a defect in the sella floor through which the tumor extends into the sphenoid sinus.

tumor is found to have penetrated far into the third ventricle and would not descend with suprasellar debulking.

MANAGEMENT OF POSTOPERATIVE COMPLICATIONS

Visual loss is the most common neurologic deficit after radical or subradical resection. The preoperative visual status is the most important determining factor for visual outcome.[20,92] Patients with total or near-total blindness do not regain useful vision, but those with scotomas and partial field cuts may well improve after surgery. Duration of preoperative visual loss is also an important prognostic factor: visual impairment that has lasted less than a year has more than three times the chance of improvement than impairment of longer than a year.[93]

With the high likelihood of stalk sectioning or injury during tumor resection, postoperative diabetes insipidus is universal[94,95] and frequently has a triphasic course. Excessive diuresis usually begins within the first 24 hours as a result of the immediate cessation of normal intra-axonal transport of antidiuretic hormone (ADH). Degeneration of the hypothalamohypophyseal tract and necrosis of pitressin–neurophysinladen axon terminals in the neurohypophysis then causes uncontrolled release of stored ADH 24–96 hours later to give paradoxic water retention.[4,96] This phase-2 response to stalk sectioning must be kept in mind when administering pitressin analogs to avoid causing water intoxication and lethal brain edema. The initial diabetes insipidus is best managed with small doses of intravenous DDAVP (desmopressin), which has a therapeutic effect lasting up to 18 hours. When the final, permanent diuretic phase of diabetes insipidus sets in, usually in a few days when the patient is more alert, DDAVP can be given by nasal spray. It is interesting that 10–15% of patients after stalk sectioning will resume partial production of ADH within 3 years, and their pitressin requirement may lessen. This is most likely the result of formation of new neurovascular units in the magnocellular portion of the supraoptic and paraventricular nuclei of the hypothalamus.[95,97]

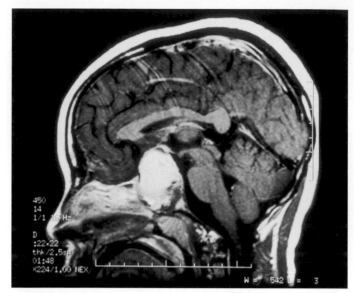

Figure 39.27 Post-contrast sagittal MRI of a child with craniopharyngioma showing the lower pole of the tumor has eroded into and massively expanded the sphenoid sinus.

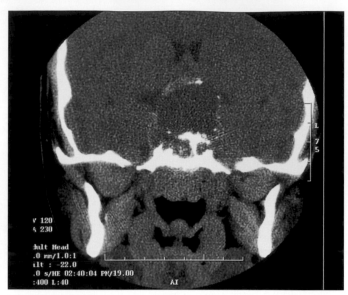

Figure 39.29 Coronal CT of a child with a solid craniopharyngioma, showing "fluffy–flaky" erosion of the sella floor and dorsium sellae, with adjacent calcification.

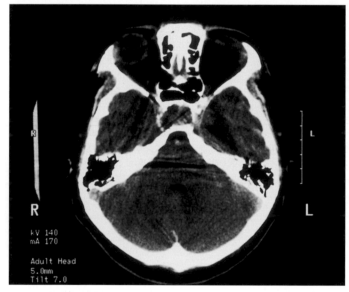

Figure 39.28 Axial CT of a child with a solid craniopharyngioma, showing calcium deposits either in the walls of the cavernous sinuses or actually within the sinuses.

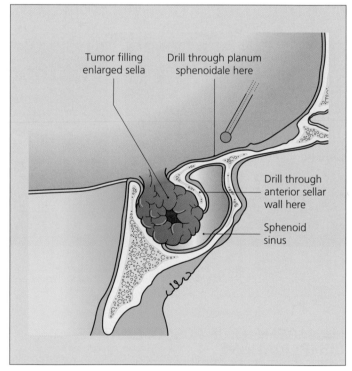

Figure 39.30 Subfrontal–transsphenoidal approach. Sagittal view shows large intrasellar and intrasphenoid tumor. The direction of drilling through the planum sphenoidale to gain entrance into the sphenoid sinus and access to the anterior sellar floor is indicated.

Stress doses of corticosteroid can be tapered to normal maintenance dosage in the form of oral cortisone acetate after the first 4–5 days. Dexamethasone used prophylactically for brain edema can also be tapered off completely according to the anticipated time-course of postsurgical edema. Post-stalk-sectioning hypothyroidism requiring replacement occurs in 60–80% of patients.[94] Follicle-stimulating hormone (FSH) and luteinizing hormone (LH) deficiencies are permanent. Children are begun on estrogen and testosterone replacement when the appropriate pubertal ages are reached, to impart secondary sexual characteristics. Testosterone is given to adult males to maintain libido. Ovulation in adult females can be induced by a costly process of priming ovarian follicular growth with human menopausal gonadotropins (Pergonal, containing FSH and LH) and then stimulating the follicles with a burst of human chorionic gonadotropin (possessing strong LH activity).[98] Patients with preserved pituitary stalk have been known to regain various endocrine functions,[94] but recovery of the exquisitely sensitive LHRH pacemaker function in the arcuate nucleus, vital to the induction of ovulation, has not been observed to date.

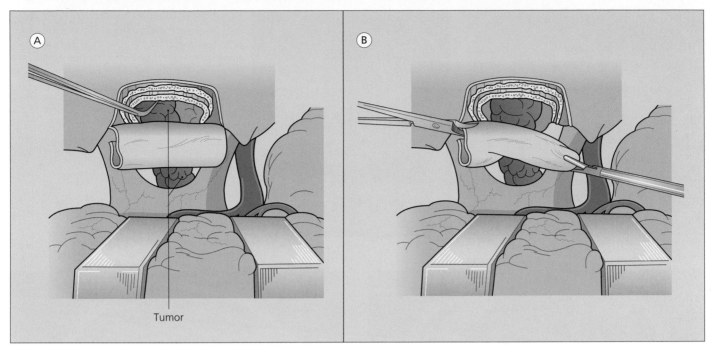

Figure 39.31 Subfrontal–transsphenoidal approach. **(A)** Exenteration of sella with microcurette scraping against bony sellar floor. **(B)** Intrasellar tumor is pushed into the interoptic space. If necessary, the remaining tuberculum sellae dura may be excised to improve exposure.

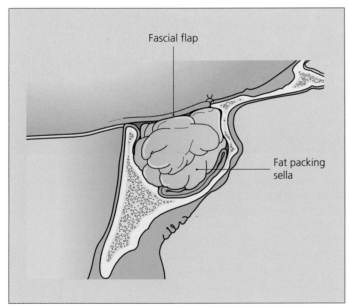

Figure 39.32 The sella–sphenoid confluent space is packed with free fat graft and overlaid with a fascial flap that is sutured to the anterior free dural edge.

The growth rate of most children remains low after stalk section. Growth hormone (GH) therapy is usually started 6–9 months after surgery.[99] Because estrogen and testosterone are known to accelerate closure of the epiphyseal plates of long bones in children, they are postponed until some growth has been made up by GH therapy for several years, sometimes in spite of considerable psychosocial difficulties experienced by the hypogonadal adolescent patient. The initial 6–9 months wait before starting GH therapy is imposed to select out children who continue to grow normally despite the absence of GH.[100–106] In a few of these children, growth is attributed to hyperinsulinemia secondary to hyperphagia and weight gain,[100,101] but in others the growth is related to normal or supranormal levels of insulin-like growth factors (IGF-I and IGF-II).[107] IGFs are probably stimulated by increased insulin secretion,[108,109] but increased prolactin secretion from residual pituitary tissue caused by reduced prolactin-inhibiting factor output from the injured hypothalamus may also boost IGF production activity.[106]

Serious hypothalamic syndromes, such as loss of thirst sensation, dysthermia, and sleep disorders, are now seldom seen in radical excisions. More likely are minor hypothalamic syndromes such as memory deficits and appetite changes. Detailed neuropsychological evaluation in children following surgical treatment has shown significant decrease in verbal and visuospatial memory scores in the face of normal general cognitive functions.[110] The pattern of memory deficits indicates specific impairment in retrieval mechanisms whereas encoding and storage are better preserved. Injury to the fornices, mamillary bodies, and the dorsal medial thalamus may be responsible.[111] Interestingly, memory and general cognitive performance scores are unaffected in adults after radical tumor resection, and there are actually reports of improvement in specific areas such as cognitive speed and verbal IQ.[112]

In children and young adults it is also common to see some degree of weight gain 1–6 months after surgery.[26] Morbid obesity, defined as body mass index [BMI = weight/(height^2)] > 3 SD, is seen in 30–45% of children after craniopharyngioma surgery.[113–115] There is a correlation between obesity and the size of the tumor, the use of the translamina terminalis approach, and the presence of serious neuropsychological syndromes. The etiology of the postresection obesity is probably multifactorial. There is always an increased desire to eat. Severely affected children also have bizarre food-seeking behaviours and eating habits. Serum leptin, which normally inhibits appetite via hypothalamic receptors, has

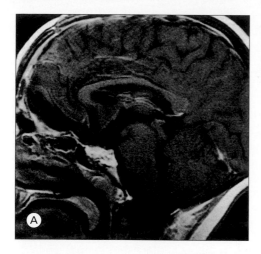
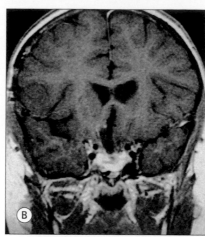

Figure 39.33 Postoperative MRI of the case shown in Figure 39.26, sagittal **(A)** and coronal **(B)** views. Note total excision of tumor by the subfrontal transsphenoidal route, loss of the tuberculum sellae "angle," and survival of fat graft within the sella-sphenoid space. Note resumption of air filling in the sphenoid sinus indicative of mucosal preservation.

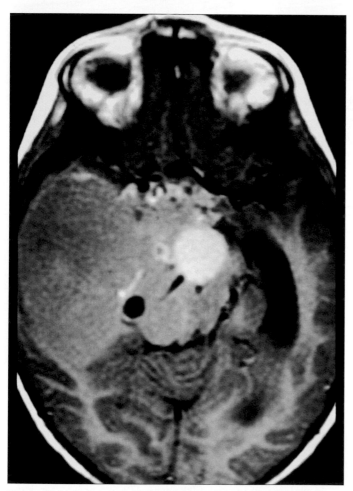

Figure 39.34 Postcontrast axial MRI of a child with a giant mixed cystic–solid craniopharyngioma, showing large rambling cyst extending far into the right posterior choroid fissure. This case necessitated a two-stage resection: a right subfrontal approach followed by a right subtemporal–pterional approach.

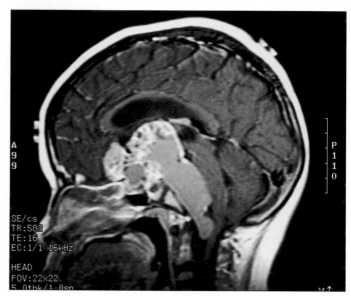

Figure 39.35 Postcontrast sagittal MRI of a child with a giant mixed cystic–solid craniopharyngioma, showing a large posterior extension of a cyst far down into the posterior fossa behind the clivus, reaching down to the C2 level, displacing the entire brainstem and the upper cervical spinal cord. This case necessitated a two-stage resection: a right subfrontal approach followed by a left retrosigmoid–far lateral clival–cervical approach.

been consistently shown to be elevated in obese children after craniopharyngioma resection, suggesting that there is a central insensitivity to leptin secondary to hypothalamic injury. This in turn leads to a failure in the down-regulation of appetite and hence central hyperphagia.[108,116,117] In addition to leptin, raised serum insulin levels have also been found in obese patients after surgery.[108,109] Insulin is a strong stimulus for eating behaviours and also induces lipogenesis in selective far depots. Its augmented secretion appears to be related to hyperactive central vagal output from the injured medial basal hypothalamus,[118–120] because vagotomy in obese hyperphagic animals abruptly reduces insulin production and appetite.[121,122]

Finally, central hyperphagia has recently been postulated to result from injury to the serotoninergic eating inhibitory pathways originating from the anterior nucleus and preoptic area of the anterior hypothalamus. Weight gain usually stabilizes after hyperphagia subsides, but strict behavioral modification, stringent exercise programs, and psychologic counseling must be enforced to avoid morbid obesity. The use of dextroamphetamine to treat hyperphagia and obesity in these children has shown some initial promise.[123]

Another interesting neurobehavioral syndrome, particularly following translamina terminalis resection of large tumors, is abulia minor, characterized by psychomotor retardation, flattening of affect, lack of enthusiasm and spontaneity of action and thoughts, loss of adventitious body motions and gesticulation, and reduction of exploratory behaviors.[124] Children thus affected are unmotivated in play and learning and consequently have extremely poor school performance. The neuropathologic basis for abulia is not known for certain, but it may be related to injury of the mesolimbic pathways projecting from the rostral midbrain to the medial septal nuclei, nucleus accumbens, and anterior cingulate gyrus[33,67,68] by way of the medial septal area, just underneath the deep subfrontal brain retractors.[124]

POSTOPERATIVE FOLLOW-UP

Postoperative CT with and without contrast should be obtained within 24 hours after surgery (when contrast enhancement of surgically traumatized brain is minimal) to detect residual tumor and hence rule out false cure. Signal artifacts sometimes last as long as 10 weeks on the gadolinium-enhanced MRI, which makes MRI a less desirable test for this particular period. Presence of unsuspected residual tumor on the "next-day" CT should prompt a second-look operation within 1–2 weeks, i.e. before exuberant scarring makes reoperation difficult. If the "next-day" CT shows no residual tumor, or if the second attempt at total resection accomplishes its goal, the next CT and MRI can be obtained in 3–6 months. Thereafter, a yearly CT and MRI should be adequate.

Complete endocrine evaluation should be repeated 6 months after surgery to monitor thyroid and adrenocortical functions. Cortisone replacement is almost certainly permanent if stalk section was performed, but if the stalk was anatomically preserved, one may carefully withdraw cortisone in hospital and restudy the ACTH reserve to see if continued full replacement is necessary or whether the dose can be reduced. Excessive cortisone intake contributes potently to hyperphagia and must be categorically ruled out. Because of the recovery capacity of the magnocellular system of the supraoptic and paraventricular nuclei, the DDAVP requirement must also be re-evaluated 1–2 years after surgery even if total stalk section has been performed. At least 9 months should elapse before GH treatment is initiated, to determine whether adequate growth continues as a result of sustained IGF levels. A low postoperative GH level has no bearing on the growth curve after craniopharyngioma resection.[102,103,107]

Tests of visual acuity and fields should be repeated twice yearly. This is most useful in cases of known residual or recurrent tumor, when a subtle change in vision may herald regrowth of a previously quiescent tumor before the increase in tumor size can be appreciated on imaging studies. At each clinical follow-up, the patient's neurobehavioral status is briefly evaluated as part of the routine. All growth indices are measured for children. The body weight and height are accurately documented since they remain the best indicators of abnormal eating behaviors, which are never truthfully reported by the patient and are often overlooked by the parents. Descriptions of the meal contents, timing, and patterns, as well as of eating habits, are best obtained from witnesses (siblings, friends), and are evaluated to distinguish between central hyperphagia, psychogenic polyphagia, and excessive corticosteroid intake. An abridged neuropsychologic minibattery should include verbal recall test, complex figure duplication and graphic recall to assess spatial orientation and nonlogic memory, respectively, object similarities and differences, and proverb interpretation. The patient's psychomotor activity level, mood, willingness to participate in work and recreation, and enthusiasm for social interaction are also recorded. A full neuropsychologic battery should be repeated on children 6 months to 1 year after surgery to plan school re-entry levels and long-term educational goals.

REFERENCES

1. Cobb CA, Youmans JR. Brain tumors of disordered embryogenesis in adults. In: Youmans JR (ed.). *Neurological Surgery*. 2nd edn. Philadelphia, PA: WB Saunders Co; 1976: 2899–935.

CLINICAL PEARLS

- Craniopharyngiomas are rare tumors of childhood, constituting about 8–10% of all childhood brain tumors.

- They probably derive from embryonic ectoblastic cell rests along the migration path of the hypophysiopharyngeal duct.

- They are predominately solid but almost always have a cystic component. Almost all childhood crangiopharyngiomas have calcium detectable by CT, a key diagnostic clue.

- Children with crangiopharyngiomas commonly present with hydrocephalus, growth retardation, and obesity. Adults present with visual symptoms.

- Large cystic tumors can be treated with β-emitting radionuclide colloids such as ^{90}Y or ^{32}P.

- Smaller solid tumors or recurrences can be treated with stereotactic radiosurgery.

- Total resection, if possible, is associated with the best long-term results, with 80–90% 10-year disease free survival.

- Unilateral subfrontal resection is favored by the author, with or without the translaminar terminalis approach. Large tumors which extend into the sella or sphenoid sinus will require a combined subfrontal–trans-sphenoidal approach. Two-stage fronto-temporal and posterior fossa craniotomies are necessary for exceedingly large and sprawling tumors.

2. Kernohan JW. Tumors of congenital origin. In: Minckler J (ed.). *Pathology of the Nervous System*. New York, NY: McGraw-Hill; 1971: 1927–37.

3. Matson DD. *Neurosurgery in Infancy and Childhood*. 2nd edn. Springfield, IL: Charles C Thomas Publisher; 1969: 544–74.

4. Carmel PW. Craniopharyngiomas. In: Wilkins RH, Rengachary SS (eds). *Neurosurgery*. New York, NY: McGraw-Hill; 1985: 905–16.

5. Koos WT, Miller MJ. *Intracranial Tumors of Infants and Children*. Stuttgart: Thieme; 1971: 188–213.

6. Banna M, Hoare RD, Stanley P, Till K. Craniopharyngiomas in children. *J Pediatr* 1973; 83: 781–5.

7. Carmel PW, Antunes JL, Chang CH. Craniopharyngiomas in children. *Neurosurgery* 1982; 11: 382–9.

8. Hoffman HJ, Hendrick EB, Humphreys RP, Buncic JR, Armstrong DL, Jenkins RDT. Management of craniopharyngioma in children. *J Neurosurg* 1977; 27: 218–27.

9. Erdheim J. Über Hypophysenganggeschwulste und Hirncholesteatome. *Sitzungsberichte der mathematisch-naturwissenschaftlichen Klasse der kaiserlichen Akademie der Wissenschaften, Abteilung* LLL. 1904; 113: 537–726.

10. Goldberg GM, Eshbaugh DE. Squamous cell rests of the pituitary gland as related to the origin of craniopharyngiomas. *Arch Pathol* 1960; 70: 293–9.

11. Pertuiset B. Craniopharyngiomas. In: Vinken PH, Bruyn FW (eds.). *Tumors of the Brain and Skull, Part II. Handbook of Clinical Neurology*, Vol. 19. Amsterdam: North-Holland; 1975: 531–71.

12. Tiberin P, Goldberg GM, Schwartz A. Craniopharyngiomas in the aged. *Neurology* 1958; 8: 31–54.

13. Luse SA, Kernohan JW. Squamous-cell rests of the pituitary gland. *Cancer* 1955; 8: 623–8.

14. Kahn EA, Gosch HH, Seger JF, Hicks SP. Forty-five years experience with the craniopharyngiomas. *Surg Neurol* 1973; 1: 5–12.

15. Till K. Craniopharyngioma. *Childs Brain* 1982; 9: 179–87.

16. Sekine S, Shibata T, Kokubu A, *et al*. Craniopharyngiomas of adamantinomatous type harbor β-catenine gene mutations. *Am J Pathol* 2002; 161: 1997–2001.

17. Rienstein S, Adams EF, Pilzer D, Goldring AA, Goldman B, Friedman E. Comparative genomic hybridization analysis of craniopharyngiomas. *J Neurosurg* 2003; 98: 162–4.

18. Lefranc F, Chevalier C, Vinchon M, *et al*. Characterization of the levels of expression of retinoic acid receptors galectin-3, macrophage migration inhibiting factor, and p53 in 51 adamantinomatous craniopharyngiomas. *J Neurosurg* 2003; 98: 145–53.

19. Bollati A, Giunta F, Lenzi A, Marina G. Third ventricle intrinsic craniopharyngioma. *J Neurosurg Sci* 1973; 17: 316–17.

20. Cashion EL, Young JM. Intraventricular craniopharyngioma: report of two cases. *J Neurosurg* 1971; 4: 84–7.

21. Van den Bergh R. The transventricular approach in craniopharyngioma of the third ventricle: neurosurgical and neuropathological aspects. *Neurochirurgie* 1970; 16: 51–65.

22. Olivecrona H. The surgical treatment of intracranial tumors. In: Olivecrona H, Tonnis W (eds). *Handbuch der Neurochirurgie*. Heidelberg: Springer-Verlag; 1967; IV: 1–301.

23. Svien HJ. Surgical experience with craniopharyngiomas. *J Neurosurg* 1965; 23: 148–55.

24. Krayenbühl H, Yasargil MC. Radiological anatomy and topography of the cerebral arteries. In: Vinken PH, Bruyn GW (eds). *Vascular Diseases of the Nervous System, Part I. Handbook of Clinical Neurology*, Vol. 2. Amsterdam: North-Holland; 1972: 65–101.

25. Lazorthes G. *Vascularisation et Circulation Cérébrales*. Paris: Masson; 1961: 14–30.

26. Pang D. Craniopharyngiomas. In: Deutsch M (ed.). *Management of Childhood Brain Tumors*. Norwell, MA: Kluwer Publishers; 1990: 285–307.

27. Kramer S, Southard M, Mansfield CM. Radiotherapy in the management of craniopharyngiomas: further experiences and late results. *Am J Roentgenol Radiat Ther Nucl Med* 1968; 103: 44–52.

28. Northfield DWC. *The Surgery of the Central Nervous System*. Oxford: Blackwell Publications; 1973: 179–83.

29. Bailey P, Buchanon DN, Bucy PC. *Intracranial Tumors of Infancy and Childhood*. Chicago, IL: University of Chicago Press; 1939: 361–8.

30. Cabezudo JM, Perez C, Vaguero J, DeSola GR, Bravo G. Pubertas praecox in craniopharyngioma. *J Neurosurg* 1981; 55: 127–31.

31. Zachmann M, Illig R. Precocious puberty after surgery for craniopharyngioma. *J Pediatr* 1979; 95: 86–8.

32. Fisher CM. Abulia minor vs. agitated behavior. *Clin Neurosurg* 1983; 31: 9–31.

33. Iversen SD, Koob GF. Behavioral implications of dopaminergic neurons in the mesolimbic system. *Adv Biochem Psychopharmacol* 1977; 16: 209–14.

34. Lindvall O, Bjorklund A. The organization of the ascending catecholamine neuron system in the rat brain. *Acta Physiol Scand* 1974; 412(suppl.): 1–49.

35. Banna M. Craniopharyngiomas in adults. *Surg Neurol* 1973; 1: 202–4.

36. Bartlett JR. Craniopharyngioma—an analysis of some aspects of symptomatology, radiology, and histology. *Brain* 1971; 94: 725–32.

37. Kahn EA, Cosby EC. Korsakoff's syndrome associated with surgical lesions involving the mamillary bodies. *Neurology* 1972; 22: 117–25.

38. Rougerie J, Fardeau M. *Les Craniopharyngiomes*. Paris: Masson et Cie; 1962.

39. Russel RW, Pennybacker JB. Craniopharyngiomas in the elderly. *J Neurol Psychiatr* 1961; 24: 1–13.

40. Shapiro K, Till K, Grant N. Craniopharyngioma in childhood. *J Neurosurg*. 1979; 50: 617–23.

41. Sweet WH. Radical surgical treatment of craniopharyngioma. *Clin Neurosurg* 1976; 23: 52–79.

42. Sweet WH. Recurrent craniopharyngiomas: therapeutic alternatives. *Clin Neurosurg* 1980; 27: 206–29.

43. Symon L, Sprich W. Radical excision of craniopharyngioma. *J Neurosurg* 1985; 62: 174–81.

44. Fahlbusch R, Honegger J, Paulus W, Huk W, Buchfelder M. Surgical treatment of craniopharyngiomas experience with 168 patients. *J Neurosurg* 1999; 90: 237–50.

45. Katz EL. Late results of radical excision of craniopharyngiomas in children. *J Neurosurg* 1975; 42: 86–90.

46. Matson DD, Crigler JF. Management of craniopharyngioma in childhood. *J Neurosurg* 1969; 30: 377–90.

47. Villani RM, Tomei G, Bello L, *et al*. Long-term results of treatment for craniopharyngioma in children. *Child Nerv Syst* 1997; 13: 397–405.

48. Raghavan R, Dicke Jr WT, Margraf LR, *et al*. Proliferative activity in craniopharyngiomas clinicopathological correlations in adults and children. *Surg Neurol* 2000; 54: 241–8.

49. Nishi T, Kuratsu JI, Takeshima H, Saito Y, Kochi M, Ushio Y. Prognostic significance of the MIB-1 labeling index for patient with craniopharyngioma. *Int J Mol Med* 1999; 3: 157–61.

50. Cabezudo JM, Vaguero J, Areitia E, Martinez R, DeSola RG, Bravo G. Craniopharyngiomas: a clinical approach to treatment. *J Neurosurg* 1981; 55: 371–5.

51. Kobayashi T, Kageyama N, Ohara K. Internal irradiation for cystic craniopharyngioma. *J Neurosurg* 1981; 55: 896–903.

52. Lichter AS, Wara WM, Sheline GE, Townsend JJ, Wilson CB. The treatment of craniopharyngiomas. *Int J Radiat Oncol Biol Phys* 1977; 2: 675–83.

53. Manaka S, Teramoto A, Takakura K. The efficacy of radiotherapy for craniopharyngiomas. *J Neurosurg* 1985; 62: 648–56.

54. McKissock W, Ford RK. Results of treatment of the craniopharyngiomas. *J Neurol Neurosurg Psychiatr* 1966; 29: 475 (Abstract).

55. Merchant TE, Kiehna EN, Sanford RA, *et al*. Craniopharyngioma: The St. Jude Children's Research Hospital Experience 1984–2001. *Int J Radiation Oncology Biol Phys* 2002; 53: 533–42.

56. Backlund EO. Studies on craniopharyngiomas, III: stereotaxis treatment with intracystic yttrium-90. *Acta Chir Scand* 1973; 139: 237–47.

57. Harris JR, Levene MB. Visual complications following irradiation for pituitary adenomas and craniopharyngiomas. *Radiology* 1976; 120: 167–71.

58. Martin AM, Johnston JS, Henry JM, Stoffel TJ, Di Chiro G. Delayed radiation necrosis of brain. *J Neurosurg* 1977; 47: 336–45.

59. Cavazzuti V, Fischer EG, Welch H, Belli JA, Winston KR. Neurological and psychophysiological sequelae following different treatment of craniopharyngioma in children. *J Neurosurg* 1983; 59: 409–17.

60. Chadduck WM, Roberts M. Long term survival with craniopharyngioma: report of patient in 29th year after treatment, seen for a second intracranial tumor. *J Neurosurg* 1966; 25: 312–14.

61. Waga S, Handa H. Radiation induced meningioma: with review of literature. *Surg Neurol* 1976; 5: 215–19.

62. Kranzinger M, Jones N, Rittinger O, *et al*. Malignant glioma as a secondary malignant neoplasm after radiation therapy for craniopharyngioma report of a case and review of reported cases. *Onkologie* 2001; 24: 66–72.

63. Hoff JT, Patterson RH. Craniopharyngiomas in children and adults. *J Neurosurg* 1972; 36: 299–302.

64. Sung DI, Chang CH, Harisiadis L, Carmel PW. Treatment results of craniopharyngiomas. *Cancer* 1981; 47: 847–52.

65. Backlund EO. Studies on craniopharyngiomas, IV: stereotaxis treatment with radiosurgery. *Acta Chir Scand* 1973; 139: 248–50.

66. Larrson B, Liden K, Sarby B. Techniques for irradiation of small intracranial structures through the intact skull. *Proceedings of the Ninth Symposium Neuroradiologium, Gothenburg*, April; 1979: 14–16.

67. Leksell L. *Stereotaxis and Radiosurgery*. Springfield, IL: Charles C Thomas Publisher; 1981: 1–69.

68. Leksell L, Backlund EO, Johansson L. Treatment of craniopharyngiomas. *Acta Chir Scand* 1967; 133: 345–50.

69. Rubin P, Casarett GW. *Clinical Radiation Pathology*. Philadelphia, PA: WB Saunders Co; 1968; 34–50.

70. Backlund EO. Stereotaxic treatment of craniopharyngioma. *Acta Neurochir Suppl* 1974; 21: 177–83.

71. Plowman PN, Wraith C, Royle N, Grossman AB. Stereotactic radiosurgery IX craniopharyngioma durable complete imaging responses and indications for treatment. *Br J Neurosurg* 1999; 13: 352–8.

72. Mokry M. Craniopharyngiomas a six year experience with gamma knife radiosurgery. *Stereotact Funct Neurosurg* 1999; 72 (suppl. 1): 140–9.

73. Chung WY, Pan DH, Shiau CY, Guo WY, Wang LW. Gamma knife radiosurgery for craniopharyngiomas. *J Neurosurg* 2000; 93 (suppl. 3): 47–56.

74. Backlund EO. Solid craniopharyngiomas treated by stereotactic radiosurgery. *INSERM Symposium (#12)* 1979; 340: 271–7.

75. Backlund EO. Studies on craniopharyngiomas, II: treatment by stereotaxis and radiosurgery. *Acta Chir Scand* 1973; 139: 225–36.

76. Backlund EO. Stereotactic treatment of craniopharyngiomas—15 years experience. *Presented at the 32nd Annual Meeting of the Scandinavian Neurosurgical Society;* September 5, 1980; Linkoping, Sweden. Abstract.

77. Ulfarsson E, Lindquist C, Roberts M, *et al*. Gamma knife radiosurgery for craniopharyngiomas: long-term results in the first Swedish patients. *J Neurosurg* 2002; 97(suppl. 5): 613–22.

78. Voges J, Sturm V, Lehrke R, Treuer H, Gauss C, Berthold F. Cystic craniopharyngioma: long-term results after intracavitary irradiation with stereotactically applied colloidal beta-emitting radioactive sources. *Neurosurgery* 1997; 40: 263–9; discussion 269–70.

79. Pollock BE, Lunsford LD, Kondziolka D, Levine G, Flickinger JC. Phosphorus-32 intracavitary irradiation of cystic craniopharyngiomas: current technique and long-term results. *Int J Radiat Oncol Biol Phys* 1995; 33: 437–46.

80. Yu X, Liu Zonghui, Li Shiyue. Combined treatment with stereotactic intracavitary irradiation and gamma knife surgery for craniopharyngiomas. *Stereotact Funct Neurosurg* 2000; 75: 117–22.

81. Chiou SM, Lunsford LD, Niranjan A, Kondziolka D, Flickinger JC. Stereotactic radiosurgery of residual or recurrent craniopharyngioma, after surgery, with or without radiation therapy. *Neuro-oncology* 2001; 3: 159–66.

82. Blackburn TPD, Doughty D, Plowman PN. Stereotactic intracavitary therapy of recurrent cystic craniopharyngioma by instillation of ^{90}yttrium. *Br J Neurosurg* 1999; 13: 359–65.

83. Mottolese C, Stan H, Hermier M, Berlier P, Convert J, Frappaz D, Lapras C. Intracystic chemotherapy with bleomycin in the treatment of craniopharyngiomas. *Child's Nerv Syst* 2001; 17: 724–30.

84. Hader WJ, Steinbok P, Hukin J, Fryer C. Intratumoral therapy with bleomycin for cystic craniopharyngiomas in children. *Pediatr Neurosurg* 2000; 33: 211–18.

85. Savas A, Arasil E, Batay F, Selcuki M, Kanpolat Y. Intracavitary chemotherapy of polycystic craniopharyngioma with bleomycin. *Acta Neurochir (Wien)* 1999; 141: 547–9.

86. Jackacki RI, Cohen BH, Jamison C, *et al*. Phase II evaluation of interferon-α-2a for progressive recurrent craniopharyngiomas. *J Neurosurg* 2000; 92: 255–60.

87. Lippens RJ, Rotteveel JJ, Otten BJ, Merx H. Chemotherapy with adriamycin (doxorubicin) and CCNU (lomustine) in four children with recurrent craniopharyngiomas. *Eur J Paediatr Neurol* 1998; 2: 263–8.

88. Kenny FM, Preeyasombat C, Migion CH. Cortisol production rate, II: normal infants, children, and adults. *Pediatrics* 1966; 37: 34–42.

89. Fischer EG, Welch K, Belli JA, *et al*. Treatment of craniopharyngioma in children. *J Neurosurg* 1985; 62: 496–501.

90. Carmel PW, Antunes JL, Ferrin M. Collection of blood from the pituitary stalk and portal veins in monkeys, and from the pituitary sinusoidal system of monkey and man. *J Neurosurg* 1979; 50: 75–80.

91. Long DM, Chou SN. Transcallosal removal of craniopharyngiomas within the third ventricle. *J Neurosurg* 1973; 39: 563–7.

92. Abrams LS, Repka MX. Visual outcome of craniopharyngioma in children. *J Pediatr Ophthalmol Strabismus* 1997; 34: 223–8.

93. Artero JMC, Crespo JV, Zabolgoita GB. Status of vision following surgical treatment of craniopharyngiomas. *Acta Neurochir (Wien)* 1984; 73: 165–77.

94. Honegger J, Buchfelder M, Fahlbusch R. Surgical treatment of craniopharyngiomas: endocrinological results. *J Neurosurg* 1999; 90: 251–7.

95. Lehrnbecher T, Muller-Scholden J, Danhauser-Leistner I, Sorensen N, von Stokhausen HB. Perioperative fluid and electrolyte management in children undergoing surgery for craniopharyngiomas. A 10 year experience in a single institution. *Childs Nerv Syst* 1998; 14: 276–9.

96. Shucart WA, Jackson I. Management of diabetes insipidus in neurosurgical patients. *J Neurosurg* 1976; 44: 65–70.

97. Antunes, JL, Carmel PW, Zimmerman EA, Ferin M. Regeneration of the magnocellular system of the rhesus monkey following hypothalamic lesions. *Ann Neurol*. 1979; 5: 462–9.

98. Glass RH. Infertility. In: Yen SSC, Jaffe RB (eds). *Reproductive Endocrinology: Physiology, Pathophysiology and Clinical Management*. Philadelphia, PA: WB Saunders Co; 1978: 398–417.

99. Price DA, Wilton P, Jonsson P, Albertsson-Wikland K. Growth hormone treatment in children with prior craniopharyngioma: an analysis of Pharmacia and Upjohn International Growth Database (KIGS) from 1988 to 1996. *Horm Res* 1998; 49: 97.

100. Ayral D, Talot L, David M, Lecornu M, François R. Etude de la croissance paradoxale de certains enfants après chirurgie hypothalamo-hypophysaire en dépit de l'absence d'hormone de croissance. *Pediatrie* 1980; 35: 389–401.

101. Costin G, Hogut MD, Philips LS, Daughaday WH. Craniopharyngioma: the rate of insulin in promoting postoperative growth. *J Clin Endocrinol Metab* 1976; 42: 370–9.

102. Finkelstein JW, Kream J, Ludan A, Hellman L. Sulfation factor (somatomedin): an explanation for continued growth in the absence of immunoassayable growth hormone in patients with hypothalamic tumor. *J Clin Endocrinol Metab* 1972; 35: 13–37.

103. Job JC, Lambertz J, Sizonenko PC, Rossier A. La croissance des enfants atteints de craniopharyngiome: vitesse de croissance et resultats des dosages d'hormone de croissance dans le plasma avant et après intervention chirurgicale. *Arch Fr Pediatr* 1970; 27: 341–53.

104. Thomsen MJ, Conte FA, Kaplan SK, Grumbach MM. Endocrine and neurological outcome in childhood craniopharyngioma: a review of the effect of treatment in 42 patients. *J Pediatr* 1980; 97: 728–35.

105. Bucher H, Zapf J, Torresani T, Prader A, Froesch ER, Illig R. Insulin-like growth factors I and II, prolactin, and insulin in 19 growth hormone-deficient children with excessive, normal, and decreased longitudinal growth after operation for craniopharyngioma. *N Engl J Med* 1983; 309: 1142–6.

106. Hogeveen M, Noordam C, Otten B, Wit JM, Massa G. Growth before and during growth hormone treatment in children operated for craniopharyngioma. *Horm Res* 1997; 28: 258–62.

107. Pang D. Surgical management of craniopharyngioma. In: Sekhar LN, Janecka IP (eds). *Surgery of Cranial Base Tumors*. New York, NY: Raven Press; 1993: 787–807.

108. Pinto G, Bussières L, Recasens C, Souberbielle JC, Zerah M, Brauner R. Hormonal factors influencing weight and growth patterns in craniopharyngioma. *Horm Res* 2000; 53: 163–9.

109. Tiulpakov An, Mazerkina NA, Brook CG, Hindmarsh PC, Peterkova VA, Gorelyshev SK. Growth in children with craniopharyngioma following surgery. *Clin Endocrinol (Oxf)* 1998; 49: 733–8.

110. Carpentieri SC, Waber DP, Scott RM, et al. Memory deficits among children with craniopharyngiomas. *Neurosurgery* 2001; 49: 1053–8.

111. Donnet A, Schmitt A, Dufour H, Grisoli F. Neuropsychological follow-up of twenty two adult patients after surgery for craniopharyngioma. *Acta Neurochir (Wien)* 1999; 141: 1049–54.

112. Honegger J, Barocka A, Sadri B, Fahlbusch R. Neuropsychological results of craniopharyngioma surgery in adults: a prospective study. *J Neurosurg* 1998; 50: 19–29.

113. Duff JM, Meyer FB, Ilstrup DM, Laws Jr ER, Schleck CD, Scheithauer BW. Long-term outcomes for surgically resected craniopharyngiomas. *Neurosurgery* 2000; 46: 291–305.

114. Muller HL, Bueb K, Bartels U, et al. Obesity after childhood craniopharyngioma – German multicenter study on pre-operative risk factors and quality of life. *Klin Pädiatr* 2001; 213: 244–49.

115. DeVile CJ, Grant DB, Hayward RD, Kendall BE, Neville BGR, Stanhop R. Obesity in childhood craniopharyngioma: relation to post-operative hypothalamic damage shown by magnetic resonance imaging. *J Clin Endocrinol Metab* 1996; 81: 2734–7.

116. Roth C, Wilken B, Hanefeld F, Schroter W, Leonhardt U. Hyperphagia in children with craniopharyngioma is associated with hyperleptinaemia and a failure in the downregulation of appetite. *Eur J Endocrinol* 1998; 138: 89–91.

117. Brabant G, Horn R, Mayr B, von zur Muhlen A, Honegger J, Buchfelder M. Serum leptin levels following hypothalamic surgery. *Horm Metab Res* 1996; 28: 728–31.

118. York D, Bray GA. Dependence of hynothalamic obesity on insulin, the pituitary and the adrenal gland. *Endocrinology* 1972; 90: 885–94.

119. Jeanrenaud B. Hyperinsulinemia in obesity syndromes: Its metabolic consequences and possible etiology. *Metabolism* 1978; 27: 1881–92.

120. Lustig RN, Rose SR, Bughen GA, et al. Hypothalamic obesity caused by cranial insult in children: altered glucose and insulin dynamics and reversal by a somatostatin agonist. *J Pediatr* 1999; 135(pt 1):162–8.

121. Inouc S, Gray G. An autonomic hypothesis for hypothalamic obesity. *Life Sci* 1979; 25: 561–6.

122. Jeanrenaud B. An hypothesis on the acitology of obesity: dysfunction of the central nervous system as a primary cause. *Diabetologia* 1985; 28: 502–13.

123. Mason PW, Krawiecki N, Meacham LR. The use of dextroamphetamine to treat obesity and hyperphagia in children treated for craniopharyngioma. *Arch Pediatr Adolesc Med* 2002; 156: 887–92.

124. Ungerstedt U. Stereotaxic mapping of the dopamine pathways in the rat brain. *Acta Physiol Scand* 1971; 367(suppl.): 1–48.

125. Coffey RJ, Lunsford LD. Stereotactic radiosurgery using the 201 cobalt-60 source gamma knife. *Neurosurg Clin North Am* 1990; 1: 955–90.

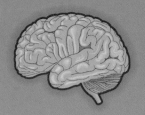

TUMORS AND CYSTS OF THE THIRD VENTRICLE

40

Georg Fries and Axel Perneczky

Tumors and cysts of the third ventricle present a therapeutic challenge to the neurosurgeon as a result of their deep-seated location adjacent to sensitive neural structures and cerebrospinal fluid (CSF) pathways. Most of these lesions are histopathologically benign. Table 40.1 summarizes a 10-year series of third ventricle tumors and cysts operated on in our neurosurgical department; about 90% of third ventricular lesions are benign and only 10% are malignant. Nevertheless, in both benign and malignant lesions, their special location within the third ventricle may cause acute and severe neurologic deterioration, including sudden death from increased intracranial pressure following obstruction of the CSF pathways. CSF flow may be obstructed through one or both foraminae of Monro, or through the aqueduct of Sylvius, which may result in acute unilateral, bilateral, or triventricular hydrocephalus. Such a threatening situation can even occur with small third ventricular lesions. Therefore, timely

and accurate diagnostic imaging regarding the lesions of the third ventricle and adequate surgical treatment are mandatory for virtually all of these lesions, independent of whether they are tumors or cysts.

PATHOLOGY

Tumors

Various tumors can appear in the third ventricle. The walls, contents and surrounding structures of the third ventricle arise from a multitude of different anatomical regions, with variable histological origins. The roof of the third ventricle contains part of the choroid plexus, from which plexus papillomas or plexus carcinomas may arise. Pineal tumors (see Chapter 33), such as pineocytomas or pineoblastomas, arise primarily from the posterior part of the third ventricle and can easily cause obstruction of the aqueduct of Sylvius. Astrocytomas, ependymomas, subependymomas and central neurocytomas may grow from the walls of the third ventricle and obstruct the flow of CSF. Metastatic tumors from lung, breast and gastrointestinal cancers (see Chapter 31) may migrate to the walls of the third ventricle. It is common to all of these lesions that they form a space-occupying pathology within a relatively small space. Thus, tumor invasion or compression of sensitive neural or endocrine structures such as the optic chiasm, fornix, thalamus, hypothalamus, pituitary stalk, or brainstem may occur at an early stage of the disease.[1–4]

In addition to mass lesions growing directly within the third ventricle or invading its walls, several tumors, such as craniopharyngiomas, pituitary adenomas, meningiomas, chordomas, or other cranium-base tumors, may affect the third ventricle from the "outside" (Figure 40.1). In general, these tumors arise from sellar or parasellar skull-base structures and extend upward through the floor of the third ventricle into its cavity. Following destruction of the floor of the third ventricle, these tumors may cause neurologic and endocrine impairment as well as acute hydrocephalus by obstructing the aqueduct of Sylvius or the intraventricular foramen of Monro.[5]

Colloid cysts

Colloid cysts of the third ventricle are located anteriorly at the level of the foramen of Monro in the coronal plane. Colloid cysts may be attached to the roof or floor of the third ventricle, the columns of the fornix, or the choroid plexus. The size of colloid cysts may range from a few millimeters to several centimeters

Lesion	Benign	Malignant	Total
Cysts	**53**	**–**	**53**
Arachnoid cysts	22	–	22
Colloid cysts	19	–	19
Choroid plexus cysts	5	–	5
Cysts of unknown origin	7	–	7
Tumors	**71**	**14**	**85**
Craniopharyngeoma	25	–	25
Astrocytoma	10	3	13
Pituitary adenoma	8	–	8
Ependymoma	5	2	7
Germinoma	6	–	6
Pineocytoma	5	–	5
Metastasis	–	5	5
Meningioma	3	–	3
Plexuspapilloma	3	–	3
Subependymoma	2	–	2
Central neurocytoma	2	–	2
Plexus carcinoma	–	1	1
Oligodendroglioma	1	–	1
Teratoma	–	1	1
Glioblastoma	–	1	1
Tuberous sclerosis	1	–	1
Pineoblastoma	–	1	1

Table 40.1 Surgical series demonstrating the frequency and status of third ventricular lesions

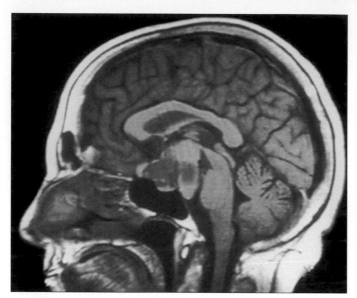

Figure 40.1 Sagittal T1-weighted MRI showing a large craniopharyngioma extending into the third ventricle.

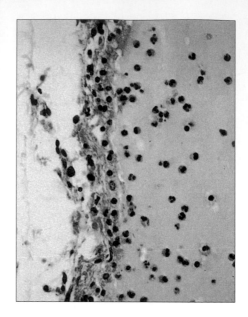

Figure 40.3 Photomicrograph of a colloid cyst demonstrating a fine fibrous capsule, epithelial layer and amorphous contents. Sparse cellular debris is seen within the central portion.

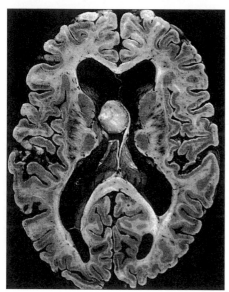

Figure 40.2 Gross transverse pathological specimen demonstrating a 2.5-cm colloid cyst in its characteristic position at the level of the foramen of Monro. Note the diffuse enlargement of lateral ventricles.

(Figure 40.2). With refinements in diagnostic imaging and increased accessibility of this imaging, the number of incidentally diagnosed small, asymptomatic colloid cysts is constantly increasing.[6] Histologically, the cysts demonstrate either a single layer of pseudostratified columnar epithelium, with or without cilia, or cuboidal low columnar epithelium.[7] Mucous goblet cells are commonly found, with a mucin-positive mucicarmine on periodic acid–Schiff staining. The epithelium and the fibrous capsule surrounding it together form the wall of the cyst; the amorphous material that comprises the content of the cyst is believed to be a result of cellular discharge of mucin and cellular desquamation (Figure 40.3). The consistency of the cyst contents varies considerably among individual cysts, from liquid to viscous, semisolid or solid. This observation is important when considering various strategies for surgical treatment.[1,6,8–17]

Suprasellar arachnoid cysts

Suprasellar arachnoid cysts become symptomatic when they obstruct CSF flow through the foraminae of Munro or the third ventricle. It is believed that suprasellar arachnoid cysts arise from arachnoid duplications at the level of the membrane of Liljequist.[18–20] Suprasellar arachnoid cysts can reach an enormous size before becoming symptomatic (Figure 40.4). The enlarging arachnoid cyst may extend from the floor or walls of the third ventricle and subsequently occlude the foraminae of Munro, the aqueduct of Sylvius, or both. This can cause chronic or acute hydrocephalus with increased intracranial pressure not only through obstruction of CSF flow but also secondary to compression from the enlarging arachnoid cyst. CSF similar to that found in the ventricles comprises the contents of arachnoid cysts. Histologically, the walls of arachnoid cysts consist of sparsely vascularized layers of arachnoid membrane often enmeshed with additional fibrotic tissue that forms gradually over time. This additional fibrotic tissue frequently affects the surgical manipulation of arachnoid cysts. During surgery, suprasellar arachnoid cyst walls may be seen and these can feel quite firm.

DIAGNOSTIC IMAGING

Historically, pneumencephalography was important for the diagnosis of tumors and cysts of the third ventricle. Today, noninvasive imaging techniques such as computed tomography (CT) and magnetic resonance imaging (MRI) form the basis for diagnoses of tumors and cysts of the third ventricle.[21–28] Both imaging modalities provide information regarding the presence or absence of ventriculomegaly and hydrocephalus (Figures 40.5 and 40.6). On CT, colloid cysts appear as round or oval lesions in the anterior and superior areas of the third ventricle at the level of the foramen of Monro. The attenuation coefficient relative to brain tissue may range from hypodense to hyperdense. Usually, there is no, or minimum, contrast enhancement in the wall of the colloid cysts.

MRI may provide important additional information and thus reduce the differential diagnosis among tumors and colloid cysts

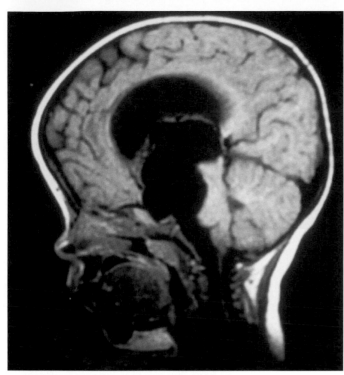

Figure 40.4 Sagittal T1-weighted MRI demonstrating a suprasellar arachnoid cyst extending into the third ventricle.

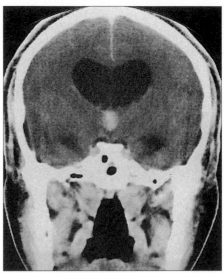

Figure 40.6 Coronal CT scan of a hyperdense colloid cyst producing symmetrical enlargement of the lateral ventricles including the temporal horns.

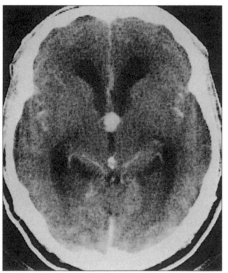

Figure 40.5 Axial CT scan showing a hyperdense colloid cyst at the level of the foramen of Monro, which is characteristic of this lesion. Note the temporal horns of the lateral ventricles are enlarged, indicating obstructive hydrocephalus.

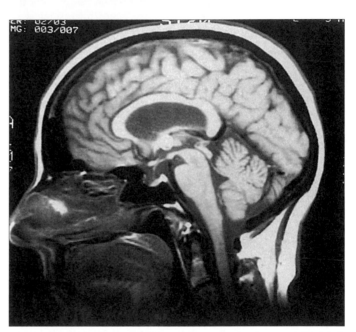

Figure 40.7 Sagittal T1-weighted MRI demonstrating increased T1 signal from a colloid cyst in the anterior third ventricle.

of the third ventricle before treatment. Characteristically, colloid cysts appear as hyperintense round lesions on T1-weighted images (Figure 40.7). Because multiplanar imaging is possible with MRI, the location and relationship of the lesion to the surrounding anatomical structures is best ascertained with these studies. MRI provides information on both the suspected histology and the exact topographical relation of the pathology to the neighboring anatomical structures. Therefore, preoperative surgical planning becomes an important step in the microsurgical treatment of patients with lesions of the third ventricle. In addition, flow-sensitive T2-weighted MRI studies provide important information about CSF flow. Noninvasive MR-angiography may replace invasive conventional angiography in many patients with tumors and

cysts of the third ventricle.[29,30] Today, conventional angiography is indicated only for large third ventricular tumors involving the cranial base or the large cerebral veins close to the third ventricle. It is not needed for surgical planning in patients with colloid cysts, arachnoid cysts, or small tumors.

PATIENT MANAGEMENT

The correct diagnosis and treatment of tumors and cysts of the third ventricle depends on careful integration of history, neurologic examination and imaging studies. A profound medical history and detailed neurologic examination is imperative, because signs of increased intracranial pressure, such as intermittent headache, change in mental status, disturbed vision, and pathologic fundoscopy with papilledema, warrant close attention.

As a result of refined microsurgical and endoscopic operative techniques which substantially reduce surgical trauma, the general tendency in neurosurgery is to recommend surgical intervention to those patients with clinical signs and symptoms and to those with incidental, asymptomatic tumors and cysts of the third ventricle.[4] Sudden death and severe neurologic deterioration as a result of acute hydrocephalus with increased intracranial pressure has been reported quite frequently, even with small third ventricular tumors and cysts.[2,4] Therefore, close follow-up and observation of asymptomatic third ventricular lesions is useful only for multi-morbid patients in poor general condition. All other patients should undergo surgical treatment, after careful surgical planning, as soon as possible.

SURGICAL TREATMENT

Endoscopic third ventriculostomy, pellucidotomy, and shunting procedures

Patients with hydrocephalic dilation of the lateral ventricles or the third ventricle, who are not eligible for acute microsurgical or endoscopic removal of their third ventricular lesion, may require immediate diversion of CSF for stabilization until a definite operation is performed. The easiest way to acquire CSF diversion is unilateral or bilateral external drainage of the lateral ventricles. Unilateral drainge carries the risk of progressing ventricular dilation of the contralateral ventricle. To prevent contralateral ventricular dilation causing further neurologic deterioration and decerebration from midline shift with a unilateral ventricular tap, endoscopic pellucidotomy can be performed. This simple technique is applied as follows: after puncture of the lateral ventricle, the septum pellucidum can be opened endoscopically between the frontal horns of the lateral ventricles to achieve a good CSF communication between both lateral ventricles.[31]

Patients with triventricular hydrocephalus caused by a cyst or tumor in the posterior part of the third ventricle occluding the aqueduct of Sylvius may be treated best with an endoscopic third ventriculostomy.[31,32] In general, endoscopic third ventriculostomy can be performed as a free-hand procedure; usually, the frontal horn of the lateral ventricle, the foramen of Monro, and the third ventricle are wide enough to navigate down to the pars membranacea of the tuber cinereum. The external landmark on the skull for burr hole trephination is the coronary suture, about 2–2.5 cm from midline. The exact position of the burr hole can be easily determined using coronary and sagittal MRI scans, with a straight line drawn from the imaginary burr hole through the foramen of Monro down to the stoma area at the floor of the third ventricle (Figure 40.8). Following trephination and opening of the dura, the frontal horn of the lateral ventricle is punctured with a Cushing needle. After withdrawal of the needle, the same trajectory is passed with the endoscope, which is navigated through the foramen of Monro, leaving the choroid plexus, thalamostriate vein, septal vein, fornix and caudate nucleus untouched. The endoscope is then fixed in the third ventricle, where in between the infundibular recess rostrally and the mamillary bodies caudally, the thinned-out floor of the third ventricle is transparent enough to give view to the basilar tip, the P1-segments of the posterior cerebral arteries, the posterior communicating arteries, the superior cerebellar arteries, the prepontine cistern, and the dorsum sellae. The stoma is created midway between the infundibular recess and the mamillary bodies anterior to the basilar tip. In most patients, the stoma is performed with a Fogarty

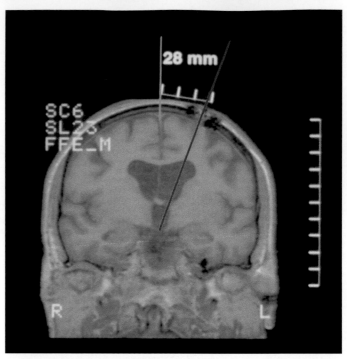

Figure 40.8 Determination of the burr hole position for endoscopic third ventriculostomy using a trajectory from the floor of the third ventricle through the foramen of Monro to the skull surface.

balloon catheter. The tip of the catheter is punctured through the third ventricle floor, and the small stoma is dilated with the inflated balloon. After the stoma has been created, the prepontine cistern in between the basilar trunk and the clivus is inspected to exclude further arachnoid membranes, which sometimes impair the CSF flow through the stoma. If such membranes exist, they are opened in the same fashion with the balloon catheter.

In patients with tumors or cysts in the anterior part of the third ventricle, endoscopic third ventriculostomy cannot be performed because the lesion obscures the endoscopic view towards the floor of the third ventricle.

Although still controversial, definitive implantation of ventriculo-atrial or ventriculo-peritoneal shunts for CSF diversion in patients with third ventricular lesions is indicated only for well-defined cases of hydrocephalus. Such situations may be caused by inflammatory or posthemorrhagic impairment of CSF resorption or by carcinomatous meningitis.

Endoscopic fenestration of suprasellar arachnoid cysts

Endoscopic fenestration is the ideal treatment for suprasellar arachnoid cysts extending into the third ventricle and causing occlusive hydrocephalus.[19,20] This minimally invasive procedure can be performed through a precoronal suture burr hole. The endoscope trocar, with channels for irrigation and instruments, is introduced transcortically into the frontal horn of the lateral ventricle. In most cases, the suprasellar arachnoid cyst is already visible through the enlarged and extremely widened foramen of Monro. The rostral part of the slightly vascularized, yet tough, cyst membrane is shrunk by coagulation with a bipolar electrode. This manipulation usually reduces the size of the cyst so that CSF flow through the foramen of Monro and into the aqueduct becomes possible. The rostral cyst membrane is then fenestrated widely under endoscopic control, so that the cyst becomes deflated. The endoscope is advanced further through the cyst towards the prepontine cistern, where the caudal part of the cyst membrane is also fenestrated. This method prevents recurrent obstruction by the cyst and supports free CSF flow from the third ventricle and the cyst into the basal cisterns.

Endoscopic and stereotactic tumor biopsies

Biopsies can determine whether microsurgical removal, radiation, chemotherapy, or a combination of these modalities is performed to treat tumors of the third ventricle. In patients with a dilated ventricular system, endoscopic biopsies are possible. For this purpose, the endoscope is introduced through a precoronal suture burr-hole into the frontal horn of the lateral ventricle and is advanced through the foramen of Monro. In patients with a small ventricular system it may be necessary to combine the endoscopic technique with frame-based or frameless stereotactic determination of the entry point, the trajectory, and the target area from where the biopsy material will be taken.

Aspiration techniques for colloid cysts

Several modalities have been reported in the aspiration of colloid cysts. Gutierrez-Lara et al.[33] reported on the free-hand aspiration of a colloid cyst. Bosch et al.,[14] in 1978, reported on the successful application of stereotactic methods for colloid cyst aspiration. In 1983, Powell et al.[34] advocated ventriculoscopy for the aspiration of colloid cysts. The simplicity of aspiration has a certain appeal;[15,35] however, there are definite disadvantages. First, the content of colloid cysts is of variable consistency and is mostly viscous, semisolid, or solid. In such cases, aspiration, whether free-hand, stereotactically guided, or endoscopic, would fail. Second, when aspiration is performed, it often remains incomplete, and recurrences are documented.[16] Third, contents spilled into the ventricular system during aspiration have been associated with ventriculitis and aqueductal stenosis.[5,36] Finally, as the surface of most colloid cysts is vascularized and attached to the choroid plexus or the cerebral veins, aspiration may induce hemorrhage, which cannot easily be controlled through a small aspiration device. For these reasons, simple aspiration of colloid cysts cannot be recommended as a routine procedure.

Microsurgical removal

Although endoscopic fenestration is the definitive treatment for suprasellar arachnoid cysts, complete removal of tumors and colloid cysts of the third ventricle through a well-planned microsurgical approach should be applied whenever feasible.[37] Generally, the microsurgical manipulation of the tumor or colloid cyst comprises three stages. First, after exposure of the tumor or cyst, its surface is coagulated. Second, the tumor or cyst is opened, and the content is debulked. Third, after collapse of the lesion, its walls are removed from the surrounding structures.

Depending on the size and the precise location of the lesion within the third ventricle, which determines the individual direction from where to approach, the most atraumatic microsurgical route should be chosen.[38] Today, a number of microsurgical approaches are well-described (e.g. the transcortical, transventricular approach through the frontal lobe, either from an ipsilateral or from a contralateral craniotomy; the transcallosal

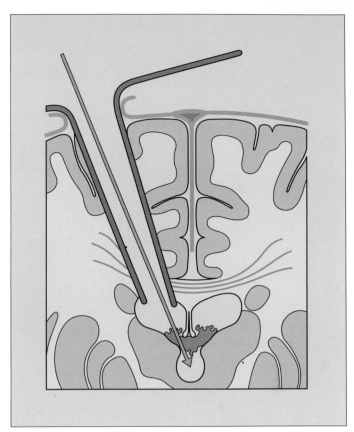

Figure 40.9 Schematic drawing of the transcortical transventricular approach to the anterior part of the third ventricle.

approach, either through the foramen of Monro or via para- or interforniceal entries; the subfrontal trans-lamina terminalis approach, either through a frontolateral supraorbital craniotomy or through a frontomedial parasagittal craniotomy; and the infratentorial supracerebellar approach from a posterior direction).

Transcortical approach

Most colloid cysts, tumors in the level of the foramen of Monro, or tumors arising from the lateral walls or the floor of the third ventricle can be removed microsurgically through the transcortical transventricular approach (Figure 40.9).[39] Anterior third ventricular lesions are approached via a precoronal suture craniotomy, whereas posterior lesions are treated from a more frontal craniotomy (Figure 40.10). Dandy, in 1930, using macrosurgery, had to resect a part of the frontal lobe for this approach.[8] Today, this has been substantially refined, using a 10–15-mm longitudinal cortical incision, which can be carried out in a transgyral or, if applicable, in a trans-sulcal fashion. In large tumors or colloid cysts, an ipsilateral approach can be performed (i.e. the approach is carried out on the side of the largest extent of the lesion); however, because of the straight working axis under the microscope, medium-sized or small tumors arising from the lateral wall of the third ventricle are usually eligible for contralateral removal.[39,40] (For example, a left-sided tumor is best removed through a right transcortical approach via the right foramen of Monro.)

The transcortical transventricular approach is ideal when the ventricles are dilated, but this approach can also be applied in patients with normally sized ventricles.

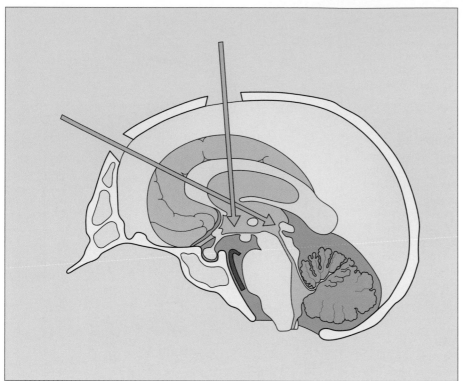

Figure 40.10 Schematic drawing of two variations of the transcortical transventricular approach. Lesions of the anterior part of the third ventricle are best approached from a precoronary craniotomy, those of the medium and posterior part require a more frontal craniotomy.

Transcallosal approach

The transcallosal approach to the third ventricle is applied in the absence of hydrocephalic dilation of the ventricles, because relatively atraumatic access between the frontal lobe and the falx is achieved with this approach.[11,41,42] The relative disadvantages are that it is somewhat more demanding technically, and injury may occur to related vascular structures such as the superior sagittal sinus, parasagittal bridging veins, and the anterior cerebral arteries. The incision in the corpus callosum should be no more than 20–25 mm to prevent disconnection symptoms. Once the corpus callosum has been divided, one of two trajectories may be taken. The first is to deviate to either side, enter the lateral ventricle, and then approach the tumor or colloid cyst through the foramen of Monro.[42] This is called the paraforniceal variation (Figure 40.11). The second is to proceed in the midline and use the interforniceal entry[11] (Figure 40.12). The advantage to the latter method is that lesions too large to be delivered through the foramen of Monro, or those located in the medium or posterior part of the third ventricle, may be removed more easily. The disadvantage is that bilateral injury to the fornix may occur, which can lead to severe recent memory deficit.[43]

To leave both fornices intact, alternative methods to enlarge the foramen of Monro posteriorly can be applied. One is to use the subchoroidal exposure of the mid-third ventricle according to Lavyne and Patterson,[13] the other is to use the transchoroidal exposure (Figure 40.13) described by Wen et al.[44] The disadvantage of both techniques is that the thalamostriate vein and the internal cerebral vein may be affected. Nevertheless, both strategies are well accepted and may be used alternatively, depending on the individual anatomic situation.

Frontal trans-lamina terminalis approach

Subfrontal or frontal paramedian interhemispheric trans-lamina terminalis approaches[45] (Figure 40.14) are applicable for small

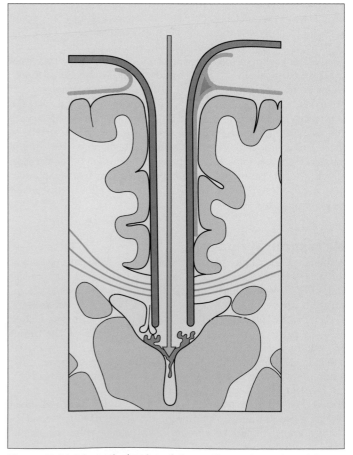

Figure 40.11 Schematic drawing of the paraforniceal variation of the transcallosal approach to the third ventricle.

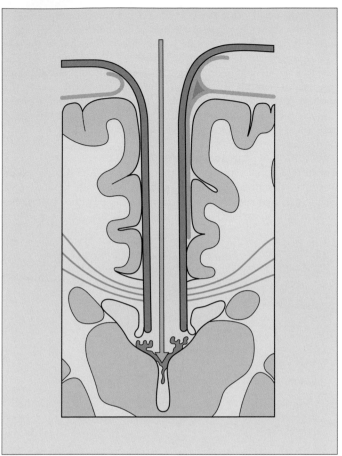

Figure 40.12 Schematic drawing of the interforniceal variation of the transcallosal approach to the third ventricle.

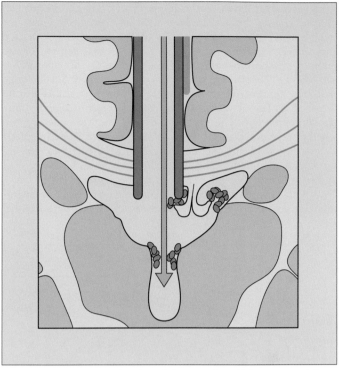

Figure 40.13 Schematic drawing of the transchoroidal exposure of the medium and posterior part of the third ventricle.

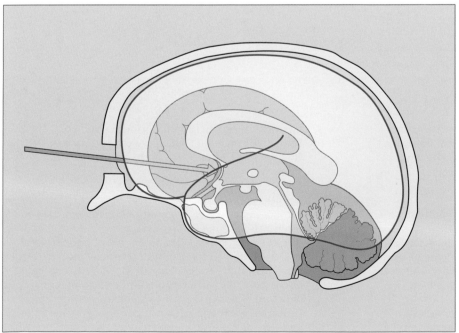

Figure 40.14 Schematic drawing of the frontal trans-lamina terminalis approach to the third ventricle, either from a paramedian interhemispheric or from a more lateral supraorbital direction.

third ventricular lesions in the anterior part of the third ventricle, especially those located in the suprachiasmatic recess, and for small lesions at the posterior roof of the third ventricle. With such approaches, sometimes anterior or posterior enlargement of the foramen of Monro, which might be necessary in other approaches and which might damage the fornix, can be avoided. Several large skull-base tumors extending into the third ventricle can also be removed via lateral subfrontal or frontal paramedian interhemispheric approaches. The exact location of the lesion determines whether a paramedian interhemispheric or more laterally placed supraorbital or pterional craniotomy will give the best access.

A kind of supraorbital subfrontal approach was first described by Fedor Krause in 1908.[46] Krause created a rather large craniotomy with a combined skin, periosteum and bone flap. This supraorbital approach provides a convenient access to the supratentorial base of the brain without too much retraction of the brain.[47]

The modern supraorbital subfrontal key-hole craniotomy, with a diameter of about 20 mm, is the latest variation of the old Krause approach. It is described in detail elsewhere.[39,48,49] The essence of this key-hole approach, which basically encompasses the frontal part of the classical pterional approach, is that the anterior part of the temporal lobe obscures access to most of the supratentorial parts of the brain base, especially to the important suprasellar space, including the third ventricle.

Infratentorial supracerebellar approach

The infratentorial supracerebellar approach (Figure 40.15), which was first described by Stein in 1971,[50] is one of the most frequently used approaches to lesions of the posterior part of the third ventricle, especially for pineal tumors (see Chapter 33). It

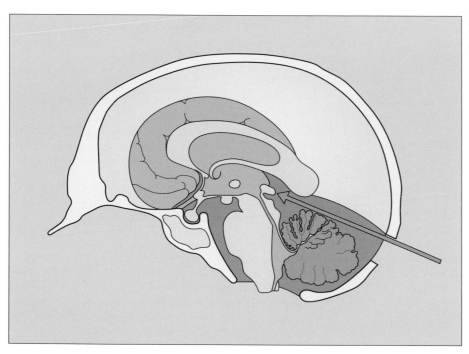

Figure 40.15 Schematic drawing of the infratentorial supracerebellar approach to the posterior part of the third ventricle.

CLINICAL PEARLS

- Tumors and cysts of the third ventricle are located near important neural structures and CSF pathways, which makes the surgical approach challenging. However, most, but not all, of the lesions in this location are pathologically benign.

- Mass lesions in the third ventricle often present with symptoms related to increased intracranial pressure as a result of obstruction of CSF pathways. Acute and severe neurological deterioration can occur because of obstructive hydrocephalus; therefore, surgical removal of these lesions is often recommended.

- Cranial MRI is the best way to diagnose these lesions. Careful neurological assessment is important to define the deficits prior to surgery. Surgical management of the hydrocephalus includes endoscopic third ventriculostomy or CSF diversion by shunting. If both foraminae of Munro are obstructed a biventricular shunt will be required.

- Surgical approaches for removal of third ventricular tumors and cysts include endoscopic biopsy/fenestration/removal, as well as standard microsurgical approaches. The three main microsurgical routes to the anterior third ventricle include the transcortical, trancallosal and trans-lamina terminalis approaches. All three require entry through a neural structure to access the third ventricle from the lateral ventricles. Each approach has its specific advantages and risks and must be applied in a case-by-case basis.

can be carried out in a sitting or a prone position. Ideally, the infratentorial supraorbital approach is applied when the tentorium is not too steep. Otherwise, the upper cerebellar vermis may obscure vision towards the cisterna veli interpositi and the posterior part of the third ventricle, unless substantial compression from the mass lesion has forced the cerebellum to move more caudal. The demanding points of the infratentorial supracerebellar approach are the venous structures, like the sinus confluens, the superior cerebellar bridging veins to the straight sinus, the vein of Galen, and the internal cerebral veins; however, the advantage is that the vein of Galen can be exposed from below, and both internal cerebral veins can be kept intact, even when large pineal tumors have to be removed.

This chapter contains material from the first edition, and we are grateful to the authors of that chapter for their contribution.

REFERENCES

1. Stookey B. Intermittent obstruction of the foramen of Monro by neuroepithelial cysts of the third ventricle: symptoms, diagnosis and treatment. *Bull Neurol Inst NY* 1934; 3: 446–500.
2. Chan RC, Thompson GB. Third ventricular colloid cysts presenting with acute neurological deterioration. *Surg Neurol* 1983; 19: 358–62.
3. Weisz RR, Faxal M. Colloid cyst of the third ventricle: a neurological emergency. *Ann Emerg Med* 1983; 12: 783–5.
4. Ryder JW, Kleinschmidt-DeMasters BK, Keller TS. Sudden deterioration and death in patients with benign tumors of the third ventricle area. *J Neurosurg* 1986; 64: 216–23.
5. Brun A, Egund N. The pathogenesis of cerebral symptoms in colloid cysts of the third ventricle: a clinical and pathoanatomical study. *Acta Neurol Scand* 1973; 49: 525–35.
6. Camacho A, Abernathey CD, Kelly PJ, et al. Colloid cysts: experience with the management of 84 cases since the introduction of computed tomography. *Neurosurgery* 1989; 24: 693–700.
7. Leech RW, Freeman T, Johnson R. Colloid cyst of the third ventricle: a scanning and transmission electron microscopic study. *J Neurosurg* 1982; 57: 108–13.
8. Dandy WE. *Benign Tumors of the Third Ventricle. Diagnosis and Treatment*. Springfield, IL: Charles C Thomas Publisher; 1933.
9. Little JR, MacCarty CS. Colloid cysts of the third ventricle. *J Neurosurg* 1974; 40: 230–5.
10. Shucart WA, Stein BM. Transcallosal approach to the anterior ventricular system. *Neurosurgery* 1978; 3: 339–43.
11. Apuzzo MLJ, Gianotta SL. Transcallosal interforniceal approach. In: Apuzzo MLJ (ed.). *Surgery of the Third Ventricle*. Baltimore, MD: Williams & Wilkins; 1987: 354–80.
12. Hirsch JF, Zouaoui A, Renier D, et al. A new surgical approach to the third ventricle with interruption of the striothalamic vein. *Acta Neurochir* 1979; 47: 135–47.
13. Lavyne MH, Patterson RH. Subchoroidal transvelum interpositum approach to mid-third ventricular tumors. *Neurosurgery* 1983; 12: 86–94.
14. Bosch DA, Rahn T, Backlund EO. Treatment of colloid cysts of third ventricle by stereotactic aspiration. *Surg Neurol* 1978; 9: 15–18.
15. Mohadjer M, Teshmar E, Mundinger F. CT-stereotaxic drainage of colloid cysts in the foramen of Monro and the third ventricle. *J Neurosurg* 1987; 67: 220–3.
16. Donauer E, Moringlane JR, Ostertag CB. Colloid cysts of the third ventricle. *Acta Neurochir (Wien)* 1986; 83: 24–30.
17. Abernathey CD, Kelly PJ, Davis DH. Treatment of colloid cysts of the third ventricle by stereotactic microsurgical laser craniotomy. *J Neurosurg* 1989; 70: 525–9.
18. Raimondi AJ, Shimoji T, Gutierrez FA. Suprasellar arachnoid cysts: surgical treatment and results. *Childs Brain* 1980; 7: 57–72.
19. Santamarta D, Aguas J, Ferrer E. The natural history of arachnoid cysts: endoscopic and cine-mode MRI evidence of a slit-valve mechanism. *Minim Invas Neurosurg* 1995; 38: 133–7.
20. Schroeder HWS, Gaab MR, Niendorf WR. Neuroendoscopic approach to arachnoid cysts. *J Neurosurg* 1996; 85: 293–8.
21. Boor S, Resch KDM, Perneczky A, et al. Virtual endoscopy (VE) of the basal cisterns: its value in planning the neurosurgical approach. *Minim Invas Neurosurg* 1998; 41: 177–82.
22. Helseth A. The incidence of primary central nervous system neoplasms before and after computerized tomography availability. *J Neurosurg* 1995; 83: 999–1003.
23. Kalender W, Vock P, Seissler W. Spiral CT scanning for fast and continuous volume data acquisition. In: Fuchs W (ed.). *Advances in CT*. Berlin, New York: Springer; 1990: 55–64.
24. Kendall B, Reider-Grosswasser I, Valentine A. Diagnosis of masses presenting with the ventricles on computed tomography. *Neuroradiology* 1983; 25: 11–22.
25. Sartor K. MR *Imaging of the Skull and Brain. A Correlative Text–Atlas*. Berlin: Springer; 1992.
26. Tsuchiya K, Hachiya Y, Mizutani Y, et al. Three-dimensional helical CT angiography of skull base meningeomas. *AJNR* 1996; 17: 933–6.
27. Vion-Dury J, Vincentelli F, Jiddane M, et al. MR images of epidermoid cysts. *Neuroradiology* 1989; 29: 333–8.
28. Young IR, Rurl M, Clarke GJ, et al. Magnetic resonance properties of hydrogen: imaging the posterior fossa. *AJNR* 1981; 2: 487–93.
29. Atlas S. *Magnetic Resonance Imaging of the Brain and Spine*, 2nd edn. New York: Lippincott-Raven Publishers; 1996.
30. Hausmann R. Imaging techniques of magnetic resonance angiography. In: Arlart IP, Bongartz GM, Marchal G (eds). *Magnetic Resonance Angiography*. New York: Springer; 1996: 35–47.
31. Fries G, Perneczky A. Intracranial endoscopy. In: Cohadon F, et al. (eds). *Advances and Technical Standards in Neurosurgery*, vol. 25. Vienna: Springer; 1999: 21–60.
32. Hopf N, Grunert P, Fries G, et al. (1999) Endoscopic third ventriculostomy: outcome analysis of 100 consecutive procedures. *Neurosurgery* 1999; 44: 795–806.
33. Gutierrez-Lara F, Patino R, Hakim S. Treatment of tumors of the third ventricle: a new and simple technique. *Surg Neurol* 1975; 3: 323–5.
34. Powell MP, Torrens MJ, Thomson JLG, et al. Isodense colloid cysts of the third ventricle: a diagnostic and therapeutic problem resolved by ventriculoscopy. *Neurosurgery* 1983; 13: 234–7.
35. Rivas JJ, Lobato RD. CT-assisted stereotaxic aspiration of colloid cysts of the third ventricle. *J Neurosurg* 1985; 62: 238–42.
36. Antunes JL, Louis KM, Ganti SR. Colloid cysts of the third ventricle. *Neurosurgery* 1980; 7: 450–5.
37. Yamamoto I, Rhoton Jr, AL, Peace DA. Microsurgery of the third ventricle: Part 1. Microsurgical anatomy. *Neurosurgery* 1981; 8: 334–56.
38. Rhoton AL Jr, Yamamoto I, Peace DA. Microsurgery of the third ventricle: Part 2. Operative approaches. *Neurosurgery* 1981; 8: 357–73.
39. Perneczky A, Müller-Forell W, van Lindert E, et al. *Keyhole Concept in Neurosurgery*. Stuttgart: Thieme; 1999.
40. Ungersböck K, Perneczky A. Intraventricular aneurysm clipped via the contralateral transcallosal approach. *Acta Neurochir* 1986; 82: 24–7.
41. Jeeves MA, Simpson DA, Geffen G. Functional consequences of the transcallosal removal of intraventricular tumours. *J Neurol Neurosurg Psychiatr* 1979; 42: 134–42.

42. Ehni G, Ehni B. Consideration in transforaminal entry. In: Apuzzo MLJ (ed.). *Surgery of the Third Ventricle*. Baltimore, MD: Williams & Wilkins; 1987: 326–53.

43. Sweet WH, Talland GA, Ervin FR. Loss of recent memory following section of the fornix. *Trans Am Neurol Assoc* 1959; 84: 76–82.

44. Wen HT, Rhoton Jr. AL, de Oliveira E. Transchoroidal approach to the third ventricle: an anatomic study of the choroidal fissure and its clinical application. *Neurosurgery* 1998; 42: 1205–19.

45. Scarff JE. Treatment of obstructive hydrocephalus by puncture of the lamina terminalis and floor of the third ventricle. *J Neurosurg* 1951; 8: 204–13.

46. Krause F. *Chirurgie des Gehirns und Rückenmarks nach eigenen Erfahrungen*, Vol. 1. Berlin, Vienna: Urban & Schwarzenberg; 1908.

47. Al-Mefty O. The supraorbital-pterional approach to skull base lesions. *Neurosurgery* 1987; 21: 474–7.

48. van Lindert E, Perneczky A, Fries G, *et al*. The supraorbital keyhole approach to supratentorial aneurysms. Concept and technique. *Surg Neurol* 1998; 49: 481–90.

49. Fries G, Perneczky A. Endoscope-assisted keyhole surgery for aneurysms of the anterior circulation and the basilar apex. *Oper Techn Neurosurg* 2000; 3: 216–30.

50. Stein BM. The infratentorial supracerebellar approach to pineal lesions. *J Neurosurg* 1971; 5: 197–202.

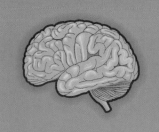

METASTATIC TUMORS OF THE SPINE

41

Richard G Perrin and Robert J McBroom

INTRODUCTION

The expression "show a little backbone" emphasizes, metaphorically, the importance of the vertebral column, while "spineless creature" evokes the devastating disability inflicted by conditions that destroy the functional and structural integrity of the spine. The management of spinal metastases – establishing a diagnosis and determining and executing the optimal treatment – is a paradigm for the management of all spinal tumors.

INCIDENCE

The most frequently occurring tumors of the spinal column are metastatic and the spine is the most common site for skeletal metastases.[1] It is estimated that between 5% and 10% of cancer patients develop symptomatic spinal metastases.[2–5]

Secondary spinal tumors most often originate from carcinomas of the breast, prostate, and lung, reflecting both the prevalence of these primary neoplasms and the propensity for carcinomas of the breast and prostate to metastasize to bone. Approximately 9% of patients with symptomatic spinal metastases present without known primary.[6–8]

Post-mortem studies have shown that secondary spinal tumors are distributed along the spinal column in approximate proportion to the bulk of the vertebrae. The lumbar region is the most common site whereas the cervical spine is least often involved.[1] Based on clinical experience, however, *symptomatic* spinal metastases most frequently affect the thoracic segments, with particular predilection for levels between T4 and T11.[7]

CLASSIFICATION

Spinal metastases (and spinal tumors in general) are classified according to anatomic location (Table 41.1).[9–11] The vast majority are extradural. Intradural extramedullary metastases are uncommon and are most often found in the thoraco-lumbar area. These so-called "drop metastases" generally represent tertiary lesions originating from cerebral secondaries that drift along the cerebrospinal fluid (CSF) to become entangled in the roots of the cauda equina.[11] Intramedullary metastases are relatively rare.

DIAGNOSIS

Symptoms and signs

Symptomatic spinal metastases produce a characteristic clinical syndrome.[6–12] Pain is the earliest and most prominent feature in 90% of patients. Local back or neck pain may be associated with band-like radicular extension indicating nerve root involvement. Pain that is described as severe and burning or dysesthetic should raise suspicion of an intradural extramedullary tumor. Local back or neck pain that is aggravated by movement about the involved segment and relieved by immobilization indicates underlying mechanical instability. Palpation of the posterior spine usually elicits local tenderness at vertebrae involved with extradural metastases.

Local back or neck pain as a result of spinal metastases may be present for weeks or months and is often initially attributed to "arthritis," "back strain," or disc disease. The correct diagnosis may be delayed until more blatant evidence of spinal cord or nerve root compromise is manifest.[13]

It is axiomatic that back or neck pain in a cancer patient heralds spinal metastasis until proven otherwise.

The back or neck pain is followed by weakness, numbness, and sphincter dysfunction. Once established, the weakness progresses relentlessly to complete and irreversible paralysis unless timely treatment is undertaken.[6]

Table 41.1 Relative frequency (%) of spinal metastases according to anatomic location

Author	Patients	ED	ID/EM	IM
Rogers (1958)[35]	17	94	6	–
Barron et al. (1959)[2]	125	98	–	1.6
Edelson et al. (1972)[43]	175	97	–	3.4
Perrin and Livingston (1981)[44]	200	94	5	0.5

ED, extradural; ID/EM, intradural/extramedullary; IM, intramedullary.

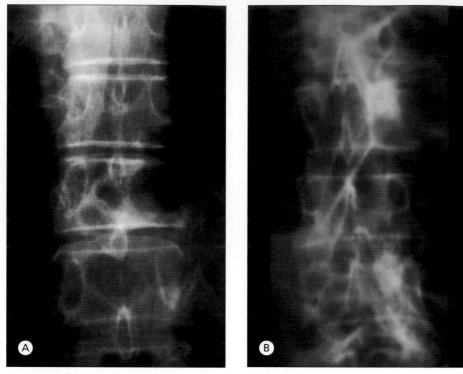

Figure 41.1 (A) Osteolytic metastasis arising from lung; **(B)** osteosclerotic metastasis arising from prostate.

Radiographic studies

Radiographic studies are essential for the diagnosis, staging, surgical planning, and follow-up of patients with spinal metastases.

Plain films

Plain X-ray studies of the spine provide a useful screening test, showing an abnormality in 90% of patients with secondary tumors of the vertebral column. Evaluation of plain X-rays should include assessment of:

1   Qualitative bony alterations (i.e. lytic, blastic, or sclerotic abnormalities). The majority of spinal metastases produce osteolytic alteration. Osteoblastic or sclerotic changes most often occur with metastases arising from breast or prostate (Figure 41.1).[14]

2   Site of involvement (i.e. posterior elements, pedicles, or vertebral body). It is uncommon for spinal metastases to involve only the posterior elements (spine and laminae). More often, the tumor focus is located in the vertebral body, causing compression of the dural sac and its contents from the front. Most often, however, spinal metastases evolve laterally, in the region of the pedicle, and extend anterolaterally or posterolaterally. Pedicle erosion is the earliest and most common abnormality seen on plain films of the spine in patients with spinal metastases. The anteroposterior radiograph of the spine normally resembles a "totem of owls" (Figure 41.2). Pedicle erosion produces a "winking owl" sign (Figure 41.3); bilateral pedicle erosion causes a "blinking owl" sign.[15]

3   Ancillary findings (i.e. paraspinal soft tissue shadow, vertebral collapse, pathological fracture dislocation, and malalignment).[7,12,15] The region of pedicle erosion is often associated with paravertebral soft tissue shadow (Figure 41.4).

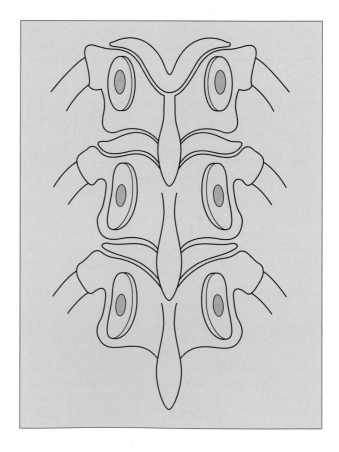

Figure 41.2 The anteroposterior radiograph of the spine resembles a "totem of owls."

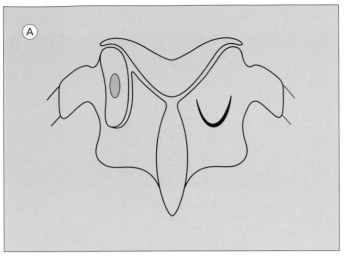

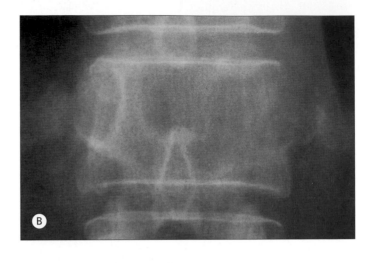

Figure 41.3 "Winking owl" sign at site of pedicle erosion.

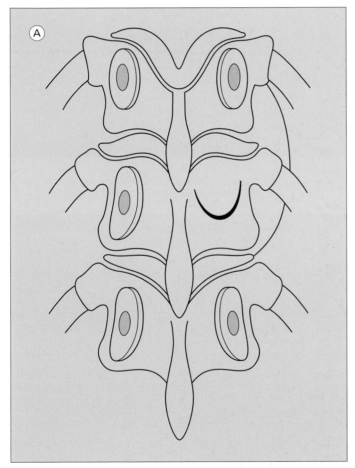

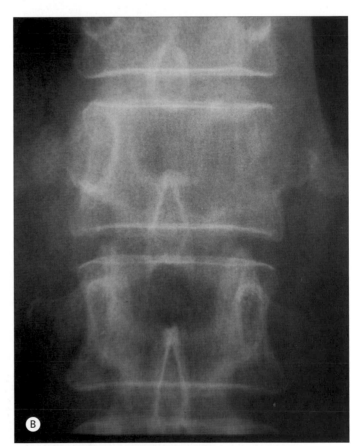

Figure 41.4 Paraspinal soft tissue shadow, associated with pedicle erosion.

Loss of structural integrity may lead to vertebral collapse with wedge compression (Figure 41.5). Further destruction of the vertebral body can result in pathologic fracture dislocation (Figure 41.6). Pathologic fracture dislocation occurs most frequently in the cervical region, where the wide range of neck movements, dependent position of the head, and lack of rib cage supporting structure all contribute to placing at risk the structural integrity of the spinal column and the anatomic alignment of the spinal canal.[12]

Bone scan
A bone scan using radioisotopes may show evidence of metastatic spinal tumor at an earlier stage than plain X-rays.[18–22] It has been estimated that 50–75% of the vertebral medullary space is

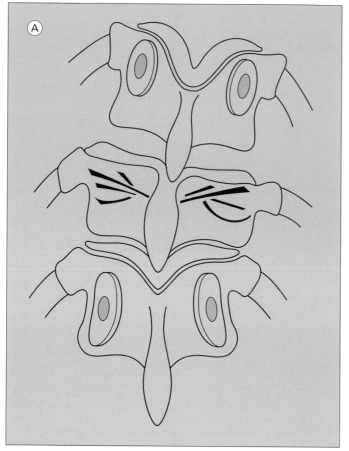

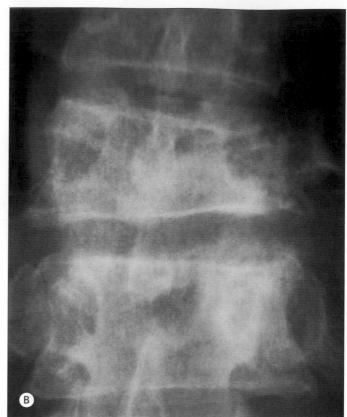

Figure 41.5 Vertebral collapse.

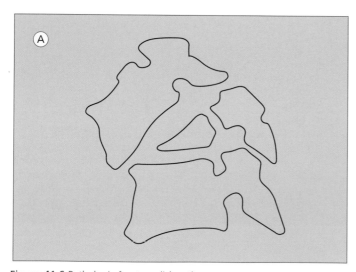

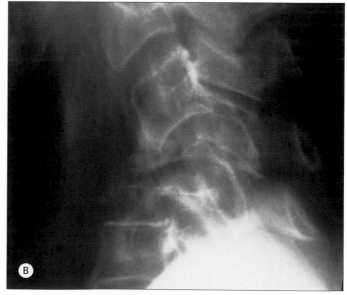

Figure 41.6 Pathologic fracture dislocation.

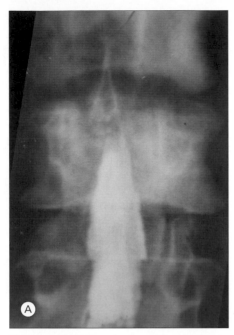

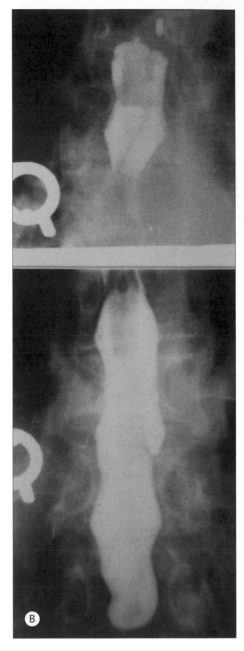

Figure 41.7 (A) Extradural myelographic block at sclerotic metastasis; **(B)** compilation of cisternal and lumbar myelograms to determine the extent of a lesion.

replaced before radiographic changes are discernible.[22] However, bone scans are relatively nonspecific – degenerative changes and infection, as well as spinal tumors, cause positive uptake.[22] The utility of bone scan is in demonstrating multiplicity of skeletal involvement, if present.

Myelography

Myelography has, in the past, been the "gold standard" for identifying the location and level of spinal cord and nerve root compromise caused by spinal tumors. Extradural, intradural extramedullary, and intramedullary spinal tumors are distinguished by characteristic myelographic patterns (Figure 41.7). Deviation of the dye column indicates the source (anterior, lateral, posterior) of the compression mass. When the level of a complete block identified by lumbar myelography is incongruent with the clinical assessment, a cisternal myelogram should be performed to determine the extent of a single lesion or to identify more proximal levels of involvement (Figure 41.7B). Magnetic resonance imaging (MRI) has largely replaced myelography as the diagnostic procedure of choice in assessing vertebral metastasis (see below).

Computed axial tomography

Computed axial tomography (CT) scans are useful to demonstrate the distribution of spinal tumors, the displacement of the spinal cord and nerve roots, the degree of bony destruction, and paraspinal extension of the lesion in the horizontal plane (Figure 41.8). CT is also effective in distinguishing benign spinal degenerative disease from neoplastic lesions.[23,24]

Magnetic resonance imaging

MRI has become the imaging modality of choice for spinal tumors, including metastases.[26–28] MRI permits display of the entire spinal

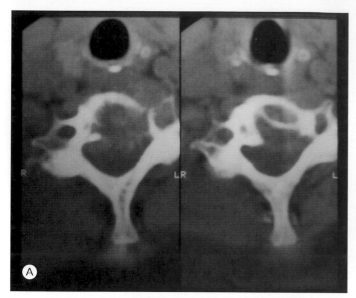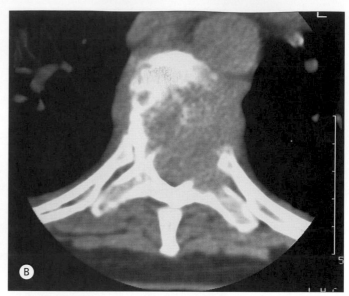

Figure 41.8 Computed tomography scan showing anterior **(A)** and anterolateral **(B)** metastases.

column in sagittal sections to confirm an isolated level of involvement, multiple levels of contiguous tumor spread, or disparate tumor foci at multiple levels (Figure 41.9). Horizontal and coronal reconstructions provide important information concerning tumor geometry – useful in planning surgical decompression, as well as in providing data about vertebral bony integrity – essential in executing the spinal reconstruction.

MRI may be contraindicated in patients with prosthetic devices and implants, in which case reliance is placed on myelography followed by CT scan.

MANAGEMENT

Treatment of patients with spinal metastases is designed to relieve pain and to preserve or restore neurologic function. The realistic objective is palliation. Nevertheless, relief from pain and preservation or restoration of neurologic function contribute immeasurably to the quality of remaining life for a cancer patient and reduces the burden of care.

Radiation versus surgery

The relative merits of therapeutic irradiation, surgery, or a combination of these treatment modalities for the management of spinal metastases has been a matter of conjecture and continuing debate. Radiation therapy is usually considered the initial treatment of choice for the majority of patients with symptomatic radiosensitive secondary spinal tumors with minimal or no neurologic deficit and is especially effective for lymphoreticular lesions.[6,29–32] Surgery is widely considered to be a treatment of last resort.[5] The generally accepted indications for surgical intervention are listed in Table 41.2.[6,11,12,15,29,31,33]

Failure of radiation therapy

Most patients referred for the surgical management of spinal metastases have relapsed during, or after radiation therapy. The

Table 41.2 Indications for surgery
Failure of radiation therapy
Diagnosis unknown
Pathologic fracture/dislocation
Paraplegia: rapidly progressing/far advanced

majority have persistent or recurring tumor causing spinal cord and/or nerve root compromise despite maximum tolerable therapeutic irradiation.

Diagnosis unknown

Surgery is indicated when the diagnosis is in doubt. Some 9% of patients with symptomatic spinal metastases present with no known primary tumor.[6–8] Surgical decompression may then be diagnostic as well as therapeutic. Surgery is also indicated when pathology other than metastatic tumor (e.g. disc protrusion, abscess, hematoma) is suspected of causing spinal cord or nerve root compromise in a cancer patient.[13]

Pathologic fracture dislocation

Pathologic fracture dislocation of the spine produces neurologic compromise by a combination of factors, including distortion caused by spinal malalignment and compression produced by extradural tumor. Surgical intervention is then required to restore spinal alignment, eliminate the compressing tumor, and stabilize the spinal column.[12,34]

Paraplegia: rapidly progressing/far advanced

Urgent surgical decompression should be considered for patients with rapidly progressing or advanced paraplegia. Therapeutic irradiation can initially aggravate the neurologic compression syndrome;[36] therefore, complete and irreversible paraplegia may supervene before the benefits of radiation therapy are manifest.

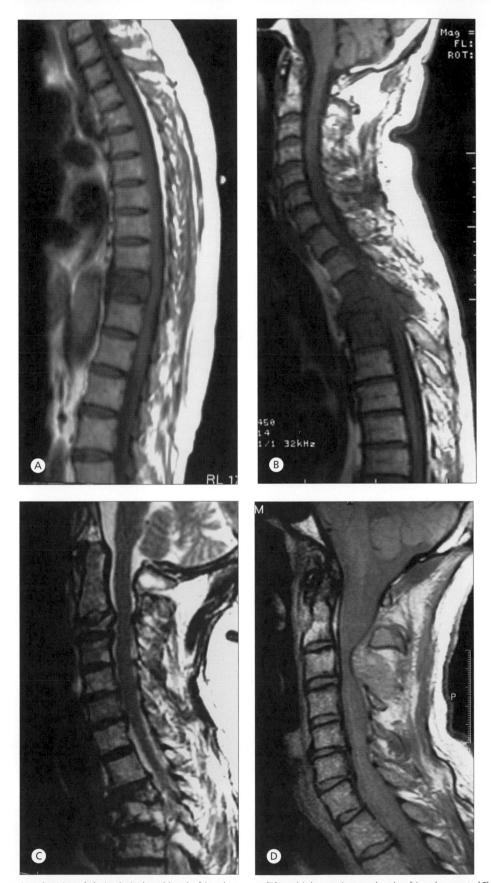

Figure 41.9 MRI of the spine showing: **(A)** single isolated level of involvement; **(B)** multiple contiguous levels of involvement; **(C)** multiple disparate levels of metastatic involvement; and **(D)** involvement of only the posterior spine and laminae.

Surgical approach

Surgery for spinal metastases is designed to *decompress* the spinal cord and nerve roots and *stabilize* the spinal column.[7,12,16,36,37] The surgical approach can be primarily anterior anterolateral or posterior posterolateral; each has its uses, and neither avenue is always appropriate. Occasionally, the two approaches may be combined. The optimal avenue, i.e. anterior, posterior, or a combination, is determined following consideration of a number of factors (Table 41.3).[38]

Tumor location

Intradural spinal metastases are usually best approached from behind.[10,11] The posterior approach using a standard laminectomy technique permits craniocaudad exposure along the length of the spinal column and provides appropriate transdural access for intradural extramedullary, as well as intramedullary metastases.

Extradural spinal metastases can be approached from the front or from the back. Occasionally they involve only the posterior spine and laminae (see Figure 41.10D), in which case decompres- sion through a posterior approach (laminectomy) is appropriate. More often the compressing mass is located in front of the dural sac (Figure 41.9B), and requires decompression through an anterior approach. Most extradural metastases, however, evolve laterally in the vertebral body, extending anterolaterally or posterolaterally (Figure 41.9C). Effective spinal decompression in these cases can be achieved through either an anterior (anterolateral) or a posterior (posterolateral) approach.

Finally, extradural metastases often extend in a napkin-ring fashion about the dural sac; in such cases the posterior approach permits more thorough circumferential decompression of the dural sac and nerve roots.

Spinal level

The anterior approach is awkward at the highest cervical (C1 and C2), high thoracic (T1–T3), and lowest lumbar (L5) and sacral segments.

A transoral approach and mandible-splitting manoeuvres have been described for anterior access to the upper cervical spine. However, the technical challenge of such procedures and the difficulties for a patient, whose physical and emotional resources are already being tested by systemic cancer, usually outweigh the benefits, and are inconsistent with the realistic aim of palliation.

The highest thoracic segments can be reached from the front by splitting the manubrium and reflecting the first and second ribs laterally.[42] More caudal exposure is limited by the heart and great vessels; furthermore, the natural thoracic kyphos restricts visualization during this approach for both decompression and instrumentation.

Decompression at the lumbosacral junction from the front is relatively straightforward. However, spinal stabilization at this level is difficult. Thus, even if adequate decompression is achieved, anterior spinal reconstruction – particularly at the

Table 41.3 Factors determining the surgical approach
Tumor location
Spinal level
Tumor extent
Bony integrity
Patient debility

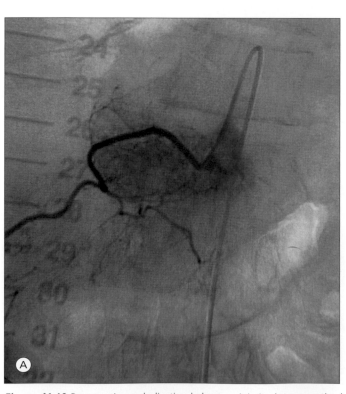
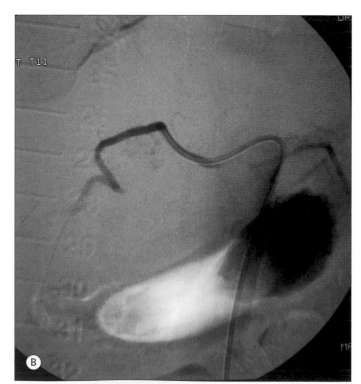

Figure 41.10 Preoperative embolization helps to minimize intraoperative blood loss: **(A)** pre-embolization; **(B)** post-embolization.

cephalad (C1 and C2) and caudad (L5 and sacrum) extremes of the spinal column – poses enormous biomechanical problems.

Tumor extent

Spinal stabilization is necessary following all anterior decompression (corpectomy) procedures and after most posterolateral decompression procedures.[15,16] Stabilization of the spine at any level is less likely to be achieved with an anterior fixation construct if the defect to be spanned encompasses two or more corpectomy segments, and it may be necessary in such cases to reinforce the anterior stabilization apparatus with a posteriorly applied device. Posterior stabilization can be achieved by sublaminar wiring fixed to rib grafts, steel rods, or methyl methacrylate struts at a minimum of two levels above and two levels below the decompression defect.

Bony integrity

Spinal stability after reconstruction depends on the integrity of the bony elements adjacent to the decompression site, which must accept, anchor, support, and maintain the fixation devices. The same biomechanical factors that render the diseased cervical spine susceptible to pathologic fracture dislocation, also jeopardize an anteriorly applied reconstruction apparatus. Fixation of a prosthesis is further limited by the diminutive size of the cervical vertebral bodies. Consequently, an anterior stabilization construct in the cervical spine should be supplemented by a posterior stabilization device or an external brace or appliance.

Patient debility

Local and systemic patient debility plays an important role in selecting the surgical approach. Posterior spinal decompression and stabilization procedures performed through a radiated field carry a high risk of wound complications, including dehiscence with or without infection.[36,39,40] For this reason (other things being equal), previously irradiated thoracic and lumbar spinal metastases are best approached from the front. However, this does not apply to the cervical region, where radiation-induced soft tissue injury, scarring, and loss of anatomical planes increase the risk of vascular and esophageal injury along the anterior avenue of dissection. Finally, some patients may be unable to tolerate the more involved transthoracic or thoracoabdominal exposures because of systemic illness or concurrent conditions.

Surgical strategies

Embolization

Spinal metastases can be highly vascular – particularly those originating from cancers of thyroid or kidney. It is advisable, in such cases, to embolize the lesions before direct surgical intervention, in an effort to minimize intraoperative blood loss (Figure 41.10).

Vertebroplasty

Methyl methacrylate percutaneous vertebroplasty is an option for palliative treatment of vertebral bony metastases without spinal canal involvement in the mid-to-lower thoracic and lumbar regions.

Posterior decompression

Posterior decompression is performed with the patient in an appropriate prone position. In the face of existing or potential spinal instability, care must be taken to avoid exacerbation of spinal malalignment. When frank pathologic fracture dislocation is present in the cervical segments, skeletal traction is applied to restore spinal alignment before surgery.

Manipulation of the diseased cervical spine during tracheal intubation may precipitate or aggravate a neurologic deficit; consequently, it may be prudent to intubate the awake patient with fiberoptic bronchoscopy.[41] Once the patient is intubated and anesthetized, skull tongs (if not already present) are applied for skeletal traction (10 pounds; 4.5 kg) during surgery (Figure 41.11A). The surgical procedure is facilitated by the use of a turning bed, such as a Stryker frame, so that after induction of anesthesia, the patient can be repositioned from supine to prone with minimal risk of exacerbating spinal malalignment (Figure 41.11B). When overt spinal instability is not a concern, the patient can be placed prone in the knee–chest position or on a suitable frame without thoracic or abdominal restriction (Figure 41.12).

The midline incision should be of sufficient length to permit decompression for at least half a segment above and half a segment below the area of spinal cord compromise. The paraspinal muscles are stripped subperiostially from the spines and laminae around the diseased area (Figure 41.13). Care must be taken to avoid inadvertently plunging through the bony laminae, which may be destroyed by tumor. A wide laminectomy is performed that extends for a half segment above and a half segment below the area of spinal cord compression. In the uncommon event that the extradural tumor is restricted to the posterior elements (as for example, in Figure 41.9C), laminectomy alone may provide adequate decompression.

In most cases, however, adequate decompression from the back requires posterolateral exposure for removal of tumor-destroyed lateral elements. This, in turn, provides anterior access to the vertebral body. Excavation of the tumor-involved vertebral body can be accomplished with cup curettes (upward-angled and downward-angled) and pituitary forceps. A downward-angled cup curette can be used to decompress the dural sac anteriorly by displacing the compression mass into the hollowed-out vertebral body (Figure 41.14). The tumor should be carefully peeled off the dural sac and root sleeves.

Encased nerve roots in the thoracic segments may be intentionally crushed if radicular pain caused by involvement of these roots is present.

The posterolateral decompression may be undertaken bilaterally to enable radical and circumferential decompression of the spinal cord and nerve roots (Figure 41.15; see also Figure 41.14).

The posterior approach is based on a standard laminectomy technique, is easily extended superiorly or inferiorly to include additional segments (as is often required), and is applicable along the length of the spinal column. Adequate posterolateral exposure provides access through the tumor-destroyed lateral elements into the vertebral body anterolaterally and permits removal of an anterior compression mass. Radical decompression circumferentially about the dural sac and root sleeves can thus be accomplished. Pulsation of the dural sac is often seen after appropriate surgery, and is an indication that adequate decompression has been achieved.

Brisk bleeding may occur during excavation of the vertebral body. This usually diminishes when the vertebral body has been gutted and can be controlled by application of thrombin-soaked pledgets.

Posterior stabilization

When spinal metastases involve only the posterior bony elements (spine and laminae) or occur exclusively within the spinal canal

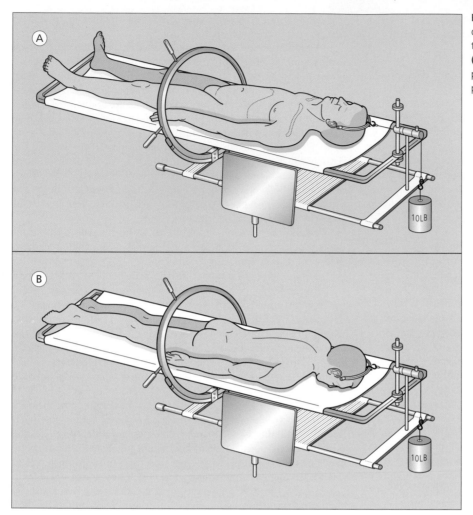

Figure 41.11 (A) Positioning for anterior decompression and stabilization with skeletal traction to resotre and maintain spinal alignment; **(B)** use of a turning bed (such as a Stryker frame) permits repositioning of the patient from supine to prone.

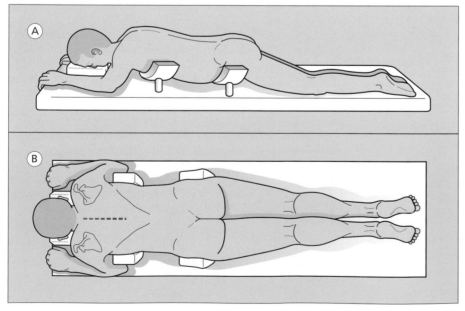

Figure 41.12 Prone positioning when overt spinal instability is not a concern.

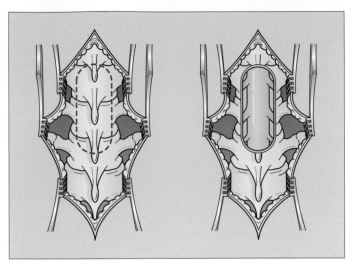

Figure 41.13 Posterior exposure is achieved by stripping muscles subperiosteally from the spines and laminae around the disease area. Exposure must extend for at least a half segment above and a half segment below the area of cord compression.

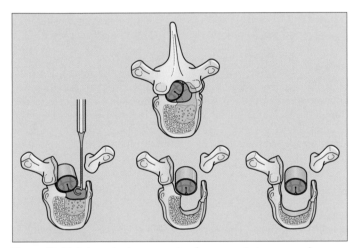

Figure 41.14 Adequate decompression from a posterior approach usually requires posterolateral exposure. Removal of tumor-destroyed elements provides access anteriorly into the vertebral body. A compression mass can be displaced into the hollowed-out vertebral body, using a downward-angled cup curette.

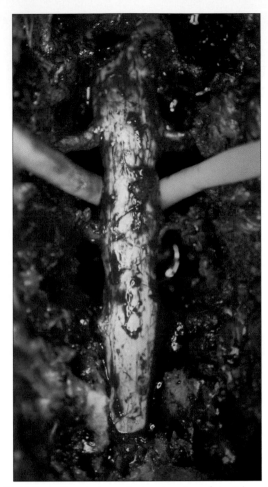

Figure 41.15 Operative photograph showing circumferential decompression of the dural sac and nerve roots through the posterolateral approach.

(without bony involvement), a laminectomy without spinal recon-struction may be adequate. However, in most cases an adequate posterior decompression procedure for spinal metastases (postero-lateral decompression) precipitates or aggravates spinal instability and must therefore be followed by spinal stabilization.

Spinal instrumentation is used to secure and maintain normal spinal alignment with rigid internal fixation. The goal is to provide immediate spinal stability that will remain intact for the patient's lifetime.

Posteriorly applied spinal reconstruction involves laminar fixation to bone grafts, steel rods, or methyl methacrylate struts. Meticulous care must be taken with the sublaminar wiring to avoid dural laceration and spinal cord injury. Preoperative assess-ment of the spinal canal by radiograph and CT scan helps to determine if there is adequate extradural space for the passage of sublaminar wires.

Intraoperatively, the entry and exit points of each sublaminar wire trajectory are prepared by removing the overlapping inferior laminar edge and associated ligamentum flavum (Figure 41.16). The doubled end of the stainless steel wire is curved to facilitate sublaminar passage; the leading tip is bent back somewhat to help one feel its location and to ensure its proper emergence at the exit site (Figure 41.16A). Intimate contact must be maintained between the sublaminar surface and the wire during its passage (Figure 41.16B). The wire should be firmly twisted or cinched in place immediately after sublaminar passage so that it maintains snug and firm contact with the lamina, thus preventing displace-ment of the sublaminar loop against the dural sac and its contents (Figure 41.16C). The firmly secured wires are then fixed to appropriately contoured bone, steel rod, or methyl methacrylate struts (Figure 41.16D). Autogenous bone (e.g. rib, iliac crest, fibula) should be used for bony arthrodesis when the patient is expected to enjoy prolonged survival. If bone struts are used, the contact surfaces between the bone graft and spinal elements (spines and laminae) should be roughened to promote fusion. Segmental instrumentation with steel rods or loops or methyl methacrylate struts is usually more appropriate when palliation is the realistic goal. Use of a rectangular loop prevents both vertical

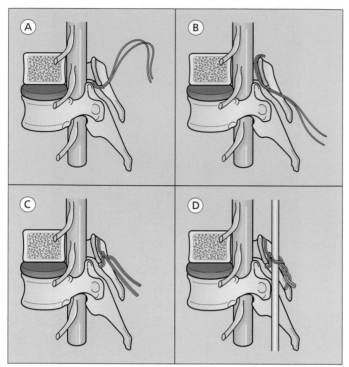

Figure 41.16 (A) Curving the doubled end of stainless steel wire facilitates sublaminar passage; the leading tip is bent back further to assist in its location and proper emergence at the exit site. **(B)** Intimate contact must be maintained between the sublaminar surface and length of wire during and after passage. **(C)** The wire should be firmly secured and placed by twisting or cinching to maintain snug and firm contact about the lamina to prevent displacement of the sublaminar loop. **(D)** The firmly secured wires are fixed to appropriately contoured stabilization constructs.

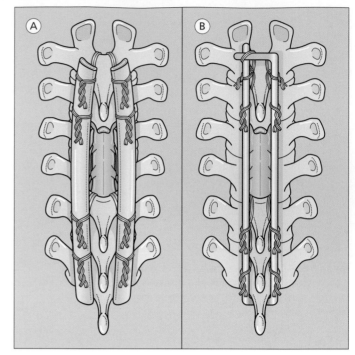

Figure 41.17 Fixation at two levels above and two levels below the decompressed segment to: **(A)** rib struts; **(B)** steel rods/rectangle.

and rotational displacement. If methyl methacrylate is used, the struts can be applied while malleable, thus enhancing the fit and providing intimate articulation with the spinal surface. Whatever supporting material is used (bone, steel, or methyl methacrylate), it is essential to secure multiple levels of fixation to the spine, and at a minimum of two levels above and two levels below the unstable segment (Figures 41.17, 41.18).

Anterior decompression

Anterior (anterolateral) decompression is performed with the patient in an appropriate supine position. The anterior avenue used depends on the level of spinal involvement. Care must be taken, especially in the cervical region, to avoid exacerbation of spinal malalignment.

CERVICAL (C3–C7) Spinal metastases affecting the cervical segments are most often associated with existing or potential spinal instability. Patients presenting with frank pathologic fracture dislocation are treated preoperatively with skeletal traction to restore spinal alignment. As with posterior decompressions, consideration should be given to intubating the awake patient with fiberoptic bronchoscopy, followed by application of skull tongs for intraoperative traction. When anterior and posterior procedures are performed under the same anesthetic, surgery is facilitated by use of a turning bed such as a Stryker frame (see Figure 41.11).

Neck dissection may be carried out from the right side or the left. The recurrent laryngeal nerve is at risk during a right-sided approach, and on the left side the long thoracic duct is in jeopardy. Preoperative evaluation of vocal cord function is essential when circumstances suggest that a patient's vocal cord function is already compromised and helps to determine the appropriate side for neck dissection.

A skin incision along the anterior border of the sternocleidomastoid muscle provides an appropriate approach to the anterior cervical spine (Figure 41.19). The platysma is divided in line with the skin incision and the anterior border of the sternocleidomastoid is cleared. The cervical fascia is divided and a plane is developed between the carotid sheath and its contents laterally and the trachea and esophagus medially. It is often necessary to ligate and divide the superior thyroid artery and vein, and it may be necessary to divide the omohyoid muscle to achieve sufficient longitudinal exposure. Adequate access is thus gained to the vertebral bodies (and anterior spinal canal) from C3 through C7. A diseased vertebra is often identified by gross paraspinal tumor extension, which causes discoloration and deformity of the anterior longitudinal ligament. Intraoperative X-ray is used to confirm the spinal level.

Further dissection should be performed, using the operating microscope to permit precise technique. The medial border of the longus colli muscle is detached across the area of the diseased vertebral body and adjacent disc spaces bilaterally. Resection of the vertebral body is facilitated by first excising the intervertebral disc above and below the diseased segment. The tumor-destroyed vertebral body is removed with the aid of curettes, drill, and suction (Figure 41.20). Care must be taken to avoid injuring the vertebral arteries that may be buried in the tumor or tethered to lateral bone fragments. The posterior longitudinal ligament should be excised and the anterior dural sac cleared to ensure complete removal of any epidural tumor extension.

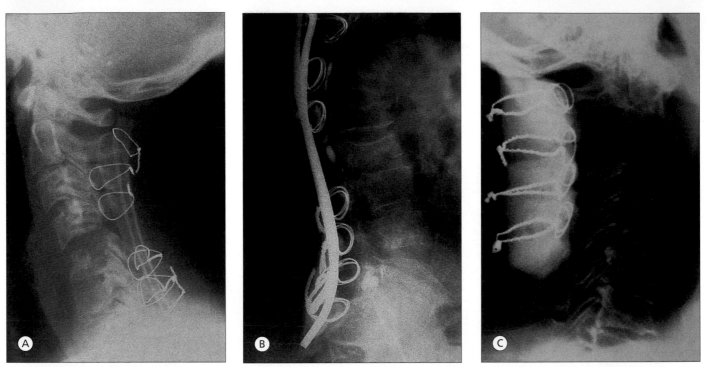

Figure 41.18 Postoperative radiographs showing segmental wiring to: **(A)** autogenous bone (rib struts); **(B)** steel rod; and **(C)** methyl methacrylate strut.

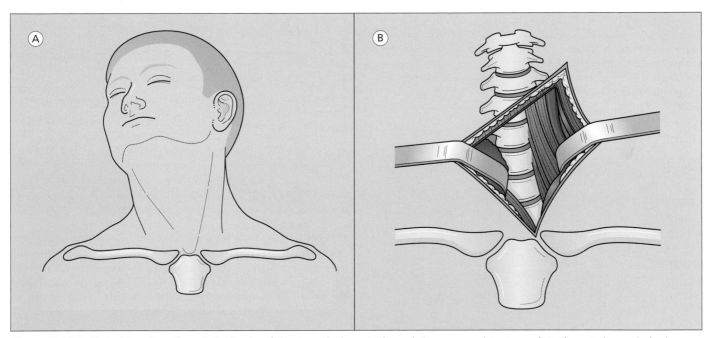

Figure 41.19 A skin incision along the anterior border of the sternocleidomastoid muscle is an appropriate approach to the anterior cervical spine.

THORACIC (T1–T3) Anterior exposure of the highest thoracic segments is achieved through a midline sternotomy that extends through the second intercostal space (Figure 41.21).[42] The dissection begins with exposure of the lower cervical spine (as described above) and is carried inferiorly by dividing the omohyoid muscle. The manubrium sterni is divided in the midline and then to the second intercostal space with an oscillating saw. The soft tissues beneath the sternum are dissected and divided, with care taken to avoid injury to the internal mammary vessels and long thoracic duct (on the left side). A small sternal retractor assists in exposing the retrosternal space. The great vessels are identified down to the aortic arch and the dissection plane is established between the trachea and esophagus (medially) and the great vessels (laterally). Exposure of the upper thoracic segments is limited by the aortic arch and the oblique view of the upper thoracic spine coursing posteriorly to follow the natural kyphotic

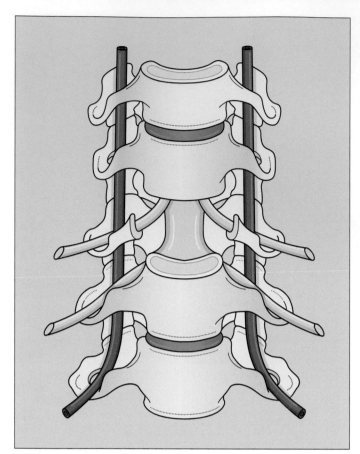

Figure 41.20 For resection of the vertebral body the intervertebral disc is excised above and below the affected segment, which is then removed with curettes, drill, and suction. The posterior longitudinal ligament is removed to ensure thorough decompression of the dural sac and root sleeves.

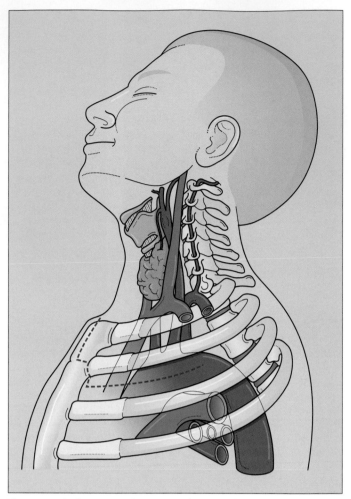

Figure 41.22 The aorta and great vessels anteriorly, the oblique view of the upper thoracic spine posteriorly, along the natural kyphotic curve of the upper thoracic spine limit the exposure.

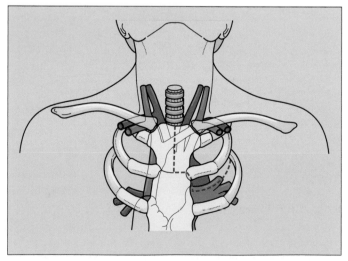

Figure 41.21 Anterior exposure of the highest thoracic segments is achieved by extending the anterior neck approach inferiorly through a midline sternotomy, and along the second intercostal space.

curve (Figure 41.22). The diseased vertebral body is removed as described above.

THORACIC (T4–T11) Spinal metastases involving T4 through T11 can be approached anteriorly through the chest. The location of the major bony destruction or spinal cord compression determines the side on which the thoracotomy should be carried out. When the spinal disease is symmetrical, a right-sided thoracotomy is performed so that the instrumentation used for spinal stabilization will be remote from the aorta.

A double-lumen endotracheal tube or bronchial blocker is used whenever possible, so that the exposed lung can be deflated. The anesthetized patient is arranged in the lateral decubitus position and then rolled posteriorly 20° to aid in visualization beyond the midline of the spine (Figure 41.23A). The operating table is extended approximately 20° with the apex at the level of the spinal pathology to facilitate surgical exposure.

The skin incision begins anteriorly and, following the path of the sixth or seventh rib, courses posteriorly and superiorly, midway between the medial border of the scapula and the line of spinous processes. The skin, subcutaneous tissues, latissimus dorsi,

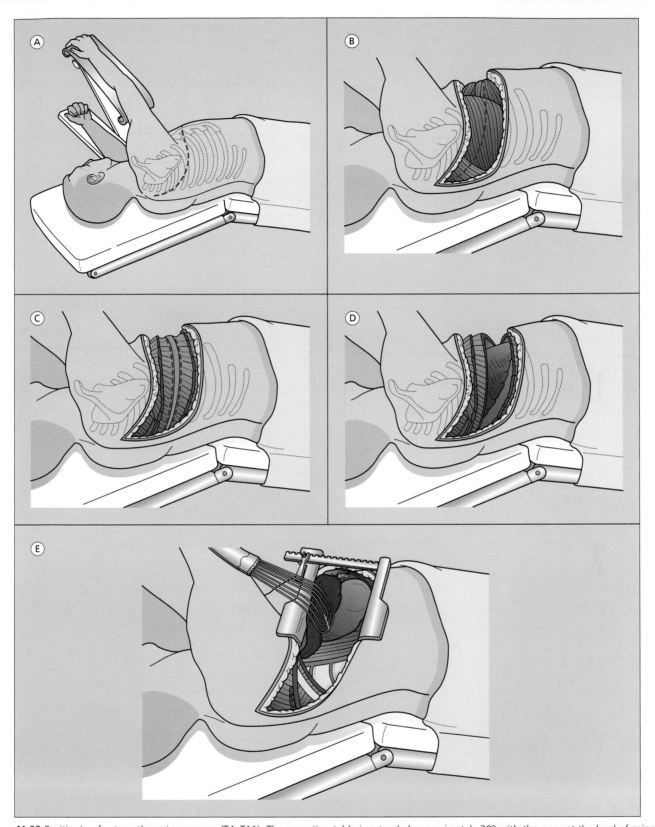

Figure 41.23 Positioning for transthoracic exposure (T4–T11). The operating table is extended approximately 20° with the apex at the level of spinal pathology. **(A)** The anesthetized patient is arranged in the lateral decubitus position and rolled posteriorly 20° to aid visualization beyond the midline of the spine. **(B)** A skin and muscle "flap" is raised to provide access to the bony thorax and ribs. **(C)** The chest is entered and the appropriate rib is exposed subperiosteally and then divided. **(D)** The parietal pleura is divided and the lung is deflated. **(E)** The anterior and lateral surfaces of the vertebral bodies are exposed. The level of disease involvement is usually marked by discoloration or deformity.

and serratus anterior are divided along the line of the incision, raising a skin and muscle "flap," which provides immediate access to the lateral bony thorax and the third through eighth ribs (Figure 41.23B). Adequate access to the upper thoracic spine may require mobilization of the scapula.

The chest is entered along the rib corresponding to the segment two levels above the spinal pathology. The appropriate rib is exposed subperiosteally, with care being taken to avoid the neurovascular bundle that lies immediately beneath it (Figure 41.23C). The rib is divided near the costochondral junction anteriorly and behind the angle of the rib posteriorly, and is excised. The underlying parietal pleura is divided and the lung is deflated, then retracted anteriorly and medially (Figure 41.23D,E).

The level of disease involvement is usually identified by local discoloration or deformity. Confirmation of the correct level is obtained by counting the ribs from above and from below. Review of the preoperative chest X-ray is essential to exclude supernumerary, bifid, or absent ribs.

The parietal pleura overlying the lateral surface of the vertebral bodies is divided longitudinally. The intervertebral discs are identified and exposed to make it easier to find the segmental arteries and veins, which cross the middle of the vertebral bodies and must be sequentially ligated and divided. The segmental vessel at the level of the spinal tumor is frequently the most difficult to find. Once the segmental vessels are divided, the aorta and vena cava are gently retracted to expose the anterior and lateral surfaces of the vertebral bodies. Exposure of the vertebral bodies must extend for one intact vertebra above and below the diseased segment.

Adequate decompression of the dural sac and nerve roots involves removal of the tumor-destroyed vertebral body (corpectomy). The intervertebral discs above and below the diseased segment are excised, delineating the longitudinal extent of the surgical decompression. The affected bone is removed down to the posterior longitudinal ligament using curettes, drill, and suction. The posterior longitudinal ligament is excised and the dura is exposed to permit removal of extradural tumor extension (Figure

41.24). Careful removal of the pedicle (which is often destroyed by tumor) allows exposure of the inferiorly coursing segmental root sleeve. The dural root sleeves are rather delicate along the thoracic segments. If a sleeve is inadvertently torn, the defect should be closed under magnification. Oversewing the repaired defect with a muscle pledget helps to ensure a water-tight closure.

The transthoracic approach permits decompression, under direct vision, of approximately two-thirds of the dural sac circumference around the anterior and lateral spinal canal (Figures 41.24, 41.25). Nerve roots on the side opposite the surgical exposure are hidden from view. Attempts at blind circumferential decompression may result in dural laceration and nerve root injury, and in a CSF which is very difficult to repair.

THORACOLUMBAR (T12–L2) The side on which to perform the thoracotomy is determined by the local spinal pathology. When the disease is symmetrical the left side is chosen, as the spleen is

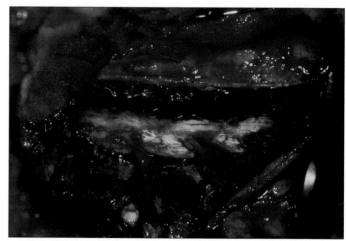

Figure 41.25 Intraoperative photograph showing anterolateral decompression of the dural sac and root sleeves.

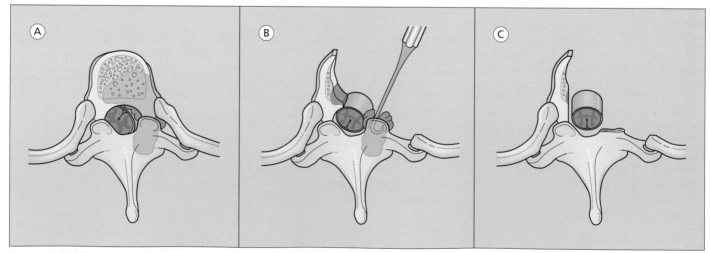

Figure 41.24 (A) Resection of the vertebral body is facilitated by first excising the intervertebral disc above and below the diseased segment(s) and then removing the destroyed vertebral body. The posterior longitudinal ligament is excised and the dura is exposed for removal of extradural tumor extension. **(B)** Removal of the pedicle exposes the inferiorly coursing segmental root sleeve. **(C)** Anterior thoracolumbar exposure permits decompression of the anterior and lateral spinal canal around approximately two-thirds of the dural sac circumference.

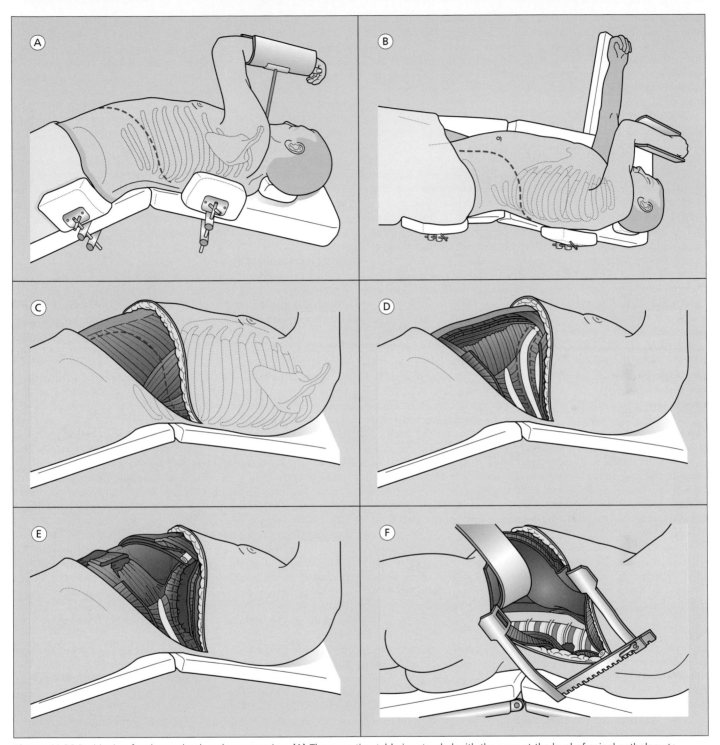

Figure 41.26 Positioning for thoracolumbar decompression. **(A)** The operating table is extended with the apex at the level of spinal pathology to facilitate the surgical exposure. The patient is placed in the lateral decubitus position and rolled posteriorly 20° to aid in visualization of the contralateral portion of the spinal canal. **(B)** The skin incision is made along the course of the tenth rib, anteromedially crossing the costal cartilage and proceeding along the lateral edge of the rectus sheath. **(C)** The latissimus dorsi overlying the tenth rib is divided. **(D)** The external oblique is separated to expose the rib, which is separated from its cartilage attachment anteriorly and divided posterior to the angle of the rib. **(E)** The parietal pleura is incised to expose the superior surface of the diaphragm. The peritoneum is bluntly dissected from the posterior surface of the transversus abdominis so that the anterior abdominal wall muscles can be safely divided. **(F)** The posterior diaphragm is divided medially to gain access to the psoas muscle, which is retracted laterally to expose the spine. The diaphragm is exposed by bluntly dissecting the peritoneum from its inferior surface and is then divided near its peripheral attachment.

easier to mobilize than the liver. A double-lumen endotracheal tube or bronchial blocker is usually not necessary. The patient is placed in the lateral decubitus position and then rolled posteriorly 20° to facilitate visualization of the contralateral portion of the spinal canal. The operating table is extended with the apex at the level of the spinal pathology to facilitate the surgical exposure (Figure 41.26A).

The skin incision is made along the course of the tenth rib. The incision crosses the costal cartilage anteromedially and proceeds along the lateral edge of the rectus sheath (Figure 41.26B). Posterolaterally, the latissimus dorsi overlying the tenth rib is divided and the external oblique is separated in line with its fibers to expose the tenth rib (Figure 41.26C). The tenth rib is separated from its cartilage attachment anteriorly and divided posterior to the angle of the rib (Figure 41.26D). The parietal pleura is incised and the superior surface of the diaphragm is visualized. The retroperitoneal space is identified by cutting the costal cartilage of the tenth rib. Once in the retroperitoneal space, the peritoneum is bluntly dissected from the posterior surface of the transversus abdominis. The muscles of the anterior abdominal wall can then be divided safely (Figure 41.26E).

The diaphragm is exposed by bluntly dissecting the peritoneum from its inferior surface. The diaphragm is then divided in a semicircular fashion near its peripheral attachment (Figure 41.26F). This incision should not stray into the center of the diaphragm because of the risk of denervating the muscle and the reduced healing capacity of the central tendon. Only a cuff of muscle (approximately 2 cm) is left attached to the rib to facilitate closure. The posterior portion of the diaphragm is divided medially to gain access to the psoas muscle so it can be retraced laterally to expose the vertebral body.

The intervertebral discs are identified to facilitate isolation, ligation, and division of the segmental vessels. The aorta and vena cava are then retracted to expose the anterior and lateral surfaces of the vertebral bodies. The spinal level is confirmed by identifying the convergence of the twelfth rib and the first lumbar transverse process.

Decompression of the dural sac and nerve roots then proceeds with excision of the intervertebral disc above and below the diseased segment, removal of the tumor-destroyed vertebral body, excision of the posterior longitudinal ligament, and exposure of the dural sac and segmental root sleeve as described above (Figure 41.27).

LUMBAR (L3–L5) The side of approach is usually determined by local spinal pathology. The patient is positioned supine and then rolled through 30° to facilitate retraction of the peritoneal contents (Figure 41.28). The operating table is extended at the level of the spinal pathology.

The skin incision is made obliquely across the anterior abdominal wall (Figure 41.29). It extends from midway between the twelfth rib and superior iliac crest superiorly to just above the pubic rami at the lateral edge of the rectus sheath inferiorly. Each muscle layer of the abdominal wall is divided sequentially in line with the skin incision. Before the transversus abdominis muscle is divided the peritoneum must be bluntly dissected from its posterior surface to avoid inadvertent entry into the peritoneal cavity (Figure 41.30). The retroperitoneal space is exposed by sweeping the peritoneum and fat off the inner surfaces of the ilium and psoas. Care must be taken not to extend the dissection posterior to the psoas, as this would jeopardize the lumbosacral plexus. During exposure the ureter is retracted anteriorly and

medially with the peritoneum. The spinal level is confirmed by identifying the prominence of the sacrum or by intraoperative radiography. The intervertebral discs are identified to facilitate localization and subsequent ligation and division of the segmental vessels.

To expose L5, the iliolumbar vein, which is usually a very large vessel that joins the posterior aspect of the common iliac vein, should be identified and ligated. Controlling this vessel is frequently the most difficult part of the dissection.

Decompression of the dural sac and nerve roots proceeds with excision of the intervertebral disc above and below the diseased segment. The tumor-destroyed vertebral body is removed, the posterior longitudinal ligament is excised, and the dural sac and nerve roots are exposed as described above. Since the approach for the lumbar segments is more truly anterior, it is possible to expose and visualize the root sleeves bilaterally.

Anterior stabilization

Adequate procedures for anterior spinal decompression involve vertebral corpectomy at one or more levels and therefore *must* be followed by spinal stabilization. The variety of anterior spinal instrumentation devices and techniques that have been described suggests that there is no single superior method to secure and maintain normal spinal alignment for both immediate and long-term stability.

Autogenous bone should be used to secure bony arthrodesis if prolonged survival is anticipated. A tricorticate segment of iliac crest is usually an appropriate graft. After decompression of the dural sac and nerve roots and realignment of the spine, vertebral height is restored, using skeletal traction in the cervical segments and a vertebral spreader in the thoracic and lumbar spine. This tightens the lax and redundant soft tissues about the corpectomy segment and permits placement of the graft under compressive forces. The iliac crest strut is tailored to fit the corpectomy defect and is keyed into place, resting on the vertebral end plates above and below (Figure 41.31). Obliquely oriented screws can be inserted through the graft and into the vertebral bodies above and below to increase the compression of the graft and its stability. Neutralization of the forces across the bone graft can be achieved by applying an anterior spinal plate to the vertebral bodies above and below the spanned segment and securing it with three screws. Postoperatively, an appropriate external brace is used for 3 months to protect the stabilization construct while bony arthrodesis occurs.

A preformed titanium mesh cage may be used to supplement autogenous bone grafts (Figure 41.32). The titanium cage provides immediate structural support while the bone graft will permit bony arthrodesis. The bone graft may be morselized bone harvested from the iliac crest, or morselized rib which is removed during transthoracic exposure. The cage eliminates the need for a structurally strong iliac crest, and is therefore useful in patients who have significant osteopenia. The cage must be anchored with additional anterior instrumentation. The Kaneda Instrumentation may be used in the thoracolumbar spine (Figure 41.33). Compression is applied across the cage in order to secure it in position (Figure 41.34).

The use of bone graft is inappropriate for most patients with symptomatic spinal metastases. Structurally intact autogenous bone is often not available, bone graft is incorporated slowly in a milieu characterized by residual tumor, osteoporosis, and changes caused by irradiation, and an external support is required for a minimum of 3 months. Consequently, it is generally more appro-

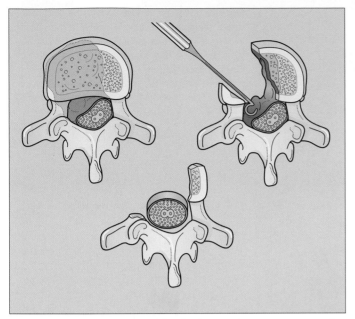

Figure 41.27 Decompression of the dural sac and nerve roots proceeds with excision of the intervertebral disc above and below the diseased segment, removal of the tumor-destroyed vertebral body, excision of the posterior longitudinal ligament, and exposure of the dural sac and segmental root sleeve.

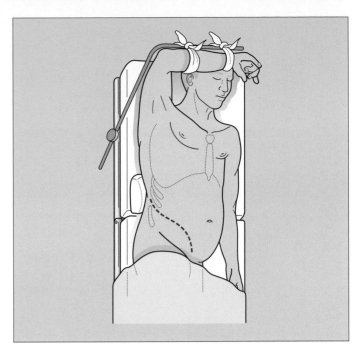

Figure 41.29 An oblique skin incision across the anterior abdominal wall extends (superiorly) from midway between the twelfth rib and superior iliac crest to (inferiorly) just above the pubic rami at the lateral edge of the rectus sheath.

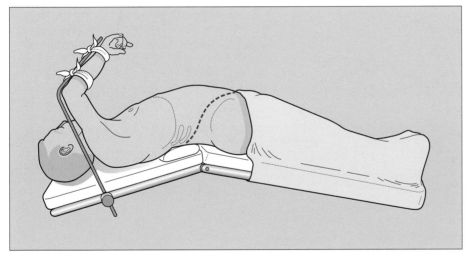

Figure 41.28 Position of the patient for transabdominal anterior approach to the spine. The operating table is extended with apex at the level of the spinal pathology. The patient is arranged supine and then rolled through up to 30° to aid in retraction of the peritoneal contents.

priate to use a synthetic construct, which can provide immediate spinal stabilization, thus eliminating the need for prolonged external orthotics.

A simple and effective prosthetic fixation system is derived from a tailored AO (Arbeitsgemeinschaft für Osteosynthesefragen) construction plate and screws, augmented with methyl methacrylate (the Wellesley Wedge).[16] A stainless steel construction plate (3.5 mm wide for the cervical spine and 4.5 mm wide for the thoracic and lumbar spine) is contoured to size, with dimensions determined intraoperatively, to fit the decompression defect (Figure 41.35). The U-shaped plate is secured to the vertebrae above and below with fully threaded cancellous screws. The plate can be extended for more than one vertebral segment above and below the decompression defect, depending on the local skeletal architecture. Each cervical vertebra can accommodate only one or two screws. In the upper thoracic spine two screws are inserted into each vertebral body. In the lower thoracic and lumbar spine fixation with three screws can be achieved (Figure 41.36). Improved screw purchase can be obtained by preinjecting the holes with low-viscosity methyl methacrylate, provided the drill has not perforated the far cortex. Once the plate has been secured, methyl methacrylate in malleable form is used to fill the defect bracketed by the plate. The cement is inspissated through the empty screw holes and around the screw heads to prevent its dislodgement from the plate. During polymerization of the methyl methacrylate, the dura is protected by a fat graft and

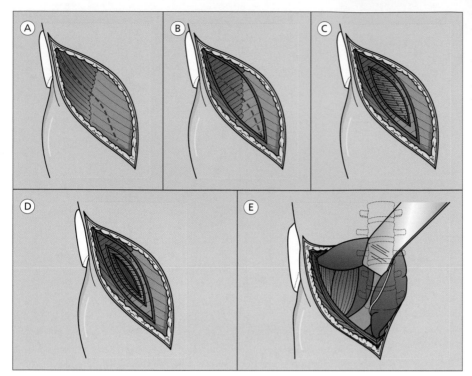

Figure 41.30 Each muscle layer of the abdominal wall is sequentially divided in line with the skin incision: **(A)** external oblique; **(B)** internal oblique; **(C)** transversus. **(D)** The peritoneum must be bluntly dissected from the posterior surface of the transversus abdominis before this muscle is divided to prevent inadvertent entry into the peritoneal cavity. **(E)** The retroperitoneal space is exposed.

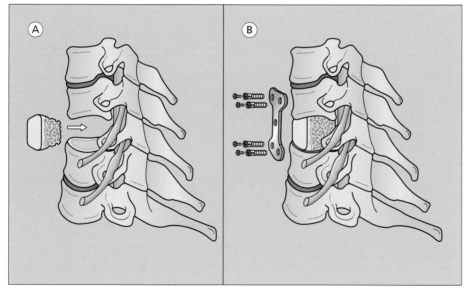

Figure 41.31 (A) An autogenous iliac crest strut is tailored to fit the defect and is keyed into place, resting on the vertebral end plates. **(B)** Neutralization of forces across the bone graft can be achieved with an anterior spinal plate secured to the vertebral bodies above and below the spanned segment.

constant irrigation with cool normal saline. The fat graft is left in place to reduce postoperative scar formation. The Wellesley Wedge provides a simple, safe, and effective means of spinal stabilization, particularly in the thoracic and lumbar regions (Figure 41.37).

Because the cervical vertebrae are smaller, the cervical spine poses a challenge in securing and preserving stability of the spinal column. Furthermore, the cervical spine's mobility makes stability difficult to maintain. Consequently, it is often advisable to supplement the anterior spinal instrumentation with a posterior stabilization procedure. By the same token, when adequate anterior spinal decompression results in resection of two or more vertebral thoracic or lumbar (corpectomy) levels, it is advisable to reinforce the anterior stabilization construct with a posteriorly applied device.

The fifth lumbar vertebra can be excised through an anterior approach. However, spinal reconstruction with fixation to the sacrum is tenuous at best. Therefore, tumors involving L5 are initially managed through a posterior approach. Once stable fixation is obtained (posteriorly), anterior spinal decompression (L5 corpectomy) can be carried out at a second stage.

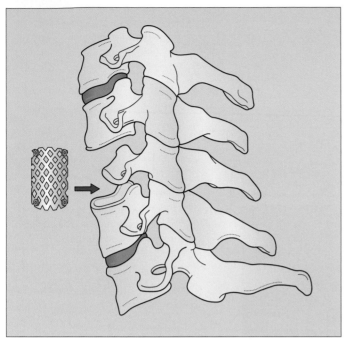

Figure 41.32 A preformed titanium cage may be used to supplement autogenous bone grafts.

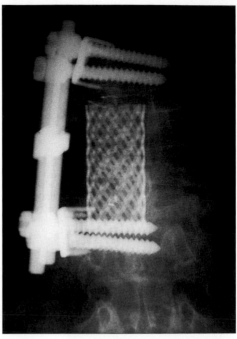

Figure 41.34 Postoperative radiograph showing the titanium cage with instrumentation.

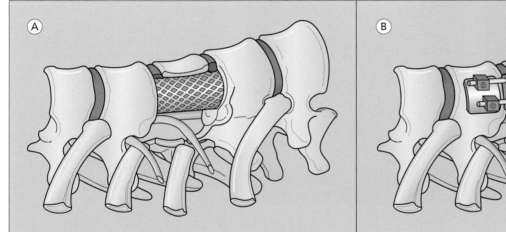

Figure 41.33 Titanium mesh cage in the thoracic spine **(A)**, anchored with Kaneda instrumentation **(B)**.

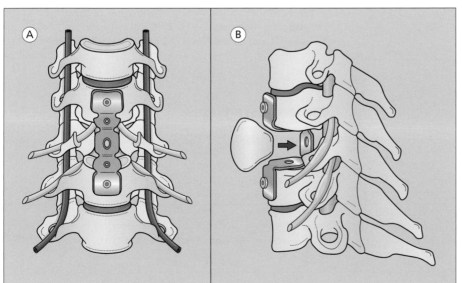

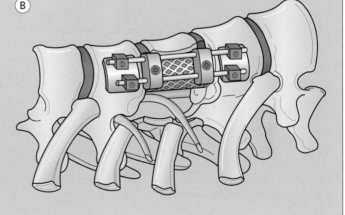

Figure 41.35 A simple and effective prosthetic fixation system is shown (the Wellesley Wedge). **(A)** The stainless steel plate is contoured to size with dimensions determined intraoperatively to fit the decompression defect and the plate is secured to the vertebra above and below with fully threaded cancellous screws. **(B)** Methyl methacrylate in malleable form fills the defect bracketed by the plate.

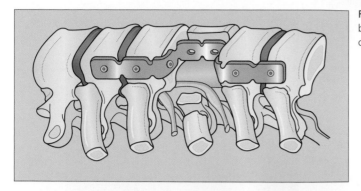

Figure 41.36 The Wellesley Wedge can be applied to replace the vertebral bodies of C3–L4. The tailored plate is inserted anteroposteriorly in the cervical spine, and is oriented laterally in the thoracic and lumbar levels.

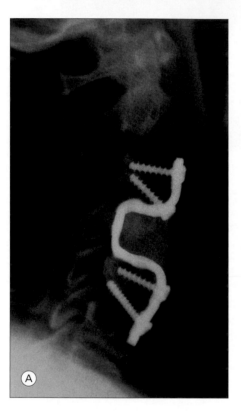

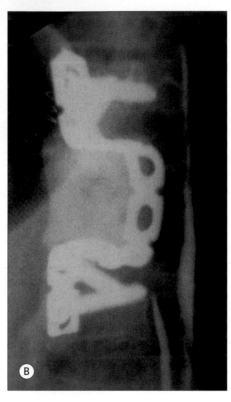

Figure 41.37 Postoperative radiographs showing an anterior fixation construct (Wellesley Wedge) in **(A)** the cervical spine and **(B)** the thoracolumbar spine.

Table 41.4 Outcome determinants
Degree of deficit
Duration of symptoms
Tumor type
Tumor location
Stage of the disease

RESULTS

The prognosis for patients with symptomatic spinal metastases is variable, given the heterogeneity of this patient population. The outcome of treatment depends on a number of factors (Table 41.4).

Degree of deficit

The degree of neurologic deficit at the time of treatment is the most reliable prognostic factor. Patients who are ambulatory do best, whereas patients with complete paralysis below the level of spinal cord compression do worst and have a poor chance of recovering useful motor function.

Duration of symptoms

Recovery from spinal cord compression depends on the rate of onset and duration of symptoms. Long duration of symptoms and slowly evolving paraplegia are relatively favorable prognostic factors.

Tumor type

The biologic properties of the culpable primary tumor, including growth characteristics and radiation sensitivity, are factors that should determine method of management as well as the results of treatment and length of survival. Spinal metastases of reticuloendothelial origin have a relatively favorable outcome, whereas those arising from carcinoma of the lung carry a poor prognosis.

Tumor location

Intradural spinal metastases are uncommon and carry a poor prognosis. Intradural extramedullary metastases, in particular, are associated with a virulent clinical syndrome and rapid deterioration to fatal outcome.

Advanced disease

The degree of debility will determine the feasibility of surgery. Local and systemic factors influence the approach adopted and the surgical strategies employed.

SUMMARY

Metastatic tumors of the spine are the most common neoplasms of the vertebral column and represent an ominous complication of systemic cancer. The relative merits of therapeutic irradiation, surgical intervention, or a combination of these treatment modalities remain a matter of debate.

Surgical strategies should provide for *both* decompression of the spinal cord and nerve roots, *as well as* stabilization of the spinal column.

A multidisciplinary approach with collaboration among neurosurgeon, oncologist, and orthopaedic surgeon is advisable to achieve optimal outcome in the management of patients with symptomatic spinal metastases.

CLINICAL PEARLS

- Spinal metastases are the most common tumors of the vertebral column

- The vast majority (95%) are extradural; intradural extramedullary metastases are most often tertiary "drop metastases" from cerebral secondary sites. Intramedullary metastases are rare.

- The characteristic clinical syndrome begins with pain (90%) followed by weakness, numbness, and sphincter dysfunction, all of which are relentlessly progressive.

- *Back or neck pain in a cancer patient heralds spinal metastasis until proven otherwise.*

- Plain films are abnormal in 90% of cases; a "winking owl" sign is the most common finding.

- MRI is the imaging method of choice.

- Indications for surgery include: failed radiation therapy, diagnosis unknown, pathologic fracture dislocation, and paraplegia (rapidly progressing/far advanced).

- Surgical strategies must provide *both* decompression of the spinal cord and nerve roots, *as well as* stabilization of the spinal column.

- Surgical approach depends on a number of interrelated factors: tumor location, spinal level, tumor extent, bony integrity, and patient debility.

- Outcome depends on: degree of deficit, duration of symptoms, tumor type, tumor location, advanced disease.

REFERENCES

1. Willis RA. *The Spread of Tumors in the Human Body*, 3rd edn. London: Butterworths; 1973.
2. Barron KD, Hirano A, Araki S, Terry RD. Experiences with metastatic neoplasms involving the spinal cord. *Neurology (Minneap)* 1959; 9: 91–106.
3. Clarke E. Spinal cord involvement in multiple myelomatosis. *Brain* 1986; 79: 332–48.
4. Galaski CSB. Skeletal metastases and mammary cancer. *Ann R Coll Surg Engl* 1972; 50: 3–28.
5. Sundaresan N, Digiacinto GV, Hughes JEO, Cafferty M, Vllejo A. Treatment of neoplastic spinal cord compression: results of a prospective study. *Neurosurgery* 1991; 29: 645–50.
6. Botterell EH, Fitzgerald GN. Spinal cord compression produced by extradural malignant tumors. *Can Med Assoc J* 1959; 80: 791–6.
7. Livingston KE, Perrin RG. Neurosurgical management of spinal metastases. *J Neurosurg* 1978; 49: 839–43.
8. Macdonald DR. Clinical manifestations. In: Sunderesan N, Schmidek H, Schiller A, Rosenthal A (eds). *Tumors of the Spine: Diagnosis and Clinical Management*. Philadelphia: WB Saunders Co.; 1990; 6–21.
9. Chade HO. Metastatic tumors of the spine and spinal cord. In: Vinken, PJ, Bruyn GW (eds). *Handbook of Clinical Neurology*. Amsterdam: North-Holland Publishing Co.; 1976; 415–33.
10. Murphy KC, Feld R, Evans WK, *et al.* Intramedullary spinal cord metastases from small cell carcinoma of the lung. *J Clin Oncol* 1983; 1: 99–106.
11. Perrin RG, Livingston KE, Aarabi B. Intradural extramedullary spinal metastasis. *J Neurosurg* 1982; 56: 835–7.
12. Perrin RG, Livingston KE. Neurosurgical treatment of pathological fracture-dislocation of the spine. *J Neurosurg* 1980; 52: 330–4.
13. Goodkin R, Carr B I, Perrin RG. Herniated lumbar disc disease in patients with malignancy. *J Clin Oncol* 1987; 5: 667–71.
14. Shoskes DA, Perrin RG. The role of surgical management for symptomatic spinal cord compression in patients with metastatic prostate cancer. *J Urol* 1989; 142: 337–9.
15. Perrin RG, McBroom RJ. Surgical treatment for spinal metastases: the posterolateral approach. In: Sundaresan N, Schmidek H, Schiller A, Rosenthal A (eds). *Tumors of the Spine: Diagnosis and Clinical Management*. Philadelphia: WB Saunders Co.; 1990; 305–15.
16. Perrin RG, McBroom RJ. Spinal fixation after anterior decompression for symptomatic spinal metastasis. *Neurosurgery* 1988; 22: 324–7.
17. Belliveau RE, Spencer RP. Incidence and sites of bone lesions detected by 99mTc-polyphosphate scans in patients with tumors. *Cancer* 1975; 36: 359–63.

18. Fletcher JW, Solaric-George E, Henry RE, *et al*. Radioisotope detection of osseous metastases. *Arch Intern Med* 1975; 135: 553–7.

19. Low JC. The radionuclide scan in bone metastasis. In: Weiss L, Gilbert HA (eds). *Bone Metastasis*. Boston: GK Hall & Co; 1981: 231–44.

20. McNeil BJ. Rationale for the use of bone scans in selected metastatic primary bone tumors. *Semin Nucl Med* 1978; 8: 336–45.

21. Edelstyn GA, Gillespie PJ, Grebbell FS. The radiological demonstration of osseous metastases:experimental observations. *Clin Radiol* 1967; 18: 158–62.

22. O'Mara RE. Bone scanning in osseous metastatic disease. *JAMA* 1974; 229: 1915.

23. O'Rourke T, George CB, Redmond J, *et al*. Spinal computed tomography and computed tomographic metrizamide myelography in the early diagnosis of metastatic disease. *J Clin Oncol* 1986; 4: 576–83.

24. Redmond J, Spring DB, Munderloh SH, *et al*. Spinal computed tomography scanning in the evaluation of metastatic disease. *Cancer* 1984; 54: 253–8.

25. Brunberg JA, Dipietro MA, Venes JL, *et al*. Intramedullary lesions of the pediatric spinal cord: correlation of findings from MR imaging, intraoperative sonography, surgery, and histologic study. *Radiology* 1991; 181: 573–9.

26. Jaeckle KA. Neuroimaging for central nervous system tumors. *Semin Oncol* 1991; 18: 150–7.

27. Lisbona R, Rosenthall L. Role of radionuclide imaging in osteoid osteoma. *Am J Roentgenol* 1979; 132: 77–80.

28. Sze G. Magnetic resonance imaging in the evaluation of spinal tumors. *Cancer* 1991; 67: 1229–41.

29. Dunn RC Jr, Kelly WA, Wohns RN, Howe JF. Spinal epidural neoplasia: a 15-year review of the results of surgical therapy. *J Neurosurg* 1980; 52: 47–51.

30. Friedman M, Kim THE, Panahon AM. Spinal cord compression in malignant lymphoma: treatment and results. *Cancer* 1976; 37: 1485–91.

31. Gilbert RW, Kim JH, Posner JB. Epidural spinal cord compression from metastatic tumor: diagnosis and treatment. *Ann Neurol* 1978; 3: 40–51.

32. Maranzano E, Latini P, Checcaglini F, *et al*. Radiation therapy in metastatic spinal cord compression. *Cancer* 1991; 67: 1311–17.

33. Delaney TF, Oldfield EH. Spinal cord compression. In: DeVita VT, Hellman S, Rosenberg SA (eds). *Cancer: Principles and Practice of Oncology*, 3rd edn. New York: JB Lippincott; 1989: 1978–85.

34. Perrin RG, Livingston KE. Pathological fracture dislocation of the cervical spine. In: Tator CH (ed.). *Early Management of Acute Spinal Cord Injury*. New York: Raven Press; 1982; 365–72.

35. Rogers L. Malignant spinal tumors and the epidural space. *Br J Surg* 1958; 45: 416–22.

36. Heller M, McBroom RJ, MacNab T, Perrin RG. Treatment of metastatic disease of the spine with posterolateral decompression and Luque instrumentation. *Neuro-Orthopedics* 1986; 2: 70–4.

37. Perrin RG, McBroom RJ, Perrin RG. Metastatic tumors of the cervical spine. In: Black P (ed.). *Clinical Neurosurgery*. Baltimore: Williams & Wilkins; 1991; 740–55.

38. Perrin RG, McBroom RJ. Anterior versus posterior decompression for symptomatic spinal metastasis. *Can J Neurol Sci* 1987; 14: 75–80.

39. Macedo N, Sundaresan N, Galicich JH. Decompressive laminectomy for metastatic cancer: what are the current indications? *Proc Am Soc Clin Oncol* 1985; 4: 278.

40. Martenson JA, Evans RG, Lie MR, *et al*. Treatment outcome and complications in patients treated for malignant epidural spinal cord compression. *J Neuro-oncol* 1985; 3: 77–84.

41. Tindall S, Perrin RG. Anesthesia for surgical management of spinal metastases. *Prob Anesth* 1991; 5: 80–90.

42. Darling GE, McBroom RJ, Perrin RG. Modified anterior approach to the cervical thoracic junction. *Spine* 1995; 20: 1519–21.

43. Edelson RN, Deck MDF, Posner JB. Intramedullary spinal cord metastases: clinical and radiographic findings in nine cases. *Neurology* 1972; 22: 1222.

44. Perrin RG, Livingston KE. Intradural-extramedullary metastases. Presentation at the *Annual Meeting of the Neurosurgical Society of America*, Pebble Beach, CA, 17 March 1981.

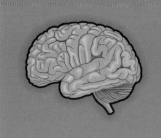

SPINAL INTRADURAL EXTRAMEDULLARY TUMORS

42

Jacques Brotchi

Intradural, extramedullary tumors constitute two-thirds of all spinal neoplasms. Schwannomas (neurilemomas) and meningiomas make up approximately 90% of the total and occur in equal numbers.[1,2] The remaining 10%, which will not be described in this chapter, are divided amongst a host of clinical entities, including ependymoma (filum terminale), dermoid, epidermoid, angioma, lipoma, metastatic carcinoma, arachnoid cyst, ependymoma, chordoma, lymphoma, melanoma, myxoma, and sarcoma.

Epidemiologic studies suggest that primary spinal tumors occur with an approximate annual incidence of 2 per 100 000 population. However, with the increasing availability of new radiological tools such as magnetic resonance imaging (MRI), spinal cord tumors are discovered more frequently.

Approximately 20% of all central nervous system tumors lie within the spinal canal. Estimates of location suggest that 25% are extradural, 50% are intradural and extramedullary, and 25% are intramedullary.[3] Based upon this information, a neurosurgeon should anticipate an incidence of at least one intradural extramedullary tumor per 100 000 population per annum. Since schwannomas and meningiomas make up approximately 90% of all intradural extramedullary tumors, the emphasis of this chapter will be devoted to the management of these two neoplasms.

CLINICAL PRESENTATION

Most intradural extramedullary neoplasms present with progressive, slowly evolving neurologic signs and symptoms. Pain is the primary symptom in initial presentation of intradural extramedullary tumors.[4-6] The pain is often radicular in nature but can occur in a diffuse, nondescript pattern. The pain is generally described as a dull, aching sensation with occasional sharp inflections. It is uncommon for patients to report burning or similar dysesthetic sensations, as is common in intramedullary neoplasms. Nocturnal pain may be prominent, as may exacerbation on assuming a recumbent position. This type of presentation is often relieved by resuming an upright position. The radicular pain is often worse at night and may completely disappear during the day. Paresthesias are also common, with descriptions of "numbness and tingling."

Weakness is the most readily identified objective symptom and sign. It typically follows the sensory symptoms but may, on occasion, occur as the primary complaint. Weakness is often associated with hyperreflexia and spasticity in the affected extremities. Flexor spasms or muscle cramps may develop as weakness and spasticity increase. In addition to these upper motor neuron signs, lower motor neuron symptomatology can also be identified, including hyporeflexia, atrophy and fasciculations along the innervation of the affected level. Specific segmental weakness can also occur. Patients may present with a partial or complete Brown–Séquard syndrome because of the frequent asymmetric location of meningiomas and schwannomas. Later symptoms and signs include autonomic dysfunction, bladder and bowel disturbances. Urinary and fecal incontinence or retention are most common, while sexual dysfunction is infrequently identified. Rarely, clinicians will observe spinal deformities. It has become uncommon for these disturbances to develop as a result of early diagnosis by modern neuroimaging techniques, such as MRI and computed tomography (CT).

The clinical presentation is useful in determining the exact level and location of the spinal lesion. A careful history may provide clues as to the exact location of the lesion within the spinal canal. For example, lesions occurring in the posterior aspect of the spinal cord will produce posterior column dysfunction, such as joint position and vibratory sensation loss. Anterior lesions will spare the posterior column function while causing weakness and loss of sensation below the level of the abnormality. Anterior lesions may also affect the spinocerebellar tracts, resulting in uncoordinated and ataxic gait, unrelated to the degree of long tract (motor) dysfunction. Lesions lying at the anterolateral aspect of the spinal cord will demonstrate classic Brown–Séquard symptoms. The speed with which neurologic deficits occur in spinal intradural extramedullary tumors is predictive of eventual outcome. Lesions that create sudden loss of function are most commonly the result of immediate neurovascular compromise. The ischemia created by a vascular insult is almost always irreversible and function is poorly recoverable. Fortunately, sudden paralysis is a rare presentation. Classically, the symptoms are slowly progressive over weeks to months or even years, and then they are most likely the result of slow compressive effects on the neural elements themselves. In these cases, an excellent recovery after surgical decompression of the mass lesion heralds a very satisfying neurologic recovery. Often, severe neurologic injury will recover completely with surgical extirpation of the mass. Nevertheless, it is advantageous to make the diagnosis on the initial radicular symptoms, or at the beginning of spinal cord dysfunction, to prevent permanent neurological dysfunction.

NEURORADIOLOGICAL INVESTIGATIONS

Plain spine roentgenograms have been overlooked in recent years as a source of valuable information in the assessment of spinal tumors. As lesions have been identified earlier in their course with

MRI and CT myelography, plain spine roentgenography has become less useful. However, the classic descriptions of bony destruction warrant reiteration. Classically, approximately half of all neurogenic tumors and 10% of meningiomas will present with changes in the bone, including erosion of the pedicles, scalloping of vertebral bodies, or neural arches. The presence of expanded neuroforamina and a widened spinal canal may also be helpful in identification of these lesions by plain X-ray or CT. Calcification in long-standing tumors is common.

Lumbar puncture is seldom performed, but when undertaken in patients with intradural extramedullary tumors often demonstrates an elevated protein level. CT with contrast usually shows marked enhancement of the tumor and associated erosion of the bone. A dumb-bell-shaped enhancement pattern is typical of schwannomas. Before the development of MRI, CT myelography was considered the most useful diagnostic procedure for the demonstration of intradural extramedullary masses. However, at present, MRI has largely supplanted CT myelography as the definitive diagnostic approach.[7–9]

Increasingly, MRI has become the primary diagnostic modality in the assessment of intradural extramedullary lesions.[10–12] MRI evaluation should include views in all three planes (sagittal, axial and coronal) both with and without administration of paramagnetic contrast agents such as Gd-DTPA (gadolinium). The majority of schwannomas (74%) are isointense to spinal cord on T1-weighted images, while a minority (26%) are hypointense.[13] On T2-weighted images, schwannomas are usually hyperintense. These lesions usually enhance intensely and fairly homogeneously with gadolinium, but may also enhance heterogeneously. Peripheral enhancement has also been reported.[14] Meningiomas usually have a broad-based dural attachment and frequently show a linear enhancement pattern called "the dural tail sign." Meningiomas do not have a central area of decreased signal on T2-weighted images, but this is frequently seen in schwannomas.[14]

SURGICAL MANAGEMENT

The day before surgery, we discuss with the neuroradiological team the detailed position of the tumor and its relationship with the spinal cord. It is mandatory to know if the tumor is anterior, posterior, or on which side lateral to the spinal cord and/or nerve roots (Figure 42.1). Surgical approaches are mostly dependent on the presumed diagnosis, and on the location of the tumor within the spinal canal (postero-lateral or antero-lateral). Moreover, in the case of hourglass-shaped schwannomas, it is sometimes safer to perform a posterior surgical approach followed by an antero-lateral approach, either at the same sitting or in a second stage procedure (Figures 42.2–42.7). That decision is often made prior to commencing the first surgery. But in many cases, hourglass-shaped tumors may be removed in one stage through a posterior approach. When the tumor is anteriorly placed, such as with meningiomas, a more lateral surgical approach should be planned.

The patient is placed under general endotracheal anesthesia. Electrophysiologic monitoring is employed.[15] Somatosensory evoked potentials and motor evoked potentials are monitored throughout the procedure by a specially trained neurologist or neurophysiologist. Changes in the baseline recording will alert the surgeons to stop their surgical manipulation. Often, a change will occur if excessive traction or compression occurs while removing the tumor. The surgeon will be alerted and will cease the manipulation and permit the recordings to return to baseline; the surgery may then re-commence. Most schwannomas may be removed through a posterior midline approach. In the case of an anteriorly placed meningioma, it is necessary to make a more lateral surgical approach; for example, through a costovertebral or costopedicular trajectory. The key point is that the surgeon desires to take an approach that will avoid any retraction on the spinal cord.

An initial lateral radiograph is obtained with a marker placed on the skin surface to localize the level of the tumor more

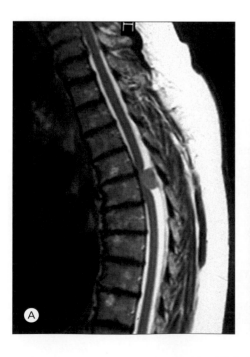
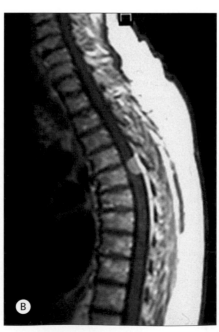

Figure 42.1 Thoracic meningioma. Sagittal T2-weighted image (WI) **(A)** and gadolinium-enhanced T1WI **(B)**. This posterior mid-thoracic meningioma is almost isointense on T2WI, isointense on T1WI and enhances strongly and homogeneously after gadolinium injection. The tumor displaces the spinal cord anteriorly.

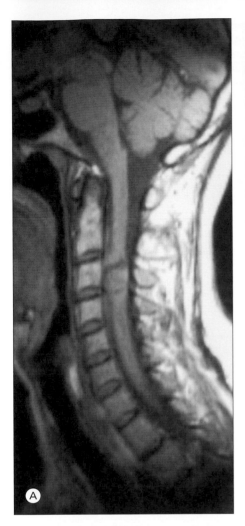

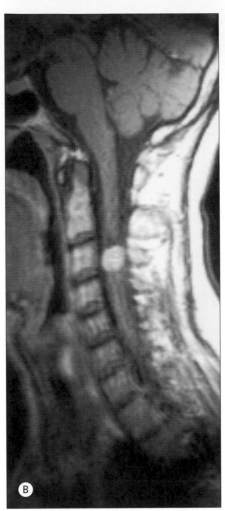

Figure 42.2 Cervical schwannoma: sagittal T1 **(A)** and gadolinium-enhanced T1WI **(B)**. A round mass is found at the level of C3 with well-defined borders. The lesion is isointense to the cord but is surrounded by a hypointense rim. After contrast injection, intense contrast uptake is seen.

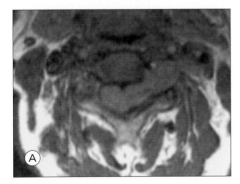

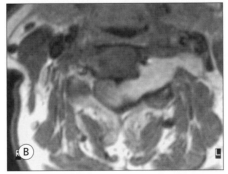

Figure 42.3 Cervical schwannoma (same case as in Figure 42.2): axial images without **(A)** and with **(B)** gadolinium injection. The extramedullary location and extension within the left, enlarged, neural foramina is much better appreciated on those axial views.

accurately. An attempt is made to limit the surgical exposure to the focal point of the tumor. Typically, only two vertebral levels need to be exposed, as it is rare for these tumors to extend much beyond one or two vertebral segments. Subperiosteal dissection is carried sharply down to the laminae on one side. The spinous process is cut at its base and the paraspinous musculature is then swept laterally, keeping the interspinous ligament intact.

Surgery is performed with the aim of minimizing bone removal. With a lateral tumor, the laminectomy is more generous on the side of the tumor while respecting the contralateral hemi-lamina and articular processes. We perform a laminectomy for

most tumors, except for very laterally displaced tumors in which a hemi-laminectomy may be sufficient to provide adequate exposure.

The dura mater is opened in a longitudinal fashion over the tumor and not simply on the midline, except in posterior located lesions. The margins of the dura mater are reflected laterally with silk sutures. The tumor is visualized and the arachnoid is opened immediately over it. In antero-lateral displaced lesions, division of the dentate ligament is helpful. Tenting sutures hold the dentate ligament to the opposite dura, which rotates and keeps the spinal cord away, giving more access to the intradural extramedullary

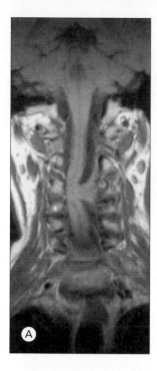
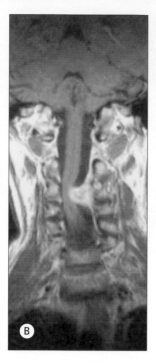
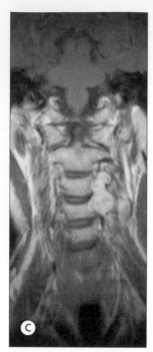

Figure 42.4 Cervical schwannoma: coronal T1 (A) and gadolinium-enhanced coronal slices (B,C): the lesion is isosignal to the cord and displaces the cord to the right. The most anterior image (C) shows the associated bony erosion.

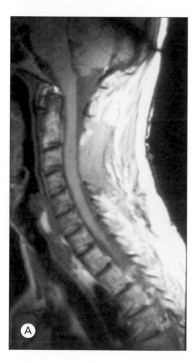

Figure 42.5 Cervical schwannoma: postoperative control MRI performed after the first surgical step with removal of the intra-canal component. (A) Sagittal T1WI image and (B) axial gadolinium T1WI.

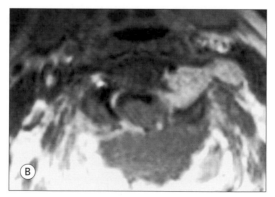

space. The tumor surface is cauterized with bipolar cautery to improve hemostasis as the resection proceeds. Cottonoid pledgets are placed at the superior and inferior aspects of the neoplasm to decrease the migration of blood products into the subarachnoid space. Inevitably, some surgical debris will seep into the subarachnoid space and will require irrigation with normal saline solution to decrease the risk for postoperative aseptic meningitis. The tumor is then entered and debulked with sharp and blunt dissection techniques or with the cavitronic ultrasonic aspiration device (CUSA). Traction may be placed on the tumor, if neces-

sary, but never on the spinal cord. An intracapsular debulking is performed before complete tumor removal. As the center of the tumor is removed, the capsule falls in upon itself and is mobilized from the surrounding neural elements and dural margin. Upon completion of the intracapsular resection, the capsule is carefully dissected free with bipolar and microscissor dissection. Schwannomas rarely adhere to the spinal cord. Most meningiomas stay extrapial and also do not adhere to the spinal cord (Figures 42.8–42.13). It is rare to have adhesions or spinal cord invasion, but in some rare circumstances schwannomas may extend, in part,

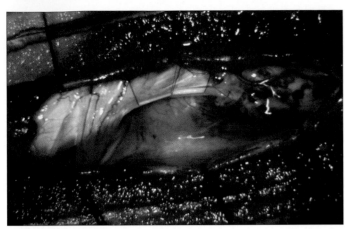

Figure 42.6 Left hourglass cervical schwannoma. The dentate ligament has been cut. It is held by sutures to the opposite dura mater, giving sufficient room for surgery.

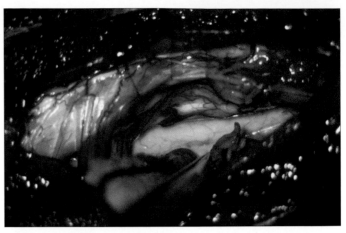

Figure 42.7 Left hourglass cervical schwannoma. First surgical step: most of the intradural part of the schwannoma has been removed. See the anterior surface of the spinal cord compressed by the tumor and the clean surgical field.

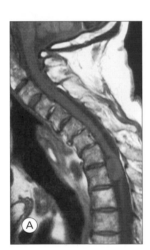
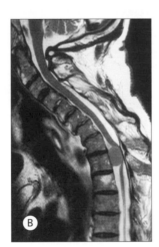
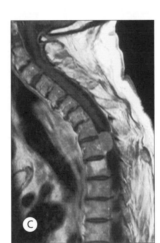

Figure 42.8 Upper anterior thoracic meningioma: sagittal T1 (A), T2 (B) and gadolinium T1 (C) images: the meningioma is seen as a round mass with sharp borders, isosignal to the cord on T1WI, almost isointense on T2WI and enhances mildly and homogeneously after contrast injection.

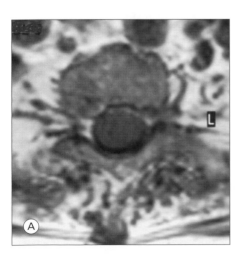
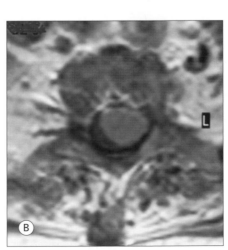

Figure 42.9 Upper anterior thoracic meningioma: axial T1WI without (A) and with (B) gadolinium injection. The tumor occupies almost the entire canal compressing the cord and distorting it to the right.

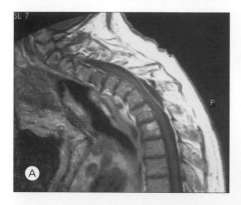

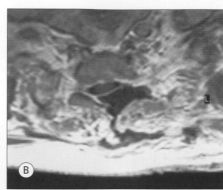

Figure 42.10 Upper anterior thoracic meningioma: postoperative control MRI performed 1 week after surgery: Sagittal (A) and axial (B) gadolinium-enhanced T1WI. Total resection of the tumor; the spinal cord has already recovered a normal location.

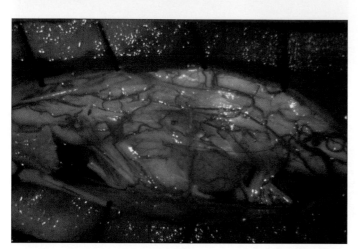

Figure 42.11 Left anterolateral thoracic meningioma. A transpedicular approach offers a good view of the tumor and compressed spinal cord.

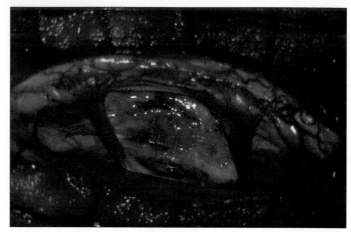

Figure 42.13 Same case as Figures 42.8 and 42.12: complete removal of the meningioma. The spinal cord is still rotated away by sutures in the dentate ligament, demonstrating access to anterior dura where the tumor was attached.

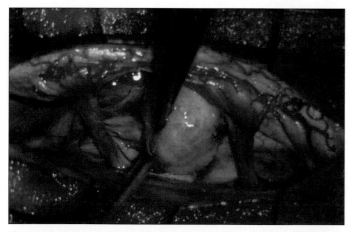

Figure 42.12 Same case as Figure 42.8. After division of the dentate ligament, the spinal cord is held by sutures placed in the ligament and sutured to the opposite dura mater and slightly rotated to gain sufficient access for surgical removal. Microsurgery is performed between the posterior rootlets which are preserved.

in an intramedullary way. In schwannomas that jut into the spinal cord, surgery is conducted as it would be for an intramedullary tumor.[16] In schwannomas, it is safe to cut the nerve root or rootlet from which the tumor arises. This rarely leaves any neurological deficit in the patient as the rootlet is often sensory in origin, and

often dysfunctional. In cervical hourglass-shaped tumors it is sometimes necessary to add an anterolateral approach after removal of the intraspinal lesion. It is also possible to perform the operation through solely the anterolateral approach.[17]

In meningiomas, it is important to coagulate the dura mater attachment. Indeed, cauterization instead of resection of the meningioma matrix does not increase the recurrence rates. However, re-operation and the resultant arachnoid scarring makes surgery much more difficult. The aim should be complete removal during the first surgery. When incomplete removal occurs, 50% tumor recurrence at 1 year is reported in the literature.[18] All vasculature on or adjacent to the spinal cord should be preserved and protected. Only vessels that supply the tumor may be sacrificed. Upon completion of the tumor removal, the spinal cord is often found to return immediately to a more normal anatomic position. However, with long-standing neoplasms, the spinal cord may be thinned to a ribbon-like shape and unable to regain its former bulk. Once satisfied that a gross total resection of the tumor has been accomplished, meticulous hemostasis is obtained with bipolar cautery. The wound is irrigated with copious amounts of normal saline solution and the arachnoid is repositioned over the spinal cord and reapproximated with interrupted 6-0 nonabsorbable sutures. This maneuver helps to prevent the spinal cord from scarring to the dura mater. This is also recommended for intramedullary tumors.[19] The dura mater is then closed in a watertight fashion with running 5-0 non-absorbable sutures. Prior to the final suture placement, the thecal sac is re-expanded with sterile normal saline solution to aid in the prevention of epidural hemorrhage. Hemostasis can be achieved with simple re-expansion of the thecal sac to tamponade the epidural venous channels. The paraspinous musculature and fascial tissues are then closed in anatomic layers with interrupted absorbable sutures. Clips are used to approximate the skin.

RESULTS

Short-term outcome in the surgical treatment of intradural extra-medullary neoplasms is generally excellent, with very gratifying improvement of neurologic function, as the rule.[20] Depending on the severity of the initial presentation, and there is no evidence of vascular injury during the operation, excellent improvement in neurologic function can be anticipated. Most patients will return to normal or near normal status. Physical therapy and occupational therapy are considered to be standard postoperative treatments to optimize the neurologic recovery period. An initial surge of neurologic improvement is witnessed in the first 6 weeks following surgical intervention, and dramatic results can often occur. However, long-term recovery can continue for up to a year. The risk of recurrence is estimated to be less than 10% in gross total resections of schwannomas but may jump 20% at 5 years in meningiomas.[18] In subtotal resection, or in "en plaque" meningiomas that cannot be completely removed, then a symptomatic recurrence rate of approximately 80% can be expected.[18] As a general rule, recurrences of most intradural extramedullary tumors are treated by repeat surgical intervention. Postresection, radiation therapy is controversy and no clear consensus is expressed in the literature on that matter. A follow-up MRI study is recommended at 6 months, then 1 year after surgery. If the MRI does not demonstrate obvious recurrence, a follow-up study is scheduled after 2 years. If this subsequent study does not demonstrate tumor recurrence, a follow-up study at 5 years is recommended.

Complications related to surgical intervention for intradural extramedullary tumors include standard risks, such as hemorrhage, infection, cerebrospinal fluid leak. The most significant and troublesome complications consist of new significant neurologic deficits, which often do not resolve. Sensorimotor deficits are more likely to recover than bladder or bowel/autonomic dysfunction. These intraoperative injuries are typically related to vascular insult of the spinal cord or manipulation of the neural elements.

Cerebrospinal fluid leaks represent one of the more dreaded complications since treatment may be problematic. If a leak occurs through the wound site, then standard treatment includes revision of the wound or lumbar drainage for several days . If a persistent leak occurs despite treatment, then revision of the surgical wound is warranted. In dumb-bell-shaped tumors that develop pleural or retroperitoneal cerebrospinal fluid fistulae, a trial with chest tube drainage is performed. However, this maneuver is often unsuccessful and open repair is required.

CONCLUSIONS

The surgical management of spinal intradural extramedullary neoplasms has become simplified in the past 10 years. The excellent surgical outcomes obtained today are primarily related to the early diagnosis achieved with new neuroradiological

CLINICAL PEARLS

- Surgery is the gold standard in the treatment of intradural extramedullary tumors.

- MRI study in three planes and careful preoperative planning with regard to the location and size of the tumor will dictate the most appropriate surgical approach.

- An intracapsular tumor debulking is performed to achieve safe tumor removal.

- Traction on the spinal cord should be avoided at all times.

- In antero-lateral lesions, division of the dentate ligament is helpful in rotating the spinal cord away from the surgeon and providing superior access to the intradural extramedullary space.

diagnostic studies (MRI) and to improved surgical techniques. In addition, intraoperative electrophysiologic monitoring has been exceedingly valuable in predicting, detecting and preventing neurological injury. In summary, neurosurgeons today can anticipate a very satisfying surgical result in the treatment of intradural extramedullary neoplasms.

This chapter contains material from the first edition, and I am grateful to the author of that chapter for his contribution.

ACKNOWLEDGMENTS

I also wish to thank Dr Danielle Balériaux for her great help with the neuroradiological images and Dr Daniele Morelli for his technical support.

REFERENCES

1. Levy W, Latchaw J, Hahn J, et al. Spinal neurofibromas: a report of 66 cases and a comparison with meningiomas. *Neurosurgery* 1986; 18: 331–4.

2. Namer IJ, Pamir MN, Benli K, Saglam S, Erbengi A. Spinal meningiomas. *Neurochirurgia* 1987; 30: 11–15.

3. McCormick P, Post K, Stein B. Intradural extramedullary tumors in adults. *Neurosurg Clin North Am* 1990; 1: 591–608.

4. Abernathey CD, Onofrio BM, Schneithauer BW, Pairolero PC, Shives TC. Surgical management of giant sacral schwannomas. *J Neurosurg* 1986; 65: 286–95.

5. Dodge HW Jr, Svien H, Camp J, Craig W. Tumors of the spinal cord without neurologic manifestations producing low back and sciatic pain. *Proc Staff Meet Mayo Clin* 1951; 26: 88.

6. Horrax G, Poppen JL, Wu WQ, Weadon PR. Meningiomas and neurofibromas of the spinal cord: certain clinical features and end results. *Surg Clin North Am* 1949; 29: 659–65.

7. Blews D, Wang H, Ashok J, et al. Intradural spinal metastases in pediatric patients with primary intracranial neoplasms: Gd-DTPA-

enhanced MR vs CT myelography. *J Comput Assist Tomogr* 1990; 14: 730–5.

8. Scotti G, Scialfa G, Colombo N, *et al*. MR imaging of intradural extramedullary tumors of the cervical spine. *J Comput Assist Tomogr* 1985; 9: 1037–41.

9. Sze G. Magnetic resonance imaging in the evaluation of spinal tumors. *Cancer* 1991; 67: 1229–41.

10. Takemoto K, Matsumura Y, Hashimoto H, *et al*. MR imaging of intraspinal tumors–capability in histological differentiation and compartmentalization of extramedullary tumors. *Neuroradiology* 1988; 30: 303–9.

11. Parizel P, Baleriaux D, Rodesch G, *et al*. Gd-DTPA-enhanced MR imaging of spinal tumors. *AJR* 1989; 152: 1087–96.

12. Dillon W, Normal D, Newton T, *et al*. Intradural spinal cord lesions: Gd-DTPA-enhanced MR imaging. *AJNR* 1989; 170: 229–37.

13. Hu HP, Huang QL. Signal intensity correlation of MRI with pathological findings in spinal neurinomas. *Neuroradiology* 1992; 34: 98–102.

14. Sze G. Neoplastic disease of the spinal cord. In: Atlas SW (ed.). *Magnetic Resonance Imaging of the Brain and Spine*. Philadelphia: Lippincott Williams & Wilkins; 2002: 1715–67.

15. Deletis V. Intraoperative monitoring for the functional integrity of the motor pathway. In: Devinsky O, Beric A, Dogali M (eds). *Advances in Neurology*. New York: Raven Press; 1994: 201–14.

16. Fischer G, Brotchi J. *Intramedullary Spinal Cord Tumors*. Stuttgart: Thieme; 1996: 80–1.

17. Lot G, George B. Cervical neuromas with extradural components: surgical management in a series of 57 patients. *Neurosurgery* 1997; 41: 813–22.

18. Klekamp J, Samii M. Surgical results for spinal meningiomas. *Surg Neurol* 1999; 52: 552–62.

19. Brotchi J. Intrinsic spinal cord resection. *Neurosurgery* 2002; 50: 1059–63.

20. Ciapetta P, Domenicucci M, Raco M. Spinal meningiomas: prognosis and recovery factors in 22 cases with severe motor deficits. *Acta Neurol Scand* 1988; 77: 27–30.

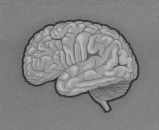

INTRAMEDULLARY TUMORS AND TUMORS OF THE CAUDA EQUINA

43

Kent C New and Allan H Friedman

Over the past 30 years, technological advances have aided the diagnosis and treatment of intramedullary spinal cord tumors. Magnetic resonance imaging (MRI) has enhanced our ability to detect these lesions, and microsurgical techniques have better enabled us to resect some of these tumors surgically.

Intramedullary spinal cord tumors comprise 4–10% of all central nervous system tumors. They account for about 25% of adult intradural spinal tumors, but in children, in whom the incidence of meningiomas and neurofibromas is low, they account for 50% of intradural spinal tumors.[1] Gliomas, particularly ependymomas and astrocytomas, are the most commonly encountered intramedullary spinal cord tumors (Table 43.1).[2] Ependymomas are slightly more common than astrocytomas in adults, but astrocytomas are more prevalent in children and adolescents. Anaplastic astrocytomas and glioblastomas account for approximately 10% of spinal cord gliomas. Hemangioblastomas account for 3–4% of intramedullary spinal cord tumors.

Tumors that rarely occur within the spinal cord include primary tumors such as gangliogliomas, oligodendrogliomas, and melanomas, as well as metastatic tumors. Benign tumors such as lipomas, dermoids, epidermoids, cavernous angiomas, and schwannomas have been noted. Intramedullary mass lesions can result from inflammatory processes, such as sarcoidosis, infection, and multiple sclerosis and may be difficult to differentiate from intrinsic tumors[3,4] both clinically and radiologically.

Table 43.1 Intramedullary spinal tumors

Most common tumors	Less common tumors	Expansile nontumorous lesions
Ependymoma	Oligodendroglioma	Multiple sclerosis
Astrocytoma	Ganglioglioma	Infections
Hemangioblastoma	Malignant glioma	Abscess
	Schwannoma	Sarcoidosis
	Melanoma	
	Metastatic tumors	
	Teratoma	
	Neuroenteric cyst	
	Dermoid tumor	
	Epidermoid tumor	
	Lipoma	
	Cavernous angiomas	

INTRAMEDULLARY TUMORS

Ependymomas

Ependymomas are the most common intramedullary spinal cord tumors encountered in the adult population (Figure 43.1). These tumors appear to be discrete with little invasive potential. The gray to purple tumor tissue readily separates from the adjacent white spinal cord. The tumor is frequently capped by a cyst over its cranial pole; less frequently there is a cyst below its caudal pole. Histologic examination most often reveals an epithelial ependymoma comprised of sheets of cells broken up by pseudorosettes (anuclear zones comprised of cytoplasmic processes surrounding blood vessels). True rosettes are rarely seen. The occasional tanycytic ependymoma contains free-standing anuclear areas of fibrillary processes reminiscent of an astrocytoma. In fact, this histology may lead to the erroneous diagnosis of an astrocytoma. Myxopapillary ependymomas are virtually restricted to the cauda equina and filum terminale.

Intramedullary ependymomas occur anywhere along the spinal cord, although they have a slight propensity to appear in the cervical region. They are heralded by a slow, insidious clinical course, usually evolving for years prior to diagnosis. On MRI, the tumor appears as a well-circumscribed, gadolinium-enhancing mass capped by a nonenhancing cyst.

The primary treatment of intramedullary spinal cord ependymoma is surgical resection. Authors report complete resection in 50–100% of these lesions. The resection rate has improved with advances in microsurgical techniques.[2,5–7] Although approximately 50% of patients develop new neurologic deficits immediately after surgery, the deficits are transient in all but 5–10% of patients. The patients' postoperative neurologic function is most strongly influenced by their preoperative state.[2] Marked neurologic improvement of a long-standing preoperative neurologic deficit is rare.[7] If the surgeon achieves gross total resection, the rate of recurrence is 5–10% over a 5-year follow-up period.[8] Radiation therapy is reserved for patients in whom gross total resection cannot be achieved.[8,9] Even in this group, the efficacy of radiation therapy is suggested but not proven by the available literature.

Astrocytomas

Ninety per cent of spinal cord astrocytomas are well differentiated. These "benign" lesions can be divided into two types: diffusely infiltrating and pilocytic. Infiltrating astrocytomas consist of cells that permeate a localized portion of the spinal cord,

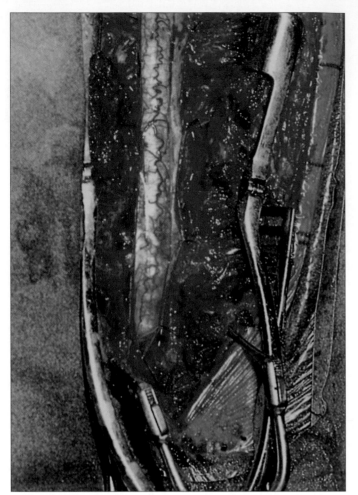

Figure 43.1 Ependymoma: intraoperative view. This 52-year-old female had a 3-year history of episodic radicular burning pain. Following laminectomies, her spinal cord was found to be enlarged by an ependymoma and its adjacent cyst. Note the stretched appearance of the vessels on the dorsum of the spinal cord.

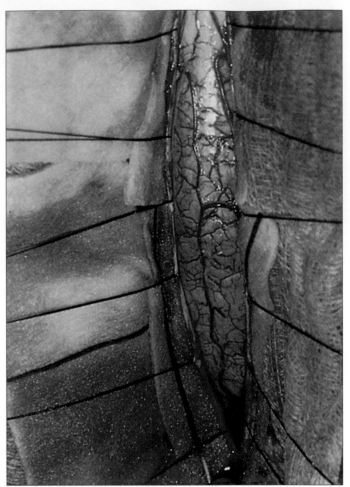

Figure 43.2 Astrocytoma: intraoperative view. This 14-year-old presented with a 6-year history of scoliosis and 4 months of progressive leg numbness. At the time of surgery, his conus medullaris was found to be enlarged by an infiltrating astrocytoma.

causing a restricted swelling. Although the heart of these tumors appears to consist of a pure population of tumor cells, these cells intermingle with the normal spinal cord around the tumor's periphery. Pilocytic astrocytomas are similar to their cranial counterparts (Figure 43.2). They are relatively discrete lesions composed of compact fascicles of elongated cells separated by loose areas of stellate cells and microcysts. Pilocytic astrocytomas are frequently associated with large cysts that in extreme cases span the entire spinal cord. Ten per cent of intramedullary astrocytomas are malignant.[5]

The progressive neurologic deficit produced by an intramedullary astrocytoma may unfold slowly.[10] One long-term follow-up study documenting the natural history of childhood spinal cord astrocytomas demonstrated an 80% 5-year survival rate and 55% 10-year survival rate. It should be noted that others have not reported such an optimistic prognosis.[11,12] In adults the natural history of the disease varies greatly, and authors have reported 5-year survival rates between 57% and 86%.[13,14] Malignant astrocytomas are associated with a relentlessly progressive course with average postoperative survival of 6 months in adults and 13 months in children.[15]

On a myelogram an intramedullary spinal cord astrocytoma appears as a focal swelling of the spinal cord. Infiltrating fibrillary astrocytomas present as diffuse and nonenhancing masses when imaged on MRI (Figure 43.3). The MRI scan may demonstrate cysts within the infiltrating tumor. Pilocytic astrocytomas enhance densely with gadolinium on MRI scan (Figure 43.4). These tumors are usually associated with a large peritumoral cyst that is often several times as large as the tumor nodule.

The optimal therapy for intramedullary spinal cord tumors has yet to be determined. Surgical therapy is apparently not beneficial when treating malignant spinal cord astrocytomas.[16] Many childhood tumors appear to be amenable to surgical excision;[11,17] short-term follow-up of surgical therapy for astrocytomas presenting during childhood and adolescence demonstrates good results, but long-term follow-up remains to be published in detail.[18] The results of surgical therapy for low-grade spinal cord astrocytomas in adults are not as good;[2,16,19] surgery is associated with a significant incidence of neurologic worsening and long-term follow-up demonstrates a high incidence of tumor recurrence.[2] The available literature has failed to demonstrate a significant correlation between prognosis and degree of surgical resection.

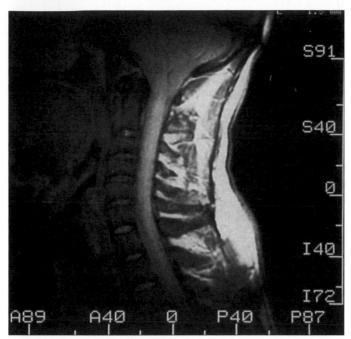

Figure 43.3 MRI (TR 2000, TE 35) demonstrates a diffuse infiltrating astrocytoma of the cervical spinal cord. This lesion did not enhance with gadolinium.

Radiation therapy is difficult to assess for juveniles because these patients have such a variable long-term survival rate when untreated. Radiation therapy appears to be effective in impeding tumor growth in adults.[8,14] Chemotherapy for spinal cord astrocytomas has shown some promise in children,[20] but has been less well studied in adults.[21]

Metastatic tumors

As patients with metastatic malignancies are living longer, metastatic tumors of the spinal cord are becoming more common, now comprising approximately 5% of all spinal cord tumors.[22] The most common primaries are lung cancer, breast cancer, and lymphoma.[21] Spinal cord metastasis can produce symptoms without significantly enlarging the spinal cord, and therefore are notoriously difficult to detect by radiologic techniques.[23] Gadolinium-enhanced MRI appears to be the best method of detecting these lesions.[24] Most patients are treated with radiation as surgery usually results in subtotal resection. Chemotherapy is recommended for patients with associated carcinomatous meningitis.[21] Survival is approximately 5% at 1 year.[25]

Hemangioblastomas

Hemangioblastomas are slow-growing neoplasms that make up approximately 5–10% of intramedullary spinal cord tumors and usually present as slowly enlarging masses or, rarely, subarachnoid hemorrhage.[22,26] These highly vascular tumors appear in the spinal cord either as a solid mass or as a nodule in a cyst (Figures 43.5, 43.6) and are comprised of clumps of yellow lipid-laden cells separated by pink vascular tissue. In the cystic variety, it is usually the cyst that makes up the majority of the mass and causes the neurologic symptoms. The nodule within the cyst has a propensity to appear on the dorsum of the spinal cord and can be identified by the tortuous arteries and varices emerging from its surface. One-quarter to one-third of patients with intramedullary spinal cord hemangioblastomas have other manifestations of von Hippel–Lindau disease.[27]

The tumor cyst shows a higher protein content than cerebrospinal fluid on the MRI (Figure 43.7). The elusive tumor nodule can be located on a gadolinium-enhanced MRI scan. If the tumor nodule is resected, the tumor can be cured. The gadolinium-

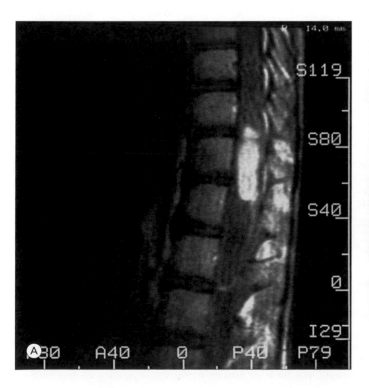

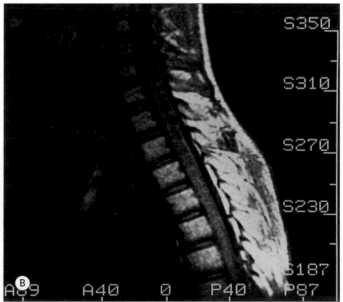

Figure 43.4 (A) MRI (TR 500, TE 20) contrasted with gadolinium demonstrating a well-circumscribed astrocytoma within the spinal cord. **(B)** The cyst associated with this tumor extends up into the cervical spinal cord.

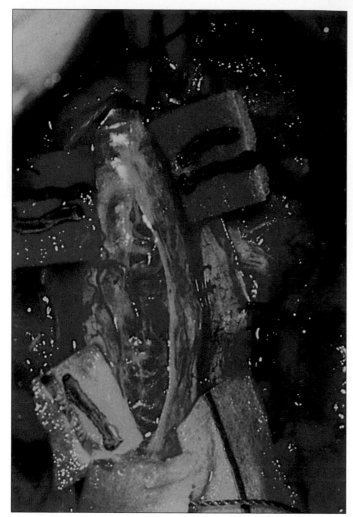

Figure 43.5 Hemangioblastoma: intraoperative view. A 26-year-old presented with progressive leg numbness and weakness. This intraoperative photograph demonstrates venous varices emanating from the dorsum of an intramedullary solid spinal cord hemangioblatoma.

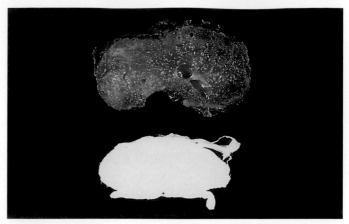

Figure 43.6 Following resection of this lesion, the patient had no new neurologic deficit. For comparison, an axial cross-section of the resected tumor (top) is shown with a cross-section of a normal spinal cord obtained from an autopsy of a different patient.

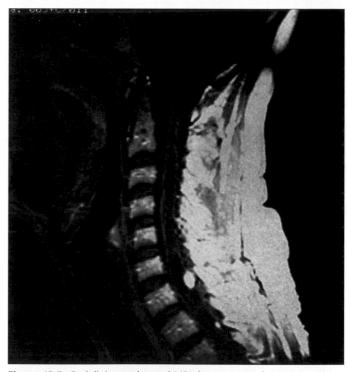

Figure 43.7 Gadolinium-enhanced MRI demonstrates the two tumor nodules and the extensive cyst of this spinal hemangioblastoma.

enhanced MRI scan often demonstrates asymptomatic tumors in patients with von Hippel–Lindau disease.

Lipomas

Lipomas of the spinal cord are most often intimately related to the substance of the cord (Figure 43.8). These lesions are usually not amenable to complete resection.

Schwannomas

Schwannomas are usually found on spinal nerve roots, but may occur completely within the substance of the spinal cord.[28]

CLINICAL PRESENTATION

Early diagnosis of an intramedullary spinal cord tumor is a challenge for the clinical neurologist.[29] The earliest manifestations of an intraspinal mass are nonspecific and often masquerade as a more common and benign musculoskeletal disorder. The average reported time between the onset of symptoms and the establishment of the correct diagnosis is $3^1/_2$ years.

The most common initial symptom of an intramedullary spinal cord tumor is pain. Unfortunately, the pain that accompanies these lesions is usually not distinctive and cannot be classified. Most often the pain is initially a deep, dull ache located adjacent to the affected spine. As time passes, the pain radiates either around the torso or into an extremity depending on the level of

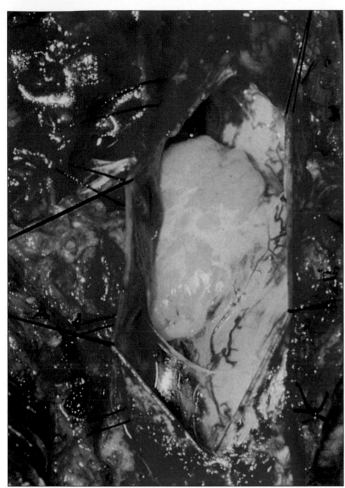

Figure 43.8 Intraoperative photograph demonstrating an exophytic lipoma infiltrating into the dorsum of the spinal cord. Although the exophytic component was resected, the intramedullary portion could only be incompletely removed.

the tumor. The pain tends to be diffuse, eschewing dermatomal boundaries. Although the discomfort occasionally fluctuates in intensity, it almost always becomes more severe with time.

Occasionally the pain takes on characteristics that should raise the suspicions of the examining physician.[30] If the pain is worse at night and awakens the patient from a sound sleep, the possibility of a spinal tumor must be considered. Unfortunately, only a minority of patients report nocturnal pain. A small group of patients report characteristic burning or intermittently lancinating pain. A patient with burning sciatic pain and a negative Lasègue's sign is likely to have a spinal cord tumor.

Some patients do not note radiating pain but report paresthesias in the dermatomes innervated by the compressed spinal cord. This zone of paresthesias tends to extend caudally with time.

Neurologic deficits may not appear until years after the onset of pain, but once present these deficits often accelerate rapidly.

A smaller group of patients present with weakness unaccompanied by numbness. This weakness may be only lower motor neuron weakness or a combination of upper and lower motor neuron weakness mimicking amyotrophic lateral sclerosis. Cervical spinal cord tumors may cause wasting confined to the patient's hands or, more rarely, the proximal musculature of the arms.

Sensory deficits are rarely an early manifestation of a spinal cord tumor, although such deficits appear as the clinical syndrome unfolds. The classic sensory deficit produced by a lesion intrinsic to the spinal cord is a dissociated, suspended sensory level that descends with time. Neurologic examination of adjacent dermatomes reveals loss of pain and temperature sensation, although touch, position, and vibratory sensation remain. Unfortunately this classic picture only occurs in approximately 20% of patients harboring intrinsic spinal cord tumors.

Incontinence is usually a late manifestation of cervical and thoracic tumors, but it occurs early in a patient who has a tumor of the conus medullaris.

Patients only rarely present with sudden neurologic deficit secondary to a hemorrhage within the tumor.

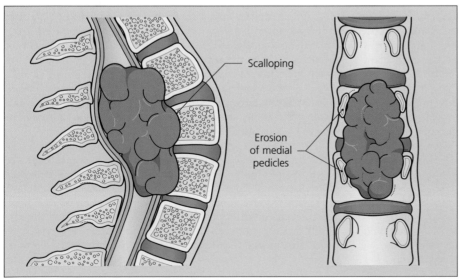

Scalloping

Erosion of medial pedicles

Figure 43.9 Although roentgenograms are a poor screening tool for the detection of an intramedullary tumor, the observant physician can sometimes note erosion of the medial pedicles and scalloping of the posterior vertebral body, which betray the presence of an intraspinal mass.

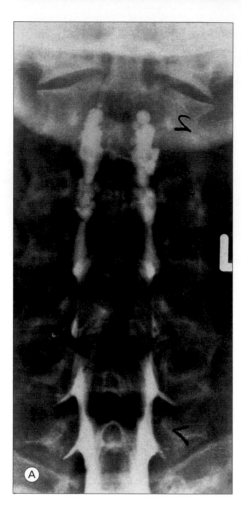

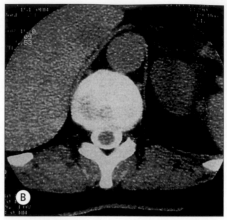

Figure 43.10 (A) Cervical myelogram demonstrating a smooth widening of the spinal cord which reveals the location of an intramedullary spinal cord tumor. **(B)** This thoracic CT myelogram better defines the enlarged spinal cord, which thins the subarachnoid space.

IMAGING

Plain roentgenograms are a poor screening tool for intramedullary spinal cord tumors, but the observant physician may detect indirect evidence of an intraspinal mass. These indirect signs include scalloping of the posterior border of the vertebral body, erosion of the medial pedicles, and thinning of the lamina (Figure 43.9). More frequently, plain roentgenograms demonstrate the nonspecific finding of scoliosis.

An intramedullary tumor can be imaged by myelography and computed tomography (CT). It appears on myelography as a non-specific widening of the spinal cord shadow seen on antero-posterior (Figure 43.10A) and lateral views. This spinal cord enlargement is demonstrated on the postmyelogram CT scan (Figure 43.10B).

MRI with and without contrast gives the physician the most information concerning intramedullary spinal cord tumors.[24,31] MRI allows the physician to see the extent of the tumor, and the gadolinium enhancement differentiates the tumor from an adjacent cyst (Figure 43.11). In the past, spinal angiography has been used to seek out the vascular nodule associated with a cystic hemangioblastoma. In most cases, the gadolinium-enhanced MRI scan obviates the need for this study.

SURGICAL MANAGEMENT[1,32,33]

Most intramedullary spinal cord tumors are approached through an incision made between the posterior columns (Figure 43.12), although occasionally the best approach is through the dorsal root entry zone or even the anterior spinal cord.[34] The posterior aspect of the spinal cord is exposed by removing the overlying lamina. When cervical laminectomies are performed, special care is taken to maintain the integrity of the facets in order to preserve spinal stability. If feasible, the lamina are removed en bloc and wired or sutured back in place at the end of the case.[35]

If the tumor is wholly contained within the spinal cord, the spinal cord is opened between the posterior columns over the length of the solid portion of the tumor. The midline is usually easily discerned. Even in a distorted spinal cord, the midline is marked by the attachment of the posterior septum of arachnoid. The surgeon confirms this plane of dissection by noting the fine vessels that pass between the posterior columns.

If the tumor is an ependymoma, the surgeon is likely to encounter a gray to purple capsule that easily separates from the softer white spinal cord. Once the posterior portion of the tumor is separated from the spinal cord, the pial edges are gently retracted using 7-0 Prolene suture. The capsule is opened and a

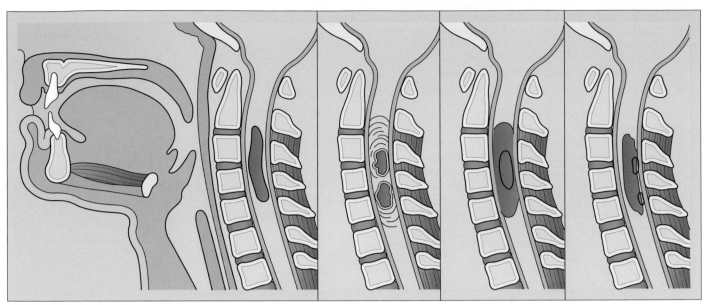

Figure 43.11 MRI is the best method for detecting intramedullary spinal tumors. These line drawings depict the MRI appearance of commonly seen intramedullary tumors (left to right): ependymoma, infiltrating astrocytoma, pilocytic astrocytoma, and hemangioblastoma.

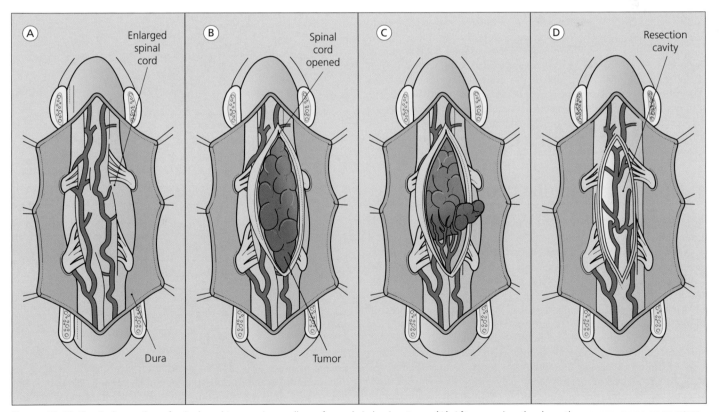

Figure 43.12 Surgical resection of spinal cord tumors is usually performed via laminectomy. **(A)** After opening the dura, the neurosurgeon encounters a spinal cord that is swollen by the intramedullary mass. **(B)** A myelotomy is made between the dorsal columns. The gray tumor separates from the white matter of the spinal cord around the periphery. **(C)** The pole of the tumor is mobilized, and blood vessels emanating from the anterior spinal artery are coagulated and cut. **(D)** Following surgery, the resection cavity is lined by shaggy-looking thinned spinal cord that usually functions quite well.

portion of the tumor's center is removed leaving 1 or 2 mm of tumor circumferentially. Overly vigorous gutting of the tumor will lead to fragmentation of the friable tumor capsule. The circumferential dissection around the waist of the tumor is continued using blunt dissection. Small feeding and draining vessels are cauterized and cut. Occasionally the plane separating the tumor from the spinal cord will be lost over a small portion of the capsule. Once the problem region has been flanked by a dissection above and below, the plane between the spinal cord and tumor in the problem area will become clearer.

Dissecting the poles of the tumor is more difficult. If a cyst is present, the end of the tumor is obvious. If there is no cyst, the tumor seems to taper into a root that blends into the spinal cord. As this cord of tumor tissue is pursued, histologic confirmation verifies that tumor and not gliotic spinal cord is being resected. Once one pole has been dissected free, it is gently retracted from its bed. Since the tumor's blood supply comes from the anterior spinal artery, vessels along the anterior aspect of the tumor are sought out, coagulated, and cut as the tumor is extracted.

If the spinal cord harbors an infiltrating astrocytoma, a tumor margin may be encountered, in which case dissection proceeds as outlined for ependymomas. One pole usually blends with the normal spinal cord. When the edge of the tumor is no longer obvious, the resection should stop. In cystic astrocytomas with a tumor nodule, the tumor is usually of a different consistency than the normal spinal cord, allowing the nodule to be grossly resected.

Hemangioblastomas have a propensity to occur at the dorsum of the spinal cord. When the lesion is associated with a large cyst, the edge of the pia around the tumor nodule is coagulated and the plaque of tumor is easily removed. When a larger solid tumor is encountered, the tumor capsule is gently coagulated with a bipolar cautery to diminish the tumor. The contracted tumor is then carefully dissected from the surrounding spinal cord; the feeding and draining vessels are coagulated and cut as they are encountered. Operating within the hemangioblastoma is treacherous, and gutting the tumor usually results in severe hemorrhage. Occasionally, a large tumor is bisected to facilitate its removal.

TUMORS OF THE CAUDA EQUINA

Primary tumors of the cauda equina are listed in Table 43.2. Ependymomas of the cauda equina have almost exclusively a myxopapillary histology.[36] Some ependymomas are quite smooth, seemingly contained by the thinly stretched filum terminale (Figure 43.13). Others are nodular, surrounding and incorporating the nerves of the cauda equina. On histologic examination, these tumors contain rings of ependymal cells that surround cores of blood vessels and mucin.

Epidermoid and dermoid tumors of the spine tend to occur at the cauda equina. Although these tumors are usually discrete, they may be bound to the surrounding nerve roots. Neurofibromas are well-circumscribed lesions involving only a single nerve root until late in their course. Meningiomas rarely occur in the lumbar spinal canal.

Clinical presentation

Pain is the most common presenting symptom of a tumor of the cauda equina and may precede any demonstrable neurologic deficits by several years (Figure 43.14).[37] For approximately 50% of patients, the pain becomes more severe at night or when the

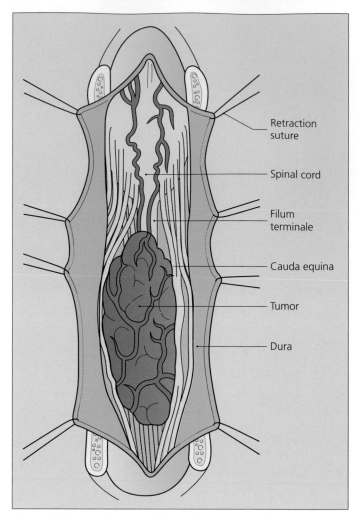

Figure 43.13 Ependymomas of the lumbar spinal canal are tenuously contained within the filum terminale. Initially, they displace the nerve roots of the cauda equina, but as the tumor enlarges the roots become encased.

Table 43.2 Tumors of the cauda equina	
Ependymoma	Lipoma
Schwannoma	Metastatic tumors
Meningioma	

patient assumes a recumbent position for any length of time. Unlike the more common musculoskeletal back pain, this pain is not relieved by shifting position while the patient remains recumbent.[38] The pain is only mitigated when the patient stands or sits up. Frequently the patient will report sleeping at night in the sitting position.

Patients with tumors of the cauda equina may present with cauda equina syndrome, which classically includes lumbar pain, urinary retention, and saddle anesthesia. More rarely, patients with tumors of the cauda equina present with painless, progressive leg weakness. Patients with myxopapillary ependymomas occa-

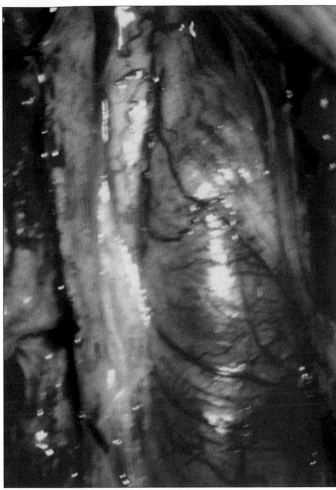

Figure 43.14 Schwannoma: intraoperative view. This patient presented with progressive radicular right leg pain. At the time of surgery, a large schwannoma was found to be compressing the conus medullaris and the nerve roots of the cauda equina.

sionally present with subarachnoid hemorrhage or papilledema, presumably the result of an increase in spinal fluid protein.

Imaging

Lumbar spine roentgenograms performed on a patient with a tumor of the cauda equina occasionally demonstrate widening of the intrapedicular distance, erosion of the posterior vertebral body, or enlargement of a neural foramen. Because of their subarachnoid location, these lesions are readily demonstrated by myelography or MRI.

Surgical management

Surgery has been reported to be successful in removing approximately 50% of myxopapillary ependymomas. Urinary retention is the most common side-effect of this procedure. It can only be assumed that newer imaging techniques that allow for earlier diagnosis and advances in microsurgical techniques will increase the number of tumors that can be completely removed. Neurofibromas usually remain discrete and can be completely removed surgically without adding to the patient's neurologic deficit.

CLINICAL PEARLS

● The most common presenting symptom of an intramedullary spinal cord tumor is pain along the spine adjacent to the tumor, which is sometimes worse at night.

● The most common intramedullary spinal cord tumor in an adult is ependymoma, followed closely by astrocytoma, which is the most common in children and adolescents. The most common tumor of the cauda equina is myxopapillary ependymoma.

● MRI performed with and without contrast enhancement is the most useful imaging modality in the evaluation of spinal cord tumors.

● Ependymomas, hemangioblastomas, and pilocytic astrocytomas of the spinal cord are frequently amenable to gross total surgical resection, while infiltrating astrocytomas and metastases usually are not.

● The prognosis in cases of spinal cord tumors is highly variable, and correlates most closely with the patient's preoperative neurologic status and tumor grade.

REFERENCES

1. McCormick PC, Stein BM. Intramedullary tumors in adults. *Neurosurg Clin North Am* 1990; 1: 609–30.
2. Fornari M, Pluchino F, Solero CL, *et al*. Microsurgical treatment of intramedullary spinal cord tumours. *Acta Neurochir Suppl* 1988; 43: 3–8.
3. Choksey MS, Powell M, Gibb WRG, *et al*. A conus tuberculoma mimicking an intramedullary tumour: a case report and review of the literature. *Br J Neurosurg* 1989; 3: 117–22.
4. Lammoglia FJ, Short SR, Sweet DE, *et al*. Multiple sclerosis presenting as an intramedullary cervical cord tumor. *Kans Med* 1989; 90: 219–21.
5. McCormick PC, Torres R, Post KD, *et al*. Intramedullary ependymoma of the spinal cord. *J Neurosurg* 1990; 72: 523–32.
6. Guidetti B, Mercuri S, Vagnozzi R. Long-term results of the surgical treatment of 129 intramedullary spinal gliomas. *J Neurosurg* 1981; 54: 323–30.
7. Schwartz TH, McCormick PC. Intramedullary ependymomas: clinical presentation, surgical treatment strategies and prognosis. *J Neuro-Oncol* 2000; 47: 211–18.
8. Isaacson SR. Radiation therapy and the management of intramedullary spinal cord tumors. *J Neuro-Oncol* 2000; 47: 231–8.
9. Shaw EG, Evans RG, Scheithauer BW, *et al*. Radiotherapeutic management of adult intraspinal ependymomas. *Int J Radiat Oncol Biol Phys* 1986; 12: 323–7.
10. Rossitch E Jr, Zeidman SM, Berger PC, *et al*. Clinical and pathological analysis of spinal cord astrocytomas in children. *Neurosurgery* 1990; 27: 193–6.
11. Reimer R, Onofrio BM. Astrocytomas of the spinal cord in children and adolescents. *J Neurosurg* 1985; 63: 669–75.

12. Hardison HH, Packer RJ, Rorke LB, *et al*. Outcome of children with primary intramedullary spinal cord tumors. *Child's Nerv Syst* 1987; 3: 89–92.

13. Sandler HM, Papadopoulos SM, Thornton AF, Jr, Ross DA. Spinal cord astrocytomas: results of therapy. *Neurosurgery* 1992; 30: 490–3.

14. McLaughlin MP, Buatti JM, Marcus RB, Jr, *et al*. Outcome after radiotherapy of primary spinal cord glial tumors. *Rad Oncol Invest* 1998; 6: 276–80.

15. Houten JK, Cooper PR. Spinal cord astrocytomas: presentation, management and outcome. *J Neuro-Oncol* 2000; 47: 219–24.

16. Cohen AR, Wisoff JH, Allen JC, Epstein F. Malignant astrocytomas of the spinal cord. *J Neurosurg* 1989; 70: 50–4.

17. Epstein F, Epstein N. Surgical treatment of spinal cord astrocytomas of childhood: a series of 19 patients. *J Neurosurg* 1982; 57: 685–9.

18. Allen JC, Lassoff SJ. Outcome after surgery for intramedullary spinal cord tumors. *Neurosurgery* 1980; 26: 1091 [Letter].

19. Cooper PR. Outcome after operative treatment of intramedullary spinal cord tumors in adults: intermediate and long-term results in 51 patients. *Neurosurgery* 1989; 25: 855–9.

20. Allen JV, Avivner S, Yates AJ, *et al*. Treatment of high-grade spinal cord astrocytoma of childhood with "8-in-1" chemotherapy and radiotherapy: a pilot study of CCG-945. *J Neurosurg* 1998; 88: 215–20.

21. Balmaceda C. Chemotherapy for intramedullary spinal cord tumors. *J Neuro-Oncol* 2000; 47: 293–307.

22. Kane PJ, El-Mahdy W, Singh A, *et al*. Spinal intradural tumours: Part II. Intramedullary. *Br J Neurosurg* 1999; 13; 558–63.

23. Winkelman MD, Adelstein DJ, Karlins NL. Intramedullary spinal cord metastasis. *Arch Neurol* 1987; 44: 526–31.

24. Sze G, Krol G, Zimmerman RD, *et al*. Intramedullary disease of the spine: diagnosis using gadolinium-DTPA-enhanced MR imaging. *Am J Roentgenol* 1988; 151: 1193–204.

25. Grem JL, Burgess J, Trump DL. Clinical features and natural history of intramedullary spinal cord metastasis. *Cancer* 1985; 56: 2305–14.

26. Neumann HPH, Eggert HR, Weigel K, *et al*. Hemangioblastomas of the central nervous system: a 10-year study with special reference to von Hippel–Lindau syndrome. *J Neurosurg* 1989; 70: 24–30.

27. Browne TR, Adams RD, Roberson GH. Hemangioblastoma of the spinal cord. *Arch Neurol* 1976; 33: 435–41.

28. Ross DA, Edwards MSB, Wilson CB. Intramedullary neurilemomas of the spinal cord: report of two cases and review of the literature. *Neurosurgery* 1986; 19: 458–64.

29. Guidetti B, Fortuna A. Differential diagnosis of intramedullary and extramedullary tumors. In: Vinken PJ, Bruyn GW (eds). *Handbook of Clinical Neurology*. Amsterdam: North-Holland; 1975; 51–75.

30. Austin GM. The significance and nature of pain in tumors of the spinal cord. *Surg Forum* 1959; 10: 782–5.

31. Scotti G, Scialfa G, Colombo N, *et al*. Magnetic resonance diagnosis of intramedullary tumors of the spinal cord. *Neuroradiology* 1987; 29: 130–5.

32. Malis LI. Intramedullary spinal cord tumors. *Clin Neurosurg* 1978; 25: 512–39.

33. Stein BM. Surgery of intramedullary spinal cord tumors. *Clin Neurosurg* 1979; 26: 529–42.

34. Ahyai A, Woerner U, Markakis E. Surgical treatment of intramedullary tumors (spinal cord and medulla oblongata): analysis of 16 cases. *Neurosurg Rev* 1990; 13: 45–52.

35. Zide BM, Wisoff JH, Epstein FJ. Closure of extensive and complicated laminectomy wounds. *J Neurosurg* 1987; 67: 59–64.

36. Sonneland PRL, Scheithauer BW, Onofrio BM. Myxopapillary ependymoma: a clinicopathologic and immunocytochemical study of 77 cases. *Cancer* 1985; 56: 883–93.

37. Fearnside MR, Adams CBT. Tumours of the cauda equina. *J Neurol Neurosurg Psychiatr* 1978; 41: 24–31.

38. Wiss DA. An unusual cause of sciatica and back pain: ependymoma of the cauda equina: case report. *J Bone Joint Surg* 1982; 64A: 772–3.

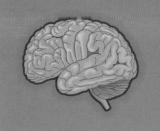

TUMORS OF THE CRANIAL BASE

44

Nevo Margalit and Chandranath Sen

Tumors of the cranial base arise from or are in the vicinity of the bony structures at the base of the brain (Table 44.1, Figure 44.1). These tumors may originate from the extracranial tissues, namely, the paranasal sinuses, pharynx, and connective tissues, secondarily invading the basal bones, meninges, and even the brain. Other tumors, such as osteosarcomas, fibrous dysplasia, chordomas, and chondrosarcoma, may arise from the basal bone and cartilage.

Primarily intracranial tumors from the meninges, blood vessels, cranial nerves, and pituitary gland may arise from and encroach upon this region. Despite their varied histology and biologic behavior, these tumors have a common feature – they are difficult to reach and involve critical structures. The base of the skull represents a transition area through which important blood vessels, like the internal carotid and vertebral arteries, enter, and the cranial nerves exit. In addition, large venous sinuses draining blood from the brain aggregate at the skull base as they exit the cranial vault. They are difficult to reach because they are located ventral to the brain and posterior to the facial skeleton and aerodigestive system (Figure 44.2).

Several advances in the last two decades have significantly improved the surgical management of such tumors. These advances include a better understanding of microsurgical anatomy, refinements in imaging techniques and neuroanesthesia, and the development of microsurgical techniques using a variety of disciplines (neurosurgery, otolaryngology, and plastic surgery). More information is still being collected regarding the biology of these

Table 44.1 Classes of skull-base tumors

Class	Examples
(a) Tumors originating external to the skull base and invading it	Malignant tumors of the paranasal sinuses and nasopharynx
(b) Primary skull-base tumors and tumor-like conditions	Osteosarcomas, fibrous dysplasia chordomas and chondrosarcomas
(c) Primary basal intracranial tumors invading the skull	Meningiomas, pituitary neoplasms and tumors arising from cranial nerves

Figure 44.1 Anatomy of the skull base.

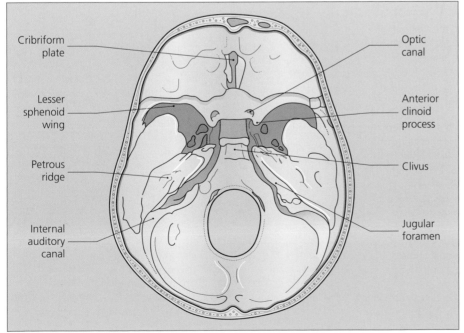

Cribriform plate

Lesser sphenoid wing

Petrous ridge

Internal auditory canal

Optic canal

Anterior clinoid process

Clivus

Jugular foramen

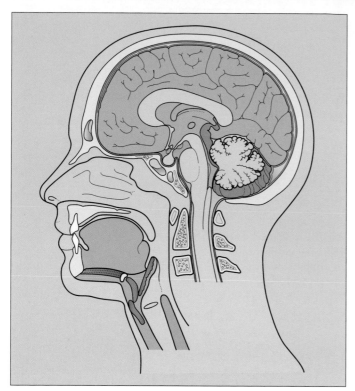

Figure 44.2 Midline sagittal section showing the anterior, middle, and posterior cranial bases and their relation to the brain and pharynx.

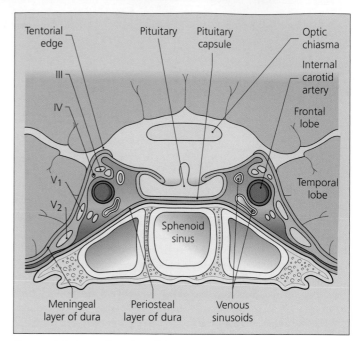

Figure 44.3 Coronal section of the parasellar region. The central portion of this region is occupied by the pituitary gland and the lateral portion is occupied by the temporal lobes. The dura of the middle cranial fossa consists of two layers, the outer periosteal and inner meningeal layers, which enclose the cavernous sinuses.

tumors. With these advances, surgical mortality has become rare and morbidity has improved, resulting in better outcome.

Radiosurgery has proved to be a valuable adjunct to the treatment of these complicated tumors.

ANATOMY OF THE CRANIAL BASE

The cranial base is divided into three portions – anterior, middle, and posterior – that correspond to the respective cranial fossa. These are further divided into two segments – midline and lateral. Numerous surgical approaches to the cranial base have been described, and such subdivisions of this area greatly facilitate evaluation of radiographic studies and selection of the appropriate surgical procedure.

The anterior cranial base[1] is made up of the frontal, ethmoid, and sphenoid bones, which form the orbital roofs laterally and the cribriform plates and roofs of the ethmoidal and sphenoidal sinuses medially. Posteriorly it is limited by the tuberculum sella and the lesser sphenoid wings. The optic canals (diverging fronto-laterally towards the orbits), the superior orbital fissures, and the anterior genu of the cavernous internal carotid arteries (ICAs) form the posterior relations of the anterior fossa. About 44 olfactory fila exit the cribriform plate, each with their own arachnoidal and dural sheaths. The orbital roofs and the anterior clinoid processes can be pneumatized to a variable degree from extensions of the frontal, ethmoidal, and sphenoidal sinuses.

The middle cranial base[2] is made up of the body and greater wings of the sphenoid and petrous temporal bones (Figure 44.3). Occupying a significant portion of this region, the cavernous sinus is situated between the temporal lobes and the pituitary gland (Figure 44.4). It consists of a mixture of venous plexus and

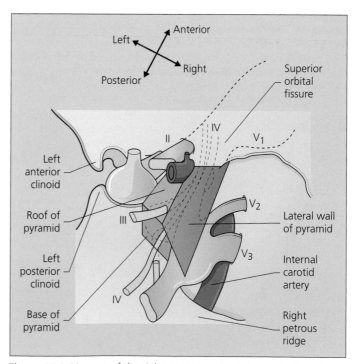

Figure 44.4 Diagram of the right cavernous sinus, demonstrating the pyramidal shape of the space (shaded) with its base towards the posterior fossa and the apex merging anteriorly with the orbital apex. The internal carotid artery exits the sinus anteriorly. Cranial nerves III, IV, and V occupy the lateral wall from above downwards, respectively, on their way to the superior orbital fissure.

sinusoids within the dural leaves, draining the brain and orbits and anastomosing with other extracranial venous networks. The ICA and the abducens nerve travel through the sinus. The oculomotor nerve pierces the roof posteriorly as it enters the cavernous sinus. Medially, the cavernous sinus is separated from the pituitary gland by a thin layer of periosteal dura (pituitary capsule). The floor is composed of dura, which rests on the lateral wall of the sphenoid sinus, and laterally the bone separates this from the infratemporal fossa.

The petrous temporal bone houses the middle and inner ear structures and the petrous segment of the ICA. The petrous ICA is made up of an initial vertical segment and then a horizontal section before it enters the cavernous sinus. The genu of the petrous ICA is near the cochlea and the geniculate ganglion of the facial nerve.

The greater wing of sphenoid lies above the infratemporal and pterygopalatine fossa, which contain the masticatory and pharyngeal muscles, cranial nerves, internal and external carotid arteries, eustachian tube, and a venous plexus that communicates through the foramina at the skull base with the cavernous sinus above.

The posterior cranial base[3] is made up of the clivus in the middle and the posterior surface of the petrous temporal bones and the occipital bones on either side. The upper portion of the clivus is formed by the sphenoid bone and the lower portion by the basiocciput. The posterior cranial base is related to the brainstem and cerebellum on its dorsal surface. Several cranial nerves exit the posterior cranial fossa. The abducens nerve leaves by piercing the meningeal layer of the dura on either side of the clivus to enter Dorello's canal, where it ascends, crosses the petrous apex, and enters the cavernous sinus. The facial and vestibulocochlear nerves enter the internal auditory canal. The jugular foramen is situated just caudal and lateral to the internal auditory canal and contains the jugular bulb and the glossopharyngeal, vagus, and accessory nerves. The hypoglosal canal is immediately medial and rostral to the occipital condyles. The articular surfaces of the occipital condyles face anterolaterally and the anterior ends point medially. The vertebral arteries exit the foramen transversarium of atlas, hug the joint capsule of the atlanto-occipital joint closely, and then enter the dura on the lateral aspect at the foramen magnum.

The venous plexus between the two layers of the clival dura is very well developed, and the superior and inferior petrosal sinuses travel between these layers to connect the cavernous sinuses to the jugular system. Ventrally, the posterior cranial base is situated over the nasopharynx, separated only by the mucosa and the constrictor.

TYPES OF TUMORS

Tumors in this region originate from three principal sources: intracranial tissues, cranial bones and cartilage, and extracranial tissues. These tumors could be further classified according to their degree of malignancy: benign tumors (most meningiomas and schwannomas), intermediate grade tumors (chordomas and chondrosarcomas), and malignant tumors (carcinoma arising from the paranasal sinuses, nasopharyngeal carcinoma, and melanoma.).

Some of the more common types are described below.

Meningioma

Forty to fifty per cent of meningiomas involve the skull base. The usual locations are the olfactory grooves, the sella and parasellar region including tuberculum sella and anterior clinoid, sphenoid wing, Meckel's cave, and the posterior fossa. The clinical presentation depends on the location of the tumor. The radiological features are typical – on computed tomography (CT) these tumors appear isodense to the brain and they enhance with contrast. Frequently calcification may be seen. On magnetic resonance imaging (MRI) the tumor is isointense to the brain on T1 and T2 and enhances with gadolinium. A dural "tail" is a typical finding although not specific for meningiomas.

Although benign in most cases, these tumors often engulf cranial nerves and blood vessels and grow through the dura mater to invade the basal bony structures and enter the orbit, paranasal sinuses, and the muscles at the base of the skull (Figure 44.5). Tumor in proximity to bone causes a hyperostotic reaction; tumor cells are frequently found within such bone. Benign meningiomas usually displace rather than invade the brain. However, because they grow slowly, there may be extensive involvement of the basal structures at the time of presentation. Malignant, atypical, and

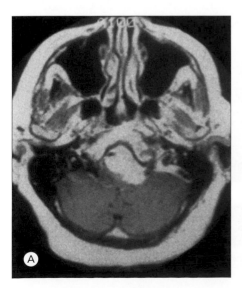
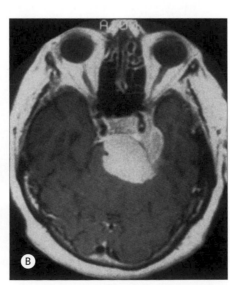

Figure 44.5 (A, B) Extensive basal meningioma that involves the cavernous sinus, clivus, and sphenoid sinus and surrounds the left internal carotid artery and basilar artery.

papillary meningiomas behave aggressively and tend to grow rapidly. The goals of surgery are to remove the tumor totally with the involved tissues, but preserving neurovascular structures. In cases where complete resection could not be achieved, adjunctive treatment is needed to prevent recurrence. Radiosurgery has shown good results in controlling tumor growth with relatively few side-effects.[4]

Schwannoma

Schwannoma is a benign neoplasm arising from the cranial nerve sheaths. The vestibular nerve is the most frequent site of origin, comprising about 10% of all primary brain tumors. Less frequently, the trigeminal, vagus, facial, glossopharyngeal, and hypoglossal nerves are sites of origin. The tumor becomes symptomatic either from dysfunction of the parent or neighboring cranial nerves or from progressive distortion of the brainstem. The tumor does not invade tissue and tends to displace cranial nerves, blood vessels, and the brain. Tumors arising from nerve sheaths may occupy more than one compartment and extend extracranially along the course of the nerve (Figure 44.6A). The tumor does not invade the bone; instead, smooth remodeling around the tumor, which is most remarkable in the region of the exit foramen of the cranial nerve, is a clue to the diagnosis (Figure 44.6B). The radiographic appearance is iso- to hypointense on CT and shows enhancement with contrast. On MRI, the tumor is isointense on T1 and hyperintense on T2; it enhances with gadolinium. Multiple nerve sheath tumors that occur in patients with neurofibromatosis-type 2 behave more aggressively and are prone to malignant transformation. In these cases a mutation in a tumor suppressor gene is found on chromosome 22 and results in inactivation of the gene. The tumors tend to be bilateral. Any young patient with a vestibular Schwannoma or a patient of any age with bilateral disease is suspected of having neurofibromatosis-2.

Esthesioneuroblastoma[5]

This is a malignant tumor arising from the olfactory epithelium on the nasal side under the cribriform plate. There are two peaks of incidence, at 30 and 60 years of age. It is slow growing and has a 20–40% metastatic potential to the regional lymph nodes, bone, and lungs. Invasion of the anterior cranial base is common by the time of presentation. Surgical resection entails en bloc removal of the tumor and surrounding tissues, including the bone of the cranial base, the dura, and the olfactory tracts. These tumors respond favorably to radiation, so surgery is followed by external beam irradiation. Large tumors can grow posteriorly, threatening the optic nerves and involving the frontal lobes (Figure 44.7). When this occurs, only piecemeal removal is possible. Local recurrence is common, even years after surgical removal.

Chordoma[6]

This tumor should be considered as a low-grade malignant tumor. It arises from the notochordal remnants that extend from the clivus to the sacrum. The average age at presentation is 40 years. The frequent presenting symptoms are multiple cranial nerve deficits – diplopia due to sixth nerve palsy, hoarseness, and

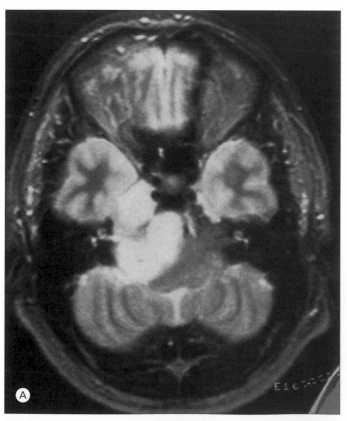
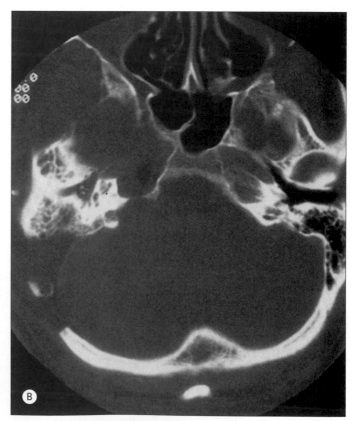

Figure 44.6 (A) MRI scan shows a large trigeminal neurinoma in the middle and posterior fossa displacing the internal carotid artery and the basilar artery. (B) CT scan shows smooth remodeling of the bone in the region of Meckel's cave.

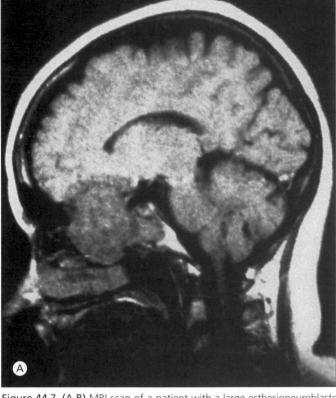

Figure 44.7 (A,B) MRI scan of a patient with a large esthesioneuroblastoma who presented with bilateral loss of vision.

dysphagia. Headache is common. About 35% of chordomas occur in the skull base, and the majority of the rest occur at the caudal end of the spine. These tumors are usually slow growing and quite large at the time of presentation. They are grayish, lobulated masses without a distinct capsule, and they contain varying amounts of calcification. Irregular bone destruction is evident on the CT scan. On MRI the tumor is isointense on T1, hyperintense on T2, and enhances variably with gadolinium. MRI is the most important imaging study to show the extent of the tumor and its relation to brain, vessels, and cranial nerves. The consistency of the tumor may vary from soft and gelatinous to hard. They are extradural in origin and tend to displace the dura. Large or recurrent tumors invade and penetrate the dura, and they may bury themselves inside the brainstem and surround important arteries and cranial nerves (Figure 44.8). It is usually possible to establish a plane of dissection around the tumor and the neurovascular structures; however, such a plane cannot be developed in the bone because of tumor infiltration. The local recurrence rate is quite high, and metastasis occurs in 10–40% of cases. In a large epidemological series recently published, the median survival was 6.29 years; 5- and 10-year survival rates were 67.6% and 39.9%, respectively.[7] Chordomas are relatively radioresistant to conventional radiation, and aggressive surgical resection is the initial therapy of choice that will predict the best long-term outcome.[8] However, patients receiving postoperative proton-beam therapy experienced better long-term results.[9] There are no histologic indicators to predict the aggressiveness of a particular case. Older series found histological subtypes to be predictors of outcome but this is not true in the larger, better-controlled recent series. A correlation between tumor doubling time and KI67LI was found for both chordoma and chondrosarcoma and this marker could be used to predict tumor behavior in a specific patient.[10]

Chondrosarcoma

Like chordomas, these are slow-growing, malignant neoplasms. They are believed to originate in the primitive mesenchymal cell rests in the cartilaginous matrix at the skull base. They are more frequent in males. In the past, these tumors were regarded as very similar to chordomas but recent studies have shown significant differences: chondrosarcoma are rarer, tend to have a better prognosis, are less aggressive, and their recurrence rate is lower. The 5- and 10-year local control rates were 99% and 98% respectively, and the 5- and 10-year disease-specific survival rates were both 99% and 93%,[11] respectively and 84% in another series.[12] The radiographic appearance is similar to chordomas – bone erosion on CT (Figure 44.9), hypointense on T1, hyperintense on T2, and enhancement with gadolinium. They involve the middle, anterior, and posterior cranial base in decreasing order of frequency. The parasellar and petrous apices are the most common sites (Figure 44.10). These tumors are primarily extradural with dural invasion occurring at a later stage or after previous surgery. They can be graded histologically to indicate their relative biologic aggressiveness; a subtype, mesenchymal chondrosarcoma, is an aggressive tumor with less favorable prognosis. Radical surgical excision is the treatment of choice; however, this is done in a piecemeal fashion to preserve the important neurovascular structures. Local recurrence rate is high and is usually the ultimate cause of the patient's death.

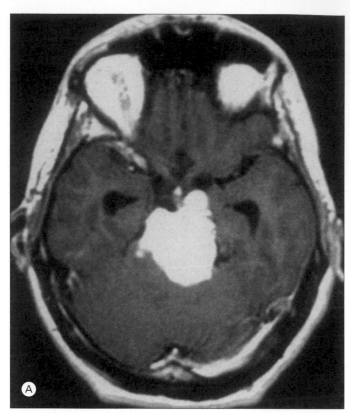

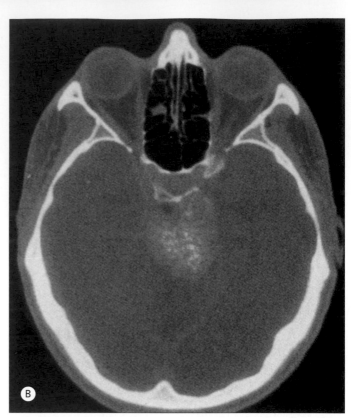

Figure 44.8 (A) MRI scan with gadolinium in a 22-year-old patient with a large clivus chordoma. **(B)** CT scan with bone algorithms shows fine calcification within the tumor.

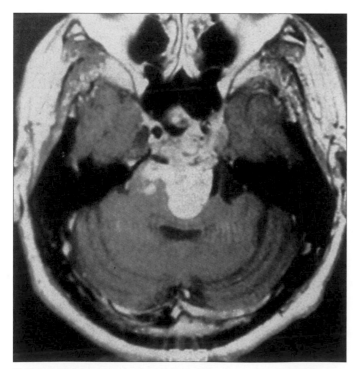

Figure 44.9 MRI scan of a young man with a large chondrosarcoma invaginating the clivus and extending into the sphenoid and cavernous sinus. Radiologically, a chondrosarcoma is indistinguishable from a chordoma.

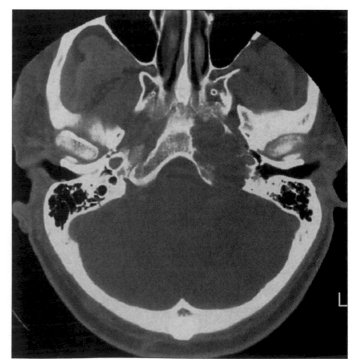

Figure 44.10 CT scan of a patient with a chondrosarcoma shows irregular bone destruction in the region of the petroclival synchondrosis. The scalloping of the bone margins is typical of this tumor.

Adenoid cystic carcinoma

This malignant neoplasm arises from the major and minor salivary glands or the sinonasal tracts, and affects patients in their fourth to sixth decades. The natural course of the disease is relentless progression and local invasion. Its high propensity for perineural extension, distant from the primary gross location, is a significant limiting factor in its surgical treatment. A recent study has found that even after an aggressive resection the local recurrence rate is high.[13] The bones may be involved even if there is no radiographic evidence; however, usually irregular bone destruction is noted on the CT scans. Metastasis is a late finding in the disease. Because of its protracted course, follow up of more than 5 years is required for prognostication. Despite incomplete excision, long periods of survival are not uncommon. Multiple treatments for recurrent disease are justified to provide symptomatic relief.

Nasopharyngeal carcinoma[14]

This type of tumor commonly occurs in Oriental people. The average age of the patient at presentation is 45 years, and males are more frequently affected. There is a high incidence of invasion of the skull base, and spread to the cervical lymph nodes occurs early in the course of the disease. Three histologic types exist, whose biologic behavior and prognosis vary. These are the keratinizing squamous cell, nonkeratinizing squamous cell, and undifferentiated type (types 1, 2 and 3 respectively in the World Health Organization classification). Types 2 and 3 are strongly associated with exposure to Epstein–Barr virus and carry a better prognosis than the keratinizing squamous cell variety. Type 3, the undifferentiated type, is by far the most common, more so in the endemic areas. The keratinizing squamous carcinoma (World Health Organization type 1) is not radiosensitive and has a 5-year survival rate of 20%. Radiation is the initial treatment for the nonkeratinizing and undifferentiated types, with surgery reserved for recurrent disease. Surgery plays a greater role, however, in the treatment of the keratinizing squamous cell carcinoma.

Paragangliomas

These tumors arise from the paraganglia of the head and neck and belong to a family of tumors that originate from cells called APUD cells (from Amine Precursor Uptake and Decarboxylation). In contrast to other tumors from this family, only 4% of cases will have the clinical syndrome of excessive catecholamine release. Of this group, the glomus jugulare and tympanicum are of interest to the cranial base surgeon. These tumors are multicentric in 10% of cases and appear at different times in the patient's life. Before surgery, CT is performed to assess the bone destruction and MRI shows the extent of the tumor and the intracranial involvement with typical salt-and-pepper appearance. Angiography helps to confirm the diagnosis and to assess the collateral venous circulation in case the jugular vein will be sacrificed. It is also used for preoperative embolization to reduce blood loss in surgery. These tumors are vascular and their response to radiation is variable. The average age at the time of presentation is 45 years, and females are more frequently affected. These tumors are generally regarded as benign and slow growing, progressively involving critical structures in the temporal bone. The initial presentation is pulsatile tinnitus, which progresses to conductive hearing loss and cranial neuropathies of nerves VII through XII as the tumor grows. Intracranial extension occurs in larger tumors. The tumor also extends for distances inside the lumen of the sigmoid and transverse sinuses and the internal jugular vein. Involvement of the ICA and the caudal cranial nerves is the major cause of surgical morbidity. Surgical excision is the primary treatment.

Craniopharyngioma

This benign tumor arises from the anterior superior area of the pituitary. It commonly involves the pituitary stalk and is adherent to the hypothalamus. Histologicaly this is an epithelial tumor with stratified epithelium lining cystic areas with calcification in the wall and cholesterol crystals in the cyst fluid. In most cases, the tumor has a cystic component. This tumor has two ages of peak incidence – childhood between 5 and 10 years and another peak around the 6th decade. On CT, the tumor shows calcifications in almost all childhood cases and in about half of the adult cases. These tumors present with visual disturbances in adults and with headache, nausea and vomiting due to high intracranial pressure in children. In both age groups, it is critical to check for endocrinological disturbances and correct them before surgery. These patients are assumed to be hypo-adrenal and are treated with hydrocortisone in addition to the "usual" dose of dexamethasone. After surgery, the patient is followed for diabetes insipidus; and some cases may need lifelong treatment with vasopressin because of injury to the pituitary stalk. The overall survival varies between the age groups – in children 5-year survival is around 90% whereas in adults it is 60% and after the age of 65 years it drops to 34%.[15]

In cases where complete resection cannot be achieved, adjuvant treatment may be offered. Radiation therapy, radiosurgery and direct administration of radionuclides or chemotherapeutic agent into the tumor cyst have been shown to be effective in preventing recurrence or the growth of a residual tumor. The most frequently used agent is bleomycin injected repeatedly into the tumor cyst through an omaya reservoir (a small reservoir connected to a ventricular catheter, allowing injection in or drainage out).[16]

RADIOGRAPHIC EVALUATION

Current progress in treating tumors at the cranial base is partly attributed to advances in imaging techniques. Radiographic imaging is essential for diagnosing the tumor and, more importantly, estimating accurately the extent of the disease to facilitate surgical planning. Neuronavigational systems help plan the approach or identify important landmarks during the procedure. Intraoperative imaging will help to assure the completeness of the tumor resection. The goals of radiographic evaluation of skull-base lesions are (1) to screen for base of the skull involvement, (2) to determine the extent of bony involvement, (3) to determine the relationship of the soft tissue structures in the region of the tumor (i.e. whether there is invasion or displacement of the brain, pituitary, arteries, and extracranial soft tissues), and (4) to determine the vascular anatomy in the vicinity of the tumor and, in case of involvement of major vessels by the tumor, to determine the collateral channels and the circulatory reserve. It is also possible to predict the histology of the lesion based on characteristic changes produced by the lesion.

Computed tomography

A high-resolution CT scanner is essential for minute details. The area of the tumor is scanned in 1.5- to 3-mm slices parallel to the planum sphenoidale. To obtain an overview of the region and identify associated abnormalities, such as hydrocephalus, the remainder of the head is scanned in 10-mm slices. Axial scans are always supplemented with coronal scans of the same thickness; these are performed with the gantry and head angled to provide a true coronal view, which is preferable to a computer-reformatted study. The scanning is carried out before and after intravenous contrast medium has been administered and using bone and soft-tissue algorithms. This provides an accurate delineation of the bone and shows to a degree the relation of soft tissue to the tumor. Thus, the study of the lesion in two planes gives a three-dimensional evaluation. Software for three-dimensional reconstruction is currently available and is helpful in some cases. The CT scan is the most sensitive way of detecting minute amounts of calcification in the tumor (see Figure 44.8B). It provides the best possible view of the type of bony involvement – e.g. irregular bone destruction as in a malignant tumor (see Figure 44.10), smooth remodeling of bone as in a neurilemoma (see Figure 44.6), or hyperostosis (Figure 44.11) – and its extent and relation to the various foramina, paranasal sinuses, and the labyrinth, which is important for planning surgical resection. The major drawback of the CT scan is its inability to depict the vascular relations of the tumor. The development of CT angiography has greatly improved the ability to show the vascular anatomy in the base of the skull and this modality may replace the more invasive angiography in certain cases.

Magnetic resonance imaging

Currently MRI is the best technique available for studying the relation of the tumor to soft tissue. It has excellent contrast resolution, and a magnet of high field strength yields high-quality images. Like CT, MRI is performed in thin slices in the axial, coronal, and sagittal planes. Intravenous gadolinium further enhances the contrast of the lesion. MRI enables the tumor to be distinguished from the neurovascular structures, fat, and extracranial soft tissues. It allows the surgeon to determine whether a distinct plane exists between the tumor and the brain or if the tumor has invaded the brain or soft tissues (Figure 44.12). When an important blood vessel, such as the ICA, or the vertebrobasilar system is in close proximity to the tumor, the status of the parent vessel or its major branches (i.e. whether they are completely surrounded by the tumor) is best determined by MRI (Figure 44.13). A similar assessment of the venous sinuses can also be made. The limitation of MRI seems to be its inability to differentiate specks of calcification from flowing blood in tumor vessels; thus, a densely calcified tumor may appear to be very vascular. Consequently, CT and MRI provide complementary information. Magnetic resonance angiograms and venograms (MRA and MRV) are new imaging techniques using special software to show blood vessels in the arterial system or the venous system. As for CT angiography, these may replace the formal more invasive angiography in demonstrating major arteries or in showing the venous anatomy and the patency of the sinuses before surgery. MRI is now being used as an intraoperative imaging system. Intraoperative imaging may help tailor the resection of skull-base tumors.[17,18]

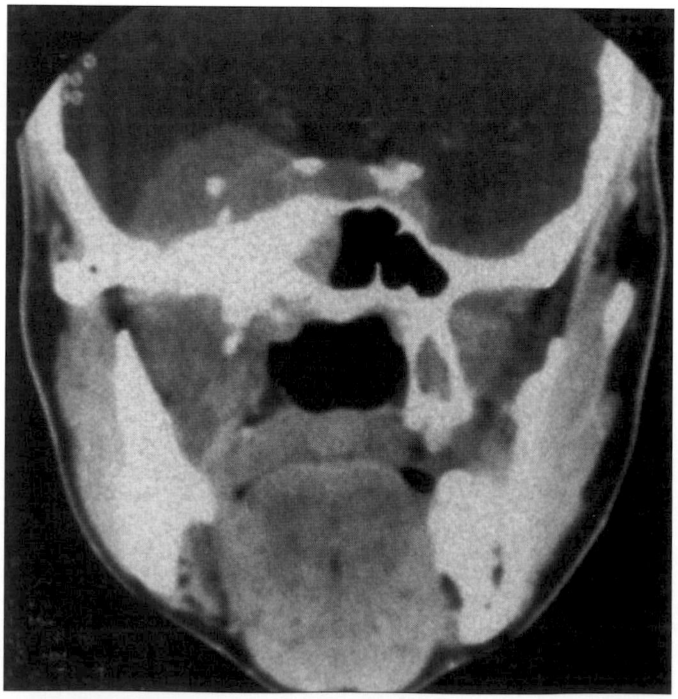

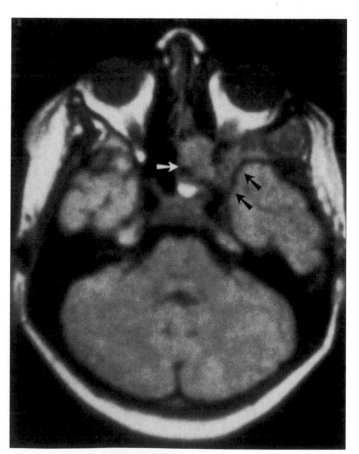

Figure 44.11 Coronal CT scan of a patient with an extensive meningioma of the middle fossa and extracranial region shows severe hyperostotic bone involvement.

Figure 44.12 MRI scan of a patient with a juvenile angiofibroma occupying the nasopharynx and extending into the sphenoid sinus, superior orbital fissure, and the anterior cavernous sinus (arrows).

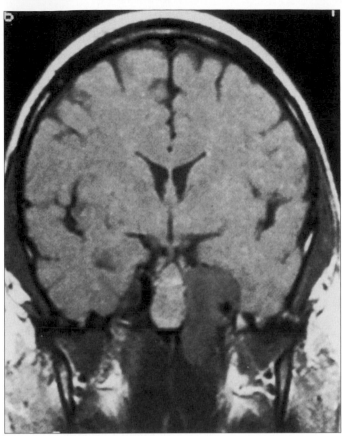

Figure 44.13 MRI scan of a patient with a chondrosarcoma surrounding the internal carotid artery without compromise of the lumen on arteriography.

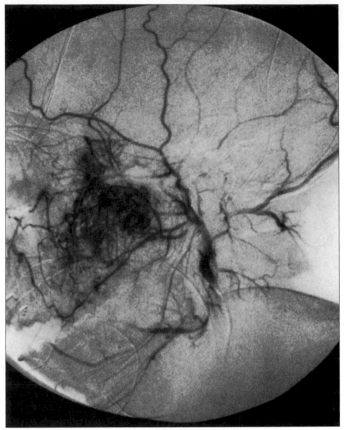

Figure 44.14 The same patient as in Figure 44.12. External carotid arteriogram showing typical hypervascularity of the tumor.

Cerebral angiography

Although MRI has limited its use, conventional arteriography is still important for investigating tumors at the cranial base. Arteriography is better able to define the relationship of the major arteries and their branches to the tumor. When there is encasement, arteriography enables the length of involvement, the caliber of the lumen, and the status of the vessel wall to be evaluated. It is also used to determine a tumor's vascularity and the angio-architecture, which can sometimes indicate the type of tumor in question, e.g. juvenile angiofibroma (Figure 44.14), meningioma, glomus tumor, etc. Simple displacement, as opposed to constriction with irregularity of the vessel wall in a particular segment, can indicate whether the vessel can be separated from the tumor without injuring it. Because of the heavy bony overlay in the region of the skull base, the subtraction technique is essential when studying the angiograms. Important drainage veins and their patency should be known preoperatively so they will not be compromised. This is especially important with tumors in the vicinity of the sigmoid sinus and jugular bulb, in which case dominance of the jugular bulb and adequacy of communication between the transverse sinuses must be assessed (Figure 44.15). Free communication between the various sinuses at the torcula exists in 57% of patients, while the remainder have some type of anomaly.[19]

The collateral arterial circulation can be estimated by observing the presence and size of the anterior and posterior communicating arteries and the pattern of flow with cross compression of the ICA. An accurate knowledge of the cerebral circulatory reserve is

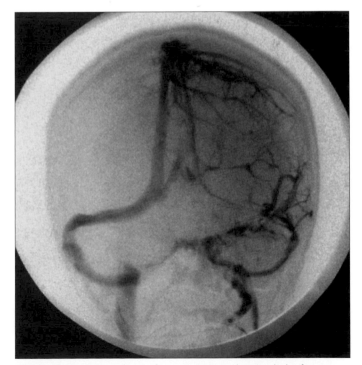

Figure 44.15 Venous phase of an arteriogram showing lack of communication between the transverse sinuses on either side with the superior sagittal sinus draining into the right transverse sinus.

extremely important because the ICA is frequently involved in the skull base by the tumor. In certain cases, the vessel may need to be sacrificed, if there is a malignant tumor or the tumor and vessel are inseparable (with a meningioma). In other instances the artery may be injured and need to be occluded temporarily for repair. The consequences of such a course of action must be predetermined. The balloon test occlusion is used for this purpose and forms part of the arteriographic examination. The test tries to predict which of the patients will not tolerate temporary or permanent carotid occlusion.[20] Thus, patients who fail the clinical test and those who show critical reduction in blood flow need some type of vascular reconstructive procedure to maintain their cerebrovascular reserve in case of injury to or sacrifice of the artery. This revascularization is usually carried out under barbiturate and hypothermic brain protection. In patients with adequate collaterals, the artery may be ligated in such a way that there is no blind stump to act as an embolic source. Knowledge of the extent and source of the blood supply to the tumor is also important. In addition to its diagnostic importance, it is helpful to perform superselective catheterization of the feeding vessels preoperatively and embolize them to reduce intraoperative blood loss and facilitate surgical removal. Despite significant advances in this field, certain vessels cannot be safely embolized, especially if they are small and arise directly from the ICA or the vertebrobasilar system.

SURGICAL MANAGEMENT

Anesthesia and monitoring

The length and complexity of the operative procedures require constant communication between the surgeon and anesthesiologist and the use of sophisticated anesthetic techniques. These techniques include management of intracranial hypertension, brain relaxation, brain protection during vascular occlusion and reconstruction, and intraoperative electrophysiologic monitoring of brain and cranial nerve function. Finally, after the long operation, a smooth and rapid emergence from anesthesia with a wakeful patient allows for a neurologic evaluation. Because the surgeon needs to work beneath the brain, brain retraction is a major cause of morbidity. Several techniques to cause brain relaxation are used, including patient positioning, hyperventilation, loop and osmotic diuretics, and cerebrospinal fluid (CSF) drainage. CSF drainage is performed using a lumbar sub-arachnoid drain or ventricular catheter. A lumbar drain is used in the absence of a significant intradural mass or brain distortion. The drain is usually inserted by the neuro-anesthesiologist after induction and intubation, and gradual withdrawal of fluid is carried out during the operation as required. When needed, the ventricular catheter is inserted by the surgeon at the beginning of the case.

In addition to the cerebral metabolic lowering effects of the anesthetic technique, the brain can also be protected from ischemia by administering sodium thiopental to electroencephalographic burst suppression, the induction of pre-ischemic hypothermia, and avoiding hyperglycemia with glucose-containing solutions. These measures are instituted before vascular clamping and are continued until the blood flow is re-established. Methods of monitoring vital functions follow standard American Society of Anesthesiology guidelines in addition to radial artery catheterization and insertion of a Foley catheter. Sequential pneumatic compression stockings of the lower extremities are used to reduce the incidence of deep vein thrombosis.

It is necessary to estimate closely the amount of blood lost during surgery so that appropriate intraoperative fluid replacement can occur. Hemodilution-related coagulopathy can be a significant problem and appropriate preventative measures must be used. Fresh frozen plasma, packed red blood cells, platelets, magnesium and calcium replacement are based on laboratory blood tests performed at regular intervals. Toward the end of the operative procedure, the anesthesiologist can help the surgeon achieve a dry vascular bed by raising the mean arterial blood pressure to anticipated awake levels prior to closure. A crucial issue is the control of blood pressure during both the procedure and the emergence from anesthesia. During emergence from anesthesia and neurologic assessment prior to extubation, aggressive hemodynamic control using short- and intermediate-acting agents is of extreme importance. Vigilance and readiness to treat untoward hemodynamic changes *must* extend into the immediate postoperative period.

Monitoring

To some extent, the type of intraoperative electrophysiologic monitoring dictates the anesthetic technique. Brain stem auditory evoked responses (BAERs), somatosensory evoked potentials (SEPs), and motor evoked potentials (MEPs) are frequently used to continually assess important brainstem functions.[21] Retraction or direct injury by manipulation of the brain or brainstem can cause serious postoperative sequelae. Changes in the electrophysiologic recording can enable the surgeon to avoid these damaging incidents. When cranial nerve manipulation is anticipated, the spontaneous and evoked activity of the nerves are monitored to facilitate identification and reduce operative trauma. Motor nerves are best suited for such monitoring, and the anesthesiologist must refrain from using long-acting paralytic drugs and inhalational agents such as isoflurane or desflurane. When using MEPs, we use a total intravenous anesthetic technique with propofol and remifentanil without muscle relaxation.

In conclusion, a concerted effort by the surgeon, the neuroanesthesiologist, and the neurophysiologist, is essential to insure a successful operation.

Surgical principles

Adequate exposure

Many innovative operative exposures for approaching skull-base lesions have been devised. Each provides exposure of a specific region of the skull base. Thorough knowledge of the surgical anatomy is essential to maximize the benefits of a particular approach while reducing complications. The surgeon may use more than one approach simultaneously to obtain multiple viewing angles. This is necessary not only because of the restrictive nature of many of the approaches, but because a combination of approaches, at one or more than one sitting, permits more thorough removal, especially of larger tumors.

Control of important neural and vascular structures

The procedure may involve separation of the tumor from major neurovascular structures, or these structures may be encountered during surgical exposure. The surgeon must establish proximal and distal control of major vessels during these maneuvers so that inadvertent injury can be satisfactorily managed. Such control is a prerequisite during arterial grafting when an involved segment of the ICA is resected.

Staging of operations for radical surgical excision

Radical tumor removal, which includes the involved margins, is the goal of surgery. Staging may be required for several reasons. Intra- and extradural tumors may need to be removed in stages to reduce the risks of CSF leakage. Large tumors requiring tedious and lengthy dissections may need more than one operative approach. These may be tackled in stages to reduce the surgeon's fatigue and thus increase the effectiveness of the operation.

In some instances, residual tumor may be seen on postoperative imaging studies and a second operation may then be undertaken to remove the remaining tumor.

Strategies to reduce or eliminate brain retraction

Major morbidity in these operations arises from prolonged and excessive brain retraction. One of the most effective ways of reducing this is by judicial resection of nonessential bony structures or temporary displacement of the facial skeleton to improve exposure and access to a particular region. Other means of brain relaxation are also used.

Adequate reconstruction after tumor removal

The purpose of this is to prevent infection, CSF leakage, and facial disfigurement. Complete separation of the CSF, brain, and major arteries from the contaminated regions of the paranasal sinuses and pharynx must be restored at the end of the operation. Vascularized tissue is the mainstay of reconstruction, along with pieces of fat, muscle, or bone. The vascularized flaps may be local tissue, such as the galeal pericranial flap, temporalis and sternomastoid muscle transfers, or vascularized free flaps (rectus abdominis, greater omentum, etc.).

Surgical approaches

Table 44.2 lists the commonly used approaches for cranial base tumors, which are broadly divided into anterior and lateral. Some of these approaches are described below.

Anterior approaches

These are used for pathology involving the anterior cranial base as far posterior as the optic foramina. These approaches may also be used for the sella turcica, sphenoid sinus, clivus, and craniocervical junction. When these approaches are used posterior to the optic foramina, they are restricted to the median and paramedian areas, limited laterally by the exit foramina of cranial nerves VI through XII, the cavernous sinuses, and the ICAs, and caudally by the jugular bulbs and occipital condyles. Additionally, the surgeon may not have proximal control of the ICA and the vertebral arteries and thus will be unable to deal with intraoperative vascular problems. Another limitation of the anterior approaches is the paucity of reconstructive options. This can be a serious handicap if a large defect created in the skull base causes free communication between the intradural space or the great vessels with the contaminated spaces of the pharynx and paranasal sinuses. Complications such as CSF fistulae and infections can have disastrous consequences. Nevertheless, the anterior approaches are ideal for certain lesions confined to this particular anatomic region.

EXTENDED SUBFRONTAL APPROACH WITH SUPRAORBITAL OSTEOTOMIES A bicoronal incision is made from zygoma to zygoma at or behind the coronal suture to create a long pericranial flap for reconstruction. The pericranium is elevated with the scalp and reflected down to the lateral walls of the orbits. The peri-

Table 44.2 Surgical approaches to the cranial base

Approach	Principal region exposed
Intradural	
Retrosigmoid	Cerebellopontine angle
Posterior subtemporal-presigmoid-transpetrous	Petrous ridge, upper and middle clivus
Frontotemporal transsylvian	Parasellar
Transsylvian-anterior subtemporal-transcavernous	Tentorial notch, upper clivus
Anterior subtemporal-preauricular infratemporal	Upper and middle clivus
Extreme lateral transcondyle	Ventral craniocervical junction
Extradural anterior	
Transbasal	Anterior cranial base, sphenoid sinus, middle clivus, medial to petrous ICA
Extended subfrontal (with orbital osteotomy)	
Transethmoidal	Sphenoid, ethmoid sinus, middle clivus
Transsphenoidal	
Transoral (and extensions)	Midclivus, craniocervical junction
Bilateral maxillotomy	Maxillary sinus, pterygopalatine fossa
Unilateral maxillotomy	Craniocervical junction
Transcervical	Craniocervical junction
Lateral	
Subtemporal-preauricular infratemporal	Infratemporal fossa, petrous apex, middle clivus
Postauricular-infratemporal	
Transcochlear	Middle clivus
Total petrosectomy	Middle and lower clivus
Extreme lateral transcondyle	Anterior craniocervical junction

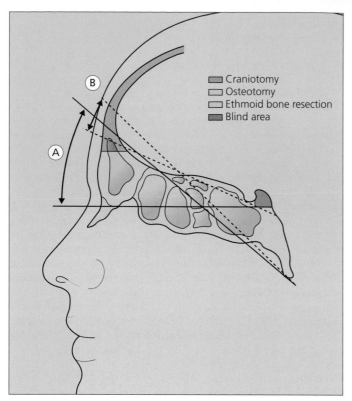

Figure 44.16 Additional room can be obtained underneath the frontal lobes by performing a supraorbital and ethmoidal osteotomy **(A)**. However, a superficially wide exposure is required for access to the deeper areas of the clivus, and the posterior clinoids are in a blind area with this approach **(B)**.

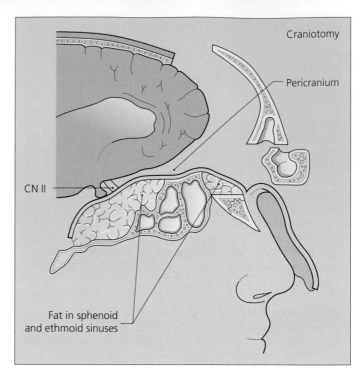

Figure 44.17 Reconstruction of the floor is performed by exenterating the sphenoidal, ethmoidal, and frontal sinuses, filling them with fat, and laying a long pericranial flap.

orbita is stripped from the roof and lateral wall of the orbit after the supraorbital nerves and vessels are freed from the foramen. A bifrontal craniotomy is performed, including the supraorbital rims, and the anterior portions of the orbital roof, which are removed with a reciprocating saw. Removal of the supraorbital rims permits an additional 2.5–3 cm of room underneath the frontal lobes, thus reducing the degree of brain retraction. The brain can be further slackened by withdrawing spinal fluid through a lumbar subarachnoid drain inserted before positioning the patient or by a ventricular catheter inserted at the beginning of the case. The olfactory nerves may be divided or may be preserved using previously described techniques.[22,23] The frontal lobes are elevated extradurally. Limited access to the anterior fossa through the frontal sinus has been described and is suitable for smaller and anteriorly located pathology. Access to the middle and posterior skull base is acquired by entering the sphenoid sinus. The planum sphenoidale and posterior ethmoidal air cells are drilled away in between the optic nerves to provide wide entry into the sphenoid sinus. The major advantage of this approach is that it allows wide exposure of the pathology with minimal brain retraction (Figure 44.16), and the basal defect can be satisfactorily reconstructed with a galeal or pericranial flap (Figure 44.17).[24] This approach is useful for both intra- and extradural tumors of the anterior base and predominantly extradural tumors of the middle and posterior cranial base. The wide exposure is particularly important when treating deep lesions. The extended subfrontal approach has been used either singly or in combination with a transfascial or lateral approach for different tumors including esthesioneuroblastomas,

meningiomas of the anterior cranial base that have extended inferiorly in the sinuses and bony structures, sinonasal carcinomas, orbital tumors, and chordomas and chondrosarcomas of the middle and posterior cranial base. In addition, it has been used for repair of CSF leaks through the anterior fossa and the sphenoid sinus.

TRANSORAL APPROACH This approach provides access to the clivus and anterior craniocervical junction through the oropharynx (Figure 44.18).[25] It is used predominantly for extradural lesions, but in specific instances, it can be used for intradural lesions.[26] It is most commonly used for basilar invagination from a variety of causes and cervicomedullary compression in rheumatoid arthritis. A special mouth gag is inserted to depress the tongue while the soft palate is retracted upward. The posterior pharyngeal wall is incised in the midline, and the prevertebral muscles are stripped and retracted laterally. The anterior tubercle of the atlas is the most important landmark to the midline, and the lateral limits of the exposure are formed by the occipital condyles and the jugular and hypoglossal foramina, which are about 18 mm to either side of the midline. The bone of the clivus, the anterior arch of C1, and the vertebral bodies are removed with a high-speed drill as needed.

After removal of the lesion, the prevertebral muscles and pharyngeal mucosa are reapproximated in layers. On occasion, a bone strut from the iliac crest may be left in the bony defect to "fill out" the space, preventing postoperative velopharyngeal insufficiency. However, this is not widely practiced because it carries a high risk of infection and dislodgment of the bone graft. Thus the approach can be extended in a longitudinal direction but is quite limited laterally. Another limitation of the approach is its depth from the surface (about 10 cm from the level of the

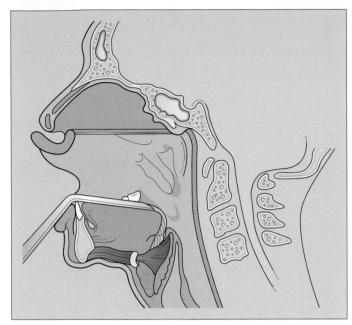

Figure 44.18 The exposure obtained by adding a bilateral maxillectomy to a standard transoral approach.

incisors in the adult). The exposure is therefore narrow and deep. Adequate reconstruction of the operative area is severely restricted, and this limitation should be seriously considered in the preoperative planning. The major advantage of the procedure is direct access to the ventral aspect of the cranio-cervical junction without need for brain retraction. Modifications such as the Le

Fort maxillotomy, mandibulotomy, and glossotomy along with division of the soft and hard palate can be added to the standard transoral approach depending on the particular lesion in question. These additions increase the longitudinal limits of the exposure, but the area is still limited laterally by the structures enumerated previously.

Lateral approaches

Understanding the three-dimensional anatomy of the temporal bone is essential for the proper selection and optimal use of the lateral approaches to the skull base (Figure 44.19). The major structures in consideration here are the petrous ICA, cochlea, labyrinth, facial nerve, and the jugular bulb and foramen. The preoperative radiographs of the patient need to be analyzed in relation to these landmarks and the appropriate surgical approach should be selected accordingly. The approach is determined by the location and extent of the tumor, whether or not there is extra-dural extension of the tumor, status of hearing, and existing cranial nerve dysfunction. Tumors in the cavernous sinus are approached through the transsylvian and subtemporal route with or without an orbito-zygomatic osteotomy. For intradural clival lesions, a few approaches are possible, including the subtemporal, pre-sigmoid transpetrosal, total petrosal, preauricular infratemporal, or extreme lateral transcondylar routes. Lateral approaches are also indicated for lesions intimately involving the ICA and for extradural tumors involving the temporal bone, infratemporal, and pterygoid regions. Table 44.3 indicates the areas of the clivus exposed by the various approaches. The advantages of the lateral approaches are several: the ipsilateral internal carotid and vertebral arteries, the internal jugular vein, and the cranial nerves can be adequately controlled during the operation; a wider exposure reduces the working depth; the plane between the brain

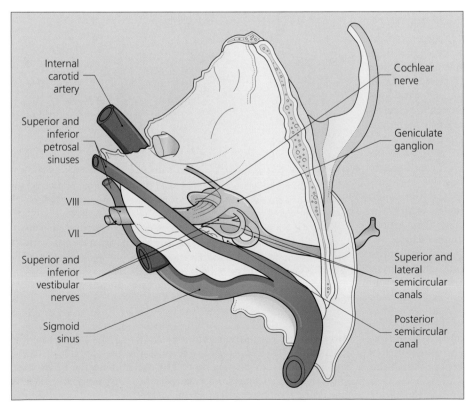

Figure 44.19 Superior view of the contents of the temporal bone. The surgical approaches to the clivus go through these structures, or in front of or behind them, depending on the status of hearing and size of the tumor.

Table 44.3 Areas of the clivus exposed by surgical approaches

Area of clivus exposed	Surgical approach
Superior clivus (above V root) and posterior clinoid	Transsylvian Subtemporal
Middle clivus (between V root and jugular bulb)	Presigmoid–subtemporal Preauricular infratemporal Transoral transpalatal or with Le Fort maxillotomy Retrosigmoid Total petrosectomy
Lower clivus (jugular bulb to foramen magnum)	Extreme lateral transcondylar Transoral

and the tumor is better defined; contaminated spaces are usually not traversed; and the options for reconstruction are numerous.

Many names have been used by different authors for the different lateral approaches to the skull base. In order to prevent confusion, one should determine which type of craniotomy is performed (fronto-temporal, temporal, suboccipital, zygomatic osteotomy) and whether the approach is anterior or posterior to the petrous bone. The anterior petrosectomy is for lesions in the petrous apex and the superior half of the clivus and the posterior petrosectomy is for lesions in the petroclival region and the cerebellopontine angle.[27] The petrous temporal bone can be drilled away in increments depending on the site and type of the lesion and the extent of exposure that is needed.

SUBTEMPORAL AND PREAURICULAR INFRATEMPORAL APPROACH According to the classification discussed above, the craniotomy is fronto-temporal and the petrosectomy is anterior.

This approach is used for extradural lesions that are predominantly unilateral, involve the middle and posterior cranial base, and may extend across the midline.[28] Certain intradural tumors can also be managed by this approach,[29] including meningiomas in the petroclival region. In some cases, the intra- and extradural portions may be removed at separate stages to reduce the chances of CSF leakage. An important reason this approach is preferable to a translabyrinthine or total petrosectomy approach is that it preserves hearing, since the approach path stays anterior to the critical portion of the temporal bone and there is no need to displace the facial nerve.

A frontotemporal craniotomy is performed and the supraorbital rim and zygomatic arch are removed (Figure 44.20). The mandibular condyle is dislocated from the joint. The greater sphenoid wing is rongeured down to unroof the foramen ovale and rotundum to allow access to the base of the pterygoid plate (Figure 44.21). The petrous ICA is completely unroofed from its entry into the skull base up to the cavernous sinus and displaced laterally after establishing control in the neck. The bone medial to the petrous ICA is part of the clivus and can be drilled away after completely displacing the ICA from the bony canal to expose the clival dura. The sphenoid sinus can also be entered by removing the bone between V2 and V3. The eustachian tube, situated immediately lateral to the petrous ICA, is transected during this approach and must be obliterated adequately to avoid a CSF fistula. Surgical exposure extends from the foramen rotundum in

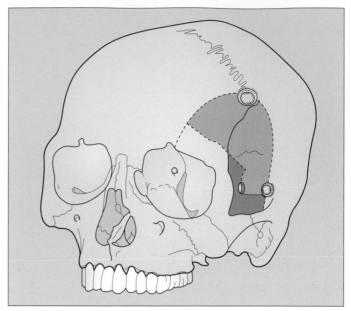

Figure 44.20 The incision, craniotomy, and orbitozygomatic bone flap are shown. The major vessels are controlled in the neck, while the needle electrodes are used for intraoperative neurophysiologic monitoring.

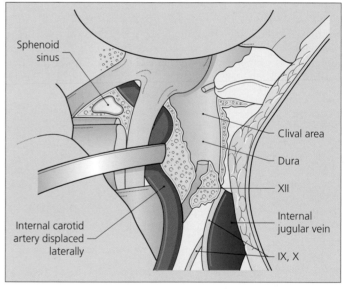

Figure 44.21 The greater sphenoid wing and the anterior portion of the petrous bone are rongeured to unroof the maxillary and mandibular nerves and the petrous internal carotid artery is completely exposed, dividing the eustachian tube. The internal carotid artery at its entry into the skull base is surrounded by a dense fibrous ring that is continuous with the periosteum; this has to be divided to mobilize the artery fully out of the bone. Removal of bone between V2 and V3 leads into the sphenoid sinus while drilling the bone medial to the internal carotid artery exposes the clival dura.

front to the hypoglossal foramen (Figure 44.22). Only the middle portion of the clivus from the level of the trigeminal root to the hypoglossal foramen is exposed. The upper clivus can be exposed only through an intradural transsylvian or subtemporal route by traversing the posterior cavernous sinus.

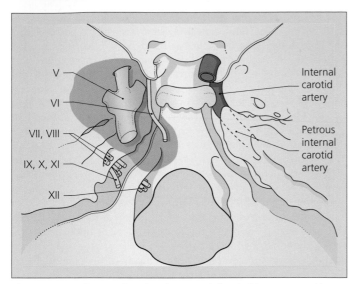

Figure 44.22 Diagram showing the area of the skull base exposed by the subtemporal and preauricular infratemporal approach.

Following removal of the tumor, the clival defect can be filled with fat while the area around the petrous ICA is covered by transposing the temporalis muscle pedicled on the coronoid process. Another option is a temporoparietal fascial flap pedicled on the superficial temporal artery. If a large defect is produced, as with malignant tumors, a vascularized free flap of the rectus abdominis or latissimus dorsi is used, deriving its blood supply from the external carotid artery or one of its branches. The orbito-zygomatic segment and craniotomy bone flap is replaced (Figure

44.23). Disadvantages of this approach include potential problems with the temporomandibular joint and destruction of the eustachian tube with conductive hearing loss (managed with a tympanostomy tube).

Kawase approach – anterior petrosectomy

This approach uses the triangle described by Kawase. It is used for lesions of the cavernous sinus as well as intra- and extradural lesions of the upper and middle clivus. The boundaries of the area that can be safely drilled are the greater superficial petrosal nerve laterally, the trigeminal impression anteriorly and the arcuate eminence posteriorly.[30] It is a more limited anterior petrosectomy approach. This approach involves a fronto-temporal craniotomy with or without zygomatic osteotomy. The middle meningeal artery is unroofed, coagulated at its entry from the foramen spinosum and cut. V3 is unroofed down to the foramen ovale. The horizontal segment of the carotid in the petrous bone is partially unroofed using a diamond burr, to gain control and to mobilize if required to access the tumor. The eustachian tube is not opened. The greater superficial petrosal nerve must be identified and either sacrificed or preserved without traction to prevent traction injury to the facial nerve. Drilling of the petrous bone is performed anterior and/or medial to the cochlea. The dura is opened over the trigeminal ganglion and root. The superior petrosal sinus is obliterated and the tentorium is incised to provide intradural access.

Combined subtemporal presigmoid retrolabyrinthine approach

This approach is used primarily to treat intradural clival tumors (e.g. meningiomas and neurilemmomas) in patients who have intact hearing.[31] The skin incision begins in the temporal region

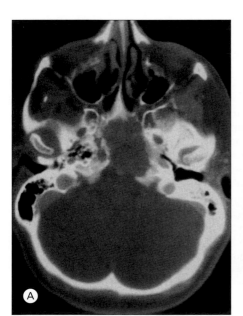
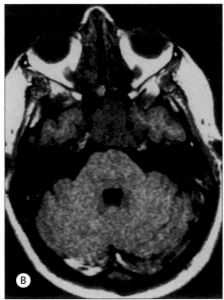
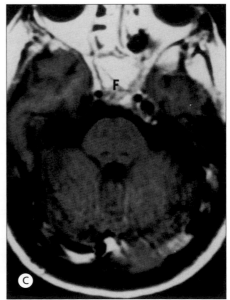

Figure 44.23 Preoperative CT **(A)** and MRI **(B)** scans showing the tumor in the clivus and left petrous apex with irregular bone destruction. The first operation was carried out through a bifrontal craniotomy and an extended subfrontal extradural approach. The tumor, which was found to be an adenoid cystic carcinoma, was very fibrous and tenacious and was only partially removed. The floor was reconstructed with a galeal pericranial flap. Two weeks after the first operation the remaining tumor around the left petrous internal carotid artery and the clivus was removed through a left subtemporal and preauricular infratemporal approach, after a left temporal craniotomy and orbitozygomatic osteotomy and resection of the mandibular condyle. The petrous internal carotid artery was completely exposed and mobilized and a gross total excision of tumor was achieved. Postoperative MRI **(C)** showing the area of tumor removal filled with fat and pericranial flap (F) (high-intensity signal).

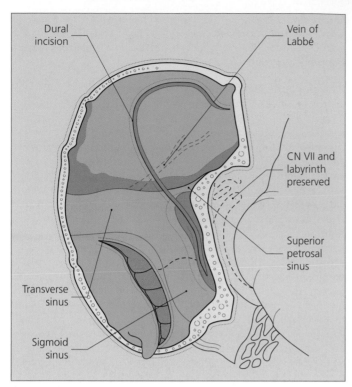

Figure 44.24 Exposure provided by the presigmoid subtemporal approach, used to reach petroclival tumors.

and curves inferiorly in the postauricular area and behind the mastoid. Following a combined temporal posterior fossa craniotomy, the sigmoid sinus and the lateral portion of the transverse sinus are completely unroofed by performing a mastoidectomy with a high-speed drill. This bone removal is carried up to the mastoid segment of the facial nerve and the semicircular canals, which are not disturbed. The dura is opened in front of the sigmoid sinus and in the temporal area (Figure 44.24). The superior petrosal sinus is ligated and divided, the incision extending medially toward the tentorial notch posterior to the entry of the trochlear nerve. The temporal lobe is elevated, protecting the veins that drain the temporal lobe, while the cerebellum is retracted posteriorly along with the sigmoid sinus to expose the tumor.

The advantage of this approach over a standard retrosigmoid approach is that the labyrinth is preserved while enough bone is removed in the petrous temporal region to bring the surgeon closer and more lateral to the tumor (Figure 44.25). Following tumor removal, the dura is closed in a watertight fashion, using a graft if necessary.

The petrous bone defect is filled with fat harvested from the abdomen. A temporal bone piece with titanium mesh plates can be used to reconstruct the craniotomy. In patients with no hearing, the approach can be further extended anteriorly into the labyrinth to provide a combined translabyrinthine and subtemporal access to the tumor.

Total petrosectomy

In contrast to the previous operation, this approach involves removal of the entire petrous temporal bone providing wider access to the intradural clivus and cerebellopontine angle. It is usually used for large petroclival meningiomas, glomus jugulare

tumors, and temporal bone carcinomas, particularly in patients with hearing loss. The surgical incision is usually a postauricular one and the external ear canal is divided and closed as a blind pouch. The ICA is uncovered as in the previous procedure, and the temporal bone is drilled down between the sigmoid sinus and the ICA. The facial nerve is completely lifted out of the temporal bone and rerouted anteriorly or posteriorly as required (Figure 44.26). The jugular bulb and the sigmoid sinus can be obliterated, if adequate communication with the opposite transverse sinus is demonstrated angiographically. When this approach is used for malignant tumors of the temporal bone, an en bloc resection that includes the cranial nerves is preferred. However, when the approach is used for benign tumors or to provide access to an intradural tumor, the bone is removed piecemeal, usually with a high-speed drill, preserving the cranial nerves anatomically. When this approach is used to gain access to a large intradural clival tumor, the tumor removal is performed at a separate stage, because of the duration and complexity of each part of the operation.

Reconstruction involves a thorough dural closure with a graft and a temporalis or sternomastoid flap to fill the defect. If the facial nerve has been transected it is also reconstructed with a greater auricular or sural nerve graft.

Extreme lateral transcondylar approach

This approach is used for intra- and extradural tumors at the lower clivus or foramen magnum, and those at C1 and C2 that are situated ventrally and ventrolaterally to the neuroaxis.[32,33] The incision is an inverted "L" shape behind the ear extending vertically downward in the upper cervical area. Craniectomy is extended in the retrosigmoid area to include the foramen magnum (C1 and C2 hemilamina and articular facets can be included when lower access is desired). The vertebral artery is isolated from the C2 or C1 foramen transversarium up to its dural entry. The joint between the occipital condyle and C1 lateral mass are fully exposed. If necessary, a portion or the entire occipital condyle may be removed. Removal of the occipital condyle and isolation of the extradural vertebral artery permits a true lateral perspective of this area. The vertebral artery is also completely released at its dural entry point to allow full mobilization and thus safe dissection from the tumor. The area of access is indicated in Figure 44.27. This approach provides access to the ventral craniocervical junction without brain retraction, and it enables the surgeon to remove all involved bone in the region of the occipital condyle, hypoglossal and jugular foramina, and the ventral clivus below the level of the jugular bulbs. If the tumor extends into the jugular foramen and the jugular bulb is either occluded or nondominant and has adequate cross-communication with its counterpart, the caudal cranial nerves can be completely skeletonized. The sigmoid sinus and the jugular vein can then be ligated and the tumor within the jugular foramen can be thoroughly removed (Figure 44.28). Following tumor removal, the dura is closed with a graft, and fat or a temporalis flap is used to obliterate the defect.

In some of the cases performed through a far lateral approach, cranio-cervical fusion is needed. The need for fusion depends on the amount of bone resected, mainly the occipital condyle, and whether the tumor itself has caused bony or joint disruption.[34] In cases where more than two-thirds of the condyle are removed or in cases of chordomas that tend to invade the joint, fusion is indicated. Metastatic tumors to the occipito-cervical area may destroy joints and will also require fusion. However, for most foramen magnum meningiomas, drilling of the condyle is limited and fusion is not needed.

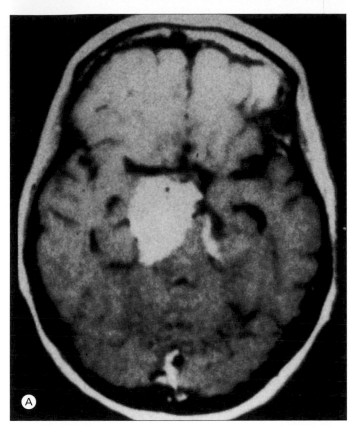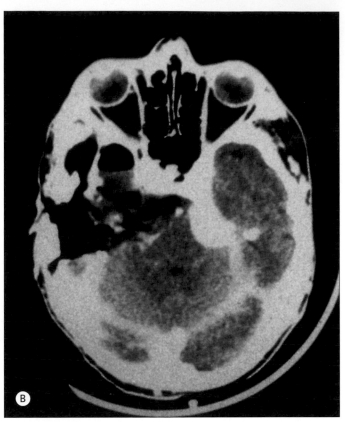

Figure 44.25 **(A)** Axial MRI showing a patient with bilateral medial tentorial meningiomas distorting the brainstem. The arrowhead points to the fetal origin of the posterior cerebral artery within the tumor. **(B)** The patient underwent a frontotemporal craniotomy, orbitozygomatic osteotomy, and removal of the supratentorial portion of the tumor. Two months later the remaining tumor, including its extension into the posterior cavernous sinus, was removed by a presigmoid subtemporal approach. A postoperative CT scan shows satisfactory tumor removal on the right.

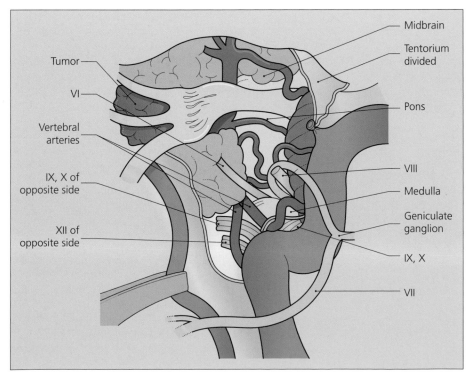

Figure 44.26 Petrosectomy approach used for a large intradural clival tumor. Note the removal of the temporal bone from the sigmoid sinus to the internal carotid artery and from the trigeminal root above to the jugular bulb below, allowing mobilization of the facial nerve. This approach provides a wide access to these extensive tumors.

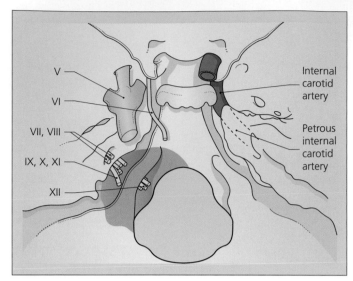

Figure 44.27 Area of access and bone removal by the extreme lateral transcondylar approach.

Postoperative care and complications

Postoperative problems are usually related to fluid and electrolyte imbalance, brain swelling, delayed vascular occlusion, CSF leaks, and, most frequently, difficulties arising as a consequence of cranial nerve palsies. Serious and irreversible complications may result if these problems are not anticipated or detected and treated early.

Although cranial-base surgery is a team effort, most of the life-threatening complications are neurologic or vascular, and thus the neurosurgeon must exercise special vigilance to prevent them.

Fluids and electrolytes

Close monitoring of the fluid balance and serum electrolytes reveals imbalances early. The follow-up should include every kind of intake and output as well as daily chemistry analysis. Fluid restriction in cases of SIADH and fluid augmentation with or without ADH in cases of diabetes insipidus are treatments that must start in an early phase of imbalance to prevent any major changes in the serum sodium level.

Imaging

A CT scan is performed on the first postoperative day to obtain a "baseline study," which reveals the presence of intracranial air, brain swelling, and hematomas as well as ventricle size, and can be compared with subsequent studies. In addition, this study allows assessment of the degree of tumor resection.

CSF leak

CSF leakage is a relatively common problem after these operations because of entry of the fluid into the paranasal sinuses, temporal air cells, or eustachian tube. Early detection helps prevent meningitis. Thorough reconstruction with vascularized tissue is a key step in preventing this problem. When the leak is

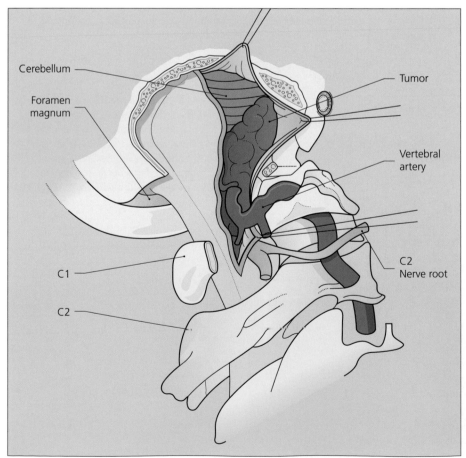

Figure 44.28 Bony removal includes partial or total condylectomy, and complete isolation of the vertebral artery up to its dural entry. The foramen magnum has been opened and a C1 hemilaminectomy has been performed. The C2 nerve root is crossing over the vertebral artery at its course between C1 and C2.

small it can usually be managed with a temporary spinal fluid drain; however, larger leaks require accurate determination of the fistula site and surgical repair. In any case of CSF leak, the question of hydrocephalus should be addressed. Ventricular enlargement may not be apparent on the scan because of the fluid escape through the leakage site.

Vascular problems

Following tumor resection the major intracranial arteries must be carefully protected from the contaminated spaces of the sinuses and the nasopharynx by vascularized tissue (e.g. temporalis muscle flap or galeal-pericranial flap) or through a vascularized tissue transfer. Postoperative angiography is recommended when the integrity of a particular vessel is in question. Occlusion of the vessel or formation of a pseudoaneurysm may thus be detected, and revascularization or obliteration of the vessel by neuroradiologic intervention may be undertaken before a catastrophic event develops.

Because the operations and confinement to bed are prolonged, deep venous thrombosis and pulmonary thromboembolism are risks. Pneumatic compression stockings and subcutaneous heparin are continued until the patient is ambulatory. Deep venous thrombosis should be detected early and anticoagulation therapy should be instituted if indicated. If this is contraindicated, insertion of a vena caval filter should be considered.

Cranial nerve problems

Cranial nerve dysfunction occurs frequently and can cause secondary problems. When either the trigeminal or the facial nerve is impaired, protection of the ipsilateral eye must involve shielding and adequate lubrication. An eyelid augmentation is necessary if prolonged difficulty is anticipated. Dysfunction of the glossopharyngeal, vagus, or hypoglossal nerves affects swallowing and airway protection. Under such circumstances, tracheostomy and feeding gastrostomy or jejunostomy are performed early – preventing aspiration and facilitating adequate nutrition and a smooth postoperative course – and can be reversed when these functions are recovered. Although nerve dysfunction is usually temporary, secondary disability is great if the nerves are affected jointly rather than individually, and grave if they are bilaterally impaired.

Infection

Fortunately, infection is infrequent considering the nature and duration of these operations. Infection can present as meningitis and intradural or extradural abscess. Its presence is heralded by fever and changes in the patient's mental status or local wound appearance. Spinal fluid examination and contrast-enhanced CT scan provide the diagnosis. Treatment involves prolonged intravenous antibiotics and debridement of an abscess if present. Removal of the bone flaps may also be necessary

When the temporomandibular joint or the masticatory muscles have been disrupted, early jaw exercises can prevent trismus and limited jaw excursion.

CONCLUSION

Tremendous progress has been made in the field of cranial base surgery, especially in the last decade. It continues to be a challenging multidisciplinary collaboration. Constant refinement and critical evaluation of the results are necessary to define the role of such treatment. Adjunctive treatment modalities need to be explored so the efficacy and safety of the management of lesions in these areas can be enhanced and supplemented.

CLINICAL PEARLS

- Meningiomas are the common tumors found at the skull base. These tumors are benign in most cases, but complete resection is difficult to achieve because of cranial nerves, blood vessels, and brainstem involvement. In some cases, adding radiation after removing the main bulk of the tumor may improve the prognosis for recurrence. Surgery must take into account the limitations of radiation in these cases – mainly the optic nerves and the brainstem.

- Cranial chordomas are typical of the clival area. These are tumors of low malignancy with low chance of distant metastasis but with locally aggressive behavior. Radical resection is the best treatment for these tumors, and even then, there is a high recurrence rate. The surgeon must remember that this is a bony tumor and remove all involved bone around the soft component. Most of the primary cases are extradural, but with recurrence, the tumor tends to be intradural and the chance for a complete resection is small.

- CSF leak is a common problem in skull-base surgery. Avoiding or correcting it requires knowledge of the anatomy of the paranasal sinuses and of their potential points of communication with the skull base. Sealing these spaces after removing a tumor should utilize a vascularized tissue. A team approach involving the neurosurgeon as well as an ear, nose, and throat surgeon that is specialized in skull-base surgery can achieve the best results.

- Cranial nerve injury is another common complication that may require a team approach for rehabilitation. Procedures like facial nerve grafting or lower cranial nerve injury resulting in swallowing problems are two of the more common examples.

- Skull-base surgery involves working in areas that are difficult to reach and are surrounded with critical structures. Improving the accessibility to these areas involves drilling away or temporarily removing bony structures and trying to avoid brain retraction. Further space is gained by brain relaxation using pharmacological agents and CSF drainage.

- Selecting the approach for resecting skull-based tumors depends on the location and extension of the tumor. Specific approaches are suitable for specific locations in every cranial fossa. In some cases, when the tumor occupies more then one cranial fossa, a combined approach could be used. When the tumor is very extensive, a staged procedure can be planned, performed in two sittings.

REFERENCES

1. Lang J. Anterior cranial base anatomy. In: Sekhar LN, Schramm VL Jr (eds). *Tumors of the Cranial Base: Diagnosis and Treatment*. Mt Kisco, NY: Futura Publishing Co.; 1987: 247–64.

2. Lang J. Middle cranial base anatomy. In: Sekhar LN, Schramm VL Jr (eds). *Tumors of the Cranial Base: Diagnosis and Treatment*. Mt Kisco, NY: Futura Publishing Co.; 1987: 313–34.

3. Lang J. Posterior cranial base anatomy. In: Sekhar LN, Schramm VL Jr (eds). *Tumors of the Cranial Base: Diagnosis and Treatment*. Mt Kisco, NY: Futura Publishing Co.; 1987: 441–60.

4. Black PM, Villavicencio AT, Rhouddou C, et al. Aggressive surgery and focal radiation in the management of meningiomas of the skull base: preservation of function with maintenance of local control. *Acta Neurochir (Wien)* 2001; 143: 555–62.

5. Batsakis JG. *Tumors of the Head and Neck—Clinical and Pathological Considerations*, 2nd edn. Baltimore: Williams & Wilkins; 1979.

6. Sen CN, Sekhar LN, Schramm VL, et al. Chordomas and chondrosarcomas of the cranial base. *Neurosurgery* 1989; 25: 931–41.

7. McMaster ML, Goldstein AM, Bromley CM, et al. Chordoma: incidence and survival patterns in the United States, 1973–1995. *Cancer Causes Control* 2001; 12: 1–11.

8. Crockard HA, Steel T, Plowman N, et al. A multidisciplinary team approach to skull base chordomas. *J Neurosurg* 2001; 95: 175–83.

9. Noel G, Habrand JL, Mammar H, et al. Combination of photon and proton radiation therapy for chordomas and chondrosarcomas of the skull base: the Centre de Protontherapie D'Orsay experience. *Int J Radiat Oncol Biol Phys* 2001; 51: 392–8.

10. Holton JL, Steel T, Luxsuwong M, et al. Skull base chordomas: correlation of tumor doubling time with age, mitosis and KI67 proliferation index. *Neuropathol Appl Neurobiol* 2000; 26: 497–503.

11. Rosenberg AE, Nielsen GP, Keel SB, et al. Chondrosarcoma of the base of the skull: a clinicopathologic study of 200 cases with emphasis on its distinction from chordoma. *Am J Surg Pathol* 1999; 23: 1370–8.

12. Crockard HA, Cheeseman A, Steel T, et al. A multidisciplinary team approach to skull base chondrosarcomas; *J Neurosurg* 2001; 95: 184–9.

13. Pitman KT, Prokopakis EP, Aydogan B, et al. The role of skull base surgery for the treatment of adenoid cystic carcinoma of the sinonasal tract. *Head Neck* 1999; 21: 402–7.

14. Weiland LH. Nasopharyngeal carcinomas. In: Barnes L (ed.). *Surgical Pathology of the Head and Neck*. New York: Marcel Dekker; 1985: 453–66.

15. Greta R, Bunin, Tanya S, et al. The descriptive epidemiology of craniopharyngioma. *Neurosurg Focus* 1997; 3: Article 1.

16. Mottolese C, Stan H, Hermier M, et al. Intracystic chemotherapy with bleomycin in the treatment of craniopharyngiomas. *Child's Nerv Syst* 2001; 17: 724–30.

17. Dort JC, Sutherland GR. Intraoperative magnetic resonance imaging for skull base surgery. *Laryngoscope* 2001; 111: 1570–5.

18. Fahlbusch R, Ganslandt O, Buchfelder M, et al. Intraoperative magnetic resonance imaging during transsphenoidal surgery. *J Neurosurg* 2001; 95: 381–90.

19. Osborn AG. *Introduction to Cerebral Angiography*. Hagerstown, MD: Harper & Row; 1980: 331.

20. Marshall RS, Lazar RM, Young WL, et al. Clinical utility of quantitative cerebral blood flow measurements during internal carotid artery test occlusions. *Neurosurgery* 2002; 50: 996–1004.

21. Moller AR. *Evoked Potentials in Intraoperative Monitoring*. Baltimore: Williams & Wilkins; 1988.

22. Spetzler RF, Herman JM, Beals S, et al. Preservation of olfaction in anterior craniofacial approaches. *Neurosurgery* 1993; 79: 48–52.

23. Sepehrnia A, Knopp U. Preservation of the olfactory tract in bifrontal craniotomy for various lesions of the anterior cranial fossa. *Neurosurgery* 1999; 44: 113–17.

24. Raveh J, Turk JB, Ladrach K, et al. Extended anterior subcranial approach for skull base tumors: long-term results. *J Neurosurg* 1995; 82: 1002–10.

25. Menezes AH, VanGilder JC. Transoral transpharyngeal approach to the anterior craniocervical junction. *J Neurosurg* 1988; 69: 895–903.

26. Crockard HA, Sen CN. The transoral approach for the management intradural lesions at the craniovertebral junction. *Neurosurgery* 1991; 28: 88–98.

27. Miller CG, van Loveren HR, Keller JT, et al. Transpetrosal approach: surgical anatomy and technique. *Neurosurgery* 1993; 33: 461–9.

28. Sekhar LN, Schramm VL, Jones NF. Subtemporal-preauricular infratemporal fossa approach to large lateral and posterior cranial base neoplasms. *J Neurosurg* 1987; 67: 488–99.

29. Sen CN, Sekhar LN. The subtemporal and preauricular infratemporal approach to intradural structures ventral to the brain stem. *J Neurosurg* 1990; 73: 345–54.

30. Kawase T, Shiobara R, Toya S. Anterior transpetrosal-transtentorial approach for sphenopetroclival meningiomas: surgical method and results in 10 patients. *Neurosurgery* 1991; 28: 869–75.

31. Al-Mefty O, Fox JL, Smith RR. Petrosal approach for petroclival meningiomas. *Neurosurgery* 1988; 22: 510–17.

32. Sen CN, Sekhar LN. An extreme lateral approach to intradural lesions of the cervical spine and foramen magnum. *Neurosurgery* 1990; 27: 197–204.

33. Sen CN, Sekhar LN. Surgical management of anteriorly placed lesions of the craniocervical junction—an alternative approach. *Acta Neurochir* 1991; 122: 108.

34. Bejjani GK, Sekhar LN, Riedel CJ. Occipitocervical fusion following the extreme lateral transcondylar approach. *Surg Neurol* 2000; 54: 109–15.

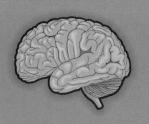

RADIATION THERAPY FOR CENTRAL NERVOUS SYSTEM TUMORS

45

Rakesh R Patel, Wolfgang A Tomé, and Minesh P Mehta

INTRODUCTION

Primary malignant tumors of the brain are relatively uncommon neoplasms, accounting for less than 2% of all malignancies diagnosed in the United States; however, because of their extremely poor overall survival, they represent a significant cause of cancer mortality. In contrast, metastatic tumors to the brain are a very commonly encountered clinical situation with the annual estimated incidence of brain metastasis in the United States in excess of 100 000 cases.[1] These patients have even poorer survival rates than those with primary brain tumors. In this chapter, we will highlight the role of radiation therapy in the management of these disease processes, including the radiobiologic rationale, and will emphasize the evolving techniques of radiation delivery as well as advances in treatment planning and subsequent clinical breakthroughs.

RADIOBIOLOGY AND THE PHYSICS OF RADIOTHERAPY

Radiation is energy that is emitted and propagated through space or a medium in the form of waves or particles, and is categorized as electromagnetic or particulate. Particulate radiation is the propagation of energy by traveling particles that are characterized by mass, momentum, and position in time; examples include electrons, protons, and α-particles. First described by Maxwell in the mid-19th century, electromagnetic radiations are transverse waves consisting of oscillating electric and magnetic fields; examples include X-rays, gamma-rays, radiowaves, visible light, ultraviolet light, and microwaves. The energy of electromagnetic radiation is often quantified as photons, or "packets" of energy.

Therapeutic radiation can be categorized by how it is produced – either high-energy machines, such as linear accelerators, can generate radiation beams; or radiation can be emitted through radioisotope decay. Most commonly, radiation therapy involves external beam treatments using X-rays or electrons, but protons, neutrons, and gamma-rays from cobalt-60 decay may also be used. The X-rays (photons) and electrons used in radiation oncology are of much higher energy than those used in diagnostic radiology, and are produced by linear accelerators. Most linear accelerators are capable of generating therapeutic X-rays and electrons of varying energies; this results in beams with different tissue-penetrating characteristics, making the treatment of malignancies in various anatomical locations possible.

Radiation can be either directly or indirectly ionizing. Directly ionizing radiations, such as protons and other charged particles, produce chemical and biologic damage by disrupting subcellular targets of the cells through which they pass. Electromagnetic X-rays and gamma-rays, which are the most commonly used, however, are indirectly ionizing. They do not produce direct damage themselves, but when absorbed in a medium, usually rich in water content, they give up their energy to produce ultra-short-lived, fast-moving charged particles and radicals that cause chemical and biologic damage. There is strong circumstantial evidence that the primary target of this biologic damage is DNA.[2]

Radiation impact at the cellular level

What happens when DNA is targeted by radiation? When cells are irradiated, many single-strand DNA breaks occur. Generally, these breaks are readily repaired using the opposite strand of the DNA as a template, and thus are of minimal biological consequence. Alternatively, double-strand DNA breaks can be biologically significant. If both strands of the DNA break directly opposite or very near to one another, then a double-strand break may occur. If the two breaks rejoin in their original configuration, then the next mitosis can proceed without difficulty. The two breaks may not reunite, leading to a deletion, or the breaks in the two chromosomes may rejoin incorrectly, giving rise to distorted chromosomes at the next mitosis.

There are two classes of distortions that occur, chromosomal and chromatid aberrations. Chromosomal aberrations occur if a cell is irradiated before the chromosomal material has been copied, and chromatid aberrations are produced if the radiation occurs after DNA has been duplicated. There are many types of chromosomal aberrations that can occur – some are lethal to the cell and some are nonlethal but are associated with carcinogenesis.

Cell death can be described as apoptotic or mitotic. Apoptosis, also called "programmed cell death," is an active process of rapid cell death resulting from the triggering of a sequence of morphologic events that culminate with the fragmentation of DNA and phagocytosis of the apoptotic cell. Certain cell types, such as lymphoid and hemopoietic cells, are particularly prone to radiation-induced apoptosis. Mitotic death occurs in the cell's attempt to divide, and is the result of damaged chromosomes. Mitotic death is the most common form of radiation-induced cell death, and in some cells is the only mode of death.

Cellular radiosensitivity to mitotic death varies with the stage of the cell cycle. Cells are most sensitive at or close to mitosis and

G2 phase, and most resistant in S phase. A family of genes, called molecular checkpoint genes, control progression through the cell cycle. These molecular checkpoint genes delay transition from G1 to S, or G2 to M, in cells that are exposed to radiation. This pause in cell cycle progression allows the chromosomes to be checked for damage and the damage to be repaired before mitosis occurs. Certain syndromes associated with a predisposition to cancer or that exhibit an exquisite radiosensitivity have been discovered to have cells with mutated genes that fail to arrest at molecular checkpoints.

THE CLINICAL ROLE OF RADIATION THERAPY

Radiotherapy is frequently employed in the management of patients with central nervous system (CNS) neoplasms (Table 45.1). It is often used postoperatively as adjunctive therapy to decrease local failure, to delay tumor progression and prolong survival as in malignant glioma, as curative treatment in diseases such as primitive neuroectodermal tumor, germ cell tumors, and pilocytic astrocytoma (unresectable or multiply recurrent), or as a therapy that halts further tumor growth as in schwannoma, meningioma, pituitary tumors, and craniopharyngioma.

Radiotherapy improves local control and survival

Radiotherapy is used in several types of brain tumors, both benign and malignant, after subtotal resection to improve local control; as a consequence, recurrence-free survival, as well as overall survival can potentially be improved[3] (Table 45.2). Composite data from 34 literature reports documenting outcomes for craniopharyngioma are presented to illustrate the reduction in local failure, which translates to a survival advantage.[4] The recurrence/relapse rate following subtotal resection alone for craniopharyngioma is 73% and drops to 17% with postoperative radiotherapy, resulting in improved 5- and 10-year survival (Table 45.3). Similarly, progression-free survival is improved with the addition of radiotherapy in cases of subtotally resected meningioma (Table 45.4).

Table 45.1 Brain tumors with a defined or possible role for radiotherapy

Low-grade astrocytoma	Vestibular and other schwannoma
Anaplastic astrocytoma	Craniopharyngioma
Glioblastoma multiforme	Pituitary tumors
Low-grade oligodendroglioma	CNS germ cell tumors
Anaplastic oligodendroglioma	Pilocytic astrocytoma
Mixed gliomas	Ganglioglioma
Ependymoma	Hemangioblastoma
Primitive neuroectodermal tumors	Hemangiopericytoma
Primary CNS lymphoma	Sarcoma
Meningioma	Choroid plexus carcinoma

Table 45.2 The curative potential of radiotherapy

Disease	Survival (no XRT)	Survival (with XRT)
PNET	< 10%	50–70%
CNS germinoma	< 5%	> 90%
Craniopharyngioma	10-year: 37%	10-year: 77%
Vestibular schwannoma	5-year PFS: > 90%	5-year PFS: > 90%
Glioblastoma	MS: 18 weeks	MS: 42 weeks

XRT, radiotherapy; CNS, central nervous system; MS, median survival; PFS, progression-free survival; PNET, primitive neuroectodermal tumor.

Table 45.3 Diminished local failure rates affect survival for craniopharyngioma after subtotal resection (STR), total resection (TR), or radiation therapy (XRT)

Treatment outcome	TR	STR	STR + XRT
5-year survival	81%	53%	89%
10-year survival	69%	37%	77%
Recurrence	29%	73%	17%

Table 45.4 Radiotherapy diminishes local failure rates for meningioma after subtotal resection (STR), total resection (TR), or radiation therapy (XRT)

Treatment outcome	TR	STR	STR + XRT
5-year progression	5%	37%	11%
10-year progression	10%	55%	23%
15-year progression	32%	91%	

Table 45.5 The effect of posterior fossa dose for medulloblastoma

Author	Year	< 50 Gy	> 50 Gy
Harisiadis[5]	1977	24%	48%
Cumberlin[6]	1979	17%	86%
Berry[7]	1981	42%	78%
Silverman[8]	1982	38%	80%
Kopelson[9]	1983	50%	78%

Gy, gray

The impact of radiation dose

An excellent case study illustrating the impact of radiotherapy dose–response effect is provided by the clinical experience with medulloblastoma (posterior fossa primitive neuroectodermal tumor). The typical treatment approach for patients with non-disseminated disease is craniospinal irradiation to 36 Gy followed by a boost to the posterior fossa to 54 Gy. The impact of posterior fossa dose on local control is presented in Table 45.5. Low doses

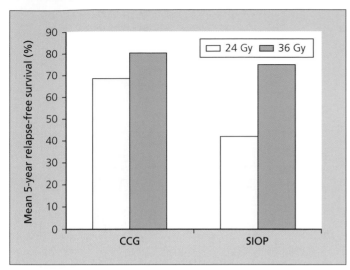

Figure 45.1 The impact of reducing craniospinal axis dose: medulloblastoma. Reduced radiation doses led to increased neuraxis failure rates in these two randomized trials.

Table 45.6 The impact of dose for low-grade glioma

Dose	n	Five-year survival	Five-year RFS	Second malignancy
0 Gy*		66%	37%	23/29 (79%)
45 Gy†	171	58%	47%	
50.4 Gy‡	101	73%		
54 Gy*		63%	44%	19/22 (86%)
59.4 Gy†	172	59%	50%	
64.8 Gy‡	102	68%		

Second malignancy, rate of malignant conversion of initial low-grade gliomas calculated as a crude (not actuarial) rate from patients undergoing reoperation; Gy, gray; RFS, relapse-free survival. *Arms from EORTC 22845 trial; †arms from EORTC 22844 trial; ‡arms from NCCTG 867251.

yield high local failure rates, whereas higher doses lead to significant reduction in posterior fossa failures. The dose to the craniospinal axis was lowered in one Children's Cancer Group (CCG) trial to 24 Gy and compared with the standard dose. Three-year analysis of the data from CCG 923 showed that the isolated neuraxis failure rate was two of 44 in the 36-Gy arm compared with 11 of 45 in the 24-Gy arm.[10] A European trial, SIOP II also demonstrated this phenomenon, with 5-year relapse-free survival of 42 versus 75% for the lower and higher dose arms, respectively (Figure 45.1).[11]

HISTOLOGIC SUBTYPES

Treatment of low-grade gliomas

Three randomized trials evaluating the role of radiotherapy for low-grade gliomas have now been completed (Table 45.6).[12–14] These trials tested the dose range from 0 to 64.8 Gy, and at the 5-year time point did not demonstrate a survival advantage. The 5-year relapse-free survival was lowest at 37% in patients who were observed and did not receive radiotherapy. In the radiation arms, 5-year relapse-free survival ranged from 44 to 50%. These differences are important in a tumor with a slow rate of growth and relatively prolonged natural history. Although a survival advantage may not necessarily be apparent at 5 years, it could in fact become significant with longer follow-up, especially given that relapse-free survival appears to be better in patients receiving up-front radiotherapy. However, no apparent dose-effect on relapse-free survival is clearly discernible. Furthermore, in the patients undergoing re-operation, the rate of malignant conversion is not different in patients who were observed compared with those who received up-front radiotherapy.

Treatment of anaplastic astrocytomas

Anaplastic astrocytoma presents an interesting paradox for the dose–response theme. To enhance the effectiveness of radiotherapy dose, several clinical trials have explored either the addition of chemotherapy, radiosensitizers, or neutrons; unfortunately, a composite analysis of the data shows poorer survival with the more aggressive approaches. Laramore has reviewed the Radiation Therapy Oncology Group's experience with conventional radiotherapy, chemo-radiotherapy and the addition of neutrons, demonstrating median survival values of 3, 2.3 and 1.7 years (Figure 45.2A). Recent analysis of a randomized trial evaluating the role of bromodeoxyuridine (Budr), a radiosensitizer, showed an inferior 1-year survival of 68% in the experimental arm, compared with 82% in the arm not receiving the sensitizer (Figure 45.2B). Similarly, the addition of PCV [procarbazine, CCNU (lomustine), and vincristine] chemotherapy has not demonstrated any convincing survival benefit for this disease, as an adjuvant to radiotherapy.[15]

Treatment of glioblastoma multiforme

For malignant brain tumors such as glioblastoma, traditional therapeutic trials have explored the 0–60 Gy dose range, hyperfractionation trials have explored doses up to 80 Gy and brachytherapy trials have reached 100–120 Gy. Although the dose–response phenomenon across this large range has not been prospectively evaluated, a review of the composite data from various clinical trials and institutional experiences suggest a shallow dose–response effect. It is therefore not surprising that whereas no-dose versus high-dose studies have shown a survival benefit (Table 45.7), clinical trials seeking to identify survival differences between dose-schedules of modest dose-variation (60–80 Gy) have not been statistically meaningful.[3] Effective improvement is not likely to be realized until substantial dose escalation can be achieved. This will require the development of techniques that maximally spare normal tissue and imaging advances that identify well-defined sub-volumes that represent the focus from which resistant clones arise, thereby permitting up-front differential boosting of these regions.

Treatment of oligodendrogliomas

Oligodendroglioma represents a unique clinical situation from the perspective of radiotherapy. These tumors are generally classified

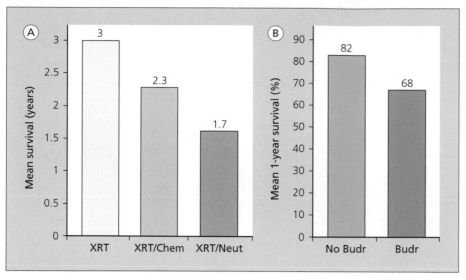

Figure 45.2 Anaplastic astrocytoma: is more worse? Median survival values of 3, 2.3 and 1.7 years with radiotherapy alone, radiotherapy plus chemotherapy, and radiotherapy plus neutron therapy **(A)**. The impact of bromodeoxyuridine (Budr) demonstrating an inferior 1-year survival of 68% compared with 82% in the arm not receiving the sensitizer **(B)**.

Table 45.7 Local control is a function of dose for glioblastoma

Dose	MS (weeks)	25% survival	P
0 Gy	18	N/A	N/A
< 45 Gy	14	N/A	ns
50 Gy	28	52	< 0.001
55 Gy	36	57	< 0.001
60 Gy	42	68	< 0.001

25% survival, 25th percentile survival; MS, median survival.

Table 45.8 Survival by histologic type following resection and radiotherapy

Tumor type	Median survival
Low-grade oligodendroglioma	~120 months
Low-grade astrocytoma	~60 months
Anaplastic oligodendroglioma	~60 months
Anaplastic astrocytoma	~36 months
Glioblastoma multiforme	~10 months

Table 45.9 Radiotherapy techniques

External beam radiotherapy	Brachytherapy
Conventional	Temporary high dose-rate
Three-dimensional conformal	Permanent low dose-rate
Radiosurgery	Intracavitary isotopes
Fractionated stereotactic radiotherapy	Isotope balloon implants
Intensity-modulated radiation therapy monoclonal antibodies	Localized radiolabeled

as low-grade or anaplastic and typically carry a more favorable prognosis than their astrocytic counterparts (Table 45.8). Recent molecular analysis suggests that subsets of these tumors are characterized by chromosomal losses on 1p and/or 19q. These tumors exhibit exquisite sensitivity to radiation and chemotherapy and preliminary reports suggest that improved survival may also be associated with such deletions.[16] Identification of the specific gene losses and their gene products may yield novel strategies to modulate the radiation responsiveness of several glial neoplasms, thereby providing a discriminant that drives therapeutic decisions.

RADIOTHERAPY TECHNIQUES

Radiation therapy can be delivered using either external beam techniques of varying degrees of sophistication, or through highly localized isotope placement, known as brachytherapy (Table 45.9). There are several different options, each with specific advantages and disadvantages. Brachytherapy approaches are most effective at delivering highly localized radiation and avoiding irradiation of normal tissue, but they are limited because of their invasive nature. External beam radiotherapy approaches have evolved and have recently become very sophisticated, enabling the radiation beam to be shaped so as to minimize normal tissue exposure. This has been achieved by improvement in tumor targeting, using sophisticated treatment planning programs capable of permitting

image-fusion of multiple different datasets, such as computed tomography (CT), magnetic resonance imaging and spectroscopy (MRI, MRS), and positron emission tomography, etc., as well as significant improvement in immobilization and localization processes, allowing a reduction in the size of the error margin that is typically built into radiotherapy treatment plans.

Stereotactic radiosurgery

Radiosurgery refers to the delivery of a single large dose of radiation to a small intracranial target, utilizing a stereotactic

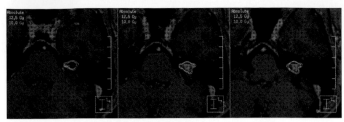

Figure 45.3 Radiosurgery. Treatment plan of a left vestibular schwannoma demonstrating 12.5 Gy and 10 Gy isodose lines.

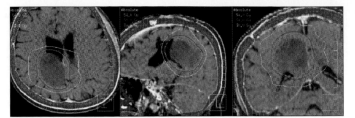

Figure 45.4 Fractionated stereotactic radiotherapy. Treatment plan of a well-circumscribed 4.5 cm lesion (red = target volume) demonstrating 30 Gy, 51 Gy, and 54 Gy isodose lines.

localization system, and maximal head immobilization, frequently achieved by using an invasive stereotactic frame. This concept is radically different from the usual fractionation approach of radiotherapy delivery. The technique was initially developed to deliver substantial doses of radiation to ablate tiny regions of brain to achieve a functional change, such as seizure control, control of tremor, trigeminal neuralgia, etc. Over the last two decades, the approach has found application in treating several CNS tumors. Currently, the most commonly used stereotactic tools for both brain tumors and functional regions include the LINAC, which uses the energy from a linear accelerator, and gamma-knife radiosurgery which uses a gamma source. The example in Figure 45.3 demonstrates the use of radiosurgery in the management of vestibular schwannoma. The radiation is conformed primarily around the tumor. Local control rates in excess of 90% are achieved.[17] Several other well-localized brain tumors are now treated with radiosurgery, either alone or as part of the boost phase of radiotherapy.

Fractionated stereotactic radiotherapy

One of the primary disadvantages of single fraction radiosurgery is the inability to exploit the various radiobiological characteristics of tumors, which make fractionation more appealing.[18] This includes the possibility of targeting the tumor in multiple phases of the cell cycle, thereby avoiding the pitfall of having all cells in a radioresistant phase, which could happen with single fraction treatment. In addition, late normal tissue effects are most sensitive to fraction size, and decreasing fraction size, which is not possible with radiosurgery to a substantial degree, would permit reduction in toxicity. On the other hand, radiosurgery, with its precision delivery and almost perfect immobilization, provides an unprecedented degree of delivery accuracy. The two concepts can therefore be merged into an option referred to as fractionated stereotactic radiotherapy (FSRT).

FSRT provides the opportunity to treat even larger tumors (up to 6 cm diameter) than is possible with radiosurgery (up to 3 cm diameter) with margins that only take uncertainties introduced through imaging and the physical penumbra into account. An example is illustrated in Figures 45.4 and 45.5, in which a well-defined 4.5-cm diameter tumor is treated with five beams, all non-coplanar, and all using the concept of "beam's eye-view," i.e. targeting the tumor along the axis where its projected diameter to the skull surface is the smallest and adding a 7-mm block margin. This permits the radiation dose to normal tissue to be minimized. FSRT can be employed with as few as 4–5, or with as many as 25–33 fractions, as dictated by the clinical scenario.[19]

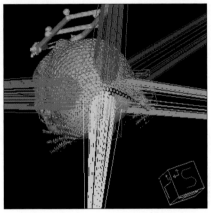

Figure 45.5 Fractionated stereotactic radiotherapy. Schematic of the five noncoplanar beams utilized for optimal target volume coverage.

Intensity-modulated radiotherapy

In the ultimate effort to improve normal tissue sparing and enhance tumor dose-conformality, the ideal approach would alter the radiation intensity across the width of the beam, such that the portions targeting larger tumor volumes deliver a higher dose, whereas other segments targeting lesser tumor burden deliver a lower dose. This approach, referred to as intensity modulated radiotherapy (IMRT), can further improve the therapeutic ratio. An example is presented in Figure 45.6. This pilocytic astrocytoma was treated to a total dose of 45 Gy and treatment planning was performed using three approaches: a standard three-field, an FSRT and an IMRT approach; the resulting dose-distributions are presented as dose–volume histograms in Figure 45.7. The IMRT plan results in the greatest sparing of normal brain tissue.

ADVANCES IN TREATMENT PLANNING

The use of image-fusion

Traditional planning in radiotherapy has relied on the treatment-planning CT scan. This has several advantages such as allowing imaging in the exact treatment position, thereby allowing easy dosimetric calculations to be performed with dose distributions in three-dimensional space. However, in many instances, superior tumor visualization is achieved with MRI. Most modern radiotherapy treatment plans now permit on-line imports of secondary image data-sets such as MRI, which can be co-registered (or fused) with the primary dataset (CT). This approach allows precise dosimetry using CT, and superior tumor definition using MRI, as illustrated in Figure 45.8. As imaging techniques become more

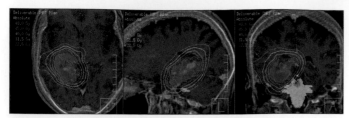

Figure 45.6 Intensity-modulated radiotherapy. Treatment plan of a left-sided lesion demonstrating conformal tight target coverage (blue) and avoidance of nearby critical structure, brainstem (yellow).

Table 45.10 Useful information in image modalities for treatment planning

Anatomical imaging modalities
CT and 3D-SPGR-T1 MRI: provides anatomical information.

Physiological or functional imaging modalities
Chemical shift imaging (CSI): can be used to determine the metabolic "fingerprint" from a region of tumor
Perfusion imaging (pMR): can be used to measure the cerebral blood volume on a voxel by voxel basis, and therefore is a measure of tumor angiogenesis
Diffusion imaging (dMR): can be used to detect areas of active cell proliferation within a tumor volume
BOLD imaging: when combined with carbogen breathing, BOLD imaging can be employed to gain an understanding of possible chronically hypoxic regions within a tumor

BOLD imaging, blood-oxygen-level-dependent imaging; SPGR-T1 MRI, spoiled gradient-T1 magnetic resonance imaging.

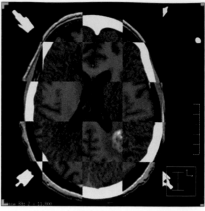

Figure 45.8 Image-fusion. In this figure, both CT and MRI are superimposed and viewed in a checkerboard format which allows visual confirmation of sound image fusion. In this example, the tumor is well-visualized on the MRI, but poorly on CT.

sophisticated, these need to be incorporated into the treatment planning process.

Implementation of advanced physiologic imaging

Methods for integrating advanced physiological imaging into radiation therapy treatment planning of brain tumors are being investigated.[20] Several examples are illustrated in Table 45.10 and

Figure 45.9. These imaging techniques may allow one to define subvolumes consisting of areas of possible chronic hypoxia, areas of high perfusion, high proliferation and areas containing high choline concentrations, thereby improving precise target volume delineation. For example, the advent of MRS now permits better definition of the chemical signatures of tumors (Figure 45.10). In normal brain, the MRS pattern typically shows a high N-acetyl aspartate (NAA) peak and lower choline and creatine peaks; in gliomas, the NAA peak is depressed, with a corresponding increase, particularly of the choline peak. Such chemical composition can be assayed voxel-by-voxel and displayed as chemical "maps." Such information can be fused to treatment-planning CT scans, allowing better tumor definition. In the future, it will be possible to make a probabilistic model that could predict possible relapse rate frequencies in varying zones, of choline concentration for example, and design radiation treatment plans with differential doses to these regions, thereby treating the highest risk areas to the highest dose. This will also help differentiate tumor regions from gliosis and necrosis, which can appear similar on standard MRI. This should in turn allow safer dose escalation studies with subsequent improved clinical outcomes.

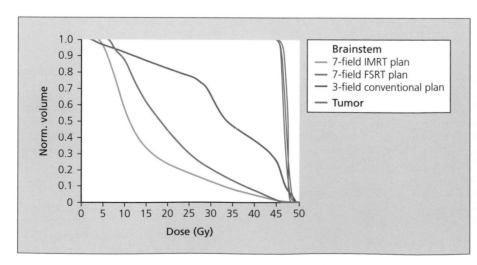

Figure 45.7 Dose–volume histogram comparisons of various techniques. Three different techniques for treating the tumor illustrated in Figure 45.6 are presented. The x-axis depicts the dose in Gy to any structure and the y-axis represents the proportionate volume for the region of interest. The tumor dose–volume histograms are illustrated by the three curves in the upper right corner, which demonstrate that the entire tumor receives at least 45 Gy, and small proportions up to 49 Gy. Tumor coverage is identical with all techniques. The dose to the brainstem however is considerably different. The dose received by 50% of the brainstem is 34 Gy, 17 Gy and 12 Gy with the three-field, FSRT and IMRT methods, respectively.

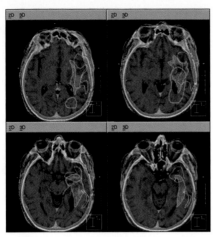

Figure 45.9 Contours from physiologic imaging modalities. Target volume delineation based on various advanced imaging modalities. Blue area, volume determined from choline maps, indicative of possible microscopic extensions of the tumor. Green area, volume of blood–brain barrier breakdown as determined from T1 MRI. This is the standard gross tumor volume. Yellow area, volume determined using pMR, indicative of areas of tumor that are well-perfused (aerobic areas of the tumor). Red area, volume determined form BOLD imaging combined with carbogen breathing, indicative of chronically hypoxic tumor regions.

RADIATION INJURY TO THE CENTRAL NERVOUS SYSTEM

The mechanism of normal tissue injury

The dose of irradiation that can be delivered to the tumor is often limited by the tolerance to radiation of the surrounding normal tissues (Figures 45. 11, 45.12). This is true in the CNS as well as in other regions of the body. The development of a normal tissue injury depends on the interaction of a number of factors, including the ability of irradiated cells to repair damage to their DNA, the total dose of radiation, the daily dose of radiation, the ability of tissues to regenerate after radiation injury, and the effect of intercurrent insults such as chemotherapy, surgery, trauma, or infections (Figure 45.13). By adjusting the total dose and the dose per fraction one can minimize the risk of normal tissue injury while maximizing the chances of achieving tumor control. In general, the use of daily doses above 2 Gy will require that the total dose be lowered to avoid late normal tissue injury. In general, radiation reactions can be broadly classified into three temporal categories: acute, subacute and delayed.

Acute reactions

Acute reactions are those that occur during and immediately following completion of a course of external beam radiation

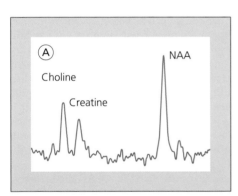

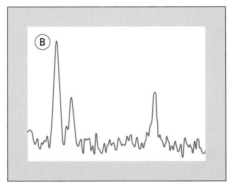

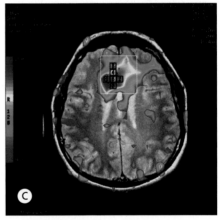

Figure 45.10 MRS for gliomas. The case for differential boosting: both normal **(A)** and tumor **(B)** spectra, as well as a tumor metabolite map **(C)**, are illustrated.

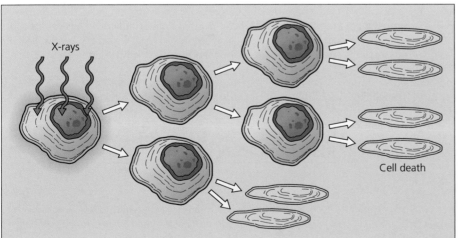

Figure 45.11 The causes and consequences of the lethal effect of ionizing radiation on normal and tumor cells are of great interest to the clinician. The loss of cell viability means a loss of capacity for sustained proliferation of the tumor with its attendant local compression/ infiltration, metabolic demands on the host, and risk of tumor dissemination. The target for the cytotoxic effects of radiation is DNA. Cell death is most commonly the result of nonrepaired double-strand breaks in the double helix. Death is manifested by an inability to carry out cell division successfully – a clonogenic death. As this cell pedigree shows, a cell may go through one or several divisions before death occurs.

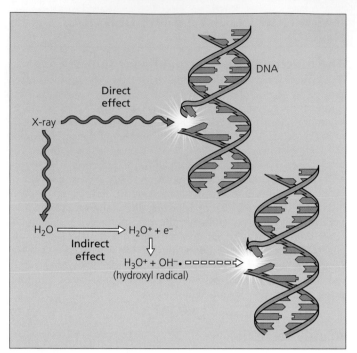

Figure 45.12 Ionizing radiation may damage DNA following ionization of purine or pyrimidine bases via a direct interaction of photons with the DNA – radiation's direct effect. The effects of radiation may be secondary to biochemical intermediates such as those produced by the interaction of radiation with water – radiation's indirect effect. The most important of the biochemical intermediates generated by radiation are hydroxyl radicals. These highly reactive compounds have an unpaired electron in the outer shell. The chemical changes wrought by free radicals produce the biologic damage leading to clonogenic death. Most radiation biologic damage is caused by the indirect effect.

therapy. Using current technologies, these reactions are usually rare and clinically readily manageable. They include acute skin reactions, typically dry desquamation and some degree of erythema, which are managed with local ointments; temporary alopecia within the radiation field is a common sequela. Fatigue may be observed with radiation therapy, but is often a function of several other variables such as age, performance status, underlying medical status, extent of brain being irradiated, etc. Acute visual complications during radiotherapy are very rare, but occasionally patients report seeing flashes of light while undergoing radiation therapy. This is believed to be secondary to retinal stimulation, secondary to a phenomenon described as Cerenkov radiation. If both ear canals are included in the radiation field, serous otitis media may develop towards the end of radiation therapy, sometimes producing muffled hearing. Nausea is uncommon unless the area postrema is treated to high doses or with large fractions. Increased intracranial pressure during radiotherapy is uncommon. This, however, may be masked as the vast majority of patients have been initiated on steroids prior to radiotherapy and are frequently maintained on steroids during radiation therapy.

Subacute reactions

Subacute reactions may occur several weeks or months after completion of radiation therapy. When large volumes of the brain are treated, especially in younger patients, lethargy and somno-

lence may be observed in approximately 3 months. In children, this is specifically described as an acute somnolence syndrome. Rarely, some patients may develop localized demyelination resulting in nausea, vomiting, ataxia, dysphasia, and cerebellar ataxia. This is usually self-limiting. If the lacrimal gland/s are included in the radiation portal, dry eye may result; similarly, a keratoconjunctivitis may develop if the cornea is not protected.

Late complications

Late complications of radiotherapy occur from several months to several years after completion of therapy. The exact incidence of these complications is unclear as a substantial proportion of patients are either short-term survivors only or have a component of both tumor progression and delayed radiation morbidity. Radiation necrosis in the absence of tumor progression is not commonly encountered when total doses are kept under 60 Gy. However, necrosis in concert with viable tumor is not uncommonly seen, especially in patients with malignant glioma. With sequential CT imaging, a mineralizing angiopathy can be identified, characterized by loss of white matter, enlarged ventricles and microcalcifications. This occurs as a consequence of radiation injury to small vessels, and clinically may result in impairment of intellectual function, especially memory and mathematical ability. In severe cases, this may result in significant dementia, ataxia, and confusion. Significant white matter atrophy may be an accompaniment on imaging studies.

The clinical sequelae of these changes are frequently manifest as neurocognitive impairment. The exact incidence of such impairment remains inadequately quantified, as many patients with malignant neoplasms frequently succumb to the disease process before neurocognitive development is impaired; therefore, the true incidence of this phenomenon is probably greater than is reported in most clinical trials. Several factors have now been identified as contributory to overall neurocognitive decline in these patients, including the tumor itself, surgery, radiation, and chemotherapy. In addition, host factors such as underlying diseases, especially those diseases characterized by microvascular changes, such as diabetes, hypertension, smoking, stroke, cardiovascular insufficiency, etc., also contribute to this. Specific radiotherapy parameters that influence the risk profile for neurocognitive decline include fraction size, total dose, and volume irradiated. Therefore, current radiotherapy paradigms, in general, avoid large fraction irradiation, with radiosurgery representing an exception to this rule. More importantly, three-dimensional and conformal techniques are evolving and hold the promise of reducing the volume of normal brain irradiated. These approaches are of significance because no effective therapy exists for the patient suffering neurocognitive decline after radiotherapy.

This chapter contains material from the first edition, and we are grateful to the authors of that chapter for their contribution.

REFERENCES

1. Greenlee RT, Murray T, Bolden S, *et al.* Cancer Statistics. *CA Cancer J Clin* 2000; 50: 7–33
2. Prise KM, Pinto M, Newman HC, Michael BD. A review of studies of ionizing radiation-induced double-strand break clustering. *Radiation Res* 2001; 156: 572–6.

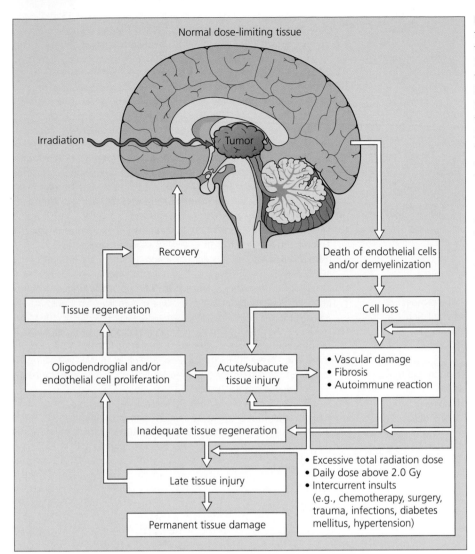

Normal dose-limiting tissue

Figure 45.13 The dose of radiation delivered to a tumor is often limited by the surrounding normal tissues' tolerance to irradiation. This normal tissue injury may be divided into acute, subacute, or late forms of injury depending on the interval between irradiation and the onset of injury. Acute injury occurs during the course of irradiation or within 4 weeks following its completion. Subacute injury occurs from 1 to 6 months after the completion of radiation therapy. Late injury occurs more than 6 months after radiation treatments have ceased. The patient generally recovers from the acute effects of irradiation, but under certain circumstances, such as in the setting of mechanical trauma, acute injury may progress to late injury. It is also possible for patients to develop late injury without ever developing clinical signs of acute injury. This most often occurs in the setting of intercurrent insults, such as surgery, or following treatments using daily doses above 2 Gy. Late radiation injury may be reversible, but it is more likely to be irreversible than acute injury

CLINICAL PEARLS

- Radiation therapy is used as an adjuvant therapy in the treatment of brain tumors. The goal of the therapy is to increase survival and decrease local recurrence in malignant tumors. In some malignant tumors, such as germinoma and primitive neuroectodermal tumors, radiation therapy is used to help effect a cure. In benign tumors, such as craniopharyngioma, it is used to improve progression-free survival.

- Stereotactic radiosurgery represents a great advance in technology. Using the precision of stereotactic methods, single-dose fraction of radiation from a linear accelerator or gamma-source can be used to ablate functional targets, such as for trigeminal neuralgia, or to control certain tumors, such as acoustic neuromas, by gamma-knife radiosurgery. Fractionated stereotactic radiosurgery has the benefit of the stereotactic precision coupled with the

multiple fractions of radiation which can destroy tumor cells through several cell cycle phases.

- Advances in radiation therapy are primarily aimed at improving the therapeutic ratio by targeting neoplastic tissue and avoiding the detrimental effects associated with radiation of normal cerebral tissue. Intensity-modulated radiotherapy uses technology which varies the intensity of the radiation across the width of the beam; i.e. it increases the dose of radiation directed at neoplastic tissue and decreases the dose to less involved regions. Other advances include "image fusion" which improves the precision of the dosimetry by combining the images from CT and MRI. The addition of images obtained from MRS will help differentiate tumor tissue from necrosis and thus hopefully improve clinical outcome.

3. Walker MD, Strike TA, Sheline GE, et al. An analysis of dose–effect relationship in the radiotherapy of malignant gliomas. *Int J Radiat Oncol Biol Phys* 1979; 5: 1725–31.

4. Mehta MP. Radiotherapy of pituitary hypothalamic tumors. In: Becker KL (ed.). *Principles and Practice of Endocrinology and Metabolism*, 3rd edn. Philadelphia: J.B. Lippincott Publishing Co.; 2001: 243–54.

5. Harisiadis L, Chang CH. Medulloblastoma in children: a correlation between staging and results of treatment. *Int J Rad Oncol Biol Phys* 1977; 2: 833–41.

6. Berry MP, Jenkin DT, Kenn CW, et al. Radiation treatment for medulloblastoma. A 21-year review. *J Neurosurg* 1981; 55: 43–51.

7. Cumberlin RL, Luk KH, Wara WM, et al. Medulloblastoma: treatment results and effects on normal tissues. *Cancer* 1979; 43: 1014–20.

8. Silverman CL, Simpson JR. Cerebellar medulloblastoma: The importance of posterior fossa dose to survival and patterns of failure. *Int J Rad Oncol Biol Phys* 1982; 8: 1869–76.

9. Kopelson G, Linggood RM, Kleinman GM. Medulloblastoma. The identification of prognostic subgroups and implications for multimodality management. *Cancer* 1983; 51: 312–19.

10. Deutsch M, Thomas PRM, Krischer J, et al. Results of a prospective randomized trial comparing standard dose neuraxis irradiation (3600cGy/20) with reduced neuraxis irradiation (2340cGy/13) in patients with low-stage medulloblastoma: a CCG/POG study. *Pediatr Neurosurg* 1996; 24: 167–77.

11. Bailey CC, Gnekow A, Jones M, et al. Prospective randomised trial of chemotherapy given before radiotherapy in childhood medulloblastoma: SIOP II. *Med Ped Oncol* 1995; 25: 166–78.

12. Shaw E, Arusell R, Scheithauer B, et al. A prospective randomized trial of low- versus high-dose radiation therapy in adults with supratentorial low-grade glioma: initial report of NCCTG-RTOG-ECOG study. *Proceedings of ASCO* 1998; 17: 401a (1545).

13. Karim A, Maat B, Hatlevoll R, et al. A randomized trial on dose response in radiation therapy of low grade cerebral glioma: EORTC 22844 study. *Int J Radiat Oncol Biol Phys* 1996; 36: 549–56.

14. Karim A, Cornu P, Bleehen N, et al. Immediate postoperative radiotherapy in low grade glioma improves progression free survival, but not overall survival: Preliminary results of an EORTC/MRC randomized Phase III study. *Proceedings of ASCO* 1998; 17: 400a (1544).

15. Laramore GE. Martz KL. Nelson JS. Griffin TW. Chang CH. Horton J. Radiation Therapy Oncology Group (RTOG) survival data on anaplastic astrocytomas of the brain: does a more aggressive form of treatment adversely impact survival? *Int J Radiat Oncol Biol Phys* 1989; 17: 1351–6.

16. Smith JS. Perry A. Borell TJ, et al. Alterations of chromosome arms 1p and 19q as predictors of survival in oligodendrogliomas, astrocytomas, and mixed oligoastrocytomas. *J Clin Oncol* 2000; 18: 636–645.

17. Kondziolka D, Lunsford L, McLaughlin M, et al. Long-term outcomes after radiosurgery for acoustic neuromas. *N Engl J Med* 1998; 339: 1426–33.

18. Fowler JF. The linear quadratic formula and progress in fractionated radiotherapy. *Br J Radiol* 1989; 62: 679–94.

19. Tomé WA, Meeks SL, Buatti JM, Bova FJ, Friedman WA, Li Z. A high-precision system for conformal intracranial radiotherapy, *Int J Radiat Oncol Biol Phys* 2000; 47: 1137–43.

20. Jaradat HA, Tomé WA, McNutt TR, Meyerand E. On the incorporation of multimodality image fusion into the radiation therapy process. *Technol Cancer Res Treat* 2003; 2: 1–11.

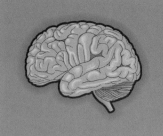

STEREOTACTIC RADIOSURGERY

46

Bruce E Pollock and Paul D Brown

In 1951, the Swedish neurosurgeon Lars Leksell conceived the idea of stereotactic radiosurgery.[1] His vision was to provide "a technique for noninvasive destruction of intracranial tissues or lesions that may be inaccessible or unsuitable for open surgery." To this end, Leksell coupled stereotactic localization with the delivery of a large, single-fraction dose of ionizing radiation.[2,3] His early devices used low energy X-rays (280 kV) to treat primarily functional disorders including obsessive-compulsive states and trigeminal neuralgia. Leksell later explored the utility of linear accelerators (LINAC) and proton beams for radiosurgery. In 1968 Leksell, in collaboration with Börje Larsson, developed the first cobalt-60 gamma unit (the Gamma-Knife, Elekta Instuments, Norcross, GA). However, only a few centers in the world performed radiosurgical operations until the 1980s. Over the past two decades, there has been an exponential growth in the number of radiosurgical sites across the world. Increased utilization of radiosurgery arose in large measure as a result of improved neuro-imaging with the introduction of computed tomography (CT) and later magnetic resonance imaging (MRI). Another critical factor linked to the advancement of radiosurgery was the growing power of modern computers. These advances have made the integration of imaging and physics dosimetry quick, accurate, accessible, and affordable for a large number of medical centers.

COMPARISON OF RADIOSURGERY AND RADIOTHERAPY

The goal of radiosurgery is to obliterate a relatively small intra-cranial target with a high, single-fraction irradiation dose while sparing adjacent and distant tissues. In contrast to conventional fractionated radiation therapy, radiosurgery does not rely on the increased radiation sensitivity of the target compared with the normal brain. Rather, radiosurgical treatment spares normal structures by physical deposition of significant doses of radiation into the target lesion with a steep decrease of the absorbed dose at the edges of the target. Stereotactic imaging and target localiz-ation using CT, MRI, and/or angiography must be fully integrated with the radiation delivery device to achieve pinpoint localization of the target. The irradiation isocenter must accurately and repeatedly coincide with the desired target. Different radiosurgical systems satisfy these essential criteria by using various technical solutions. Similarly, a variety of computer-based approaches to radiosurgical dose planning provide a three-dimensional represen-tation of isodose contours superimposed on the stereotactic images of the target and surrounding intracranial structures (Figures 46.1, 46.2).

One of the key elements in stereotactic radiosurgery (and three-dimensional conformal radiotherapy) is the use of many radiation fields distributed over space all focusing on a target. A single field (or a pair of opposed fields) will deliver the full dose to the target but will also treat a large portion of the normal tissues with the full dose. By increasing the number of fields while decreasing the dose each field delivers the high-dose region tends to conform to the target. The dose to the normal surrounding tissues is approximately equal to the prescribed dose divided by the number of fields, resulting in a significant reduction in the amount of normal tissues receiving high dose levels.

RADIOSURGICAL INSTRUMENTS

The gamma knife

Leksell and Larsson designed the first 179-source cobalt-60 (^{60}Co) gamma unit as a "practical, precise, and simple tool which could be handled by the surgeon himself."[2] The first gamma unit was

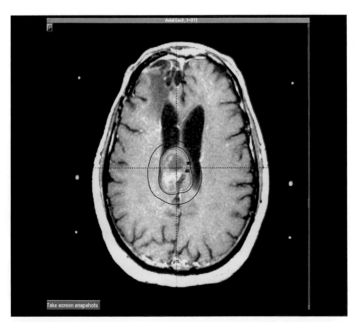

Figure 46.1 Axial post-gadolinium MRI showing the dose plan for a 52-year-old man with a recurrent Grade 3 oligodendroglioma having gamma-knife radiosurgery. The 50% isodose line covers the volume of the tumor.

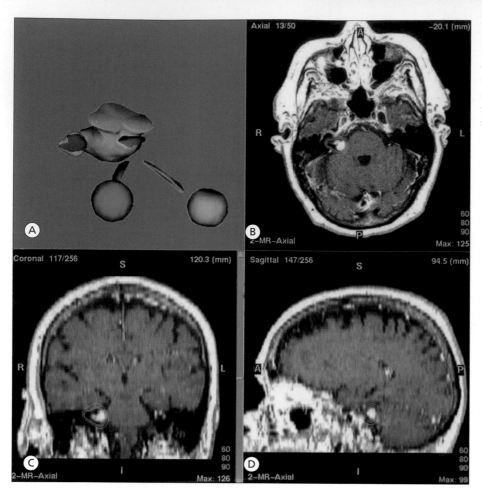

Figure 46.2 Patient with an acoustic neuroma having linear accelerator (LINAC) radiosurgery. **(A)** Three-dimensional volumetric reconstruction of the target volume (encompassed by the 80% isodose volume), brainstem, optic chiasm, optic nerves, and eyes. **(B–D)** Axial, coronal and sagittal gadolinium-enhanced T1-weighted MRI scan with 60%, 80%, and 90% isodose lines.

installed at the Sophiahemmet Hospital in Stockholm in 1968. However, the clinical usefulness of this device became widely appreciated only after the initial experience from the University of Pittsburgh was published by Lunsford and his colleagues.[4] The current version of this device contains 201 individual cobalt-60 (^{60}Co) sources which naturally decay to nickel (^{60}Ni). During this process gamma photons are released with energies of 1.17 MeV (mega-electron volts) and 1.33 MeV. The emitted photons are precisely directed through circular channels drilled into a high-density metal helmet. Each of these channels houses an individual collimator. The collimators are removable with diameters of 4, 8, 14, or 18 mm. One or more of these collimators can be removed and replaced with a plug with no aperture to block radiation from that particular source. This is often performed if it is determined that a beam passes through a radiosensitive structure. The coordinates, collimator size, and relative weighting of each isocenter are entered into the treatment-planning computer. The current generation of institutionally developed and commercially available dose-planning systems provides an interactive video display of multiplanar isodose contours superimposed on the stereotactic images, plus a three-dimensional analysis of isodose volumes in relation to adjacent intracranial structures. Since the gamma knife employs fixed sources with a constant relation to the collimator helmet and stereotactic frame, "isocenter verification films" or "port films" are unnecessary. The majority of targets are enclosed within the 40% or 50% isodose shell. The dose distribution can be modified by several variables including the

number of isocenters, the placement of isocenters, the choice of different collimator helmets, plugging individual beam channels, and weighting of isocenters. The latest version of the gamma knife (Model C) features an automatic positioning system, which is a fully motorized system that automatically sets the head-frame coordinates, repositioning the patient for each isocenter via treatment parameters transferred digitally from the operator's console. In addition to a reduction in the time needed to treat individual patients, this system minimizes the chance for human error in the setting of coordinates and has encouraged centers to use a higher number of small isocenters, thereby allowing for even more conformal radiosurgical plans.

Linear accelerator-based radiosurgery

Although LINACs have been used by radiation oncologists since the 1950s, the development of LINAC-based radiosurgical systems began in the 1980s.[5] Betti and Derechinsky,[6] Colombo and colleagues,[7,8] Hartmann and colleagues,[9] Winston and Lutz,[10] and others have contributed to the innovation and growth of this technology. The original systems generally utilized a stereotactic head-frame, floor-stand, and a 6-megavolt (MV) linear accelerator. Four or more sagittally oriented irradiation arcs are typically delivered using 12.5–30-mm circular collimators (Figure 46.3). Detection of mechanical inaccuracy is performed by a phantom-target film technique for every treatment arc. Friedman and Bova further refined LINAC-based radiosurgery by adding a high-

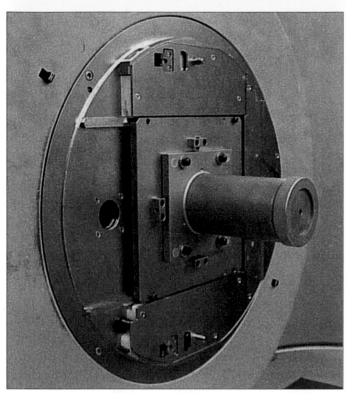

Figure 46.3 Close-up of a rigid collimator assembly attached to the faceplate of a linear accelerator. Variable diameter collimation apertures can be inserted at the end of the radiosurgery collimator.

precision attachment to control movements of the patient's head and the tertiary collimators (5–35-mm diameter) independent of potential variations in gantry or treatment-couch alignment.[11]

Linear accelerators are room-sized devices that use electromagnetic waves to accelerate a stream of electrons to nearly the speed of light. The electrons then hit a high-density metal target with most of the energy converted to heat. A small portion of the energy is converted to X-rays through the process of "bremsstrahlung" (braking radiation). This produces a polyenergetic beam of photons (X-rays) with energies in the MV range. The X-rays generated by a linear accelerator and gamma rays emitted by ^{60}Co are both photons, the only significant difference between the two is their origin. LINAC-produced photon beams of 4 MV have energies roughly equivalent to the gamma radiation emitted by ^{60}Co sources in the gamma knife, whereas LINAC-produced beams of 6–18 MV possess higher energies. The treatment plans can be individualized for each patient by adjusting the variables of a multiple arc plan. These variables include the number of arcs, the gantry start and end angles of each arc (amplitude), the couch angle (the separation between arcs), and collimation. LINAC-based radiosurgery typically employs a specialized collimation assembly that allows the placement of inserts of different diameters (range typically 5–50 mm) that define the field.

Intensity modulated radiation therapy (IMRT) is a new form of external beam treatment that is able to conform radiation to the size, shape and location of a desired target. IMRT relies on two advanced technologies, inverse treatment planning and multileaf collimator (MLC).[12,13] With IMRT treatment planning, instead of clinicians defining beam directions, beam weights, wedges, blocks, margins, then computing and displaying dose distributions to assess whether the treatment plan is acceptable, they do the opposite or "inverse" treatment planning. With inverse treatment planning sophisticated algorithms evaluate millions of possible beam arrangements, determine the clinically optimized treatment plan, and maximize the dose to the tumor while minimizing exposure to surrounding healthy tissue. The MLC is composed of computer-controlled tungsten leaves that shift to form specific patterns, selectively blocking the radiation to create beams of varying intensities. Hundreds to thousands of small, modulated radiation beams strike a tumor site with varying intensities and from many angles to attack the target in a complete three-dimensional manner; the combination of these beams produces the final dose distribution that conforms to the desired target.

Charged-particle-beam therapy and radiosurgery

The overwhelming number of patients treated with charged-particle beams have been irradiated with either protons (hydrogen nuclei) or helium ions.[14] The most attractive feature of particle beams for radiosurgery relates to the phenomenon called the Bragg-peak effect which permits increased dose at depth rather than at the surface of tissue, and the dose can be placed over a finite range in tissue. This high-dose zone can be directed accurately and precisely at the target, thereby minimizing radiation to adjacent normal structures. However, because the thickness of the unmodulated Bragg peak of proton or helium ion beams is only a few millimeters, much smaller than the usual intracranial lesion being treated, the peaks of various entering beams must be "spread out" to encompass the lesion volume. Telescoping or variable length water absorbers, fixed absorbers, and variable thickness rotating modulators within the beam path have been used in various combinations to match the dose distribution to the size and shape of the lesion being treated. Some centers have refined the beam shape further by using custom-formed collimator apertures that correspond to the shape of the target from a particular imaging projection. Additional calculations are necessary to determine the depth or range of the Bragg peak in tissues of variable density and thickness (scalp, bone, brain) to ensure appropriate beam modulation. Currently, this is accomplished most accurately by computerized analysis of beam paths through bone and soft tissue based on X-ray absorption data from CT scans. Often treatments are given over many fractions, and therefore do not fit the classic definition of radiosurgery but instead should be classified as stereotactic radiation therapy. However, because of the complexity of particle-beam-treatment planning, the need for a cyclotron to generate the protons, and the expense of these units, only a limited number of facilities around the world provide particle-beam therapy.

The CyberKnife

Adler and colleagues have developed a unique radiosurgical approach, incorporating a compact, lightweight linear accelerator mounted on a robotic arm, creating a frameless, image-guided device called the CyberKnife (Accuray, Sunnyvale, CA).[15] In this system, no head-frame is used. Instead, skeletal landmarks define stereotactic space. To achieve this purpose, radiographs of the treatment site are taken and image registration is performed to determine the target's coordinates with respect to the LINAC. The target coordinates are transferred to the robot, which directs the beam to the treatment site. Any movement of the target during treatment is detected, and this results in repositioning of the linear accelerator. For intracranial targets, patients are fitted with a non-invasive flexible mesh mask to limit large movements. This device is quite flexible and can be used to treat extracranial targets.[16]

CLINICAL RESULTS OF RADIOSURGERY

Indications

Radiosurgery is now accepted as an integral part of modern neurosurgery. As outlined earlier, radiosurgery has been utilized in the management of patients with intracranial diseases for almost 50 years. However, the most important factor associated with good outcomes after radiosurgery remains proper patient selection. As a general rule, patients with lesions > 35 mm in average diameter are typically not considered good candidates for radiosurgery. This is because patients with larger lesions often have symptoms related to mass effect. So although radiosurgery does result in growth control and size reduction in the majority of benign and malignant tumors, this is often a gradual process requiring a number of years. For such patients, surgical resection is the preferred approach, as it will decompress the adjacent neural structures in a rapid fashion. Moreover, at larger volumes the radiation fall-off into the surrounding normal tissues is not as steep and the risk of delayed radiation-related complications increases.

Table 46.1 outlines the indications for first 2117 patients undergoing radiosurgery at the Mayo Clinic, Rochester, MN, from January 1990 to December 2001. Over these 12 years, 25% had

vascular malformations, 31% had benign intracranial tumors, and 35% had malignant intracranial tumors. One hundred and eighty-seven patients (9%) underwent radiosurgery for trigeminal neuralgia. It should be understood that these percentages are not static, as the indications for radiosurgery have changed significantly over the past decade (Figure 46.4). For example, prior to 1996 no patient had radiosurgery for trigeminal neuralgia. During the following 6-year period, trigeminal neuralgia radiosurgery went from 1% (1996), to a high of 20% (1999), to 13% of our total radiosurgical volume in 2001. This initial increase followed by the later decline in utilization for this indication reflects both our early enthusiasm and later evaluation of the technique in comparison to other available surgeries for medically intractable trigeminal neuralgia.[17,18] As the debate concerning the role radiosurgery should play in patient management for a number of disorders remains intense, it is critical that the results of radiosurgery be objectively analyzed in comparison to other treatment modalities for individual indications. Table 46.2 outlines the current indications for radiosurgery according to their acceptance in patient management. In addition, radiosurgery continues to be investigated for new indications. For example, mesial temporal lobe epilepsy and large arteriovenous malformations (AVMs) (staged-volume AVM radiosurgery) are two indications currently being evaluated at a number of centers.[19–21]

Vascular malformations

Radiosurgery for patients with AVMs was one of the first indications of radiosurgery because they could be visualized, and thus targeted, based on cerebral angiography. Today, few questions remain unanswered with regard to AVM radiosurgery.

1. Numerous studies have documented that obliteration correlates with the margin dose to the malformation, not with AVM volume.[22,23]
2. Radiation-related complications are predicted by AVM location and the volume receiving some threshold dose of radiation (10 Gy volume, 12 Gy volume, or the mean dose to 20 cm^3).[24–26]
3. The hemorrhage rate after radiosurgery is either unchanged until obliteration or else some protective effect is provided compared with the natural history of untreated AVMs.[27–29]
4. Repeat radiosurgery results in complete obliteration for the majority of patients who had persistent arteriovenous shunting after their initial procedure.[30]

Table 46.1 Gamma-knife radiosurgery patients at the Mayo Clinic from January 1990 to December 2001 (n = 2117)

Indication	No. of patients (%)
Arteriovenous malformation	385 (18.2)
Dural arteriovenous fistula	133 (6.3)
Cavernous malformation	18 (0.9)
Vestibular schwannoma	216 (10.2)
Meningioma	288 (13.6)
Pituitary adenoma	122 (5.8)
Other schwannoma	29 (1.4)
Brain metastases	343 (16.2)
Glial tumor*	155 (7.3)
Hemangiopericytoma	34 (1.6)
Other tumor†	207 (9.8)
Trigeminal neuralgia	187 (8.8)

*Includes patients with astrocytoma, anaplastic astrocytoma, glioblastoma multiforme, oligodendroglioma, ependymoma, medulloblastoma, neurocytoma, and pilocytic astrocyoma.
†Includes patients with chordoma, chondrosarcoma, glomus tumor, craniopharyngioma, hemangioblastoma, and nasopharyngeal carcinoma.

Table 46.2 Indications for radiosurgery

Accepted	Controversial
Select AVMs	Cavernous malformation
Brain metastases	Dural arteriovenous fistula
Skull-base meningioma	Primary trigeminal neuralgia
Vestibular schwannoma	High-grade glioma
Recurrent pituitary adenoma	
Recurrent trigeminal neuralgia	

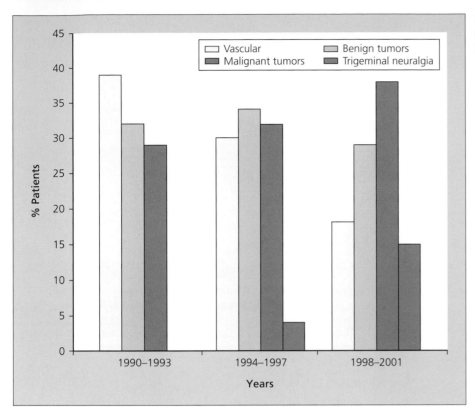

Figure 46.4 Graph showing the percentage of patients having radiosurgery for different indications from 1990 to 2001.

As a result, a great deal of information is available when counseling AVM patients regarding radiosurgery that allows comparison with either the natural history of untreated AVMs or surgical resection.

Despite the large amount of data collected to date, no grading scale was available to allow prediction of outcomes for the individual patient after radiosurgery. Moreover, although the Spetzler–Martin grading scale has become widely accepted as a method with which to predict patient outcome after surgical resection, this system does not correlate with successful AVM radiosurgery.[31] As a result, we recently developed a radiosurgery-based grading scale to predict patient outcomes after single-session AVM radiosurgery.[32] Briefly, a multivariate logistic regression analysis of factors associated with excellent outcomes (complete obliteration without new neurologic deficit) was performed for 220 patients undergoing radiosurgery at the University of Pittsburgh between 1987 and 1992 and a grading system was developed based on three preoperative AVM variables: AVM volume, patient age, and AVM location (Table 46.3). The model was then tested on a second group of 136 patients who underwent AVM radiosurgery at the Mayo Clinic between 1990 and 1997. Despite significant differences in the patient characteristics and radiosurgical dosing between the two centers, the proposed system strongly correlated with patient outcomes. Current studies are focusing on the application of this grading system to long-term outcomes taking into account the results of repeat radiosurgical procedures (Figure 46.5) as well as late complications such as cyst formation which may occur many years after an AVM patient was considered "cured" (Figure 46.6).[33]

Cavernous malformation (CM) radiosurgery remains controversial. Problems related to the assessment of the efficacy of CM radiosurgery are two-fold. First, the incidence and natural history of these lesions remains poorly understood. Second, unlike AVM

Table 46.3 Radiosurgery-based arteriovenous malformation grading system

AVM score[†]	% Excellent outcome
< 1.00	100
1.00–1.24	85
1.25–1.49	75
1.50–1.74	65
1.75–1.99	55
> 2.00	< 40

*AVM Score = (0.1) (AVM volume, cm^3) + (0.02) (Patient age, years) + (0.3) (AVM location)
[†]Frontal, temporal = 0; parietal, occipital, intraventricular, corpus callosum, cerebellum = 1; basal ganglia, thalamus, brainstem = 2.

radiosurgery, where obliteration can be confirmed with angiography, CMs often do not change appearance after radiosurgery on MRI and it is the clinical course of the patient that is followed to determine whether radiosurgery has reduced either their risk of bleeding or new neurologic events. Numerous studies have documented a decline in the annual bleeding risk after the first several years.[34–38] However, recent observations that CMs tend to bleed in "clusters" followed by more quiescent periods creates doubt that radiosurgery has any effect on hemorrhage risk for these patients.[39] Moreover, it has been noted that the risk of radiation-related complications is greater for patients with CMs

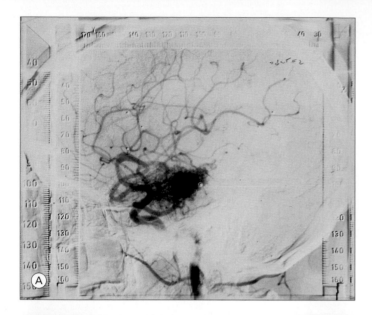

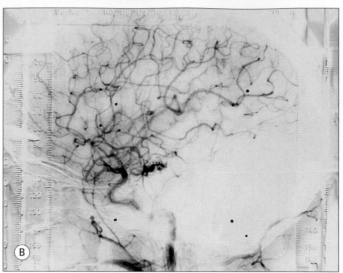

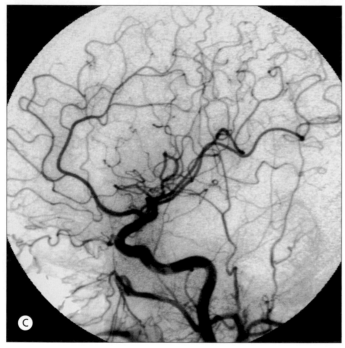

Figure 46.5 Lateral carotid angiograms of a 32-year-old man who suffered a tonic–clonic seizure and was discovered to have a left temporal AVM. **(A)** At the initial radiosurgery; **(B)** 39 months later, patient underwent repeat radiosurgery for residual AVM; **(C)** 74 months after the original radiosurgery, angiography shows complete obliteration.

compared with patients with AVMs, even when lesion size, location, and radiation dose are comparable (Figure 46.7).[34,37,38] For these reasons, and because the majority of CMs are not difficult to resect safely, the criteria for CM radiosurgery have been strict. Generally, only patients with a hemorrhagic (at least two separate bleeding episodes) CM located in a high-risk surgical location have been considered good candidates for radiosurgery. Thus, although some centers are confident that radiosurgery provides a reduction in the hemorrhage risk for CM patients,[36] it is our opinion that a prospective randomized trial is needed to understand better the safety and efficacy of CM radiosurgery.

Dural arteriovenous fistulas (DAVF) are rare lesions that typically present in adulthood and are more common in women. Most are believed to be acquired lesions secondary to thrombosis of an adjacent venous sinus. Intracranial hemorrhage is less common as

the presenting symptom in patients with DAVFs compared with patients with AVMs. One hundred and thirty-three DAVF patients have undergone radiosurgery at the Mayo Clinic.[40–42] Whenever possible, radiosurgery is combined with transarterial particulate embolization in the management of DAVFs. Radiosurgery is generally performed prior to embolization so that all the components of the DAVF are well visualized and included within the radiosurgical treatment volume. The patient then undergoes embolization (primarily through branches of the external carotid artery or other hypertrophied arteries supplying the dura) in the days following the radiosurgical procedure. This multimodality approach provides rapid improvement in the patient's symptoms and a reduction in hemorrhage risk by the embolization procedures, and long-term cure of the fistula by progressive radiosurgical obliteration of the involved vasculature. Symptom relief (pulsatile

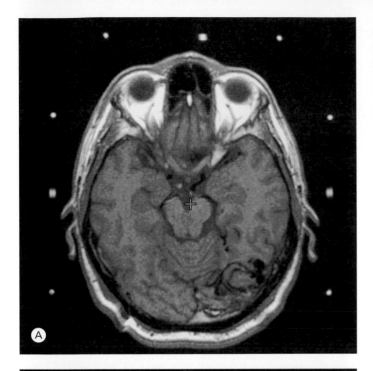

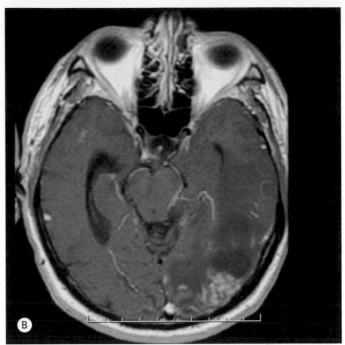

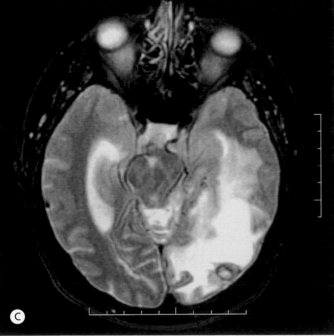

Figure 46.6 Axial MRIs of a 48-year-old man with headaches who had this left occipital AVM. **(A)** MRI at time of radiosurgery. **(B,C)** MRI 90 months after radiosurgery showing enhancement at site of the irradiated AVM, adjacent formation, extensive edema, and mass effect. The patient required craniotomy and AVM resection.

tinnitus, proptosis, chemosis) has been achieved in over 70% of our patients with this approach; no patient has suffered an intracranial hemorrhage after radiosurgery. Follow-up angiography one or more years after radiosurgery has shown that approximately three-quarters of patients had total or near-total obliteration of their DAVFs. Radiosurgery appears especially effective in the treatment of patients with DAVFs involving the cavernous sinus.[42] However, similar to CM radiosurgery, more studies are needed to determine what benefit patients derive from DAVF radiosurgery compared with other available treatments (primarily endovascular) and the natural history of these lesions.

Benign tumors

Discussions about vestibular schwannoma (acoustic neuroma) radiosurgery tend to be highly emotional and subjective. Proponents quote tumor control rates exceeding 95%, with less than 5% risk of any facial weakness or numbness.[43–46] In addition, patients have approximately a 40–60% chance of retaining their preoperative level of hearing. At our center, only five patients (2%) have shown progressive tumor enlargement after radiosurgery. Also, we have not had a single patient suffer any degree of facial weakness in the past 5 years. Critics of vestibular schwannoma radiosurgery state that the long-term tumor control rate remains

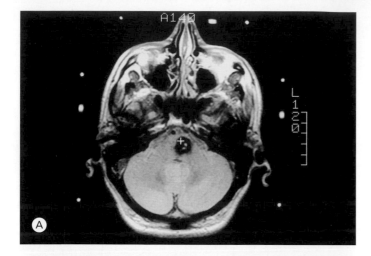

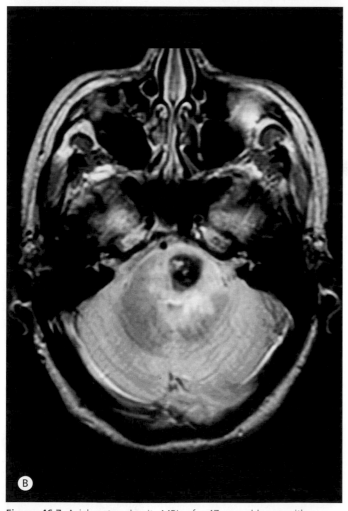

Figure 46.7 Axial proton-density MRIs of a 47-year-old man with a pontine cavernous malformation. **(A)** MRI at the time of radiosurgery. The prescription isodose volume was 3.2 cm³; the margin dose was 18 Gy. **(B)** MRI 8 months later shows adjacent edema which required corticosteroid therapy.

Table 46.4 Results of pituitary adenoma radiosurgery

	Hormone-producing adenoma	Nonhormone-producing adenoma	Nelson syndrome
No. of patients	70*	40	12
Growth control	100%	95%	80%
Endocrine cure	60%†	NA	33%‡
New anterior pituitary deficits	20%	40%	20%

*Growth hormone-producing (n = 42), adrenocorticotropin-producing (n = 15), prolactin-producing (n = 13).
†Cure defined as (1) acromegaly-fasting growth hormone level less than 2 ng/mL and normal age and sex-adjusted insulin-like growth factor (IGF-I levels), (2) Cushing's disease-24-hour UFC (urine-free cortisol) <90 µg, (3) Prolactinoma-prolactin levels < 23 ng/mL.
‡Cure defined as normal adrenocorticotropic hormone levels and improved pigmentation.

uncertain despite follow-up intervals that now extend beyond 10 years because the prescribed radiation doses have continually decreased over this interval.[47] Moreover, if the tumor progresses after radiosurgery, patients are informed that later surgical resection will be more difficult and preservation of facial movement unlikely.[48] In addition, the risk of later malignant transformation or induction of a radiation-related neoplasm is frequently cited as reasons that patients should undergo tumor resection rather than radiosurgery.[49,50] To date, comparisons between surgical resection and radiosurgery have found that patients undergoing radiosurgery have better outcomes with regards to facial function, hearing, and returning to their activities of daily living.[51,52] However, such comparisons have all been retrospectively performed and suffer the flaws of that methodology. At our center an additional 29 patients had radiosurgery for schwannomas involving other cranial nerves (trochlear, trigeminal, jugular foramen region).[53] Compared with historical controls, the morbidity associated with these cases has been lower, especially for patients with tumors of the jugular foramen region.

We have managed 288 patients with meningiomas either as a primary management strategy or as an adjunct after prior surgical resection.[54] The majority of patients had meningiomas of the skull base. Similar to other series, the tumor control rate continues to be greater than 90%.[55,56] The majority of patients with tumor progression have had atypical or malignant meningiomas. Also, patients with previous surgery appear to be at greater risk for tumor progression after radiosurgery. In an analysis of 62 patients undergoing primary radiosurgery for meningiomas at our center between 1990 and 1997, the 7-year actuarial progression-free survival was 95%.

Radiosurgery has been used for 122 patients with pituitary adenomas (Table 46.4). Over 90% of patients had undergone prior surgery; approximately 75% had tumors with extension to the cavernous sinus. Patients with large tumors distorting the optic chiasm or nerves are generally not considered to be good candidates for radiosurgery. To minimize the incidence of post-radiosurgical visual deficits, we limit the radiation dose to the

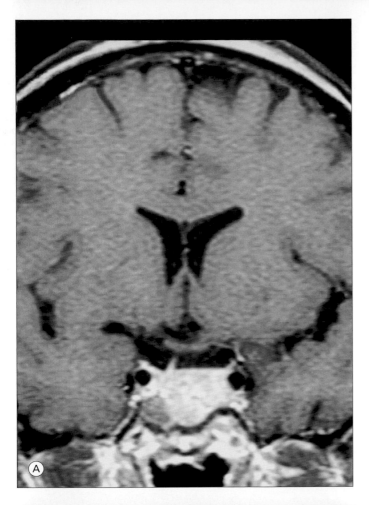

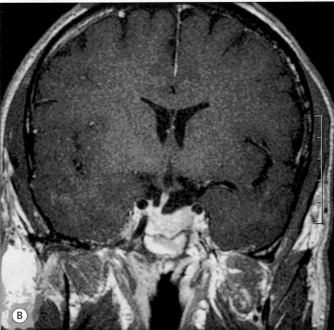

Figure 46.8 Coronal MRIs of a 44-year-old man with an enlarging non-hormone-producing pituitary adenoma after prior transsphenoidal resection. **(A)** MRI at the time of radiosurgery. The tumor volume was 9.1 cm³ and the tumor was covered with a margin dose of 18 Gy. **(B)** Fifty-eight months later, the tumor is smaller, but the patient developed complete anterior hypopituitarism.

optic nerves to < 12 Gy. Such a dose prescription has resulted in visual morbidity < 3%. The tumor growth control rate for these tumors has been greater than 90% (Figure 46.8); the highest failure rate has been for patients with adrenocorticotropic hormone-producing tumors who have undergone prior adrenalectomy. Two factors appear to correlate with endocrine cure after radiosurgery: higher radiation doses and the absence of pituitary-suppressing medications at the time of radiosurgery.[57–61]

Malignant tumors

Approximately 150 000 people are discovered to have metastatic brain disease each year in the United States. Although two randomized trials have shown that surgical resection combined with postoperative radiation therapy provides significantly longer survival compared with radiation therapy alone for patients with a solitary brain metastasis, patients with three or more tumors or those with tumors located in deep brain locations are generally not considered reasonable candidates for surgical resection. Radiosurgery provides high local tumor control rates (80–92%) (Figure 46.9) for brain metastases without the risks associated with craniotomy and tumor removal.[62–65] Comparison between surgical resection and radiosurgery for patients with a single brain metastasis have found no difference in either patient survival or tumor control.[66] The practice of neurological surgery would be significantly altered if neurosurgeons were more actively involved in the management of patients with brain metastases. Assuming that only 20% of the approximately 150 000 people developing brain metastases each year in the United States are felt to be good candidates for radiosurgery, this would result in 30 000 cases annually. This figure is roughly equal to the total number of patients treated with gliomas, meningiomas, pituitary adenomas, and schwannomas combined.

Radiosurgery has also been used extensively for glioma patients.[67–69] Unlike brain metastases, high-grade astrocytomas typically infiltrate beyond the margins defined by MRI. Consequently, focused radiation delivery will not cover a substantial portion of the tumor mass in most cases unless the area of concern is relatively small. As a result, the results of radiosurgery for high-grade gliomas have been criticized, much like the earlier works on brachytherapy, because of favorable patient selection for the procedure. Conversely, the results of radiosurgery for patients with pilocytic astrocytomas that are recurrent after prior surgery or in deep locations look promising.[70]

Trigeminal neuralgia

Sixty-three of the first 762 patients (8%) having radiosurgery at the Karolinska Institute between 1968 and 1982 had trigeminal neuralgia.[3] However, the inability to image directly the trigeminal system limited the usefulness of this procedure. However, with the advent of CT and MRI, Rand and colleagues and others proceeded to evaluate trigeminal neuralgia radiosurgery using modern techniques.[71–73] Recent series have found that approximately 40–60% of patients become pain-free and are able to discontinue their medications.[17,18,74–76] At this point, we believe radiosurgery is an ablative procedure that provides most trigeminal neuralgia patients with durable pain relief if they develop some degree of new trigeminal dysfunction.

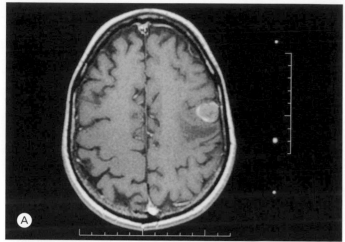

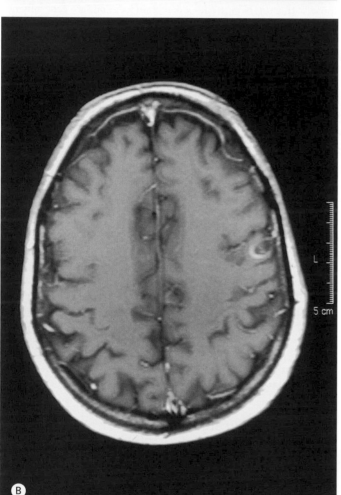

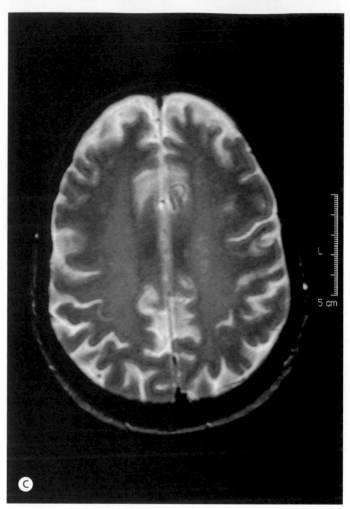

Figure 46.9 Axial MRIs of a 53-year-old man with a left frontal metastasis from non-small cell lung cancer. **(A)** MRI at the time of radiosurgery. **(B,C)** MRI 3 months later shows that the tumor is smaller and the adjacent edema has resolved

invasive nature and low associated morbidity. It is now being recognized that late complications (beyond 5 years) can occur after radiosurgery, emphasizing the continued need for diligent long-term follow-up for a large number of patients.

This chapter contains material from the first edition, and we are grateful to the author of that chapter for his contribution.

CONCLUSIONS

Radiosurgery has gained wide acceptance in both neurological surgery and radiation oncology as a safe and effective management strategy for a wide variety of disorders and is now a mandatory part of residency training for both fields. Radiosurgery appeals to patients, their physicians, and third-party payers due its non-

REFERENCES

1. Leksell L. The stereotactic method and radiosurgery of the brain. *Acta Chir Scand* 1951; 102: 316–19.
2. Larsson B. The history of radiosurgery: the early years (1950–1970), In Kondziolka D (ed.). *Radiosurgery*. Basel: Karger; 1996: 1–10.

CLINICAL PEARLS

- Patient selection is the critical factor associated with good outcomes after stereotactic radiosurgery.

- Radiosurgery does not rapidly reduce mass effect. For patients with symptomatic mass effect, surgical resection is preferable.

- Reduced morbidity after radiosurgery (single-fraction radiation delivery) is achieved by precisely conforming the dose-plan to the three-dimensional shape of the target. If a conformal dose-plan is not possible with a particular system, then radiotherapy (multiple-fraction radiation delivery) is necessary to minimize complications.

- The concern regarding whether a patient has tumor progression or simply imaging changes related to radiosurgery is typically impossible to determine from a single study. Progressive changes noted on serial imaging over time is a more sensitive indicator of radiosurgical failure than virtually any other method available.

- Centers that recognize and value the contributions of all members of the radiosurgical team (neurological surgery, radiation oncology, radiation physics, neuroradiology, and nursing) have succeeded the most in this multidisciplinary field.

3. Leksell L. Stereotactic radiosurgery. *J Neurol Neurosurg Psychiatr* 1983; 46: 797–803.
4. Lunsford LD, Coffey RJ, Flickinger JC. Stereotactic gamma knife radiosurgery: initial North American experience in 207 patients. *Arch Neurol* 1990; 47: 169–75.
5. Heifetz MD, Wexler M, Thompson R. Single-beam radiotherapy knife: a practical theoretical model. *J Neurosurg* 1984; 60: 814–18.
6. Betti OO, Derechinsky VE. Hyperselective encephalic irradiation with linear accelerator. *Acta Neurochir* 1984; 33(suppl.): 385–90.
7. Colombo F, Benedetti A, Pozza F, *et al*. External stereotactic irradiation by linear accelerator. *Neurosurgery* 1985; 16: 154–60.
8. Colombo F, Benedetti A, Pozza F, *et al*. Linear accelerator radiosurgery of three-dimensional irregular targets. *Stereotact Funct Neurosurg* 1990; 54/55: 541–6.
9. Hartmann G, Schlegel W, Sturm V, *et al*. Cerebral radiation surgery using moving field irradiation at a linear accelerator facility. *Int J Radiat Oncol Biol Phys* 1985; 11: 1185–92.
10. Winston KR, Lutz W. Linear accelerator as a neurosurgical tool for stereotactic radiosurgery. *Neurosurgery* 1988; 22: 454–64.
11. Friedman WA, Bova FJ. The University of Florida radiosurgery system. *Surg Neurol* 1989; 32: 334–42.
12. Cardinale RM, Benedict SH, Wu Q, *et al*. A comparison of three stereotactic radiotherapy techniques; ARCS vs. noncoplanar fixed fields vs. intensity modulation. *Int J Radiat Oncol Biol Phys* 1998; 42: 431–6.
13. Shiu AS, Kooy HM, Ewton JR, *et al*. Comparison of miniature multileaf collimation (MMLC) with circular collimation for stereotactic treatment. *Int J Radiat Oncol Biol Phys* 1997; 37: 679–88.

14. Levy RP, Fabrikant JI, Frankel KA, *et al*. Charged-particle radiosurgery of the brain. *Neurosurg Clin N Am* 1990; 1: 955–90.
15. Adler RJ Jr, Murphy MJ, Chang SD, *et al*. Image-guided robotic radiosurgery. *Neurosurgery* 1999; 44: 1299–307.
16. Ryu SI, Chang SD, Kim DH, *et al*. Image-guided hypo-fractionated stereotactic radiosurgery to spinal lesions. *Neurosurgery* 2001; 49: 838–46.
17. Pollock BE, Phuong LK, Foote RL, *et al*. High-dose trigeminal neuralgia radiosurgery associated with increased risk of trigeminal dysfunction. *Neurosurgery* 2001; 49: 58–64.
18. Pollock BE, Phuong LK, Gorman DA, *et al*. Stereotactic radiosurgery for idiopathic trigeminal neuralgia. *J Neurosurg* 2002; 97: 347–53.
19. Kondziolka D. Functional radiosurgery. *Neurosurgery* 1999; 44: 12–22.
20. Régis J, Bartolomei F, Metellus P, *et al*. Radiosurgery for trigeminal neuralgia and epilepsy. *Neurosurg Clin N Am* 1999; 10: 359–77.
21. Pollock BE, Kline RW, Stafford SL, *et al*. The rationale and technique of staged-volume arteriovenous malformation radiosurgery. *Int J Radiat Oncol Biol Phys* 2000; 48: 817–24.
22. Flickinger JC, Pollock BE, Kondziolka D, *et al*. A dose–response analysis of arteriovenous malformation obliteration by radiosurgery. *Int J Radiat Oncol Biol Phys* 1996; 36: 873–9.
23. Karlsson B, Lax I, Soderman M. Can the probability for obliteration after radiosurgery for arteriovenous malformations be accurately predicted? *Int J Radiat Oncol Biol Phys* 1999; 43: 313–19.
24. Flickinger JC, Kondziolka D, Lunsford LD, *et al*. Development of a model to predict permanent symptomatic post-radiosurgery injury for arteriovenous malformation patients. *Int J Radiat Oncol Biol Phys* 2000; 46: 1143–8.
25. Lax I, Karlsson B. Prediction of complications in gamma knife radiosurgery of arteriovenous malformations. *Acta Oncol* 1996; 35: 49–56.
26. Voges J, Treuer H, Lehrke R, *et al*. Risk analysis of linac radiosurgery in patients with arterio-venous malformations (AVM). *Acta Neurochir* 1997; 68: 118–23.
27. Friedman WA, Blatt DL, Bova FJ, *et al*. The risk of hemorrhage after radiosurgery for arteriovenous malformations. *J Neurosurg* 1996; 84: 912–19.
28. Karlsson B, Lindquist C, Steiner L. The effect of gamma knife surgery on the risk of rupture prior to AVM obliteration. *Minim Invas Neurosurg* 1996; 39: 21–27.
29. Pollock BE, Flickinger JC, Lunsford LD, *et al*. Hemorrhage risk after stereotactic radiosurgery of cerebral arteriovenous malformations. *Neurosurgery* 1996; 38: 652–61.
30. Maesawa S, Flickinger JC, Kondziolka D, *et al*. Repeated radiosurgery for incompletely obliterated arteriovenous malformations. *J Neurosurg* 2000; 92: 961–70.
31. Pollock BE, Flickinger JC, Lunsford LD, *et al*. Factors associated with successful arteriovenous malformation radiosurgery. *Neurosurgery* 1998; 42: 1239–47.
32. Pollock BE, Flickinger JC. A proposed radiosurgery-based grading system for arteriovenous malformations. *J Neurosurg* 2002; 96: 79–85.
33. Pollock BE, Brown RD, Jr. Management of cysts arising after radiosurgery of intracranial arteriovenous malformations. *Neurosurgery* 2001; 49: 259–65
34. Amin-Hanjabi S, Ogilvy CS, Candia GJ, *et al*. Stereotactic radiosurgery for cavernous malformations: Kjellberg's experience with proton beam therapy in 98 cases at the Harvard cyclotron. *Neurosurgery* 1998; 42: 1229–38.
35. Chang SD, Levy RP, Adler JR Jr, *et al*. Stereotactic radiosurgery of angiographically occult vascular malformations: 14-year experience. *Neurosurgery* 1998; 43: 213–21.

36. Hasegawa T, McInerney J, Kondziolka D, *et al*. Long-term results after stereotactic radiosurgery for patients with cavernous malformations. *Neurosurgery* 2002; 50: 1190–7.

37. Karlsson B, Kihlström L, Lindquist C, *et al*. Radiosurgery for cavernous malformations. *J Neurosurg* 1998; 88: 293–7.

38. Pollock BE, Garces YI, Stafford SL, *et al*. Stereotactic radiosurgery of cavernous malformations. *J Neurosurg* 2000; 93: 987–91.

39. Barker FG II, Amin-Hanjabi S, Butler WE, *et al*. Temporal clustering of hemorrhages from untreated cavernous malformations of the central nervous system. *Neurosurgery* 2001; 49: 15–25.

40. Friedman JA, Pollock BE, Nichols DA, *et al*. Results of combined stereotactic radiosurgery and transarterial embolization for dural arteriovenous fistulae of the transverse and sigmoid sinuses. *J Neurosurg* 2001; 94: 886–91.

41. Link MJ, Coffey RJ, Nichols DA, *et al*. The role of radiosurgery and particulate embolization in the treatment of dural arteriovenous fistulas. *J Neurosurg* 1996; 84: 804–9.

42. Pollock BE, Nichols DA, Garrity JA, *et al*. Stereotactic radiosurgery and particulate embolization of cavernous sinus dural arteriovenous fistulae. *Neurosurgery* 1999; 45: 459–67.

43. Foote KD, Friedman WA, Buatti JM, *et al*. Analysis of risk factors associated with radiosurgery for vestibular schwannoma. *J Neurosurg* 2001; 95: 440–9.

44. Kondziolka D, Lunsford LD, McLaughlin MR, *et al*. Long-term outcomes after radiosurgery for acoustic neuromas. *N Engl J Med* 1998; 339: 1426–33.

45. Prasad D, Steiner M, Steiner L. Gamma surgery for vestibular schwannomas. *J Neurosurg* 2000; 92: 745–59.

46. Petit JH, Hudes RS, Chen TT, *et al*. Reduced-dose radiosurgery for vestibular schwannomas. *Neurosurgery* 2001; 49: 1299–306.

47. Sekhar LN, Gormley WB, Wright DC. The best treatment for vestibular schwannoma (acoustic neuroma): microsurgery or radiosurgery? *Am J Otol* 1996; 17: 676–82.

48. Slattery WH III, Brackmann DE. Results of surgery following stereotactic irradiation for acoustic neuromas. *Am J Otol* 1995; 16: 315–19.

49. Shin M, Ueki K, Kurita H, *et al*. Malignant transformation of a vestibular schwannoma after gamma knife radiosurgery. *Lancet* 2002; 360: 309–10.

50. Shamisa A, Bance M, Nag S, *et al*. Glioblastoma multiforme occurring in a patient treated with gamma knife surgery. *J Neurosurg* 2001; 94: 816–21.

51. Pollock BE, Lunsford LD, Kondziolka D, *et al*. Outcome analysis of acoustic neuroma management: a comparison of microsurgery and stereotactic radiosurgery. *Neurosurgery* 1995; 36: 215–23.

52. Roijen LV, Nijs HGT, Avezaat CJJ, *et al*. Costs and effects of microsurgery versus radiosurgery in treating acoustic neuroma. *Acta Neurochir* 1997; 139: 942–8.

53. Pollock BE, Foote RL, Stafford SL. Stereotactic radiosurgery: the preferred management for patients with non-vestibular schwannomas? *Int J Radiat Oncol Biol Phys* 2002; 52: 1002–7.

54. Stafford SL, Pollock BE, Foote RL, *et al*. Meningioma radiosurgery: tumor control, outcomes, and complications in 190 consecutive patients. *Neurosurgery* 2001; 49: 1029–38.

55. Chang SD, Adler JR Jr. Treatment of cranial base meningiomas with linear accelerator radiosurgery. *Neurosurgery* 1997; 41: 1019–27.

56. Lee JY, Ninanjan A, McInerney J, *et al*. Stereotactic radiosurgery providing long-term tumor control of cavernous sinus meningiomas. *J Neurosurg* 2002; 97: 65–72.

57. Landolt AM, Dieter H, Nicoletta L, *et al*. Stereotactic radiosurgery for recurrent surgically treated acromegaly: comparison with fractionated radiotherapy. *J Neurosurg* 1998; 88: 1002–8.

58. Pollock BE, Nippoldt TB, Stafford SL, *et al*. Stereotactic radiosurgery for patients with hormone producing pituitary adenomas: factors associated with endocrine normalization. *J Neurosurg* 2002; 97: 525–30.

59. Sheehan JM, Vance ML, Sheehan JP, *et al*. Radiosurgery for Cushing's disease after failed transsphenoidal surgery. *J Neurosurg* 2000; 93: 738–42.

60. Landolt AM, Haller D, Lomax N, *et al*. Octreotide may act as a radioprotective agent in acromegaly. *J Clin Endocrinol Metab* 2000; 85: 1287–9.

61. Landolt AM, Lomax N. Gamma knife radiosurgery for prolactinomas. *J Neurosurg* (suppl. 3) 2000; 93: 14–18.

62. Brown PD, Brown CA, Pollock BE, *et al*. Stereotactic radiosurgery for patients with radioresistant brain metastases. *Neurosurgery* 2002; 51: 656–67.

63. Kondziolka D, Patel A, Lunsford LD, *et al*. Stereotactic radiosurgery plus whole brain radiotherapy versus radiotherapy alone for patients with multiple brain metastases. *Int J Radiat Oncol Biol Phys* 1999; 45: 427–34.

64. Sneed PK, Lamborn KR, Forstner JM, *et al*. Radiosurgery for brain metastases: is whole brain radiotherapy necessary. *Int J Radiat Oncol Biol Phys* 1999; 43: 549–58.

65. Weltman E, Salvajoli JV, Brandt RA, *et al*. Radiosurgery for brain metastases: a score index for predicting prognosis. *Int J Radiat Oncol Biol Phys* 2000; 46: 1155–61.

66. Muacevic A, Kreth FW, Horstmann GA, *et al*. Surgery and radiotherapy compared to gamma knife radiosurgery in the treatment of solitary cerebral metastases of small diameter. *J Neurosurg* 1999; 91: 35–43.

67. Kondziolka D, Flickinger JC, Bissonette DJ, *et al*. Survival benefit of stereotactic radiosurgery for patients with malignant glial neoplasms. *Neurosurgery* 1997; 41: 776–85.

68. Nwokedi EC, DiBiase SJ, Jabbour S, *et al*. Gamma knife stereotactic radiosurgery for patients with glioblastoma multiforme. *Neurosurgery* 2002; 50: 41–46.

69. Shrieve DC, Alexander E III, Wen PY, *et al*. Comparison of stereotactic radiosurgery and brachytherapy in the treatment of recurrent glioblastoma multimorme. *Neurosurgery* 1995; 36: 275–84.

70. Hadjipanayis CG, Kondziolka D, Gardner P, *et al*. Stereotactic radiosurgery for pilocytic astrocytomas when multimodality therapy is necessary. *J Neurosurg* 2002; 97: 56–64.

71. Kondziolka D, Lunsford LD, Flickinger JC, *et al*. Stereotactic radiosurgery for trigeminal neuralgia: a multiinstutional study using the gamma unit. *J Neurosurg* 1996; 84: 940–5.

72. Rand W, Jacques DB, Melbye RW, *et al*. Leksell gamma knife treatment of tic douloureux. *Stereotact Funct Neurosurg* 1993; 61: 93–102.

73. Young RF, Vermeulen SS, Grimm P, *et al*. Gamma knife radiosurgery for treatment of trigeminal neuralgia: idiopathic and tumor related. *Neurology* 1997; 48: 608–14.

74. Brisman R, Khandji AG, Mooij RB. Trigeminal nerve-blood vessel relationship as revealed by high-resolution magnetic resonance imaging and its effect on pain relief after gamma knife radiosurgery for trigeminal neuralgia. *Neurosurgery* 2002; 50: 1261–6.

75. Flickinger JC, Pollock BE, Kondziolka D, *et al*. What length should be irradiated? A randomized blinded study of radiosurgery to different lengths of trigeminal nerve for trigeminal neuralgia. *Int J Radiat Oncol Biol Phys* 2001; 51: 449–54.

76. Maesawa S, Salame C, Flickinger JC, *et al*. Clinical outcomes after stereotactic radiosurgery for idiopathic trigeminal neuralgia. *J Neurosurg* 2001; 94: 14–20.

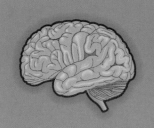

CHEMOTHERAPY OF CENTRAL NERVOUS SYSTEM TUMORS

47

S Clifford Schold Jr

Cytotoxic drugs have had a significant impact on the natural history of many forms of cancer in the last 50 years. Acute lymphocytic leukemia in children and testicular cancer, among others, have become curable diseases because of the introduction of chemotherapy. Many other forms of leukemia, most forms of lymphoma, and several solid tumors, including breast cancer and small cell lung cancer, are sensitive to conventional doses of currently available agents. On the other hand, numerous common forms of cancer have been only minimally responsive to chemotherapy. Examples include non-small cell lung cancer, melanoma, pancreatic cancer, and renal cell carcinoma. Unfortunately, the most common form of primary brain tumor, the glioblastoma multiforme, also belongs in this unresponsive category (Figure 47.1). There have been many instances of unequivocal responses to chemotherapy among patients with anaplastic gliomas (including glioblastomas), and other forms of central nervous system (CNS) tumors are clearly sensitive to chemotherapy. Nevertheless, the impact of chemotherapy on the most common and malignant forms of brain tumor has still been minimal.

Discovery of new forms of chemotherapy remains a major area of emphasis in cancer research. This has led to new treatments for CNS tumors in the last decade and will undoubtedly lead to more effective treatments in the near future. In this chapter, I will review and discuss the process of evaluation of new chemotherapeutic agents, the agents themselves, the current status of chemotherapy of CNS tumors, and some special problems with respect to the chemotherapy of brain tumors.

CLINICAL TRIALS

Formal clinical trials are both expensive and complicated. Before embarking on a trial, there should be a reasonable and answerable question of sufficient interest to justify application of the necessary resources. This is a potential problem for the development of new treatments for CNS tumors since the pharmaceutical companies do not consider this a lucrative market. The pharmaceutical industry is most likely to develop

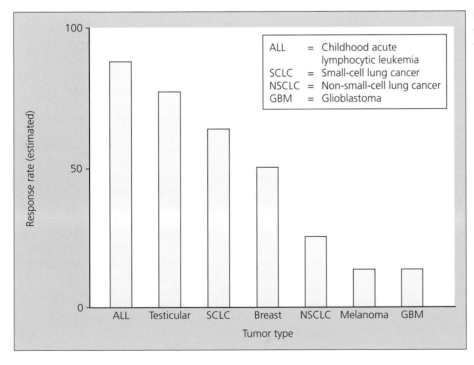

Figure 47.1 Estimated response rates to conventional chemotherapy of a variety of common forms of cancer.

new agents for brain tumors if those agents are thought to have wider applicability.

It is extremely important that the precise objectives of a trial be specified and that there be in-depth statistical input into its design. This increases the likelihood of the study resulting in a new or deeper understanding of a disease process or its treatment. Too many poorly designed and inconclusive studies have been conducted and published on the chemotherapy of CNS tumors. This both clutters the literature and confuses the reader who is not intimately involved in the field.

There is a standardized sequence for evaluating new cancer chemotherapeutic agents in people, which allows progressive and continuous assessment of toxicity and efficacy. These stages are referred to as phase I, II, III, and IV trials (Figure 47.2).

Phase I

Phase I trials are designed to identify the qualitative *toxicity* of new chemotherapeutic agents and to determine the maximum tolerated dose in humans. These are the first trials done in people with a new drug, and in oncology they are generally conducted with patients whose disease is considered refractory to standard forms of therapy (they may be conducted in normal volunteers in the development of less toxic forms of therapy). It is unusual for standard phase I trials to be performed in patients with CNS tumors because the confounding variable of intracranial disease would make identification of neurologic toxicity difficult. However, in specialized situations, such as intracarotid drug administration and other targeted routes of delivery, it is important to conduct the phase I trials in patients being treated for CNS disease to identify toxicity associated with a particular route or drug formulation.

Phase II

Phase II trials are the initial tests of a drug's *activity* against specific diseases. The doses and schedules are determined by experience in the phase I trial, and the treated population is made as homogeneous as possible. Consequently, with an adequate number of patients, such a trial allows one to estimate the response rate of a specific form of cancer to a specific drug using a particular dose and schedule. In brain tumor trials, patients with anaplastic gliomas of all types are frequently included in individual phase II trials, and then the analysis is carried out separately for the glioblastomas and the non-glioblastoma anaplastic gliomas.

Phase III

Phase III trials are the definitive tests of a drug's *efficacy* in a specific disease. They are generally randomized trials in which the new agent is compared against a treatment of known efficacy in the disease. A much larger number of patients is required for phase III trials than for phase II trials because of the statistical comparison to a control arm, but the phase III trial is virtually the only way to be certain of a new drug's role in the treatment of a disease. They are the most expensive trials and are undertaken only if there was promising evidence of activity in the phase II trials.

Phase IV

Phase IV are so-called post-marketing or surveillance trials. They are conducted after the agent has received the necessary approvals to enter the marketplace. They have two broad purposes. The first is to identify any toxicity, particularly *long-term toxicity* that was not detected in the pre-approval trials. The second is to *expand the possible indications* and uses of the agent. Once the drug is approved investigators have more latitude in exploring its use in different diseases, such as relatively uncommon forms of brain tumor, and alternative dosages, schedules, and routes.

An important question in the conducting of these trials is what level of activity in a phase II trial justifies advancing the treatment to a phase III trial, a much longer and more expensive enterprise. This decision rests primarily on the activity of the control or standard drug in a phase II setting in a disease. If the phase II level of activity of the new drug is comparable to or exceeds that of the historic results with a standard drug and if the toxicity is not excessive, it is reasonable to proceed with the phase III trial. Clearly, this level of activity in a phase II setting varies widely with the disease under consideration, and it emphasizes the importance of selecting the appropriate population for the phase II trial.

DRUGS IN USE IN NEURO-ONCOLOGY

Alkylating agents

The most common and effective drugs in the treatment of gliomas are the nitrosoureas and the methylating agents (Figure 47.3). These compounds act by alkylating tumor DNA at the O^6-position of guanine, thereby interfering with DNA replication. The alkyl group produced by many nitrosoureas is chloroethylguanine, and methylation at the O^6-position of guanine is produced by the related agents procarbazine and temozolomide. The most common drugs in this class for the treatment of gliomas are BCNU (carmustine), CCNU (lomustine), procarbazine, and temozolomide. A number of other nitrosoureas have been introduced into clinical trials, including PCNU, ACNU, and methyl-CCNU, but none has shown clear superiority to the widely available agents. It has also been possible to formulate BCNU into a biodegradable polymer in the form of a wafer so that the drug can be applied locally at the time of surgical resection.[1] This results in higher local concentration of the drug with reduced systemic exposure.

In the widely quoted trial of therapy for adults with anaplastic gliomas conducted by the Brain Tumor Study Group (BTSG) in the 1970s,[2] BCNU increased the percentage of survivors at

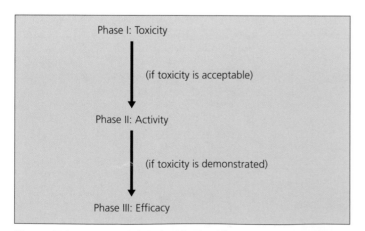

Phase I: Toxicity

↓

(if toxicity is acceptable)

Phase II: Activity

(if toxicity is demonstrated)

↓

Phase III: Efficacy

Figure 47.2 Sequence of clinical evaluation of new anticancer agents.

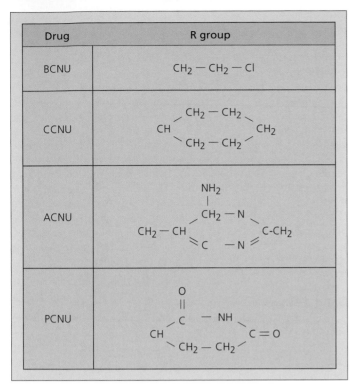

Drug	R group
BCNU	$CH_2 - CH_2 - Cl$
CCNU	
ACNU	
PCNU	

Figure 47.3 Structures of nitrosoureas in common use.

18 months after diagnosis in comparison to patients treated with radiotherapy alone. This study defined BCNU as the standard against which newer forms of therapy are compared, although the results were modest at best. Procarbazine was shown in a later study by the BTSG not to be significantly different from BCNU, and therefore it also is presumed to have some efficacy in the treatment of this group of diseases.[3] Although CCNU has never been compared directly with BCNU, its pharmacologic similarity and its ease of administration (since it is taken orally) have led many neuro-oncologists to use it in preference to BCNU. More recently, the orally administered methylating agent temozolomide has been shown to have comparable or better activity.[4] In many hands, it is now the drug of choice for anaplastic gliomas.

The other major class of alkylating drugs is the mustard derivatives, the most common examples of which are cyclophosphamide and L-phenylalanine mustard (melphalan). These drugs also alkylate DNA, but they do so at a different site and hence their spectrum of activity is different from that of the nitrosoureas. Cyclophosphamide has shown activity against recurrent gliomas at high doses, and melphalan appears to have activity against oligodendroglial tumors and neuronal tumors, such as medulloblastoma and pineoblastoma.

Cisplatin and carboplatin

Cis-diaminedichloroplatinum II (cisplatin) is a DNA-intercalating agent that has shown impressive antitumor activity in a number of human cancers, including germ cell tumors, head and neck tumors, and small-cell lung tumors. Cisplatin, at least when given by the intra-arterial route, has activity against both recurrent glioma and newly diagnosed anaplastic glioma.[5] It is also effective against intracranial germ cell tumors. Its analogue carboplatin also

has efficacy against some forms of brain tumors and is often preferred because of a more manageable toxicity profile.

Antimetabolites

The classic antineoplastic agents are the antimetabolites, which are analogs of normal metabolites that function by serving as artificial and imperfect substrates for natural metabolic reactions. The most widely used of these agents are methotrexate, a folic acid antagonist, 5-fluorouracil, 6-mercaptopurine, and cytosine arabinoside (ara-C). The antimetabolites as a class are relatively inactive against CNS tumors, at least when used as single agents. They are cell-cycle-specific agents that are most effective against tumors with a high growth fraction.

Natural products and biologics

There are several natural product drugs that have been used in the treatment of brain tumors and other forms of cancer. These include taxol, the vinca alkaloids (vincristine and vinblastine), the topoisomerase I inhibitor irinotecan (CPT-11), the topoisomerase II inhibitors etoposide (VP-16) and veniposide (VM-26), and the antitumor antibiotics such as adriamycin and actinomycin D. These drugs are usually large, complex molecules that penetrate the blood–brain barrier poorly. They have been of interest because the multidrug-resistant (MDR) phenotype appears to produce cross-resistance to many of these natural product anticancer drugs. Some forms of interferon, retinoic acid, and the anti-angiogenic agent thalidomide have also shown activity against gliomas. Novel and more specific potential anti-neoplastic agents, such as epidermal growth factor receptor antagonists, are the current most active focus of investigation, and they offer the promise of individualizing therapy for specific tumors.

CHEMOTHERAPY OF INDIVIDUAL TUMOR TYPES

Astrocytic tumors

The drugs that have been used most extensively in the treatment of astrocytic tumors are the nitrosoureas, procarbazine, temozolomide, cisplatin/carboplatin, and, to a lesser extent, other alkylating drugs. BCNU is the only drug that has shown unequivocal efficacy in improving survival of patients with newly diagnosed anaplastic gliomas. It is usually given intravenously at a dose of 200 mg/m^2 every 6 weeks. Temozolomide is currently favored by many because of its comparable activity and ease of administration. It is usually given at a dose of 200 mg/m^2 orally on days 1–5 of each 28-day cycle.

Oligodendroglial tumors

There is now substantial reported experience with the combination of CCNU, procarbazine, and vincristine ("PCV") in the treatment of oligodendroglial tumors, and it appears that this form of glioma is more sensitive to chemotherapy than the more common astrocytic tumors.[6] Temozolomide has also produced responses in an impressive percentage of patients. Standard practice is evolving toward the use of chemotherapy in preference to radiotherapy in the treatment of these tumors. Specific mutational patterns (mainly deletions on the 1p chromosome) in oligodendroglial tumors predict for drug sensitivity.[7]

Medulloblastomas

Packer and colleagues have shown that a combination of cisplatin, vincristine, and CCNU has substantially delayed recurrence in children with high-risk medulloblastoma.[8] Other forms of chemotherapy have activity as well.

Primary CNS lymphomas

Primary CNS lymphomas are generally highly sensitive to corticosteroids and radiotherapy, but despite this therapeutic sensitivity, the prognosis for patients with this disease is quite poor. Consequently, there has been substantial interest in using chemotherapeutic agents, and it appears that recurrent CNS lymphoma will respond to high-dose methotrexate as well as to other drug combinations that are effective in systemic lymphoma.[9] Since this is a chemosensitive tumor, most current trials use chemotherapy prior to or instead of radiation, which had been the standard form of treatment for this tumor.

Germ cell tumors

The most common germ cell tumor of the CNS is the pure germinoma. This is a highly radiosensitive tumor that generally does not require chemotherapy. However, other cellular elements in a germ cell tumor, such as endodermal sinus tumor, teratoma, or choriocarcinoma, are associated with a worse prognosis, and these are often treated with a combination of radiotherapy and chemotherapy. Cisplatin and its derivatives are the most active agents in the treatment of intracranial germ cell tumors, as they are in the treatment of germ cell tumors that appear elsewhere in the body.

Ependymal tumors

It also appears that ependymal tumors in the brain and spinal cord respond to conventionally administered cisplatin or carboplatin, but again it is not clear whether the addition of chemotherapy at the time of diagnosis will materially affect the outcome.

Meningiomas, chordomas, neuromas

There are several relatively common extra-axial intracranial tumors for which chemotherapy is employed when surgery (and occasionally radiotherapy) have failed. Unfortunately, there is very little evidence of any activity of standard drugs in this setting.

SPECIAL PROBLEMS

Individualizing therapy

A major problem in the treatment of human cancer is that it has not been possible to predict reliably the response of an individual patient to a particular treatment. One can make general statements about the probability of response based on the histologic type of tumor, the extent of disease, and certain demographic features, such as the age of the patient. However, with few exceptions it has not been possible to assay an individual tumor in some sense and select the most appropriate therapy, as is done in microbiology. Consequently, for example, a small percentage of children with acute lymphoblastic leukemia do not respond to conventional chemotherapy, just as a small percentage of patients with anaplastic glial tumors respond dramatically to standard systemic chemotherapy at conventional doses. A reliable method to make these determinations in advance would have a profound impact on the treatment of patients suffering from these diseases.

If the primary mechanism of action of a chemotherapeutic agent is known, the mechanisms of resistance to this action have been determined, and it is possible to assay a tumor or a portion of a tumor for mechanisms of resistance, it may be possible to tailor therapy to individual cases. For example, it is thought that the primary biochemical mechanism of resistance to the nitrosoureas is a protein (O^6-alkylguanine-DNA alkyltransferase or AGT) that removes the alkyl adduct formed by the drug on the guanine base of the tumor DNA. If this repair protein is present in high levels, tumors are relatively resistant to nitrosoureas, but if the tumor is AGT-deficient it is very sensitive to the cytotoxic effects of these alkylating drugs.[10] An assay of this type can be performed on resected tissue to guide the choice of therapeutic agent to be used. Other specific biochemical and molecular characteristics might be used to individualize therapy.

Drug delivery

A unique aspect of the chemotherapy of tumors in the brain is the physiologic blood–brain barrier. Generally speaking, chemotherapy is ineffective in the treatment of CNS tumors. To what extent is this failure a result of inadequate drug delivery to the brain and spinal cord because of this barrier? On the one hand, lipid-soluble agents, i.e. those that are able to penetrate the barrier, are the most effective drugs in the treatment of CNS tumors. On the other hand, the barrier is clearly disrupted in many of these tumors, at least as measured by contrast enhancement on computed tomography (CT) or magnetic resonance imaging (MRI). The question is important because its resolution will herald the strategy of new therapeutic developments by emphasizing either new methods of delivery or totally new agents.

It appears that the answer will not be simple. There is experimental and clinical evidence that there is considerable variability in capillary permeability among and within primary CNS tumors,[11] and it is likely that the biochemical sensitivity of these tumors is similarly variable. To the extent that capillary permeability, blood flow, and biochemical sensitivity of individual tumors can be measured, it will become possible to select treatment rationally on the basis of measurable traits.

Evaluating response

Another peculiar and difficult problem in the treatment of CNS tumors is the determination of response to therapy. This was accomplished largely on clinical grounds in the early co-operative trials, and more recently assessment of treatment response has been based on a combination of clinical factors and imaging data from CT or MRI. Unfortunately, there are complexities even with the sophisticated imaging equipment available. First, these tumors are often irregular and highly infiltrative with indistinct margins, so attempts to determine tumor volume are subject to considerable measurement error. Second, contrast enhancement on CT or MRI lacks specificity, so in the setting of recurrent disease after primary treatment it is not always possible to distinguish active disease from gliosis or necrosis. This of course makes precise determination of a change in tumor volume after treatment nearly impossible. Third, the clinical neurologic status of a patient may not be reflected in the change on the imaging study. Patients can be considerably worse despite little change on CT or MRI, parti-

CLINICAL PEARLS

- The most common chemotherapeutic agents in use for the treatment of gliomas are BCNU (carmustine), CCNU (lomustine), procarbazine, and temozolomide.

- Chemotherapy has had minimal impact on the most common and malignant forms of primary brain tumor.

- Oligodendroglial tumors, particularly those with a 1p deletion, are usually highly sensitive to chemotherapy.

- Medulloblastomas, primary CNS lymphomas, and intracranial germ cell tumors are sensitive to different chemotherapeutic regimens.

- An accurate histologic diagnosis is currently the most important factor in selecting chemotherapy. In the future, specific molecular and biochemical features of an individual tumor will guide therapy.

cularly those with very large tumors. On the other hand, tumors in relatively silent areas of the brain can show considerable change without any effect on the neurologic examination. Furthermore, established neurologic deficits tend to remain fixed despite reversal of the pathologic process, so it is usually not reasonable to require improvement in the neurologic examination in the definition of response. Finally, all of these things can be profoundly affected by a change in the dose of corticosteroids being administered to the patient.

Because of the uncertainty surrounding the assessment of response in CNS tumors, study design and reports of clinical trials must include precise definitions. The variability in reported response rates in different trials probably largely reflects different definitions of response to therapy.

REFERENCES

1. Brem H, Piantadosi S, Burger PC, *et al*. Placebo-controlled trial of safety and efficacy by biodegradable polymers of chemotherapy for recurrent gliomas. *Lancet* 1995; 345: 1008–12.
2. Walker MD, Alexander E III, Hunt WE, *et al*. Evaluation of BCNU and/or radiotherapy in the treatment of anaplastic gliomas. *J Neurosurg* 1978; 49: 333–43.
3. Green SB, Byar DP, Walker MD, *et al*. Comparisons of carmustine, procarbazine, and high-dose methylprednisolone as additions to surgery and radiotherapy for the treatment of malignant glioma. *Cancer Treat Rep* 1983; 67: 1–12.
4. Yung WKA, Prados MD, Yaya-Tur R, *et al*. Multicenter phase II trial of temozolomide in patients with anaplastic astrocytoma or anaplastic oligoastrocytoma at first relapse. *J Clin Oncol* 1999; 17: 2762–71.
5. Dropcho EJ, Rosenfeld SS, Morawetz RB, *et al*. Pre-radiation intracarotid cisplatin treatment of newly diagnosed anaplastic gliomas. *J Clin Oncol* 1992; 10: 452–8.
6. Paleologos N, Cairncross JG. Treatment of oligodendroglioma: an update. *J Neuro-Oncol* 1999; 1: 61–8.
7. Ino Y, Beteusky RA, Zlatescu MC, *et al*. Molecular subtypes of anaplastic oligodendroglioma: implications for patient management at diagnosis. *Clin Cancer Res* 2001; 7: 839–45.
8. Packer RJ, Goldwein J, Nicholson HS, *et al*. Treatment of children with medulloblastomas with reduced-dose craniospinal radiation therapy and adjuvant chemotherapy: a Children's Oncology Group study. *J Clin Oncol* 1999; 17: 2127–36.
9. Abrey LE, DeAngelis LM, Yahalom J. Long-term survival in primary CNS lymphoma. *J Clin Oncol* 1998; 16: 859–63.
10. Jaeckle KA, Eyre HJ, Townsend JJ, *et al*. Correlation of tumor O^6-methylguanine-DNA methyltransferase levels with survival of malignant astrocytoma patients treated with *bis*-chloroethylnitrosourea (BCNU). *J Clin Oncol* 1998; 16: 3310–15.
11. Groothuis DR, Vriesendorp FJ, Kupfer B, *et al*. Quantitative measurements of capillary transport in human brain tumors by computed tomography. *Ann Neurol* 1991; 30: 581–8.

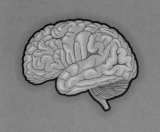

DEGENERATIVE SPONDYLOLISTHESIS

48

Bernard H Guiot and Ehud Mendel

INTRODUCTION

Spondylolisthesis refers to the forward displacement of one vertebra relative to another. Five types of listhesis have been described according to the Wiltse–Newman–MacNab classification system and include isthmic, degenerative, dysplastic, traumatic, and pathologic forms.[1] Degenerative spondylolisthesis was first described by Junghans in 1931 as a specific form of listhesis associated with an intact neural arch.[2]

Degenerative spondylolisthesis typically occurs at the level of L4–L5. It is then most likely at L3–L4, followed by L5–S1.[3] Older people are most commonly affected; the average age at presentation being 60 years. It is four times more likely to occur in women than men.[3] A clear explanation for this large difference between the genders is lacking. Certainly, parity has been associated with an increased incidence of spondylolisthesis. However, it is not known which of the features of pregnancy predisposes to slippage. Ligamentous laxity, increased weight bearing and abdominal muscle weakness have all been considered as contributing factors, yet nulliparous women have been found to have twice the rate of listhesis when compared with men, suggesting that other variables are implicated in the genesis of degenerative spondylolisthesis.[4] These have generally focused on disc dysfunction and changes in lamina and facet inclination.

Penning and Blickman[5] have suggested that degenerative spondylolisthesis arises as a result of hypermobility at the level of the disc. This dysfunction produces instability at the disc space and brings about the listhesis. According to this model of spondylolisthesis, facet and ligamentum flavum hypertrophy occur as a secondary phenomenon to prevent further slipping, which in turn results in spinal stenosis. Nagaosa and colleagues[6] however concluded from their review of pre- and post-slip X-rays of the spine that disc dysfunction is not significantly different in cases with and without slippage. Furthermore, the hypermobility required for facet hypertrophy is generally not seen in cases of degenerative spondylolisthesis. Indeed, McGregor and colleagues[7] have shown that there is a trend towards hypomobility when a slip is present.

An alternative view of degenerative spondylolisthesis suggests that changes in facet inclination and alignment predispose to slippage. Nagaosa and colleagues[6] reported that horizontalization of the lamina and the facet joints occurs before listhesis is seen. The facet joints have also been noted to become more sagittally aligned, particularly at the L4 and L5 levels.[8,9] The increased sagittal alignment may predispose to listhesis, where individuals with facet angles exceeding 45° have a 25-fold greater risk of developing degenerative spondylolisthesis.[8] There is however considerable controversy as to whether the change in facet alignment is the cause of the slip or rather its result. Love and co-workers[10] proposed that the change in facet alignment occurs as a result of remodeling associated with an underlying arthritic process in the facet joint. The higher joint angles arise due to wear on the anterior aspect of the facet, which is the area that offers the greatest resistance to flexion.[11,12] In turn, the increased facet angle may lead to slippage. Nagaosa's group[6] reported that while an increased sagittal alignment of the facet occurred more frequently in people with spondylolisthesis, a significant proportion (40%) of people did not demonstrate this feature. It remains that the importance of facet sagittal alignment is uncertain.

From a mechanical standpoint, degenerative spondylolisthesis is more likely to occur at the L4–L5 segment. The L5 vertebral body is characterized by large transverse processes, which support strong muscular and ligamentous attachments. In addition, the coronal orientation of the L5–S1 facets increases translational stability at that level. The relative immobility of L5–S1 in the face of lumbar lordosis results in a build-up of rotational and shear stress at L4–L5. The weaker muscular and ligamentous attachments at L4, coupled with sagittal facet orientation at L4–L5, results in a region less capable of resisting the stresses that predispose to spondylolisthesis.

CLINICAL PRESENTATION

Patients with degenerative spondylolisthesis frequently complain of intermittent low back pain. However, they generally present with symptoms consistent with neurogenic claudication. Thus, they experience leg pain, numbness and weakness that increase with walking and are relieved by rest. Flexion is also known to provide relief by increasing the anteroposterior diameter of the spinal canal. Activities such as bicycling, or walking uphill may therefore be well tolerated. Occasionally, patients present with radicular pain resulting from compression by the degenerative facet. The L5 root is most commonly affected, followed by the L4 root. On examination the patient may maintain a flexed position either when standing or walking. Range of motion of the lumbar spine is generally normal. The sensory and motor examinations are usually unremarkable, particularly when patients present with neurogenic claudication. Peripheral pulses must be palpated to exclude a vascular etiology.

NATURAL HISTORY

Degenerative spondylolisthesis is usually associated with low grade (I–II) slips. Progression of more than 5% occurs in 30% of cases over a 5-year period but is not correlated with clinical changes. The overall slip rarely attains 50%.[13] The disc space usually narrows progressively with time, a factor that is likely to contribute to additional stability at the affected segment.[14]

IMAGING

Plain X-ray

Multiple views are obtained during the work-up of degenerative spondylolisthesis. These include standing lateral, anteroposterior, oblique, and flexion/extension views of the lumbar spine. Standing studies may be helpful in demonstrating a slip that is difficult to visualize on supine films. In the upright position, the forces resulting from weight bearing are directed through the affected spinal level and may increase the extent of listhesis. Flexion/extension maneuvers may also produce changes in the degree of slip and thus provide information regarding stability at the affected segment. Oblique views should be included to exclude a defect in the pars interarticularis.

Spondylolisthesis can be graded using the Myerding method (Table 48.1).[15] A grade (between I and IV) is assigned based on the percentage of slip that has occurred across the level of the listhesis. A grade I spondylolisthesis is defined as a slip up to the first-quarter of the superior endplate of the vertebral body below the listhesis (Figure 48.1). Subsequent grades correspond to increases in slip by quarterly increments along the superior endplate of the inferior vertebral body.

Magnetic resonance imaging

Magnetic resonance imaging (MRI) has the highest diagnostic specificity and sensitivity of any spinal imaging modality. It allows for excellent visualization of the thecal sac and the nerve roots as well as the disc and ligamentous structures and hence is optimal for the evaluation of neural compression. Significant deformity may limit the information obtained through MRI and necessitate an alternative study, such as myelography and computed tomography (CT) scan.

Computed tomography myelography

This study was the gold standard until the advent of MRI. It continues to be useful in select cases where MR is contraindicated or in those patients with a clinical picture of degenerative spondylolisthesis but in whom the MRI fails to demonstrate the abnormality. The ability to reconstruct the CT images in multiple planes is most helpful, particularly where significant three-dimensional deformity is present.

TREATMENT

The North American Spine Society Task Force on Clinical Guidelines[16] has produced a document based on an extensive review of the literature to assist multidisciplinary spine-care professionals in the treatment of degenerative spondylolisthesis. The recommendations made are summarized below.

Nonoperative care

Three phases of specialized nonoperative care are outlined. The patient is entered into the appropriate phase based on the clinical condition.

Initial phase

This phase is appropriate for patients who have experienced an acute onset of pain, either as a first-time event or as a recurrence of an existing problem. Little or no deconditioning has occurred. The goal of this phase is symptom control to promote rapid return to premorbid activity. Treatment duration is typically 8 weeks and consists of the following:

- nonpharmacologic pain control modalities;
- manipulations;
- thermal (hot/cold) modalities;
- massage;
- electrical stimulation;
- ultrasound;
- activity modification;
- work modification;
- stretching and mobilizing exercises;
- bracing;
- traction;
- pharmacologic pain control modalities;
- nonsteroidal anti-inflammatory agents;
- steroidal anti-inflammatory agents, oral or epidural;
- analgesics;
- muscle relaxants.

Table 48.1 Myerding grading for spondylolisthesis	
Grade	Percent slip
I	0–25
II	25–50
III	50–75
IV	75–100

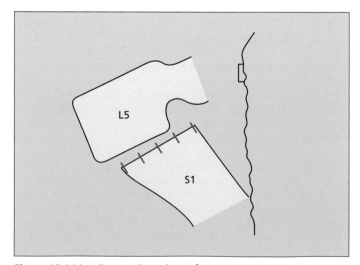

Figure 48.1 Myerding grading scheme for spondylolisthesis.

Secondary phase

This phase is appropriate for patients who have had a partial response to the initial therapy. These patients have typically been injured for several months and are limited in their daily activities. They may begin to demonstrate mental health problems and psychosocial barriers. Their physical examination shows early deconditioning characterized by loss of motion and loss of strength. Treatment duration is typically 8 weeks and consists of the following:

- nonpharmacological pain control modalities;
- de-emphasize passive modalities;
- activity resumption;
- pharmacological pain control modalities;
- de-emphasize narcotics;
- de-emphasize tranquilizers;
- nonsteroidal anti-inflammatory agents;
- epidural, facet joint, and selective nerve root injections;
- mental health intervention;
- behavior modification;
- medication;
- exercise;
- physical therapy;
- aerobic conditioning.

Tertiary phase

This phase is appropriate for patients with physical and psychological changes of chronic pain. Previous attempts at nonoperative and operative treatments have all proven ineffective. The goal of this phase is a return to productivity in the professional and personal arena. The patient's premorbid level of function may not be reached. Treatment duration is typically 10 weeks and consists of the following:

- interdisciplinary programs;
- includes physical therapy, occupational therapy, nursing, psychology, and multidisciplinary medical specialties;
- chronic pain management;
- functional restoration;
- behavior techniques;
- nonpharmacological pain control modalities;
- limited passive modalities;
- TENS (transcutaneous electrical nerve stimulation);
- pharmacological pain control modalities;
- de-emphasize habituating medications;
- nonsteroidal anti-inflammatory medications;
- epidural, facet joint, and selective nerve root injections;
- mental health intervention;
- behavioral modification;
- medication.

Operative intervention

Surgery is indicated in those patients who demonstrate progressive neurological deficit or who have failed to improve with nonoperative treatment. Specifically, those people with persistent pain, either radicular or claudicatory, that interferes with professional and personal activity as well as quality of life should be considered for surgery. Many procedures that have been described for the management of degenerative spondylolisthesis, including spinal decompression alone, decompression with fusion and decompression with instrumented fusion. Unfortunately, considerable controversy exists in the selection of the operation.

Posterior decompression

Decompression is indicated for those patients with radicular or claudicatory symptoms who have failed to improve with conservative measures. The goal of surgery is to relieve compression on the neural elements without destabilizing the functional unit. Ideally, laminoforaminotomies can be performed at multiple levels to effect the decompression. Kleeman and colleagues[17] report on 54 patients who underwent a 'port hole' decompression for spinal stenosis, and obtained good to excellent results in 88% of people. Only 15 patients within their cohort had an associated degenerative spondylolisthesis, and outcomes in this population were not significantly different from the rest of the group. Most importantly, the degree of listhesis remained stable in 13 of 15 (87%) of patients. Epstein[18] reported on 290 patients with degenerative spondylolisthesis treated with laminectomies and fenestration procedures. Patients were followed for an average of 10 years; 82% enjoyed a good to excellent outcome, whereas 18% had fair or poor results. Only eight (2.7%) required secondary fusion for progressive listhesis or instability. Others have been less successful at relieving symptoms with minimal posterior bony decompressions. Good to excellent results were obtained by Lombardi and colleagues in only 33% of patients.[19] Turner and associates[20] report an average success rate of 64%. Thus, more extensive bony removal may be required, which can be accomplished by pedicle to pedicle bony removal (Figure 48.2), or alternatively by undercutting the facet (Figure 48.3). It is important to decompress the L5 nerve root in the L5–S1 foramen, which is the most common site of compression resulting in the characteristic radicular pain.

Posterior decompression and fusion

Posterior spinal decompression alone has been shown to be quite successful at relieving the symptoms associated with spinal stenosis and nerve root compression, although debate continues surrounding the extent of bony resection that is optimal. There is significant concern that wide laminectomies and generous facetectomies required for adequate relief of neural compression will lead to spinal instability. Attempts have been made to

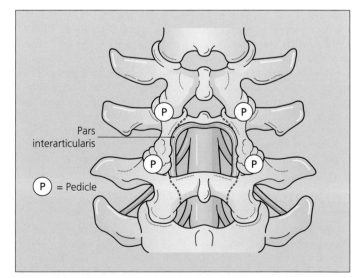

Figure 48.2 Wide decompression of the spinal canal is performed from pedicle to pedicle. This may result in instability if the facet joints are sagittally aligned.

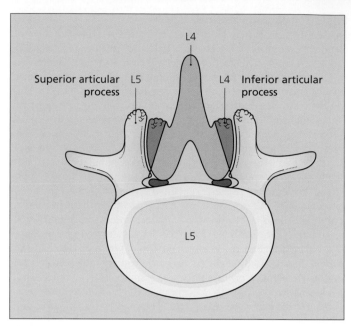

Figure 48.3 A narrow midline decompression is performed and the facets are undercut in order to alleviate the lateral recess stenosis.

quantify the amount of bone removal that can be safely undertaken,[21] but facet alignment has not been considered in this determination. Sagittal orientation of the facet joints, which predisposes to spondylolisthesis, is likely to increase the risk of instability postoperatively as well.

Several studies have looked at outcomes following decompression without and with fusion. Herkowitz and Kurz[22] found that patients obtained significantly better results for low back and leg pain when posterolateral fusions were undertaken. Mardjetko and colleagues[23] found that decompression alone was associated with a 69% rate of satisfaction as compared with 90% in patients who had also had a fusion. The issue of instrumentation in conjunction with fusion has also been examined. Booth and co-workers[24] noted a satisfactory outcome in terms of back and leg pain in 86% of patients with low complication rates. Mardjetko's group[23] found that fusion rates were higher in instrumented patients as compared with noninstrumented patients, although the difference did not reach statistical significance. Furthermore, there was no difference in clinical outcome. Bridwell and colleagues[25] showed that patients who achieved fusion with or without instrumentation reported better rating of improvement and decreased progression of listhesis. These results however proved statistically significant in the instrumented group only.

CONCLUSIONS

Much controversy surrounds the surgical management of degenerative spondylolisthesis. Posterior decompression, either limited or more extensive, has been shown to yield satisfactory results. There is evidence from a number of studies to suggest that fusion improves success rates in terms of low back and leg pain. Instrumentation yields higher fusion rates but this does not appear to translate into better outcomes.

CLINICAL PEARLS

- Degenerative spondylolisthesis refers to the forward displacement of one vertebra relative to another, where the neural arch is intact.

- It is most common in women and typically presents in the elderly.

- The underlying cause of degenerative spondylolisthesis is not well understood. It has been postulated that disc dysfunction or abnormal lamina/facet inclination leads to the progressive slip.

- Treatment is controversial and may include nonoperative modalities, surgical decompression with or without fusion and instrumented fusion.

This chapter contains material from the first edition, and we are grateful to the authors of that chapter for their contribution.

REFERENCES

1. Wiltse LL, Newman PH, MacNab I. Classification of spondylosis and spondylolisthesis. *Clin Orthop* 1976; 117: 23–9.
2. Junghans H. Spondylolisthesen ohne Spalt im Zwischergelenkstuclz ("Pseudospondylolisthen"). *Arch Orthop Unfallchirurgie* 1931; 29: 118–27.
3. Rosenberg NJ. Degenerative spondylolisthesis: predisposing factors. *J Bone Joint Surg (Am)* 1975; 57-A: 467–74.
4. Sanderson PL, Fraser RD. The influence of pregnancy on the development of degenerative spondylolisthesis. *J Bone Joint Surg (Br)* 1996; 78-B: 951–4.
5. Penning L, Blickman LR. Instability in lumbar spondylolisthesis: a radiographic study of several concepts. *Am J Radiol* 1980; 134: 293–301.
6. Nagaosa Y, Kikuchi S, Haue M, Sato S. Pathoanatomic mechanisms of degenerative spondylolisthesis: a radiographic study. *Spine* 1998; 23: 1447–51.
7. McGregor AH, Cattermole HR, Hughes S. Global spinal motion in subjects with lumbar spondylosis and spondylolisthesis. *Spine* 2001; 26: 282–6.
8. Boden SD, Riew KD, Yamaguchi K, *et al.* Orientation of the lumbar facet joints: association with degenerative disc disease. *J Bone Joint Surg (Am)* 1996; 78-A: 403–11.
9. Grobler LJ, Robertson PA, Novotny JE, Pope MH. Etiology of spondylolisthesis: assessment of the role played by lumbar facet joint morphology. *Spine* 1993; 18: 80–91.
10. Love TW, Fagan AB, Fraser RD. Degenerative spondylolisthesis; developmental or acquired. *J Bone Joint Surg (Br)* 1999; 81-B: 670–4.
11. Farfan HF. The pathological anatomy of degenerative spondylolisthesis: a cadaver study. *Spine* 1980; 5: 412–18.
12. Taylor JR, Twomey LT. Age changes in lumbar zygopophyseal joints: observations on structure and function. *Spine* 1986; 11: 739–45.
13. Matsunaga S, Sakou T, Morizono Y, Masuda A, Demirtas AM. Degenerative spondylolisthesis: pathogenesis and natural course of slippage. *Spine* 1990; 15: 1204–10.

14. Robertson PA, Grobler LJ, Novotny JE, Katz JN. *Spine* 1993; 18: 1483–90.
15. Myerding HW. Spondylolisthesis. *Surg Gynecol Obstet* 1932; 54: 371–7.
16. North American Spine Society. *Phase III Clinical Guidelines for Multidisciplinary Spine Care Specialists*. North American Spine Society; 2000.
17. Kleeman TJ, Hiscoe AC, Berg EE. Patient outcome after minimally destabilizing lumbar stenosis decompression. *Spine* 2000; 25: 865–70.
18. Epstein NE. Decompression in the surgical management of degenerative spondylolisthesis: advantages of a conservative approach in 290 patients. *J Spinal Disord* 1998; 11: 116–22.
19. Lombardi J, Wiltse L, Reynolds J, Widell EH, Spencer C. Treatment of degenerative spondylolisthesis. *Spine* 1985; 10: 821–7.
20. Turner JA, Ersek M, Herron L, Deyo R. Surgery for lumbar stenosis: attempted meta-analysis of the literature. *Spine* 1992; 17: 1–8.
21. Abumi K, Panjabi M, Kramer KM. Biomechanical evaluation of lumbar spinal stability after graded facetectomies. *Spine* 1990; 15: 1142–7.
22. Herkowitz HN, Kurz LT. Degenerative lumbar spondylolisthesis with spinal stenosis; a prospective study comparing decompression with decompression and intertransverse process arthrodesis. *J Bone Joint Surg (Am)* 1991; 73: 802–8.
23. Mardjetko SM, Connolly PJ, Shott S. Degenerative lumbar spondylolisthesis, a meta-analysis of literature 1970–1992. *Spine* 1994; 19: 2256S–65S.
24. Booth KC, Bridwell KH, Eisenberg BA, Baldus CR, Lenke LG. Minimum 5-year results of degenerative spondylolisthesis treated with decompression and instrumented posterior fusion. *Spine* 1999; 24: 1721–7.
25. Bridwell KH, Sedgewick TA, O'Brien MF, Lenke LG, Baldus C. The role of fusion and instrumentation in the treatment of degenerative spondylolisthesis with spinal stenosis. *J Spinal Disord* 1993; 6: 461–72.

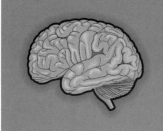

LUMBAR DISC HERNIATION

49

Christopher E Wolfla

INTRODUCTION

Lumbar disc herniation represents one of the most common problems that a neurosurgeon will be called upon to evaluate. It is estimated that 50% of working adults will experience back pain in any given year.[1] Of that number, many will be found to harbor a herniated lumbar disc. Neurosurgeons, while having extensive training in the management of disorders of the brain and peripheral nervous system, nevertheless spend the majority of their career treating patients with spinal disorders. Of those patients, more than 50% will harbor diseases of the lumbar spine, including lumbar disc herniation. Furthermore, over 296 000 intervertebral disc operations are performed in the United States per year.[2] Exceptional familiarity and expertise in the management of lumbar disc herniation is essential to the successful practice of neurological surgery.

NORMAL ANATOMY OF THE LUMBAR SPINE

The intervertebral disc is composed of three parts: the annulus fibrosus, the nucleus pulposus, and the cartilaginous end plates (Figure 49.1).[3–5] The annulus fibrosus is a tough outer ring composed of 10 to 12 concentric layers of fibrous tissue and fibrocartilage (Figure 49.2). It is reinforced ventrally by the anterior longitudinal ligament and dorsally by the posterior longitudinal ligament (Figures 49.2, 49.3). The nucleus pulposus, contained within this outer ring and slightly dorsal to the midpoint (Figure 49.2), is a remnant of the notochord and composed of a softer form of cartilage. In the child, the nucleus pulposus is semiliquid, but it becomes more solid and fibrous with age. Each lumbar intervertebral disc is bonded to the vertebral body above it by a thin plate of hyaline cartilage, and to the vertebral body below it by a similar thin plate of hyaline cartilage (Figure 49.1).

The bony arch that encircles the spinal canal posteriorly is formed by the two pedicles, two laminae, and the spinous process (Figure 49.2). The laminal arches of adjacent vertebrae are connected by an elastic yellow ligament, the ligamentum flavum (Figure 49.1). The caudal end of the spinal cord, the conus medullaris, extends down to about the level of the L1 vertebra. It is continuous inferiorly with a thin band called the filum terminale. The spinal canal in the lumbar area also contains the lumbar and sacral sensory and motor nerve rootlets, which in the aggregate are referred to as the cauda equina (Figure 49.2). These nerve roots lie within a cylindrical sac of dura mater and arachnoid and are bathed by the cerebrospinal fluid contained within the lumbar subarachnoid cistern.

At each spinal level, on each side, a nerve root containing both motor and sensory components exits from the dural sac. It then lies adjacent to the dural sac laterally before it turns further laterally to exit from the bony spinal canal one vertebral level below where it exited the dural sac. Therefore, the left L5 nerve root, which exits from the bony spinal canal through the left L5–S1 intervertebral foramen (just caudal to the left L5 pedicle), leaves the dural sac at about the level of the L4–5 intervertebral disc (Figure 49.4).

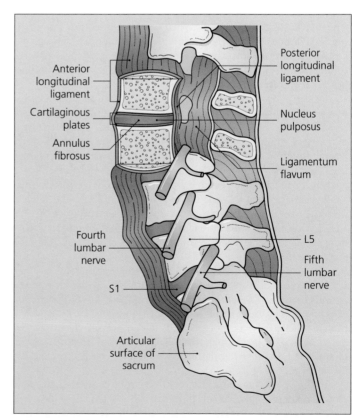

Figure 49.1 Sagittal view of the lumbar spine, with some components removed to better demonstrate the anatomy. (Modified from Keim.[16])

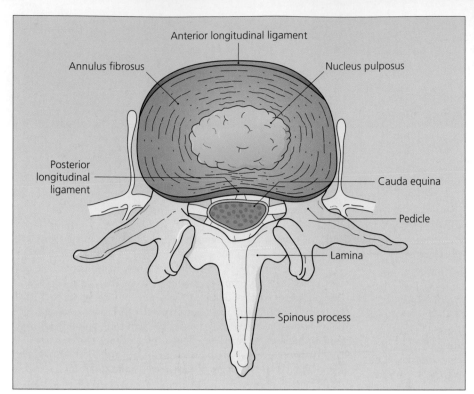

Figure 49.2 Axial view of the lumbar spine, showing an intervertebral disc, the contents of the spinal canal, and the elements of the dorsal bony arch.

Labels on figure:
Anterior longitudinal ligament
Annulus fibrosus
Nucleus pulposus
Posterior longitudinal ligament
Cauda equina
Pedicle
Lamina
Spinous process

PATHOPHYSIOLOGY

The nucleus pulposus may herniate in any direction out of its normal confines. If it herniates superiorly or inferiorly through the cartilaginous plate into the adjacent vertebral body, it is referred to as a Schmorl's nodule. Generally these are incidental findings noted radiographically or at autopsy.

Probably because the nucleus pulposus is situated somewhat posteriorly, and because the posterior longitudinal ligament reinforces the annulus fibrosus in the midline posteriorly, the majority of clinically significant disc herniations occur in a postero-lateral direction. The nucleus pulposus first herniates into tears in the concentric rings of the annulus fibrosus (Figure 49.5A), eventually causing the remaining outer rings to bulge focally (disc protrusion) (Figure 49.5B). If the process continues, the nuclear material may then escape from the disc (disc extrusion) to lie just anterior to the posterior longitudinal ligament (subligamentous disc herniation), or to lie free in the spinal canal (free fragment disc herniation) (Figure 49.5C).

The usual posterolateral disc herniation compresses the ipsilateral nerve root at its exit from the dural sac, rather than in the neural foramen. Therefore, a posterolateral left L4–5 disc herniation compresses the left L5 nerve root (Figure 49.4). However, if the disc herniation is more lateral, it compresses the ipsilateral nerve root exiting through the adjacent neural foramen. A far lateral left L4–5 disc herniation, for example, compresses the left L4 nerve root (Figure 49.6).

In the above scenarios, discrete nerve root compression causes radicular symptoms and signs in the distribution of a specific nerve root. A centrally located disc herniation of significant size may involve several elements of the cauda equina on both sides of the midline, producing spinal stenosis symptoms or even the equina syndrome, as described below.

In recent years, research has focused on the anatomical and molecular substrate of the radicular pain produced by lumbar disc herniation. While it appears that mechanical compression of the nerve root does play a role in the generation of this pain, other factors may be equally important. In particular, inflammation caused by biochemical mediators released by the injured intervertebral disc may play an important role in the clinical features of disc herniation.[6]

CLINICAL PRESENTATION

Syndromes

The clinical presentation of the patient with a herniated lumbar disc typically falls into one or more of the following categories: radiculopathy, neurogenic claudication, or cauda equina syndrome.

Radiculopathy is the most common syndrome associated with lumbar disc herniation, usually resulting from a posterolateral (Figure 49.7) or lateral (Figure 49.6) disc herniation impinging on a single nerve root. This results in pain, numbness, and/or weakness in the distribution of that nerve root.

When secondary to disc herniation, the syndrome of neurogenic claudication is most commonly associated with a large central lumbar disc herniation with resultant central spinal stenosis. Patients with neurogenic claudication, while frequently asymptomatic at rest, typically complain of bilateral lower extremity pain that begins after a reproducible period of exertion and increases the farther they walk or the longer they stand. Numbness and, later, weakness, may develop if the patient continues to stand or walk. A brief period of sitting alleviates the symptoms.

The cauda equina syndrome may result from a very large central lumbar disc herniation that compresses the entire bundle of rootlets traversing the region of the herniation (Figure 49.8).

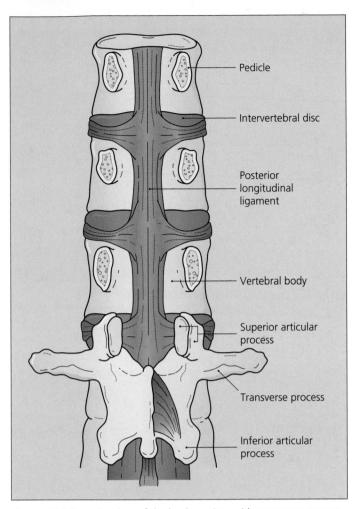

Figure 49.3 Posterior view of the lumbar spine, with some components removed to show the posterior surface of the vertebral bodies and intervertebral discs, reinforced by the posterior longitudinal ligament. (Modified from Keim.[16])

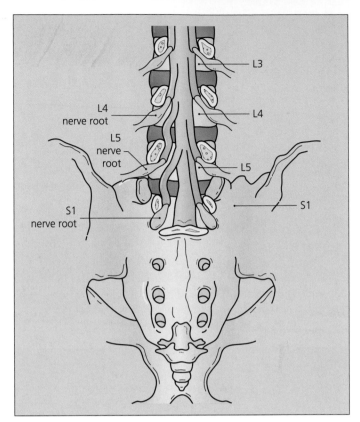

Figure 49.4 Posterior view of the lower lumbar spine. A disc protrusion at L4–5 on the left results in compression of the L5 nerve root where it leaves the dural sac, but before it exits from the spinal canal. (Modified from Keim.[16])

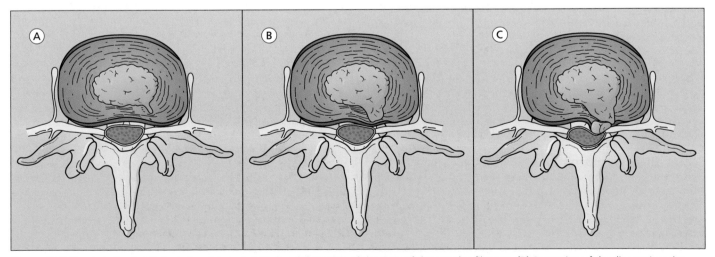

Figure 49.5 Stages in the herniation of an intervertebral disc. **(A)** Tearing of the rings of the annulus fibrosus. **(B)** Protrusion of the disc against the nerve root. **(C)** Extrusion of part of the nucleus pulposus, with further nerve root compression.

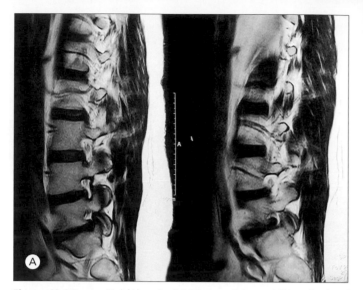

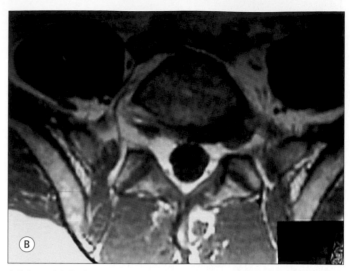

Figure 49.6 Parasagittal **(A)** and axial **(B)** views from an MRI study, showing a left lateral ("far lateral") herniation of the L5–S1 intervertebral disc causing compression of the left L5 nerve root in the neural foramen.

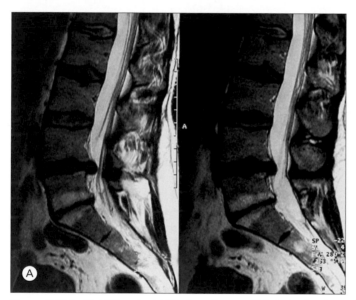

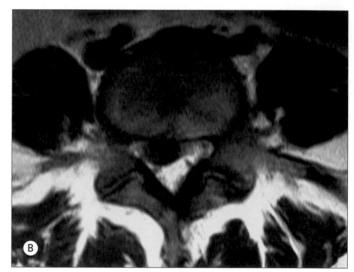

Figure 49.7 Sagittal **(A)** and axial **(B)** views from an MRI study, showing a right paracentral herniation of the L4–5 intervertebral disc causing compression of the right L5 nerve root.

While radiculopathy may coexist, the patient complains of perineal numbness, inability to void secondary to flaccid bladder, and/or incontinence. Recognition of this syndrome is paramount as its presence demands urgent work-up and treatment.

Signs and symptoms

Pain is the complaint that most commonly causes the patient to seek medical attention. Back pain, while probably the most common symptom of lumbar disc herniation, is also perhaps the least useful symptom in making the diagnosis. The differential diagnosis of back pain is enormous, with lumbar disc herniation being the cause in only a fraction of cases. Interestingly, while back pain is a nearly ubiquitous finding early in the course of disc herniation, it may resolve or nearly resolve later in the course

of the disease only to be replaced by extremity weakness and numbness.

The character of the back pain may give some clue as to the underlying disease process. Pain improved by back flexion suggests a component of lumbar spinal stenosis, while pain exacerbated by back flexion suggests instability or advanced disc degeneration. In contrast, pain with simulated axial loading, pain with simulated rotation, and other nonorganic physical signs suggest that the patient is showing psychologic distress out of proportion to the organic back disorder.[7]

Leg pain is also a common finding in lumbar disc herniation. While hip and buttock pain are frequent complaints, their presence rarely helps to localize the problem. Pain that is primarily localized to the hip, in particular, must be differentiated from hip joint pathology, especially if there is radiation to the groin.

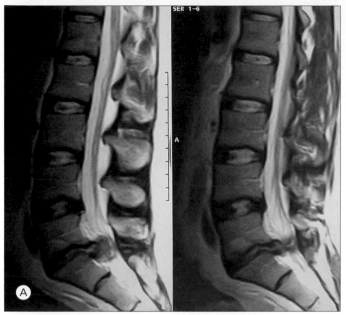
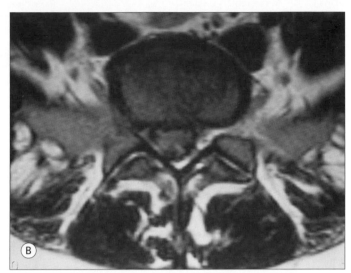

Figure 49.8 Sagittal **(A)** and axial **(B)** views from an MRI study, showing an enormous central herniation of the L5–S1 intervertebral disc causing compression of the entire thecal sac and distal cauda equina.

Table 49.1 Examination of patient

Standing	Sitting on table	Lying on table
Body build, posture	Straight leg raising	Supine
Deformities, pelvic obliquity, spine alignment	Popliteal compression test	Straight leg raising test:
Paravertebral muscle spasm, spinal tenderness	Knee jerks, ankle jerks	1 Flex hip with knee extended (sciatic nerve stretch)
Spinal column movements:	Anterior sensation	2 Flex hip with knee flexed
flexion, extension, lateral bending, and	Strength of hip flexion, knee extension and	Prone
rotation	flexion, foot dorsiflexion, great toe extension,	Spine extension
Posterior sensation	and foot plantarflexion	Hip extension
Walking on toes (tests plantarflexion of feet)		
Walking on heels (tests dorsiflexion of feet		
and extension of great toes)		
Stepping onto step		

The most common type of radicular leg pain is "sciatica," a deep, occasionally stabbing pain felt in the posterior thighs and calves. This pain tends to be worst when standing or walking and best when the patient is lying down with the legs elevated and knees bent. More severe radicular pain is generally better localized, and may be accompanied by numbness in an identifiable nerve root distribution. It is this type which is of most value in localizing the problem. Leg pain exacerbated by coughing or the Valsalva maneuver is also suggestive of radiculopathy.[8]

Physical examination includes an assessment of the patient's neurologic status as well as the status of all supporting structures (Table 49.1). Lower extremity neurologic findings, while not always present, may be particularly helpful in confirming the diagnosis of radiculopathy and localizing the source. Common findings on the neurological examination, as well as patterns of pain, for the three most commonly found radiculopathies are detailed in Table 49.2. The sensory examination, being dependent on patient interpretation, is the most subjective portion of the neurologic examination. The strength examination, while less subjective, relies on consistent patient effort. The reflex examination is the least subjective portion of the examination, though usually not helpful in the presence of a suspected L5 radiculopathy. Leg pain brought on by, or exacerbated by, the straight leg raising test is suggestive of radiculopathy. Back pain exacerbated by the straight leg raising test is non-specific. Rectogenital examination is mandatory when cauda equina syndrome is suspected.

DIAGNOSTIC STUDIES

Static radiographs of the lumbosacral spine and pelvis are obtained to rule out other causes of pain in the back and leg, such as fracture, neoplasia, infection, ankylosing spondylitis, or degenerative hip arthritis. Dynamic radiographs of the lumbar spine, typically lateral flexion and extension views, are obtained to detect any evidence of instability, including spondylolisthesis

Table 49.2 Typical clinical features of unilateral lumbar herniated nucleus pulposus

Disc	Nerve root	Pain	Paresthesias, numbness	Weakness	Reflexes
L3–4	L4	Lower back buttock lateral/anterior thigh, anterior leg	Anterior thigh, anterior leg	Quadriceps femoris femoris (extension of knee)	Knee jerk diminished or absent
L4–5	L5	Lower back, buttock, lateral thigh, anterolateral calf, occasionally groin	Anterolateral calf to great toe	Extensor hallucis longus (extension of great toe)	Usually no changes
L5–S1	S1	Lower back, buttock, lateral thigh and calf	Lateral calf to small toe	Gastrocnemius (plantarflexion of ankle)	Ankle jerk diminished or absent

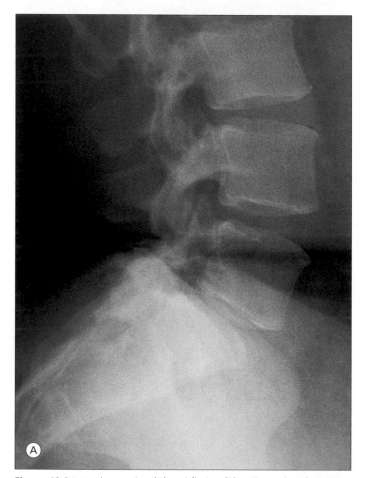

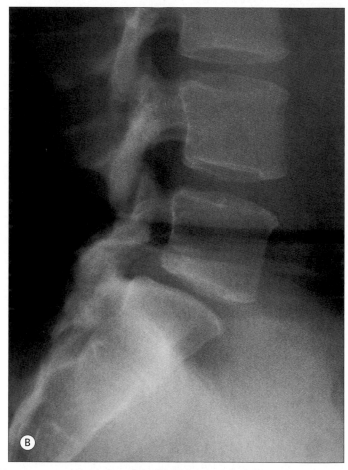

Figure 49.9 Lateral extension **(A)** and flexion **(B)** radiographs of a patient with a paracentral herniation of the L5–S1 intervertebral disc. Anterior sagittal plane translation at L5–S1 is observed in flexion, with reduction in extension.

(Figure 49.9). If the back and leg symptoms continue despite nonoperative therapy, and surgical treatment is contemplated, the underlying process can be delineated with a magnetic resonance imaging (MRI) study of the lumbar spine (Figures 49.6–49.8) or a lumbar myelogram with a delayed computed tomography (CT) scan (Figures 49.10, 49.11). Occasionally an electromyogram/nerve conduction study may be necessary, particularly when L5 radiculopathy cannot be distinguished from peroneal neuropathy on clinical grounds.

TREATMENT

As would be expected for a common, debilitating condition, many treatment options exist for lumbar disc herniation. Treatment options generally fall into one of two categories, nonsurgical or surgical.

Nonsurgical treatment of lumbar disc herniation should be considered at the onset of symptoms in most cases. Notable exceptions include those patients presenting with the cauda equina

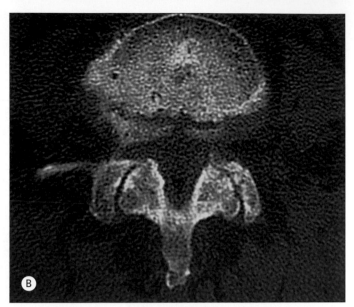

Figure 49.10 Same patient as in Figure 49.11. Axial MRI **(A)** and CT **(B)** views at the level of the L5–S1 disc. The MRI demonstrates a right paracentral disc herniation as well as significant hyperintense synovial fluid within the L5–S1 facet joints. The CT scan demonstrates advanced degenerative arthritis of the L5–S1 facet joints.

syndrome and/or profound motor weakness. Approximately 90% of patients will experience resolution of symptoms within 1 month without surgical treatment.[1] Medical therapy consists of nonsteroidal anti-inflammatory medications and occasionally oral corticosteroids on a short, tapering schedule. Narcotic pain medications are generally best avoided. If necessary for control of severe acute pain, they should be prescribed in the lowest effective dose for short periods of time. Muscle relaxers should likewise be avoided. Bed rest, while formerly a common treatment, is not advantageous.[9,10]

Manual therapies, such as back exercises, supervised physical therapy, and chiropractic, may be beneficial in reducing the period of disability, though data on efficacy are sparse. Likewise, epidural corticosteroid injections may produce dramatic relief of symptoms in selected patients, though the effect is variable and frequently temporary.[11]

Patients who have failed a reasonable trial of nonoperative treatment for lumbar disc herniation may consider surgical treatment. When planning surgical treatment, one must take into account all aspects of the patient's disease. For the patient with a typical unilateral paracentral disc herniation, a preponderance of leg pain, and a neurologic examination consistent with a discrete radiculopathy at the appropriate level, a standard partial hemilaminectomy and discectomy is an appropriate surgical treatment. Alternative or adjunctive surgical procedures, however, merit consideration in certain situations. Lateral or foraminal disc herniations require either a posterolateral approach to the herniation or significantly more extensive resection of the medial portion of the facet joint, possibly including complete unilateral facetectomy. As this is a potentially destabilizing procedure, consideration may be given to a concurrent arthrodesis.[12] Likewise, patients harboring large midline disc herniations producing neurogenic claudication or cauda equina syndrome may require a concurrent full laminectomy and discectomy for decompression of the neural elements. As this is also a potentially destabilizing procedure, consideration may be given to a concurrent arthrodesis. There is

some evidence to suggest that the surgical outcome is better if surgery is performed within 8 months of the onset of leg pain.[13]

The standard surgical treatment of a posterolateral lumbar disc herniation consists of a partial hemilaminectomy at the involved interspace on the appropriate side, with removal of the herniated disc material as well as any loose cartilage from within the disc space. Decompression of the affected nerve root is the primary goal (Figure 49.12). This may be accomplished in several ways, including open (under direct vision or using the operating microscope) and endoscopic. Regardless of the technique utilized, patients are generally allowed to ambulate on the day of surgery and may be discharged when pain is controlled with oral medications and when they are able to eat, void, and ambulate with

CLINICAL PEARLS

- Lumbar disc herniation is one of the most frequently encountered diagnoses in neurosurgical practice.

- Syndromes produced by lumbar disc herniation include radiculopathy, neurogenic claudication, and the cauda equina syndrome.

- Signs and symptoms resolve without surgical treatment in the majority of patients.

- Surgical treatment must be tailored to the individual underlying disease process.

- The majority of patients who do not improve with nonsurgical treatment experience a favorable outcome with appropriate surgical intervention.

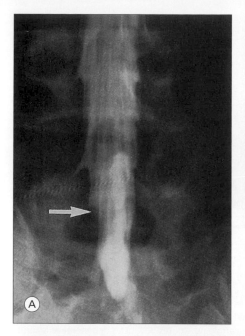
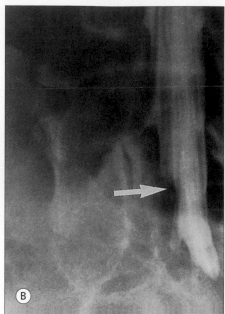
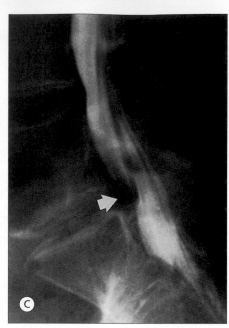

Figure 49.11 (A) Anteroposterior, **(B)** oblique, and **(C)** lateral views of a lumbar myelogram, showing a herniation of the L5–S1 invertebral disc, impinging on the S1 nerve root (arrow) **(D)**.

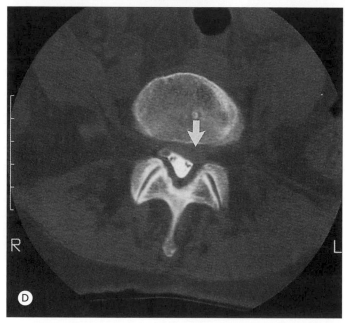

minimal assistance, usually with 24 hours. The patient usually recovers sufficiently to return to work 4–6 weeks later.

About 75–80% of patients treated for a lumbar disc herniation by a partial hemilaminectomy and discectomy will have excellent or good relief of symptoms. For patients with moderate or severe sciatica, surgical treatment may be associated with greater improvement than nonsurgical treatment at 5 years.[14] Relief of leg pain symptoms may occur slightly more commonly than relief of back pain symptoms.[15] Treatment failure suggests the need for additional studies to rule out recurrent herniation, infection, or underlying spinal instability, as well as to confirm that the appropriate level was surgically treated. Overall, about 15% of patients with a lumbar disc herniation will later have another disc herniation, either at the same location or at a different spinal level.

This chapter contains material from the first edition, and I am grateful to the authors of that chapter for their contribution.

REFERENCES

1. Bigos S, Bowyer O, Braen G, *et al. Acute Low Back Problems in Adults. Clinical Practice Guideline, Quick Reference Guide Number 14.* Rockville, MD: US Department of Health and Human Services, Public Health Service, Agency for Health Care Policy and Research, AHCPR Pub. No. 95–0643; December 1994.
2. Hall MJ, Owings MF. *2000 National Hospital Discharge Survey. Advance Data from Vital and Health Statistics*, no. 329. Hyattsville, MD: National Center for Health Statistics; 2002.

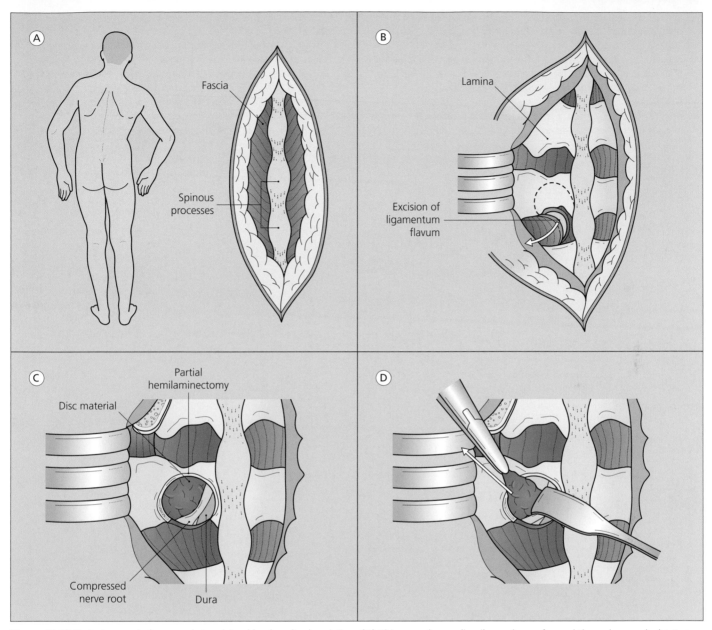

Figure 49.12 Posterior surgical approach to a lateral lumbar disc herniation. **(A)** This procedure ordinarily can be performed through a much shorter incision than that shown, with only unilateral exposure. **(B)** Portions of the adjacent laminae are removed, as is the ligamentum flavum. **(C,D)** The exposed nerve root is retracted medially and the herniated disc material is removed from its location anterior to the nerve root. (Modified from Netter.[17])

3. Coventry MB, Ghormley RK, Kernohan JW. The intervertebral disc: its microscopic anatomy and pathology. *J Bone Joint Surg* 1945; 27: 105–12, 233–47, 460–74.

4. DePalma AF, Rothman RH. *The Intervertebral Disc*. Philadelphia: WB Saunders Co.; 1970.

5. Spurling RG. *Lesions of the Lumbar Intervertebral Disc With Special Reference to Rupture of the Annulus Fibrosus With Herniation of the Nucleus Pulposus*. Springfield, IL: Charles C Thomas Publisher; 1953.

6. Saal JS. The role of inflammation in lumbar pain. *Spine* 1995; 20: 1821–7.

7. Waddell G, McCullough JA, Kummel E, Venner RM. Nonorganic physical signs in low-back pain. *Spine* 1980; 5: 117–25.

8. Vroomen PC, de Krom MC, Knottnerus JA. Consistency of history taking and physical examination in patients with suspected lumbar nerve root involvement. *Spine* 2000; 25: 91–6.

9. Malmivaara A, Hakkinen U, Aro T, *et al*. The treatment of acute low back pain – bed rest, exercises, or ordinary activity? *N Engl J Med* 1995; 332: 351–5.

10. Hagen KB, Hilde G, Jamtvedt G, Winnem MF. The Cochrane review of bed rest for acute low back pain and sciatica. *Spine* 2000; 25: 2932–9.

11. Carette S, Leclaire R, Marcoux S, *et al*. Epidural corticosteroid injections for sciatica due to herniated nucleus pulposus. *N Engl J Med* 1997; 336: 1634–40.

12. Bennett GJ, Serhan HA, Sorini PM, Willis BH. An experimental study of lumbar destabilization, restabilization and bone density. *Spine* 1997; 22: 1448–53.

13. Nygaard OP, Kloster R, Solberg T. Duration of leg pain as a predictor of outcome after surgery for lumbar disc herniation: a prospective cohort study with 1-year follow up. *J Neurosurg* 2000; 92(2 Suppl.): 131–4.

14. Atlas SJ, Keller RB, Chang Y, *et al*. Surgical and nonsurgical management of sciatica secondary to a lumbar disc herniation: five-year outcomes from the Maine lumbar spine study. *Spine* 2001; 26: 1179–87.

15. Asch HL, Lewis PJ, Moreland DB, *et al*. Prospective multiple outcomes study of outpatient lumbar microdiscectomy: should 75 to 80% success rates be the norm? *J Neurosurg* 2002; 96 (Spine 1): 34–44.

16. Keim HA. Low back pain. *Clin Symp* 1973; 25: 1–32.

17. Netter FH. *The CIBA Collection of Medical Illustrations, Volume I. Nervous System, Part II: Neurologic and Neuromuscular Disorders.* West Caldwell, NJ: CIBA Pharmaceutical Co; 1986; 197.

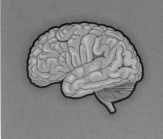

LUMBAR STENOSIS

50

Robert F Heary and Christopher M Bono

INTRODUCTION

Lumbar stenosis is a descriptive term denoting narrowing of the spinal canal. In some individuals, this can be associated with the characteristic clinical signs and symptoms of neurogenic claudication. Typically, neurogenic claudication refers to activity-related leg and buttock pain. By convention, this is referred to as lumbar spinal stenosis.[1–3] Stenosis can be divided into two main types: congenital/developmental and acquired.[1,2,4–7] Common to both types is reduced space available for the neural elements. While this, by itself, may not be solely responsible for neurologic compromise, it is thought to be a major predisposing factor. The actual pathomechanism is probably a combination of mechanical compression and vascular insufficiency.[8–12]

While the diagnosis is a clinical one, physical findings should be correlated with appropriate imaging studies. Both nonoperative and operative treatments are useful.[13–22] In properly selected cases, various methods of surgical decompression can lead to good results.[17,23–26] The role of fusion is less clear; however, fusion is advocated in cases of segmental instability.[16,27,28] Effective management of lumbar stenosis relies on a full understanding of this information. It is the authors' intent to review the outcomes of both surgical and nonsurgical treatment.

ETIOLOGY AND PATHOGENESIS OF LUMBAR STENOSIS

Congenital or developmental stenosis

Narrowing of the spinal canal and neuroforamina can arise from congenital or developmental conditions. Recently, the distinction between these two terms has been the focus of some discussion. "Congenital" implies that the stenosis is present at birth, while "developmental" denotes that which develops with growth. Patients with diastrophic dysplasia are not necessarily born with stenosis, but can develop degenerative-like enlargements of the facets that may cause neural impingement.[29] In contrast, patients with achrondroplasia are born with dimensional spinal canal narrowing, though clinical symptoms usually present in the third or fourth decades from secondary degenerative changes.[30,31] Idiopathic types of narrowing have also been recognized which are not associated with any particular developmental syndrome. These can display familial patterns; therefore, suggesting a genetically inherited form.[7] Though there is some confusion in the literature, the term developmental stenosis should not be confused with acquired stenosis.

The characteristic feature of congenital lumbar stenosis is shortened pedicles.[32] This decreases the anteroposterior spinal canal diameter as well as the space available for the exiting nerve roots. Most authors hold that this anatomic finding alone does not usually cause symptoms. Further stenosis from degenerative changes is thought to be necessary to surpass the compensatory threshold of the cauda equina, and thus, give rise to neurogenic claudication or radiculopathic complaints[7,32] (Figure 50.1).

Acquired lumbar stenosis

The most common type of lumbar stenosis arises from degenerative spinal disease. Degenerative lumbar stenosis is one of the "products" of the degenerative cascade.[1,2,33] A single motion segment in the lumbar spine is made up of three "joints": the intervertebral disc and two zygapophyseal facet joints. Mild disc degeneration alters the mechanics of this three-joint intervertebral complex. As the disc loses its ability to withstand axial and translational forces, greater loads are placed on the facet joints. The facet joints then begin to undergo arthritic changes akin to other larger joints in the body such as the hip or knee joints. Consecutively, these changes include synovitis, articular cartilage degeneration and synovial tag formation, followed by capsular laxity, joint subluxation and articular surface enlargement. The last change is believed to be the facet joint's attempt to stabilize itself with increased surface area.

Facet incompetence places further stresses on the intervertebral disc. Subsequent degeneration leads to so-called internal disc disruption in which the nucleus pulposus is broken down and resorbed. Eventually, osteophytes develop and project from the endplates to stabilize the motion segment. These osteophytes can be differentiated from traction spurs, as described by McNab, which arise at the insertion of the annulus fibers along the vertebral body. Occurring earlier in the degenerative cascade, traction spurs are located at a distance from the endplate and are not likely to affect overall stability.

Degenerative changes do not necessarily cause symptoms. Degenerative changes can be detected in a large proportion of asymptomatic individuals by plain films, myelography, computed tomography (CT) scans, and magnetic resonance imaging (MRI).[34–37] However, in some individuals, these changes can result in symptomatic degenerative disc disease, dynamic or static lumbar instability, or degenerative scoliosis. Neurogenic claudication associated with lumbar stenosis can occur with each of these disorders.

Various degenerative changes can cause neural impingement. A bulging posterior annulus or posterior vertebral body osteophyte

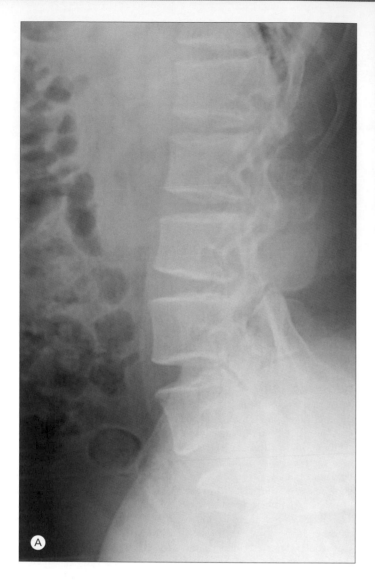

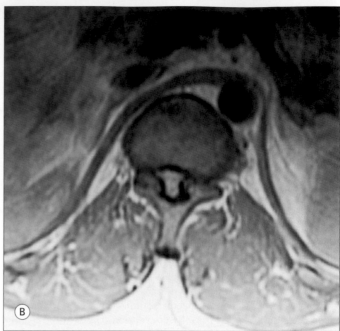

Figure 50.1 Imaging studies from a 32-year-old achondroplastic dwarf who developed progressive neurogenic claudication over a 5-year period which eventually required surgical decompression. **(A)** Plain film lateral radiograph – characteristic appearance of foreshortened pedicles. **(B)** MRI (axial T2-weighted) – L1 vertebra – even in the rostral lumbar spine, significant stenosis is present as a result of ligamentum flavum hypertrophy and short pedicles seen in congenital stenosis.

can cause central compression of the ventral dural sac. Lateral disc osteophytes might narrow the intervertebral foramina. Facet joint hypertrophy can affect both the central and lateral canals. Overgrowth of the inferior articular process can encroach upon the lateral recess and central canal, while an enlarged superior articular process can impinge the exiting nerve root within the neural foramen. As a general rule, central canal stenosis is associated with compression by the inferior facets and lateral recess, or foraminal, stenosis is associated with compression by the superior facets (Figure 50.2).

As the disc space narrows, the facet joints sublux slightly. This contributes to an overall decreased area for the exiting nerve roots and might predispose to nerve root redundancy within the dural sac.[12] The relative decrease in intervertebral distance can also lead to infolding of the ligamentum flavum. The ligamentum flavum will often become hypertrophied, and occasionally, even calcified.[4,38]

Other less common disorders can cause acquired lumbar stenosis. Hyperostotic bone disease can result in bony proliferation in nonarticular regions of the posterior vertebral body which may in turn lead to symptomatic lumbar stenosis.[39] Ossification of the yellow ligament has also been a reported cause of stenotic

symptoms.[5] The clinical features and treatment are principally the same as for degenerative stenosis. However, in these other disorders, the dura may frequently adhere to the ossified structures. In more severe cases, the dura may be absent altogether, making surgical decompression more difficult.

The exact mechanism of neural dysfunction remains speculative. A majority of spine surgeons believe that it is primarily from mechanical compression. This line of thinking forms the rationale for conventional surgical treatment. Some surgeons have suggested that a vascular etiology is responsible. This may be a form of venous congestion or arterial insufficiency causing neural ischemia.[9] The actual pathomechanics is probably a complex interaction of these processes.[8–12]

CLINICAL PRESENTATION AND PHYSICAL EVALUATION

Clinical features

Patients typically present with fatigue of the lower extremities with ambulation. This can be bilateral or unilateral and may or may not be associated with pain, numbness, or weakness.

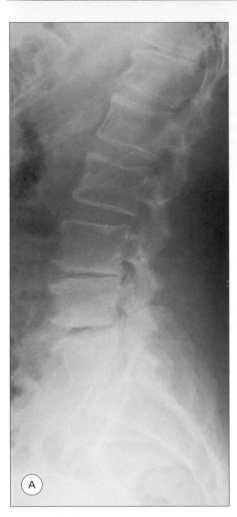

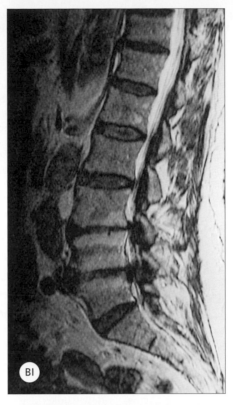

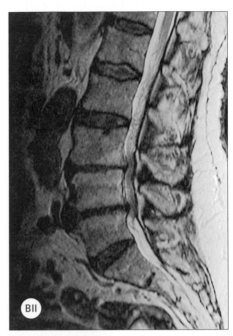

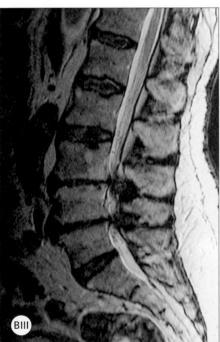

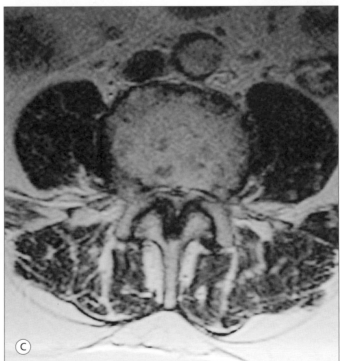

Figure 50.2 Preoperative imaging studies of a 77-year-old former boxer with severe degenerative changes in the lumbar spine and neurogenic claudication which limited his walking to 25 steps. **(A)** Plain film lateral radiograph – severe multilevel degenerative changes are evident. **(B)** MRI (sagittal T2-weighted) – view of three adjacent parasagittal cuts shows severe central and lateral stenosis **(BI–BIII)**. **(C)** MRI (axial T2 weighted) – combination of intervertebral disc bulging from ventral, zygapophyseal facet joint hypertrophy causing lateral narrowing, and ligamentum flavum hypertrophy contributing to dorsal impingement into the spinal canal.

Frequently, signs and symptoms may not be present at rest. As the dimensions of the canal and neural foramina are wider with spinal flexion, patients often report better stamina while walking stooped over, leaning on a shopping cart, or bicycling. Claudicant pain is relieved by flexing the spine. The seated position accomplishes flexion of the lumbar spine while standing and walking produce a relative extension in the lumbar spine. As such, patients with lumbar spinal stenosis will usually develop their symptoms when standing or walking and will sit down, intermittently, to relieve the symptoms. Another frequent neurologic complaint is gait instability, which may be the result of diminished proprioception from the lower extremities.

It is important to attempt to distinguish between neurogenic claudication and vascular claudication. Vascular claudication results from vascular insufficiency of the lower extremities and will usually manifest as pain in the calf region that is exacerbated with walking and relieved with rest. Neurogenic claudication may have similar symptoms; however, it will often include pain in the buttocks or posterior thigh regions. In cases of lateral recess stenosis, particularly if there is a component of spondylolisthesis, the neurogenic claudication may be impossible to distinguish from vascular claudication by taking a medical history alone (Figure 50.3).

Back pain is a frequent symptom in lumbar spinal stenosis. It is generally thought to relate to the underlying spondylosis. Interestingly, back pain often resolves after a simple decompressive laminectomy. This suggests that a form of neurogenic back pain may also be responsible. Claudicant buttock pain might be construed as back pain by some individuals. This may account for some of the reported relief in clinical series. Despite this, a predominance of back pain is associated with poorer results after surgery.[3]

Katz et al.[3] analyzed the diagnostic predictive value of various symptoms for degenerative lumbar stenosis. Pain below the buttocks was the most sensitive predictor but was only minimally specific. Resolution of pain with sitting was the most specific predictor but was among the least sensitive. Pain in the lower extremities (below the knees) also demonstrated poor sensitivity. Interestingly, the classic claudicant findings of activity-related symptom exacerbation with walking was 71% sensitive but only 30% specific. The major flaw of this study was that the ultimate "accuracy" of the diagnosis was based on clinical judgement, as there is no diagnostic gold standard for degenerative lumbar stenosis.

Less frequently, patients complain of urinary or bowel dysfunction. Bladder symptoms are more frequent.[40,41] Unfortunately, lumbar spinal stenosis tends to occur in the elderly population. In this group, urinary symptoms of frequency and urgency can occur in males as a result of prostatic enlargement or in females because of weakening of the perineal floor. These same complaints can result from spinal stenosis. The most common complaint in degenerative lumbar stenosis is a feeling of incomplete voiding. Frank urinary incontinence, small urinary stream, urinary retardation, and protracted voiding time may also be reported. Importantly, these complaints can be present in patients with normal bladder function. Urinary incontinence is the most specific predictor for lumbar stenosis. In patients with lumbar stenosis and bladder complaints, the practitioner should consider obtaining urodynamic studies to document the dysfunction preoperatively.[40,41]

Priapism is a rare but well-documented complaint in patients with lumbar spinal stenosis.[42–44] Baba et al.[42] reported nine patients with claudicant priapism that occurred during walking. As the same activity-related pathomechanism is probably responsible, it appears to respond well to surgical decompression.[42,44]

A complete medical history should be obtained for each patient. Especially when surgery is being considered, medical comorbidities should be noted, as they may be associated with a poorer surgical outcome.[45] A sense of the patient's overall well-being should also be assessed, as well as the psychological history. Concomitant peripheral or central nervous disorders, such as multiple sclerosis or other demyelinating diseases, should be noted as they can coexist with lumbar spinal stenosis. They may mask or exacerbate symptoms and should be differentiated as best as possible prior to treatment.

As patients with the acquired form of stenosis are often older at the time of surgery, any additional systemic medical problems need to be clarified prior to determining whether the patient is a surgical candidate. In the developmental/congenital form of stenosis, surgical intervention is usually performed at an earlier stage in life.

Physical findings

Distal pedal pulses should be evaluated to discriminate between neurogenic and vascular claudication. This is particularly true if the history is not able to distinguish adequately between these two diagnoses. If there is concern regarding the possibility of a vascular component to the claudication complaints, then noninvasive blood flow studies in a vascular laboratory are indicated. As the presence of spinal deformities (i.e. kyphosis or scoliosis) can affect surgical decision-making, the patient's overall body habitus and posture should be noted.

A complete neurologic examination should be performed. This includes an evaluation of perianal sensation. Patients may present with motor or sensory deficits; however, a high proportion of patients with lumbar spinal stenosis will have no focal findings. The straight leg test is usually negative. A wide-based gait is a highly specific (97%) positive predictor for lumbar stenosis. Other important predictors are an abnormal Romberg test (91% specific, 39% sensitive), muscle weakness (78% specific, 47% sensitive), and vibration deficits (81% specific, 53% sensitive).[3] Reflexes are typically hypoactive or absent but they may also be normal. Hyperreflexia is not usually seen in these patients and its presence suggests upper motor neuron involvement of an unrelated cause.

By the nature of the disease, neurologic findings may be clinically senescent at rest during a physical examination. Methods of eliciting specific deficits have been devised to localize the level of stenotic lesions, particularly in those with more than one involved level. Sato and Kikuchi[8] used a gait-load test in patients with two-level stenosis. This test involves walking with the patient until symptoms worsen. A quick neurologic examination is then performed with the intent to isolate a focal motor or sensory change. This information is then correlated with radiographic findings to determine the more symptomatic stenotic region. Although good results have been documented with decompression of the one symptomatic level,[8] we have not found this particular test to be valuable in clinical practice.

DIAGNOSTIC EVALUATION

Plain roentgenograms can demonstrate spondylosis, i.e. degenerative changes. These include anterior, lateral and less-well-

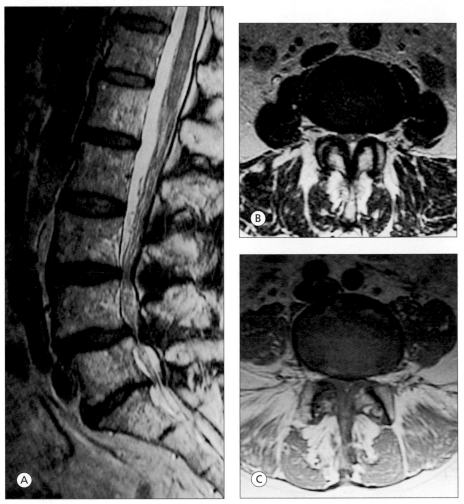

Figure 50.3 MRI of a 75-year-old former operating room nurse. **(A)** MRI (sagittal T2-weighted) – marked canal compromise. **(B)** MRI (axial T2-weighted) – trefoil appearance of spinal canal is visualized. **(C)** MRI (axial proton density image) – both central and foraminal narrowing is evident.

visualized posterior vertebral body osteophytes. Narrowing of the facet joints is best noted on oblique views. Segmental instability can be recognized as listhesis of one vertebra on the other. This can be dynamic or static. Dynamic instability is best demonstrated on lateral flexion/extension films. Spondylolisthesis is characterized by anterolisthesis of the cranial vertebra on its caudal counterpart. This is most common at the L4–L5 segment but it may occur at other levels.[27] Spondylolisthesis is frequently associated with spinal stenosis (Figure 50.4). Cauda equina compression is exacerbated by the neural arch offset. The foramina are compromised as the inferior articular processes of the upper level sublux forward on the superior articular processes of the lower level.

The overall spinal alignment should be noted in both the coronal and sagittal planes. Degenerative scoliosis is frequently complicated by spinal stenosis (Figure 50.5). Kyphosis should also be appreciated as such deformities can progress in patients who are treated with laminectomy without fusion. Canal compromise is difficult to appreciate on plain films and is better assessed with advanced neuroimaging studies.

Myelograms have fallen out of favor because of the invasiveness of the procedure, though they still have utility in some cases. In patients with hardware, particularly stainless-steel implants, the quality of CT and MRI scans can be obscured by artifacts, while myelography remains relatively unaffected. Likewise, myelography may be preferable for delineating lateral recess stenosis where the presence of cortical bone in the neural foramen makes MRI less valuable. The limitations of myelography include that it is a two-dimensional examination, though plain film tomography can still be performed in some centers. Also, it only allows visualization of intradural structures, so that the nerve roots may be poorly contrasted within the neural foramina. The major advantage of myelography over other modalities is that it reflects the dynamic mechanical flow of cerebrospinal fluid within the dural sac.

For some spine surgeons, CT scanning remains the imaging modality of choice.[46,47] It gives excellent bony resolution with fairly good visualization of the soft tissues. Canal dimensions can be best measured on bone windows of CT scan images. Osteophytes and facet hypertrophy can be readily appreciated. As it is

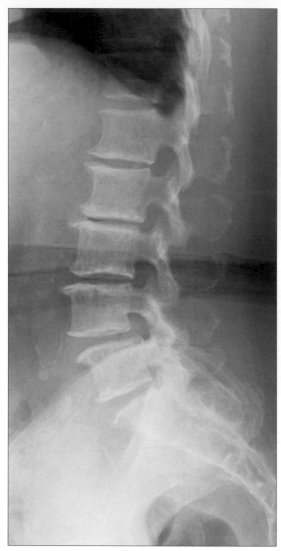

Figure 50.4 A 72-year-old woman with a combination of spinal stenosis and spondylolisthesis; at the L4–L5 level, an 8-mm anterolisthesis is present; no motion occurred on flexion/extension lateral views.

of the spinal canal. As the cerebrospinal fluid has a bright signal on T2-weighted images, this imaging sequence can create a myelogram-like effect. The classic MRI description of lumbar spinal stenosis is a trefoil appearance on axial views as a result of a bulging intervertebral disc ventrally, hypertrophied facet joints laterally, and ligamentum flavum hypertrophy dorsally.

The disadvantages of MRI have been recognized. MRI can overestimate the degree of lateral recess stenosis because of the low signal intensity, especially on T2-weighted images, created by sclerotic osteophytes off the posterior vertebral body.[46] It is also difficult to interpret images taken from a scoliotic spine as the plane of the images cannot be adjusted to the plane of the vertebral bodies. This is a potential advantage of CT scanning, in which the imaging plane can be modified. Furthermore, as with CT scans, hardware artifacts can obscure spinal detail, though this is less problematic with titanium implants. While both CT and MRI scans are useful in determining the regions and amounts of lumbar stenosis, these parameters are not predictive of the severity of the clinical presentation.[47,49] Similarly, the degree of radiographically detected postoperative stenosis after decompressive surgery does not accurately correlate with clinical outcomes.[50]

NONOPERATIVE TREATMENT

Noninterventional treatment of lumbar spinal stenosis is essentially observation of its natural history.[13,51–53] Between 15 and 43% of patients report some relief with a course of medications and rehabilitation, while the majority of patients (50–70%) report no improvement. Between 15 and 27% of patients worsen over time. The outcome of noninterventional management is not directly related to the radiographic severity of the stenosis.[13] However, scoliosis is associated with a significantly higher rate of failure with conservative modalities than other forms of degenerative lumbar stenosis.[13] In general, the beneficial results of nonoperative treatment tend to deteriorate within 6 months.

Nonoperative management can include one or more of the following components: medications, bracing, physical therapy and injections. Useful first-line pharmaceuticals include nonsteroidal anti-inflammatory medications. If pain becomes less bearable, a mild narcotic may be prescribed with caution, as the sedating effects can be significant in the elderly population. Some practitioners recommend a short course of oral steroids for acute episodes; however, the efficacy of this practice has not been clearly demonstrated. Importantly, none of these agents affect the natural history of lumbar spinal stenosis.

Bracing has been advocated for the nonoperative treatment of lumbar stenosis. A lumbar corset is probably the most commonly prescribed device.[20] In a small series of patients, use of a corset was associated with modest improvements in walking endurance and significantly reduced pain. The mechanism of this relief is unknown, as corsets have minimal effect on intersegmental lumbar motion.[54] It is more likely that subjective feelings of increased stability are at play. Alternatively, most lumbar braces place the lumbar spine into a flexed posture which will enlarge the dimensions of the bony spinal canal.

Physical therapy can have temporary beneficial effects for patients with lumbar stenosis. Programs should focus on flexibility, strengthening and aerobic conditioning. Bodack and Monteiro[19] recommend flexion exercises to stretch the posterior lumbar paraspinal muscles. These movements tend to increase the dimensions of the spinal canal and the neural foramina. The

performed in a supine position, CT scanning may underestimate the degree of stenosis in mild or moderate cases compared with myelography obtained in the standing position with the spine in extension.[48] The addition of intrathecal contrast to a CT scan can be of benefit to identify areas of limited cerebrospinal fluid flow and this is a useful adjunct if MRI cannot be obtained. Similarly, a myelogram, with a post-myelogram CT scan, is an excellent method to diagnose foraminal stenosis. Listhesis is poorly visualized with axial CT scans. To appreciate the degree of spondylolisthesis, sagittal reformations of the CT scans are needed.

In the authors' opinion, MRI is the modality of choice for lumbar spinal stenosis. In addition to adequate visualization of the bony structures, though not as defined as on CT scans, MRI allows superior delineation of the soft tissues. These include the ligamentum flavum, the intervertebral discs, and synovial redundancy around the facet joints. Facet cysts, or synovial cysts, which are not well visualized by other modalities, are easily seen with MRI. Furthermore, MRI allows true sagittal, coronal and axial imaging

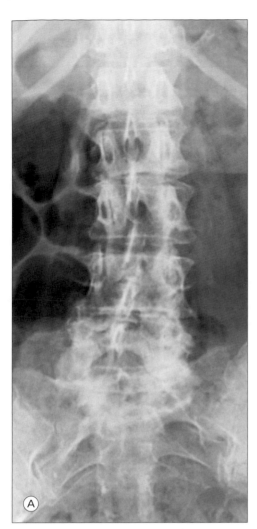
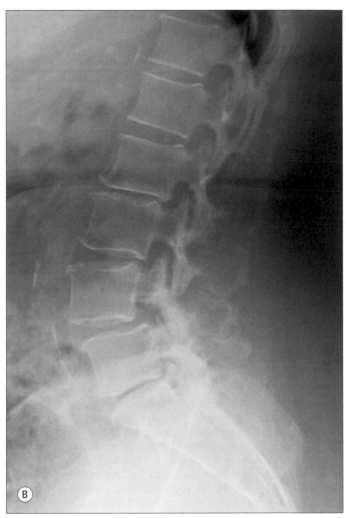

Figure 50.5 Plain film radiographs of a 65-year-old female physician. **(A)** Anteroposterior view – mild scoliosis with facet joint degenerative changes are seen. **(B)** Lateral view – typical degenerative changes frequently seen with stenosis.

physical therapy regimens utilized for spondylolisthesis patients focus on flexion exercises and these regimens have the most success for patients with spinal stenosis as well. Extension-based exercise regimens, which are commonly used to treat patients with herniated lumbar intervertebral discs, will often worsen the symptoms in patients with stenosis. As such, it is important to oversee the treatment program to confirm that the correct exercises are being carried out.

Aerobic conditioning is also important. Traditional walking exercises may be difficult for stenotic patients to perform. Stationary bicycling is excellent for improving overall aerobic endurance. The flexed posture of the lumbar spine on a bicycle helps to prevent the onset of neurogenic claudication. This allows the lumbar spinal stenosis patient the opportunity to improve conditioning while not acutely exacerbating their symptoms. Aquatic therapy and swimming have also been advocated.[55]

Epidural steroid injections are commonly performed for the treatment of symptomatic lumbar stenosis with neurogenic claudication. The effectiveness of epidural steroid usage has not been agreed upon.[13,21,22,56] Ciocon et al.[21] found that a combina-

tion of xylocaine and Depo-medrol provided effective pain reduction for up to 10 months in an elderly population. The effects on walking distance were not reported. In a three-armed randomized, prospective study, Fukasaki et al.[56] found epidural steroid injections of methylprednisolone (with local anesthetic) to be no more effective than local anesthetic alone in improving walking endurance. Importantly, the placebo group, who were treated with saline epidural injections, had significantly less improvement than either of the treatment groups. At 3 months, all three groups had similar results, with approximately 6% of patients reporting sustained gains in walking distances. Other studies have indicated that nonoperative treatment in conjunction with epidural steroid injections can help to avoid surgery in a large number of patients.[22] At best, injections can be expected to provide short-term symptomatic relief; however, it is doubtful that they have any long-term effects on the natural history of the disease.

Injections may be delivered to the central canal epidural space or selectively around a particular nerve root. Fluoroscopy in the interventional radiology suite or operating room can be a useful adjunct in appropriate delivery of the medication. Selective nerve

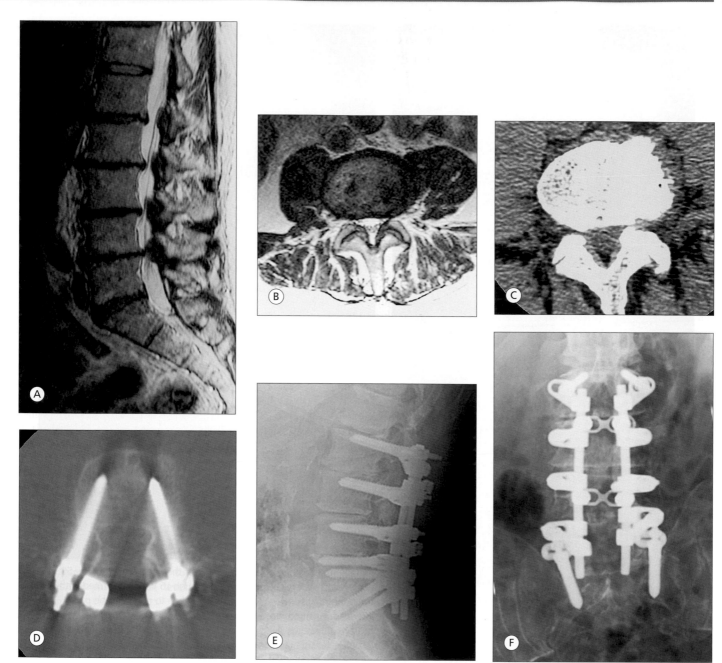

Figure 50.7 A 70-year-old retired businessman with lumbar spinal stenosis which markedly limited his walking distance; symptoms were predominantly leg pain with walking as a result of lateral recess stenosis. **(A)** MRI (sagittal T2-weighted) – moderate narrowing in the midline noted. **(B)** MRI (axial T2-weighted) – proportionally much more impingement at the foraminal level. **(C)** CT scan (axial bone windows) – demonstrates the lateral recess stenosis due to hypertrophy of the superior articular processes (located laterally). **(D)** CT scan (axial bone windows) – postoperative view after aggressive decompression was followed by pedicle screw stabilization. **(E)** Plain film lateral radiograph (1-year postoperatively) – good alignment with no signs of hardware failure and reasonable maintenance of sagittal plane balance. **(F)** Plain film anteroposterior aligned spine following aggressive laminectomies for lateral recess stenosis; stabilization and fusion were performed because of the extent of resection of the pars interarticularis and the inferior facet joints bilaterally; the patient has resumed walking distances greater than 1 mile (1.6 km).

technique resulted in less back pain than laminectomy while neural complications were higher after the laminotomies. Importantly, greater relief of radicular complaints was documented in the laminectomy group. While no cases of instability occurred in the laminotomy group, 50% of patients with preoperative degenerative spondylolisthesis had a mild increase in slip, despite *in situ* fusion. This is compared with a 61% incidence of mild or moderate slip in the laminectomy group. These results were not statistically analyzed or correlated to clinical outcome. As most reports of limited resection techniques do not document the incidence of postoperative instability, the relative worth of preserving the midline structures must be weighed against the higher neural complication rate and the increased operative time required to perform the procedure.

CLINICAL PEARLS

- Lumbar stenosis is a descriptive term denoting narrowing of the spinal canal. In symptomatic patients it is associated with activity-related leg, calf, and buttock pain. There are two main types: congenital (due to anatomic limitations such as short pedicles) and acquired (often due to degenerative spine disease).

- The clinical features include pain, numbness, and weakness that are worse with ambulation and improve on rest. It is important to distinguish between vascular claudication from vascular insufficiency and neurogenic claudication from lumbar stenosis. The symptoms may be similar. Back pain and posterior thigh pain are usually associated with lumbar stenosis. On examination there may be motor, sensory, or reflex neurological deficits in patients with lumbar stenosis. A decrease in distal pedal pulses and vascular studies showing insufficiency are typical of vascular claudication.

- MRI has evolved to be the single imaging modality of choice because of its ability to delineate soft tissue, CSF spaces, severity of neural compression, and disc disease. Myelography in selected patients can provide very useful information on the mechanical flow of CSF fluid in the thecal sac and lateral recess stenosis and in patients with hardware in the spine. CT scanning is excellent for bone resolution. The combination of myelography followed by CT scan is excellent for assessing the degree of foraminal stenosis and nerve root compression.

- Nonoperative treatment includes physical therapy, administration of nonsteroid anti-inflammatory drugs, aerobic conditioning, and epidural injections, and is useful in about 15–40% of all patients. The natural history of the disease is associated with deterioration of symptoms and is not necessarily related to the radiological severity of the disease.

- Operative treatment is indicated in patients with progressive neurological deficits or lifestyle-limiting symptoms for which conservative therapy has failed after 6 months. A decompressive laminectomy of affected segments, with or without foraminotomies, continues to yield the best surgical benefit for most patients. Patients, however, may still deteriorate over time. The precise role/benefit of fusion in addition to decompression for this disease is yet to be elucidated.

CONCLUSIONS

Symptomatic lumbar stenosis can occur from acquired or congenital/developmental etiologies. While the exact pathogenesis is still unclear, it appears that mechanical compression plays a major role in a fairly large proportion of patients. This is evident in the reasonably good results from decompressive surgery. Nonoperative care has a role and should be initiated upon presentation. With failure of conservative treatment, surgical treatment can be considered. Careful preoperative planning involves correlation of the radiographically involved levels with the clinical findings. A decompressive laminectomy, with or without foraminotomies, continues to be the most reliable method for neural decompression with good surgical results documented. Unfortunately, many of these results deteriorate over time. The role of more limited resection techniques, as well as the addition of fusion or instrumentation to standard laminectomy techniques, remains to be elucidated. Meticulous surgical technique as well as scrupulous patient selection and counseling are important measures to improving operative outcomes.

This chapter contains material from the first edition, and we are grateful to the authors of that chapter for their contribution.

REFERENCES

1. Kirkaldy-Willis WH. The relationship of structural pathology to the nerve root. Spine 1984; 9: 49–52.
2. Kirkaldy-Willis WH, Wedge JH, Yong-Hing K, Reilly J. Pathology and pathogenesis of lumbar spondylosis and stenosis. Spine 1978; 3: 319–28.
3. Katz JN, Dalgas M, Stucki G, et al. Degenerative lumbar spinal stenosis. Diagnostic values of the history and physical examination. Arthritis Rheum 1995; 38: 1236–41.
4. Specchia N, Pagnotta A, Gigante A, Logroscino G, Toesca A. Characterization of cultured human ligamentum flavum cells in lumbar spine stenosis. J Orthop Res 2001; 19: 204–300.
5. Kurihara A, Tanaka Y, Tsumura N, Iwasai Y. Hyperostotic lumbar spinal stenosis. A review of 12 surgically treated cases with roentgenographic survey of ossification of the yellow ligament at the lumbar spine. Spine 1988; 13.
6. Dauser RC, Chandler WF. Symptomatic congenital spinal stenosis in a child. Neurosurgery 1982; 11.
7. Postacchini F, Massobrio M, Ferro L. Familial lumbar stenosis: case report of three siblings. J Bone Joint Surg 1985; 67-A: 321–3.
8. Sato K, Kikuchi S. Clinical analysis of two-level compression of the cauda equina and the nerve roots in lumbar spinal canal stenosis. Spine 1997; 22: 1898–903.
9. Iwamoto H, Kuwahara H, Matsuda H, Nortage A, Yamano Y. Production of chronic compression of the cauda equina in rats for use in studies of lumbar spinal canal stenosis. Spine 1995; 20: 2750–7.
10. Kauppila LI, Karhumen PJ, Lahdenranta U. Intermittent medullary claudication: postmortem spinal angiographic findings in two cases and in six controls. J Spinal Disord 1994; 7: 242–7.
11. Naylor A. Factors in the development of the spinal stenosis syndrome. J Bone Joint Surg 1979; 61-B: 306–9.
12. Tusji H, Tamaki T, Itoh T, et al. Redundant nerve roots in patients with degenerative lumbar spinal stenosis. Spine 1985; 10: 72–82.

13. Simotas AC. Nonoperative treatment for lumbar spinal stenosis. *Clin Orthop* 2001; 384: 153–61.

14. Katz JN, Lipson SJ, Larson MG, McInnes MM, Fossel AH, Liang MH. The outcome of decompressive laminectomy for degenerative lumbar stenosis. *J Bone Joint Surg Am* 1991; 73: 809–16.

15. Katz JN, Lipson SJ, Chang LC, Levine SA, Fossel AH, Liang MH. Seven to 10 year outcome of decompressive surgery for degenerative lumbar spinal stenosis. *Spine* 1996; 21: 92–8.

16. Katz JN, Lipson SJ, Lew RA, et al. Lumbar laminectomy alone or with instrumented or noninstrumented arthrodesis in degenerative lumbar spinal stenosis. Patient selection, costs, and surgical outcomes. *Spine* 1997; 22: 1123–31.

17. Mariconda M, Zanforlino G, Celestino GA, Brancalcone S, Fava R, Milano C. Factors influencing the outcome of degenerative lumbar spinal stenosis. *J Spinal Disord* 2000; 13: 131–7.

18. Mariconda M, Fava R, Gatto A, Longo C, Milano C. Unilateral laminectomy for bilateral decompression of lumbar spinal stenosis: a prospective comparative study with conservatively treated patients. *J Spinal Disord Tech* 2002; 15: 39–46.

19. Bodack MP, Monteiro M. Therapeutic exercise in the treatment of patients with lumbar spinal stenosis. *Clin Orthop* 2001; 384: 144–52.

20. Prateepavanich P, Thanapipatsiri S, Santisatisakul P, Somshevita P, Charoensak T. The effectiveness of lumbosacral corset in symptomatic degenerative lumbar spinal stenosis. *J Med Assoc Thai* 2001; 84: 572–6.

21. Ciocon JO, Galindo-Giocon D, Amaranath L, Galindo D. Caudal epidural blocks for elderly patients with lumbar canal stenosis. *J Am Geriatr Soc* 1994; 42: 593–6.

22. Radu AS, Menkes CJ. Update on lumbar spinal stenosis. Retrospective study of 62 patients and review of the literature. *Rev Rheum Engl Ed* 1998; 65: 337–45.

23. Tsai RY, Yang RS, Bray RS. Microscopic laminotomies for degenerative lumbar spinal stenosis. *J Spinal Disord* 1998; 11: 389–94.

24. Silvers HR, Lewis PJ, Asch HL. Decompressive lumbar laminectomy for spinal stenosis. *J Neurosurg* 1993; 78: 695–701.

25. Postacchini F, Cinotti G, Perugia D, Gumina S. The surgical treatment of central lumbar stenosis. Multiple laminotomy compared with total laminectomy. *J Bone Joint Surg Br* 1993; 75: 386–92.

26. McGullen GM, Bernini PM, Bernstein SH, Tosteson TD. Clinical and roentgenographic results of decompression for lumbar spinal stenosis. *J Spinal Disord* 1994; 7: 380–7.

27. Herkowitz HN, Kurz LT. Degenerative lumbar spondylolisthesis with spinal stenosis. A prospective study comparing decompression with decompression and intertransverse process arthrodesis. *J Bone Joint Surg* 1991; 73-A: 802–8.

28. Fischgrund JS, Mackay M, Herkowitz HN, Brower R, Montgomery DM, Kurz LT. Volvo award winner in clinical studies: degenerative lumbar spondylolisthesis with spinal stenosis: a prospective, randomized study comparing decompressive laminectomy and arthrodesis with and without spinal instrumentation. *Spine* 1997; 22: 2807–2801.

29. Remes V, Tervahartiala P, Poussa M, Peltonen J. Thoracic and lumbar spine in diastrophic dysplasia: a clinical and magnetic resonance imaging analysis. *Spine* 2001; 26: 187–95.

30. Fortuna A, Ferrante L, Acqui M, Santoro A, Mastronardi L. Narrowing of thoraco-lumbar spinal canal in achondroplasia. *J Neurosurg Sci* 1989; 33: 185–96.

31. Lonstein JE. Treatment of kyphosis and lumbar stenosis in achondroplasia. *Basic Life Sci* 1988; 48: 283–92.

32. Arnoldi CC, Brodsky AE, Cauchoix J, et al. Lumbar spinal stenosis and nerve root entrapment syndromes. *Clin Orthop* 1976; 115.

33. Lee CK, Rauschning W, Glenn W. Lateral lumbar spinal canal stenosis: classification, pathologic anatomy and surgical decompression. *Spine* 1988; 13: 313–20.

34. Boden SD, Davis DO, Dina TS, Patronas NJ, Wiesel SW. Abnormal magnetic resonance scans of the lumbar spine in asymptomatic subjects. A prospective investigation. *J Bone Joint Surg* 1990; 72-A: 403–8.

35. Fullenlove TM, Williams AJ. Comparative roentgen findings in symptomatic and asymptomatic backs. *Radiology* 1957; 68: 572–4.

36. Kitselberger WE, Witten RM. Abnormal myelograms in asymptomatic patients. *J Neurosurg* 1968; 28: 204–6.

37. Wiesel SW, Tsourmas N, Feffer HL, Citrin CM, Patronas N. A study of computer-assisted tomography. I. The incidence of positive CAT scans in an asymptomatic group of patients. *Spine* 1984; 9: 549–51.

38. Baba H, Maezawa Y, Furosawa N, Imura S, Tomita K. The role of calcium deposition in the ligamentum flavum causing a cauda equina syndrome and lumbar radiculopathy. *Paraplegia* 1995; 33: 219–23.

39. Leroux JL, Legeron P, Moulinier L, et al. Stenosis of the lumbar spinal canal in vertebral ankylosing hyperostosis. *Spine* 1992; 17: 1213–18.

40. Kawaguchi Y, Kanamori M, Ishihara H, et al. Clinical symptoms and surgical outcome in lumbar spinal stenosis patients with neuropathic bladder. *J Spinal Disord* 2001; 14: 404–10.

41. Smith AY, Woodside JR. Urodynamic evaluation of patients with spinal stenosis. *Urology* 1988; 32: 474–7.

42. Baba H, Furosawa N, Tanaka Y, Imura S, Tomita K. Intermittent priapism associated with lumbar spinal stenosis. *Int Orthop* 1994; 18: 150–3.

43. Baba H, Maezawa Y, Furawa N, Kawahara N, Tomita K. Lumbar spinal stenosis causing intermittent priapism. *Paraplegia* 1995; 33: 338–45.

44. Maurice-Williams RS, Marsh HT. Priapism as a feature of claudication of the cauda equina. *Surg Neurol* 1985; 23: 626–8.

45. Katz JN, Stucki G, Lipson SJ, Fossel AH, Grobler LJ, Weinstein JN. Predictors of surgical outcome in degenerative lumbar spinal stenosis. *Spine* 1999; 24: 2229–33.

46. Spivak JM. Degenerative lumbar spinal stenosis. *J Bone Joint Surg* 1998; 80: 1053–66.

47. McAfee PC, Ullrich CG, Yuan HA, Sherry RG, Lockwood RK. Computed tomography in degenerative spinal stenosis. *Clin Orthop* 1981; 161: 221–34.

48. Saint-Louis LA. Lumbar spinal stenosis assessment with computed tomography, magnetic resonance imaging, and myelography. *Clin Orthop* 2001; 284: 122–36.

49. Jonsson B, Annertz M, Sjoberg C, Stromqvist B. A prospective and consecutive study of surgically treated lumbar spinal stenosis: Part I: clinical features related to radiographic findings. *Spine* 1997; 22: 2932–7.

50. Herno A, Partanen K, Talaslahati T, et al. Long-term clinical and magnetic resonance imaging follow-up assessment of patients with lumbar spinal stenosis after laminectomy. *Spine* 1999; 25: 1533–7.

51. Johnsson KE, Rosen I, Uden A. The natural course of lumbar spinal stenosis. *Clin Orthop* 1992; 279: 82–96.

52. Atlas SJ, Deyo RA, Keller RB, et al. The Maine lumbar spine study, Part III. 1-year outcome of surgical and nonsurgical management of lumbar spinal stenosis. *Spine* 1996; 21: 1787–94.

53. Onel D, Sari H, Donmez C. Lumbar spinal stenosis: clinical/radiologic therapeutic evaluation in 145 patients: conservative treatment of surgical intervention? *Spine* 1993; 18: 291–8.

54. Lantz SA, Schultz AB. Lumbar spine orthosis wearing. *Spine* 1986; 11: 838.

55. Fritz JM, Erhard RE, Vignovic M. A nonsurgical treatment approach to patients with lumbar spinal stenosis. *Phys Ther* 1997; 77: 962–73.

56. Fukasaki M, Kobayashi I, Hara T, Sumikawa K. Symptoms of spinal stenosis do not improve after epidural steroid injection. *Clin J Pain* 1998; 14: 148–51.

57. Burton CV, Kirkaldy-Willis WH, Yong-Hing K, Heithoff KB. Causes of failure of surgery on the lumbar spine. *Clin Orthop* 1981; 157: 191–9.

58. Verbiest H. Results of surgical treatment of idiopathic developmental stenosis of the lumbar vertebral canal. *J Bone Joint Surg* 1977; 59-B: 181–8.

59. Hansraj KK, Cammisa FP, O'Leary PF, *et al*. Decompressive surgery for typical lumbar spinal stenosis. *Clin Orthop* 2001; 384: 10–17.

60. Iguchi T, Kurihara A, Nakayama J, Sato K, Kurosaka M, Yamasaki K. Minimum 10-year outcome of decompressive laminectomy for degenerative lumbar spinal stenosis. *Spine* 2000; 25: 1754–9.

61. Lee CK. Accelerated degeneration of the segment adjacent to a lumbar fusion. *Spine* 1988; 13: 375–7.

62. Frazier DD, Lipson SJ, Fossel AH, Katz JN. Associations between spinal deformity and outcomes after decompression for spinal stenosis. *Spine* 1997; 22: 2025–9.

63. Johnsson KE, Willner S, Johnsson K. Postoperative instability after decompression for lumbar spinal stenosis. *Spine* 1986; 11: 107–10.

64. Grobler LJ, Robertson PA, Novotny JE, Ahern JW. Decompression for degenerative spondylolisthesis and spinal stenosis at L4–5. The effects of facet joint morphology. *Spine* 1993; 18: 1475–83.

65. White AA, Panjabi MM. *Clinical Biomechanics of the Spine*. Philadelphia: Lippincott-Raven; 1990

66. Abumi K, Panjabi MM, Kramer KM, Duranceau J, Oxland T, Crisco JJ. Biomechanical evaluation of lumbar spinal stability after graded facetectomies. *Spine* 1990; 15: 1142–7.

67. Benz RJ, Ibrahim ZG, Afshar P, Garfin SR. Predicting complications in elderly patients undergoing lumbar decompression. *Clin Orthop* 2001; 384: 116–121.

68. Sanderson PL, Wood PL. Surgery for lumbar spinal stenosis in old people. *J Bone Joint Surg Br* 1993; 75: 393–7.

69. Robertson PA, Grobler LJ, Novotny JE, Katz JN. Postoperative spondylolisthesis at L4–5. The role of facet joint morphology. *Spine* 1993; 18: 1483–90.

70. Fox MW, Onofrio BM, Hanssen AD. Clinical outcomes and radiological instablity following decompressive lumbar laminectomy for degenerative spinal stenosis: a comparison of patients undergoing concomitant arthrodesis versus decompression alone. *J Neurosurg* 1996; 85: 793–802.

71. McCulloch JA. Microdecompression and uninstrumented single-level fusion for spinal canal stenosis with degenerative spondylolisthesis. *Spine* 1998; 23: 2243–52.

72. O'Leary PF, McCance SE. Distraction laminoplasty for decompression of lumbar spinal stenosis. *Clin Orthop* 2001; 384: 26–34.

73. Sanderson PL, Getty CJ. Long-term results of partial undercutting facetectomy for lumbar lateral recess stenosis. *Spine* 1996; 21: 1352–6.

74. Kleeman TJ, Hiscoe AC, Berg EE. Patient outcomes after minimally destabilizing lumbar stenosis decompression: the "Port-Hole" technique. *Spine* 2000; 25: 865–70.

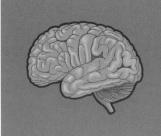

TRIGEMINAL NEURALGIA

51

Gerald A Grant and John D Loeser

Trigeminal neuralgia, also known as *tic douloureux*, is an excruciatingly painful condition that is most common in people aged 50–70 years. It is a stereotyped, repetitive, unilateral, electric-shock-like facial pain triggered by non-noxious stimulation with clear pain-free intervals.[1–5] The incidence of trigeminal neuralgia is 4–5 per 100 000 population (median age 67 years).[6] It involves the right side of the face more often than the left side, at a ratio of about 3:2. Women are more often affected than men in a ratio that has varied from 2:1 to 4:3 in reported series.[7]

ETIOLOGY AND PATHOGENESIS

Tic douloureux can be caused by any of a number of conditions affecting the ipsilateral trigeminal system.[10] In the vast majority, the etiology seems to be compression of the trigeminal nerve at its exit from the pons by an adjacent artery or vein that has elongated and kinked to become wedged against the nerve. In about 1–2% of cases, the pain results from a benign tumor in the cerebellopontine angle, such as a meningioma, epidermoid tumor, or acoustic neuroma, or even an arteriovenous malformation.[8] Other authors have indicated that 1–8% of patients with trigeminal neuralgia have multiple sclerosis.[9–13] Therefore, infrequently, trigeminal neuralgia may be the presenting symptom of multiple sclerosis.[14] A variety of other rare etiologic associations have been reported, but all of these together probably do not account for more than a few percent of cases. In a significant number of patients, the etiology of the tic douloureux is not apparent.

The pathogenesis of trigeminal neuralgia remains uncertain, as are the mechanisms by which treatments are effective. For example, some authors have postulated that nerve root demyelination resulting from neural compression by a blood vessel or tumor or resulting from multiple sclerosis is an important feature, perhaps permitting ephaptic transmission or ectopic impulse generation between adjacent denuded axons. Both peripheral and central mechanisms are most likely required for the production of tic douloureux. Calvin and colleagues presented a comprehensive theory which utilizes two known physiological mechanisms: the trigeminal dorsal root reflex and repetitive firing of extra action potentials from a focal region of altered axonal size or myelination.[15] Altered central connectivity and neuronal hyperactivity caused by deafferentation (centralist concept) as well as changes in the trigeminal myelin and axons can lead to altered peripheral sensitivity to chemical and mechanical stimuli (peripheralist concept).[15,16] However, as attractive as such ideas are, no theory has yet been postulated that explains all aspects of tic douloureux, such as the pain-free periods, which may last for months or years

early in the course of the condition, the triggering of tic pain by non-noxious stimuli, the separation of the trigger areas from the painful region, and the response to anticonvulsants. Elimination of root compression by adjacent vessels does not take into account the effectiveness of numerous other surgical procedures, most of which injure the root or ganglion, but decompression of the root may relieve pain by facilitating remyelination.

CLINICAL FEATURES

Tic douloureux is diagnosed on the basis of the patient's history (Table 51.1). The International Headache Society defined trigeminal neuralgia as a "sudden, usually unilateral, severe, brief, stabbing, and recurrent pain in the distribution of one or more branches of the fifth cranial nerve."[17,18] The three divisions of the trigeminal nerve are the ophthalmic, maxillary, and mandibular. For the accurate diagnosis of facial pain, a detailed knowledge of the anatomy of the fifth cranial nerve is essential. By definition, the pain of tic douloureux is confined to the distribution of one trigeminal nerve (Figure 51.1) and more commonly affects the lower part of the face than the upper.[16] The maxillary division of the fifth cranial nerve (V2) is the site of pain alone or in combination with other divisions, most commonly the mandibular division (V3) in 45% of cases. The ophthalmic division (V1) is

Table 51.1 International Headache Society criteria for trigeminal neuralgia

Paroxysmal attacks of frontal pain which last a few seconds to less than 2 minutes
Pain has at least four of the following characteristics: distribution along one or more divisions of the trigeminal nerve; sudden, intense, sharp, superficial, stabbing or burning in quality; pain intensity severe; precipitation from trigger areas or by certain daily activities such as eating, talking, washing the face or cleaning the teeth; between paroxysms the patient is entirely asymptomatic.
No neurological deficit
Attacks are stereotyped in the individual patient
Exclusion of other causes of facial pain by history, physical examination, and special investigation when necessary.

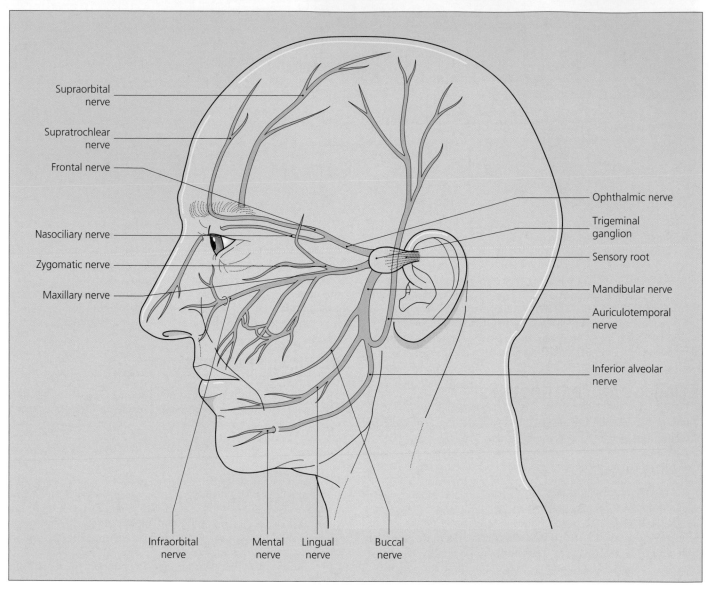

Supraorbital nerve

Supratrochlear nerve

Frontal nerve

Nasociliary nerve

Zygomatic nerve

Maxillary nerve

Ophthalmic nerve

Trigeminal ganglion

Sensory root

Mandibular nerve

Auriculotemporal nerve

Inferior alveolar nerve

Infraorbital nerve

Mental nerve

Lingual nerve

Buccal nerve

Figure 51.1 The peripheral and central aspects of the trigeminal nerve and its branches.

least affected in trigeminal neuralgia (Figure 51.2). A small number of patients have a pain syndrome in the territory of the nervus intermedius, glossopharyngeal, or vagus nerves. The pain of untreated tic douloureux occurs unpredictably and is sudden in onset, severe in degree, and short in duration. Often the patient can experience many paroxysms of pain within a single hour, and such bouts may go on for days, with some fluctuation in frequency from hour to hour and day to day. Early in the course of the syndrome, pain-free periods lasting months are common, but as time goes on these natural remissions tend to become less frequent and less prolonged. Although tic pain is ordinarily spontaneous in onset, it can frequently be triggered by a non-noxious stimulus, such as touching the skin on that side of the face, chewing, swallowing, or talking. Some patients are sensitive in certain areas of the face, called trigger zones, which when touched cause an attack of pain. Even a gentle breeze can trigger pain in some patients. The pain has been described as lancinating, lightning-like, or electrical in quality, and has been likened to the pain experienced when a dentist drills into the pulp of a tooth.[7]

The patient may wince in response to the pain, hence the name tic douloureux. A history of bilateral tic pain can be elicited in 3% of patients, although no patient has bilateral tic pain during one episode.[16]

Often the patient who develops tic douloureux sees the dentist first, because lancinating lower facial pain seems to be arising from a certain tooth or teeth. Dentists are often fixated on peripheral lesions as the etiology for pain. A diseased tooth in the upper jaw can cause headache on the same side, which may radiate into the orbit or face. A diseased tooth in the lower jaw may cause considerable pain in the distribution of the mandibular division of the nerve, including pain deep in the ear. In addition, dental pain is much more common than tic douloureux. Teeth may be extracted or other dental procedures performed without providing any relief of the pain of tic douloureux. The patient may also consult more than one physician before the correct diagnosis is made. In the majority of patients, the trigeminal neuralgia is idiopathic in that there is no identifiable cause.[8] However, the presence of sensory loss mandates a thorough search for structural

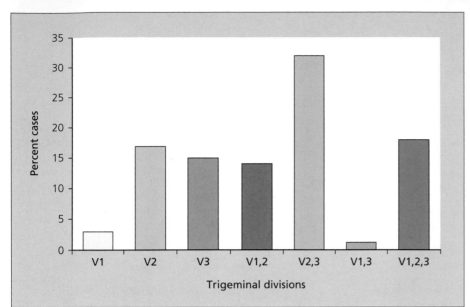

Figure 51.2 Distribution of pain among divisions of the trigeminal nerve in patients with tic douloureux (Figure 2, Loeser[16]).

pathology. Patients with idiopathic trigeminal neuralgia can develop more atypical features with time in the absence of efficacious therapy. In all likelihood, this development coincides with ongoing neuropathic injury. Pain that is continuous, lacks a shock-like quality, or is associated with objective evidence of cranial nerve dysfunction should raise the suspicion of diseases other than trigeminal neuralgia. However, the most likely cause of this type of pain is a prior ablative procedure that damages the trigeminal nerve. Atypical facial pain is described as deep, burning and continual. There is no jabbing onset as occurs in tic douloureux. The pain can radiate behind the ear, down onto the neck, or across to the opposite maxillary area. These patients, in contrast, often clutch their face, unlike the patient with tic douloureux who shields her face but is very careful not to actually touch it (Table 51.2). Myofascial pains involving the muscles of mastication and temporomandibular joint pain occur predominantly in the lateral face. They are also described as aching, burning, or cramping pains, and are often associated with tenderness to palpation of involved muscles.[16]

Deviations from the typical picture of tic douloureux can occur, although the more unusual features the patient manifests, the less likely is a favorable response to either medical or surgical therapies. Furthermore, surgical procedures that damage the trigeminal nerve can produce changes in the findings and in the patient's symptoms. Nerve damage over time can lead to a burning component of the pain, although these iatrogenically acquired changes in the pain syndrome do not alter the original diagnosis. It is therefore essential to ascertain what the symptoms were prior to any intervention.

DIAGNOSIS

The diagnosis of tic douloureux is based on the history; no diagnostic studies available will confirm its presence. The neurological examination is ordinarily normal except for mild sensory changes in a minority of patients in the region of their pain, with the exception that those few patients with multiple sclerosis or a large structural lesion such as a tumor in the cerebellopontine angle usually have altered trigeminal sensation and other evidence that heralds the underlying disorder. Likewise, diagnostic radiologic studies such as computed tomography or magnetic resonance imaging are normal in the usual patient with tic douloureux, but they are performed to identify the exceptional patient with a recognizable etiologic condition such as those just mentioned.[7] Patients with a Chiari malformation may also develop trigeminal neuralgia, thought to be the result of venous or arterial compression of the cranial nerves along with the tonsillar ectopia. Advances in magnetic resonance angiography have improved the sensitivity and specificity of diagnosing neurovascular compression of the nerve by evaluating the anatomical relationships of the arterial and venous structures with the trigeminal nerve at the root entry zone in the cerebellopontine angle.[16] However, so far these studies have been more used as a preoperative adjunct than for diagnostic purposes.[19]

TREATMENT

Despite the relative lack of understanding of pathophysiological mechanisms of trigeminal neuralgia, very effective medical and surgical treatments have been developed. Although generally effective treatments are available for tic douloureux, none are successful in all cases. Few or no randomized trials exist comparing medical, surgical, and interventional techniques and therefore treatment decisions for these patients with neuropathic pain can be challenging and are largely empiric. Furthermore, the individual patient frequently requires more than one form of treatment during the course of the disease. The psychosocial and behavioral response patterns of patients with chronic facial pain are similar to those of other patients with chronic pain.

In those few patients with an abnormality along the path of the trigeminal nerve that can be detected radiologically, such as a neoplasm in the cerebellopontine angle, the treatment is directed against the lesion that has been demonstrated. This approach ordinarily will also relieve the tic douloureux. However, the overwhelming majority of patients do not fall into this category and must be treated in other ways.

Table 51.2 Differential diagnosis of facial pain

Condition	Trigeminal neuralgia	Atypical facial pain	Migrainous facial pain	Acute herpes zoster
Age/Sex	Over 50 years 60% F	30–50 years 75% F	Typically, 40–50 age range; M = F	> 70 years F > M
Site	V2 or V3 most common alone or in combination but limited to distribution of trigeminal nerve (intraoral or extraoral), unilateral	Deep non-muscular areas of face, maxillary or whole face, unilateral or bilateral, does not follow nerve distribution	Anywhere in face. Deep eye pain, sinus pain or toothache	Herpetic lesions in the distribution of trigeminal nerve; V1 most common, most severe in eyebrow; facial or deep ear pain often precedes vesicular eruption
Character	Sudden severe, brief lancinating, electric shock-like, no allodynia	Throbbing, deep, diffuse, nagging, aching, burning, cramping; may have allodynia	Throbbing or pulsatile, lacrimation or conjunctival injection (cluster headache), no allodynia	Burning, tingling in quality; itching, dysesthesia, may have allodynia
Severity	Severe	Moderate to severe	Moderate	Severity varies
Duration	Seconds to minutes	Seconds to minutes or continuous	15 minutes to several hours	Continuous. Pain may precede vesicular eruption
Periodicity	Pain-free between attacks, long periods of no pain	Continuous background pain or dysesthesia; less likely to have complete pain remission, interferes with sleep	Often nocturnal or early morning	Continuous pain until vesicles heal, may then develop post-herpetic neuralgia
Provoking factors	Non-noxious stimulation of discrete trigger zones in face or in buccal mucosa, hot/cold fluids in mouth or chewing	Stress, fatigue	Alcohol, hormone replacement therapy, seasonal, cold, warm	Skin stimulation by clothing or touch

Medication

The initial treatment of patients with trigeminal neuralgia is pharmacologic. Drugs with anticonvulsive properties rather than analgesic ones are most effective. There are a limited number of controlled trials that have studied the pharmacologic treatment for trigeminal neuralgia. The anticonvulsants carbamazepine, phenytoin, and gabapentin have been found to reduce or control the pain of tic douloureux. Likewise, oxcarbazepine, lamotrigine, and baclofen are said to have beneficial effects in the treatment of tic douloureux.

Carbamazepine is considered the first-line treatment for patients with trigeminal neuralgia and is ordinarily begun at a dosage of 200 mg/day, being increased as tolerated to 200 mg three or four times a day, or more. Over 70% of patients report symptomatic improvement, although it is not an analgesic and must be taken regularly to maintain its efficacy. The goal is to reach the smallest dose that provides adequate pain relief. At high doses, the patient may experience the side effects of lethargy, sluggish thinking, and imbalance.[7] Doses higher than 1800 mg have not been more effective.[20] Carbamazepine may also interfere with the production of blood elements and may alter hepatic function. Therefore, a patient being treated with carbamazepine should have periodic complete blood counts and hepatic function studies. Oxcarbazepine is another anticonvulsant that has become quite attractive recently since it is dosed less frequently and has fewer side effects than carbamazepine but has the same efficacy.

Phenytoin is ordinarily begun at a dosage of 100 mg three times a day. Intravenous phenytoin has been used in some patients for acute exacerbations with frequent, easily triggered, high-intensity pain attacks. Approximately 25% of patients obtain satisfactory pain relief although, unlike epilepsy, relief of tic douloureux pain has been shown to correlate with phenytoin blood levels. Gabapentin has also shown promise in relieving many forms of neuropathic pain.[21]

Any of these three medicines is used alone at first, and is increased as needed to control the facial pain. With time, a patient may need progressively larger dosages to provide the same degree of relief. The development of toxicity may necessitate a reduction in the dosage, and the occurrence of some other significant side effect may require cessation of the medication altogether and lead patients to consider other forms of treatment. In this case, a second drug may be added to or substituted for the first. At times, it may be necessary to use all three. Approximately two-thirds of patients with tic douloureux are adequately managed on anti-epileptic drugs, but one-third of these cannot tolerate the side effects of these medications. Therefore, about one-half of the patients with tic douloureux are candidates for surgery.

Surgical treatment

Medical management should always precede a surgical procedure and no surgical procedure is warranted unless pharmacologic therapy has failed either because of inadequate pain relief or unacceptable side-effects. The three primary surgical treatments are gangliolysis, stereotactic radiosurgery, and suboccipital craniectomy with microvascular decompression (Table 51.3).

Table 51.3 Surgical management of trigeminal neuralgia

Radiofrequency gangliolysis
Balloon gangliolysis
Glycerol gangliolysis
Gamma-knife radiosurgery
Microvascular decompression
Trigeminal rhizotomy
Trigeminal tractotomy

Gasserian gangliolysis

Trigeminal gangliolysis avoids the risks of a craniotomy and its objective is to destroy selectively the A-δ and C fibers (nociceptive) while preserving the A-α and β fibers (touch). It can be repeated easily if the pain recurs, and is associated with minimal morbidity. In the gangliolysis procedure, the gasserian ganglion and adjacent sensory root of the trigeminal nerve are injured, with the expectation that a more permanent effect can be achieved than following a neurectomy because neural regeneration is less likely to occur in these areas than in the peripheral trigeminal branches. In the past, an anterior trigeminal rhizotomy was performed by exposing and dividing or otherwise injuring part or all of the main trigeminal sensory root adjacent to the gasserian ganglion.[4,5] The radiofrequency gangliolysis procedure is performed by inserting a needle through the cheek into the third division of the trigeminal nerve at the foramen ovale, and then advancing the needle under fluoroscopic guidance into the gasserian ganglion and sensory root (Figure 51.3). [3,20,22–24] The entry point is 2.5 cm lateral to the corner of the mouth in the occlusal plane and the needle is aimed toward the intersection of the coronal plane halfway between the external auditory meatus and the lateral canthus and the sagittal plane centered at the pupil. The needle is advanced through the foramen ovale at the petrosphenoid junction and positioned at the level appropriate for the affected trigeminal branch. The third, second, and first divisions can then be stimulated in sequence by slowly advancing the needle tip. Generally, the mandibular division of the root is encountered 1 cm after penetration of the foramen ovale, V2 is located at 2 cm, and V1 is at 3 cm and at the level of the clivus. Once the needle is ideally situated, the patient is awakened and the relevant nerve root is stimulated to confirm stimulus-provoked cutaneous paresthesia in the painful trigeminal division. Contractions of the masseter and pterygoid muscles can occur at a low stimulation threshold with a medial trajectory. The patient is then reanesthetized and the neural destruction is produced by using a radiofrequency current to create a thermal lesion. Gangliolysis can also be performed under general anesthesia using a Fogarty catheter balloon to damage the ganglion mechanically, or by injecting glycerol into the cistern of the trigeminal ganglion. The goal is to produce the least neurological deficit that will control the patient's pain.

Gangliolysis by any method produces pain relief for a longer period than by the injection or avulsion of a peripheral branch. Radiofrequency gangliolysis offers an 80% chance of 1-year pain relief and a 50% chance of 5-year success.[16,25] Approximately 5–10% will not obtain relief initially or will have an early

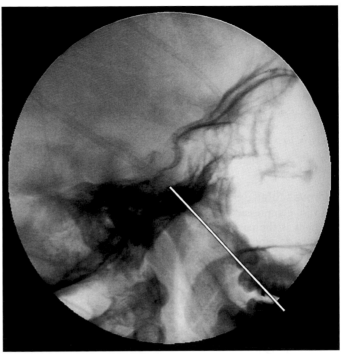

Figure 51.3 Percutaneous trigeminal/gasserian rhizolysis. Lateral fluoroscopic skull image shows the needle is inserted through the cheek into the third division of the trigeminal nerve at the foramen ovale and is advanced into the gasserian ganglion and sensory root. The fibers of V3, then V2, and finally V1 are encountered in sequence as the needle is advanced toward the clivus.

recurrence of pain; during the 5 years after the procedure, about 25% will experience recurrence.[26,27] The complication rate of radiofrequency gangliolysis is 0.5–1% and can include meningitis, damage to other cranial nerves, corneal anesthesia, masseter weakness, and anesthesia dolorosa (total sensory loss). Anesthesia dolorosa is the most dreaded complication of ablative lesions of the trigeminal nerve and refers to pain in an anesthetic region. Unfortunately, no pharmacologic or ablative surgical treatment is effective for this complication.[20]

Balloon compression is performed under general anesthesia. Using fluoroscopic control, a large 14-gauge guide needle is inserted until it just penetrates the foramen ovale and the balloon is slowly inflated. Balloon compression is technically easier than radiofrequency thermocoagulation, which produces similar results and does not require patient participation; however, bradycardia should be anticipated during the procedure. Some authors believe that the risk of corneal hypoesthesia and anesthesia dolorosa is lower with balloon compression and therefore is the procedure of choice in patients with ophthalmic division involvement or in patients who are not good awake surgical candidates for radiofrequency gangliolysis.

Glycerol gangliolysis is less often performed today than the radiofrequency or balloon gangliolysis. Because the location of the glycerol cannot be precisely targeted after injection, the results are somewhat unpredictable; however, overall there is a lower incidence of sensory loss and anesthesia dolorosa than with the radiofrequency lesion. With glycerol gasserian rhizolysis, the long-term results are not quite as good: there is a 5–15% incidence of early failure and about a 20–30% incidence of later failure.[26,27]

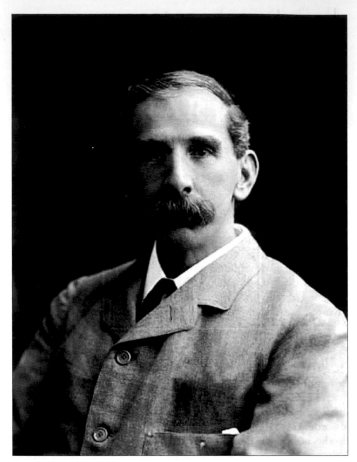

Figure 52.2 Sir Victor Horsley (courtesy of the National Library of Medicine).

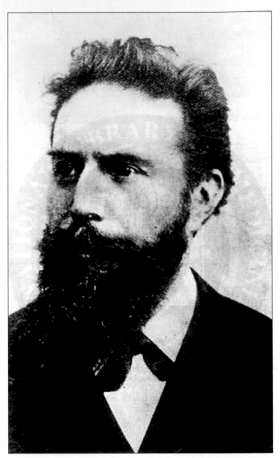

Figure 52.3 Wilhem-Conrad Roentgen (courtesy of the National Library of Medicine).

to develop the first true human stereotactic system in 1947[7] (Figure 52.4). The technique allowed the reference of any point to deep intracranial landmarks, which, in turn, were less anatomically variable than external osseous structures. In 1952 Spiegel and Wycis also published the first human stereotactic atlas – the map necessary for intracranial navigation.[8] With a navigational system and a guiding map, human stereotactic neurosurgery was born. The first stereotactic operation by Spiegel and Wycis was a thalamotomy for depression.[7] Others soon followed with their own modifications. Lars Leksell, working in Sweden, published a description of his arc quadrant apparatus in 1949.[9] In 1950 Tailarach developed a device with a fixed grid system in Paris.[10] The following year Riechert and Wolff of Germany described a device with a phantom base which allowed the mechanical determination of the frame settings.[11] Narabayashi, working independently in post-war Japan, developed his own system in 1951.[12] Over the next decade dozens of systems were designed and custom built (Figure 52.5). However, as a result of various factors, including development time and expense, only 10–20 commercially available systems remain commonly employed today (Figure 52.6). Each of these systems has its own benefits and limitations but, for the most part, they accomplished what their creators envisioned: reaching their intracranial targets with great precision and minimal morbidity.

Human stereotactic procedures gained momentum when it was demonstrated that stereotactic pallidotomy guided by pneumoencephalography or positive-contrast ventriculography was a safer and more effective treatment for the motor manifestations of Parkinson's disease than other more invasive methods. Other less common stereotactic applications, however, preceded the treatment of movement disorders. These included the surgical treatment of pain and psychiatric disorders. In fact, Spiegel and Wycis first used their Cartesian-based stereotactic frame to create a deep-brain lesion by instilling alcohol into the medial globus pallidus in a patient with Huntington's chorea.[7,13] Between 1960 and 1970, more than 40 000 stereotactic procedures were performed worldwide.[14] With the advent of L-Dopa in 1968, however, the number of stereotactic procedures dropped dramatically and, with rare exception, stereotactic surgery became a forlorn talent.[15] The few remaining stereotactic operations were performed for deep-seated biopsies, volumetric tumor resections and stereotactic radiosurgery.

While initially extremely effective in the majority of patients, neurologists began to note the long-term effects of dopamine and its agonists by the mid-1980s. They began to reconsider surgery as a complement to medical therapy for intractable cases. The reincarnation of both functional and morphological stereotactic neurosurgery that has occurred over the past 15 years can be attributed to several factors. With respect to functional neurosurgery, Lauri Laitinen's rediscovery of Leksell's pallidotomy published in 1992 demonstrated encouraging surgical results.[16] Refinements of physiological localization techniques, as well as improvements in implantable hardware for stimulation, have greatly improved the safety profile of functional neurosurgery.

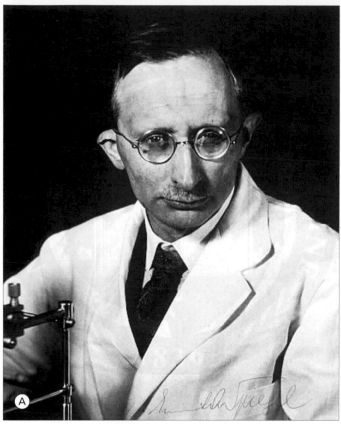 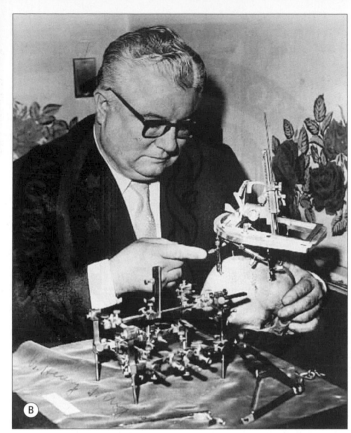

Figure 52.4 (A) Ernst Spiegel (courtesy of the National Library of Medicine). **(B)** Henry Wycis with early stereotactic instruments (courtesy of the National Library of Medicine).

Furthermore, the potential advantages of chronic electrical stimulation, including its adjustability and reversibility, have become more attractive. Neuroimaging, in the form of computed tomography (CT) and magnetic resonance imaging (MRI), has continually and dramatically improved the neurosurgeon's ability to target directly the structure of interest. In addition, the introduction of three-dimensional volumetric anatomic and functional imaging into the stereotactic database has further increased the safety and utility of stereotactic neurosurgery. Radiosurgery began to be applied for a variety of common neurosurgical disorders, with encouraging results and patient enthusiasm over its minimal invasiveness. The resultant renaissance, in turn, has fueled other areas of stereotactic neurosurgery, including image-guided techniques and spinal stereotaxy. The continual refinement and user-friendliness of these methodologies have broadened the scope and acceptance of the stereotactic technique. While the interfaces of modern frame-based and frameless navigational systems are becoming ever more intuitive and transparent, an understanding of the fundamentals of stereotaxy is imperative in minimizing possible errors, as well as in providing an impetus for further progress.

BASIC PRINCIPLES

As briefly described in the previous section, the historical foundation of the stereotactic approach rests on the stereotactic frame. There are several purposes of a stereotactic frame. First, a frame establishes a coordinate system in relation to the frame. This provides a means of co-registering the physical coordinate space with atlases and various imaging spaces. Second, it provides a means of introducing surgical instruments within that coordinate system. For those frames that are rigidly affixed to the skull, it additionally ensures the stability of the coordinate system in relation to such fixed structures as the patient's skull.

Prior to the fusion of ventriculography with stereotaxy by Spiegel and Wycis, a frame placed on a patient's head provided a reference with respect to extracranial landmarks, similar to the animal apparatus of Horsely and Clark. Unfortunately, these landmarks were too crude and variable for human use. By employing intracranial landmarks, such as the foramen of Monro and pineal gland, any intracranial point could be targeted with respect to these intracranial markers. To improve subcortical localization further, Talairach in Paris began using the anterior and posterior commissures, which are the most common intracranial landmarks in modern use. Prior to the advent of CT and MRI, direct visualization of subcortical structures was not possible. Targeting of such structures had to rely on indirect atlas-based measurements from known intracranial landmarks, such as the anterior and posterior commissures. Dozens of human atlases have since been constructed, some of which will be discussed in a subsequent section. For functional neurosurgical procedures, further refinement of targeting variability inherent even when using intracranial references, such as the anterior and posterior commissures, can be achieved with electrophysiological mapping.

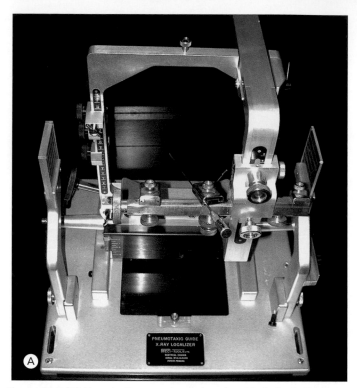
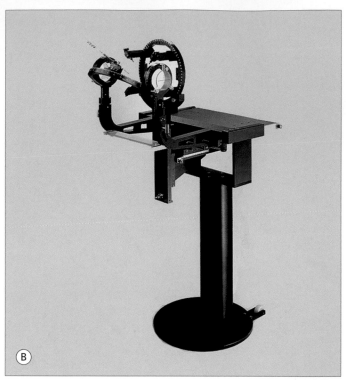

Figure 52.5 (A) Stereotactic apparatus designed and built for Dr Eric Peterson at the University of Ottawa, Canada (courtesy of Dr Erico Cardoso). **(B)** Stereotactic apparatus designed and built for Dr Patrick J. Kelly at the Mayo Clinic (courtesy of Compass International).

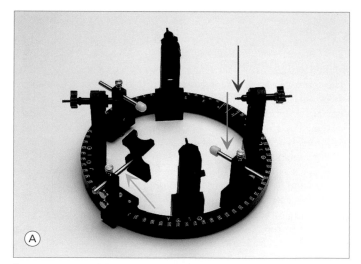
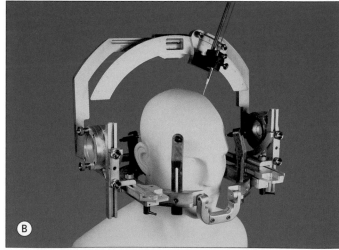

Figure 52.6 Two of the more commonly-employed modern stereotactic frames. **(A)** Compass stereotactic headframe with four skull pins (red arrow), ear stabilization bars (green arrow) and nasal support (light blue arrow) (courtesy of Compass International, Rochester, MN). **(B)** Radionics stereotactic headframe with stereotactically guided probe attached to the arc-quadrant assembly (courtesy of Radionics, Burlington, MA).

COORDINATE SYSTEMS

The goal of stereotactic surgery is to target a point or volume in space precisely via a predefined minimally invasive trajectory. The target location is not absolute; it is always situated in reference to some other intra- or extracranial site(s). For example, the center of a right frontal tumor may be 2 cm from midline, 3 cm posterior to the inner table of the skull, and 1 cm dorsal to the base of the anterior fossa. Similarly, that same tumor may be some three-dimensional distance from fiducial markers present on the skin surface or on an externally applied headframe. Thus, all points within a given volume can be related to other sites within that same volume providing that there is a constant frame of reference.

Establishment of a frame of reference requires a minimum of one point per dimension. Operative space, therefore, requires a minimum of three noncolinear points to establish a three-dimensional reference system. The majority of commercially available stereotactic systems require a minimum of an additional fourth point to estimate the error of image co-registration. An infinite variety of reference systems can be devised. The most intuitive system provides three planes traversing each other at right angles, with the point of intersection being defined as the origin. A point of interest can then be defined as being a certain distance along each of these planes, commonly referred to as x, y and z (Figure 52.7). As alluded to in the Introduction, this rectangular system is also referred to as the Cartesian co-ordinate system. By convention, the x-dimension typically denotes right–left, the y-dimension denotes anterior–posterior, and the z-dimension denotes superior–inferior. All Cartesian-based coordinate systems must be in one of two arrangements: left-handed or right-handed (Figure 52.8). Which arrangement is used is irrelevant as long as it is recognized and is consistent.

In addition to Descartes' method, a point within a plane may be described as being a certain distance and angle from a predetermined origin, commonly annotated as r (radius) and θ (theta). Extending this polar plane into three dimensions, either a cylindrical or a spherical system can be established (Figure 52.9). In a cylindrical coordinate system the third dimension is delineated by specifying a distance along an additional axis (z) perpendicular to the original polar plane. In a spherical system, an additional angle perpendicular to the original polar plane is defined, allowing a point to be characterized by a distance and two angles from the origin (e.g. r, θ, and φ). Conversion from one coordinate system to another, a process called transformation, is straightforward because the systems are mathematically equivalent. This process permits the integration of patient-specific imaging coordinate systems and atlases, with the physical operating space defined by the stereotactic coordinate system. An iterative process can transform not just points in space, but entire volumes. This becomes extremely useful in the surgical or radiosurgical treatment of tumors, vascular malformations, and other conditions where the target is best defined as a volume.

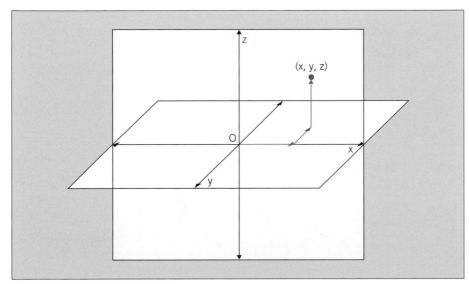

Figure 52.7 A standard rectangular Cartesian coordinate system. The location of a point (red) within the coordinate system can be denoted as the distance along each of three dimensions (x, y and z) from the origin of the system (O).

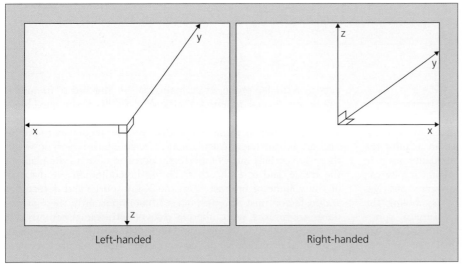

Figure 52.8 Left-handed and right-handed Cartesian coordinate systems. If one's thumb points in the x-direction, and the index finger points in the y-direction, then the z-direction can be determined by the middle digit of the corresponding hand, e.g. the right hand for a right-handed coordinate system.

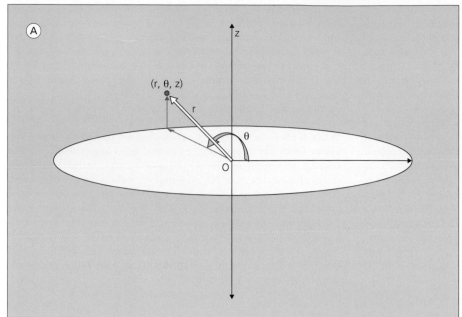

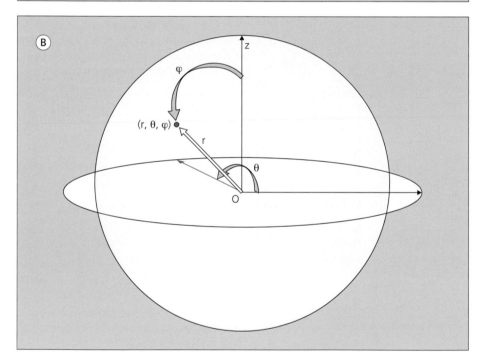

Figure 52.9 (A) Cylindrical coordinate system. The location of a point (red) within the coordinate system can be denoted as the distance from the origin of the system (O) denoted by *r*, the distance from the plane of the origin (*z*), and the angle from the origin (θ) expressed in radians or degrees. **(B)** Spherical coordinate system. The location of a point (red) within the coordinate system can be denoted as the distance from the origin of the system (O) denoted by *r*, and the angles from the origin in two planes (θ, φ) expressed in radians or degrees.

STEREOTACTIC IMAGING

Various anatomical and functional neuroimaging modalities are currently available. Each modality is based upon an inherent coordinate system particular to the device used to acquire the images. The oldest, yet least direct, imaging modality used in stereotactic procedures is ordinary radiography. Radiography can take many forms, including pneumoencephalography, positive-contrast ventriculography and angiography. By assembling the frame from radiopaque materials, the location of surgical points of interest, such as the anterior and posterior commissures, can be calculated in stereotactic space. Once an operative target is determined, a radiation beam, or instrument such as a biopsy needle, lesioning probe, or catheter, can be directed to its target. There are several inherent limitations of this technique. First, because each radiograph compresses three-dimensional space into a two-dimensional plane, more than one projection is required. Second, for the target calculations to be straightforward, however, these projections must be perfectly perpendicular to the plane of the frame, and to each other. Third, depending on the distance of the volume of interest from the X-ray source and detector, a scaling factor must be determined. Most importantly, these procedures are invasive with inherent risks of intracranial hemorrhage, headache, infection, nausea and vomiting. Prior to the widespread availability of affordable digital computers, these calculations were intricate, time-consuming and prone to human error.

The development of CT scanning in the early 1970s by Godfrey Hounsfield and Allan Cormack propelled the field of stereotactic neurosurgery to, quite literally, a new dimension.[17] Rather than inferring the location of the anterior and posterior commissures based on ventricular anatomy, it now became possible to visualize these structures directly. The stereotactic targeting accuracy of CT and MRI has proven to be comparable to ventriculography.[18–22] There was little need for invasive ventriculography or pneumoencephalography (with their associated risks and possible distortions due to cerebrospinal fluid loss). Furthermore, given that a CT scanner inherently consists of a computer, three-dimensional distances between visible structures could be easily calculated. The location of a given intracranial structure can, therefore, be defined with respect to the stereotactic frame, allowing for identification of multiple targets.

With the advent of MRI, the stereotactic era was catapulted to a new summit. The first MRI scanner was made commercially available by the Fonar Corporation (Melville, NY) in 1980. The additional advantages of using MRI as opposed to CT scans or ventriculography in stereotactic surgery include the increased tissue contrast of the lesion or target and therefore the ability to visualize subcortical targets directly, as well as the ability to obtain directly nonreformatted multiplanar images. One disadvantage of MRI stereotaxis, however, is the potential for anatomic inaccuracy as a result of ferromagnetically induced inhomogeneities of the magnetic field. With the nonferromagnetic construction materials used in many of the newer frames, as well as the lack of any ferromagnetic material during frameless procedures, the distortions induced by modern MRI scanners can be minimized.[23,24] Fortunately, distortions are inherently minimal at the center of the frame where the majority of functional neurosurgical targets are located. However, greater attention must be paid when targeting a lesion at the periphery of the frame.[25,26]

While anatomic imaging endows the physician with the ability to visualize the structure of the human brain directly, functional neuroimaging allows for the visualization of actual brain function. Of the more commonly employed functional imaging techniques, electroencephalography (EEG) and magnetoencephalography (MEG) directly measure neuronal electrical activity with a high temporal resolution. Imaging techniques such as positron emission tomography (PET), single-photon emission computed tomography (SPECT), functional MRI, and optical imaging measure regional blood flow changes and thus deduce neuronal activity.[27–31] The results of this information can be employed to determine the optimal surgical route, or even whether surgery should be undertaken in the first place. Ideally, this information can be integrated into the stereotactic database resulting in a fused "functional–anatomic" image-guided surgical procedure, as is briefly described in the following section.

IMAGE CO-REGISTRATION

The anatomic imaging space must be correlated to the physical operating space to maximize the utility of the imaging data. In simpler terms, the preoperative images must be aligned to the patient's head during surgery so that the surgeon has a better idea of what should be treated and what should best be left alone. In addition to the anatomic imaging, functional imaging modalities, such as PET, functional MRI, or MEG, can also be co-registered and incorporated into the stereotactic imaging database.[32–36] This allows for simultaneous visualization of the pathological and functionally eloquent brain tissue, thereby minimizing risks while maximizing benefit (Figure 52.10).

These image co-registration procedures can be accomplished in one of several ways, including point-based approaches, surface methods and interactive techniques.[37–41]

Frame-based systems

To co-register a set of anatomic images to the stereotactic frame, several orthogonally oriented reference plates are placed at the periphery of the frame base. Each reference plate contains fiducial rods, usually in a "letter-N" arrangement (Figure 52.11). When an image is obtained through any plane, the cylindrical rods appear to be circles or ovals in a "picket-fence" distribution (Figure 52.12). Reference plate arrays for various imaging modalities are commercially available for many stereotactic systems (Figure 52.13). Some frame systems, like the Leksell model G, allow for the determination of the x, y and z coordinates of any intracranial point directly from the CT or MRI computer console (Figure 52.14). A separate computer system is only required when the base of the frame is not parallel to the scanning plane, necessitating additional calculations. For the majority of other systems, a dedicated computer system performs the calculations necessary for co-registration.

Frameless cranial systems

Over the past decade frameless systems have surpassed frame-based techniques in popularity and versatility (Figure 52.15). These systems employ fiducial markers that either affix temporarily to the skin or are implanted into the outer table of the skull. The markers are visible on the imaging modality being employed and by determining the physical location of these fiducial markers, the corresponding points on the image can be aligned with the physical operating space (Figure 52.16). Other methods include digitizing the surface contour of a portion of the patient's head and aligning this surface with that derived from the imaging studies.[41] The surface digitization can be performed by physically tracing the skin surface using a trackable pointer, or by laser scanning of the actual surface without any physical contact with the skin (e.g. Medtronic, Minneapolis, MN or BrainLab, Heimstetten, Germany).[38,40] The result is the ability to then physically touch a point beneath the surface and visualize the corresponding point on the imaging studies. This method obviates the need to affix any skin markers prior to imaging acquisition but is somewhat less accurate.[38,41–44]

Recent advances in computer imaging technology have resulted in software algorithms permitting image fusion across modalities. Thus, a high resolution MRI performed days to weeks prior to surgery, for example, can be "fused" with a stereotactic CT performed on the day of surgery. Prior to the development of these algorithms, the acquired images were co-registered to the physical stereotactic operative space by employing the physical fiducial localizer attached to the frame, applied skin fiducial markers, or skin surface. The new software techniques can co-register various anatomic and functional imaging data (e.g. CT, MRI, functional MRI, PET, etc.) by employing one of several advanced mathematical algorithms, such as the mutual information-based algorithm, the time-weighted alternation method, as well as the uniformity index matching technique.[45–47] Preoperative planning can now, for example, be performed based on the frameless MRI data, and co-registered to the frame-based

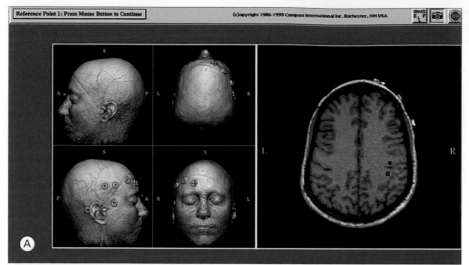

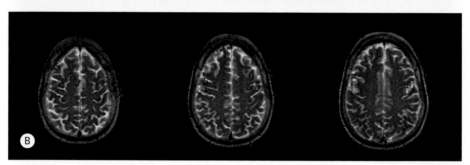

Figure 52.10 (A) Motor (solid circle) and sensory (empty square) cortices of the left hand localized using preoperative magnetoencephalography and incorporated into the intraoperative stereotactic database. **(B)** Preoperative functional magnetic resonance localization of the facial motor cortex bilaterally in a patient asked to smile.

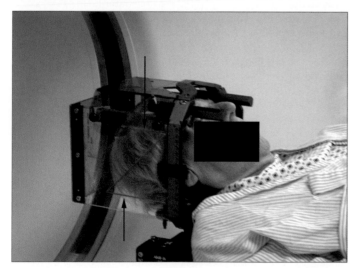

Figure 52.11 Leksell Model G frame with attached reference plates containing fiducial rods in a "letter-N" arrangement (arrows) within the CT gantry.

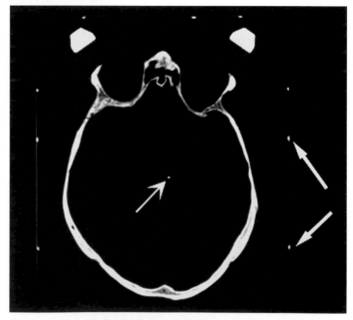

Figure 52.12 A CT slice leveled to display bone windows demonstrating a cross-section of nine fiducial rods (straight tip arrows) in a "picket-fence" distribution. Note the metallic deep-brain-stimulating electrode tip (concave tip arrow) surrounded by the fiducial rods.

CT acquisition. This process minimizes operating room or radiosurgical suite downtime and avoids the necessity of frame reapplication by separating the two phases of the stereotactic surgery process: image acquisition and actual surgery. These techniques have primarily been applied to radiosurgery.[48–51] However, applications for neurosurgical interventions have also been developed and are continually refined. In fact, several reports have described the use of image fusion in functional neurosurgery, and image fusion for deep-brain targets is routinely used at our home institutions when performing functional procedures (see section entitled Subthalamic nucleus deep-brain stimulation).[52–54]

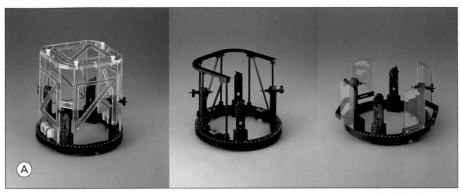

Figure 52.13 (A) An example of reference plate arrays for MRI, CT, and angiography (left, middle, right) for the Compass stereotactic system (courtesy of Compass International, Rochester, MN). (B) CT (left) and MR (right) reference plate arrays for the Leksell stereotactic system.

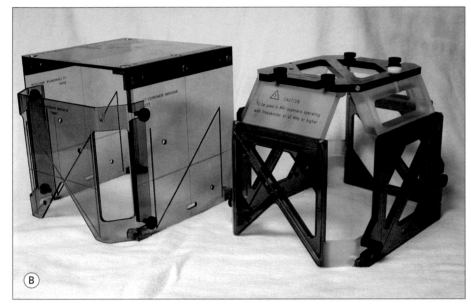

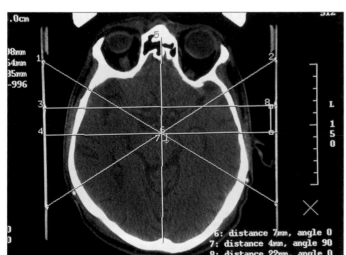

Figure 52.14 A noncontrast head CT in a patient with a deep-brain-stimulating electrode within the left subthalamic nucleus. The overlaid drawings are easily performed directly on the computer console of the CT scanner. The origin of the Leksell stereotactic system is on the right superior-posterior corner of the frame. The center of the frame is then denoted as being 100 mm anterior, 100 mm to the left, and 100 mm inferior to the origin (x, y and z = 100,100,100). The intersection of lines 1, 2 and 4 denotes the frame center. The three-dimensional coordinates of the deep-brain-stimulating lead are 104, 93, 122.

Frameless spinal systems

Although the vast majority of stereotactic procedures have been developed and used for cranial applications, there has been a recent extension of basic navigational principles to other areas of the body, including the spine.[55–60] In essence, the basic principles of stereotaxy can be, and have been, applied to areas of the body where precise localization is deemed necessary, and a navigational frame of reference can be established. The rationale for employing stereotactic principles in the surgical treatment of spinal disorders includes error rates of pedicle screw placement as high as 30%, especially in the thoracic spine, as well as the distorted anatomy that may be encountered during deformity correction procedures.[61–66] Additional spinal applications include image-guided cervical instrumentation, such as atlanto-axial transarticular screw placement, transoral odontoid resection, and lateral mass screw placement.[67–70] A spinal reference frame can be established in any one of several ways. The most basic method includes physically touching several well-defined bony landmarks, such as the tips of the spinous and transverse processes, with a digitizing pointer (described in the section "Digitizer technologies"). The corresponding points are selected on the preoperative imaging and the imaging space is co-registered with the physical operative space by a computer-based mathematical transformation algorithm, identical to the process involved in cranial registration. A second method involves co-registration based on a surface fitting

Table 52.1 Types of stereotactic frames

Frame type	Examples
Simple orthogonal systems	Hayne–Meyers,[83] Spiegel–Wycis,[7] Talairach[82]
Burr-hole-mounted systems	Austin–Lee,[84] Navigus,[a] Sterotactic Guide[b]
Arc-quadrant systems	Leksell,[b] Compass,[c] Laitinen,[d] Sugita Type II,[e] CRW[f]
Arc-phantom systems	Riechert/Mundinger,[g] Sugita Type I[e]
Computer-based systems	Majority of modern stereotactic systems

a. Image-Guided Neurologics, Melbourne, FL.
b. Electa, Stockholm, Sweden.
c. Compass International, Rochester, MN.
d. Sanstrom Trade and Technology Welland, Ontario, Canada.
e. Mizuho Ikakogyo, Tokyo, Japan.
f. Radionics, Burlington, VT.
g. Stryker Leibinger, Freiberg, Germany.

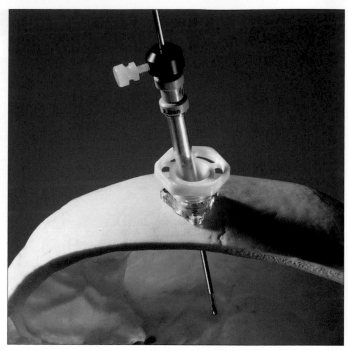

Figure 52.17 A burr hole-mounted system (Image-Guided Neurologics) allowing for two angular degrees of freedom.

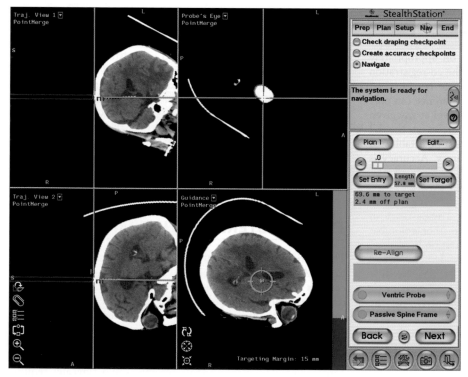

Figure 52.18 Trajectory views generated by the StealthStation frameless system during an Ommaya reservoir placement demonstrating the optimal path towards the ipsilateral foramen of Monro. Note the 6.96-cm distance from the outer table of the skull to target.

simple orthogonal systems, the surgeon can place the entry site over nonessential cortex and direct the probe to its target under radiographic guidance. Using CT or MRI with a modern computer system, for example, a trajectory intersecting a given target (Figure 52.18) can be reached at a specified depth by using either direct depth calculations from the imaging studies, or by repeatedly re-acquiring the images for a real-time update of the position of the probe tip. Recently, the integration of these devices with frameless stereotaxy has made planning and real-time updates more convenient (Figure 52.19). The major disadvantage of such a system is that a slight error in the angle of trajectory can result in a large linear error at the depths of the brain. Therefore, these systems have primarily been used for localizing larger targets, not requiring extreme precision.

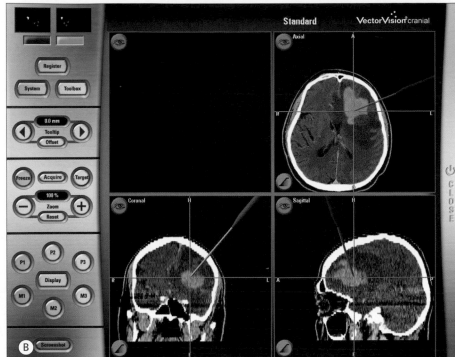
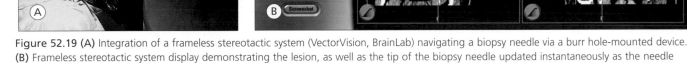

Figure 52.19 (A) Integration of a frameless stereotactic system (VectorVision, BrainLab) navigating a biopsy needle via a burr hole-mounted device. **(B)** Frameless stereotactic system display demonstrating the lesion, as well as the tip of the biopsy needle updated instantaneously as the needle advances through the mass.

Lars Leksell first described the more elegant arc-quadrant system in 1949.[9] Based on the center-of-sphere concept, the probe is rotated about the vertical (arc) and horizontal (quadrant or collar) axes and is advanced to a depth always equal to the radius of the sphere defined by the arc-quadrant system (Figure 52.20). Targeting can be achieved in one of two ways: either the arc-quadrant can be moved in three-dimensional space with respect to a fixed patient head, or the patient's head can be moved with respect to a stationary arc-quadrant (Figure 52.21). The advantage of this design is that any intracranial site can be accessed with great mechanical precision via any entry point, allowing a surgeon to reach the target while minimizing exposure of eloquent brain tissue. Some systems, such as the Leksell system, permit the targeting to be performed directly on the CT or MRI consoles with minimal calculations. This is directly related to the ingenious fiducial rod arrangement on the reference plates, discussed in the section entitled "Image co-registration." The disadvantages of an arc-quadrant system are that it is somewhat more cumbersome to use and can partially obstruct the operative field.

An arc-phantom system allows for the required complex trigonometric calculations to be performed by a simple mechanical analog computer: the phantom. Once the image-defined x, y, z target(s) is selected on the phantom, the tip of the probe is used to touch the phantom target by directing the aiming device. The aiming device is then transferred to the patient's base ring and the probe is lowered to a predetermined depth within the patient's brain. Slight angular errors, however, can result in significant targeting inaccuracies.

Electronic computer-based systems have evolved in tandem with the computer revolution. Complex calculations can now be

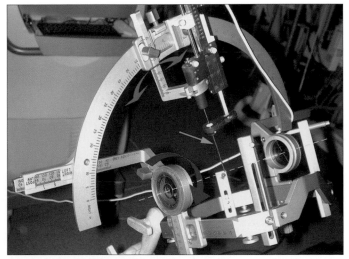

Figure 52.20 The Leksell Model G stereotactic frame and arc assembly demonstrating the center-of-sphere principle. The probe (green arrow) is rotated about the vertical (arc, blue arrows) and horizontal (quadrant or collar, red arrows) axes and advanced to a depth always equal to the radius of the sphere defined by the arc-quadrant system. Thus the same target (located at the center of the arc in the medial–lateral dimension, and at the dashed yellow line in the superior–inferior and dorsal–ventral dimensions) can be reached from a wide range of trajectories. Alternatively, the probe tip position is maintained despite adjustments of the arc and collar angles.

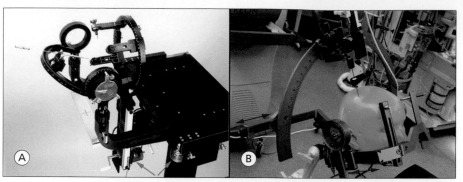

Figure 52.21 In the Compass (**A**) stereotactic systems targeting is achieved by moving the cranium in three dimensions (red arrows) with respect to the arc-quadrant assembly. Note two of three computer-controlled stepper-motors (green arrows) which move the assembly. In the Leksell stereotactic system (**B**) targeting is achieved by moving the arc-quadrant assembly in three dimensions (red arrows) with respect to the cranium secured to the frame.

performed almost instantaneously, thereby allowing the surgeon to focus on the surgery rather than on the mathematics. Computer-driven visual enhancements have augmented the surgeon's ability to comprehend the anatomy in ways that were previously unimaginable. The major drawback of these systems is that complete reliance on them can be very disappointing in the event of computer failure or malfunction. Thus a manual back-up system, allowing for straightforward mechanical targeting, should always be available.

DIGITIZER TECHNOLOGIES

Determining the location of a pointer in the physical space of the operating room can be accomplished by any of several different digitization technologies. The most elementary, of course, is a mechanical probe which is brought to its target by a carrier directly attached to a stereotactic frame (Figure 52.22). Frameless systems, on the other hand, employ more advanced and computer-driven digitizer technologies, including passive articulated arms, active robotic arms, active or passive infrared light-based systems, sonic triangulation methods, passive stereoscopic video or "machine vision" techniques, as well as magnetic-field technologies. Many of these technologies can be integrated with the operating microscope, enabling the stereotactic localization of the focal point of the microscope by overlaying this point onto the preoperative imaging studies.[85–88] Each digitization technique exhibits certain advantages and disadvantages (Table 52.2) but when optimized, their accuracy is comparable.[89–92]

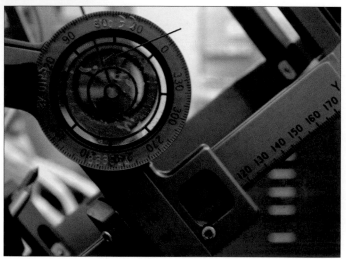

Figure 52.22 A mechanical probe (red arrow) is brought to its target by a carrier attached to the stereotactic frame/arc-quadrant assembly. The stereotactic target is visualized at the intersection of the near (in-focus, circular) and far (out-of-focus, linear X) radicules with the probe tip arriving in between the radicules.

Illustrative examples

Passive articulating arms were among the first frameless digitizer technologies to emerge on the commercial market. A popular system, the ISG Viewing Wand System (ISG Technologies,

Table 52.2 Advantages and disadvantages of various digitizer technologies

System	Advantages	Disadvantages
Frame-based probe	No line-of-sight limitation, high mechanical accuracy, simple	Requires placement of a frame, bulky, restrictive
Passive articulated arm	Simple, no line-of-sight limitations	Bulky, restrictive
Active robotic arm	Target a point in stereotactic space by mechanical/computer-driven means	Bulky, restrictive
Active infrared	Accurate, less bulky	Clear line-of-sight, attached cord
Passive infrared	Cordless, convenient	Clear line-of-sight, more expensive
Ultrasonic	Inexpensive, no line-of-sight requirement	Affected by drafts and by noise in the operating room
Machine vision	Allows any identifiable pointing device to be used	Clear line-of-sight, computationally intensive
Magnetic	Inexpensive, no line-of-sight requirement	Accuracy affected by neighboring metallic objects

Mississauga, Ontario, Canada) employed a passive localizing arm composed of two articulating segments and six joints, giving it a length of 60 cm and six degrees of freedom (FARO Medical Technologies, Miami, FL). Each joint possessed an electro-potentiometer, the analog output of which, when digitized by a computer, allowed 30 angular measurements per second. By knowing the fixed geometry of the arm, along with the angle of each joint, the computer calculated the tip of the arm in physical space. Co-registered with preoperative imaging, the frameless system was employed by numerous groups for a wide range of neurosurgical applications.[40,93–98]

Passive infrared systems employ wireless pointing devices equipped with an array of shiny reflective spheres. As a result of their ease-of-use and versatility they are becoming the most commonly employed frameless stereotactic systems in use today. Two to three high-resolution stereoscopic charge-coupled device (CCD) cameras surrounded by multiple infrared emitters detect the reflection of the infrared light off the spheres and, using triangulation techniques, determine the location of each sphere. Because the position and orientation of these spheres is fixed with respect to one another, the tip location of an instrument can be calculated with respect to the sphere array. Once the tip location is identified, the computer overlays this position onto preoperative images via co-registration techniques described in the previous section. Some systems allow the sphere array to be attached to any rigid surgical instrument during surgery, and after minimal end-user manipulation, the instrument is co-registered to the physical operative space (e.g. VectorVision, BrainLab, Heimstetten, Germany). Thus a suction tip, bipolar forceps, ventricular catheter, endoscope, surgical microscope, or a biopsy needle can all be used, alone or in combination, to target an intracranial or spinal lesion (Figure 52.23). The result is a system which is not mechanically constrained or cumbersome. However, the position of the cameras must be such that they are able to view the operative field.

ACCURACY

Before one can measure "accuracy," one must first define it. Maciunas et al. identified two essential components of accuracy: bias and precision (Figure 52.24).[99,100] Bias measures the spatial error a given system exhibits when attempting to find a point in space, while precision measures reproducibility, or the ability to return to any previous location. Both elements are essential in determining accuracy.

Overall stereotactic accuracy, also called application accuracy, is a measure of how well a stereotactic system localizes a point in space when used under real-world conditions. Application accuracy is affected by several factors, including imaging quality, mathematical calculations, and, of course, mechanical accuracy – the ability of the system to bring the tip of an instrument to a given coordinate within its range. The application accuracy is the vector sum of the independent sources of error, and thus, minimizing all sources of error is obligatory. It must be realized, however, that mean accuracy, commonly reported by device manufacturers, is typically only a description of mechanical accuracy. Furthermore, what a neurosurgeon really needs to know is not the mean error between the location of the target and the probe, but rather the magnitude of the largest error.

Of equal importance, is an understanding of the anatomic accuracy of the stereotactic process, especially when it relates to functional neurosurgical procedures. Numerous studies have demonstrated the significant interindividual variability that exists between anatomical structures and the corresponding functionally relevant areas.[101–104] Thus while the anterior and posterior commissures are more precise than external skull landmarks, functionally relevant areas, such as the globus pallidus, thalamic nuclei, or the corpus of Luysıi (i.e. subthalamic nucleus), are not always perfectly related to the intercommissural line. In fact, several studies have demonstrated that direct MR-based anatomic targeting of functional targets requires significant physiological refinement in the form of microelectrode recording, micro- or macrostimulation.[101–103,105–108] While the final clinical relevance of physiological confirmation has not been definitively proven, the majority of centers performing functional neurosurgical procedures do not solely rely on anatomic targeting and employ some form(s) of physiologic confirmation. Thus even in an ideal world where the application accuracy of a stereotactic system is flawless, and the probe reaches the intended anatomic target perfectly, the intended functional and clinically relevant target may be several millimeters away, resulting in a suboptimal clinical outcome.

Actual measurement of application accuracy is a daunting task. An ideal evaluation would involve measuring the three-dimensional distance from a probe to its intended intracranial

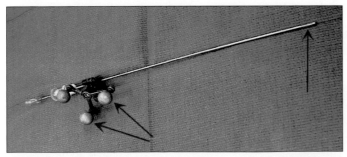

Figure 52.23 Nashold-type stereotactic biopsy needle with reflective spheres (red arrows) attached via a clamp and co-registered almost instantaneously during surgery. Note the side-cutting exposed 1-cm tip (blue arrow).

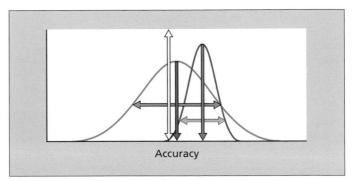

Figure 52.24 Accuracy has two components: bias and precision. Bias denotes the difference between the mean (vertical solid lines) and the true value (yellow line), while precision is denoted by the standard deviation (dashed horizontal lines). Bias measures the spatial error a given system exhibits when attempting to find a point in space. Precision measures reproducibility, or the ability to return to any previous location. Thus while stereotactic system A, denoted graphically in green, is less biased, system B, denoted graphically in blue, is more precise.

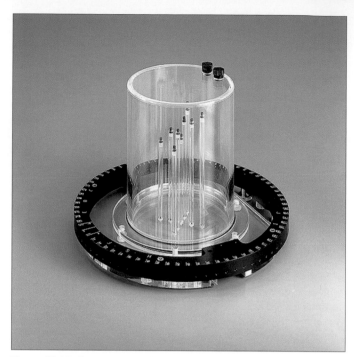

Figure 52.25 Phantom secured to the Compass stereotactic frame. The phantom houses several rods with known tip locations which serve to verify the accuracy of the stereotactic system (courtesy of Compass International, Rochester, MN).

target in a real-world setting. While several studies examining various stereotactic frame-based and frameless systems have been performed, each has its advantages and disadvantages.[24,100,109–111] Without reviewing each individual study's weaknesses, several points can be made. First, while using a phantom is a good approximation of intracranial contents, it may nevertheless, be subject to different imaging distortions than a human brain (Figure 52.25). Second, the true accuracy is dependent upon various intra-operative factors such as positioning, patient cooperation during image acquisition, re-application of the arc-quadrant apparatus in frame-based procedures, the weight and possible bending of an instrument attached to the arc, and a host of other factors that are only realized in individual patient cases. The ideal study examining overall application accuracy has yet to be performed. The application accuracy of the more common stereotactic frames is reported to range from a mean of 0.9 mm to 1.9 mm with the

maximal application error ranging from 1.3 to 5.0 mm (slice thickness 1–2 mm).[24,100,109–114] The application accuracy of frameless stereotactic systems ranges between 0.7 mm to 3.9 mm, with a maximal application error of 9.5 mm.[90,110–114] It is important to note, however, that the largest contribution to application accuracy is not the particular frameless digitizer technology, but rather the imaging resolution and accuracy of the co-registration.[115]

HUMAN STEREOTACTIC ATLASES

Both geographic drawings and maps relay information about the shape of a sea or land mass; a map, however, provides additional critical information – measurements and distances between these terrestrial objects in some frame of reference. Similarly, while anatomical drawings of the human brain have existed for several centuries, precise size measurements of subcortical structures, and their relationship to each other had not been performed until the twentieth century. In 1908 Horsley and Clarke used their stereotactic frame to derive a Cartesian-based atlas of the monkey cerebellum in relation to external anatomical landmarks – the inferior orbital rims and the external auditory meatus.[116] However, external anatomical references proved too variable for human use. It was not until the middle of the century that Spiegel and Wycis first used a stereotactic device in humans.[7] The reference frame was based on the calcified pineal gland and the foramen of Monro visualized on pneumoencephalography. Within 5 years, they had published the first Cartesian-based stereotactic atlas of the human brain.[8] Others soon followed suit, replacing the intracranial landmarks upon which the atlases were based to the anterior and posterior commissures, as suggested by Talairach et al.[117] This set of reference points is the most commonly employed system in use today. Stereotactic atlases have since appeared for deep cerebral structures, intracerebral vasculature, cerebellum, and spinal cord.[118–124]

The purpose of these atlases is to provide the dimensions of various structures, and the distances between them. These measurements can be scaled to conform to an individual patient's anatomy. For example, a commonly employed atlas is based on an intercommissural distance of 24 mm.[119] Thus if a particular patient's anterior to posterior commissure length is 30 mm, then the distances between various structures needs to be augmented by 125%. These scaling operations can easily be performed by modern computers. Not only can software be used to scale and display a particular atlas section for a given patient (Figure 52.26),

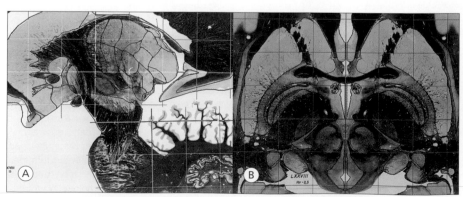

Figure 52.26 (A) Sagittal (13 mm lateral to midline) and **(B)** axial (3.5 mm ventral to midcommissural line) sections of the Schaltenbrand–Warhen atlas with blue nuclear tracing overlaid onto the pathological slices (courtesy of Thieme, Stuttgart and New York and Kent Ridge Digital Labs, Singapore. Adapted by Nowinski et al. from ref. 126).

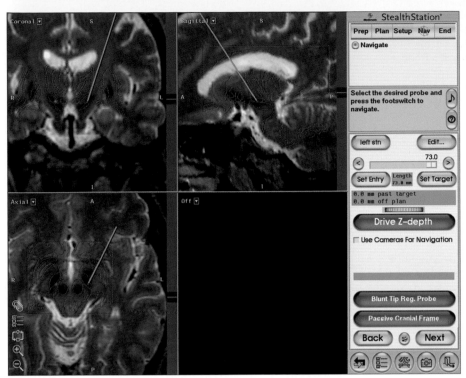

Select the desired probe and
press the footswitch to
navigate.

left stn   Edit...

73.0
Set Entry Length Set Target
73.8 mm

0.0 mm past target
0.0 mm off plan

Drive Z-depth

Use Cameras For Navigation

Blunt Tip Reg. Probe

Passive Cranial Frame

Back   Next

Figure 52.27 The surgical target (e.g. the subthalamic nucleus) and its trajectory are visualized on a fused anatomic–atlas image in the three standard imaging planes. The neuronavigational system facilitates interactive operative planning.

but the atlas sections can also be automatically overlaid onto the patient's actual CT or MRI scans. In turn, the surgical target can be determined from the combined anatomic–atlas image in stereotactic coordinates directly on the neuronavigational system (Figure 52.27). The fusion of these data greatly facilitates operative planning.

Atlases, however, harbor significant disadvantages. Besides the technical imperfections of certain atlases, such as the uneven spacing between slices in the Schaltenbrand–Wahren publication, atlases are inherently only an approximation of the true neuro-anatomy of an individual patient[119] (Figure 52.28). Although atlases based on intracranial landmarks are far more accurate than those based on extracranial landmarks, the interindividual variability is, nevertheless, significant for most functional neurosurgical applications.[108] Additionally, while newer computer-based atlases capable of nonlinear transformation and segmentation are being tested, no clinical evidence exists to confirm their validity. As such, some form of physiological confirmation, either microelectrode recording or microstimulation/macrostimulation is deemed mandatory by the majority of stereotactic neurosurgeons. However, atlases have maintained a significant role in the modern treatment of functional disorders as a helpful adjunct to neuroimaging and neurophysiological localization techniques.

PHYSIOLOGICAL TARGET REFINEMENT

As mentioned in the previous section, the inherent anatomic variability of the human brain occasionally necessitates additional target verification. Physiological target confirmation is usually reserved for functional neurosurgical procedures where the goal of intervention is to alter the patient's physiological functioning. While there are various forms of noninvasive functional target localization, including functional MRI, MEG and PET, these

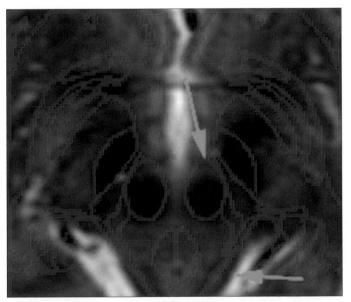

Figure 52.28 Axial slice from the Schaltenbrand–Wahren atlas[126] 3.5 mm ventral to the midcommissural plane overlaid on to corresponding MRI scan. Note the fit imperfections at the anterior border of the red nucleus and the posterior edge of the midbrain (green arrows).

modalities currently lack the spatial resolution deemed necessary for the majority of functional neurosurgical procedures.[125–127] More invasive procedures involve microinjection of various substances, such as GABA agonists, or electrical recording and stimulation.[128–133] Electrical modalities, such as micro- or semi-microelectrode recording, micro- or macrostimulation, are especially helpful. This makes intuitive sense given that the human brain is, in its most elementary function, an electrical organ. Microelectrode recording is typically performed using an electrode with carrier tube diameter of 350 μm, a 1- to 3-μm tip, and an impedance ranging from 0.5 to 3 MOhms at a frequency of 1000 Hz. After the signal is filtered and amplified (Figure 52.29), the electrode is capable of distinguishing the firing characteristics of a single cell (Figure 52.30). Microelectrode recording can be used to identify the boundaries of various nuclear structures – critical information for the functional neurosurgeon (Figure 52.31). In addition, thalamic recordings, for example, can identify the receptive fields of individual cells.[134,135] Semi-microelectrodes, with a much lower impedance and, therefore, a lower discriminatory capability, can record the activity of a cluster of several thousand cells. While much less sensitive to individual cells than a microelectrode, semi-microelectrodes may supply enough physiologically-based localizing information at a fraction of the time and cost.

Microstimulation of amplitudes up to 100 μA also affects a similarly-sized group of cells and is usually performed via the same microelectrode used for recording. Macrostimulation, on the other hand, is believed to stimulate structures up to 3 mm away from the electrode and usually ranges from 1 to 1.5 mm in tip diameter.[135,136]

The exact form of physiological confirmation depends on the procedure being performed and the preference of the surgeon performing it. The extent of physiological confirmation ranges from none to a combination of microelectrode recoding and micro- and macrostimulation.[130,137–142] The relative advantages and disadvantages of each electrophysiologic method are described in Table 52.3. A common combination includes microelectrode recording to identify the borders of a particular subcortical structure followed by macrostimulation via either the final deep-brain stimulation lead or lesioning probe to confirm the appropriate neurophysiological response.

The use of microelectrode recording in routine clinical use is controversial. While no doubts exist as to its research utility, a considerable debate rages as to its ability to improve clinical outcomes without increasing morbidity.[106,108,143–149] Although the majority of experienced centers utilize microelectrode recording for localization, some centers report excellent results with macrostimulation alone.[150–152]

APPLICATIONS OF STEREOTACTIC SURGERY

Stereotaxy is employed when precise localization of a target is essential. With the current trend towards minimally-invasive surgery, stereotactic procedures are becoming more common. Almost every neurosurgical operation has been performed using the stereotactic method. Overall cost, time consumption, surgeon's comfort level and experience, size of lesion, and lesion location are all factors responsible for a surgeon's preference to

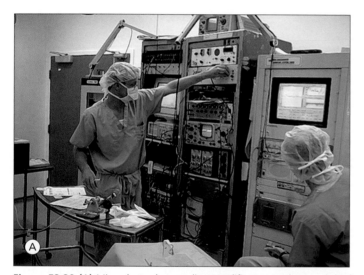
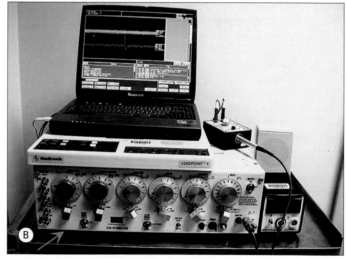

Figure 52.29 (A) Microelectrode recording amplifiers, recorders, and displays in a full rack configuration. **(B)** Compact laptop-based microelectrode recording system sitting atop a microstimulator unit (green arrow).

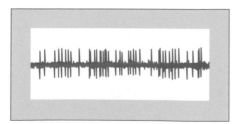

Figure 52.30 Microelectrode recording trace demonstrating the firing characteristics of a single subthalamic nucleus cell.

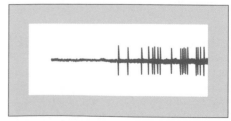

Figure 52.31 Microelectrode recording trace beginning in the relatively acellular zona incerta. Note the larger background noise indicated by the thicker baseline upon entry into the more cellular subthalamic nucleus.

Table 52.3 Comparison of electrophysical subcortical mapping techniques

	Microelectrode recording (MER)	Semi-MER	Microstimulation	Macrostimulation
Time required	Long	Medium	Medium	Short
Estimated current spread	20–200 μm	< 1 mm	200–1000 μm	2–3 mm
Record/stimulate from same tip	Yes	Yes	Yes	No
Cost	High	Medium	Medium	Low

utilize stereotaxy. Table 52.4 is a listing of the more common applications of stereotactic surgery. The recent advances in frameless technology have had a revolutionary impact on the prevalence of stereotaxy in the neurosurgical operating room. The continually improving user-friendliness and versatility of these systems has greatly facilitated their use for procedures traditionally performed nonstereotactically. In addition, several studies have demonstrated the efficacy and cost effectiveness of a variety of stereotactically assisted procedures.[153–157] Over the past 5 years, the authors have witnessed a significant rise in the number of stereotactic operations at their respective institutions (unpublished observations). This trend will continue as surgeons, and the public, strive towards less invasive approaches to treat common neurosurgical disorders.

SELECTED STEREOTACTIC PROCEDURES IN CURRENT USE

Morphologic surgery

Stereotactic biopsy/radiosurgery

Until the recent frameless revolution one of the most common indications for morphological stereotactic surgery was a stereotactic needle biopsy. A similar procedure, stereotactic radiosurgery, is analogous in that radiation beams, rather than biopsy needles, are directed at the target. A somewhat more sophisticated radiosurgical technique, known as the gamma knife, was developed by Lars Leksell in 1967 in Sweden, and currently consists of 201 intersecting cobalt-60 radiation beams focused on a target[158–160] (Figure 52.32). Computer software aids in surgical planning by calculating the stereotactic coordinates of the lesion, the necessary collimators, and the radiation exposure time necessary to administer a certain dose (Figure 52.33).

The advent of CT, and later, MRI, resulted in a significant increase in the number of these procedures for several reasons. First, direct visualization of the lesion greatly facilitates its targeting. By attaching a frame with reference plates containing fiducial rods, the neurosurgeon or radiation oncologist is able to visualize and localize the lesion with respect to the fiducial rods. After co-registering the image data set to the physical space, as described in a previous section of this chapter, a biopsy probe or radiation beam is directed at the lesion. Second, the increased prevalence of imaging has resulted in the discovery of many incidental masses which are subsequently biopsied, and possibly radiated. Third, the advances in frameless stereotactic technologies have further facilitated routine brain biopsies (Figure 52.34). Stereotactic biopsy allows the physician to ascertain the histologic or microbiologic nature of a brain lesion with an accuracy of well

Table 52.4 Common applications of stereotactic surgery

Cranial stereotactic surgery
Craniotomy/needle biopsy/therapeutic aspiration
  Tumor
    Transphenoidal approaches
    Insular lesions
    Lesions in deep/eloquent areas
  Vascular malformation
  Benign lesions (e.g. colloid cyst)
  Infectious lesion
  Third ventriculostomy
  Endoscopically assisted surgery
  Brachytherapy
  Catheter placement

Spinal stereotactic surgery
Pedicle screw placement, especially for deformity corrective surgery
  Cervical
  Thoracic
  Lumbar
Atlantoaxial transarticular screw placement
Transoral odontoid resection
Cervical lateral mass screw placement
Anterior cervical instrumentation

Functional neurosurgery
Lesions and deep-brain stimulation
  Movement disorders
    Pallidum, thalamus, subthalamic nucleus
  Pain
    Periaqueductal grey, periventricular grey, medial lemniscus, sensory nucleus of the thalamus
  Psychiatric disorders
    Cingulate gyrus
    Anterior internal capsule

Epilepsy surgery
Depth electrode placement for monitoring
Amygdalo-hippocampectomy
Cortical resections
Subthalamic nucleus or anterior thalamic stimulation

over 90%. The reported permanent morbidity is less than 3%, with a mortality rate under 2%.[161–167] Depending on several factors, including the size and location of the lesion, as well as the patient's age and overall medical condition, some lesions, such as vestibular schwannomas, arteriovenous malformations, and

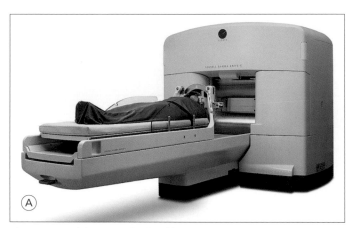
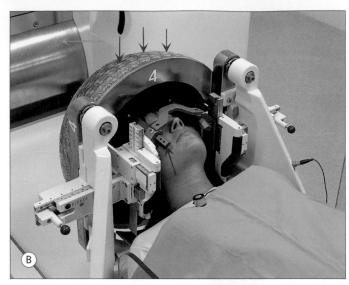

Figure 52.32 (A) Gamma-knife table and chamber housing the cobalt-60 radiation sources (courtesy of Elekta Instruments, Norcross, GA). **(B)** Patient with stereotactic headframe in place (blue arrow). Note hemispheric dome containing 201 4-mm collimators (red arrows pointing to individual collimators). The radiation (stored behind shielded doors denoted by the green arrows) passes through each of the collimators and is focused on the target by the three-dimensional coordinate settings on the stereotactic frame (courtesy of Elekta Instruments, Norcross, GA).

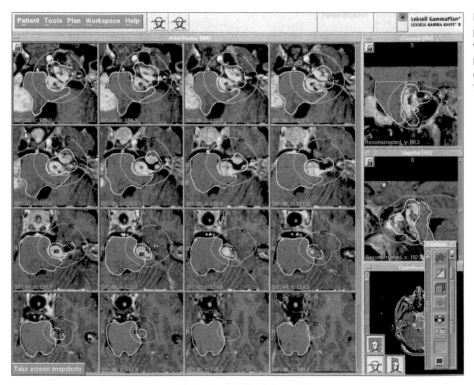

Figure 52.33 Screen snapshot of Leksell software planning the radiosurgical treatment of a left vestibular schwannoma (outlined in yellow) in a patient with neurofibromatosis type II. Note the deformed brainstem outlined in pink (courtesy of Theodore Schwartz, MD).

skull-base meningiomas are treated very effectively with radiosurgery.[168–177]

Volumetric tumor resection

The stereotactic technique is not only helpful for biopsies of deeply situated lesions, but is increasingly being used for craniotomies for lesional resections. As discussed in the previous section on Applications of stereotactic surgery, the advent and further improvement of frameless stereotactic neuronavigational systems has greatly increased the use of stereotaxy in everyday neurosurgery. There are several advantages in employing the stereotactic technique. First, it commonly minimizes the size of the skin incision and craniotomy. Second, the direct guidance to deeper subcortical masses reduces disruption of the neighboring white matter tracts. This can be accomplished in one of several ways. The most current technique employs a computer reconstruction of the axial MRI acquisition with a reformatted trajectory view. By pointing a probe in either a frame-based or frameless

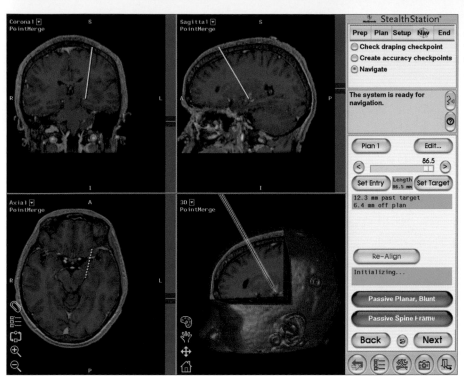

Figure 52.34 Brain biopsy of enhancing left medial hippocampal lesion. Surgical trajectory is visualized on the three standard orthogonal MR views, as well as the reconstructed three-dimensional view.

system, the precise trajectory to target can be obtained and followed surgically through the subcortical white matter. An older, yet very effective, technique is to place a catheter or probe to the target using either a frame-based or frameless system. The surgeon then dissects along the catheter or probe until reaching the lesion, at which point it is resected in the standard fashion.[178] Stereotaxy, in general, provides a comforting reassurance to the neurosurgeon that the target will be reached with minimal disruption of normal tissue.

Once the lesion is identified, the ideal route is chosen to avoid eloquent cortex. Preoperative functional imaging, such as MEG or functional MRI, may be directly incorporated into the stereotactic database, resulting in the ability to view simultaneously the functionally and anatomically relevant brain regions.[179–181] In addition, stereotaxy may improve completeness of resection by identifying the lesional margins. In practice, however, this is an unrealistic expectation for several reasons. First, an experienced surgeon will rely on his or her visual and tactile feedback in establishing the borders of the mass. Second, as a result of cerebrospinal fluid shifts and collapse of surrounding brain tissue the intraoperative borders of a lesion of any significant size or depth will change during the course of surgery. Therefore an intracranial point identified on the preoperative MRI data set will no longer correspond to the actual anatomy and may be misaligned by up to several centimeters.[182–186] Some workers have dealt with this "brain shift" problem using various techniques and with varying degrees of success. An early technique involved using cylindrical retractors to "immobilize" surrounding brain tissue and minimize shift.[187] Others outlined the extent of the lesion by stereotactically placing catheters at the perimeter of the lesion prior to the start of actual surgical resection. As the brain shifted, the catheters, or the injected dye, shifted in concert, thereby maintaining their relative position to the lesional borders.[188] Over the past decade the development of intraoperative real-time

imaging has emerged. These technologies include two- and three-dimensional ultrasound coupled to the neuronavigational sytem, as well as intraoperative MRI scanners.[189–197] Although these advances address the serious issue of brain shift, they possess several disadvantages. An ultrasound image lacks the contrast and

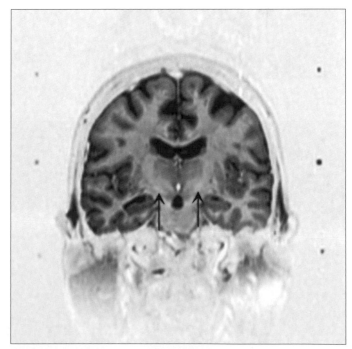

Figure 52.35 Bilateral subthalamic nuclei (arrows) are visible on this T2-weighted inversion recovery coronal MRI.

detail of MRI, while intraoperative MRI requires dedicated non-ferromagnetic instruments and a costly machine devoted to the operating theatre. The advantages and disadvantages of each modality must be carefully weighed prior to embarking on a particular path towards the minimization of brain shift error.

Functional neurosurgery

Subthalamic nucleus deep-brain stimulation

Since its introduction into clinical practice by Benabid, Pollak and others in 1993/94, chronic high-frequency stimulation of the subthalamic nucleus (STN) has been shown to be a safe and effective method for treating medically refractory idiopathic Parkinson's disease.[198,199] Recent clinical studies have shown the

efficacy of chronic STN stimulation in alleviating all cardinal motor manifestations of Parkinson's disease, including tremor, rigidity, bradykinesia, on/off fluctuation, oral control, gait and balance difficulty, and dyskinesia.[200–210]

As mentioned previously, the authors are unaware of any surgical group performing subthalamic surgery, either lesioning or stimulation, without the use of a stereotactic frame. Once the frame is applied using local anesthetic, either an MRI or a CT is obtained. Direct visualization of the STN is then possible using MRI (Figure 52.35). Alternatively, an MRI is obtained some time prior to surgery and fused to a CT obtained once the frame has been secured to the skull (Figure 52.36).[53,211] This minimizes scanning time with the frame in place, and reduces the possibility of nonlinear magnetic spatial distortion. The targets are then chosen by one or a combination of methods, including direct MRI-based

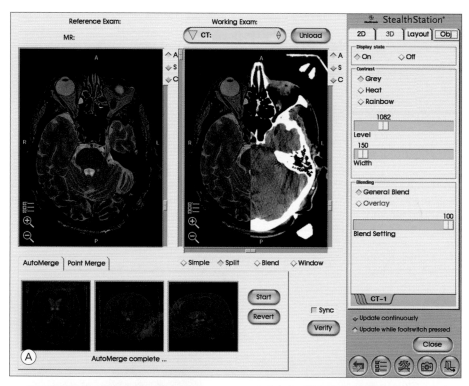

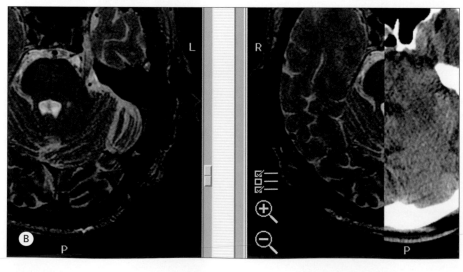

Figure 52.36 (A) Image fusion between a preoperative MRI (left) and an intraoperative CT with stereotactic frame in place (right) performed automatically by the neuronavigational system (StealthStation, Medtronic Surgical Navigation Technologies, Louisville, CO). (B) Magnified image of (A). Note the accuracy of the fusion process evident by the posterior bony skull interface, the fourth ventricle, and the co-registered cursor placed between the basilar artery and the ventral pons.

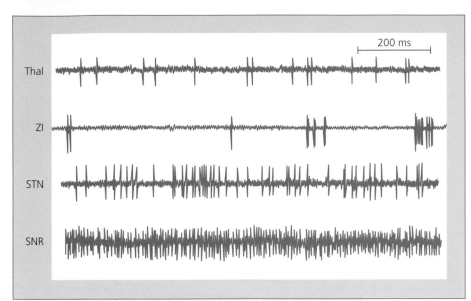

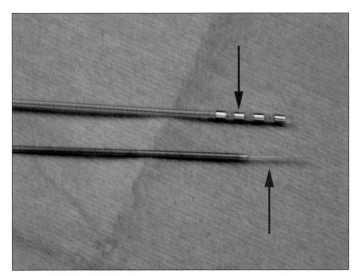

Figure 52.38 Cylindrical contact of quadripolar macroelectrode (blue arrow) with a 1.27-mm diameter compared with the ultra-fine microelectrode tip (red arrow).

targeting, atlas-based methods, and indirect mid-commissural-based localization.[115] Once the stereotactic coordinates of the STN are selected, bilateral prefrontal burr-holes are placed. The anatomical targeting is confirmed by microelectrode or semi-microelectrode recording in the majority of, but not all, centers.[106,108,150,212–214] Using microelectrode recording, various nuclear structures are traversed, each with a characteristic firing pattern (Figure 52.37). In addition, microelectrode recording can detect movement-related cellular responses in the dorsolateral aspect of the STN.[107,130,215] The preliminary location for the deep-brain-stimulating macroelectrode (Figure 52.38) is selected to encompass the longest trajectory through the STN, as determined by microelectrode recording (Figure 52.39). The implanted electrode is quadripolar, each cylindrical contact being 1.5 mm in length with varying interspacing. Depending on the particular model, the total contact span is either 7.5 or 10.5 mm.

Macrostimulation through the deep-brain-stimulating electrode then confirms the proximity of the various contacts to the internal capsule anterolaterally and the medial lemniscus posteriorly. Given that typical chronic stimulation amplitudes range from 2 to 4 volts, parasthesias or motor contractions encountered above 4–5 volts are deemed acceptable. Besides for ascertaining side-effect thresholds, immediate improvement in tremor, as well as rigidity, are often noted. Some of these positive results may be noted from the insertional effects of the deep-brain-stimulating lead prior to any test stimulation, a phenomenon termed by many as the "microsubthalamotomy effect." Once the deep-brain-stimulating lead is in the appropriate location, it is secured to a burr-hole cap using fluoroscopy to minimize migration (Figure 52.40). The majority of STN stimulation surgery is performed bilaterally, either simultaneously or in stages. The pulse generators are then implanted in the infraclavicular region (Figure 52.41).

The primary advantages of neurostimulation over lesioning include reversibility and adjustability. By selecting different contacts with varying electrical parameters (amplitude, frequency, and pulse width), optimal clinical responses can be elicited while minimizing side-effects. The drawbacks of stimulation, on the other hand, include hardware infection/malfunction, as well as the costs associated with the device. No significant risk of hemiballismus exist with either treatment modality.[198,216] Judging by the number of published reports, it appears that the majority of centers performing STN surgery employ neurostimulation. While surgical teams attempt to maximize the number of electrical contacts within the STN, it appears that the optimal contact location is at its dorsolateral border, or perhaps in the immediate vicinity of the dorsal fiber tracts.[53,217,218] The precise mechanism by which high-frequency STN stimulation results in a clinical effect similar to ablative surgery remains speculative.[217,219–222] Clinical results, as measured by improvement in the motor-subscores of the Unified Parkinson's Disease Rating Scale (UPDRS-III), demonstrate an approximate improvement of 60% in the off-medication state. When comparing the effects of stimulation in the on-medication state, results are more variable, ranging from no improvement to 50%. Mean levodopa reduction is in the 50% range.[205,217,223–227] These improvements are remarkable considering all attempts at medical management in this cohort

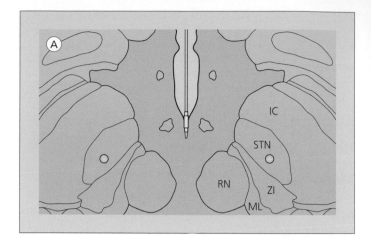

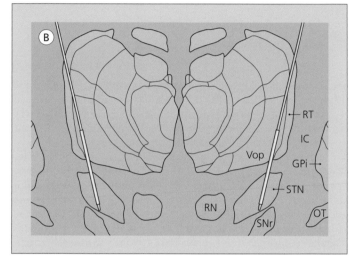

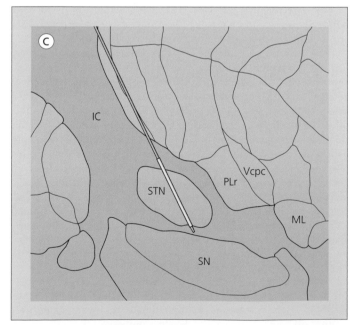

Figure 52.39 Annotated axial **(A)**, coronal **(B)**, and sagittal **(C)** Morel[127] atlas sections with a superimposed quadripolar lead within the subthalamic nucleus.

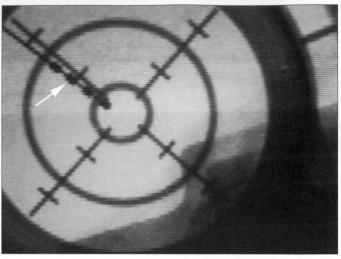

Figure 52.40 Fluoroscopic image of deep-brain-stimulating macroelectrode (arrow pointing to one of the four cylindrical contacts) being advanced to its target at the center of the radicules mounted on the stereotactic frame/arc assembly.

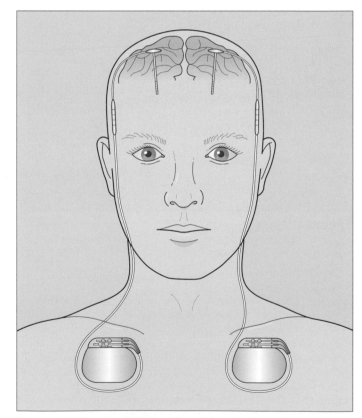

Figure 52.41 Drawing depicting bilateral deep-brain-stimulator implants, including the pulse generators inserted in the infraclavicular region (courtesy Medtronic, Minneapolis, MN).

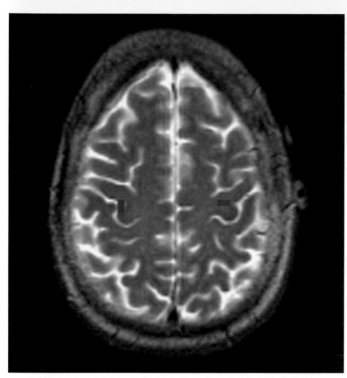

Figure 52.42 Pre-operative functional MRI obtained using a bilateral thumb movement task. Note the precentral gyrus is highlighted in red by an increase in the blood oxygen level-dependent (BOLD) signal during the motor task.

of surgical patients have been largely unsuccessful. Additionally, the majority of studies examining the neuropsychiatric consequences of STN stimulation reveal no significant effects.[225,228–232] However, reports of long-term clinical results are, as yet, unavailable.

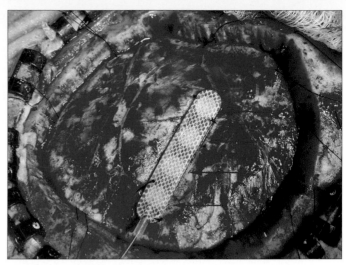

Figure 52.44 Quadripolar paddle electrode (blue arrows showing the electrical contacts) sutured to the outer layer of the dura overlying the motor cortex.

Epidural motor cortex stimulation

Over the past 30 years a wide variety of surgical procedures have been employed for the treatment of chronic neuropathic pain refractory to medical treatment. Ablative lesioning procedures as well as electrical stimulation at different locations within the peripheral and central nervous system have been utilized, with varying results. In 1993 Tsubokawa and co-workers first reported chronic stimulation of the precentral gyrus for thalamic pain.[233] Since then numerous centers throughout Japan and Europe have reported results for a variety of chronic refractory neuropathic pain conditions, including atypical facial pain, post-stroke pain, and other forms of deafferentation pain.[234–239] An improvement of at least 50% on a visual analog scale is generally regarded as a

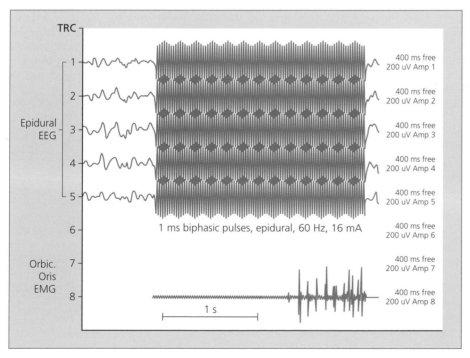

Figure 52.43 Electroencephalographic (EEG) and electromyographic (EMG) tracings obtained during transdural stimulation of the facial motor cortex using a bipolar stimulator. Note the EEG artifact during the 2.5 s of stimulation (upper traces), as well as the delayed onset of EMG activity within the orbicularis oris muscle approximately 1500 ms after the start of stimulation.

surgical success. Based on very limited case-series data, it appears that motor cortex stimulation is somewhat more effective and certainly less invasive than thalamic sensory nucleus (Vc) stimulation.[240–242] As such, the authors believe that epidural motor cortex stimulation should be attempted prior to other forms of brain stimulation for most forms of refractory chronic neuropathic pain.

The majority of groups performing this procedure obtain some form of pre-operative functional imaging study to determine the location of the central sulcus (Figure 52.42). This information is then incorporated into a stereotactic system, fusing the preoperative functional information to the anatomic imaging. Surgery is usually performed with the patient awake. After stereotactic image co-registration, a small craniotomy is performed centered over the motor cortex and physiological mapping commences. The authors typically obtain somatosensory evoked potentials, with the electrical stimulus being generated over the painful body area. In addition, transdural stimulation using a standard cortical stimulator (Ojemann, Radionics, Burlington, MA) is used to confirm the location of the motor cortex contralateral to the painful body area (Figure 52.43). The epidural quadripolar paddle electrode (Model 3587A Resume II, Medtronic, Minneapolis, MN) is then placed epidurally over the motor cortex and repeat testing is performed (Figure 52.44). After confirmation of the lead position, the paddle electrode is sutured to the dura and externalized via a separate stab incision. Postoperative testing then commences, generally for up to 1 week. The stimulation amplitude is kept below 75% of the motor contraction threshold. For example, in performing surgery to treat anesthesia dolorosa, if facial contraction is noted at 9 volts, postoperative stimulation is kept below 7 volts. Additionally, unlike deep-brain stimulation for movement disorders, the stimulation frequency is typically below 100 Hz. Various parameters are tested and the pulse generator is implanted (Model 7425 Itrel® 3 Neurostimulator, Medtronic, Minneapolis, MN) if the patient experiences more than 50% pain relief as determined by the visual analog scale. Interestingly, positive clinical effects last for a period significantly longer than the actual stimulation period, and thus stimulation is administered intermittently for brief periods of time. Unlike with other forms of neurostimulation, such as thalamic or spinal cord stimulation, the patient typically senses very little when the stimulator is on. This fact can be exploited to determine the extent of the placebo effect because the patient can be blinded as to whether the stimulator is on or off. Complications that may be encountered include infection and hardware malfunction. Seizures are very rare.[234,238,242,243]

Overall, epidural motor cortex stimulation is a safe and effective therapy in a select group of patients suffering from neuropathic pain resistant to all other medical management. However, larger studies examining long-term clinical results and effects of stimulation are lacking.

FUTURE DIRECTIONS

The future of stereotactic neurosurgery appears very bright. Many ideas which were "revolutionary" only a few years ago have matured into practical and commonly used applications today. These advancements have been fueled by the perpetual drive to intervene surgically in a less invasive and more precise fashion.

Higher field magnets and improved frame materials promise to improve significantly the accuracy of spatial localization of deep-brain targets. Advanced methods of functional imaging, and their seamless incorporation into the stereotactic database, will facilitate wider acceptance into general neurosurgical practice. Along with affordable intraoperative anatomical and functional imaging, surgery in and around eloquent areas will become safer and more radical. To minimize the costs of real-time intraoperative imaging, mathematical algorithms capable of predicting nonlinear deformation will allow the surgeon to account for brain shift during surgery. Furthermore, if the past 20 years are any indication, the computational power required to perform these complex analyses will continue to become ever more affordable. Coupled with smaller and more powerful computers, micro-robotic or even nano-robotic devices will, in the not-so-distant future, be implanted intracranially to perform various remote tasks with greater precision. Surgery may one day be assisted by an expert in a particular subspecialty operating via a robotic intermediary from thousands of miles away. Indeed, this is currently being developed for gastrointestinal and urologic surgery.[244–247] The hardware and software necessary for such a "virtual" endeavor, including live audio, video, and tactile feedback, will also greatly facilitate surgical training, much like modern-day airline pilots. Today's stereotactic systems and principles are already a well-established component of many neurosurgical residency training programs.

In the realm of functional neurosurgery, advances in electronics and battery technology virtually assure further miniaturization of today's implanted pulse generators. Stimulator devices programmable via remote televideo equipment will one day fit into a burr-hole without additional extension leads or bulky electronic pacemakers. In addition, the union of stimulating electrodes coupled to recording microelectrodes via an intervening microprocessor will enable neurostimulation therapies to be delivered automatically on physiological demand. The additional fusion of automated stimulation technologies to chemoinfusion systems will allow novel targeting of selected neural substrates. Furthermore, targeted gene therapy constructs and chemotherapeutic agents directed to a very specific location are already beginning to revolutionize the treatment of neurological disease.[248,249] The currently primitive field of molecular neuro-oncology will yield great dividends in the near future. In summary, unanticipated advances in science and technology both within the neurosurgical field and outside of it are likely to alter the course of our specialty in as yet unfathomable ways.

This chapter contains material from the first edition, and we are grateful to the authors of that chapter for their contribution.

REFERENCES

1. Gildenberg PL. Whatever happened to stereotactic surgery? *Neurosurgery* 1987; 20: 983–7.
2. *Merriam-Webster Collegiate Dictionary*. Springfield, MA: Merriam-Webster, Inc.; 2001.
3. Kandel EI, Schavinsky YV. Stereotaxic apparatus and operations in Russia in the 19th century. *J Neurosurg* 1972; 37: 407–11.
4. Clarke R, Horsley R. On a method of investigating the deep ganglia and tracts of the central nervous system (cerebellum). *Br Med J* 1906; 2: 1799–800.
5. Röntgen WC. On a new kind of rays. *Nature* 1896; 53: 274–6.
6. Picard C, Olivier A, Bertrand G. The first human stereotaxic apparatus. The contribution of Aubrey Mussen to the field of stereotaxis. *J Neurosurg* 1983; 59: 673–6.

CLINICAL PEARLS

- Human stereotactic neurosurgery began when Spiegel and Wycis integrated a Cartesian-based stereotactic instrument with ventriculography in 1947. Lars Leksell described his arc-quadrant apparatus, which allowed any intracranial point to be targeted from any angle, in 1949.

- The rapid decline of stereotactic procedures began in 1968 with the advent of levodopa, which was used to treat Parkinson's disease. Stereotactic surgery was reinvigorated over the past one or two decades when the shortcomings of levodopa were realized. In addition, the evolution of frameless stereotaxy has greatly contributed to the "stereotactic renaissance."

- The integration of noninvasive anatomical imaging, such as CT and MRI, as well as functional imaging modalities into the stereotactic database, have greatly facilitated surgical planning and execution.

- Frameless cranial and spinal stereotactic systems running on affordable computer hardware have made stereotaxy a practical necessity in modern neurosurgery.

- While the accuracy of these systems varies, being primarily limited by imaging resolution and co-registration, it rivals the accuracy of frame-based systems.

- Physiological target refinement is widely employed to assist in functional neurosurgical procedures. Various physiological techniques have further been developed, including microelectrode recording, micro- and macrostimulation.

- Ablative surgery for movement disorders has largely been supplanted by chronic electrical stimulation in many regions of the world. Stimulation offers the advantages of being reversible, and adjustable.

- With rapid advances in computer-based technologies, the field of stereotactic surgery will continue to flourish making the understanding of its basic principles mandatory for the contemporary neurosurgeon.

7. Spiegel E, Wycis H, Marks M, Lee A. Stereotaxic apparatus for operations on the human brain. *Science* 1947; 106: 349–50.

8. Spiegel E, Wycis H. *Stereoencephalotomy: Part I – Methods and Stereotaxic Atlas of the Human Brain.* New York: Grune & Stratton; 1952.

9. Leksell L. A stereotactic apparatus for intracerebral surgery. *Acta Chir Scand* 1949; 99: 229–33.

10. Hecaen H, Talairach J, David M, Dell M. Coagulations limitées du thalamus dans les algies du syndrome thalamique. *Rev Neurol (Paris)* 1949; 81: 917–31.

11. Riechert T, Wolff M. Uber eine neues Zielgerat zur intracraniellen electriche Ableitung und Ausschaltung. *Arch Psych Z Neurol* 1951; 186: 225–30.

12. Narabayashi H. Stereotaxic instrument for operation on the human basal ganglia. *Psychiatr Neurol Japan* 1952; 54: 669–71.

13. Nashold BS. The history of stereotactic neurosurgery. *Stereotact Funct Neurosurg* 1994; 62: 29–40.

14. Nashold BS Jr. Stereotactic neurosurgery: the present and future. *Am Surg* 1970; 36: 91–3.

15. Kelly PJ. Stereotactic surgery: what is past is prologue. *Neurosurgery* 2000; 46: 16–27.

16. Laitinen LV, Bergenheim AT, Hariz MI. Leksell's posteroventral pallidotomy in the treatment of Parkinson's disease. *J Neurosurg* 1992; 76: 53–61.

17. Hounsfield GN. Computerized transverse axial scanning (tomography). 1. Description of system. *Br J Radiol* 1973; 46: 1016–22.

18. Alterman RL, Kall BA, Cohen H, Kelly PJ. Stereotactic ventrolateral thalamotomy: is ventriculography necessary? *Neurosurgery* 1995; 37: 717–21.

19. Hariz MI, Bergenheim AT. A comparative study on ventriculographic and computerized tomography-guided determinations of brain targets in functional stereotaxis. *J Neurosurg* 1990; 73: 565–71.

20. Hariz MI, Bergenheim AT. Clinical evaluation of computed tomography-guided versus ventriculography-guided thalamotomy for movement disorders. *Acta Neurochir Suppl (Wien)* 1993; 58: 53–5.

21. Tasker RR, Dostrovsky JO, Dolan EJ. Computerized tomography (CT) is just as accurate as ventriculography for functional stereotactic thalamotomy. *Stereotact Funct Neurosurg* 1991; 57: 157–66.

22. Yuan S, Zhang J, Gu M, et al. A new method to localize brain nuclei for surgery in extrapyramidal disease. *Stereotact Funct Neurosurg* 1995; 65: 47–53.

23. Burchiel KJ, Nguyen TT, Coombs BD, Szumoski J. MRI distortion and stereotactic neurosurgery using the Cosman–Roberts–Wells and Leksell frames. *Stereotact Funct Neurosurg* 1996; 66: 123–36.

24. Steinmeier R, Rachinger J, Kaus M, Ganslandt O, Huk W, Fahlbusch R. Factors influencing the application accuracy of neuronavigation systems. *Stereotact Funct Neurosurg* 2000; 75: 188–202.

25. Yu C, Apuzzo ML, Zee CS, Petrovich Z. A phantom study of the geometric accuracy of computed tomographic and magnetic resonance imaging stereotactic localization with the Leksell stereotactic system. *Neurosurgery* 2001; 48: 1092–8.

26. Mizowaki T, Nagata Y, Okajima K, et al. Development of an MR simulator: experimental verification of geometric distortion and clinical application. *Radiology* 1996; 199: 855–60.

27. Orrison WW Jr. Magnetic source imaging in stereotactic and functional neurosurgery. *Stereotact Funct Neurosurg* 1999; 72: 89–94.

28. Schulder M, Maldjian JA, Liu WC, et al. Functional image-guided surgery of intracranial tumors located in or near the sensorimotor cortex. *J Neurosurg* 1998; 89: 412–18.

29. Fried I, Nenov VI, Ojemann SG, Woods RP. Functional MR and PET imaging of rolandic and visual cortices for neurosurgical planning. *J Neurosurg* 1995; 83: 854–61.

30. Xiong J, Nickerson LD, Downs JH III, Fox PT. Basic principles and neurosurgical applications of positron emission tomography. *Neurosurg Clin N Am* 1997; 8: 293–306.

31. Tatlidil R, Xiong J, New P, West A, Fox P. Language mapping in pretreatment planning of patients with cerebral arteriovenous malformation: a PET study. *Clin Nucl Med* 2000; 25: 591–5.

32. Jannin P, Morandi X, Fleig OJ, *et al.* Integration of sulcal and functional information for multimodal neuronavigation. *J Neurosurg* 2002; 96: 713–23.

33. Bittar RG, Olivier A, Sadikot AF, Andermann F, Pike GB, Reutens DC. Presurgical motor and somatosensory cortex mapping with functional magnetic resonance imaging and positron emission tomography. *J Neurosurg* 1999; 91: 915–21.

34. McDonald JD, Chong BW, Lewine JD, *et al.* Integration of preoperative and intraoperative functional brain mapping in a frameless stereotactic environment for lesions near eloquent cortex. Technical note. *J Neurosurg* 1999; 90: 591–8.

35. Rezai AR, Hund M, Kronberg E, *et al.* The interactive use of magnetoencephalography in stereotactic image-guided neurosurgery. *Neurosurgery* 1996; 39: 92–102.

36. Kamiryo T, Cappell J, Kronberg E, *et al.* Interactive use of cerebral angiography and magnetoencephalography in arteriovenous malformations: technical note. *Neurosurgery* 2002; 50: 903–10.

37. West JB, Fitzpatrick JM, Toms SA, Maurer CR Jr, Maciunas RJ. Fiducial point placement and the accuracy of point-based, rigid body registration. *Neurosurgery* 2001; 48: 810–16.

38. Raabe A, Krishnan R, Wolff R, Hermann E, Zimmermann M, Seifert V. Laser surface scanning for patient registration in intracranial image-guided surgery. *Neurosurgery* 2002; 50: 797–801.

39. Kall BA, Goerss SJ, Stiving SO, Davis DH, Kelly PJ. Quantitative analysis of a noninvasive stereotactic image registration technique. *Stereotact Funct Neurosurg* 1996; 66: 69–74.

40. Golfinos JG, Fitzpatrick BC, Smith LR, Spetzler RF. Clinical use of a frameless stereotactic arm: results of 325 cases. *J Neurosurg* 1995; 83: 197–205.

41. Pelizzari CA, Chen GT, Spelbring DR, Weichselbaum RR, Chen CT. Accurate three-dimensional registration of CT, PET, and/or MR images of the brain. *J Comput Assist Tomogr* 1989; 13: 20–6.

42. Adler JR. Image-based frameless stereotactic radiosurgery. In: Maciunas RJ (ed.). *Interactive Image-Guided Neurosurgery.* Park Ridge, IL: American Association of Neurologic Surgeons; 1993: 81–9.

43. Bucholz R, Macneil W, Fewings P, Ravindra A, McDurmont L, Baumann C. Automated rejection of contaminated surface measurements for improved surface registration in image guided neurosurgery. *Stud Health Technol Inform* 2000; 70: 39–45.

44. Schmerber S, Chassat F. Accuracy evaluation of a CAS system: laboratory protocol and results with 6D localizers, and clinical experiences in otorhinolaryngology. *Comput Aided Surg* 2001; 6: 1–13.

45. Lee JS, Chee Y, Kim B, *et al.* Display of coregistered cross-modality images using time-weighted alternation method. *Stud Health Technol Inform* 1997; 39: 349–53.

46. Meyer CR, Boes JL, Kim B, *et al.* Demonstration of accuracy and clinical versatility of mutual information for automatic multimodality image fusion using affine and thin-plate spline warped geometric deformations. *Med Image Anal* 1997; 1: 195–206.

47. Pfluger T, Vollmar C, Wismuller A, *et al.* Quantitative comparison of automatic and interactive methods for MRI-SPECT image registration of the brain based on 3-dimensional calculation of error. *J Nucl Med* 2000; 41: 1823–9.

48. Julow J, Major T, Emri M, *et al.* The application of image fusion in stereotactic brachytherapy of brain tumours. *Acta Neurochir (Wien)* 2000; 142: 1253–8.

49. Lattanzi JP, Fein DA, McNeeley SW, Shaer AH, Movsas B, Hanks GE. Computed tomography-magnetic resonance image fusion: a clinical evaluation of an innovative approach for improved tumor localization in primary central nervous system lesions. *Radiat Oncol Investig* 1997; 5: 195–205.

50. Alexander E, III, Kooy HM, van Herk M, *et al.* Magnetic resonance image-directed stereotactic neurosurgery: use of image fusion with computerized tomography to enhance spatial accuracy. *J Neurosurg* 1995; 83: 271–6.

51. Kooy HM, van Herk M, Barnes PD, *et al.* Image fusion for stereotactic radiotherapy and radiosurgery treatment planning. *Int J Radiat Oncol Biol Phys* 1994; 28: 1229–34.

52. Duffner F, Schiffbauer H, Breit S, Friese S, Freudenstein D. Relevance of image fusion for target point determination in functional neurosurgery. *Acta Neurochir (Wien)* 2002; 144: 445–51.

53. Lanotte MM, Rizzone M, Bergamasco B, Faccani G, Melcarne A, Lopiano L. Deep brain stimulation of the subthalamic nucleus: anatomical, neurophysiological, and outcome correlations with the effects of stimulation. *J Neurol Neurosurg Psychiatry* 2002; 72: 53–8.

54. Murata J, Sawamura Y, Kitagawa M, Saito H, Kikuchi S, Tashiro K. [Minimally invasive stereotactic functional surgery using an intravenous anesthetic propofol and applying Image Fusion and AtlasPlan]. *No To Shinkei* 2001; 53: 457–62.

55. Blomgren H, Lax I, Naslund I, Svanstrom R. Stereotactic high dose fraction radiation therapy of extracranial tumors using an accelerator. Clinical experience of the first thirty-one patients. *Acta Oncol* 1995; 34: 861–70.

56. Dickman CA, Sonntag VK. Posterior C1–C2 transarticular screw fixation for atlantoaxial arthrodesis. *Neurosurgery* 1998; 43: 275–80.

57. Foley KT, Smith MM. Image-guided spine surgery. *Neurosurg Clin N Am* 1996; 7: 171–86.

58. Herline AJ, Stefansic JD, Debelak JP, *et al.* Image-guided surgery: preliminary feasibility studies of frameless stereotactic liver surgery. *Arch Surg* 1999; 134: 644–9.

59. Sama AA, Khan SN, Girardi FP, Cammisa FP Jr. Computerized frameless stereotactic image guidance in spinal surgery. *Orthop Clin North Am* 2002; 33: 375–80, vii.

60. Uematsu M, Shioda A, Suda A, *et al.* Intrafractional tumor position stability during computed tomography (CT)-guided frameless stereotactic radiation therapy for lung or liver cancers with a fusion of CT and linear accelerator (FOCAL) unit. *Int J Radiat Oncol Biol Phys* 2000; 48: 443–8.

61. Weinstein JN, Spratt KF, Spengler D, Brick C, Reid S. Spinal pedicle fixation: reliability and validity of roentgenogram-based assessment and surgical factors on successful screw placement. *Spine* 1988; 13: 1012–18.

62. Cinotti G, Gumina S, Ripani M, Postacchini F. Pedicle instrumentation in the thoracic spine. A morphometric and cadaveric study for placement of screws. *Spine* 1999; 24: 114–19.

63. Esses SI, Sachs BL, Dreyzin V. Complications associated with the technique of pedicle screw fixation. A selected survey of ABS members. *Spine* 1993; 18: 2231–38.

64. Gertzbein SD, Robbins SE. Accuracy of pedicular screw placement in vivo. *Spine* 1990; 15: 11–14.

65. Liljenqvist UR, Halm HF, Link TM. Pedicle screw instrumentation of the thoracic spine in idiopathic scoliosis. *Spine* 1997; 22: 2239–45.

66. Xu R, Ebraheim NA, Ou Y, Yeasting RA. Anatomic considerations of pedicle screw placement in the thoracic spine. Roy–Camille technique versus open-lamina technique. *Spine* 1998; 23: 1065–8.

67. Bolger C, Wigfield C, Melkent T, Smith K. Frameless stereotaxy and anterior cervical surgery. *Comput Aided Surg* 1999; 4: 322–7.

68. Bolger C, Wigfield C. Image-guided surgery: applications to the cervical and thoracic spine and a review of the first 120 procedures. *J Neurosurg* 2000; 92(Suppl. 2): 175–80.

69. Pollack IF, Welch W, Jacobs GB, Janecka IP. Frameless stereotactic guidance. An intraoperative adjunct in the transoral approach for ventral cervicomedullary junction decompression. *Spine* 1995; 20: 216–20.

70. Welch WC, Subach BR, Pollack IF, Jacobs GB. Frameless stereotactic guidance for surgery of the upper cervical spine. *Neurosurgery* 1997; 40: 958–63.

71. Dandie GD, Fehlings MG. Image-guided cervical instrumentation. In: Germano IM (ed.). *Advanced Techniques in Image-Guided Brain and Spine Surgery*. New York: Thieme; 2002: 176–81.

72. Ondra SL, Karahalios D. Image guidance for scoliosis. In: Germano IM (ed.). *Advanced Techniques in Image-Guided Brain and Spine Surgery*. New York: Thieme; 2002: 191–6.

73. Patel NP, Lim JY, Kim KD, Johnson JP. Image-guided lumbar instrumentation. In: Germano IM (ed.). *Advanced Techniques in Image-Guided Brain and Spine Surgery*. New York: Thieme; 2002: 197–206.

74. Youkilis AS, Papadopoulos SM. Thoracic instrumentation. In: Germano IM (ed.). *Advanced Techniques in Image-Guided Brain and Spine Surgery*. New York: Thieme; 2002: 182–90.

75. Bloch O, Holly LT, Park J, Obasi C, Kim K, Johnson JP. Effect of frameless stereotaxy on the accuracy of C1–2 transarticular screw placement. *J Neurosurg* 2001; 95(Suppl. 1): 74–9.

76. Glossop ND, Hu RW, Randle JA. Computer-aided pedicle screw placement using frameless stereotaxis. *Spine* 1996; 21: 2026–34.

77. Kalfas IH, Kormos DW, Murphy MA, *et al.* Application of frameless stereotaxy to pedicle screw fixation of the spine. *J Neurosurg* 1995; 83: 641–7.

78. Foley KT, Simon DA, Rampersaud YR. Virtual fluoroscopy: computer-assisted fluoroscopic navigation. *Spine* 2001; 26: 347–51.

79. Lefkowitz MA, Foley KT. Computer-assisted image-guided fluoroscopy (virtual fluorosocopy). In: Germano IM (ed.). *Advanced Techniques in Image-Guided Brain and Spine Surgery*. New York: Thieme; 2002: 207–17.

80. Rampersaud YR, Foley KT, Shen AC, Williams S, Solomito M. Radiation exposure to the spine surgeon during fluoroscopically assisted pedicle screw insertion. *Spine* 2000; 25: 2637–45.

81. Choi WW, Green BA, Levi AD. Computer-assisted fluoroscopic targeting system for pedicle screw insertion. *Neurosurgery* 2000; 47: 872–8.

82. Talairach J, Hecaeh H, David M, *et al.* Rechèrches sur la coagulation therapeutique des structures sous-corticales chez l'homme. *Rev Neurol* 1949; 81: 4–24.

83. Hayne R, Meyers R. An improved model of a human stereotaxic instrument. *J Neurosurg* 1950; 7: 463–6.

84. Austin G, Lee A. A plastic ball-and-socket type of stereotaxic director. *J Neurosurg* 1958; 15: 264–8.

85. Benardete EA, Leonard MA, Weiner HL. Comparison of frameless stereotactic systems: accuracy, precision, and applications. *Neurosurgery* 2001; 49: 1409–15.

86. Haberland N, Ebmeier K, Hliscs R, *et al.* Neuronavigation in surgery of intracranial and spinal tumors. *J Cancer Res Clin Oncol* 2000; 126: 529–41.

87. Eljamel MS. Frameless stereotactic neurosurgery: two steps towards the Holy Grail of surgical navigation. *Stereotact Funct Neurosurg* 1999; 72: 125–8.

88. Hirschberg H. Implementation of a stereotactic microscope using an optically coupled tracking system. *Stereotact Funct Neurosurg* 1996; 66: 96–101.

89. Li Q, Zamorano L, Jiang Z, *et al.* Effect of optical digitizer selection on the application accuracy of a surgical localization system–a quantitative comparison between the OPTOTRAK and flashpoint tracking systems. *Comput Aided Surg* 1999; 4: 314–21.

90. Takizawa T. Isocentric stereotactic three-dimensional digitizer for neurosurgery. *Stereotact Funct Neurosurg* 1993; 60: 175–93.

91. Germano IM, Villalobos H, Silvers A, Post KD. Clinical use of the optical digitizer for intracranial neuronavigation. *Neurosurgery* 1999; 45: 261–9.

92. Benardete EA, Leonard MA, Weiner HL. Comparison of frameless stereotactic systems: accuracy, precision, and applications. *Neurosurgery* 2001; 49: 1409–15.

93. Hodaie M, Musharbash A, Otsubo H, *et al.* Image-guided, frameless stereotactic sectioning of the corpus callosum in children with intractable epilepsy. *Pediatr Neurosurg* 2001; 34: 286–94.

94. Sandeman D, Moufid A. Interactive image-guided pituitary surgery. An experience of 101 procedures. *Neurochirurgie* 1998; 44: 331–8.

95. Sipos EP, Tebo SA, Zinreich SJ, Long DM, Brem H. *In vivo* accuracy testing and clinical experience with the ISG Viewing Wand. *Neurosurgery* 1996; 39: 194–202.

96. McDermott MW, Gutin PH. Image-guided surgery for skull base neoplasms using the ISG viewing wand. Anatomic and technical considerations. *Neurosurg Clin N Am* 1996; 7: 285–95.

97. Doshi PK, Lemmieux L, Fish DR, Shorvon SD, Harkness WH, Thomas DG. Frameless stereotaxy and interactive neurosurgery with the ISG viewing wand. *Acta Neurochir Suppl (Wien)* 1995; 64: 49–53.

98. Sandeman DR, Patel N, Chandler C, Nelson RJ, Coakham HB, Griffith HB. Advances in image-directed neurosurgery: preliminary experience with the ISG Viewing Wand compared with the Leksell G frame. *Br J Neurosurg* 1994; 8: 529–44.

99. Maciunas RJ, Galloway RL Jr, Latimer J, *et al.* An independent application accuracy evaluation of stereotactic frame systems. *Stereotact Funct Neurosurg* 1992; 58: 103–7.

100. Maciunas RJ, Galloway RL Jr, Latimer JW. The application accuracy of stereotactic frames. *Neurosurgery* 1994; 35: 682–94.

101. Alterman RL, Sterio D, Beric A, Kelly PJ. Microelectrode recording during posteroventral pallidotomy: impact on target selection and complications. *Neurosurgery* 1999; 44: 315–21.

102. Guridi J, Gorospe A, Ramos E, Linazasoro G, Rodriguez MC, Obeso JA. Stereotactic targeting of the globus pallidus internus in Parkinson's disease: imaging versus electrophysiological mapping. *Neurosurgery* 1999; 45: 278–87.

103. Lozano AM, Hutchison WD, Tasker RR, Lang AE, Junn F, Dostrovsky JO. Microelectrode recordings define the ventral posteromedial pallidotomy target. *Stereotact Funct Neurosurg* 1998; 71: 153–63.

104. Starr PA, Vitek JL, DeLong M, Bakay RA. Magnetic resonance imaging-based stereotactic localization of the globus pallidus and subthalamic nucleus. *Neurosurgery* 1999; 44: 303–13.

105. Bejjani BP, Dormont D, Pidoux B, *et al.* Bilateral subthalamic stimulation for Parkinson's disease by using three-dimensional stereotactic magnetic resonance imaging and electrophysiological guidance. *J Neurosurg* 2000; 92: 615–25.

106. Benazzouz A, Breit S, Koudsie A, Pollak P, Krack P, Benabid AL. Intraoperative microrecordings of the subthalamic nucleus in Parkinson's disease. *Mov Disord* 2002; 17 Suppl 3: S145–9.

107. Starr PA, Christine CW, Theodosopoulos PV, *et al.* Implantation of deep brain stimulators into the subthalamic nucleus: technical approach and magnetic resonance imaging-verified lead locations. *J Neurosurg* 2002; 97: 370–87.

108. Zonenshayn M, Rezai AR, Mogilner AY, Beric A, Sterio D, Kelly PJ. Comparison of anatomic and neurophysiological methods for subthalamic nucleus targeting. *Neurosurgery* 2000; 47: 282–92.

109. Li QH, Zamorano L, Pandya A, Perez R, Gong J, Diaz F. The application accuracy of the NeuroMate robot – A quantitative comparison with frameless and frame-based surgical localization systems. *Comput Aided Surg* 2002; 7: 90–8.

110. Roessler K, Ungersboeck K, Dietrich W, *et al.* Frameless stereotactic guided neurosurgery: clinical experience with an infrared based pointer device navigation system. *Acta Neurochir (Wien)* 1997; 139: 551–9.

111. Vinas FC, Zamorano L, Buciuc R, *et al.* Application accuracy study of a semipermanent fiducial system for frameless stereotaxis. *Comput Aided Surg* 1997; 2: 257–63.

112. Willems PW, Noordmans HJ, Berkelbach van der Sprenkel JW, Viergever MA, Tulleken CA. An MKM-mounted instrument holder for frameless point-stereotactic procedures: a phantom-based accuracy evaluation. *J Neurosurg* 2001; 95: 1067–74.

113. Meeks SL, Bova FJ, Wagner TH, Buatti JM, Friedman WA, Foote KD. Image localization for frameless stereotactic radiotherapy. *Int J Radiat Oncol Biol Phys* 2000; 46: 1291–9.

114. Roessler K, Ungersboeck K, Aichholzer M, *et al.* Frameless stereotactic lesion contour-guided surgery using a computer-navigated microscope. *Surg Neurol* 1998; 49: 282–8.

115. McInerney J, Roberts DW. Frameless stereotaxy of the brain. *Mt Sinai J Med* 2000; 67: 300–10.

116. Horsley V, Clarke R. Structure of the cerebellum examined by a new method. *Brain* 1908; 31: 45–124.

117. Talairach J, Tournoux P, Tournoux P, Corredor H, Kvasina T. *Atlas d'Anatomie Stereotaxique*. Paris: Masson; 1957.

118. *Introduction to Stereotaxis with an Atlas of the Human Brain.* Stuttgart: Georg Thieme; 1959.

119. Schaltenbrand G, Wahren W. *Atlas for Stereotaxy of the Human Brain*. New York: Georg Thieme; 1977.

120. Morel A, Magnin M, Jeanmonod D. Multiarchitectonic and stereotactic atlas of the human thalamus. *J Comp Neurol* 1997; 387: 588–630.

121. Szikla G, Bouvier G, Hori T. *In vivo* localization of brain sulci by arteriography: a stereotactic anatomoradiological study. *Brain Res* 1975; 95: 497–502.

122. Nadvornik P, Petr R, Nemecek S, Schindlery C, Beran J. [Stereotaxic atlases of the cerebellar medulla]. *J Hirnforsch* 1965; 8: 67–91.

123. Afshar F, Dykes E, Watkins ES. Three-dimensional stereotactic anatomy of the human trigeminal nerve nuclear complex. *Appl Neurophysiol* 1983; 46: 147–53.

124. Nadvornik P. Woroschiloff's locating device for interventions on the spinal cord and its influence on spinal stereotaxis. *Appl Neurophysiol* 1985; 48: 247–51.

125. Kim SG, Ogawa S. Insights into new techniques for high resolution functional MRI. *Curr Opin Neurobiol* 2002; 12: 607–15.

126. Harrison RV, Harel N, Panesar J, Mount RJ. Blood capillary distribution correlates with hemodynamic-based functional imaging in cerebral cortex. *Cereb Cortex* 2002; 12: 225–33.

127. George JS, Aine CJ, Mosher JC, *et al.* Mapping function in the human brain with magnetoencephalography, anatomical magnetic resonance imaging, and functional magnetic resonance imaging. *J Clin Neurophysiol* 1995; 12: 406–31.

128. Levy R, Lang AE, Dostrovsky JO, *et al.* Lidocaine and muscimol microinjections in subthalamic nucleus reverse Parkinsonian symptoms. *Brain* 2001; 124: 2105–18.

129. Pahapill PA, Levy R, Dostrovsky JO, *et al.* Tremor arrest with thalamic microinjections of muscimol in patients with essential tremor. *Ann Neurol* 1999; 46: 249–52.

130. Sterio D, Zonenshayn M, Mogilner AY, *et al.* Neurophysiological refinement of subthalamic nucleus targeting. *Neurosurgery* 2002; 50: 58–67.

131. Iansek R, Rosenfeld JV, Feniger H, Huxham F. Physiological localisation in functional neurosurgery for movement disorders: a simple approach. *J Clin Neurosci* 2000; 7: 29–33.

132. Tasker RR, Lenz F, Yamashiro K, Gorecki J, Hirayama T, Dostrovsky JO. Microelectrode techniques in localization of stereotactic targets. *Neurol Res* 1987; 9: 105–12.

133. Beric A, Sterio D, Dogali M, Alterman R, Kelly P. Electrical stimulation of the globus pallidus preceding stereotactic posteroventral pallidotomy. *Stereotact Funct Neurosurg* 1996; 66: 161–9.

134. Hua SE, Garonzik IM, Lee JI, Lenz FA. Microelectrode studies of normal organization and plasticity of human somatosensory thalamus. *J Clin Neurophysiol* 2000; 17: 559–74.

135. Tasker RR, Davis KD, Hutchinson WD, Dostrovsky JO. Subcortical and thalamic mapping in functional neurosurgery. In: Gildenberg PL, Tasker RR (eds). *Textbook of Stereotactic and Functional Neurosurgery*. New York: McGraw-Hill; 1998: 883–910.

136. Ranck JB Jr. Which elements are excited in electrical stimulation of mammalian central nervous system: a review. *Brain Res* 1975; 98: 417–40.

137. Duma CM, Jacques D, Kopyov OV. The treatment of movement disorders using Gamma Knife stereotactic radiosurgery. *Neurosurg Clin N Am* 1999; 10: 379–89.

138. Garonzik IM, Hua SE, Ohara S, Lenz FA. Intraoperative microelectrode and semi-microelectrode recording during the physiological localization of the thalamic nucleus ventral intermediate. *Mov Disord* 2002; 17 Suppl 3: S135–44.

139. Kall BA, Goerss SJ, Kelly PJ. A new multimodality correlative imaging technique for VOP/VIM (VL) thalamotomy procedures. *Stereotact Funct Neurosurg* 1992; 58: 45–51.

140. Young RF, Shumway-Cook A, Vermeulen SS, *et al.* Gamma knife radiosurgery as a lesioning technique in movement disorder surgery. *J Neurosurg* 1998; 89: 183–93.

141. Young RF, Vermeulen S, Posewitz A, Shumway-Cook A. Pallidotomy with the gamma knife: a positive experience. *Stereotact Funct Neurosurg* 1998; 70 Suppl. 1: 218–28.

142. Young RF, Jacques S, Mark R, *et al.* Gamma knife thalamotomy for treatment of tremor: long-term results. *J Neurosurg* 2000; 93 Suppl. 3: 128–35.

143. Palur RS, Berk C, Schulzer M, Honey CR. A metaanalysis comparing the results of pallidotomy performed using microelectrode recording or macroelectrode stimulation. *J Neurosurg* 2002; 96: 1058–62.

144. Eskandar EN, Shinobu LA, Penney JB Jr, Cosgrove GR, Counihan TJ. Stereotactic pallidotomy performed without using microelectrode guidance in patients with Parkinson's disease: surgical technique and 2-year results. *J Neurosurg* 2000; 92: 375–83.

145. Hariz MI, Fodstad H. Do microelectrode techniques increase accuracy or decrease risks in pallidotomy and deep brain stimulation? A critical review of the literature. *Stereotact Funct Neurosurg* 1999; 72: 157–69.

146. Hariz MI, Bergenheim AT, Fodstad H. Crusade for microelectrode guidance in pallidotomy. *J Neurosurg* 1999; 90: 175–9.

147. Tsao K, Wilkinson S, Overman J, Koller WC, Batnitzky S, Gordon MA. Pallidotomy lesion locations: significance of microelectrode refinement. *Neurosurgery* 1998; 43: 506–12.

148. Carlson JD, Iacono RP. Electrophysiological versus image-based targeting in the posteroventral pallidotomy. *Comput Aided Surg* 1999; 4: 93–100.

149. Vesper J, Klostermann F, Stockhammer F, Funk T, Brock M. Results of chronic subthalamic nucleus stimulation for Parkinson's disease: a 1-year follow-up study. *Surg Neurol* 2002; 57: 306–11.

150. Voges J, Volkmann J, Allert N, et al. Bilateral high-frequency stimulation in the subthalamic nucleus for the treatment of Parkinson disease: correlation of therapeutic effect with anatomical electrode position. *J Neurosurg* 2002; 96: 269–79.

151. Niranjan A, Jawahar A, Kondziolka D, Lunsford LD. A comparison of surgical approaches for the management of tremor: radiofrequency thalamotomy, gamma knife thalamotomy and thalamic stimulation. *Stereotact Funct Neurosurg* 1999; 72: 178–84.

152. Akbostanci MC, Slavin KV, Burchiel KJ. Stereotactic ventral intermedial thalamotomy for the treatment of essential tremor: results of a series of 37 patients. *Stereotact Funct Neurosurg* 1999; 72: 174–7.

153. Kelly PJ. State of the art and future directions of minimally invasive stereotactic neurosurgery. *Cancer Control* 1995; 2: 287–92.

154. Kaakaji W, Barnett GH, Bernhard D, Warbel A, Valaitis K, Stamp S. Clinical and economic consequences of early discharge of patients following supratentorial stereotactic brain biopsy. *J Neurosurg* 2001; 94: 892–8.

155. Dorward NL, Paleologos TS, Alberti O, Thomas DG. The advantages of frameless stereotactic biopsy over frame-based biopsy. *Br J Neurosurg* 2002; 16: 110–18.

156. Bhardwaj RD, Bernstein M. Prospective feasibility study of outpatient stereotactic brain lesion biopsy. *Neurosurgery* 2002; 51: 358–61.

157. Polinsky MN, Geer CP, Ross DA. Stereotaxy reduces cost of brain tumor resection. *Surg Neurol* 1997; 48: 542–50.

158. Niranjan A, Lunsford LD. Radiosurgery: where we were, are, and may be in the third millennium. *Neurosurgery* 2000; 46: 531–43.

159. Leksell L. Sterotaxic radiosurgery in trigeminal neuralgia. *Acta Chir Scand* 1971; 137: 311–14.

160. Leksell L. Stereotactic radiosurgery. *J Neurol Neurosurg Psychiatr* 1983; 46: 797–803.

161. Paleologos TS, Dorward NL, Wadley JP, Thomas DG. Clinical validation of true frameless stereotactic biopsy: analysis of the first 125 consecutive cases. *Neurosurgery* 2001; 49: 830–5.

162. Nicolato A, Gerosa M, Piovan E, et al. Computerized tomography and magnetic resonance guided stereotactic brain biopsy in nonimmunocompromised and AIDS patients. *Surg Neurol* 1997; 48: 267–76.

163. Di Lorenzo N, Esposito V, Lunardi P, Delfini R, Fortuna A, Cantore G. A comparison of computerized tomography-guided stereotactic and ultrasound-guided techniques for brain biopsy. *J Neurosurg* 1991; 75: 763–5.

164. Hall WA, Liu H, Martin AJ, Truwit CL. Comparison of stereotactic brain biopsy to interventional magnetic-resonance-imaging-guided brain biopsy. *Stereotact Funct Neurosurg* 1999; 73: 148–53.

165. Plunkett R, Allison RR, Grand W. Stereotactic neurosurgical biopsy is an underutilized modality. *Neurosurg Rev* 1999; 22: 117–20.

166. Fritsch MJ, Leber MJ, Gossett L, Lulu BA, Hamilton AJ. Stereotactic biopsy of intracranial brain lesions. High diagnostic yield without increased complications: 65 consecutive biopsies with early

postoperative CT scans. *Stereotact Funct Neurosurg* 1998; 71: 36–42.

167. Hall WA. The safety and efficacy of stereotactic biopsy for intracranial lesions. *Cancer* 1998; 82: 1749–55.

168. Flickinger JC, Kondziolka D, Niranjan A, Lunsford LD. Results of acoustic neuroma radiosurgery: an analysis of 5 years' experience using current methods. *J Neurosurg* 2001; 94: 1–6.

169. Kondziolka D, Lunsford LD, Flickinger JC. Gamma knife radiosurgery for vestibular schwannomas. *Neurosurg Clin N Am* 2000; 11: 651–8.

170. Kondziolka D, Lunsford LD, McLaughlin MR, Flickinger JC. Long-term outcomes after radiosurgery for acoustic neuromas. *N Engl J Med* 1998; 339: 1426–33.

171. Kondziolka D, Lunsford LD. The case for and against AVM radiosurgery. *Clin Neurosurg* 2001; 48: 96–110.

172. Flickinger JC, Kondziolka D, Lunsford LD, et al. A multi-institutional analysis of complication outcomes after arteriovenous malformation radiosurgery. *Int J Radiat Oncol Biol Phys* 1999; 44: 67–74.

173. Pollock BE, Flickinger JC, Lunsford LD, Bissonette DJ, Kondziolka D. Hemorrhage risk after stereotactic radiosurgery of cerebral arteriovenous malformations. *Neurosurgery* 1996; 38: 652–9.

174. Nicolato A, Foroni R, Alessandrini F, Bricolo A, Gerosa M. Radiosurgical treatment of cavernous sinus meningiomas: experience with 122 treated patients. *Neurosurgery* 2002; 51: 1153–9.

175. Kobayashi T, Kida Y, Mori Y. Long-term results of stereotactic gamma radiosurgery of meningiomas. *Surg Neurol* 2001; 55: 325–31.

176. Pendl G, Eustacchio S, Unger F. Radiosurgery as alternative treatment for skull base meningiomas. *J Clin Neurosci* 2001; 8 Suppl. 1: 12–14.

177. Muthukumar N, Kondziolka D, Lunsford LD, Flickinger JC. Stereotactic radiosurgery for tentorial meningiomas. *Acta Neurochir (Wien)* 1998; 140: 315–20.

178. Moore MR, Black PM, Ellenbogen R, Gall CM, Eldredge E. Stereotactic craniotomy: methods and results using the Brown–Roberts–Wells stereotactic frame. *Neurosurgery* 1989; 25: 572–7.

179. McDonald JD, Chong BW, Lewine JD, et al. Integration of preoperative and intraoperative functional brain mapping in a frameless stereotactic environment for lesions near eloquent cortex. Technical note. *J Neurosurg* 1999; 90: 591–8.

180. Hund M, Rezai AR, Kronberg E, et al. Magnetoencephalographic mapping: basic of a new functional risk profile in the selection of patients with cortical brain lesions. *Neurosurgery* 1997; 40: 936–42.

181. Rezai AR, Hund M, Kronberg E, et al. The interactive use of magnetoencephalography in stereotactic image-guided neurosurgery. *Neurosurgery* 1996; 39: 92–102.

182. Skrinjar O, Nabavi A, Duncan J. Model-driven brain shift compensation. *Med Image Anal* 2002; 6: 361–73.

183. Ferrant M, Nabavi A, Macq B, Jolesz FA, Kikinis R, Warfield SK. Registration of 3-D intraoperative MR images of the brain using a finite-element biomechanical model. *IEEE Trans Med Imaging* 2001; 20: 1384–97.

184. Hata N, Nabavi A, Wells WM, III, et al. Three-dimensional optical flow method for measurement of volumetric brain deformation from intraoperative MR images. *J Comput Assist Tomogr* 2000; 24: 531–8.

185. Nimsky C, Ganslandt O, Cerny S, Hastreiter P, Greiner G, Fahlbusch R. Quantification of, visualization of, and compensation for brain

shift using intraoperative magnetic resonance imaging. *Neurosurgery* 2000; 47: 1070–9.

186. Hill DL, Maurer CR Jr, Maciunas RJ, Barwise JA, Fitzpatrick JM, Wang MY. Measurement of intraoperative brain surface deformation under a craniotomy. *Neurosurgery* 1998; 43: 514–26.

187. Kelly P. Stereotactic resection: general principles. In: *Tumor Stereotaxis*. Philadelphia, PA: W.B. Saunders Co.; 1991: 272–3.

188. Hirschberg H, Samset E. Intraoperative image-directed dye marking of tumor margins. *Minim Invasive Neurosurg* 1999; 42: 123–7.

189. Nimsky C, Ganslandt O, Tomandl B, Buchfelder M, Fahlbusch R. Low-field magnetic resonance imaging for intraoperative use in neurosurgery: a 5-year experience. *Eur Radiol* 2002; 12: 2690–703.

190. Nimsky C, Ganslandt O, Hastreiter P, Fahlbusch R. Intraoperative compensation for brain shift. *Surg Neurol* 2001; 56: 357–64.

191. Fahlbusch R, Ganslandt O, Nimsky C. Intraoperative imaging with open magnetic resonance imaging and neuronavigation. *Childs Nerv Syst* 2000; 16: 829–31.

192. Hall WA, Liu H, Martin AJ, Truwit CL. Intraoperative magnetic resonance imaging. *Top Magn Reson Imaging* 2000; 11: 203–12.

193. Tronnier VM, Wirtz CR, Knauth M, *et al*. Intraoperative diagnostic and interventional magnetic resonance imaging in neurosurgery. *Neurosurgery* 1997; 40: 891–900.

194. Roberts DW, Lunn K, Sun H, *et al*. Intra-operative image updating. *Stereotact Funct Neurosurg* 2001; 76: 148–50.

195. Unsgaard G, Ommedal S, Muller T, Gronningsaeter A, Nagelhus Hernes TA. Neuronavigation by intraoperative three-dimensional ultrasound: initial experience during brain tumor resection. *Neurosurgery* 2002; 50: 804–12.

196. Comeau RM, Sadikot AF, Fenster A, Peters TM. Intraoperative ultrasound for guidance and tissue shift correction in image-guided neurosurgery. *Med Phys* 2000; 27: 787–800.

197. Jodicke A, Deinsberger W, Erbe H, Kriete A, Boker DK. Intraoperative three-dimensional ultrasonography: an approach to register brain shift using multidimensional image processing. *Minim Invasive Neurosurg* 1998; 41: 13–19.

198. Benabid AL, Pollak P, Gross C, *et al*. Acute and long-term effects of subthalamic nucleus stimulation in Parkinson's disease. *Stereotact Funct Neurosurg* 1994; 62: 76–84.

199. Pollak P, Benabid AL, Gross C, *et al*. [Effects of the stimulation of the subthalamic nucleus in Parkinson disease]. *Rev Neurol (Paris)* 1993; 149: 175–6.

200. Figueiras-Mendez R, Marin-Zarza F, Antonio MJ, *et al*. Subthalamic nucleus stimulation improves directly levodopa induced dyskinesias in Parkinson's disease. *J Neurol Neurosurg Psychiatr* 1999; 66: 549–50.

201. Gentil M, Garcia-Ruiz P, Pollak P, Benabid AL. Effect of stimulation of the subthalamic nucleus on oral control of patients with parkinsonism. *J Neurol Neurosurg Psychiatr* 1999; 67: 329–33.

202. Krack P, Benazzouz A, Pollak P, *et al*. Treatment of tremor in Parkinson's disease by subthalamic nucleus stimulation. *Mov Disord* 1998; 13: 907–14.

203. Kumar R, Lozano AM, Kim YJ, *et al*. Double-blind evaluation of subthalamic nucleus deep brain stimulation in advanced Parkinson's disease. *Neurology* 1998; 51: 850–5.

204. Kumar R, Lozano AM, Montgomery E, Lang AE. Pallidotomy and deep brain stimulation of the pallidum and subthalamic nucleus in advanced Parkinson's disease. *Mov Disord* 1998; 13 Suppl. 1: 73–82.

205. Limousin P, Krack P, Pollak P, *et al*. Electrical stimulation of the subthalamic nucleus in advanced Parkinson's disease. *N Engl J Med* 1998; 339: 1105–11.

206. Moringlane JR, Ceballos-Baumann AO, Alesch F. Long-term effect of electrostimulation of the subthalamic nucleus in bradykinetic-rigid Parkinson's disease. *Minim Invasive Neurosurg* 1998; 41: 133–6.

207. Pollak P, Benabid AL, Limousin P, *et al*. Subthalamic nucleus stimulation alleviates akinesia and rigidity in parkinsonian patients. *Adv Neurol* 1996; 69: 591–4.

208. Rodriguez MC, Guridi OJ, Alvarez L, *et al*. The subthalamic nucleus and tremor in Parkinson's disease. *Mov Disord* 1998; 13 Suppl. 3: 111–18.

209. Yokoyama T, Sugiyama K, Nishizawa S, Yokota N, Ohta S, Uemura K. Subthalamic nucleus stimulation for gait disturbance in Parkinson's disease. *Neurosurgery* 1999; 45: 41–7.

210. Vesper J, Klostermann F, Stockhammer F, Funk T, Brock M. Results of chronic subthalamic nucleus stimulation for Parkinson's disease: a 1-year follow-up study. *Surg Neurol* 2002; 57: 306–11.

211. Aziz TZ, Nandi D, Parkin S, *et al*. Targeting the subthalamic nucleus. *Stereotact Funct Neurosurg* 2001; 77: 87–90.

212. Starr PA, Christine CW, Theodosopoulos PV, *et al*. Implantation of deep brain stimulators into the subthalamic nucleus: technical approach and magnetic resonance imaging-verified lead locations. *J Neurosurg* 2002; 97: 370–87.

213. Bejjani BP, Dormont D, Pidoux B, *et al*. Bilateral subthalamic stimulation for Parkinson's disease by using three-dimensional stereotactic magnetic resonance imaging and electrophysiological guidance. *J Neurosurg* 2000; 92: 615–25.

214. Hutchison WD, Allan RJ, Opitz H, *et al*. Neurophysiological identification of the subthalamic nucleus in surgery for Parkinson's disease. *Ann Neurol* 1998; 44: 622–8.

215. Abosch A, Hutchison WD, Saint-Cyr JA, Dostrovsky JO, Lozano AM. Movement-related neurons of the subthalamic nucleus in patients with Parkinson disease. *J Neurosurg* 2002; 97: 1167–72.

216. Alvarez L, Macias R, Guridi J, *et al*. Dorsal subthalamotomy for Parkinson's disease. *Mov Disord* 2001; 16: 72–8.

217. Zonenshayn M, Sterio D, Kelly P, Rezai A, Beric A. Optimal active contact location within the subthalamic nucleus (STN) in the treatment of idiopathic Parkinson's disease. *Surgical Neurology* (in press).

218. Yokoyama T, Sugiyama K, Nishizawa S, *et al*. The optimal stimulation site for chronic stimulation of the subthalamic nucleus in Parkinson's disease. *Stereotact Funct Neurosurg* 2001; 77: 61–7.

219. Benabid AL, Benazzous A, Pollak P. Mechanisms of deep brain stimulation. *Mov Disord* 2002; 17 Suppl. 3: S73–4.

220. Beurrier C, Bioulac B, Audin J, Hammond C. High-frequency stimulation produces a transient blockade of voltage-gated currents in subthalamic neurons. *J Neurophysiol* 2001; 85: 1351–6.

221. Dostrovsky JO, Lozano AM. Mechanisms of deep brain stimulation. *Mov Disord* 2002; 17 Suppl. 3: S63–8.

222. Vitek JL. Mechanisms of deep brain stimulation: excitation or inhibition. *Mov Disord* 2002; 17 Suppl. 3: S69–2.

223. Capus L, Melatini A, Zorzon M, *et al*. Chronic bilateral electrical stimulation of the subthalamic nucleus for the treatment of advanced Parkinson's disease. *Neurol Sci* 2001; 22: 57–8.

224. Molinuevo JL, Valldeoriola F, Tolosa E, *et al*. Levodopa withdrawal after bilateral subthalamic nucleus stimulation in advanced Parkinson disease. *Arch Neurol* 2000; 57: 983–8.

225. Moro E, Scerrati M, Romito LM, Roselli R, Tonali P, Albanese A. Chronic subthalamic nucleus stimulation reduces medication requirements in Parkinson's disease. *Neurology* 1999; 53: 85–90.

226. Ostergaard K, Sunde N, Dupont E. Effects of bilateral stimulation of the subthalamic nucleus in patients with severe Parkinson's disease and motor fluctuations. *Mov Disord* 2002; 17: 693–700.

227. Simuni T, Jaggi JL, Mulholland H, *et al*. Bilateral stimulation of the subthalamic nucleus in patients with Parkinson disease: a study of efficacy and safety. *J Neurosurg* 2002; 96: 666–72.

228. Pillon B. Neuropsychological assessment for management of patients with deep brain stimulation. *Mov Disord* 2002; 17 Suppl. 3: S116–22.

229. Perozzo P, Rizzone M, Bergamasco B, *et al*. Deep brain stimulation of the subthalamic nucleus in Parkinson's disease: comparison of pre- and postoperative neuropsychological evaluation. *J Neurol Sci* 2001; 192: 9–15.

230. Alegret M, Junque C, Valldeoriola F, *et al*. Effects of bilateral subthalamic stimulation on cognitive function in Parkinson disease. *Arch Neurol* 2001; 58: 1223–7.

231. Saint-Cyr JA, Trepanier LL, Kumar R, Lozano AM, Lang AE. Neuropsychological consequences of chronic bilateral stimulation of the subthalamic nucleus in Parkinson's disease. *Brain* 2000; 123 (Pt 10): 2091–108.

232. Pillon B, Ardouin C, Damier P, *et al*. Neuropsychological changes between "off" and "on" STN or GPi stimulation in Parkinson's disease. *Neurology* 2000; 55: 411–18.

233. Tsubokawa T, Katayama Y, Yamamoto T, Hirayama T, Koyama S. Chronic motor cortex stimulation in patients with thalamic pain. *J Neurosurg* 1993; 78: 393–401.

234. Carroll D, Joint C, Maartens N, Shlugman D, Stein J, Aziz TZ. Motor cortex stimulation for chronic neuropathic pain: a preliminary study of 10 cases. *Pain* 2000; 84: 431–7.

235. Nguyen JP, Keravel Y, Feve A, *et al*. Treatment of deafferentation pain by chronic stimulation of the motor cortex: report of a series of 20 cases. *Acta Neurochir Suppl (Wien)* 1997; 68: 54–60.

236. Herregodts P, Stadnik T, De Ridder F, D'Haens J. Cortical stimulation for central neuropathic pain: 3-D surface MRI for easy determination of the motor cortex. *Acta Neurochir Suppl (Wien)* 1995; 64: 132–5.

237. Nguyen JP, Lefaucher JP, Le Guerinel C, *et al*. Motor cortex stimulation in the treatment of central and neuropathic pain. *Arch Med Res* 2000; 31: 263–5.

238. Saitoh Y, Shibata M, Hirano S, Hirata M, Mashimo T, Yoshimine T. Motor cortex stimulation for central and peripheral deafferentation pain. Report of eight cases. *J Neurosurg* 2000; 92: 150–5.

239. Ebel H, Rust D, Tronnier V, Boker D, Kunze S. Chronic precentral stimulation in trigeminal neuropathic pain. *Acta Neurochir (Wien)* 1996; 138: 1300–6.

240. Katayama Y, Yamamoto T, Kobayashi K, Kasai M, Oshima H, Fukaya C. Motor cortex stimulation for post-stroke pain: comparison of spinal cord and thalamic stimulation. *Stereotact Funct Neurosurg* 2001; 77: 183–6.

241. Levy RM, Lamb S, Adams JE. Treatment of chronic pain by deep brain stimulation: long term follow-up and review of the literature. *Neurosurgery* 1987; 21: 885–93.

242. Kumar K, Toth C, Nath RK. Deep brain stimulation for intractable pain: a 15-year experience. *Neurosurgery* 1997; 40: 736–46.

243. Bezard E, Boraud T, Nguyen JP, Velasco F, Keravel Y, Gross C. Cortical stimulation and epileptic seizure: a study of the potential risk in primates. *Neurosurgery* 1999; 45: 346–50.

244. Rassweiler J, Frede T. Robotics, telesurgery and telementoring – their position in modern urological laparoscopy. *Arch Esp Urol* 2002; 55: 610–28.

245. Ballantyne GH. Robotic surgery, telerobotic surgery, telepresence, and telementoring. Review of early clinical results. *Surg Endosc* 2002; 16: 1389–402.

246. Cheah WK, Lee B, Lenzi JE, Goh PM. Telesurgical laparoscopic cholecystectomy between two countries. *Surg Endosc* 2000; 14: 1085.

247. Lee BR, Png DJ, Liew L, *et al*. Laparoscopic telesurgery between the United States and Singapore. *Ann Acad Med Singapore* 2000; 29: 665–8.

248. During MJ, Kaplitt MG, Stern MB, Eidelberg D. Subthalamic GAD gene transfer in Parkinson disease patients who are candidates for deep brain stimulation. *Hum Gene Ther* 2001; 12: 1589–91.

249. Lonser RR, Corthesy ME, Morrison PF, Gogate N, Oldfield EH. Convection-enhanced selective excitotoxic ablation of the neurons of the globus pallidus internus for treatment of parkinsonism in nonhuman primates. *J Neurosurg* 1999; 91: 294–302.

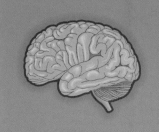

MEDICAL AND SURGICAL TREATMENT OF EPILEPSY

53

Jeffrey G Ojemann

Epilepsy is a common disorder of the nervous system, characterized by the recurrence of unprovoked seizures. A seizure is a symptom; it is the clinical manifestation of bursts of firing of a population of cortical neurons. Many normal neurons are recruited into abnormal firing patterns initiated by abnormal "irritable" neurons. The resulting attack results in sudden, transient events that can be motor, sensory, or psychic in nature. Seizures are usually self-limited, probably because this repeated synchronous burst firing makes major metabolic demands that cannot be sustained for long periods. After a seizure, the neurons enter a depressed state, often clinically manifested as a "post-ictal" period that can be characterized by drowsiness or even a focal deficit (i.e. a Todd's paralysis).

Epilepsy is a disorder of repetitive seizures; two or more seizures are required to make the diagnosis. The neuronal dysfunction that gives rise to seizures can result not only from direct neuronal injury, but also from physiologic derangements such as toxins, electrolyte abnormalities, hypoxia, infection, or fever. These causes should be treated directly. The diagnosis of epilepsy is not made in the setting of metabolic or other active derangements that may be responsible for the seizure.[1] The national prevalence (active cases in a given year) of epilepsy is probably 0.5–0.8%.[1–3] Incidence rates (new cases per year) are bimodal in age distribution, with higher rates in children and the elderly. Epilepsy may be idiopathic (no identifiable risk factor), cryptogenic (associated with central nervous system pathology, but unknown etiology) or symptomatic (known structural abnormality).

Identified risk factors include: congenital malformations, moderate to severe head injury (especially penetrating head injury), stroke, encephalitis, arteriovenous malformations, tumors, bacterial meningitis, Alzheimer's disease, and certain drug use such as alcohol or heroin. The risk for idiopathic epilepsy (no identifiable risk factor) is increased in relatives of probands with idiopathic epilepsy, suggesting a genetic component. Epilepsy resulting from stroke makes up much of the increased incidence in the elderly. The lifetime incidence of epilepsy in the United States is estimated at 3–4%.[2]

EVALUATION AND NATURAL HISTORY

The differential diagnosis of an epileptic event includes syncope, pseudoseizures, breath holding spells, panic attack, and paroxysmal rapid eye movement (REM) sleep behavior.[1] Syncopal etiologies can include vasovagal responses, cardiac events, cerebrovascular accidents, and hypotension. Episodes of vestibular disorder can also present as paroxysmal events. Pseudoseizures, non-epileptic events that often have a psychiatric etiology, can be difficult to diagnose, and can mimic frontal lobe epilepsy which can have a psychogenic "appearance."

A careful history, focusing on both the manifestations of the seizure (if observed) and any prodrome leading up to the event, can often make the diagnosis. Auras, at the onset of a seizure, may reflect the area of seizure origin with sensory changes, epigastric sensations, or psychic phenomena (such as feelings of déjà vu) and suggest a localization-related seizure. Although often non-focal, or characterized by lethargy, the post-ictal neurologic examination can direct localization if a focal deficit is found, including motor deficits, speech disturbance, or visual field deficits. Further evaluation includes general physical examination with special attention to signs of injury, cardiopulmonary dysfunction and cutaneous lesions (neurophakomas).

Another important factor in the evaluation of a seizure is a history of trauma. Post-impact seizures do not carry an increased long-term risk of recurrence, although seizures later following head trauma are generally treated (see below). Provoked seizures include stimulant or other substance abuse, withdrawal from alcohol or sedatives, hypoglycemia, electrolyte abnormalities, hypoxia, and fever. These etiologies should be considered in the initial evaluation of a seizure. For provoked seizures (fever, hyponatremia, drug use, or withdrawal) then treatment of the underlying etiology is often sufficient.

Structural imaging (magnetic resonance imaging; MRI) is recommended for evaluation of epilepsy, especially focal seizures, although lesions can manifest clinically as a generalized seizure. Seizures may be the presenting symptoms for a variety of cortical lesions such as tumors, cortical dysplasia, arteriovenous malformations, or cavernous malformations. Treatment of seizures is recommended if a lesion is present.

The initial evaluation may also include an electroencephalogram (EEG). When positive, the EEG is useful for the classification of the seizure disorder, which is useful in determining the appropriate antiepileptic drug. However, a routine EEG is abnormal in only 50–60% of those that later go on to develop epilepsy, thus the predictive value in excluding epilepsy is quite poor. If EEG and MRI are not diagnostic, continuous video monitoring with EEG can be helpful. The best uses of video EEG include evaluation for possible surgery to treat medially intractable epilepsy or to make the diagnosis of epilepsy when other etiologies are suspected. This is particularly true when pseudoseizures are suspected, although differentiating some syncopal

Table 53.1 Nomenclature of the International Classification of Epileptic Seizures; based on: The International Classification of Epileptic Seizures. *Epilepsia* 1981; 22: 489–501

I   Partial seizures (seizures beginning locally)

  A Simple partial seizures.

  B Complex partial seizures (with impairment of consciousness; may sometimes begin with simple symptomatology)

    1 Simple partial onset followed by impairment of consciousness

      (a) With simple partial features followed by impaired consciousness

      (b) Without automatisms

    2 With impairment of consciousness at onset

      (a) With impairment of consciousness only

      (b) With automatisms

  C Partial seizures evolving to secondarily generalized seizures

---

II   Generalized seizures

  A Absence seizures

    1. Typical absence

    2. Atypical absence

  B Myoclonic seizures

  C Clonic seizures

  D Tonic seizures

  E Tonic-clonic seizures

  F Atonic seizures

III   Unclassified epileptic seizures

---

events or panic attacks from seizure may also be helped by continuous monitoring until such events in question are captured.

The risk of recurrence after a first, non-febrile, seizure has been estimated by a variety of studies, and is approximately 40% at long-term follow-up.[1,4] If risk factors are present, such as an abnormal EEG, abnormal findings on neurologic examination, or structural abnormalities on imaging, treatment may be initiated after a single seizure. After two or more unprovoked seizures, a diagnosis of epilepsy is made. Using this working definition, a 65–80% 1-year control rate is anticipated. Patients who have many seizures before initiation of therapy are more likely to have refractory epilepsy. Persistent seizures were higher in patients with symptomatic or cryptogenic epilepsy than in those with idiopathic epilepsy.[5] Long-term remission has been estimated at 76% on a 15-year follow-up.[6] This is consistent with estimates that 20–30% of those diagnosed with epilepsy will progress to develop chronic epilepsy.[1]

TYPES OF SEIZURES

Seizures are classified according to the International Classification of Seizures[7] as listed in Table 53.1.

Partial seizures often arise from a focal cortical region. The EEG can reveal focal abnormalities (Figure 53.1 – temporal lobe seizures) either during inter-ictal recordings or during the recording of a seizure. A *simple* partial seizure that arises in the motor cortex may be characterized only by motor movements, such as face twitching or hand jerking. *Complex* partial seizures are focal seizures that involve impairment of consciousness. Over 50% of seizure types are partial seizures and two-thirds of these are

complex partial seizures.[3] Complex partial seizures may involve automatisms which are appear purposeful but are unconscious, actions such as lip-smacking, grabbing movements, vacant staring, scratching, etc. These can involve more elaborate activities including wandering, fugue-type states and even rage behavior, but cannot sustain goal-directed activity such as in crimes. Partial seizures may start with an aura, an initial feeling during the beginning of a seizure.

When simple or complex partial seizures evolve into tonic-clonic seizures, they are known as *secondarily generalized seizures*. These seizures are referred to as partial seizures with secondary generalization to distinguish them from primary generalized seizures that involve the bilateral cortex simultaneously at the onset.

Generalized convulsive seizures are characterized, electrically, by bilaterally synchronous epileptiform activity. Clinically, they may manifest as generalized tonic-clonic seizures/convulsions with bilateral tonic-clonic movements, tonic seizures, with bilateral tonic activity, or as myoclonic seizures with bilateral clonic movements at the seizure onset.

Generalized nonconvulsive seizures also characterized, electrically, by bilaterally synchronous epileptiform activity, and may manifest as atonic or absence seizures. Atonic seizures are characterized by an abrupt loss of body tone. These can behave as "drop attacks" with serious risk of bodily injury.

Absence seizures are typically brief, with unresponsiveness and a cessation of movement with a return to baseline immediately following the seizure. The person may often resume previous activity immediately following one or several absence seizures. Some absence seizures have a characteristic generalized, bilaterally synchronous 3-Hz spike-and-wave appearance on EEG.

Some specific syndromes

Benign childhood epilepsy with centrotemporal spikes (i.e. rolandic epilepsy) is the most common benign childhood epileptic syndrome. It has its onset in early school years and has a partial onset, usually beginning in the face and sometimes generalizing to tonic-clonic seizures. The seizures almost always occur in sleep. Treatment may not be necessary, as the seizures will remit, but drugs useful in focal and generalized tonic-clonic seizure may be used (see below).

Childhood absence epilepsies are short duration seizures (petit mal) with brief impairment of consciousness, and rapid recovery. If prolonged, automatisms (such as licking, chewing, lip-smacking, fumbling of fingers, scratching, and walking aimlessly) can occur. Such automatisms are characteristic of complex partial seizures as well and must be distinguished from them. These absence seizures can continue into adulthood. Unlike partial seizures, the EEG shows generalized, bilateral, synchronous 3-Hz spike-and-wave patterns. In contrast, the EEG for a complex partial seizure shows focal epileptiform discharges (Figure 53.1). Recovery following seizure is longer for complex partial seizures and there is no aura with absence seizures compared with the frequent occurrence of a preceding aura in complex partial seizures.

Juvenile myoclonic epilepsy begins in teenage years and is an inherited condition in children who are otherwise neurologically normal. It is characterized by myoclonus (jerking activity), generalized tonic-clonic seizures and occasionally absence seizures. This is effectively treated medically. Lifetime treatment is often necessary.

Infantile spasms (West syndrome) occur early in life (4–6 months of age). Spasms are seizures characterized usually by

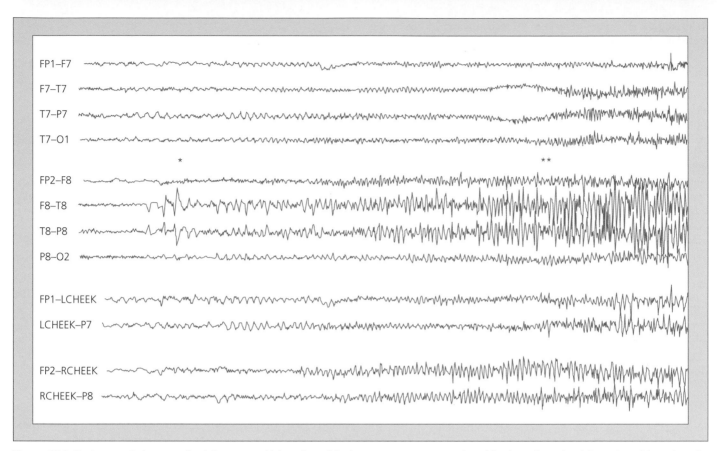

Figure 53.1 Electroencephalograpy of a right temporal lobe seizure (bipolar montage – even-numbered leads are from the right scalp, odd-numbered from the left). The complex partial seizure begins with an abnormal discharge at T8 (*). Note reversal of waveform comparing F8–T8 to T8–P8. The seizure propagates to involve all of the right temporal leads (**).

flexion of the trunk, and are usually symmetric. The seizures occur in clusters with each seizure being rapid, often a 1–2-second spasm. The inter-ictal EEG shows a pattern of hypsarrhythmia (a mixture of asynchronous high-voltage spikes and slow waves). Infantile spasms may also occur in a setting of focal lesions that often does not have a focal clinical or EEG appearance in the very young. For this reason, imaging is imperative in these children. Resection of a focal lesion leads to good outcome. Prognosis is related to etiology. Those of idiopathic origin who respond to therapy have the best prognosis, whereas those with severe diffuse encephalopathy do poorly.

Lennox–Gastaut syndrome consists of multiple seizure types, tonic, tonic-clonic, atonic, atypical absence seizures, and mental retardation. Seizures occur multiple times a day and the EEG shows slow spike-and-wave discharges. Treatment is difficult, typically medication and vagus nerve stimulation have been used. Non-structural infantile spasm often develops into a Lennox–Gastaut picture.

MEDICAL TREATMENT

Antiepileptic medications (AEDs) are the mainstay of treatment for most epilepsy (Table 53.2). Several agents have been used for decades as initial treatment for partial seizures and secondarily generalized seizures, including phenytoin, carbamazepine, and

Table 53.2 Drugs for partial seizures (see specific package inserts for specifics of indications and dosing). Generic names are listed with brand names in parentheses

Phenytoin (Dilantin®)
Carbamazepine (Tegretol®)
Valproic acid/sodium valproate (Depakote®)
Topiramate (Topamax®)
Lamotrogine (Lamictal®)
Zonisamide (Zonegran®)
Levetiracetam (Keppra®)
Gabapentin (Neurontin®)
Tiagabine (Gabitril®)
Oxcarbazepine (Trileptal®)
Felbamate (Felbatol®)
Vigabatrin (Sabril®)

valproic acid. Phenytoin (Dilantin®) is loaded with a 15–18 mg/kg dose and then sustained with maintenance doses. Steady-state occurs in about 5 days. Carbamazepine (Tegretol®) is dosed with subsequent escalation because of initial auto-induction. Carbamazepine interacts with several common drugs, which is especially a problem in the elderly. Valproic acid (Depakote®) is dosed at 15 mg/kg/day and does not have self-induction of metabolism. Valproic acid is also effective for a variety of generalized epilepsy syndromes.

Many newer agents are used as first-line agents or as stand-alone therapy (monotherapy), especially in epilepsy centers. An initial drug is selected appropriate for the specific epilepsy syndrome diagnosed. Monotherapy is effective in 80% of cases.[5] Although newer agents have helped to reduce seizure frequency with less toxicity, the rate of complete seizure control has not changed, and failure of two or more appropriate medications is usually sufficient to deem epilepsy as medically refractory.[5]

No specific drug has been determined to be superior for monotherapy, although both phenytoin and carbamazepine are superior to barbiturates for monotherapy for reasons of side-effects, not efficacy.[8] Localization-related seizure can be effectively treated singly or with add-on agents, as listed in Table 53.2. Gabapentin and levetiracetam are primarily renally metabolized and have a more favorable drug-interaction profile than other agents. Topiramate is an effective agent in localization-related seizures. It has specific side-effects of kidney stones, language and cognitive impairment, and weight loss that limit its use.

Valproic acid and lamotragine are useful not only for localization-related epilepsy, but also in juvenile myoclonic epilepsy, and other myoclonic syndromes.

Felbamate is another drug that is very effective for monotherapy in localization-related seizures and is also used in Lennox–Gastaut syndrome, however its widespread use has been limited by the significant risk of aplastic anemia.

Absence seizures are typically treated with either valproic acid, lamotrogine,[5] or ethosuxamide, however should convulsive seizures develop in those with absence, a drug such as phenytoin must be added to ethosuxamide.

Therapeutic level ranges have been established for a variety of drugs. Serum levels can be helpful in guiding treatment, but clinical manifestations of toxicity and efficacy should also be considered. Both aplastic anemia and hepatic failure can occur with many AEDs, so routine monitoring of cell count and hepatic enzyme levels are typically carried out with long-term AED therapy, although the value of such screening laboratory work has been questioned.[1]

AEDs have many side-effects. All may cause hypersensitivity. These idiosyncratic side-effects especially may be seen in carbamazepine, ethosuximide, lamotrogine, oxcarbazepine, phenobarbital, phenytoin, and primidone[1] with reactions including rash, eosinophilia, fever, or a full-blown Stevens–Johnson syndrome. Dose-dependent side-effects also occur, many are sedating. Hyponatremia and diplopia with carbamazepine, ataxia with phenytoin, and language impairment with topiramate are of obvious signficance to neurosurgical settings.

COMMON DRUG INTERACTIONS

Several AEDs (phenytoin, carbamazepine, phenobarbital, primidone, felbamate, oxcarbazepine, and topiramate) decrease the effects of several common drugs by enzymatic induction (Table 53.3). In

Table 53.3 Some common drug interactions (partial list)

Drugs that increase phenytoin and carbamazepine levels
Cimetadine (Tagamet®)
Chloramphenicol (Chloromycetin®)
Disulfirarn (Antabuse®)
Erythromycin
Isoniazid (INH®)
Propoxyphene (Darvon – affects carbamazepine)
Verapamil
Fluoxetine (Prozac) and other SSRIs

Drugs that decrease total phenytoin level but increase free phenytoin level
Valproic acid
Salicylates

Drugs with decreased efficacy by phenytoin, carbamazepine, and other AEDs that affect the p450 system:
Digitoxin (Digitalis®)
Oral contraceptives
Warfarin (Coumadin®)
Vitamin K
Chloramphenicol
Doxycycline (Vibramycin®)

many cases, this must be explicitly considered. Some of these drugs may also increase phenytoin and carbamazepine levels by enzyme inhibition (Table 53.3). Valproate has interactions with phenytoin that decrease the total phenytoin level but increases *free* phenytoin levels through competitive protein binding, resulting in an effective increase in phenytoin delivery to the brain. Aspirin and other salicylates have a similar effect. Lamotrigine levels can be increased by valproate, and valproate levels are increased by both aspirin and lamotrigine. This is not a comprehensive list of interactions as the hepatically metabolized drugs affect the isoenzymes of the cytochrome p450 system, leading to many drug interactions. Many of the newer AEDs also affect these isoenzymes, however, gabapentin and levetiracetam are primarily metabolized renally and do not seem to have the same drug-interaction profiles as the other AEDs.

TREATMENT OF CHILDHOOD SYNDROMES

Certain syndromes specific to childhood have special treatment options.[10] Neonatal seizures often have a metabolic origin. Phenytoin or phenobarbital are often used and the need reassessed after 2 weeks. Infantile spasms (see above) often respond to adrenocorticotropic hormone (ACTH), or prednisone treatment. ACTH treatment caries considerable risks of severe infection and is a very expensive therapy. Juvenile myoclonic epilepsy and morning myoclonus syndromes are treated indefinitely, whereas the benign focal epilepsies of childhood will often remit and no treatment is an option. Lennox–Gastaut syndrome is often refractory. Although several AEDs are used, the ketogenic diet is another option. In this treatment, a very strict diet of high fat foods, with low protein and carbohydrate, forces a switch in metabolism to a starvation state with the production of ketone bodies. The resulting ketosis appears to be important in the effect on seizures, although the mechanism is unknown. The ketogenic diet is often limited by compliance and side-effects from an extreme high-fat diet.

EPILEPSY AND WOMEN

Several issues arise specific to women with epilepsy. In some cases, seizures predictably occur around menses. The exact relationship is unclear and has prompted many investigations into the relationship between hormones and seizures. Eliminating menses does not reduce seizures. The decreased efficacy of oral contraceptives with enzyme-inducing AEDs is of obvious significance.

Approximately 0.5% of all pregnant woman have epilepsy.[10] The effect of pregnancy is variable, with about one-third experiencing an increase in seizure frequency during pregnancy, one-half with no change, and the remainder with a decrease. The risk of major malformations in the offspring of mothers with epilepsy receiving AEDs ranges from 4 to 8% compared with 2–4% in the general population,[11] and may be less than the risk of malformations in mothers with other chronic illness, such as diabetes.[1] Cleft lip or palate and heart defects are the most common defects seen in infants of mothers taking AEDs. Specific syndromes have been attributed to AEDs; so-called fetal AED syndrome is characterized by minor facial and finger abnormalities and may be related to a decrease in IQ. However the specificity of the syndrome to AEDs has not held up in larger studies. The incidence of this is unclear and may not, in fact, be higher in women receiving AED treatment. The incidence of birth defect seems to be reduced by monotherapy. Neural tube defects occur in 1–2% of pregnancies when the mother is on valproic acid, and in approximately 0.5% of pregnancies involving carbamazepine administration. Folate supplementation is essential in all women of reproductive age taking AEDs, because it has been found that the use of folic acid reduces the incidence of fetal malformations. Vitamin K is recommended in the last 6 weeks of pregnancy and to the newborn to avoid hemorrhagic complications that may be associated with the fetal exposure to enzyme-inducing drugs that does occur. The teratogenicity of newer AEDs is unknown at this time. Despite these risks, AEDs should be continued during pregnancy as the risk of seizures to mother and fetus are greater than the risk of AED effects to the fetus.[1]

TREATMENT OF STATUS EPILEPTICUS

Seizures that are unremitting over 30 min are classified as status epilepticus. Intermittent seizures without interval recovery also constitute status epilepticus. This represents a medical emergency as repetitive seizures can lead to irreversible brain damage and the associated anoxia can also cause permanent sequelae or even death. Waiting the full 30 min to initiate treatment may not be advisable, and it can be initiated after 5 min of unremitting seizures. Table 53.4 outlines the steps required in management of status epilepticus. The primary goal is supporting airway, ventilation, and blood pressure. Possible etiologies should be empirically treated, so glucose and intravenous thiamine are administered. Intravenous lorazepam is an excellent agent for rapid cessation (2 mg/min, up to 8 mg with a pediatric loading dose of 0.05–0.15 mg/kg). Following lorazepam infusion, intravenous fosphenytoin is given up to 18 mg/kg PE (phenytoin

Table 53.4 Protocol for treatment of status epilepticus

1 Maintain airway, support respiration and blood pressure.
2 Place an intravenous line (i.v.) and draw blood for AED levels, glucose, serum chemistries, hematology and toxicology. Keep line open with normal saline (avoid dextrose solutions, which may cause precipitation of AEDs, particularly phenytoin). Treat hypoglycemia and give i.v. thiamine.
3 Administer lorazepam, 2 mg/min, up to 8 mg for adults; pediatric dose is 0.05–0.15 mg/kg; or rectal valium if i.v. is unavailable.
4 Follow benzodiazepine infusion with fosphenytoin, up to 18 mg/kg PE, while monitoring ECG and blood pressure. Anticipate treatment of potential hypotension and cardiac arrhythmia.
5 If seizures persist, proceed to i.v. phenobarbital. Next agents will be general anesthetics (pentobarbital coma, propofol, or midazolam infusion) with intensive-care unit/anesthesia support. Respiratory depression is more likely when added to the benzodiazepines; consider intubation when proceeding to use barbiturates.
6 When control has been achieved, institute maintenance doses of the preferred antiepileptic drug.

equivalent). Fosphenytoin (Cerebyx®) is a water-soluble phosphorylated prodrug of phenytoin. It is preferable over phenytoin for status epilepticus as it does not produce phlebitis, as does intravenous phenytoin, and can be given rapidly, although the potential side-effects, as with phenytoin, of hypotension and cardiac arrhythmia must still be anticipated. This gives longer antiepileptic coverage than the benzodiazepines.

Persistent seizures require barbiturates, and then general anesthesia (pentobarbital coma, propofol, or midazolam). Intubation should be considered early if significant barbiturates or any general anesthesia is required.

Although in some cases of chronic epilepsy the etiology of status epilepticus is not in doubt, and is most often the result of AED noncompliance, computed tomography scan and/or lumbar puncture should quickly be performed to evaluate for other etiologies of severe cases of status epilepticus. In nonconvulsive seizures, status epilepticus (e.g. of absence or of complex partial seizures) may be misdiagnosed as psychiatric illness, such as fugue state. The EEG will make the diagnosis. These conditions are treated in the same way as status epilepticus of convulsive seizures.

DISCONTINUING ANTIEPILEPTIC MEDICATION

The decision to discontinue AEDs after chronic use is an individual one, with some data available on remission. In patients who have been seizure free for at least 2 years, have a normal EEG, a normal IQ and neurologic examination with a single type of seizure, the recurrence rate for seizures when not taking AEDs is 39% for adults and 31% for children.[12] These data are not pertinent for specific cases where the epilepsy may be treated by another means, e.g. self-limited benign epilepsies of childhood or in patients who have successful treatment of a structural seizure focus, and may be able to wean medication sooner than 2 years in some cases. Medication should not be stopped abruptly and patients should be counseled about the increased risk of recurrent seizures when not on AEDs.[5]

QUALITY OF LIFE ISSUES (INCLUDING DRIVING)

Driving is a common issue facing both people with epilepsy and health-care providers. Epilepsy patients do not differ in safety compared with those with other chronic illnesses. In the USA the rules and recommendations vary from state to state. Most require 3–12 months of freedom from seizures, with no requirement for physician reporting in most (but not all) states. Although strict guidelines do not exist, people with epilepsy should avoid occupations where having a seizure would pose a danger to the patient or co-workers. Heights and dangerous machinery should be avoided. Discrimination based solely on a disability is illegal. Local epilepsy associations and the Epilepsy Foundation of America offer specific information on employment. Cognitive and behavioral problems are higher in children with epilepsy than in the normal population and some children with epilepsy need special education resources to avoid social and employment maladaptation in adult life. Participation should be allowed in most sports, although potentially dangerous situations such as skydiving and scuba diving should be avoided. Supervised swimming is generally safe.[1]

PROPHYLACTIC USE OF AEDS

As head injury is a predisposing factor, prophylaxis after trauma has been used. Severe head injury, penetrating trauma, and focal deficits increase the risk. However, the benefit of prophylactic AEDs is controversial. Although there is evidence of benefit in the early post-traumatic period (first week), prophylactic use of AEDs does not prevent the later development of epilepsy and has not been shown to be beneficial for long-term prophylaxis.[13]

Intracranial operations that damage the cortex (but not cerebellum, brainstem, basal ganglia, or thalamus) increase the risk of seizures. Prophylactic AEDs are often used, common practice maintains AEDs for 3–6 months postoperatively although there is no evidence of a benefit from AEDs used as long-term prophylaxis[14] and it may be reasonable to discontinue prophylaxis after the initial postoperative period.

DEFINING INTRACTABILITY

Intractability is typically established after two or three drugs have been attempted over 1 year. The rate of intractability is estimated at 20–30% of those with epilepsy, higher in those with mental retardation (45%). In those with more than 20 seizures before treatment, 51% were intractable. Established drugs (e.g. phenytoin and carbamazepine) are equivalent to new drugs in efficacy. In an evaluation of the efficacy of multiple-agent therapy,[5] 47% were seizure free on one AED, only 14% became seizure free on a second agent and 3% achieved seizure freedom on combination treatment. Thus seizure freedom is unlikely once two agents have been tried.

The specific determination of medical intractability, and consideration for other options such as surgical resection of seizure focus, is highly individual. For some patients, rare seizures are acceptable; in others one or two per year cause significant impairment of career goals or other quality of life issues. In addition, the presence of a lesion amenable to surgical treatment may allow a less strict determination of true intractability. Extending treatment beyond two agents is not likely to result in remission[5] and experimental drug therapies and surgical options should be considered.

SURGICAL TREATMENT

The goal of surgical treatment is the removal of a focal source for intractable seizures. This requires identification of an isolated surgical focus and assessment of the risks of deficit following surgery. In some cases where resection is not possible, palliative surgical measures are available. In general, seizures associated with a structural lesion are the best candidates for surgical treatment, the patient with seizures originating from a tumor or arteriovenous malformation being the most straightforward of this category.

In the evaluation of the medically intractable patient, MRI and EEG can identify many candidates for resective surgery, with good chances of seizure freedom (Table 53.5).[15] Partial seizures with temporal lobe origin (Figure 53.1) in whom inter-ictal EEG (Figure 53.2A) and MRI (Figure 53.2B) all point to unilateral mesial temporal origin are good candidates for temporal lobectomy. Seizure-free outcome in up to 75% or more has been reported. Resection for temporal lobe epilepsy has been demonstrated to be effective in a randomized study[16] and is the therapy with the best chance for seizure freedom in patients with medically refractory temporal lobe seizures deemed to be surgical candidates.

Several variations of temporal lobectomy are used. Recently, selective procedures that resect the amygdala and hippocampus, sparing as much lateral temporal cortex as possible, have been used, with good outcome in patients with congruent EEG and MRI. In patients with possible dual pathology, more common in pediatric series, the selective procedures are targeted toward a narrower population. The surgical approach varies depending on how the hippocampal complex is approached. In a standard anterior temporal lobectomy, the lateral aspect of the anterior temporal lobe is resected, entering the temporal horn along the lateral aspect. The hippocampus and amygdala are then evident as soon as the ventricle is entered (Figure 53.3). The hippocampus is then resected posteriorly at least 1.5 cm to 3.5 cm from the pes, or anterior portion, of the hippocampus. The lateral amygdala is additionally removed. The exact extent of resection can be modified by intraoperative electrical recordings,[17] although some surgeons perform a standard operation in all cases. Selective amygdalohippocampectomies can be performed through a small lateral cortical window, through a subtemporal cortical resection that enters the ventricle through the inferior temporal or fusiform gyri, or superiorly, through a Sylvian fissure approach.

In patients with tumors or other structural lesions, resection of the lesion often results in seizure freedom. However, the rate of seizure freedom seems to improve if recordings directly from the brain surface (electrocorticography, or ECoG) are obtained, either through intraoperative measurements or invasive monitoring with implanted electrodes. Sometimes brain adjacent to pathology is involved (Figure 53.4). Especially in the temporal lobe, a neocortical focus can be associated with mesial temporal seizures. These cases of so-called "dual pathology" can require resection of both the lesion and the affected mesial temporal regions to be effectively treated.

In some cases, the EEG and MRI do not provide sufficient localization. In patients with partial seizures where a focal origin is suspected, additional information can allow surgical resection.

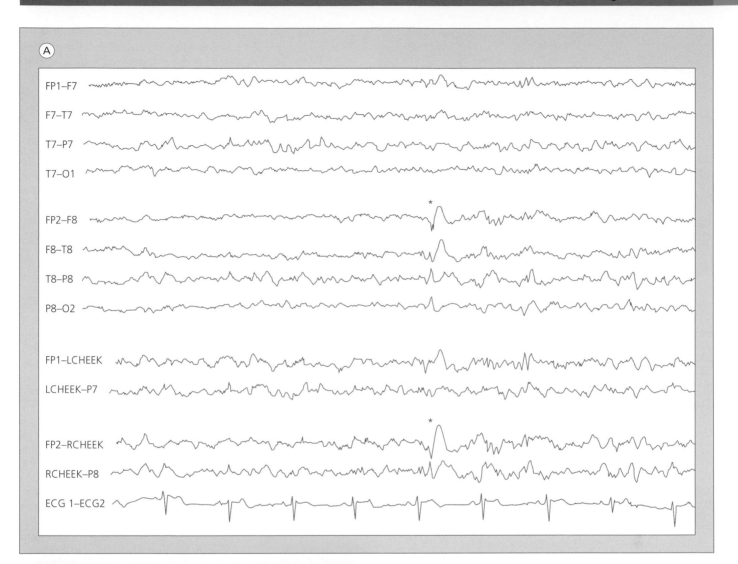

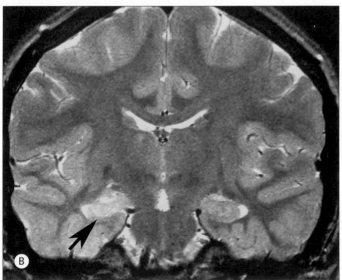

Figure 53.2 **(A)** Interictal EEG from a patient with right temporal lobe seizures and mesial sclerosis. Abnormal discharge is seen in the right temporal region (*). The EEG returns to normal following the "spike." **(B)** Coronal T2-weighted MRI showing increased signal and atrophy of the right hippocampus (arrow). This is a typical appearance of mesial temporal sclerosis. When combined with an EEG as in **(A)**, temporal lobectomy offers an excellent chance of seizure freedom.

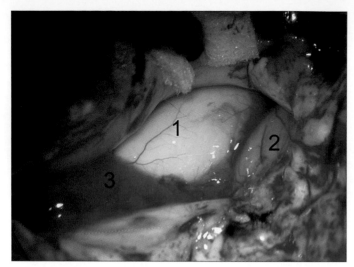

Figure 53.3 Intraoperative photograph of the left temporal horn. The lateral temporal lobe has been resected showing the relationship of the head of the hippocampus (1) and the lateral amygdala (2) that protrudes on the roof of the temporal horn. The choroid plexus (3) is draped over the remainder of the hippocampal formation.

Video EEG monitoring is performed in most candidates for seizure surgery. By injecting tracer during a seizure, ictal single photon emission computed tomography (SPECT) can identify the regional blood flow increase associated with a focal seizure, especially when compared with a resting SPECT study in a subtraction image. Positron emission tomography (PET) can demonstrate regions of decreased glucose metabolism that may be associated with seizure foci. Newer ligand PET scans, such as flumazenil-PET, are still at the experimental stage but offer hope of identifying foci, especially in the case of normal MRI and focal seizures. The cerebral amytal (Wada) test is used both to lateralize language and memory and can help in lateralization of seizure focus as well.

When the surface EEG does not localize seizure onset, or where there is other conflicting information (including seizure semiology, neuropsychological assessment, and any neurological deficits), invasive monitoring is often performed prior to any resective surgery. Strip electrodes can be placed in the subdural space through burr holes. Typically, these are used to cover bilateral mesial and subtemporal regions when temporal lobe epilepsy is present but the lateralization is unclear. If larger areas are covered, then a craniotomy is performed with placement of a subdural grid of electrodes, typically an 8 cm by 8 cm array. Electrodes passed into the interhemispheric, subtemporal, or orbitofrontal regions are especially likely to give information not evident on surface EEG. ECoG is then recorded during inter-ictal and ictal events (Figure 53.5). After sufficient localization, if a focal source of seizures is found, resective surgery can be performed.

Despite the various methods to localize a seizure focus, resections of "nonlesional" epilepsy (i.e. seizure foci without apparent structural abnormality) generally carry no greater than 50% chance of seizure freedom after surgery, although seizure-free rates of 70% have been reported if inter-ictal and ictal EEG are well lateralized.[18] Hippocampal sclerosis, or cortical dysplasia, can often be found pathologically, despite normal MRI studies, suggesting that "nonlesional" surgery may often be targeting focal lesions. Temporal lobectomy in the absence of MRI abnormalities can lead to successful outcome. Consideration of the possibility of both

mesial and lateral temporal foci may maximize outcome. Nonlesional resections outside the temporal lobe are considered less likely to achieve seizure freedom (although success of 50% seizure freedom is reported). If multilobar resection is pursued, the success rate is lower still (Table 53.5). Nevertheless, isolated seizure foci, thoroughly investigated, can be effectively treated with resection of extratemporal foci.

When surgery approaches likely motor or speech areas of the cortex, the risk of deficit must be weighed against the relative chance of good outcome with respect to seizure. Attention to mapping the motor and language cortex, either intraoperatively or through implanted electrodes, can minimize the risks. If seizures do appear to arise from critical cortex then multiple subpial transections can be considered. This procedure involves parallel transection of the crown of the cortical gyrus, and is associated with low complication rates. However, seizure control is not as good as with resective surgery, and the recurrence rate is higher.

If seizures can be lateralized, but not localized within a given hemisphere, consideration is given to a hemispherectomy.[19] Ideally, this is in a patient with evidence of significant or even complete dysfunction of the offending hemisphere, as in a patient with a large perinatal infarction. In this setting, resection and/or disconnection of one hemisphere offers as much as a two-thirds chance of seizure freedom (Table 53.5) with little new deficit. Patients who are ambulatory prior to hemispherectomy generally remain so postoperatively. The major considerations are establishing that structural and electrical abnormalities are strictly unilateral and that the hemisphere is not responsible for critical functions such as language. Spastic hemiparesis and visual field deficits should be expected postoperatively, if not already present in the candidate for hemispherectomy.

Early variations of hemispherectomy included the anatomic hemispherectomy. This met with many severe complications, including superficial siderosis, and functional hemispherectomy became more common, with resection of central cortex and disconnection of the frontal lobe, occipital lobe, and corpus callosum. Recent refinements have led to use of a hemispherotomy. Resection of the temporal lobe is followed by disconnection of cortex. This is performed by entering the ventricle and disconnecting the mesial wall of the ventricle down to the corpus callosum. This provides for functional isolation of the entire cortex (Figure 53.6).

Several palliative procedures are available in patients without focal onset amenable to surgery. In patients with severe generalized seizures, especially drop attacks, division of the corpus callosum may offer benefit. Generally the anterior two-thirds of the corpus callosum are divided through an interhemispheric approach. This can convert sudden drop attacks into seizures in

Table 53.5 Outcome from resective surgery for epilepsy

Surgery	Seizure-free	Improved	Not improved
Selective amygdalohippocampectomy	69%	22%	9%
Extratemporal lobectomy	45%	35%	20%
Hemispherectomy	67%	21%	12%
Corpus callosotomy	8%	61%	31%

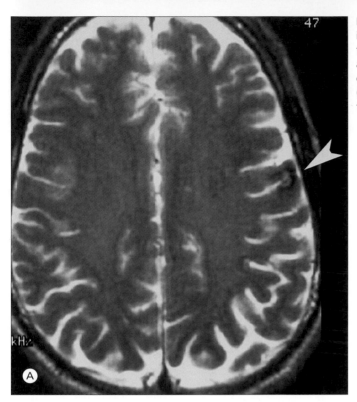

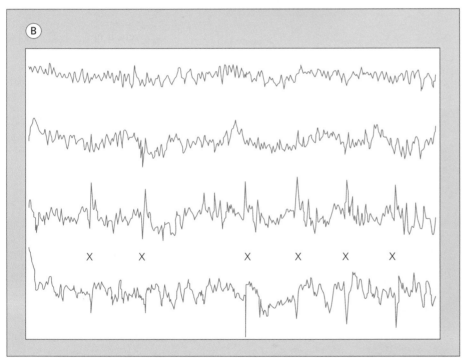

Figure 53.4 (A) Axial T2 MRI of a patient with intractable focal seizures involving aphasia and mouth motor seizures. A cavernous malformation in the posterior frontal lobe is seen (arrowhead). Surgery to resect the lesion and surrounding epileptinogenic focus was performed with awake mapping of language. **(B)** Electrocorticography from brain tissue adjacent to lesion in **(A)**. Spike activity from the third tracing (X) indicates a region included, with the cavernous malformation, in the resection.

which the patient has warning and can avoid severe injury. Although seizure freedom is not expected after such a procedure, a considerable reduction in the severity of seizures is common, with approximately 60–65% improvement (Table 53.5).

Vagus nerve stimulation has emerged as a surgical treatment approved for treatment of partial seizures. Vagus nerve stimulation is unlikely to provide seizure freedom but often gives a 50%

reduction in seizure frequency, making it particularly attractive to those with intractable epilepsy who are not candidates for resective surgery. Its efficacy is comparable to newer AEDs.[20] The electrodes are implanted around approximately 3 cm of exposed vagus nerve. Implantation is always performed on the left vagus nerve to avoid cardiac effects. Difficulties with chronic cough and hoarseness are common in the initial use of the stimulator, but

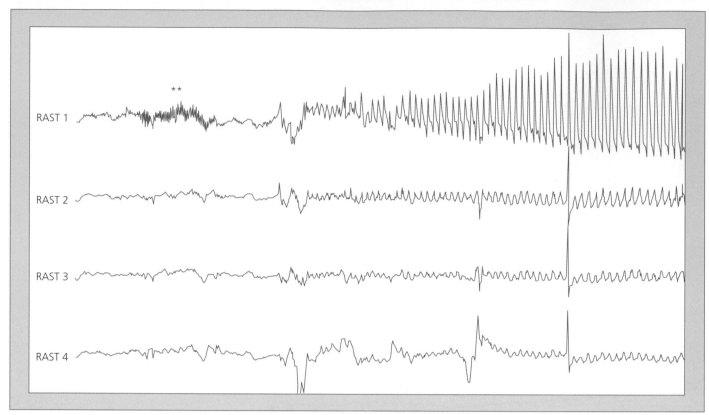

Figure 53.5 Electrocorticography from a subdural electrode placed subtemporally. The first lead is over the parahippocampus, the fourth is proximal and overlies the inferior temporal gyrus. The seizure starts with a high-frequency "buzz" (******) and develops into a higher amplitude activity maximal over the medial temporal electrode.

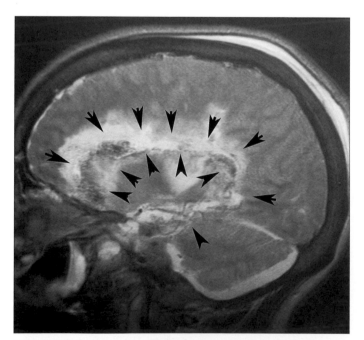

Figure 53.6 Parasagittal T2 weighted MRI postoperative from a disconnective hemispherotomy. The hemisphere is disconnected circumferentially (arrowheads), preventing propogation of any abnormal activity from the hemisphere. The mesial cortex and corpus callosum are also disconnected as part of the surgery.

typically subside. The risks of vocal cord paralysis and damage to surrounding structures are similar to other surgeries of the cervical region.

SUMMARY

Epilepsy is a common disease of the central nervous system. Initial evaluation includes assessment for possible underlying etiologies. Medical therapy is successful in controlling seizures in the majority. The side-effect profile of many of these medications is complex. In those who do not achieve seizure freedom with medication, surgery is considered. In selected cases, resection of seizure foci can offer high rates of seizure freedom.

This chapter contains material from the first edition, and I am grateful to the author of that chapter for his contribution.

REFERENCES

1. Leppik IE. *Contemporary Diagnosis and Management of the Patient with Epilepsy*, 5th edn. Newtown, PA: Handbooks in Health Care; 2001.
2. Hauser WA. In: Engel J Jr, Pedley TR (eds). Incidence and prevalance. In: *Epilepsy: A Comprehensive Textbook*. Philadelphia: Lippincott-Raven Publishers; 1997: 47–58.

CLINICAL PEARLS

- Epilepsy is a common disorder of the central nervous system which represents firing of a population of cortical neurons; two or more seizures are required to make the diagnosis. The prevelance of epilepsy is about 0.5–0.8%. Approximately 20–30% of those diagnosed with epilepsy will develop chronic epilepsy.

- Partial seizures arise from focal cortical areas. Simple partial seizures that arise in motor cortex are characterized by abnormal movements of a limb or face. Complex partial seizures are focal seizures that involve an impairment in consciousness. Absence seizures are characterized by unresponsiveness associated with a lack of movement, with return of function after the seizure. Generalized seizures often evolve into tonic-clonic movement of the limb with impairment of consciousness. Electrically, there is bilateral synchronous epileptiform activity with generalized seizures.

- Antiepileptic medications are the mainstay of treatment but these drugs have therapeutic ranges and side-effects. Monotherapy is effective in 80% of patients with epilepsy. Status epilepticus, or unremitting seizures for over 30 minutes, is a neurological emergency that can lead to irreversible damage or death. The primary goal is airway protection, ventilation, and treatment with intravenous drugs. A benzodiazepine followed by fosphenytoin (18 mg/kg) is the best first-line therapy. Persistent status epilepticus may require barbiturates or general anesthesia.

- Intractability is defined as failure to control the seizures with medicine, typically after two or more drugs have been tried. Seizure freedom is rare once two agents have been unsuccessfully tried. Surgical treatment is an option when there is an identified focal structural or electrical lesion causing the epilepsy.

- Temporal lobectomy to treat epilepsy originating in the temporal lobe associated with a structural lesion or hippocampal sclerosis is highly successful in children and adults, with acceptable morbidity. Nonlesion resections outside the temporal lobe can also be successful. A hemispherectomy is appropriate in patient who have lateralized epilepsy and has significant impairment of the offending hemisphere. Vagus nerve stimulation is a palliative treatment for partial seizures without a focal onset. It is unlikely to achieve seizure freedom but can give approximately a 50% reduction in seizures in properly selected patients.

3. Hauser WA, Annegers JF, Kurland LT. Incidence of epilepsy and unprovoked seizures in Rochester, Minnesota: 1935–1984. *Epilepsia* 1993; 34: 453–68.

4. Hauser WA, Rich SS, Annegers JF, *et al*. Seizure recurrence after a first unprovoked seizure: an extended follow-up. *Neurology* 1990; 40: 1163–70.

5. Kwan P, Brodie MJ. Early identification of refractory epilepsy. *N Engl J Med* 2000; 342: 314–19.

6. Annegers JF, Hauser WA, Eiveback LR. Remission of seizures and relapse in patients with epilepsy. *Epilepsia* 1979; 20: 729–37.

7. Commission on Classification and Terminology of the International League Against Epilepsy. Proposal for revised clinical and electroencephalographic classification of partial seizures. *Epilepsia* 1981; 22: 489–501.

8. Mattson RH, Cramer JA, Collins JF, *et al*. Comparison of carbamazepine, phenobarbital, phenytoin, and primidone in partial and secondarily generalized tonic-clonic seizures. *N Engl J Med* 1985; 313: 145–51.

9. Crumrine PK. Antiepileptic drug selection in pediatric epilepsy. *J Child Neurol* 2002; 17: 2S2–2S8.

10. Report of the Quality Standards Subcommittee of the American Academy of Neurology. Practice parameter: management issues for women with epilepsy (summary statement). *Neurology* 1998; 51: 944–8.

11. Holmes LB, Harvey EA, Coull BA, *et al*. The teratogenicity of anticonvulsant drugs. *N Engl J Med* 2001; 344: 1132–8.

12. Report of the Quality Standards Subcommittee of the American Academy of Neurology. Practice parameter: a guideline for discontinuing antiepileptic drugs in seizure-free patients (summary statement). *Neurology* 1996; 47: 600–2.

13. Temkin NR, Dikmen SS, Wilensky AJ, *et al*. A randomized, double-blind study of phenytoin for the prevention of post-traumatic seizures. *N Engl J Med* 1990; 323: 497–502.

14. Temkin NR. Prophylactic anticonvulsants after neurosurgery. *Epilepsy Currents* 2002; 2: 105–7.

15. Wiebe S, Blume WT, Girvin JP, Eliasziw M. Effectiveness and Efficiency of Surgery for Temporal Lobe Epilepsy Study Group. A randomized, controlled trial of surgery for temporal-lobe epilepsy. *N Engl J Med* 2001; 345: 311–18.

16. Engel J Jr, Van Ness PC, Rasmussen TB, Ojemann LM. Outcome with respect to epileptic seizures. In Engel J Jr (ed.). *Surgical Treatment of the Epilepsies*, 2nd edn. New York: Raven Press, Ltd; 1993: 609–21.

17. Ojemann GA. Surgical therapy for medically intractable epilepsy. *J Neurosurg* 1987; 66: 489–99.

18. Holmes MD, Born DE, Kutsy RL, Wilensky AJ, Ojemann GA, Ojemann LM. Outcome after surgery in patients with refractory temporal lobe epilepsy and normal MRI. *Seizure* 2000; 9: 407–11.

19. Ojemann JG. Surgical treatment of pediatric epilepsy. *Semin Neurosurg* 2002; 13: 71–80.

20. Cramer JA, Ben Menachen E, French J. Review of treatment options for refractory epilepsy: new medications and vagal nerve stimulation. *Epilepsy Res* 2001; 47: 17–25.

INDEX

H